CONTENTS

CONTRIBUTORS

James R. Andrews, Ph.D.
Department of Communicative Disorders
Northern Illinois University
DeKalb, Illinois

Charles I. Berlin, Ph.D.
Louisiana State University Medical Center
Kresge Hearing Research Center of the South

Lois Bloom, Ph.D.
Teachers College of Columbia University
New York, New York

Richard M. Flower, Ph.D.
Emeritus Professor
University of California Medical School
  at San Francisco

James F. Jerger, Ph.D.
Baylor College of Medicine
Houston, Texas

Raymond D. Kent, Ph.D.
Department of Communication Disorders
University of Wisconsin-Madison

Patricia K. Kuhl, Ph.D.
Department of Speech and Hearing Sciences
University of Washington
Seattle, Washington

Leonard L. LaPointe, Ph.D.
Department of Speech and Hearing Science
Arizona State University
Tempe, Arizona

Fred D. Minifie, Ph.D.
Department of Speech and Hearing Sciences
University of Washington
Seattle, Washington

David Prins, Ph.D.
Department of Speech and Hearing Sciences
University of Washington
Seattle, Washington

Lorraine Olson Ramig, Ph.D.
Department of Communication Disorders
  and Speech Science
University of Colorado
Boulder, Colorado

Robert J. Shprintzen, Ph.D.
Center for Craniofacial Disorders
Montefiore Medical Center
Bronx, New York

Brad Stach, Ph.D.
California Ear Institute at Stanford
Palo Alto, California

Kenneth N. Stevens, Ph.D.
Research Laboratory of Electronics
Massachusetts Institute of Technology
Cambridge, Massachusetts

Carol Stoel-Gammon, Ph.D.
Department of Speech and Hearing Sciences
University of Washington
Seattle, Washington

Judith R. Stone, Ph.D.
Department of Speech and Hearing Sciences
University of Washington
Seattle, Washington

Linda Swisher, Ph.D.
Department of Speech and Hearing Science
University of Arizona
Tucson, Arizona

Orlando L. Taylor, Ph.D.
Howard University
Washington, D.C.

PREFACE

This book introduces students to the field of communication sciences and disorders. This field deals with the enormously complex behaviors associated with normal speech, language, and hearing as they change throughout life and with the variety of communication disorders resulting from biological, environmental, and behavioral factors. As complicated as the field may sound, communication sciences and disorders can be understood by studying its component parts.

Consequently, this book was designed by a small group of consultants (Drs. James Jerger, Ray Kent, Fred Minifie, Leonard LaPointe, and Sadanand Singh) who listed the component parts that need to be understood by students. The consultants developed lists of scholars who might be asked to write seminal chapters on each of the component parts. As the table of contents shows, some of the nation's outstanding scholars in communication sciences and disorders write about their specialties. While there are many other outstanding scholars who might have contributed to this volume, the contributors represent some of the outstanding clinical practitioners, scientists, and academicians in the field. The authors of these chapters were specifically asked to write from the perspective of "where the student sits" and not from the perspective of "writing to impress their colleagues." Thus, the chapters provide a simple but comprehensive introduction to each area of specialty. By design, these chapters are written to provide a thought provoking, and in some cases challenging, introduction to this field. We believe that good students who are provided with a comprehensive and stimulating introduction to this field will find challenges and opportunities that can sate their career appetites, whether in the areas of clinical audiology or speech-language pathology, in basic research in communication sciences and disorders, or in a combination of such interests. By exposing students to outstanding scholars, to their ideas, and to the perspectives these scholars have about their specialties, students may focus on relevant and challenging ideas as they pursue career interests.

Perhaps no aspect of human behavior is more complex than communication. Consider the following. Communication, if viewed from a purely biological perspective, involves the use of the brain in:

- ◆ cognitive activities during the generation of thought;
- ◆ the formulation of appropriate linguistic constructions for conveying our ideas to another person;

◆ controlling the intricate patterning and recruitment of muscles used in speech production. These muscles are spatially distributed throughout the body (abdomen, thorax, larynx, head and neck areas), and contractions must be precisely timed and synchronized for normal speech to occur;

◆ the generation and regulation of air flows within the vocal tract during speech production;

◆ the generation, resonation, and transmission of the complex sound patterns used in speech production;

◆ the reception and transmission of complex speech sounds within the ear;

◆ the transduction of sound energy into neural patterns within the cochlea and the eighth cranial nerve;

◆ processing and decoding of the neural patterns resulting from stimulation of the auditory system; and

◆ cognitive assignment of linguistic form and meaning to the patterns received within the central nervous system from auditory neural stimulation.

If viewed from a behavioral or environmental perspective, the brain is involved in communication by:

◆ processing information that allows the linguistic knowledge of the talker to be presented in a way that complies with the linguistic constraints of the listener;

◆ comparing information relevant to communication from the various sensory modalities (auditory, visual, olfactory, tactile, and proprioceptive), all of which may influence the precise message conveyed. Consider, for example, the effects of body language, and facial expression on communication;

◆ evaluating the pragmatic demands for communication considering the context or environment in which communication is taking place (Is communication taking place in the home, on the street, at work, in a clinic, in a school, etc.?);

◆ determining the psychological and psycholinguistic factors influencing communication;

◆ assessment of sociolinguistic and cultural effects on communication;

◆ considering the age, gender, and role (position) of the talker and the listener participating in communicative interaction; and

◆ considering the cumulative effects of previous experience and/or events affecting communicative interaction by the participants.

By considering this short and oversimplified list of ways in which the brain participates in communication, it is clear that communication is a complicated activity. The wonder is not that people sometimes have communication disorders, but that anyone is able to communicate normally. Perhaps even more perplexing are the problems of attempting to understand the nature, severity, and treatment of communication disorders, their etiologies, how they may be diagnosed, clinical intervention strategies, available clinical technologies, the efficacy of clinical treatment approaches, and so forth.

To understand communication and its disorders, a student must approach the topic systematically. By integrating the information presented in this book, the reader can develop a foundation for understanding the basic issues that influence the field of communication sciences and disorders. No attempt has been made to present sufficient information in each chapter to allow the reader to obtain state-of-the-art understanding of the particular area being addressed. That level of understanding will come from more advanced courses. Indeed, many of the chapter titles in this book will become titles for advanced courses offered in the curricula of most of the educational programs in this academic discipline.

To organize the material covered in this introductory text into a sequence compatible with the way most introductory courses in this field are taught, we conducted a survey of professors teaching such courses. In addition to asking for their critique of the philosophy and organization of this textbook, we asked them to submit an outline for the introductory course offered at their university. Based on their responses, we have ordered the chapters in this book in roughly the "modal outline" provided by these instructors. Obviously, each professor must teach the content covered in this book in the order that makes sense to him or her.

As a student, how should you read this book? If you are reading the book without the assistance and guidance of a professor, you may benefit from reading the book from start to finish, relying on the organization imposed by the editor to guide you through the topics. However, if your professor has a different organization in mind and proposes a different sequence of chapters, follow his or her guidance. There are some "bells and whistles" built into the book to help you glean the relevant information from each chapter. First, the chapter title should direct your thinking to a specific content area covered in the chapter, and the abstract will provide a gloss coverage of the topic. The bulleted topics at the beginning of each chapter will highlight the things you should learn by reading the chapter. The chapters have been written to summarize current thinking on a topic, without many citations of where the ideas came from. although we acknowledge the importance of providing attribution to the scientific papers from which these ideas were gleaned, we have found that texts replete with reference citations are more cumbersome, less readable, and often miss reaching the student in a directly communicative way. However, we do include a list of supplementary references at the end of each chapter.

In each chapter, the authors define each new term at first mention. In this way, you can start at the beginning of the book and work your way through the text without relying on a dictionary. Definitions of these terms are also in a glossary at the end of each chapter, should you forget one of the definitions. We have used photographs, figures, and tables throughout each chapter to present material that is more easily pictured than described by text. Examples from case studies, supplementary commentary, and anecdotal observations are included in boxed inserts to highlight ideas discussed in text. Each of the chapters includes a summary of the essential ideas discussed in the chapter. Some of the chapters have sample problems that you may address as you attempt to galvanize the important ideas gleaned from the chapter. Finally, an index at the end of the book will help you identify the pages on which important terms, topics, or ideas are covered.

Special thanks must be given to the many students with whom the authors have been associated. Those students were the inspiration for this book. The textbook, if successful, will make the first exposure to this field even more exciting for the next generation of students than it has been for the students who preceded them. The success of this book wil be measured, not by the number of books sold, but by the quality of students recruited into the field.

Special thanks and acknowledgment are also merited by several people involved in the development of this textbook. Marie Linvill, who served as publisher of this book for Singular Publishing Group, Inc., maintained a steady control, gave helpful editorial suggestions, and provided useful guidance throughout the development of this text. Artistic input and formatting of the book were the province of Angie Singh, whose wise judgment and enthusiastic flair brought a special feeling to this book. Finally, and most important, Dr. Sadanand Singh's vision brought this book into being. His unstinting support and unprecedented generosity as the Chairman of Singular Publishing Group has allowed this to be a quality project from start to finish.

Introduction to the Professions

RICHARD M. FLOWER, PH.D.

After reading this chapter, you should be able to answer the following questions:

◆ Who are speech-language pathologists and what do they do?

◆ How are speech-language pathologists and audiologists credentialed?

◆ Where do speech-language pathologists and audiologists work?

◆ Who are the colleagues with whom speech-language pathologists and audiologists work?

This chapter introduces you to the professions of speech-language pathology and audiology. Speech-language pathologists and audiologists provide essential services concerned with one of the most vital of all human processes: communication with other people. Although established more recently than many human services professions, speech-language pathology and audiology offer virtually limitless opportunities for caring people who wish to devote their careers to an ever-expanding field of study and service.

✦ THE DISCIPLINE AND THE PROFESSIONS

Human communication is the highest achievement in human evolution. It is the ability to formulate and use language; the ability to speak with sufficient clarity to be understood by other people; and the ability to hear and understand what other people say. When communication is impaired by speech, language, and hearing disorders, the consequences may be devastating. This book has been written to introduce you to the discipline of communication sciences and disorders and to the professions of speech-language pathology and audiology.

A discipline is usually defined as a specialized area of study that requires mastery of a distinct body of knowledge. Furthermore, it involves approaches to investigation that differ in focus from the approaches used by other disciplines. Thus, students of the discipline of communication sciences and disorders are concerned with theoretical and applied knowledge about human communication, including:

1. The physical and behavioral bases of communication processes.

2. The acquisition and degradation of those processes.

3. The precise description of normal and aberrant communication and of other factors directly related to communication.

4. The amelioration of disordered communication.

The complexity of human communication and its disorders demands study from many different points of view. Therefore, students of this discipline draw on many other disciplines — anatomy, physiology, psychology, sociology, and the neurosciences — to acquire understanding and advance knowledge. Some students identify themselves as members of the professions of speech-language pathology and audiology, but others identify themselves as members of other professions.

Professions usually are defined on the basis of both what their practitioners know and what they do. The professions of speech-language pathology and audiology, therefore, can be briefly defined as the application of the discipline of communication sciences and disorders to:

1. The provision of clinical services for children and adults with speech, language, and hearing disorders.

2. The conduct of research aimed at expanding knowledge about human communication, communication disorders, and effective strategies for diagnosis and treatment.

3. The education and supervision of students engaged in the study of human communication sciences and disorders.

The succeeding chapters in this book will examine the many areas embraced by the discipline of human communication sciences and disorders. This chapter describes the professions of speech-language pathology and audiology which derive from that discipline.

◆ SPEECH-LANGUAGE PATHOLOGISTS AND AUDIOLOGISTS: WHO THEY ARE AND WHAT THEY DO

The professions of speech-language pathology and audiology have developed more recently than many human services professions. Nevertheless references to concerns for children and adults with speech, language, and hearing problems and for the amelioration of those problems are found throughout recorded history. The first written allusion to a communication disorder is often attributed to the Old Testament. When God commissions Moses to lead the children of Israel, Moses protests:

> But Moses said, "Oh Lord, I have never been a man of ready speech, never in my life, not even now that Thou has spoken to me, I am slow and hesitant of speech." The Lord said to him . . . "Go now; I will help your speech and tell you what to say." (4 Exod. 10–12).

Aristotle (1910) wrote in his *History of Animals*:

Viviparous quadrupeds utter vocal sounds of different kinds, but they have no power of converse. In fact, this power, or language is peculiar to man. For while the capability of talking implies the capability of uttering sounds, the converse does not hold good. Men that are deaf are in all cases also dumb; that is, they can make vocal sounds but cannot speak. Children, just as they have no control of other parts, so have no control, at first, over the tongue; but it is so far imperfect, and only frees and detaches itself by degrees, so that in the interval children for the most part lisp and stutter. (p. 126)

Ultimately, concern for helping children and adults overcome communication disorders emerged from two different perspectives. Physicians experimented with medical treatment while educators examined methods of "teaching" speech, language, and hearing handicapped children. Significant historical differences exist in the antecedents of speech-language pathology and audiology in Europe and the United States. In Europe, except for the education of hearing-impaired children, most services developments occurred in the medical arena. Initially, the providers of speech, language, and hearing services were physicians. Gradually, these physicians trained assistants who carried out prescribed remedial programs. In the United States, services developed primarily in the educational system, emphasizing the use of special "teachers" for children with communication disorders.

Although some international differences remain, dissimilarities among the services provided and the individuals providing those services have steadily diminished. Many European countries now provide an array of services through their educational systems. In the United States, a significant contingent of speech-language pathologists and audiologists now works within the health care system.

Probably the most significant milestone in the development of these professions in the United States was the formation, in 1926, of the organization that eventually became the American Speech-Language-Hearing Association (ASHA). The organization

1. provided definitions of the professions;

2. specified the preparation required for entry into the professions and established standards for university programs that offer such preparation;

3. promoted the recognition of the professions by governmental agencies, private groups that support human services, and the general public;

4. provided opportunities for continuing education; and

5. offered guidelines for ethical practice.

At first, ASHA was comprised primarily of professionals interested in speech and language disorders. Gradually they were joined by clinicians and researchers primarily interested in hearing handicapped children and adults. For many years, ASHA espoused the position that speech-language pathology and audiology constituted different areas of practice within a single profession. Steadily, the range of professional services grew and requirements for educational preparation increased. Eventually, therefore, ASHA's official position changed to recognize that speech-language pathology and audiology were best considered separate professions. Nevertheless, as the professions primarily concerned with communication disorders, they maintain substantial areas of common interest.

Although the formation of ASHA represented an historic professional milestone, the major impetus for the expansion of clinical services occurred during the 1940s. Some of America's larger school districts established limited special services for children with speech disorders during the first two decades of the 20th century, but services for adults were seldom available. During World War II and in the immediately succeeding years, our nation recognized its responsibility to provide rehabilitative services to the men and women who were injured while serving their country. This recognition led to the institution of speech, language, and hearing services in military hospitals during the war and, afterward, in Veterans Administration medical centers. When the individuals who staffed military programs returned to civilian life, many worked toward the development of comparable services in medical centers and community agencies.

During the three decades following World War II, there emerged increasing concerns for disabled children. These concerns were reflected in a philosophy which held that all children, regardless of their disabilities, should receive whatever assistance was required to achieve their potential. Consequently, there was also a steady expansion of speech, language, and hearing services in the public schools.

All of these developments substantially increased the demand for qualified speech-language pathologists and audiologists, and that demand led to growth in the number and size of university programs devoted to preparing students to enter these professions.

Few, if any, human services professions have experienced such rapid increases in size and scope of services during the 20th century. Although not all members of the professions of speech-language pathology and audiology choose to belong to ASHA, its growth in membership during the 50 years between 1943 and 1993 from less than 600 members to over 70,000 suggests the magnitude of the profession's expansion.

Speech-Language Pathology

The responsibilities of speech-language pathologists differ depending on their areas of major interest and the settings in which they work. The brief profiles that follow suggest the range of those responsibilities.

W.V. is a speech-language specialist in a suburban school district. She meets twice weekly with 35 elementary school age children who are otherwise able to progress in regular classes. Among them are children with problems in language development, children who produce the speech sounds of the language inaccurately, children who stutter, and children with chronic voice problems. Some of these children show identifiable organic deficits; others do not. In addition to the children she sees regularly, she conducts diagnostic studies on other children referred by teachers, administrators, health workers, psychologists, and parents. One of the things she particularly enjoys about her job is working in "team" efforts with other professionals to obtain information about the children she sees and, in turn, to provide information about speech and language and make suggestions for overall management.

G.L. began her career as a speech-language pathologist on the staff of a medical center. After several years of regular contacts with the physicians and other human services professionals who referred patients, she decided to establish a private practice. Her office is in a building in a neighborhood where many human services professionals maintain offices. She has exclusive use of a small suite of two rooms, but she shares reception and other office facilities with a group of psychologists and social workers who also are in private practice. Although she sees patients with a variety of communication problems for diagnosis and treatment, she has established a particular reputation for her skill in treating adults with voice problems. Many otolaryngologists (ear-nose-throat specialists) refer these patients to her. She is especially interested in problems encountered by professional voice users — singers, actors, certain executives, and so on — and particularly enjoys working with them. As her practice has grown, she now employs two other speech-language pathologists on a part-time basis to assist her in providing treatment services.

J.S. is a speech-language pathologist on the staff of a rehabilitation center that operates as a component of the county hospital system in a major urban area. The center serves both children and adults, most of whom have grave disabilities. Most of his patients have acquired speech and language disorders as a result of head injuries or strokes, although he also sees children with other neurological problems. He has been particularly interested in developing and teaching people to use augmentative and assistive communication systems. Such systems usually are based on applications of computer technology. They enable people to communicate when severe problems in muscular control preclude the production of intelligible speech. All of his patients are also treated by rehabilitation specialists representing other professions such as physical and rehabilitation medicine (a medical specialty), physical therapy, occupational therapy, social work, biomechanics, and vocational counseling. As a result he is in daily contact, both incidentally and through formal treatment planning meetings, with a variety of other professionals as well as with his colleagues in the speech-language clinic. J.S. was born in Puerto Rico and came to the United States with his family when he was 8 years old. His fluency in Spanish gives him considerable advantage because the rehabilitation center serves a substantial Hispanic population.

T.R. teaches a special day class for children with severe language disorders sponsored by a local public school system (with supplementary funding from the state education department). His class of six children ranges in age from 7 to 10. None of the children could succeed in regular classes, although they all spend a few hours each week participating in activities with
(continued)

peers from those classes. His students come by bus from neighborhoods throughout the community. The goal of the program is to help them develop sufficient language facility to spend increasing amounts of the school day in regular classes. Nevertheless, because of the severity of their problems, it is likely that they will require some special assistance throughout their school careers. With a teaching assistant, he provides complete educational programs, working not only on spoken language but written language as well. In so far as possible, he offers the overall educational experiences provided to normal children of the same age.

V.L. is the speech-language consultant to an "infant/toddler" program sponsored jointly by the school district and health department of a moderate size urban community. This program identifies infants who are at developmental risk because of low birth weight, illness, maternal substance abuse, HIV infection, or other prenatal conditions. Together with physicians, nurses, psychologists, social workers, and other human services professionals she conducts diagnostic studies, participates in planning intervention, counsels parents, demonstrates speech and language stimulation procedures, and provides other follow-along services. Her own experiences in growing up as an African-American in a low-income neighborhood in the city where she now works have led her to be particularly interested in discovering effective means of compensating for the problems children and families confront in these circumstances.

R.G. works as the speech-language consultant to a special program in a university medical center devoted to the diagnosis and treatment of oral and facial deformities. She also serves as the coordinator of that program. She sees patients who have cleft palate or other congenital malformations, patients who have suffered severe facial injuries, and patients who have experienced surgical removal of oral and facial tissues as a part of cancer treatment. Her work with all patients occurs in concert with plastic surgeons and other physicians, dentists, professionals who design and develop prosthetic appliances, audiologists, and social workers among other professionals. She collaborates with these specialists in her daily activities as well as meeting with them as a group once each month to establish diagnoses and formulate treatment plans. She is actively involved in several cooperative research projects. She also is the principal investigator in an experimental project that applies new imaging technologies to observe normal and abnormal movement of the soft palate and related structures during speech production.

Definition

The most frequently quoted source of definitions of professions and occupations is the *Dictionary of Occupational Titles* published by the United States Department of Labor (1991). Its definition of speech-language pathologist is:

- ✦ Specializes in diagnosis and treatment of speech and language problems, and engages in scientific study of human communication.
- ✦ Diagnoses and evaluates speech and language skills as related to educational, medical, social, and psychological factors.
- ✦ Plans, directs, or conducts habilitative and rehabilitative treatment programs to restore communicative efficiency of individuals with communication problems of organic and nonorganic etiology.
- ✦ Provides counseling and guidance and language development therapy to handicapped individuals.
- ✦ Reviews individual files to obtain background information prior to evaluation to determine appropriate tests and to ensure that adequate information is available.
- ✦ Administers, scores, and interprets specialized hearing and speech tests.
- ✦ Develops and implements individualized plans for assigned clients to meet individual needs, interests and abilities.
- ✦ Evaluates and monitors individuals.
- ✦ Reviews treatment plans, and assesses individual performance to modify, change, or write new programs.
- ✦ Maintains records as required by law, establishment's policy, and administrative regulations.
- ✦ Attends meetings and conferences and participates in other activities to promote professional growth.
- ✦ Instructs individuals to monitor their own speech and provides ways to practice new skills. May act as consultant to educational, medical and other professional groups.

◆ May conduct research to develop diagnostic and remedial techniques.
◆ May serve as consultant to classroom teachers to incorporate speech and language development activities into daily schedule.
◆ May teach manual sign language to students incapable of speaking.
◆ May instruct staff in use of special equipment designed to serve handicapped. (p. 62)

Scope of Practice

Professions are also defined by *scope of practice* statements. Such statements are always included in laws that license a person to practice a profession. They also are used to determine whether a particular service is appropriately provided by a particular professional (as, for example, in determining whether or not a professional should be paid for a service he or she has provided). In 1989 the American Speech-Language-Hearing Association (1990) adopted the following definition of the scope of practice of speech-language pathologists:

The practice of speech-language pathology includes:

◆ screening, identifying, assessing and interpreting, diagnosing, rehabilitating, and preventing disorders of speech (e.g., articulation, fluency, voice) and language;
◆ screening, identifying, assessing and interpreting, diagnosing, and rehabilitating disorders of oral-pharyngeal function (e.g., dysphagia) and related disorders;
◆ screening, identifying, assessing and interpreting, diagnosing, and rehabilitating cognitive/communicative disorders;
◆ assessing, selecting and developing augmentative and alternative communication systems and providing training in their use;
◆ providing aural rehabilitation and related counseling services to hearing impaired individuals and their families;
◆ enhancing speech-language proficiency and communication effectiveness (e.g., accent reduction);
◆ screening of hearing and other factors for the purpose of speech-language evaluation and/or the initial identification of individuals with other communication disorders. (pp. 1–2)

No one speech-language pathologist could possibly be expert in all areas within the defined scope of practice. Nevertheless, the statement indicates the wide variety of activities pursued by members of this profession. Individual practitioners tend to concentrate in particular areas of practice as determined by their interests, education, and experience and the settings in which they work.

Audiology

The brief profiles that follow suggest the range of activities pursued by members of the profession of audiology.

E.G. directs the audiology clinic in a large university medical center. Her responsibilities include oversight of a diagnostic and rehabilitation program; teaching medical students and residents who are preparing for practice in such specialty areas as otolaryngology and pediatrics; and conducting research. Her current research deals with a newly developed approach to identifying hearing loss in newborn infants. Because language development begins during the first year of life, it is important to identify hearing loss at the earliest possible age. The approach she is studying involves the recently discovered phenomenon of otoacoustic emissions. When the ear is stimulated by sound, it not only receives those sounds, but also emits sounds that can be recorded. When a small microphone is inserted into the infant's ear and controlled auditory stimuli are introduced, these so-called evoked acoustic emissions can be recorded. The technique seems to offer great promise for testing the hearing of individuals who are unable to make voluntary responses to sound and is, therefore, an important area of research.

When D.U. finished her graduate work in audiology, she accepted a position as an audiologist with a partnership of four otolaryngologists. Eventually, she became interested in the possibilities of independent private practice. After receiving a small business loan to cover the cost of the equipment and facilities she required, she opened her own office. She had many anxious moments during the next 3 years, but by "moonlighting" in various otolaryngologists' offices she was able to support herself while her practice developed. She now has a thriving practice, providing a wide range of audiology services to both children and adults. Although the majority of her patients are
(continued)

referred by physicians, she also sees many patients on referrals from schools, community agencies, and other human services professionals, as well as patients who come to her directly without any referral. (Many of the latter come because friends or family members who are former patients have recommended her.) She provides diagnostic services, counsels patients and their families, and dispenses hearing aids. D.U. has become particularly interested in providing services related to the new programmable hearing aids. These hearing aids enable a wider range of adjustments than were possible with previous instruments. Because these hearing aids are much more versatile and, after appropriate instruction, generally lead to greater user satisfaction, D.U. derives particular pleasure from this part of her practice.

G.W. is the audiology consultant for a county school system. He is responsible for a hearing conservation program, which involves screening the hearing of all children in the school district at least once every 3 years. He also maintains a complete diagnostic facility located in the school district administrative office building. Here he provides complete testing for children who are identified as possibly having hearing impairments during the screening program and regularly retests children who have shown hearing loss on previous tests. He also sees children on referral from teachers, school nurses, physicians, and parents. He counsels parents and consults with teachers and other school personnel regarding the children he sees. When children seem to be appropriate candidates for hearing aid use, he assists in selection of the appropriate aids, teaches them to use the hearing aids; orients their teachers, parents, and classmates; and checks regularly to ensure that the hearing aid is functioning properly. It often is necessary for him to work with public and private community agencies to assist families in obtaining needed medical services and purchasing hearing aids when financial resources are limited. He also is responsible for the selection and maintenance of the amplification systems used in the county's special classes for hearing-impaired children.

C.D. is the audiologist in a special clinical-research program. This program is concerned with the development of surgically implanted instruments that provide direct stimulation to the auditory nerve. Currently, such instruments are applied only in instances where patients have no usable hearing even with the assistance of the most powerful wearable hearing aids. Among her responsibilities are participating in the selection of appropriate patients through conducting an extensive test battery (a battery which also constitutes part of the protocol for important research studies), counseling patients and their families about the possible benefits that may be derived, working with the design engineer in making necessary adjustments once the instrument has been implanted, conducting intensive auditory training programs for newly implanted patients, and providing regular follow-up services to obtain precise data about whatever benefits accrue.

D.W. has entered into a partnership with two other audiologists to establish a company that provides audiology services to industry. When industries require personnel to work in noisy environments, they must be concerned about the effects of high levels of noise on their employees' hearing. D.W.'s company works on contract with several industries to provide a wide range of services. They operate a mobile hearing testing van which provides hearing screening for all personnel at regular intervals. They conduct sound surveys to determine the probable risk to workers of various work environments. They advise managers about steps that can be taken to reduce noise levels. They assist in the selection of noise protection equipment that can be used by individual workers, dispense such equipment, and instruct workers in its use. When workers suffer hearing loss, they make referrals to appropriate rehabilitation facilities. D.W. and his partners employ two paraprofessionals to assist them, especially in providing hearing screening services.

Definition

The *Dictionary of Occupational Titles* (United States Department of Labor, 1991) offers the following definition of audiologist:

✦ Determines type and degree of hearing impairment and implements habilitation and rehabilitation services for patient.

✦ Administers and interprets variety of tests such as air and bone conduction, and speech reception and discrimination tests, to determine type and degree of hearing impairment, site of damage, and effects on comprehension of speech.

✦ Evaluates test results in relation to behavioral, social, educational and medical information obtained from parents, families, teachers, speech pathologists, and other professionals to determine communication problems related to hearing disability.

✦ Plans and implements prevention, habilitation or rehabilitation services, including hearing aid selection and orientation, counseling, auditory training, lip reading, language habilitation, speech conservation, and other treatment programs developed in consultation with . . . other professionals.

✦ May refer patient to physician or surgeon if medical treatment is determined necessary.

✦ May conduct research in physiology, pathology, biophysics, or psychophysics of auditory systems, or design and develop clinical and research procedures and apparatus.

✦ May act as consultant to educational, medical, legal, and other professional groups.

✦ May teach art and science of audiology and direct scientific projects. (p. 61)

Scope of Practice

In 1989, the American Speech-Language-Hearing Association (1990) adopted the following scope of practice statement for the profession of audiology:

The practice of audiology includes:

✦ facilitating the conservation of auditory system function; developing and implementing environmental and occupational hearing conservation programs.

✦ screening, identifying, assessing and interpreting, diagnosing, preventing and rehabilitating peripheral and central auditory system dysfunctions;

✦ providing and interpreting behavioral and (electro) physiological measurements of auditory and vestibular functions.

✦ selecting, fitting and dispensing of amplification, assistive listening and alerting devices and other systems (e.g. implantable devices) and providing training in their use.

✦ providing aural rehabilitation and related counseling services to hearing impaired individuals and their families; and

✦ screening of speech-language and other factors affecting communication function for the purposes of an audiologic evaluation and/or initial identification of individuals with other communication disorders. (p. 2)

◆ SERVICES PROVIDED BY SPEECH-LANGUAGE PATHOLOGISTS AND AUDIOLOGISTS

The services provided by individual speech-language pathologists and audiologists depend in some measure on the settings in which they work. Nevertheless, most provide some version of the following services:

Screening

This service involves use of a standardized procedure to identify individuals who may have communication disorders and should be seen for full diagnostic studies. Screening may be directed toward a general population or specific "high-risk" groups. For example, if we wish to identify hearing-impaired children at the earliest possible date, we may apply a hearing screening procedure to all infants in a newborn nursery. Or, because we know that a high percentage of congenital or early-acquired hearing impairments are associated with some definable "risk" conditions, we may screen only children who present those conditions (e.g., a family history of hearing impairment, very low birth weight, certain infections in utero or during early infancy, etc.).

Diagnosis/Evaluation

Children and adults who show symptoms of communication disorders on the basis of screening tests, who raise the concern of their families or of other professionals, or who themselves become concerned should be seen for detailed studies. These studies seek to determine whether or not a potentially handicapping problem is present; describe the nature and extent of the disorder; suggest the next steps in further diagnostic studies or treatment; establish baselines against which the outcomes of intervention can be determined; and formulate advice to the patient, the family, and the other professionals participating in the patient's care.

Treatment/Therapy

Speech-language pathologists and audiologists provide services aimed at assisting patients to achieve communication that more nearly approximates normal, compensate for irremedial impairments, and reduce attitudinal barriers to better communication.

Counseling

Often the difference between counseling and treatment is indistinguishable. But two types of other counseling services can be differentiated: services that help patients recognize other areas in which they need assistance (e.g., the need for psychotherapy, vocational guidance, or special education), and services that help families and other "significant others" to play their roles in communicating with the patient and implementing other treatment goals.

Consultation

These services are directed toward other professionals. Speech-language pathologists and audiologists participate in two types of consultation. One type is offered to help other professionals participate more effectively in the care of specific patients. The other is more general, aimed at furthering their overall understanding of communication disorders and of the role of the particular professional in assisting children and adults with speech, language, and hearing problems. For example, speech-language pathologists may consult with classroom teachers about the management of a particular child. Or they may consult with teachers on more general issues such as the identification of children with communication disorders, the relationship between problems in spoken and written language, or planning language development activities to be carried out in the classroom.

◆ CREDENTIALS

In the United States, virtually all professions have adopted methods of assuring the public that their practitioners have completed appropriate preparation and are providing competent services in an ethical manner. At one time no such assurance was available to people with speech, language, and hearing problems. Elocution teachers — whose primary occupation was preparing refined young ladies and gentlemen to deliver recitations — offered instruction to children and adults with speech and language disorders, and sometimes even to hearing-impaired children. Often these teachers had no understanding of the real nature of those disorders. In other instances, people who themselves had — at least in their view — overcome communication disorders worked with children and adults with similar communication disorders, using methods they considered to have "cured" themselves. Some even offered courses by correspondence. When a few universities began to offer courses in speech-language pathology, it became apparent that some form of credentialing should be instituted to recognize the qualifications of people who had completed appropriate preparation to provide speech, language, and hearing services. Eventually three different forms of credentialing emerged: certification by the American Speech-Language-Hearing Association, certification by state departments of education, and state licensure.

ASHA Certification

The only nationally applicable credentials for the practice of the professions of speech-language pathology and audiology are the Certificates of Clinical Competence (CCCs) offered by the American Speech-Language-Hearing Association. These certificates do not grant the legal right to practice, but they are, nevertheless, used to define qualified providers of speech, language, and hearing services in many regulations adopted by public and private agencies.

ASHA grants two certificates, one in audiology (CCC-A) and one in speech-language pathology (CCC-SLP). Although each certificate has different requirements, the same general pattern is followed. The full text of current requirements for the CCCs appears in Appendix A. Briefly, the requirements include: (a) completion of a master's degree in speech-language pathology or audiology at a university whose program has been accredited by ASHA's Education and Training Board; (b) completion of coursework in areas related to "basic communication processes" (e.g., anatomy and physiology, acoustics, linguistics, human development); (c) coursework in the "major professional area" (i.e., speech-language pathology or audiology); (d) coursework in the "minor professional area" (i.e., to qualify for certification in speech-language pathology one must complete some coursework in audiology, or to qualify for certification in audiology one must complete some coursework in speech-language pathology); (e) completion of clinical practice under supervision; (f) completion of a Clinical Fellowship Year consisting of 9 months of full-time professional work under the sponsorship of a certified speech-language pathologist or audiologist; and (g) passing the National Examination in Speech-Language Pathology or the National Examination in Audiology.

Consumers of professional services not only deserve some assurance that the provider has appropriate qualifications, they also deserve some assurance that the services are provided in an ethical manner. Therefore, all holders of ASHA Certificates of Clinical Competence must subscribe to the ASHA Code of Ethics (see Appendix B).

School Credentials

In the United States, most matters related to regulation of services provided in the public schools are controlled at the state, rather than the national, level. These regulations also include the definition of qualifications for the providers of services in schools. As a result, there are significant differences among states in requirements for credentials for all professionals who work in the schools, including speech-language pathologists and audiologists (although relatively few states define qualifications for school audiologists).

During the first two decades of the 20th century, as local school districts recognized the need for providing special services to children with communication disorders, universities instituted programs to prepare the providers of those services. Gradually, special credentials were awarded by state departments of education to the graduates of those programs. Initially, these credential holders were considered to be specialized teachers. Thus credentials for serving children with communication disorders were considered supplementary to general education credentials. (In most instances, school language, speech, and hearing specialists completed all requirements for general classroom teaching as well as special courses dealing with communication disorders.) Gradually, this situation changed so that most states now award credentials authorizing specialists to work exclusively in this field.

Substantial differences remain among the 50 states in requirements for school language, speech, and hearing specialist credentials. Although most states require completion of a master's degree or an equivalent amount of graduate study, some still award credentials on completion of a bachelor's degree. ASHA standards have exerted some influence on school credential requirements in some states, but many still do not exact equivalent requirements. As a result of these idiosyncracies, school language, speech, and hearing specialists may encounter problems in moving from one state to another. Nevertheless, in most instances, holders of ASHA's CCC usually can obtain at least temporary credentials in any state, especially if they have completed some clinical practice in a school setting. These temporary credentials allow school employment pending completion of all requirements imposed by a particular state.

State Licensure

Most states ensure provider qualifications through state licensure. Licensure grants holders the legal right to practice a profession.

Conversely, unlicensed individuals who provide professional services are breaking the law. The first state licensure law in speech-language pathology and audiology was enacted in 1969. Subsequently licensure laws have been enacted in most, but not all, states. In a few instances, close relationships have been established between licensure standards and school credential requirements, but generally school language, speech, and hearing specialists are exempted from licensure requirements.

Fortunately, when licensure laws were enacted the ASHA Certificates of Clinical Competence were available as a nationally applicable model; thus, virtually all states adopted similar requirements. In some states holders of the CCCs qualify virtually automatically for licensure. In other states applicants must demonstrate completion of all state requirements, but those requirements closely approximate ASHA certification requirements. Some states grant reciprocity to individuals who are licensed in other states; others do not. But, even when reciprocity is not granted, general adherence to the ASHA certification model facilitates becoming licensed in another state.

State licensure laws not only define qualifications for entry into professions, they also establish some standards for the quality of the services professionals provide. The state agencies that administer licensure programs develop procedures for receiving and investigating allegations of incompetence or deleterious or unethical professional conduct. Disciplinary actions usually occur only in instances of egregious misconduct, but the mere fact that consumer complaints can be officially registered offers some protection.

◆ PROFESSIONAL SETTINGS FOR THE PRACTICE OF SPEECH-LANGUAGE PATHOLOGY AND AUDIOLOGY

An outstanding feature of the professions of speech-language pathology and audiology is the wide variety of settings in which services are provided. Some members of these professions spend their entire careers in one setting. Others transfer full-time employment from one setting to another. Still others work simultaneously in two or more settings. The majority of speech-language pathologists and audiologists are employed in the following settings:

Schools

The public schools constitute the largest single work setting for speech-language pathologists. Most speech-language pathologists in schools are engaged in providing what is usually termed "designated services." They work with students who spend the major portion of the school day in either regular classes or special day classes (e.g., classes for children with learning disabilities, developmental disabilities, or hearing impairments). However, some school districts provide special day classes for children with severe language disorders and assign speech-language pathologists to work full-time with those classes. Some school districts also provide audiology services and either employ one or more audiologists or contract services from other agencies or private practitioners.

Private schools also may offer speech-language pathology and audiology services either by employing such professionals or contracting their services. These schools may be designed to serve all children or to work with particular groups of handicapped children.

Although most educators agree that children usually are best served in day schools, residential schooling occasionally is required. Residential schools may be either public or private. Again, speech-language pathologists and audiologists often are included on their staffs. For example, most states provide one or more residential schools for deaf children. Those schools virtually always offer speech-language pathology and audiology services.

Health Services

Health care institutions probably constitute the second most prevalent work setting for speech-language pathologists and audiologists. Some institutions offer only one type of health care. However, there is a growing trend to provide a wide range of services within a single institution. Thus, many of the following services may be offered within the same complex.

Although still a vital aspect of health care, *acute inpatient hospitals,* because theirs is the most costly form of care, accommodate proportionately fewer and fewer patients. Admissions usually are restricted to patients undergoing major surgery and those requiring closely supervised intensive medical treatment. Audiologists often are called on to see patients in this setting. Speech-language pathologists may see hospital inpatients less frequently, but they do provide some vital services. They may offer initial diagnostic evaluations, short-term treatment, and most importantly counsel patients' families and assist in planning for the treatment that will take place following discharge. Increasingly, speech-language pathologists are serving inpatients with problems in swallowing as a result of whatever condition precipitated hospital admission (e.g., head trauma) or as a result of necessary surgical intervention (e.g., in the treatment of head and neck cancers).

Intermediate and long-term care facilities serve patients who do not require the level of care afforded by acute inpatient hospitals but still are not able to return home. Patients may be admitted to these facilities temporarily to complete convalescence, for extended stays when long-term treatment is required, or some patients may remain for the rest of their lives. Both speech-language pathologists and audiologists frequently serve patients in this setting.

Again because of the rising costs of health care, more and more services are provided in *ambulatory care centers*. In this instance, patients come to the center from their homes or from residential facilities to receive whatever services they need. A significant portion of speech-language pathology and audiology services are provided in these centers. When patients do not require inpatient care, but are unable to be transported to ambulatory care centers, they may be served by *home health agencies*. Occasionally such agencies offer audiology services. The majority offer speech-language pathology services.

Public health departments and *neighborhood health centers* may employ speech-language pathologists and audiologists to conduct screening programs. Some also provide treatment. Public health departments may assume responsibility for audiology services to school districts.

Industrial health programs serving industries that expose workers to high levels of noise often employ audiologists. These audiologists conduct regular hearing screening, provide more extensive hearing evaluations, offer rehabilitation services, and recommend and provide equipment to reduce the risks of noise exposure.

Speech-language pathologists and audiologists may be employed by a variety of *medical group practices*. These groups may be corporations of private medical practitioners (either practitioners of the same specialty such as otolaryngology or practitioners of various specialties) or health maintenance organizations that provide prepaid health care services and other organizations providing so-called "managed care."

Rehabilitation Services

A significant segment of speech-language pathology and audiology services is provided in *rehabilitation facilities,* which may accommodate either or both inpatients and outpatients. These facilities may be closely allied with health care institutions or they may be quite separate. *Rehabilitation* workshops prepare disabled individuals for work in business and industry and provide long-term employment for those who are unable to succeed in competitive employment. *Independent living centers* generally are geared to serving severely disabled individuals, helping them achieve the maximum possible level of independence in society.

Mental Health/Developmental Disabilities Services

As the name implies, mental health services accommodate children and adults with emotional and behavioral problems. Developmental disabilities include congenital and early acquired neurological problems, autism, as well as what was once called "mental retardation." Services may be provided in *inpatient care and treatment centers, day care and treatment centers,* and *outpatient mental health centers* (which may be called child guidance centers or child development centers). Special *high-risk infant/toddler programs* serve very young children who are considered likely to encounter developmental problems because of various physical or social factors. All these facilities and programs may employ speech-language pathologists and audiologists.

It may be optimistic to include them as mental health services, but nevertheless *facilities for juvenile offenders* serve many young people with developmental problems, particularly problems in language. A growing number of these facilities are including speech-language pathologists on their staffs.

Community Agencies and Services

Most communities now provide a variety of *child care centers.* Although their major purpose is to care for children while parents are working, they also may provide a wide range of health- and education-related services. Among the most notable early childhood programs is *Project Head Start* designed to provide early educational and health services to children from economically disadvantaged families. Many communities also provide services for older adults through *Senior Centers.* A wide range of speech-language pathology and audiology services may be provided within these community agencies.

Freestanding *speech and hearing centers* are found in many communities throughout the United States. These centers focus specifically on providing services to children and adults with speech, language, and hearing problems.

College and University Speech and Hearing Clinics

College and university speech and hearing clinics have long played an important role in the delivery of speech, language, and hearing services. Most often found in institutions preparing students to enter the professions of speech-language pathology and audiology, these clinics are established primarily to provide observational and clinical practice experiences for their students. Nevertheless, they do serve substantial numbers of children and adults with communication disorders.

Community colleges also may provide speech, language, and hearing services. Although these programs often serve only regularly enrolled students, some community colleges provide actual treatment services to disabled individuals (e.g., stroke patients) and some provide "high tech" centers which include specialized services to severely handicapped individuals such as selection and training in the use of electronic augmentative and alternative communication devices.

Private Practice

A growing number of speech-language pathologists and audiologists are venturing into the independent practice of their professions. Sometimes these private practitioners form partnerships, either with other members of their own professions or with members of related professions. Their services may be paid for by fees paid by their patients or their families or by public or private health insurance programs. Many private practitioners also contract to provide services to a variety of health care, rehabilitation, and educational institutions and programs.

SPEECH-LANGUAGE PATHOLOGY AND AUDIOLOGY IN THE SPECTRUM OF HUMAN SERVICES PROFESSIONS

Speech, language, and hearing problems often are associated with other, and sometimes multiple, physical, emotional, social, educational and vocational problems. Thus, assisting children and adults with communication disorders frequently involves the collaboration of members from different human services professions. Participating in these "team" efforts can be a highly gratifying aspect of the practice of the professions of speech-language pathology and audiology. Colleagues come from the health professions, the education professions, the rehabilitation professions, and the mental health and social services professions.

The Health Professions

Many speech and language disorders and virtually all hearing disorders are manifestations of underlying anatomic and physiologic problems. Therefore, the treatment of children and adults with communication disorders often involves close cooperation between speech-language pathologists and audiologists and health professionals.

Patients with speech, language, and hearing disorders often are referred by *physicians* for diagnostic and treatment services. In turn, speech-language pathologists may initiate referrals to physicians to assist in carrying out diagnostic and treatment programs. Such cooperative endeavors may involve practitioners of general medicine, or, more frequently, practitioners of medical specialties. Certain specialties are most likely to be involved in the care of patients with communication disorders.

Audiologists work closely with *otolaryngologists* because practitioners of that specialty are most likely to be concerned with patients with hearing impairments. Otolaryngologists also serve patients with voice disorders and, as head and neck surgeons, carry out procedures (e.g., in the treatment of cancers of the head and neck) that must be followed by rehabilitation programs provided by speech-language pathologists.

Pediatricians figure prominently among the medical referral sources to both speech-language pathologists and audiologists. Parents are most likely to consult pediatricians regarding their apprehensions concerning children's development, including speech and language acquisition. Pediatricians also treat most young patients with the middle ear infections that can reduce hearing acuity.

Neurologists see both children and adults whose central nervous system deficits interfere with language acquisition and use. They also figure prominently in the treatment of stroke patients, a group that forms a major segment of the adult population served by speech-language pathologists.

Both audiologists and speech-language pathologists see patients on referral from *neurosurgeons.* Audiologists may assist in the diagnosis of tumors involving the acoustic nerve and may even participate in monitoring certain central nervous system functions during surgery. Speech-language pathologists may see patients who show communication disorders following brain surgery.

Speech-language pathologists also sometimes work cooperatively with *plastic surgeons.* Such cooperation is most likely to occur in the treatment of patients with cleft palate, but may also involve patients with anatomic defects resulting from other congenital malformations or trauma.

Hearing loss figures prominently among occupation-related physical impairments. Therefore, audiologists often work closely with specialists in *occupational medicine.*

In many settings, speech-language pathologists and audiologists work more closely with health care professionals who are not physicians. Many of these health care workers are *nurses.* With the growing complexity of America's health care system, nurses continue to assume larger roles in that system. Graduate nurses are assuming increasingly independent responsibilities in hospitals. They often are the best source of information about individual patients. They can be of vital assistance in interpreting recommendations to families, and they often are in charge of planning programs for patients following discharge — an extremely important issue for patients who require continuing rehabilitation services.

Public health nurses carry important responsibilities in providing services to children — particularly to infants and preschoolers. They play a dominant role in the health care system of both urban centers and rural areas. Some public health programs send nurses into homes to provide direct care and counseling to families, and therefore they can be valuable allies in instances where family contacts are tenuous. In some communities, and in some school districts, public health nurses carry the responsibility for hearing screening programs.

Occupational health nurses are important colleagues of audiologists who work in industrial settings. Regrettably, recent years have seen the erosion of school nursing services provided in many school districts. Nevertheless, *school nurses* remain an essential link between school language, speech, and hearing specialists and physicians and other health care professionals and facilities.

Speech-language pathologists often find themselves in collegial relationships with *dentists.* Some speech problems characterized by inaccurate productions of particular speech sounds may result from dental malocclusions, leading to cooperative endeavors with orthodontists. When orthodontists believe that aberrant tongue patterns contribute to malocclusions, they may also refer patients to speech-language pathologists to institute retraining programs. Collaborative efforts between dentists and speech-language pathologists virtually always characterize the treatment of children and adults with cleft palate and other craniofacial anomalies. Dentists also may construct and fit prostheses for patients with anatomical defects resulting from congenital conditions or trauma — prostheses that also facilitate speech production.

The Education Professions

Increasingly federal and state laws and regulations and local school district regulations and policies require that all professional personnel serving the same child work together in achieving an accurate evaluation and planning an appropriate educational program. When children have communication disorders, speech-language pathologists and audiologists virtually always participate in that evaluation and planning. Usually these responsibilities are carried by professionals employed by a school district, but professionals employed elsewhere in the community may also be involved.

Because children spend the largest segment of the school day with classroom teachers, teacher collaboration is essential. Teachers are a vital link in the identification of children with speech, language, and hearing problems; are a source of important information; and provide valuable assistance in helping children carry over newly mastered communication skills into realistic social situations.

Most children served by language, speech, and hearing specialists come from regular classes, but when children are enrolled in special classes (e.g., for children with learning disabilities), close cooperation with special education teachers is particularly important. Recent years have given rise to a movement emphasizing educating children with various disabilities in the "least restrictive environment" (i.e., classes offering the most possible contact with normal contemporaries). As a result most disabled children today spend only portions of the school day with various special educators, rather than being placed in full-time special classes or special schools. Because this trend may increase the number of specialists serving a particular child there is an even greater need for collaboration.

School districts also employ individuals from the health care, mental health, and social services professions. Their collaborations with school speech, language, and hearing specialists are essentially similar to the collaborations that occur in other settings.

The Rehabilitation Specialties

Rehabilitation medicine is the medical specialty concerned with assisting patients in overcoming disabilities resulting from congenital deficits, illnesses, or injuries. Particularly during the early stages of rehabilitation programs they may carry the major responsibility for initiating and coordinating all treatment services.

Speech-language pathologists providing services in rehabilitation programs usually work closely with *physical therapists* and *occupational therapists*. Physical therapists are primarily concerned with the amelioration and prevention of impairments affecting posture, ambulation, and hand and arm mobility and dexterity. Traditionally, occupational therapists have been concerned with assisting disabled children and adults to master the activities of daily living and in providing programs to counteract the deleterious effects of inactivity during hospitalization or institutionalization. In recent years the scope of practice of occupational therapists has expanded beyond these areas. For example, they may work with speech-language pathologists in evaluating and adapting various communication devices.

Vocational guidance specialists also may be important allies to speech-language pathologists and audiologists who serve adolescents and adults. Communication disorders have obvious implications for occupational success. Therefore, patients with speech, language, and hearing problems often require vocational guidance and may require special vocational education, reeducation, or training programs.

The Mental Health and Social Services Professions

Psychiatry is the dominant medical specialty in the field of mental health. A few psychiatrists have become interested in speech, language, and hearing problems and collaborate with speech-language pathologists and audiologists in diagnostic and treatment programs.

No other profession has been more closely linked with the development of the field of speech-language pathology and audiology than has *psychology*. Close collaborations between these professions are maintained in virtually all work settings, both in establishing diagnoses and in carrying out treatment, therapeutic, and counseling programs.

Social service is a profession with an ever-expanding scope of practice. Social workers can be found in most work settings served by speech-language pathologists and audiologists. They are an important source of patient information; they help in finding and guiding patients toward sources of needed services; they assist in solving the economic problems that may interfere with patients receiving the services they require, and otherwise facilitate patients securing needed services. In recent years, social workers are increasingly providing psychotherapy and counseling, often as private practitioners.

As their scope of practice continues to expand and as new techniques are applied to the diagnosis and treatment of communication disorders, more and more professions will be represented among the colleagues of speech-language pathologists and audiologists. The quality of services available to children and adults with speech, language, and hearing disorders may depend to a significant degree on engaging the cooperation of an ever-widening cadre of professionals and, most importantly, on the amicability of working relationships among those professionals.

✦ SUMMARY

The discipline of human communication sciences and disorders and the professions of speech-language pathology and audiology are devoted to the study and treatment of children and adults with speech, language, and hearing disorders. Speech, language, and hearing enable people to communicate with one another. These processes are vital not only to social interaction, but also to cognition and learning. Because communication disorders have such far-reaching implications, this discipline and these professions figure prominently among the most important areas of scholarship and human services.

Practitioners of the professions of speech-language pathology and audiology provide a broad array of services. They must hold one or more of three types of credentials: Certificates of Clinical Competence awarded by the American Speech-Language-Hearing Association, licenses granted by state agencies, or credentials as school speech-language-hearing specialists awarded by state departments of education. They work in many different settings: in public and private schools, medical and other health services agencies, rehabilitation facilities, mental health/developmental disabilities agencies, other community agencies, colleges and universities, and private practices.

Because of the complexity of communication disorders, speech-language pathologists and audiologists work closely with the members of many other professions in serving their patients. These colleagues include members of the health professions, the education professions, the rehabilitation professions, and the mental health and social services professions.

The future holds bright promises for growth in the professions of speech-language pathology and audiology: growth in the number of practitioners of these professions; growth in the spectrum of settings in which speech-language pathologists and audiologists are employed and in their scope of practice; and growth in the knowledge base and the technologies that will continually improve the effectiveness of diagnosis and treatment of communication disorders.

◆ REFERENCES

American Speech-Language-Hearing Association. (1990). Scope of practice, speech-language pathology and audiology. *Asha, 32*(Suppl. 2), 1–2.

Aristotle. (1910). *The works of Aristotle* (Vol. 4). (J. A. Smith & W. D. Ross, Trans.). Oxford: Clarendon Press.

Exodus, 4, 10–12. *The New English Bible.* Oxford: Oxford University Press.

United States Department of Labor. (1991). *Dictionary of occupational titles* (4th ed., rev.). Washington, DC: U.S. Government Printing Office.

◆ SUGGESTED READINGS

American Speech-Language-Hearing Association. (1993). Preferred practice patterns for the professions of speech-language pathology and audiology. *Asha, 35*(Suppl. 11).

Butler, K. G. (Ed.). (1986). *Prospering in private practice: A handbook for speech-language pathology and audiology.* Rockville, MD: Aspen.

Flower, R. M. (1984). *Delivery of speech-language pathology and audiology services.* Baltimore, MD: Williams & Wilkins.

Lynch, C., & Welsh, R. (1993). Characteristics of state licensure laws. *Asha, 35*(3), 130–141.

McLauchlin, R. M. (Ed.). (1986). *Speech-language pathology and audiology: Issues and management.* Orlando, FL: Grune & Stratton.

Miller, R. M., & Groher, M. E. (1990). *Medical speech pathology.* Rockville, MD: Aspen.

Neidecker, E. A., & Blosser, J. (1992). *School programs in speech-language: Organization and management.* Englewood Cliffs, NJ: Prentice-Hall.

Slater, S. (1992). 1991 salaries on the rise for ASHA members. *Asha, 34*(3), 13–17.

Slater, S. (1992). Portrait of the professions. *Asha, 34*(8), 61–65.

Wood, M. L. (1991). *Private practice in communication disorders.* San Diego, CA: Singular Publishing Group.

✦ APPENDIX A

IMPLEMENTATION PROCEDURES FOR THE STANDARDS FOR THE CERTIFICATES OF CLINICAL COMPETENCE

The Standards for the Certificates of Clinical Competence are shown in italics. The Clinical Certification Board's implementation procedures are shown in regular print under each related standard.

Adopted October 23, 1988
Effective for Applications
for Certification Postmarked
on January 1, 1993,
and Thereafter[1]

The American Speech-Language-Hearing Association issues Certificates of Clinical Competence to individuals who present evidence of their ability to provide independent clinical services to persons who have disorders of communication. Individuals who meet the standards specified by the Association's Council on Professional Standards may be awarded a Certificate of Clinical Competence in Speech-Language Pathology (CCC-SLP) or a Certificate of Clinical Competence in Audiology (CCC-A). Individuals who meet the standards in both professional areas may be awarded both certificates.

STANDARD I: DEGREE

Applicants for either certificate must have a master's or doctoral degree.

Implementation:
Verification of the graduate degree on an official university transcript is required of all applicants prior to issuance of

the certificates. If the degree is not readily available, verification from the official university designee is required. Applicants may apply for certification upon completion of coursework and practicum with the recommendation of the program director. The program director should indicate the date the degree will be conferred. Individuals educated in foreign countries must verify the graduate degree with an official transcript evaluation from an educational evaluation service. A list of companies providing this service is available upon request from the National Office.

Effective January 1, 1994, all graduate coursework and graduate clinical practicum required in the professional area for which the Certificate is sought must have been initiated and completed at an institution whose program was accredited by the Educational Standards Board of the American Speech-Language-Hearing Association in the area for which the Certificate is sought.
Implementation:
Effective January 1, 1994, all applicants[2] must satisfactorily complete 21 graduate semester credit hours of coursework and 250 graduate clock hours of clinical practicum from an ESB-accredited program. These graduate semester hours and graduate clinical practicum hours must be in the area for which certification is sought.

If the master's degree is received at an ESB-accredited program and if the program director verifies that all coursework and practicum requirements have been met, approval of academic coursework and clinical practicum is automatic. In addition, the application must be received by the National Office within 3 years after the awarding of the degree.

The following applicants must complete the full application form and receive a Clinical Certification Board evaluation of their academic coursework and clinical practicum: (a) those who apply more than 3 years after receiving their master's degrees from an ESB-accredited program; (b) those who were graduate students and who were continuously enrolled in an ESB program that had its accreditation withdrawn during the applicant's enrollment; (c) those who satisfactorily completed 21 graduate semester credit hours of coursework and 250 graduate clock hours of clinical practicum in the area for which certification is sought at an ESB-accredited program but (1) received graduate degrees from programs not

---

[1]Applications postmarked January 1, 1991, and prior to January 1, 1993, may be submitted demonstrating compliance with either the current academic coursework and clinical practicum requirements for the Certificates of Clinical Competence (RCCCs) or the new academic coursework and clinical practicum standards for the Certificates of Clinical Competence (SCCCs). Upon initial application, all applicants must (a) complete all academic coursework requirements, (b) complete all clinical practicum requirements, and (c) obtain the graduate program director's signature as verification of completion of coursework and clinical practicum. Applications postmarked January 1, 1993, and thereafter must (a) demonstrate compliance with the new SCCCs and (b) obtain the graduate program director's signature as verification of satisfactory completion of coursework and clinical practicum.

If the Master's Degree is received at a program accredited by the Educational Standards Board (ESB) of ASHA, approval of academic coursework and clinical practicum will be automatic. ESB graduates whose applications are postmarked January 1, 1993, and thereafter must apply within 3 years of graduation in order to receive the automatic approval of academic coursework and clinical practicum. If an ESB graduate applies more than 3 years after the graduation date, the applicant must complete the entire application, which will be evaluated by the CCB.

---

[2]"All applicants" includes individuals who meet all certification requirements, including the graduate work at an ESB-accredited program.

accredited by ESB; (2) received graduate degrees in related areas; or (3) received graduate degrees from institutions in foreign countries; (d) those who were graduate students in a program in the ESB accreditation process, and (e) those who were enrolled in a program that was awarded candidacy status for accreditation during their course of study.

Satisfactory completion of both undergraduate and graduate academic coursework and clinical practicum requirements must be verified by the ESB-accredited program director's signature.

STANDARD II: ACADEMIC COURSEWORK
(75 Semester Credit Hours)

Applicants for either Certificate must have earned at least 75 semester[3] credit hours that reflect a well-integrated program of study dealing with (a) the biological/physical sciences and mathematics; (b) the behavioral and/or social sciences, including normal aspects of human behavior and communication; and (c) the nature, prevention, evaluation, and treatment of speech, language, hearing, and related disorders. The coursework should address, where appropriate, issues pertaining to normal and abnormal human development and behavior across the life span and to culturally diverse populations.
Implementation:
Applicants should demonstrate that their coursework addressed issues of normal/abnormal human behavior and development across the life span as well as issues pertaining to culturally diverse populations.

All coursework must be applicable toward the university's degree program.

At least 27 of the 75 semester credit hours must be in Basic Science Coursework (see Standard II-A).

At least 36 of the 75 semester credit hours must be in Professional Coursework (see Standard II-B).
Implementation:
At least 27 semester credit hours must be in Basic Sciences and 36 must be in Professional Coursework. The remaining 12 semester credit hours may be distributed between these two areas.

A specific course may usually be credited to no more than two categories. If a course is split in three categories, a course description form from the *Membership and Certification Handbook* must be submitted. This form must be accompanied by an official course description from the university's course catalogue. However, the content of at least 1 semester credit hour of the course must address the area in which partial credit is requested.

Up to 6 graduate semester credit hours for a thesis or dissertation may be accepted in the Basic Science and/or Professional Coursework category. An abstract must be submitted with the application verifying the thesis/dissertation content placement. Academic credit that is associated with

thesis or dissertation and for which graduate credit was received may apply in the Professional area, but may not be counted as meeting any of the minimum requirements, including the 21 graduate semester credit hours in the professional area for which the certificate is sought. For applicants seeking certification in speech-language pathology, minimum requirements are defined as 6 semester credit hours in speech disorders; 6 semester credit hours in language disorders; 3 semester credit hours in hearing disorders and hearing evaluations; and 3 semester hours in habilitative/rehabilitative procedures with individuals who have hearing impairments. For applicants seeking certification in audiology, minimum requirements are defined as 6 semester credit hours in hearing disorders and hearing evaluation; 6 semester credit hours in habilitative/rehabilitative procedures with individuals who have hearing impairment; 3 semester hours in speech disorders; and 3 semester credit hours in language disorders.

STANDARD II-A: BASIC SCIENCE COURSEWORK
(27 of 75 Semester Credit Hours)

Applicants for either Certificate must earn at least 27 semester credit hours in the basic sciences.

At least 6 semester credit hours must be in the biological/physical sciences and mathematics.
Implementation:
Coursework may include a variety of areas under the biological/physical sciences and mathematics areas. However, there must be one course in the biological/physical science area and one course in college-level mathematics, which may include courses in statistics. Remedial courses (skill improvement courses), historical mathematics courses, and methodology courses (such as methods of teaching mathematics) may not be used to satisfy this requirement.

At least 6 semester credit hours must be in the behavioral and/or social sciences.
Implementation:
The content of coursework in behavioral and/or social sciences should include study that pertains to understanding normal/abnormal human behavior, development across the life span, social interaction, and issues of culturally diverse populations.

At least 15 semester credit hours must be in the basic human communication processes, to include coursework in each of the following three areas of speech, language, and hearing: the anatomic and physiologic bases; the physical and psychophysical bases; the linguistic and psycholinguistic aspects.[4]

---

[3]One quarter credit hour is equivalent to two thirds of a semester credit hour.

[4]The three broad categories of required education, and the examples of areas within these classifications, are not meant to be analogous to or imply specific course titles or to be exhaustive.

Implementation:

The 15 semester credit hours should be in courses that provide information applicable to the normal development and use of speech, language, and hearing, including:

(1) At least one course in anatomic and physiologic bases for the normal development and use of speech, language, and hearing, for example, anatomy, neurology, and physiology of speech, language, and hearing mechanisms.

(2) At least one course in the physical basis and processes of the production and perception of speech, language, and hearing, for example, acoustics or physics of sound, phonology, physiologic and acoustic phonetics, perceptual processes, and psychoacoustics.

(3) At least one course in the linguistic and psycholinguistic variables related to normal development of speech, language, and hearing—for example, linguistics (historical, descriptive, sociolinguistics, urban language), psychology of language, psycholinguistics, language and speech acquisition, and verbal learning and verbal behavior.

This coursework should include emphasis on the normal aspects of human communication to give the student a wide exposure to diverse kinds of information in the content areas stated above.

Although coursework in the disorders area may contain review content in basic human communication processes, this content cannot be used to meet the 15 semester credit hour requirement in the basic human communication processes.

Some of these 15 semester credit hours may be obtained in courses that are taught in departments outside the speech-language pathology and audiology programs. Courses designed to improve the speaking and writing ability of the student cannot be used to meet the 15 semester credit hour requirement in the basic human communication processes.

STANDARD II-B: PROFESSIONAL COURSEWORK
(36 of 75 Semester Credit Hours)

Applicants for either certificate must earn at least 36 semester credit hours in courses that concern the nature, prevention, evaluation, and treatment of speech, language, and hearing disorders. Those 36 semester credit hours must encompass courses in speech, language, and hearing that concern disorders primarily affecting children as well as disorders primarily affecting adults. At least 30 of the 36 semester credit hours must be in courses for which graduate credit was received, and at least 21 of those 30 must be in the professional area for which the certificate is sought.

Implementation:

There must be at least 30 graduate semester credit hours in speech-language pathology or audiology, and 21 of the hours must be in the professional area for which the certificate is sought.

Receipt of graduate credit must be verified on an official transcript.

Certificate of Clinical Competence in Speech-Language Pathology (CCC-SLP)

At least 30 of the 36 semester credit hours of professional coursework must be in speech-language pathology. At least 6 of the 30 must be in speech disorders, and at least 6 must be in language disorders.

Implementation:

In addition to the 6 semester credit hours required in speech disorders and 6 required in language disorders, the 30 semester credit hours should include information on the understanding, evaluation, treatment, and prevention of communication disorders across all age spans in a variety of disorders, as follows:

(1) Understanding of speech and language disorders, such as various types of communication disorders, their manifestations, and their classifications.

(2) Evaluation skills such as procedures, techniques, and instrumentation used to assess the speech and language status of children and adults, and the basis of disorders of speech and language.

(3) Management procedures, such as principles in remedial methods used in habilitation and rehabilitation for children and adults with various disorders of communication, as well as prevention of communication disorders.

(4) Evaluation and management procedures that do not pertain specifically to speech disorders or language disorders and are within ASHA's current Scope of Practice for Speech-Language Pathology. Note: Courses in this category may not fulfill the 6 semester credit hour minimums for speech disorders or language disorders.

At least 6 of the 36 semester credit hours of professional coursework must be in audiology. At least 3 of the 6 must be in hearing disorders and hearing evaluation, and at least 3 must be in habilitative/rehabilitative procedures with individuals who have hearing impairment.

Implementation:

It is highly recommended that at least 3 semester credit hours in audiology be taken at the graduate level for the minor professional area.

To meet the minimum aural habilitation/rehabilitation requirement, coursework must emphasize evaluation and management procedures for speechreading, auditory training, speech/language habilitation/rehabilitation, and other communication systems for the hearing impaired. A course pertaining exclusively to acquisition of and facility with manual communication systems does not meet the minimum requirement but may be included in the total 36 semester credit hours needed in professional coursework.

When more than the required 3 semester credit hours of habilitative/rehabilitative procedures have been earned, up to 6 semester credit hours in that category may be counted in the major professional area for certification in speech-language pathology. However, these hours may not be counted toward meeting the 6 semester hour minimum requirements in speech-language pathology or the 6 semester hour minimum requirements in language disorders.

A maximum of 6 academic semester credit hours associated with clinical practicum may be counted toward the minimum of 36 semester credit hours of professional coursework, but those hours may not be used to satisfy the minimum of 6 semester credit hours in speech disorders, 6 hours in language disorders, or 6 hours in audiology, or in the 21 graduate credits in the professional area for which the certificate is sought.

Implementation:

Academic credit that is associated with clinical practicum and for which graduate credit was received may apply in the professional area but may not be counted as meeting any of the minimum requirements, including the 21 graduate semester credit hours in the professional area for which the certificate is sought. Academic credit that is obtained from practice teaching or practicum work in other professions will not be counted toward the requirements.

Certificate of Clinical Competence in Audiology (CCC-A)

At least 30 of the 36 semester credit hours of professional coursework must be in audiology. At least 6 of the 30 must be in hearing disorders and hearing evaluation, and at least 6 must be in habilitative/rehabilitative procedures with individuals who have hearing impairment. Credits in courses that concern the nature, prevention, evaluation, and treatment of speech and language disorders associated with hearing impairment may be counted.

Implementation:

The 30 semester credit hours of professional coursework required for the Certificate of Clinical Competence in Audiology should include information on hearing disorders, hearing evaluations, habilitative/rehabilitative procedures, and preventive methods, including the study of auditory disorders and habilitative/rehabilitative procedures across the life span, as follows:

(1) Auditory disorders, such as the nature and cause of pathologies of the auditory system; evaluation of auditory disorders, including assessment of the peripheral and central auditory system; the effects of auditory disorders on communication; instruction in electrophysiological measurements; and vestibular and balance testing.

(2) Habilitative/rehabilitative and preventive procedures, such as selection and use of appropriate amplification instrumentation for the hearing impaired; both individual and group evaluation of instruments using state-of-the-art instrumentation to assess real ear function of amplification; evaluation of speech and language problems of the hearing impaired; and management procedures for speech and language habilitation and/or rehabilitation of the hearing impaired, including but not exclusive to speechreading, auditory training, and manual communication. A course pertaining exclusively to acquisition of and facility with manual communication systems cannot be counted toward meeting the 6 semester hour minimum requirement in habilitation/

rehabilitation but may be included in the total 36 semester credit hours needed in professional coursework.

(3) Conservation of hearing, such as environmental noise control and identification audiometry.

(4) Instrumentation, such as calibration techniques and characteristics of amplifying systems.

At least 6 of the 36 semester credit hours of professional coursework must be in speech-language pathology. At least 3 of the 6 must be in speech disorders, and at least 3 must be in language disorders. This coursework in speech-language pathology must concern the nature, prevention, evaluation, and treatment of speech and language disorders not associated with hearing impairment.

Implementation:

It is highly recommended that at least 3 semester credit hours in speech-language pathology be taken for graduate credit.

When only the minimum requirement of 6 semester credit hours is met, such study must concern the nature, prevention, evaluation, and treatment of speech and language disorders not associated with hearing impairment.

A maximum of 6 academic semester credit hours associated with clinical practicum may be counted toward the minimum of 36 semester credit hours of professional coursework, but those hours may not be used to satisfy the minimum of 6 semester credit hours in hearing disorders/evaluation, 6 hours in habilitative/rehabilitative procedures, or 6 hours in speech-language pathology, or the 21 graduate credits in the professional area for which the certificate is sought.

Implementation:

Academic credit that is associated with clinical practicum and for which graduate credit was received may apply, but may not be counted as meeting any of the minimum requirements, including the 21 graduate semester credit hours in the professional area for which the certificate is sought. Academic credit that is obtained from practice teaching or practicum work in other professions will not be counted toward the requirement.

Standard III: Supervised Clinical Observation and Clinical Practicum
(375 Clock Hours)

Applicants for either certificate must complete the requisite number of clock hours of supervised clinical observation and supervised clinical practicum that are provided by the educational institution or by one of its cooperating programs.

Implementation:

Applicants should be assigned practicum only after they have had sufficient coursework to qualify for such experience.

The supervision must be provided by an individual who holds the Certificate of Clinical Competence in the appropriate area of practice.

Implementation:

All observation and clinical practicum hours must be supervised by individuals who hold a current CCC in the area in which the observation and practicum hours are being obtained.

Persons holding a CCC in speech-language pathology may supervise all speech-language pathology evaluation and treatment services, nondiagnostic audiologic screening for the purpose of performing a speech and/or language evaluation or for the purpose of initial identification of individuals with other communicative disorders, and aural habilitative and rehabilitative services.

Persons holding a CCC in audiology may supervise audiologic evaluations, amplification (hearing aid selection and management), speech and/or language screening for the purpose of initial identification of individuals with other communicative disorders, and aural habilitative and rehabilitative services.

Although there may be some practicum supervision overlap, the supervision of clock hours in the minor area should be conducted by individuals who are certified in the minor area. Therefore, a speech-language pathologist should not supervise all of the hours obtained in aural rehabilitation.

A supervisor with current CCCs must be on site at all times. Only a currently certified clinician may supervise student practicum at on- and off-campus sites. Supervision of the clinical practicum must include direct observation, guidance, and feedback by the currently certified supervisor to facilitate development of the student's clinical competence.

STANDARD III-A: CLINICAL OBSERVATION
(25 Clock Hours)

Applicants for either certificate must complete at least 25 clock hours of supervised observation prior to beginning the initial clinical practicum.

Implementation:

Observations serve as a preparatory experience prior to beginning direct clinical practicum with individuals who have communication disorders.

Those 25 clock hours must concern the evaluation and treatment of children and adults with disorders of speech, language, or hearing.

Implementation:

Actual observations or videotapes may be used for observation purposes.

A student clinician must observe a total of 25 clock hours of evaluation and management. These observations should be relative to, but precede, clinical assignment with specific types of communication disorders, for example, articulation, language, fluency, voice, hearing impairment. The observation experience must be under the direct supervision of a qualified clinical supervisor who holds ASHA certification in the appropriate area.

Supervision may include simultaneous observations with the student or the submission of written reports or summaries by the student for supervisor monitoring, review, and approval.

STANDARD III-B: CLINICAL PRACTICUM
(350 Clock Hours)

Applicants for either certificate must complete at least 350 clock hours of supervised clinical practicum that concern the evaluation and treatment of children and adults with disorders of speech, language, and hearing. No more than 25 of the clock hours may be obtained from participation in staffings in which evaluation, treatment, and/or recommendations are discussed or formulated, with or without the client present.

Implementation:

Direct supervised clinical practicum involves direct time spent in actual evaluation or treatment with clients who present communication disorders. Time spent with the client or caretaker engaging in information giving, counseling, or training for a home program may be counted as direct contact time if the activities are directly related to evaluation and treatment. Ancillary activities such as writing lesson plans, scoring tests, transcribing language samples, and preparing treatment activities and materials may not be counted. Meetings with practicum supervisors may not be counted under the 25 clock hours for staffing.

At least 250 of the 350 clock hours must be completed in the professional area for which the certificate is sought while the applicant is engaged in graduate study.

Implementation:

As of January 1, 1994, all 250 graduate clinical practicum hours in the area in which certification is sought must be initiated and completed at programs that are accredited by ESB during the applicant's enrollment.

At least 50 supervised clock hours must be completed in each of three types of clinical setting.

Implementation:

The clinical settings may be within the organizational structure of the training institution or include its affiliates. Such settings may include separate units/settings within an institution or its affiliates (brain injury units/stroke units/nursing homes/classrooms for severely language-impaired children), community clinics, public schools, rehabilitation centers, hospitals, and private practice settings. For the three clinical settings to be classified as different settings, the training institution must determine that the student has gained unique experiences in each one. For example, a student might have experience in an acute-care hospital as well as in a long-term-care hospital. Or the student might have experience in a school that provides itinerant services as well as in one that provides a classroom for children who present communication disorders.

Certificate of Clinical Competence in Speech-Language Pathology (CCC-SLP)

The applicant must have experience in the evaluation and treatment of children and adults, and with a variety of types and severities of disorders of speech[5], language, and hearing.

Implementation:

Clinical experience should prepare the applicant to practice in the speech-language pathology area according to ASHA's current "Scope of Practice" position statement (see *Asha, 32* [Suppl. 2], 1-2). Clinical experience should include both individual and group client contact.

At least 250 of the 350 supervised clock hours must be in speech-language pathology. At least 20 of those 250 clock hours must be completed in each of the eight categories listed below.

1. *Evaluation: Speech disorders in children*
2. *Evaluation: Speech disorders in adults*
3. *Evaluation: Language disorders in children*
4. *Evaluation: Language disorders in adults*

Implementation:

Evaluation refers to those hours in screening, assessment, and diagnosis that are accomplished prior to the initiation of a treatment program. Hours to be counted in the evaluation category may also include a formal reevaluation. Periodic assessments during treatment are to be considered treatment. The majority of evaluation hours in each category must not be in screening activities.

At least 50% of each evaluation session, including screening and identification activities, must be observed directly by the supervisor.

5. *Treatment: Speech disorders in children*
6. *Treatment: Speech disorders in adults*
7. *Treatment: Language disorders in children*
8. *Treatment: Language disorders in adults*

Implementation:

Treatment for speech and language disorders refers to clinical management, including direct and indirect services, progress monitoring activities, and counseling.

At least 25% of each applicant's total contact time in clinical treatment with each client must be observed directly by the supervisor.[6]

If a client presents communication disorders in two or more of the disorder categories, accumulated clock hours should be distributed among these categories according to the amount of treatment time spent on each. For example, if a client with both articulation and language problems received 20 hours of treatment and approximately 75% of each treatment session was spent on articulation, the clinician should record credit for 15 hours of treatment for speech disorders and 5 hours of treatment for language disorders.

---

[5]"Speech disorders" include disorders of articulation, voice, and fluency.

[6]Observations may take place on-site or by closed-circuit television. In addition to observations, it is recommended that other performance evaluations, such as conferences, audio and video recordings, written evaluations, rating instruments, inspection of lesson plans, and written reports be used in the supervisory process.

Up to 20 clock hours in the major professional area may be in related disorders.

Implementation:

Twenty clock hours may be obtained for activities related to the prevention of communicative disorders and the enhancement of speech, language, and communicative effectiveness and improved oral pharyngeal function and related disorders. Similarly, activities implemented to prevent the onset of speech/language disorders and their causes as well as efforts to advance the development and conservation of optimal communication may be counted.

At least 35 of the 350 clock hours must be in audiology. At least 15 of those 35 clock hours must involve the evaluation or screening of individuals with hearing disorders, and at least 15 must involve habilitation/rehabilitation of individuals who have hearing impairment.

Certificate of Clinical Competence in Audiology (CCC-A)

The applicant must have experience with the evaluation and treatment[7] of children and adults, with a variety of types and severities of disorders of hearing, speech, and language, and with the selection and use of amplification and assistive devices.

Implementation:

Clinical experience should prepare the applicant to practice in the area of Audiology according to ASHA's current "Scope of Practice" position statement (see *Asha, 32* [Suppl. 2], 1–2). Clinical experience should include both individual and group client contact.

Evaluation shall include collection of relevant information regarding past and present status, selection and administration of reliable evaluation procedures, interpretation of results, and appropriate referrals for additional evaluation and/or treatment based on the evaluation.

At least 50% of each evaluation session, including screening and identification activities, must be observed directly by the supervisor.

Both direct and indirect services may be counted under treatment for hearing disorders.

At least 25% of each applicant's total contact time in clinical treatment with each client must be observed directly by the supervisor.

At least 250 of the 350 supervised clock hours must be in audiology. At least 40 of those 250 clock hours must be completed in each of the first two categories listed below. At least 80 hours must be completed in categories 3 and 4 with a minimum of 10 hours in each of these categories. At least 20 of those 250 clock hours must be completed in Category 5:

1. *Evaluation: Hearing in children*
2. *Evaluation: Hearing in adults*

---

[7]"Treatment" for hearing disorders refers to clinical management and counseling, including auditory training, speech reading, and speech and language services for those with hearing impairment.

Implementation:

Applicants should demonstrate a variety of clinical experiences in screening and evaluation, including electrophysiological test measures such as ABR (excluding intraoperative monitoring) and vestibular testing.

3. *Selection and use: Amplification and assistive devices for children*
4. *Selection and use: Amplification and assistive devices for adults*

Implementation:

Applicants should demonstrate a variety of clinical experiences in selection and use of approved amplification and assistive devices including state-of-the-art measures such as real ear procedures.

5. *Treatment: Hearing disorders in children and adults*

Implementation:

Applicants should demonstrate a variety of clinical experiences in treatment of hearing disorders in children and adults.

Up to 20 clock hours in the major professional area may be in related disorders.

Implementation:

These clock hours may include but are not limited to hearing conservation programs and intraoperative monitoring.

At least 35 of the 350 clock hours must be in speech-language pathology. At least 15 of those 35 clock hours must involve the evaluation or screening of individuals with speech and language disorders unrelated to hearing impairment, and at least 15 must involve the treatment of individuals with speech and language disorders unrelated to hearing impairment.

STANDARD IV: NATIONAL EXAMINATIONS IN SPEECH-LANGUAGE PATHOLOGY AND AUDIOLOGY

Applicants must pass the National Examination in the area for which the certificate is sought.

Implementation:

The National Examinations in Speech-Language Pathology and Audiology (NESPA) are designed to assess, in a comprehensive fashion, the applicant's mastery of knowledge of professional concepts and issues to which the applicant has been exposed throughout professional education and clinical practicum. The applicant must pass the examination in the area of certification sought. The examination must be passed within 2 years after the first exam administration following the approval of the applicant's coursework and clinical practicum by the Clinical Certification Board.

An applicant who fails the examination may retake it. If the examination is not successfully passed within a 2-year period, the applicant's certification application period will

lapse. If the examination is passed at a later date, the individual may reapply for certification. Upon reapplication, the individual's application will be reviewed. Certification Standards and fees in effect at the time of reapplication will be applied.

STANDARD V: THE CLINICAL FELLOWSHIP

After completion of academic coursework (Standard II) and clinical practicum (Standard III), the applicant then must successfully complete a Clinical Fellowship.

Implementation:

The Clinical Fellowship is designed to foster the continued development and integration of the knowledge, skills, and tasks of clinical practice in speech-language pathology or audiology consistent with ASHA's current scopes of practice.

The Fellowship must be completed within 7 years of the date the academic coursework and practicum were completed. Otherwise, the individual must reapply.

Once initiated, the Clinical Fellowship must be completed within a maximum of 36 consecutive months.

Applicants must meet academic and practicum requirements in effect at the time of application or reapplication.

Because standards may change, it is to the applicant's advantage to initiate the Clinical Fellowship experience as soon as possible after the academic coursework and practicum have been completed.

The Fellowship will consist of at least 36 weeks of full-time professional experience or its part-time equivalent.

Implementation:

Full-time employment is defined as a minimum of 30 hours per week in direct patient/client contact, consultations, record-keeping, and administrative duties relevant to a bona fide program of clinical work. Part-time equivalency is defined as follows:

(1) 15–19 hours/week over 72 weeks
(2) 20–24 hours/week over 60 weeks
(3) 25–29 hours/week over 48 weeks

Professional experience of less than 15 hours/week does not meet the requirement.

The Fellowship must be completed under the supervision of an individual who holds the Certificate of Clinical Competence in the area for which certification is sought.

Implementation:

It is the applicant's responsibility to locate and obtain a qualified Supervisor for the Clinical Fellowship. In the case of multiple Supervisors, a primary Supervisor must be designated, and each Supervisor must hold the Certificate of Clinical Competence in the area in which the Clinical Fellow is working and seeking certification.

A Clinical Fellowship Registration Agreement[8] must be submitted to the Clinical Certification Board prior to or within 4 weeks of initiation of the Clinical Fellowship (CF). The CF Supervisor will then receive the Clinical Supervisor Information Packet (CSIP) from the CCB. Receipt of the CSIP by the CF Supervisor acknowledges that the CF Registration agreement has been received by the CCB. The CSIP includes Clinical Supervisor's Responsibilities, CF Instructions, CF Report, and current evaluation instrument. Failure to submit the mandatory Clinical Fellowship Registration Agreement will result in an extension of the Clinical Fellowship.

Clinical Fellowship supervision must entail the personal and direct involvement of the Supervisor in any and all ways that will permit the CF Supervisor to monitor, evaluate and improve the Clinical Fellow's performance.

The CF experience should be divided into three segments, each representing one third of the total time spent in employment (e.g., a 36-week Fellowship would be divided into three 12-week segments; a 72-week Fellowship would be divided into three 24-week segments).

The CF Supervisor must engage in no fewer than 36 supervisory activities during the CF experience. This supervision must include 18 on-site observations of direct client contact at the Clinical Fellow's work site (1 hour equals 1 on-site observation; a maximum of 6 on-site observations may be accrued in one day). At least 6 on-site observations must be accrued during each third of the experience. These on-site observations must be of the Clinical Fellow providing screening, evaluation, assessment, habilitation, and rehabilitation.

In addition, the supervision must include 18 other monitoring activities (at least 2 activities in a 4-week period). These other monitoring activities may be executed by correspondence, review of videotapes, evaluation of written reports, phone conferences with the Clinical Fellow, evaluations by professional colleagues, and so forth.

The Clinical Certification Board may allow this supervisory process to be conducted in other ways; however, this must be submitted for prior approval to the Clinical Certification Board at the time the mandatory Clinical Fellowship Registration Agreement is submitted.

The professional experience shall involve primarily clinical activities.

Implementation:

Eighty percent of the work week must be in direct clinical activities (i.e., assessment, diagnosis, evaluation, screening, treatment, report writing, family/client consultation, and/or counseling) related to the management process of individuals who exhibit communication disabilities. For example, in a 30-hour work week, at least 24 hours must consist of direct clinical activities; in a 15-hour work week, at least 12 hours must consist of direct clinical activities.

The supervisor periodically shall conduct a formal evaluation of the applicant's progress in the development of professional skills.

---

[8]Refer to the *Membership and Certification Handbook.*

Implementation:

The CF Supervisor must use the current evaluation instrument. Until January 1, 1994, the PRO Scale must be completed at least once during each of the three segments of the Fellowship. This evaluation must be shared and discussed with the Clinical Fellow, and the form must be signed and dated by both. All CF evaluations must be carried out by the primary Supervisor, who will sign the final report.

Within 1 month of the completion of the Clinical Fellowship experience, the Fellow and the Supervisor must sign and submit a Clinical Fellowship Report and the current evaluation instrument to the National Office for review by the CCB. (See the *Membership and Certification Handbook* for the required forms.)

If the Clinical Fellowship is initiated and successfully completed in a program accredited by the Professional Services Board (PSB) of ASHA, approval of the Fellowship is automatic. In such instances, the director of the PSB program must sign the Fellowship report, verifying compliance with the Clinical Fellowship requirements as stated above.

At the completion of the Clinical Fellowship, if the Supervisor does not recommend approval of the Fellowship experience, he/she must so indicate on the appropriate section of the CF report and sign the report. Then, within 30 days, the Supervisor must submit a letter of explanation and supporting documentation to the Clinical Certification Board, including a signed current evaluation instrument. This information must be shared with the Clinical Fellow.

Following a negative recommendation, the Clinical Fellow may complete an entirely new Fellowship experience and/or request a special review by the Clinical Certification Board.

In order to request a special review, the Clinical Fellow must submit the signed Fellowship report, the signed current evaluation instrument, a letter of explanation, and supporting documentation of current clinical skills within 30 days of completing the experience. It will be necessary for the Clinical Certification Board to share this information with the CF Supervisor and to solicit any additional information the Supervisor wishes to provide. The Board will then review all information submitted to determine whether the CF experience will be approved.

PROCEDURES FOR OBTAINING AND MAINTAINING THE CERTIFICATES OF CLINICAL COMPETENCE

The applicant must submit to the Clinical Certification Board a description of professional education and academic clinical practicum on the form provided for that purpose. The applicant should recognize that it is highly desirable to list upon this application form the entire professional education and academic clinical practicum training.

No credit may be allowed for courses listed on the application unless satisfactory completion is verified by an official transcript. Satisfactory completion is defined as the applicant's having received academic credit (i.e., semester hours, quarter hours, or other unit of credit) with a passing grade as defined by the training institution. If the master's degree is received from a program accredited by the Educational Standards Board (ESB) of the American Speech-Language-Hearing Association (ASHA), approval of education and academic clinical practicum requirements will be automatic.

The applicant must request that the director of the training program where the majority of graduate training was obtained sign the application. In the case where the training program is not accredited by ESB of ASHA that director (1) verifies that the applicant has met the educational and clinical practicum requirements, and (2) recommends that the applicant receive the certificate upon completion of all the requirements.

In the event that the applicant cannot obtain the signature of the director of the training program, the applicant should send with the application a letter giving in detail the reasons for the inability to do so. In such an instance, letters of recommendation from other faculty members may be submitted.

Application for approval of educational requirements and academic clinical practicum experiences should be made (a) as soon as possible after completion of these experiences, and (b) either before or shortly after the Clinical Fellowship Year is begun.

Upon completion of education and academic clinical practicum training, the applicant should proceed to obtain professional employment and a supervisor for the Clinical Fellowship. The filing of a Clinical Fellowship Registration Agreement is required.

Within one month following completion of the Clinical Fellowship, the CF and the CF supervisor must submit a Clinical Fellowship Report to the Clinical Certification Board. If the Clinical Fellowship experience was completed in a program accredited by the Professional Services Board (PSB) of ASHA, approval will be automatic. In such instance, the director of the PSB program must sign the Clinical Fellowship Report verifying compliance with requirements.

Upon approval of the academic coursework, clinical practicum hours, the Clinical Fellowship, and a passing score on the National Examination, and payment of all fees, the applicant will become certified.

A schedule of fees for certification may be obtained, and payment of these fees is requisite for the various steps involved in obtaining a certificate. Checks should be made payable to the American Speech-Language-Hearing Association.

After certification has been awarded, an Annual Certification Fee (ACF) is payable in advance each year. A certificate holder whose ACF is in arrears will be dropped from the register of certificate holders.

Appeals

In the event that at any stage the Clinical Certification Board informs the applicant that the application has been denied, the applicant has the right to request a Show Cause review. In order to initiate such a review, the applicant must write to the Chair of the Clinical Certification Board and specifically request a Show Cause review of the application. If that review results, again, in rejection, the applicant has the right to appeal the case to the Council on Professional Standards in Speech-Language Pathology and Audiology (the Standards Council) by writing to the chair of the Standards Council at the National Office of the American Speech-Language-Hearing Association. The applicant must submit a letter of intent to appeal within 30 days and a memorandum specifying the grounds of the appeal within 60 days from the date of the rejection letter. The decision of the Standards Council will be final.

OUTLINE OF THE NEW STANDARDS FOR THE CERTIFICATES OF CLINICAL COMPETENCE

Effective for Applications for Certification Postmarked January 1, 1993, and Thereafter

I: **Degree:** Applicants for either certificate must hold a master's or doctoral degree. Effective 1/1/94, all graduate coursework and clinical practicum required in the professional area for which the Certificate is sought must have been initiated and completed at an institution whose program was accredited by the ESB in the area for which the Certificate is sought.

II: **Academic Coursework:** 75 semester credit hours (s.c.h.)

A: **Basic Science Coursework: 27 s.c.h.**

- 6 s.c.h. in biological/physical sciences and mathematics
- 6 s.c.h. in behavioral and/or social sciences
- 15 s.c.h. in basic human communication processes to include the anatomic and physiologic bases, the physical and psychophysical bases, and the linguistic and psycholinguistic aspects

B: **Professional Coursework: 36 s.c.h.,** 30 in courses for which graduate credit was received and 21 in the professional area for which the Certificate is sought

CCC-SLP
30 s.c.h. in speech-language pathology
—6 in speech disorders[1]
—6 in language disorders[1]

- 6 s.c.h. in audiology
—3 in hearing disorders and hearing evaluation[1]
—3 in habilitative/rehabilitative procedures[1]

CCC-A
- 30 s.c.h. in audiology
—6 in hearing disorders and hearing evaluation[1]
—6 in habilitative/rehabilitative procedures[1]
- 6 s.c.h. in speech-language pathology, not associated with hearing impairment
—3 in speech disorders[1]
—3 in language disorders[1]

III. **Supervised Clinical Observation and Clinical Practicum:** 375 clock hours (c.h.)

A: **Clinical Observation: 25 c.h.,** prior to beginning initial clinical practicum

B: **Clinical Practicum: 350 c.h. total**
- 250 c.h. at graduate level in the area in which the Certificate is sought
- 50 c.h. in each of three types of clinical settings

CCC-SLP
- 20 c.h. in each of the following 8 categories:
  1. Evaluation: Speech[2] disorders in children
  2. Evaluation: Speech[2] disorders in adults
  3. Evaluation: Language disorders in children
  4. Evaluation: Language disorders in adults
  5. Treatment: Speech[2] disorders in children
  6. Treatment: Speech[2] disorders in adults
  7. Treatment: Language disorders in children
  8. Treatment: Language disorders in adults

- Up to 20 c.h. in the major professional area may be in related disorders

- 35 c.h. in audiology
  —15 in evaluation/screening
  —15 in habilitation/rehabilitation

CCC-A
- 40 c.h. in the first 2 categories listed below; 20 c.h. in the fifth category:
  1. Evaluation: Hearing in children
  2. Evaluation: Hearing in adults
  3. Selection and Use: Amplification and assistive devices for children*
  4. Selection and Use: Amplification and assistive devices for adults*
  5. Treatment[3]: Hearing disorders in children and adults

*At least 80 hours must be completed in categories 3 and 4 with minimum of 10 hours in each of these categories.

- Up to 20 c.h. in the major professional area may be in related disorders

- 35 c.h. in speech-language pathology unrelated to hearing impairment
  —15 in evaluation/screening
  —15 in treatment

IV: **National Examinations in Speech-Language Pathology and Audiology**

V. **The Clinical Fellowship**

---

[1] Academic credit for clinical practicum may *not* be used to satisfy these minimum requirements. However, a maximum of 6 s.ch. for practicum may be applied to the 36 s.c.h. minimum professional coursework.

[2] "Speech" disorders include disorders of articulation, voice, and fluency.

[3] "Treatment" for hearing disorders refers to clinical management and counseling, including auditory training, speech reading, and speech and language services for those with hearing impairment.

◆ APPENDIX B

CODE OF ETHICS
AMERICAN SPEECH-LANGUAGE-HEARING ASSOCIATION
January 1, 1992

PREAMBLE

The preservation of the highest standards of integrity and ethical principles is vital to the responsible discharge of obligations in the professions of speech-language pathology and audiology. This Code of Ethics sets forth the fundamental principles and rules considered essential to this purpose.

Every individual who is (a) a member of the American Speech-Language-Hearing Association, whether certified or not, (b) a nonmember holding the Certificate of Clinical Competence from the Association, (c) an applicant for membership or certification, or (d) a Clinical Fellow seeking to fulfill standards for certification shall abide by this Code of Ethics.

Any action that violates the spirit and purpose of this Code shall be considered unethical. Failure to specify any particular responsibility or practice in this Code of Ethics shall not be construed as denial of the existence of such responsibilities or practices.

The fundamentals of ethical conduct are described by Principles of Ethics and by Rules of Ethics as they relate to responsibility to persons served, to the public, and to the professions of speech-language pathology and audiology.

Principles of Ethics, aspirational and inspirational in nature, form the underlying moral basis for the Code of Ethics. Individuals shall observe these principles as affirmative obligations under all conditions of professional activity.

Rules of Ethics are specific statements of minimally acceptable professional conduct or of prohibitions and are applicable to all individuals.

PRINCIPLE OF ETHICS I

Individuals shall honor their responsibility to hold paramount the welfare of persons they serve professionally.

Rules of Ethics

A. Individuals shall provide all services competently.

B. Individuals shall use every resource, including referral when appropriate, to ensure that high-quality service is provided.

C. Individuals shall not discriminate in the delivery of professional services on the basis of race, sex, age, religion, national origin, sexual orientation, or handicapping condition.

D. Individuals shall fully inform the persons they serve of the nature and possible effects of services rendered and products dispensed.

E. Individuals shall evaluate the effectiveness of services rendered and of products dispensed and shall provide services or dispense products only when benefit can reasonably be expected.

F. Individuals shall not guarantee the results of any treatment or procedure, directly or by implication; however, they may make a reasonable statement of prognosis.

G. Individuals shall not evaluate or treat speech, language, or hearing disorders solely by correspondence.

H. Individuals shall maintain adequate records of professional services rendered and products dispensed and shall allow access to these records when appropriately authorized.

I. Individuals shall not reveal, without authorization, any professional or personal information about the person served professionally, unless required by law to do so, or unless doing so is necessary to protect the welfare of the person or of the community.

J. Individuals shall not charge for services not rendered, nor shall they misrepresent,[1] in any fashion, services rendered or products dispensed.

K. Individuals shall use persons in research or as subjects of teaching demonstrations only with their informed consent.

L. Individuals shall withdraw from professional practice when substance abuse or an emotional or mental disability may adversely affect the quality of services they render.

---

[1] For purposes of this Code of Ethics, misrepresentation includes any untrue statements or statements that are likely to mislead. Misrepresentation also includes the failure to state any information that is material and that ought, in fairness, to be considered.

PRINCIPLE OF ETHICS II _____

Individuals shall honor their responsibility to achieve and maintain the highest level of professional competence.

Rules of Ethics

A. Individuals shall engage in the provision of clinical services only when they hold the appropriate Certificate of Clinical Competence or when they are in the certification process and are supervised by an individual who holds the appropriate Certificate of Clinical Competence.

B. Individuals shall engage in only those aspects of the professions that are within the scope of their competence, considering their level of education, training, and experience.

C. Individuals shall continue their professional development throughout their careers.

D. Individuals shall delegate the provision of clinical services only to persons who are certified or to persons in the education or certification process who are appropriately supervised. The provision of support services may be delegated to persons who are neither certified nor in the certification process only when a certificate holder provides appropriate supervision.

E. Individuals shall prohibit any of their professional staff from providing services that exceed the staff member's competence, considering the staff member's level of education, training, and experience.

F. Individuals shall ensure that all equipment used in the provision of services is in proper working order and is properly calibrated.

PRINCIPLES OF ETHICS III _____

Individuals shall honor their responsibility to the public by promoting public understanding of the professions, by supporting the development of services designed to fulfill the unmet needs of the public, and by providing accurate information in all communications involving any aspect of the professions.

Rules of Ethics

A. Individuals shall not misrepresent their credentials, competence, education, training, or experience.

B. Individuals shall not participate in professional activities that constitute a conflict of interest.

C. Individuals shall not misrepresent diagnostic information, services rendered, or products dispensed

or engage in any scheme or artifice to defraud in connection with obtaining payment or reimburseme for such services or products.

D. Individuals' statements to the public shall provide accurate information about the nature and management of communication disorders, about th professions, and about professional services.

E. Individuals' statements to the public—advertising, announcing, and marketing their professional services, reporting research results, and promoting products—shall adhere to prevailing professional standards and shall not contain misrepresentations.

PRINCIPLE OF ETHICS IV _____

Individuals shall honor their responsibilities to the professions and their relationships with colleagues, students, and members of allied professions. Individuals shall uphold the dignity and autonomy of the profession maintain harmonious interprofessional and intraprofessional relationships, and accept the professions' self-imposed standards.

Rules of Ethics

A. Individuals shall prohibit anyone under their supervision from engaging in any practice that violates the Code of Ethics.

B. Individuals shall not engage in dishonesty, fraud, deceit, misrepresentation, or any form of conduct tha adversely reflects on the professions or on the individual's fitness to serve persons professionally.

C. Individuals shall assign credit only to those who have contributed to a publication, presentation, or produc Credit shall be assigned in proportion to the contribution and only with the contributor's consent.

D. Individuals' statements to colleagues about professional services, research results, and products shall adhere to prevailing professional standards and shall contain no misrepresentations.

E. Individuals shall not provide professional services without exercising independent professional judgment, regardless of referral source or prescription.

F. Individuals who have reason to believe that the Code of Ethics has been violated shall inform the Ethical Practice Board.

G. Individuals shall cooperate fully with the Ethical Practice Board in its investigation and adjudication of matters related to this Code of Ethics.

Communication and Communication Disorders in a Multicultural Society

ORLANDO L. TAYLOR, PH.D.

After reading this chapter, you will know that:

✦ The United States is becoming an increasingly diverse society.

✦ Specialists in communication and its disorders, regardless of their own cultural and ethnic roots, must be well-informed on the nature of culture and its relationship to normal and disordered communication;

✦ The development of language and cognition are influenced considerably by cultural factors;

✦ Some of the conditions that cause or predispose one to communication disorders are often related to culture; and

✦ The assessment, diagnosis, and treatment of communication disorders must take culture into account to be professionally ethical and valid.

The role of culture is essential to understanding the nature of communication disorders. Cultural considerations allow us to make several significant observations about the nature of normal and pathological communication. At a minimum these claims include the following: (1) all communication — normal and pathological — emerges out of a cultural context; (2) culture plays a central role in what a group considers to be normal, as well as abnormal, communication; (3) cultural factors may contribute to the presence and prevalence of communication disorders in a specific population; and (4) the subsequent assessment and management of communication disorders are best conducted within a cultural context.

This chapter

+ addresses the nature of cultural diversity in the United States;
+ reviews basic concepts pertaining to the nature of culture;
+ discusses some basic concepts pertaining to culture and communication; and
+ introduces some concepts that link culture to our understanding communication disorders.

The role of culture in understanding the nature of communication disorders is as old as the professions of audiology and speech-language pathology. In one of the most quoted articles in the early years of speech-language pathology, Wendell Johnson (1944) wrote that "the Indians have no word for it" — "it" being stuttering. Johnson's claim was not that nonfluent speech did not occur among Native Americans — in this case the Hopi people — but rather that the culture did not *choose* to define nonfluent speech as a problem, thus did not choose — or had no reason — to give it a label.

Johnson's observation, although more than 50 years old, provides an historical link to this chapter. That linkage revolves around the relationship between culture and communication sciences and disorders.

✦ CULTURAL DIVERSITY IN THE UNITED STATES

In its April 9, 1990 cover story, "The Changing Colors of America: Beyond the Melting Pot," *Time* (Henry, 1990) magazine proclaimed the following:

Someday soon, surely much sooner than most people who filled out their census forms last week realize, White Americans will become a minority group. Long before that day arrives, the presumption that the "typical" U.S. citizen is someone who traces his or her descent in a direct line to Europe will be part of the past. . . .

Already 1 American in 4 defines himself or herself as Hispanic or non-White. If current trends in immigration and birth rates persist, the Hispanic population will have further increased an estimated 21%, the Asian presence about 22%, Blacks almost 12% and Whites a little more than 2% when the 20th century ends. By 2020, a date no further into the future than John F. Kennedy's election is in the past, the number of U.S. residents who are Hispanic or non-White will have more than doubled, to nearly 115 million, while the White population will not be increasing at all. By 2056, when someone born today will be 66 years old, the "average" U.S. resident, as defined by census statistics, will trace his or her descent to Africa, Asia, the Hispanic world, the Pacific Islands, Arabia — almost anywhere but Europe. (p. 38)

A summary of the statistics from the 1990 U.S. Census (*Statistical Abstract of the United States,* 1992) is presented in Figure 2-1. It shows that approximately 12% of the American population of almost 250 million at that time was African American, 9% was Hispanic (Latino) American, 3% was Asian American or Pacific Islander, and 1% was Native American, Eskimo, and Aleut. More importantly, it reveals that while the White population grew by 6% between the period 1980–1990, the growth rates for people of color were much higher. For example, the Asian American population grew by 108%, the Hispanic (Latino) American population by 53%, the Native American population by 38%, and the African American population by 13%.

Other trends from the 1990 Census were as follows:

◆ Although America's suburban counties remained overwhelmingly White, people of color poured into the suburbs between 1980–1990. For example, 3.7 million more White Americans resided in suburban counties than a decade earlier, compared to 4 million more Hispanic (Latino) Americans, 2.1 million more Asian Americans, and 1.7 million more African Americans.

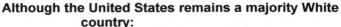

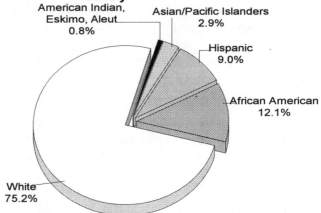

Source: Bureau of the Census, U.S. Department of Commerce

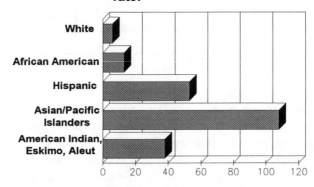

Note: Both charts above show Hispanics as a separate population category. The figures for Whites, African Americans, Asian/Pacific Islanders and American Indians, Eskimos and Aleuts are for non-Hispanic members of those groups.
Source: Bureau of the Census, U.S. Department of Commerce, 1990 (Statistical Abstract of the United States, 1992)

Figure 2–1. Cultural diversity in the 1990 U.S. Census.

♦ Minorities constituted a majority of the population in 186 counties in the United States in 1990, up from 163 a decade earlier.

♦ Fewer White Americans lived in virtually all-White counties than in 1980. In 1980, 43% of all Whites — nearly 80 million people — lived in counties where Whites comprised at least 90% of the population. Ten years later, the proportion living in such counties had declined to only 36%.

✦ If present population growth trends continue, Hispanic Americans will surpass African Americans to become the country's largest minority group sometime around the turn of the 21st century.

Several demographers have suggested that by 2010, more than one third of the American people will be non-European in ancestry. By 2050, many of the same demographers assert that upwards of one half of the U.S. population will be people of color. This "New America" where White Americans will be the "minority" is already a reality in many local communities in the United States and in the school-age populations of most urban school systems. Most of the nation's largest cities and the state of California already have populations in which people of color are a majority. The state of Texas is expected to follow suit by the year 2000.

The implications of these statistics are rather obvious. Simply stated, professionals in the fields of audiology and speech-language pathology will increasingly be called on to deliver services to increasingly diverse cultural and linguistic groups. In 1989, for example, Shewan and Malm reported that 37% of the membership of the American Speech-Language-Hearing Association (ASHA) served individuals for whom English was not a native language. Even if such diversity did not exist, one could make a strong case that cultural considerations are fundamental to understanding of normal and pathological communication because all communication is acquired and maintained within a cultural context. ASHA has embraced this notion in several of its official positions. In addition, the National Examinations in Speech-Language Pathology and Audiology contain items on cultural and linguistic diversity, and there are diversity standards for ASHA's accreditation of academic and professional service programs.

Some of the ASHA policies and positions which pertain to cultural diversity include:

Resolved, that the American Speech-Language-Hearing Association (ASHA) encourages undergraduate, graduate and continuing education programs to include specific information, course content, and/or clinical practicum which address communication needs of individuals within socially, culturally, economically and linguistically diverse populations. (*Asha*, March 1986, p. 42).

(continued)

Speech-language pathologists or audiologists who present them-selves as bilingual for the purposes of providing clinical services must be able to speak their primary language and to speak (or sign) at least one other language with native or near-native pro-ficiency in lexicon (vocabulary), semantics (meaning), phonol-ogy (pronunciation), morphology/syntax (grammar) and prag-matics (uses) during clinical management. (*Asha*, March 1989, p. 93).

Coursework should address, where appropriate, issues pertain-ing to normal and abnormal human development and behav-ior across the life span and to culturally diverse populations (Standard II: Academic Coursework Requirements for the Cer-tificate of Clinical Competence, Effective January 1, 1995). (*Asha*, January 1994, p. 63).

Although a person from any cultural or racial group can be trained to provide clinical services to individuals who come from another cultural group, cultural diversity within the communica-tion disorders workforce is a desired goal. ASHA, as well as many clinics, hospitals, colleges, universities, and other employers, has made strong statements with respect to the desirability of promot-ing cultural diversity within the professional workforce. However, the pool of persons of color for professional positions in communi-cation disorders is alarmingly small.

According to the American Speech-Language-Hearing Associ-ation, there were 59,878 individuals certified in speech-language pathology as of December 31, 1993. Yet, only 6% of this total was from groups categorized as racial/ethnic minorities: 2.43% African American, 1.56% Hispanic, 1.24% Asian—Pacific Islander, and .29% Native American. Recall that these groups represented more than 25% of the American population in 1990 and are the fastest growing groups in the United States.

✦ THE NATURE OF CULTURE

Saville-Troika (1986) defines culture as the collectivity of the shared rules for appropriate behavior (including verbal and non-verbal communication) that are learned by individuals as a conse-quence of being members of the same group or community, as well as the values and beliefs that underlie overt behaviors which are themselves shared products of group membership. In other words, culture is what individuals need to know to be functional members of a community, and to regulate interactions with other members of their community and with individuals from other cultural backgrounds. In addition to a set of behaviors, cultures also are characterized by such attributes as their social and political institutions and their technologies.

In examining this definition, one should pay particular atten tion to the fact that culture is a *learned* phenomenon. Race, by contrast, is a biological notion. Confusion between the concepts of race and culture occurs frequently; however, this confusion needs to be avoided.

Because cultures are learned, they are

1. constantly changing and evolving,

2. have internal variation, and

3. may reflect variation across groups.

It is especially important for the student of culture to recognize that many cultures may exist within a single race, language group, religion, or nationality. Moreover, within a given culture, differences typically exist as a function of age, gender, socioeconomic status, education, exposure to other cultures, and so on. Failure to recognize the notion of **intracultural variation** will lead inevitably to overgeneralizations and false stereotypes.

Another important principle to consider in understanding the nature of culture is that cultures are not discrete from one another. Indeed, they typically overlap one another. Thus, a particular cultural attribute may be shared by many cultures. For example, the game of soccer is a leisure-time sporting activity in many cultures around the world. Likewise, many cultures share a tendency for a patriarchal-oriented family structure. Despite the presence of overlaps across cultures, unique attributes (differences) typically occur within a given culture. In any event, the presence of **cultural overlaps** requires one to strive to seek *similarities*, as well as differences, between and among cultures.

Learning About Culture

Once one accepts the centrality of culture in understanding normal and pathological communication, a reasonable question that might be raised is: "How does one learn about a particular culture?" Naturally, the most convenient response would be: "Read a book or an article." Regrettably, updated and documented data are not available for many, if not most, of the cultural groups which reside in the United States. Where published data do exist, they typically do not take intracultural variation into account. For example, published data on African Americans focus disproportionately on working class individuals, and usually those residing in urban areas. Little data have been published on the African American middle class. By contrast, the White American population is usually presented as a homogenous, middle class group with little internal variation. Obviously, both views are incorrect and have led to unfortunate overgeneralizations and stereotypes.

Even if adequate and comprehensive published reports on cultural and linguistic diversity in the United States were available, anthropologists, linguists, and other students of culture generally agree that firsthand experiences are necessary to truly understand the nuances of a given culture. In fact, many believe that stereotyping and generalizations are inevitable among those who lack direct and frequent contacts with another culture.

In making direct excursions into other cultures, it is important to remember, among other things that:

◆ Feelings of apprehension, loneliness, or lack of confidence are common when visiting and experiencing another culture.
◆ Differences between cultures are often perceived as threatening.
◆ What is logical and important in a particular culture may seem irrational and unimportant to an outsider.
◆ One's own sense of cultural identity often is not evident until one encounters another culture.
◆ Understanding another culture is a continuous process.

A list of some of the more important questions to which one should seek answers (from observations, interviews, etc.) in learning about a culture is presented in Table 2–1. Examining the list of possible questions, it should become obvious that culture is a complex phenomenon which involves far more than food, dress, and music and that many aspects of a culture may be subtle, unspoken, and exist at a low level of awareness, even for its members.

Hamayan and Damico (1991) have proposed a set of continua along which cultural preferences of a group might be determined (see Table 2–2). Their view is that every individual will exhibit certain behaviors and preferences in different circumstances and at

TABLE 2-1. Questions to ask about cultures.

Family Structure	Who is considered as belonging to the family? What are the rights, roles, and responsibilities of the family members?
Life Cycle	What are the important stages, periods, and transitions in life? What behaviors are inappropriate or unacceptable for children at various ages?
Roles	What roles are available to whom? How are roles acquired?
Interpersonal Relationships	How do people greet each other? Who may disagree with whom? How are insults expressed?
Communication	What languages and dialects are spoken? What are the characteristics of speaking "well"? What roles, attitudes, and personality traits are associated with particular aspects of verbal and nonverbal behavior? How much emotional intensity is desirable in speech?
Decorum and Discipline	How do people behave at home and in public? What means of discipline are used?
Religion	What religious roles and authority are recognized? What should an outsider not know or acknowledge knowing?
Health and Hygiene	How are illness and death explained? How are specific illnesses treated? What are thought to be causes of disabilities and who should treat them?
Food	What is eaten, in what order, and how often? What are the rules for table manners, including offering foods, handling foods, and discarding foods?
Holidays and Celebrations	What holidays are observed? For what purpose? Which holidays are important for children? What cultural values are instilled in children during the holidays?

(continued)

TABLE 2-1 (continued)

Dress and Personal Appearance	What significance does dress have for social identity? What is the concept and value of beauty and attractiveness? What attributes are considered undesirable?
Values	What traits and attributes in oneself or others are important? Which values are undesirable to have? What attributes in the world are important?
History and Traditions	How are history and tradition passed on to the young? How do cultural understandings of history differ from "scientific" facts or literate history?
Education	What are the purposes of education? What kinds of learning are favored? What teaching and learning methods are used in the home? What are parental expectations for boys versus girls?
Work and Play	What behaviors are considered "work"? "Play"? What kinds of work are prestigious? Why?
Time and Space	What is considered "on time"? What is the importance of punctuality? How important is speed of performance? How are groups organized spatially by age, gender, and role?
Natural Phenomena	Who or what is responsible for rain, thunder, floods, and hurricanes? Are behavioral taboos associated with natural phenomena?
Pets and Animals	Which animals are valued and for what reasons? What animals are considered appropriate or inappropriate as pets?
Art and Music	What forms of art and music are most highly valued? What forms of art and music are considered appropriate for children to perform or appreciate?
Expectations and Aspirations	Do parents expect and desire assimilation of children to the dominant culture, language, or dialect? What cultural values are expected to be maintained despite the degree of formal education?

Source: Adapted from *A Guide to Culture in the Classroom* by M. Saville-Troike, 1978. Rosslyn, VA: National Clearinghouse for Bilingual Education.

TABLE 2–2. Continua along which cultural preferences might be determined.

Attributes	Continua
Movement	Active —— Passive
Space	Close —— Distant
Time	Strict time schedule —— No strict time schedules
Interactions	Polychronic —— Monochronic
Goal/Structures	Cooperative —— Competitive
Gender/Role	Inequality —— Equality
Role	Group —— Individual
Locus of Control	External —— Internal
Perceptual Style	Field-Dependent —— Field-Independent
Cognitive Style	Intuitive —— Reflective
Language Patterns	Mismatch —— Match
Language Loss	Extensive —— Minimal
Code Switching	Frequent —— Infrequent
Language Variance	Nonstandard —— Standard

Source: From E. V. Hamayan and J. S. Damico, *Limiting Bias in the Assessment of Bilingual Students*, 1991. Austin, TX: Pro-Ed. Reproduced by permission.

different times. Yet, they believe that specific beliefs, styles, and behaviors may predominate at a particular stage in the acquisition process.

Based on anecdotal observations and selected research findings (e.g., Kochman, 1981; Taylor, 1990), some **cultural tendencies** have been posited for several cultural groups that reside within the United States. Some of the tendencies or attributes are presented in Table 2–3 for African Americans, Hispanic Americans, Asian Americans, and Anglo-Saxon (White) Americans. In examining these tendencies, it must be recalled that none of them occurs in all individuals in a cultural group, and that some of the tendencies are seen in several other cultural groups.

It also must be remembered that terms such as Hispanic American, Asian American, or even White American grossly simplify and distort the enormous cultural variations that exist within these groups. For example, within the Hispanic American culture, differences exist between persons from Mexico and those from the Dominican Republic. Among Asian Americans, differences exist be-

TABLE 2–3. Examples of cultural tendencies of four groups of Americans.

African Americans	Asian Americans
"We" versus "I" world view	Strong family connections
Strong "in group" cultural rules	Preference toward modesty, reserve, and control
Field-dependent cognitive style	
High value on the oral tradition	Respect for silence
Emotional intensity in communication	Low regard for argumentation
	Orientation toward privacy
Respect for creativity and code switching in language	Disdain for public reprimand
Preference for retaining cultural identity	

Hispanic Americans	White (Anglo-Saxon) Americans
Unity and interdependence among members of the (extended) family	Preference for nuclear versus extended family
Respect for tradition and traditional family and social roles	Respect for individualism
	High regard for "standard English"
Physical closeness during conversation	Respect for step-by-step logic
	Preference not to show emotion
Emotional intensity in communication to demonstrate sincerity and commitment to beliefs	Respect for cultural assimilation in the U.S.
Preference for retention of the Spanish language	

tween Japanese and Chinese Americans, in addition to differences *within* these groups. Among White Americans, one can identify differences between Irish and Italian Americans. These observations are consistent with our earlier claims concerning intracultural variation and cultural overlaps.

The reader should use the tendencies presented in Table 2–3 as a vehicle for discussions and explorations with individuals from the cultural groups described. As appropriate, the list of tendencies should be modified and refined. It is important to note that although similarities are observable across the groups (e.g., the power of family relationships among Hispanics and Asian Americans), significant differences also may exist (e.g., views of assimilation versus pluralism between White Americans and African Americans). These cultural differences, if left unaddressed, can lead to discord within the society.

Nichols (1992) has proposed an intriguing model which posits underlying important philosophical attributes of world view among cultural groups which undergird important differences among them and how they behave. Nichols' notions are presented in Table 2–4.

According to Nichols, ethnic or cultural groups may be categorized according to: (a) Axiology (the nature, types, and criteria of values and value judgments, especially in ethics); (b) Epistemology (the nature and grounds for knowing); (c) Systems of Logic; and (d) Processes for linking objects together.

Although subject to the same notions of intracultural variation and cultural overlaps described above, and limited by the lack of empirical evidence, Nichols' notions provide a basis, nonetheless, for fruitful discussion and research on how different groups of individuals see and learn about the worlds in which they live, and how they organize reality within those worlds. It also helps to explain how individuals in different cultures prefer to learn and the values they place on humankind.

✦ CULTURE AND COMMUNICATION

As stated earlier, communication — in all of its forms and modalities — emanates from a cultural context. Indeed, spoken language, a universal attribute of all cultures in the world, is the principal system employed by members of cultures to express their basic thoughts, beliefs, values, and so on. Moreover, spoken language is the medium by which most of the realities of a culture are communicated among its members.

Saville-Troike (1989) states that language is an essential vehicle for establishing the boundaries of a culture, the unification of its members, and the exclusion of nonmembers. The conscious and unconscious linguistic features used by a given culture solidify categories and divisions. These rules also serve to create and reinforce social stratification within a given culture.

In short, culture cannot exist without language, because culture requires expressive means of transmittal to its membership (Taylor & Clarke, 1994). At the same time, language is dependent on culture to determine its efficacy, functionality, and utilitarianism. Moreover, language without culture would lack the influence of socialization and relationships, and would be void, without life and substance.

The concept of **speech community** is central to a discussion of the relationship between culture and communication. According to

TABLE 2–4. The philosophical aspect of cultural differences.

Ethnic Groups' World View	Axiology	Epistemology	System of Logic	Processes
European European American	**MEMBER-OBJECT** The highest value lies in the object or in the acquisition of the object.	**COGNITIVE** One knows through counting and measuring.	**DICHOTOMOUS** Either/or.	**TECHNOLOGY** All sets are repeatable and reproducible.
African African American Hispanic Arabic	**MEMBER-GROUP** The highest value lies in the interpersonal relationships between persons.	**AFFECTIVE** One knows through symbolic imagery and rhythm.	**NYAYA** The union of opposites.	**NTUOLOGY** All sets are interrelated through human and spiritual networks.
Asian Asian-American Polynesian	**MEMBER-GROUP** the highest value lies in the cohesiveness of the group.	**CONATIVE** One knows through striving toward the transcendence.	**NYAYA** the objective world is conceived independent of thought and mind.	**COSMOLOGY** All sets are independently interrelated in the harmony of the universe.
Native American	**MEMBER-GREAT SPIRIT** The highest value lies in oneness with the Great Spirit.			

Source: From E. Nichols, The philosophical aspect of cultural difference, 1992. In Report from the Working Group, *Research and training needs of minority persons and minority health issues* (Appendix C). Bethesda, MD: National Institute on Deafness and Other Communication Disorders. Copyright 1976, 1987 NINDB. Reprinted with permission.

Dell Hymes, the father of "ethnography of communication," a **speech community** consists of a collection of individuals who learn, share, and use a particular set of linguistic codes which serve to represent the universe of meanings characteristic of that culture (Hymes, 1966). Persons may share the same language code, but still not belong to the same speech community. For example, although both Parisians and many Canadians in the province of Quebec speak French, the variations of French spoken by the two groups separate them into different speech communities.

Within each speech community, subgroups also may exist which demonstrate distinctions in cultural and linguistic behavior. It also is possible to be a participant in a speech community, but to not be a member of the speech community. Several modes of communication may exist within a given speech community (e.g., verbal language, manual sign language, nonverbal language, and orthography). All modes of communication within a speech community are legitimate systems as long as they meet the needs of the users.

The concept of **communication competence** (Hymes, 1966) is another important attribute pertaining to the relationship between culture and language. Communication competence is the knowledge required of a speaker to communicate appropriately within a given speech community *and* the skills required to make use of it. This knowledge includes both linguistic and sociolinguistic rules, as well as the cultural rules and knowledge that are the bases for the content and context of communicative events and interactive processes. The knowledge within a given culture is the subject of inquiry of the ethnography of communication, which is a growing subdiscipline of anthropology that employs qualitative, culturally centered methods for identifying the communicative rules used by a cultural group.

Within every speech community, a language — and perhaps several dialects of that language — may be spoken. A **dialect** is a variety of a language associated with speakers in a particular geographical region or social group.

A rich body of literature has been published since the 1960s which describes the many dialects of English spoken in the United States. Most of these dialects are related to the influence of the language spoken by the ancestors of the speakers of the dialect (e.g., the influence of African languages on American English) or on the interactions between those ancestors and the mix of other cultures that resided in the regions where they lived.

A popular theory on the genesis of dialects is the creole theory. This theory suggests that dialects emerge as the result of an evolutionary process in which a group of speakers who speak one language comes into contact with another group of speakers who speak a different language. According to the creole theory, these speakers (usually those in the nondominant position) develop a simplified hybrid language of the two languages (a **pidgin** language). A **pidgin language** is generally thought to be spoken only in situations in which the two groups of speakers are in contact with one another, frequently for trading purpose or to conduct business. This "lingua franca" typically preserves the phonology and a simplified version of the nondominant group's first language. Each of the two groups continues to use their home language (L_1) when speaking among themselves.

Over time, pidgin languages may evolve into a full blown **creole language** which becomes the L_1 of the nondominant group and the language taught to its young. Creole languages have all of the attributes of any language system with complete phonology, grammar, and rules for discourse, pragmatics, and semantics, many of which are reflective of the many attributes of L_1. Examples of creole languages in the United States are French Cajun in Louisiana and Gullah in South Carolina.

No matter what theory one subscribes to, dialects are a reality in any multicultural society such as the United States. Dialects of a language should always be perceived as legitimate ways of speaking and not disorders of communication. Although some dialects have more prestige in the educational settings (i.e., Standard English dialects) and others are valued because of the prestige of their speakers (e.g., New England speakers), no dialect should be perceived as a disorder. While one might seek to *teach* all children to speak a Standard English dialect in the U.S. school setting, for example, such instruction should not be confused with speech-language therapy, that is, the rehabilitation of a communication disorder.

The American-Speech-Language-Hearing Association has issued an official position on language varieties. The position states, in part, the following:

> It is the position of the American Speech-Language-Hearing Association (ASHA) that no dialectal variety of English is a disorder or a pathological form of speech or language. Each social dialect is adequate as a functional and effective variety of English. Each serves a communication function as well as a social solidarity function. It maintains the communication network and the social construct of the community of speakers who use it. Furthermore, each is a symbolic representation of the historical, social, and cultural background of the speakers. (ASHA, 1983, pp. 23–25)

Examples of some of the better known English dialects in the United States are presented in Table 2–5.

TABLE 2-5. Some varieties of American English.

Dialect	Examples
Appalachian English	"He just kept a-begging and a-crying and a-wanting to go out." (He persisted in begging, crying and wanting to leave.)
Athabascan English (Alaska)	"Most time we play games." (Most of the time we play games.)
African American English Vernacular	"He be scared, but I be brave." (He is usually scared, but I am usually brave.)
General American Nonstandard English	"Don't nobody want none." (Nobody wants any.)
Keaukakha English (Hawaii)	"I no can place the name." (I cannot place that name.)
New York City Nonstandard English	"She's a good cook, your mother." (Your mother is a good cook.)
Southern American Nonstandard English	"I mon' rest." (I am going to rest.)
Spanish-Influenced English	"Carol left yesterday. I think is coming back tomorrows." (Carol left yesterday. I think she is coming back tomorrow.)

✦ CULTURE AND THE DEVELOPMENT OF LANGUAGE AND COMMUNICATION

Culture begins its influence on language and communication behavior during the early developmental stages of infancy when children acquire their indigenous language systems and the cognitive underpinnings for those systems. The elements of the cultural influence on language and communication acquisition are presented in Figure 2-2.

Developmental processes provide the essential prerequisites for understanding the nature of communicative behavior acquired by individuals in any cultural or linguistic group and the basis for establishing the norms to determine the presence of communication disorders. Two levels of development are presented in Figure 2-2. They are: (1) development within the indigenous culture and (2) optional development of the cultural, cognitive, language, and communicative rules of an external culture.

Three major outcomes of the developmental process within the indigenous culture include: (1) adult-child interaction within the

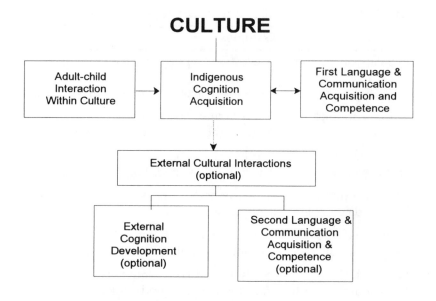

Adapted from Taylor (1986)

Figure 2-2. The influence of culture on language and communication acquisition.

culture (as well as family-child, child-child, and community-child interactions); (2) cognitive acquisition within the framework of cultural norms; and (3) the acquisition of competence iń language and communication system of the indigenous culture.

Adult-Child Interaction

The foundation for all children's cultural, cognitive, and communicative development is thought to result from their interactions with parents, other adults, siblings, and other children that occur within the sociocultural context of a specific group. These interactions, which take place in the nuclear or extended family and in the community, provide a model for the developing child for determining acceptable patterns of early socialization. The child is believed by some to develop a set of culturally and socially based concepts and thoughts (Vygotsky, 1962). Taylor and Clarke (1994) claim that this underlying conceptual development gives rise, in turn, to the acquisition of verbal and nonverbal symbols (language) and rules for using them (communication) within the rules of the indigenous culture. Through practice, increased socialization, and biological maturation, children are expected to acquire adult language and communication competence within the norms established by their cultures.

Although it is reasonable to argue that children acquire language and communicative skills in the context of a family and a community, it is by no means the case that families in all cultures are structured alike or that the roles assumed by family members (including parenting styles) and the external community are alike from culture to culture. Indeed, everything seems to point to diversity in these areas.

Crago (1992) points out that differences which exist among cultures in caregiver-child discourse may produce variations in language acquisition and developmental processes. Such variations depend on cultural values and attributes regarding caregiving and the social organization of the culture.

Westby (1986) has cited several differences in caregiver-child interactions that may have an impact on language acquisition and general development. For example, she makes the following observations to demonstrate how cultural differences in caregiver-infant interactions may have no impact on early development and language acquisition:

- ◆ Anglo mothers are inclined to rely on vocalizations and repositioning when interacting with the infant. Hopi mothers, by contrast, are inclined to rely more on active tactile movements (e.g., bouncing, juggling, and poking) in interacting with infants. (Callaghan, 1981).
- ◆ Sibling child-rearing is common in many African American, Hawaiian, Native American, and Hispanic communities. (This phenomenon probably will increase in all cultural groups in the near future as a result of the dramatic rise of single-parent mothers and fathers in many cultural groups.)
- ◆ Asian cultures are often thought to view the infant as being born independent, with the culture's responsibility being to develop the child's interdependence on the family and society. By contrast, western cultures (including White, Hispanic, and African American) are thought to view the child as being born as a dependent being, with the culture's responsibility being to teach independence and autonomy, albeit in different ways (Christopher, 1983; Kagan, Kearsley, & Zelazo, 1978).

Irrespective of the types of caregiver-child interactions that predominate in a given culture, it is probably reasonable to state that caregivers, as well as the culture at large, play an important role in providing cues to children, either directly or indirectly, concerning acceptable communicative behavior, and general behavior, within the culture. They provide the scaffolds for first language acquisition and provide the symbols that mark acceptable behavior within the culture as a function of gender, status, age, and so on.

Acquisition of the Indigenous Language/Communication System

In recent years, rather impressive data have been presented to show that language acquisition in children, irrespective of target language or dialect, has a universal quality (Bowerman, 1980). Indeed, Stockman (1986) and Vaughn-Cooke (1986) have shown that when the "mother tongue" principle (i.e., viewing the child through the lens of the language or dialect of his or her community) is employed, similar patterns of acquisition are observed across cultural groups. (Also, see Chapter 3 by Kuhl on speech perception.)

This phenomenon is observable when attributes of language such as its functions and uses are studied. Peters (1983), Stockman (1986) and Vaughn-Cooke (1986) report, for example, that when African American children's language is analyzed for its pragmatic and semantic qualities without regard to its structural qualities, their language is acquired in the same manner and with the same developmental milestones as other groups of children.

With the emergence of such research paradigms as ethnography and culturally based naturalistic observations, researchers in recent years have begun to abandon approaches to language acquisition research that focus on a single research paradigm or a common set of tasks for all children, irrespective of culture, as well as the deployment of standardized tests that make a priori assumptions about "normal language" and developmental milestones.

Language acquisition researchers with an interest in cultural diversity issues have found research paradigms that focus more on language function and meaning within a communicative context — rather than on language structure — and have been rewarded with very promising findings. Indeed, culture appears to influence a variety of communicative acts during discourse. We may define discourse as the systematic conjoining of utterances in monologue or dialogue to achieve a specific communicative purpose. These acts include: (1) opening and closing conversations; (2) taking turns and interrupting during conversations; (3) using silence as a communicative device; (4) selecting appropriate topics of conversation; (5) interjecting humor at appropriate times; (6) using laughter as a communicative device; (7) determining the appropriate amount of speech during conversations; and (8) sequencing content during discourse.

An example of cultural diversity in discourse is seen in the research on children's narratives. Narratives, which involve the translation of experiences into stories, seem to be a universal dimension of discourse. Yet, narratives seem to be structured differently by children in different cultures. Taylor and Matsuda (1988) have argued that the differing narrative strategies exhibited in children may be due, in part, to cultural differences in conceptualization, social interaction, and problem solving. Michaels (1981) is among a group of investigators who have claimed that two styles of **narrative preferences** are exhibited in cultures which influence the narrative strategy acquired by children in those cultures — topic centered and topic associating styles (see Table 2–6).

Michaels describes the **topic centered narrative style** as characterized by structured discourse on a single topic or a related group of topics with elaboration of the main topic. In the topic centered narrative style, there is little presupposition of shared knowledge between speaker and listener. This type of narrative style may well be associated with the analytical, field-independent cognitive style described in the next section of this chapter (Lee, 1987).

By contrast, in the **topic associating narrative style**, several themes — some appearing only tangentially related to one another are linked together to form a single story, with the speaker presuming shared knowledge with the listener. The topic associating narrative style may well be associated with the field-dependent cognitive style (Lee, 1987). Michaels (1981) claims that the topic centered style is characteristic of more literate cultures, whereas topic associating style is associated more with oral cultures.

Differences in narrative style may be observed among children during "sharing time" in primary grade classrooms, or among individuals of any age when asked to tell a story or to recount an experience. Topic centered stories are often perceived by speech-language pathologists and teachers as being "organized" and "focused," whereas topic associating stories are frequently perceived as being "disorganized" and "rambling." In truth, both types of stories are legitimate ways to code experiences. The values placed on them reside more in the ears of the listener than in the quality of the stories. Thus, to the person who prefers topic associating stories, topic centered stories may seem "functional," "rigid," and "boring," whereas topic associating stories may seem "comprehensive," "open," and "interesting."

Considerable research is needed on the relationship between culture and narrative style to reconcile conflicting claims on the sub-

TABLE 2-6. Two types of narrative strategies.

Topic Centered	Topic Associating
Tightly structured discourse on a single topic or series of closely related topics	A series of associated segments that may seem anecdotal in character, linked implicitly to a particular topical event or theme, but with no explicit statement or an overall theme or point
Lexically explicit referential, temporal, and spatial relationships	
No major shifts in perspective, temporal orientation, or thematic progression	Stories start with time, person and place, but temporal orientation, location, and focus often shift across segments; shifts are marked by shifts in pitch contours, tempo, and often a formulaic time marker
High degree of thematic coherence and a clear thematic progress	
Begins with temporal grounding, a statement of focus, introduction of key agents, and some indication of spatial grounding	
	Relationships between and among parts of the narrative have to be inferred by the listener
Orientation is followed by elaboration on the topic	Temporal indicators (e.g., yesterday, last night, tomorrow) occur more than once
Syntactically complete, independent clauses are marked with special intonation (high rising tone with vowel elongation) that means "more to come" and demarcates the clause as an information unit	Special intonation used to highlight discontinuity, not continuity, thereby marking the separation of narrative segments and shifts in temporal orientation, location or focus
Finishes with a punch-line sort of resolution, signaled by a markedly lower pitch or falling tone	Stories may give the impression to those who have no control over the style of having no beginning, no middle, no end, and thus no point
Stories tend to be short and concise	
	Stories tend to be long and not to be concise

Source: From H. A. Michaels, "Sharing time." Children's narrative styles and differential access to literacy, 1981. *Language and Society, 10,* 423–442.

ject. For example, it has been suggested that African American children are more likely to prefer topic associating narratives than their White counterparts. Cross' (1993) research suggests, however, that African American children, irrespective of socioeconomic status, produce more topic centered than topic associating narratives.

Finally, in any speech community, children are taught folktales, rhymes, riddles, and songs based on its belief systems and values. Such lessons serve to identify the level of cultural distinction as compared to other groups and are important tools for socialization, as well as for language acquisition.

Cognition, Culture, and Communication

All language is imposed over an underlying cognitive system. Cognition may be defined as the manner in which individuals perceive, organize and process experiences and observations within their environments (Taylor & Lee, 1987). Without a cognitive system to give rise to thoughts and ideas, there would be no language or communication, for one would have nothing to communicate about or to encode into words and sentences.

The preferred cognitive "style" or strategy employed by an individual, appears, like language, to be culturally determined. Vygotsky (1962) theorized that cognition is one of the "**cultural tools**" acquired by the child to mediate and guide thinking.

One of the popular theories relating to cognitive style is Witkin's (1967) concept of **field-dependence** and **field-independence**. This concept allows us to make some suggestions pertaining to culture, cognition, and communication. Witkin claims that although individuals possess both cognitive styles, field-independent persons tend to prefer an analytical perspective of the world. They tend to be object-oriented and to pay great attention to details. Memory for these individuals is thought to reside in the summation of parts. As stated in the previous section, the topic centered narrative style described above seems to be compatible with the field-independent cognitive style.

Field-dependent individuals, by contrast, are described as viewing the world, and their experiences in it, on a relational or contextual framework. Meaning, for these individuals, is thought to be dependent on the context in which information is presented. As such, they are sometimes thought of as being socially oriented. The topic associating narrative style seems to be compatible with the field-dependent cognitive style.

Both cognitive styles are presented by Witkin as legitimate ways of thinking, although many educators and speech-language pathologists have erroneously viewed the field-independent styles as being superior. Ramirez and Price-Williams (1974), among others, have posited that African Americans and Hispanic descendants tend to exhibit a greater preference for a relational, field-dependent cognitive style. The same researchers claim that European and Asian descendants tend to exhibit a higher preference for an analytical, field-independent cognitive style. Like ethnic claims made on virtually all other aspects of culture, the impact of socioeconomic status must be considered before valid claims can be made about preferred cognitive style. The point can be made, however, that the cognitive style acquired by a child is likely to be determined by the culture in which he or she develops.

Nichols' model, presented earlier in this chapter, also speaks to cultural differences in cognitive style. His section on epistemology, or ways of knowing, speaks directly to cognitive style. Note, for example, that Americans of European ancestry are described as having a preference for cognitive styles that focus on counting and measuring "things." This cognitive style leads naturally to the type of **positivistic**, quantitative paradigms in experimental psychology and speech-language pathology which presume certain a priori assumptions about truth and that truth is learned through empirical observations of parts to equal a whole.

By contrast, Nichols claims that persons of African American and Hispanic American cultures prefer more affective ways of knowing through symbolic imagery and rhythm. This epistemology fits more naturally in phenomenological, qualitative research paradigms used consistently with ethnographic research paradigms in anthropology. Phenomenologically based research presumes no a priori truths, and is predicated on the assumption that truth is acquired through informed observations of a culture as seen from the vantage point of the culture itself.

It should be obvious that no single cognitive style is seen within a culture. Similarly, a given cognitive style may be seen in many cultures. But, according to Nichols, a particular cognitive style tends to predominate within cultural groups. Individuals in a cultural group may acquire the preferred cognitive style of another cultural group or merge two or more cognitive styles into their own idiosyncratic style.

Second Culture and Language Acquisition

It may be claimed with some certainty that most children will acquire the culture and the associated language or dialect spoken by their home culture. This does not mean that an individual is unlikely to acquire one or more other cultures or language systems — or at least some derivative of them. Indeed, in the modern world, and especially in a multicultural society like the United States, the likelihood of becoming bicultural, multicultural, bilingual, multilingual, bidialectal, or multidialectal is increasing. The likelihood of acquiring another culture or language system is determined primarily by such factors as need, interest, and exposure.

Individuals who acquire a second language system frequently engage in **code switching** between linguistic systems, depending on the audience, setting, topic, and purpose of a communication event. This tendency is particularly important for communication disorders clinicians to know because the type of language behavior they are likely to elicit during assessments could change significantly depending on the client's perception of the communicative event, the repertoire of linguistic codes available to him or her, and the rules for using them. In addition, the treatment process must be sensitive to the needs of clients with respect to the several audiences and cultures to which they may wish or need to communicate.

Several theories have addressed the underlying processes governing second language acquisition. One such theory was proposed by Cummins (1981), who claims that a "common underlying proficiency" (CUP) undergirds an individual's acquisition of a second language (L_2). Usually the L_2, at least in the United States, is cognitive/academic language proficiency (CALP), the English language taught in schools for individuals whose L_1 is other than English. By contrast, Cummins' view is that a separate underlying proficiency (SUP) exists between the **basic interpersonal communication skills** (BICS) in L_1 and L_2 for individuals who have a competence in two languages. BICS are the visible, spoken language skills that are normally acquired by all members of a speech community.

If this theory is true, and there is some debate about its tenability, the individual learning a second language system after developing CALP in L_1 can readily apply those cognitive structures to L_2. This would explain why older persons may learn to read and to write a new L_2 faster than they can learn to speak it, that is, acquire a BICS for L_2. (Clearly, this developmental sequence is different from the one in L_1 because BICS is expected to develop before CALP.) Indeed, some L_2 adult learners may never acquire BICS for L_2.

By contrast, Cummins' theory would lead one to conclude that, if a young child is subjected to intensive L_2 instruction after acquiring BICS in L_1, but before the acquisition of CALP in L_1, he or she may experience sufficient disruption in the language acquisition process to acquire strong CALP proficiency in both L_1 or L_2. If true, this theory calls for the development of cognitive academic proficiency in L_1 before intensive instruction is instituted in CALP for L_2. A similar argument could be made for instruction in standard English for individuals who speak other English dialect varieties.

Sometimes interferences may occur between the linguistic codes used by an individual who has acquired some degree of competence in more than one language. These interferences (sometimes described as major contributors to one's accent) are *not* communication disorders. They are the normal and predictable results for an individual acquiring competence in more than one linguistic system. Although one may wish to acquire full competence in a second language or dialect, such acquisition should be seen as an educational, not a rehabilitation, goal.

Examples of the influence of one language on another resulting in linguistic interference are presented in Tables 2–7 and 2–8.

TABLE 2–7. Examples of Spanish-language influence on English phonology.

Features	Environments	Examples
/z/ phoneme	/s/ for /z/ in all positions	sip (zip); racer (razor)
/g/ phoneme	/n/ for /g/ in the word final position	sin (sing)
/θ/ phoneme	/t/ or /s/ for /θ/ in all positions	tin or sin (thin)
/ð/ phoneme	/d/ for /ð/ in all positions	den (then); ladder (lather)
/i/ phoneme	/iy/ for /i/ in all positions	cheap (chip)

TABLE 2–8. Phonological patterns of interference in three Chinese languages.

Mandarin

Substitutions:	s/θ, Z/ð, f/v
Confusions:	r/l and l/r
Omissions:	final consonants
Additions:	/ə/ in blends; belue/blue, gooda/good
Approximations:	tc/tʃ, c/s
Shortening or lengthening of vowels:	seat/sit, it/eat

Cantonese

Substitutions:	s/θ, s/z, f/v, w/v, s/ʃ, l/r, /e/ee
Omissions:	final consonants
Additions:	/ə/ in blends
Vowels:	/ɪ/, /ʌ/, /ɔ/ are difficult for Cantonese speakers

Vietnamese

Substitutions:	s/θ/, ʃ/tʃ, b/p, z/dz, d/ð, /d/dʒ/
Omissions:	final consonants and consonant blends /t/, /æ/, /ʊ/, /ə/
Vowels:	may be difficult at times

Source: From "Cross Cultural and Linguistic Considerations in Working with Asian Populations" by L. R. L. Cheng, 1987, *Asha, 29,* p. 35. Reprinted by permission of the American Speech-Language-Hearing Association.

These tables focus on Spanish and Chinese language interferences on English phonology.

The notions of **language** (dialect) **dominance** and **language** (dialect) **proficiency** are important to our understanding of the individual who may have some degree of competence in two language systems. In general, the dominant language or dialect system is usually acquired first and preferred over any other language system. Language or dialect proficiency refers to the competence with which an individual speaks a particular language or dialect. In considering the notions of second language or second dialect acquisition, it is important to remember that an individual may be dominant in one language or dialect, but not have full language proficiency in either.

Culture and Communication Disorders

The role of culture in defining communication disorders cannot be overemphasized. Scattered observations from around the world reveal that societies have different perceptions of what they consider to be pathological communication and, equally important, what to do about it when it does exist. With this notion in mind, it seems reasonable to argue that in any society a communication disorder can be defined only from the vantage point of the speech community of which a given speaker is a member.

Based on what is known currently about the relationship between culture and communication disorders, Taylor (1986) has suggested that culture may have a dominant influence on perceptions about communication disorders, including: a culture's definition of what are considered to be communication disorders and attitudes toward them; to their etiologies, incidence, and prevalence; and appropriate strategies for their diagnosis and management.

With respect to the standard list of causative factors associated with communication disorders, although many, if not most, of these causative factors exist in all world cultures, cultural factors influence the values and perceptions that interact with them. For example, a poor diet in one culture may be considered a good diet in another culture. Likewise, one's cultural view of a satisfactory social environment may be another culture's perception of a completely unacceptable social environment.

Epidemiological considerations of the causes of communication disorders deserve special attention in this discussion. Communication disorders specialists typically determine the relative importance of various diseases and syndromes as etiological factors within the framework of the prevalence of distribution in their own cultures. However, the relative importance of various diseases and syndromes as etiological factors in communication disorders may vary somewhat from culture to culture.

For example, sickle cell disease, which occurs frequently among African Americans and several other groups, may cause deafness and other communication disorders (Scott, 1986). Sickle cell disease is thought to cause hearing disorders because of the destruction of the hair cells of the inner ear following a sickle cell crisis. Yet, little research or clinical attention was directed toward this disease in the professions of speech-language pathology and audiology until recent years.

Moreover, new strains of disease could cause communication disorders to increase in future years as more immigration occurs in the United States from developing Third World countries. One such disease is schistosomiasis. Petersdorf et al. (1983) describe schistosomiasis as a water-carried parasitic disorder which affects the gastrointestinal system, the liver, the vascular system, and causes central nervous system (CNS) damage. Over 200 million persons are thought to be afflicted with this disease in more than 71 countries, virtually all in the developing world, although it is probably being brought to Europe and North America by immigrant populations. Although there are no reports in the literature on the effects of schistosomiasis on speech, language, or hearing function, it could conceivably cause such disorders because of its tendency to cause vascular obstructions and CNS damage.

Culture also influences attitudes toward communication disorders. Bebout and Arthur (1992) compared attitudes toward speech disorders held by several cultural groups (e.g., Chinese, Southeast Asian, and Hispanic) living in the United States and Canada as immigrants or foreign students with those of monolingual students who were at least second generation North Americans. The results revealed significant group differences in subjects' beliefs about the emotional health of persons with speech disorders and about the potential ability of persons with speech disorders to change their speech. For example, subjects who were born outside of North America were more likely to consider persons with speech disorders as emotionally disturbed. Foreign-born (especially Asian) subjects were more likely to believe that persons with speech disorders could improve their speech if they simply "tried harder."

The assessment and diagnosis of communication disorders must also reflect cultural considerations, particularly in the selection of valid assessment procedures and instruments to determine the presence or absence of disorders. Federal law and professional ethics require the utilization of such procedures.

Culturally valid assessment, by definition, requires the utilization of culturally sensitive instruments and other formal and informal procedures for collecting linguistic and communicative data for the purpose of determining the levels of development or the presence of abnormality. These assessments should be conducted from the vantage point of the indigenous or preferred system of communication of the person being assessed. If group comparisons are to be made, these comparisons should be made in the context of standards or norms derived from comparable groups of individuals from the same culture, linguistic group, or socioeconomic status. Taylor and Payne (1983) observe that, in order to construct culturally valid assessment instruments and procedures, controls must be implemented to prevent the emergence of several sources of potential bias: linguistic differences, format, situation, examiner, values, and directions.

Taylor (1985) has argued that culturally valid assessment procedures should:

+ Recognize that clients may perform differently under differing clinical conditions because of their cultural and language backgrounds; and
+ Recognize that different modes, channels, and functions of communication events in which individuals are expected to participate in a clinical setting may result in differing levels of linguistic or communicative performance.

Regarding management issues, it seems rather clear that effective treatment also should be developed within the context of the values, attitudes, and wishes of the indigenous culture relative to communication disorders and what to do about them. Treatment also should take into account the preferred learning style of the client and the rules of social and communicative interaction as defined by the client's indigenous cultural or linguistic group.

In a sense, all treatment encounters are cultural events. Consequently, a cultural approach to all management is desirable. In addition to the principles mentioned above for assessment, Taylor (1985) claims that clinicians should:

+ View each clinical encounter as a socially situated communicative event which is subject to the cultural rules governing such events by both the clinician and the client.
+ Recognize possible sources of conflicts in cultural assumptions and communicative norms in clients prior to clinical encounters, and take steps to prevent them from occurring during service delivery.
+ Recognize that learning and culture are ongoing processes which should result in constant reassessment and revision of ideas and greater sensitivity to cultural diversity.

Finally, culturally valid clinical treatment should utilize culturally appropriate materials, activities, and subject matter of high interest to members of the culture. These factors should be packaged in intervention strategies compatible with the preferred learning styles of the clients' culture. When "naturalistic" models are employed, care must be taken to ensure that "natural" is defined in such a way that it conforms with cultural rules governing the communicative behaviors expected for the settings, roles, and tasks associated with the communicative events in which the person receiving the service is placed.

◆ SUMMARY

As we approach the twentyfirst century, cultural considerations have become increasingly central to our understanding of normal communicative behavior and to our views on how to successfully assess, diagnose, and manage communication disorders. The role of culture in communication sciences and disorders is likely to assume even greater value in the future as the U.S. population and that of many other nations become even more culturally and linguistically diverse than they are today — and as the disciplines gain a wider presence around the world.

In this chapter, we have explored the nature of cultural diversity in the United States, the role of culture in normal communication and its acquisition, and the importance of culture in the clinical management of communication disorders. In many ways, these topics have become the most exciting and the most challenging topics in the professions of speech-language pathology and audiology. They will likely continue to be so well into the future.

◆ ACKNOWLEDGMENTS

The author acknowledges the assistance of Gwendolyn S. Bethea and Christal Evans in the preparation of this chapter.

◆ REFERENCES

ASHA, Legislative Council. (1986, March). Council report. Rockville, MD: author.

ASHA, Legislative Council. (1989, March). Council report. Rockville, MD: author.

ASHA, Legislative Council. (1994, March), Council report. Rockville, MD: author.

Bebout, L., & Arthur, B. (1992). Cross-cultural attitudes toward speech disorders. *Journal of Speech and Hearing Research, 35,* 45–52.

Bowerman, M. (1980). Language development. In H. C. Triandis & A. Heron (Eds.), *Handbook of cross-cultural psychology: Developmental psychology* (Vol. 4, pp. 93–185). Boston: Allyn and Bacon.

Bureau of the Census. (1990). *1990 U.S. Census.* Washington: Department of Commerce.

Callaghan, J. W. (1981). A comparison of Anglo, Hopi and Navajo mothers and infants. In T. M. Field, A. M. Sostek, P. Vietze, & P. H. Leiderman (Eds.), *Culture and early interactions* (pp. 115–131). Hillsdale, NJ: Lawrence Erlbaum.

Christopher, R. C. (1983). *The Japanese mind.* New York: Fawcett.

Crago, M. B. (1992). Ethnography and language socialization: A cross-cultural perspective. *Topics in Language Disorders, 12,* 28–39.

Cross, L. (1993). *Narrative styles in African American children: The effects of SES and reading bedtime stories to children.* Unpublished doctoral dissertation, University of Maryland, College Park.

Cummins, J. (1981). *Role of primary language development in promoting educational success for language minority children.* Sacramento: California State Department of Education Compendium on Bilingual Bicultural Education.

Hamayan, E. V., & Damico, J. S. (1991). *Limiting bias in the assessment of bilingual students.* Austin, TX: Pro-Ed.

Henry, W. A., III. (1990, April 9). The changing colors of America: Beyond the melting pot. *Time,* 28–31.

Hymes, D. (1966). *On communicative competence.* Paper presented at the Research Planning Conference on Language Development Among Disadvantaged Children, Yeshiva University, New York.

Johnson, W. (1944). The Indians have no word for it: Stuttering in children. *Quarterly Journal of Speech, 30,* 330–337.

Kagan, J., Kearsley, R. B., & Zelazo, P. R. (1978). *Infancy: Its place in human development.* Cambridge, MA: Harvard University Press.

Kochman, T. (1981). *Black and White: Styles and conflict.* Chicago: University of Chicago Press.

Lee, D. L. (1987). *The effects of object-oriented and socially-oriented pictures upon the elicited language of children with differing cognitive styles.* Unpublished doctoral dissertation, Howard University, Washington, DC.

Michaels, H. A. (1981). "Sharing time": Children's narrative styles and differential access to literacy. *Language and Society, 10,* 423–442.

Nichols, E. (1992). The philosophical aspect of cultural difference. In Report from the Working Group: *Research and training needs of minority persons and minority health issues* (Appendix C). Bethesda, MD: National Institute on Deafness and Other Communication Disorders.

Peters, C. (1983). *A pragmatic investigation of the speech of selected Black children.* Unpublished doctoral dissertation, Howard University, Washington, DC.

Petersdorf, R. G., Adams, R. D., Braunwald, E., Isselbacher, K. J., Martin, J. B. , & Wilson, J. D. (1983). *Harrison's principles of internal medicine.* New York: McGraw-Hill.

Ramirez, M., & Price-Williams, D. (1974). Cognitive styles of children of three ethnic groups in the United States. *Journal of Cross-Cultural Psychology, 5*, 212–219.

Saville-Troike, M. (1978). *A guide to culture in the classroom.* Arlington, VA: National Clearinghouse for Bilingual Education.

Saville-Troike, M. (1986) Anthropological considerations in the study of communication. In O. Taylor (Ed.), *Nature of communication disorders in culturally and linguistically diverse populations* (pp. 44–78). Austin, TX: Pro-Ed.

Saville-Troike, M. (1989). *The ethnography of communication: An introduction.* New York: Basil Blackwell.

Scott, D. (1986). Sickle-cell anemia and hearing loss. In F. H. Bess, B. S. Clark, & H. R. Mitchell (Eds.), *Concerns for minority groups in communication disorders* (pp. 69–73). (ASHA Reports, 16) Rockville, MD: American Speech-Language-Hearing Association.

Shewan, C., & Malm, K. (1989). The status of multilingual/multicultural service issues among ASHA members. *Asha, 31*, 78.

"Social Dialects and Implications of the Position on Social Dialects." (1983). *Asha, 25*, 23–27.

Statistical Abstract of the United States. (112th ed.) (1992). Washington, DC: The National Data Bank, U.S. Department of Commerce, Economics and Statistics Administration, Bureau of Commerce.

Stockman, I. (1986). Language acquisition in culturally diverse populations: The Black child as a case study. In O. Taylor (Ed.), *Nature of communication disorders in culturally and linguistically diverse populations* (pp. 117–155). Austin, TX: Pro-Ed.

Taylor, O. (1985). *Clinical practice as a social occasion: An ethnographic model.* Unpublished manuscript.

Taylor, O. (1986). Historical perspectives and conceptual framework for studying the nature of communication disorders in culturally and linguistically diverse populations. In O.Taylor (Ed.), *Nature of communication disorders in culturally and linguistically diverse populations* (pp. 1–8). Austin, TX: Pro-Ed.

Taylor, O. L. (1990). *Cross-cultural communication: An essential dimension of effective education.* Washington, DC: The Mid-Atlantic Equity Center.

Taylor, O. L., & Clarke, M. (in press). Culture and communication disorders: A theoretical perspective. In Kayser, H. (Ed.), *Seminars in Speech and Language.*

Taylor, O. L., & Lee, D. (1987). Standardized tests and African Americans: Communication and language issues. *Negro Education Review, 38*, 67–80.

Taylor, O. L., & Matsuda, M. M. (1988). Storytelling and classroom discrimination. In G. Smitherman-Donaldson & T. A. van Dijk (Eds.), *Discourse and discrimination* (pp. 206–220). Detroit: Wayne State University Press.

Taylor, O. L., & Payne, K. T. (1983). Culturally valid testing: A proactive approach. *Topics in Language Disorders, 3*, 8–20.

Vaughn-Cooke, F. (1986). The challenge of assessing the language of nonmainstream speakers. In O. L. Taylor (Ed.), *Treatment of communica-*

tion disorders in culturally and linguistically diverse populations (pp. 23–48). Austin, TX: Pro-Ed.

Vygotsky, L. S. (1962). *Thought and language.* Cambridge, MA: M.I.T. Press.

Westby, C. (1986). *Cultural differences in caregiver-child interaction.* Unpublished manuscript.

Witkin, H. A. (1967). A cognitive styles approach to cross-cultural research. *International Journal of Psychology, 2*(4), 233–250.

◆ RECOMMENDED READINGS

Battle, D. (1993). *Communication disorders in multicultural populations.* Boston: Andover.

Langdon, H. W., & Chen, L. L. (1992). *Hispanic children and adults with communication disorders: Assessment and intervention.* Rockville, MD: Aspen

Taylor, O. (1986). *Nature of communication disorders in culturally and linguistically diverse populations.* Austin, TX: Pro-Ed.

Taylor, O. (1986). *Treatment of communication disorders in culturally and linguistically diverse populations.* Austin, TX: Pro-Ed.

Saville-Troike, M. (1989). *The ethnography of communication: An introduction.* Oxford: Basil Blackwell.

◆ GLOSSARY

Basic interpersonal communication skills (BICS): the language skills that are normally required by all members of a speech community as a first language and used for basic social interactions with other members of the speech community.

Code switching: the act of changing from one language system or dialect to another depending on the audience, setting, topic, and purpose of a communication event.

Cognitive/academic language proficiency (CALP): the language taught in schools, which in the United States is usually English.

Creole theory: an evolutionary process in which a group of speakers develop a full-blown hybrid language based on their own language and some other language.

Communication competence: the knowledge required of a speaker to communicate appropriately within a given speech community and the skills required to make use of that knowledge.

Cultural overlaps: attributes shared by several cultures.

Cultural tendencies: behavioral attributes which are frequently, although not universally, observed among members of a culture.

Dialect: a variety of a language spoken with speakers in a particular geographical region or social group.

Field-dependent cognitive style: a way of organizing the world by focusing on the interrelatedness of the constituent parts.

Field-independent cognitive style: a way of organizing the world by focusing on its constituent parts.

Intracultural variation: the tendency for cultural groups to reflect internal variation as a function of such factors as age, gender, socioeconomic status, education, exposure to other cultures, and so on.

Language dominance: the language or dialect that an individual prefers and uses most often or in which he or she has a greater or greatest proficiency.

Language proficiency: the competence with which an individual speaks, comprehends, reads, writes, and uses a particular language or dialect.

Pidgin language: a simplified hybridization of two language systems, typically used for trading purposes or in conducting business.

Speech community: a collection of individuals who learn, share and utilize a particular set of linguistic codes which serve to represent the universe of meanings characteristic of that culture.

Topic associating narrative style: a strategy for telling stories in which several themes — some appearing tangentially related to one another — are linked together to form a single story, with the speaker presuming shared knowledge with the listener.

Topic centered narrative style: a strategy for telling stories which is characterized by structured discourse on a single topic or a related group of topics with elaboration the main topic and little presupposition of shared knowledge between speaker and listener.

Speech Perception

PATRICIA K. KUHL, PH.D.

After you have read this chapter, you should be able to:

◆ Understand why the study of speech perception is of interest to scientists, business and industry specialists, and society in general.

◆ Explain why computers cannot "understand" speech and describe the specific problems that cause difficulty for computer speech recognition.

◆ Describe the methods used to test infants' perception of speech.

◆ Trace development in infants from a "language-general" pattern of speech perception to a "language-specific" pattern of speech perception.

◆ Answer the following question with regard to speech perception in infants: What is given by nature; what is gained by experience?

◆ Describe the impact of visual information gleaned from watching the face of the talker on speech perception.

◆ Explain why scientists invent theories and describe a theory of the development of speech perception.

Language is arguably our most complex and unique behavior. As adults, we speak at a rate that results in about 15 sounds per second, a speed that exceeds the auditory system's temporal resolving power for simple sounds. Yet we listen to speech and understand it immediately. No computer system yet invented, even the fastest and most sophisticated super computers, can match the skill demonstrated by humans listening to speech, even though millions of dollars have been spent in trying to create a machine that can "understand" speech. How do we do it? What cognitive, motor, and sensory processes are involved, and how do they enable this skill? This chapter describes what we know about phonetic perception, the process of hearing and understanding the consonants and vowels that make up words. The chapter reviews studies that show that, at birth, infants have "multilingual" perceptual skills — they can hear differences between all of the sounds used to distingush words in the world's languages. However, by the time we reach adulthood, our ability to hear phonetic distinctions is severely restricted. We hear very clearly the phonetic distinctions used in our native language, but fail to hear many of the distinctions used in foreign languages. Our initial "language-universal" perceptual abilities have become "language-specific." The chapter describes when, how, and why our abilities to perceive the sounds of language undergo such a dramatic change during development.

Language acquisition poses a long-standing puzzle to scientists interested in the human mind. The puzzle is this: Infants acquire language like clockwork. Whether a baby is born in Moscow, Tokyo, Zimbabwe, or Seattle, at 3 months of age the baby will "coo," producing "oo" and "ah" sounds. At about 7 months the baby will "babble," producing long strings of syllables such as "babababa" or "mamamama." By the child's first birthday, he or she will have produced their first word ("mama" or "dada"), and by 18 months, two-word combinations such as "more juice" or "go bye-bye." By 3 years of age, children of all cultures know enough about language to carry on an intricate conversation. At this age parents report that their kids can "talk your leg off."

Language seems to appear at the appropriate time, more or less without fail. The most famous linguist of our time, Noam Chomsky, has gone so far as to suggest that language is like a reflex. According to Chomsky, language is produced by a built-in mechanism that simply makes it happen on time, much like walking or the eruption of teeth, developmental milestones that seem to occur virtually without fail.

Is there a biological mechanism that guarantees that language will occur on a fixed time schedule in infants the world over? In other words, is there a linguistic clock — some built-in mechanism provided by **nature** — that makes language simply happen at the appropriate time? What role does **nurture** play? How does linguistic input from the child's environment help bring about language? These are the questions that will be explored in this chapter.

The answer developed in the chapter can be stated simply: Language is both "given by nature" and "gained by experience." Both nature and nurture are critically important in infants' development of speech and language.

The effects of **nature** on language development can be seen in the predispositions infants are born with that support the acquisition of language. Among these infants' perceptions of speech sounds, the consonants and vowels that provide the building blocks of speech, provides evidence of infants' innate preparation for language. The effects of **nurture** on language development are illustrated by examining the impact of **language input** on the child's development of language. There is a great deal of evidence that infants and children are strongly affected by the language they listen to, and this shows the effect that the environment has on the child. One of the most dramatic examples of language input is to consider what happens when there is a lack of language input, as can be the case for certain deaf infants. A deaf infant who cannot hear language and who is not exposed to sign language will not acquire the ability to speak or to understand language. In other words, a deaf infant who is not treated in a special way (exposed to sign language early in life) will not babble at the appropriate time nor in the typical way.

Normal infants also show the effects of the environment on the language learning process. The particular language infants listen to affects the development of language at a very early age. For example, by the end of the first year, infants have begun to produce a unique set of sounds, the ones used by the particular language spoken by their parents. By the end of the second year, infants have a distinct "accent." At this age, the speech produced by American infants sounds quite different from that produced by a Russian, French, African, or Chinese infant. Even at this young age there is evidence that the language heard by the infant plays a critical role in speech and language development. At higher levels, data suggest that the specific kinds of words used by parents affect not only the kinds of words used by the child but the onset of their understanding of the related cognitive concepts. In short, there is strong evidence of the impact of linguistic input on infants' development of language.

In this chapter these issues will be addressed by examining adults' and young infants' **perception of speech**. In the case of infants, a focus on the perception of speech, rather than on the **production of speech**, allows us to examine infants at a very early age, essentially from birth on, and ask whether they respond to speech signals in a special way. Studying infants this young means that we are looking at their biological preparation for language well before they have produced their first words, even before they can understand words. The research that will be described suggests that a strong component of language is innate. However, research studies also show that, from the moment the auditory system can process sound (even in utero), listening to language plays a profound role in shaping infants' abilities. Right from the very beginning, both innate preparation and sensitivity to experience is evidenced in infants' abilities to perceive speech. Speech perception is therefore an index of the interaction of **innate predispositions** and the **effects of experience** in the development of language.

◆ INTEREST IN THE TOPIC OF SPEECH PERCEPTION

The fundamental question about the degree to which language stems from some innate mechanism or from exposure to the environment has interested speech and hearing scientists, linguists, psychologists, and philosophers for many years. More recently, however, there has been an increased interest in speech and language from a wide variety of additional members of the academic community. As depicted in Figure 3–1, interest also stems from business and industry, and from society at large. Why is this the case?

Academic interest stems from the fact that this is the "Decade of the Brain." Investigators interested in language and the brain realize that spoken language allows **brain mapping** using the new tools introduced by neuroscience. The units of language — phonemes, words, and sentences — can be manipulated to see where in the brain and how the units of language are stored. Spoken language may provide a window through which to observe the functional characteristics of the brain. What is learned may be generalized to other complex cognitive processes. This makes language and speech of interest not only to speech and hearing scientists, linguists, and psychologists, but to cognitive neuroscientists as well.

Another reason why many academicians are interested in language is that it provides an example of an activity that undergoes dramatic change during development. Research suggests that there are periods of time during development in which individuals are particularly sensitive to experience, so speech and language development raise classic issues in biology of **critical periods** for learning. Early language input to the child strongly affects speech percep-

Academic

Business

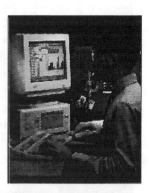

Society

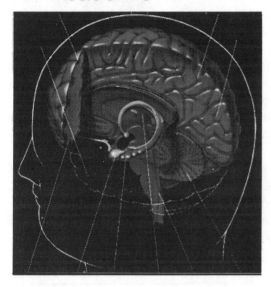

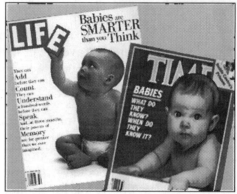

Figure 3–1. There is increased interest in humans' processing of speech and language by members of the academic community, business and industry, and society at large.

tion and speech production and this influence is exerted during the entire lifetime of the individual. We are permanently affected by the specific language environment in which we happen to be reared. Language learning thus produces permanent changes in the brain. The developmental effects of early experience make language an interesting topic to philosphers, ethologists, and biologists.

A third reason why speech is of interest is that it is not just an auditory signal. We see speech information when we watch the articulators move on the face of the talker, and experiments show that the brain takes this information into account. In other words, the brain processes not only auditory information about speech, but visual information as well. It appears, therefore, that information about speech is perceived and stored **cross-modally** by the brain. The perception of speech thus offers a way to study how the brain connects information across sensory modalities.

Business interest in speech perception stems from the fact that 10 years from now all user interfaces to computers will support speech recognition technology. Our cars and bathroom scales now talk to us, but no machine in existence today can listen to speech and "understand" it. At some point in the future, computers will have the capacity to do this, which no computer on the market today can effectively do. We will talk into our computers instead of typing the information on a keyboard, and turn on appliances and lock and unlock doors with our voices. Speech technology will be used in schools, homes, hospitals, and businesses because it will make life easier. IBM, Apple, AT&T, the government — everyone wants to "crack the speech code." In the not-too-distant future, voice-operated technology will bring information to you in a way not imagined 10 years ago. Speech recognition will be the next step in an increasingly digital world.

The interesting thing is that business interests and academic interests have never been closer. Students of speech and hearing will witness increased opportunities to work in settings other than the traditional school, clinic, or academic settings. They will be employed in business settings as well. This makes the study of speech very interdisciplinary: Computer scientists and engineers join speech scientists, linguists, psychologists, and neuroscientists in the study of speech perception.

Society's interest in speech stems from a general interest that the public has for science, especially science related to the human mind. In this "Decade of the Brain" people are interested in how the brain stores and processes information. People are especially interested in how their children's linguistic and mental abilities develop. Some parents are interested in producing a "better baby" (that is not advocated here), but most parents simply want to understand the normal process of speech and language development in their own children, so that they can contribute to this natural process in the best way possible. It is for this reason that magazine cover stories on infants have proliferated.

In summary, there is a great deal of interest in the academic community, business and industry, and society in general in the brain's ability to learn and store language information. This increased interest makes students of speech and hearing science very marketable today. Their knowledge is not only vital to the clinical treatment process and in academic institutions, but also of interest to the business community.

✦ BACKGROUND INFORMATION ON SPEECH

One of the topics discussed at great length at scientific meetings is the following: With millions of dollars being devoted to the understanding of speech by computers, why hasn't the problem been solved? Why is it that machines cannot be made to "understand" speech? As described in what follows, the answer is that speech perception requires more than analysis of a very complicated acoustic signal. It also requires an interface between the incoming information and sources of knowledge that are stored by the brain. In understanding speech, humans use a highly efficient method of analyzing the acoustic information as well as a great deal of higher linguistic and cognitive information. We acquire this higher order information by living in the world and interacting with the people and events that make up that world. The computer lacks both the sophisticated analysis techniques provided by the auditory/perceptual systems of humans and a "brain" that stores the acquired knowledge. Both may be essential before speech understanding by machines is possible. Scientists do not yet fully understand how human listeners track the acoustic signal nor how the incoming acoustic information interacts with the stored sources of knowledge, but a great deal of information has been gathered about the critical features humans attend to when analyzing speech, and how a variety of sources of knowledge can affect the interpretation of the incoming information. We turn now to a discussion of the acoustic features of speech picked up by listeners; then we will turn to the perceptual organization of that information.

The Acoustics of Speech

The production of sound by the human vocal tract has been studied extensively. An introductory description of speech acoustics is presented here to provide a foundation for the discussions of speech perception that follow. (For a more detailed description of speech acoustics, see Chapter 10 by Stevens.) As shown in Figure 3–2, the vocal tract system functions as a tube with one end closed (the glottis) and the other open (the lips). The source of sound typically is periodic vocal fold vibration at the glottis. It consists of the fundamental frequency of the talker's voice, and the fundamental's harmonics. A sound source can also be generated within the vocal tract itself. For example, an aperiodic signal (noise) can be generated at a point of constriction in the vocal tract, as in the production of a fricative sound like /s/.

Regardless of the type of sound source, the acoustic energy is modified by the shape of the vocal tract. The vocal tract acts as a filter, producing resonances (frequency regions in which the energy is passed freely) and antiresonances (frequencies in which the energy is suppressed). When producing a speech sound, the vocal tract adopts a characteristic shape, thus creating particular concentra-

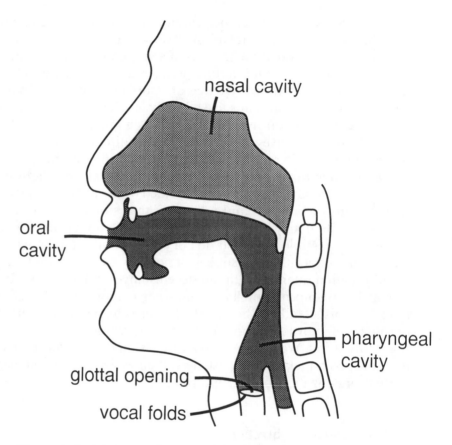

Figure 3–2. Schematic diagram of the human vocal tract.

tions of energy along the frequency scale that correspond to the resonant frequencies of the vocal tract. These regions of high energy concentration are called **formants**. When the vocal tract remains steady, as when a particular vowel sound is sustained, these resonances (and thus the formants) remain fairly constant. However, during dynamic speech production the vocal tract shape changes vary rapidly as the tongue darts from target to target. Therefore the formant frequencies almost never remain constant.

Early research on speech perception focused on single syllables, attempting to identify the acoustic information (the acoustic "cues") responsible for phonetic perception. Perception was shown to depend on formants, and particularly on the very rapid (20–100 msec) **formant transitions** that occur in speech. Figure 3–3 illustrates the vocal tract configuration for the three **point vowels** (/i, a, u/), so named because they represent acoustic and articulatory extremes. Analysis of the formant frequencies contained in these three vow-

Vocal Tract Configuration

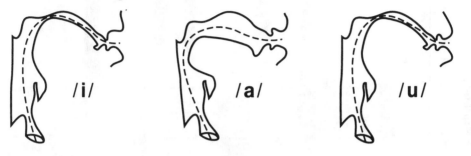

Formant Frequency Configuration

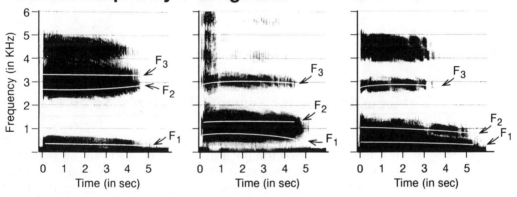

Figure 3–3. Vocal tract configurations and spectrograms of the three "point vowels," /i/, /a/, and /u/. The white lines trace the location of the formant frequencies over time.

els is accomplished by using a machine called the **sound spectrograph**. A spectrographic analysis of speech results in a display called a **sound spectrogram**, which displays the frequency content of speech over time. Figure 3–3 also shows a spectrographic display of each of the three vowels. In these displays, the formant frequencies are seen as dark bands in the spectrographic display and they are numbered consecutively from the lowest to the highest frequency.

The spectrograms in Figure 3–3 represent the acoustic results of maintaining a static vocal tract posture while sustaining a vowel sound. If a phrase is produced, the changing formant transitions reflect the altered resonances that are created as the articulators move to and from various target positions. Figure 3–4 shows a spectrographic display of the author producing the phrase "Communication Sciences and Disorders." As shown, the formant frequencies are rarely constant.

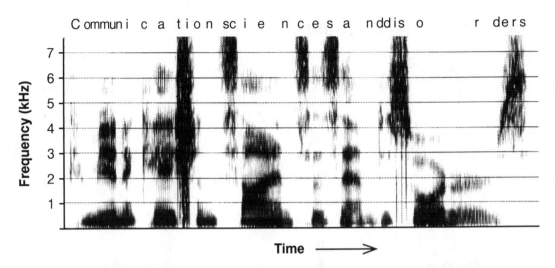

Figure 3-4. Spectrogram of the phrase, "Communication Sciences and Disorders."

Acoustic Cues for Segmental Features: Some Examples

During the past 40 years, a host of experiments on speech perception have identified the portions of the acoustic signal that govern the perception of various speech features. These studies were accomplished in four steps and always involved single isolated syllables. The four steps consisted of: (a) conducting **spectrographic analysis** of natural speech utterances differing by one linguistic feature such as /ba/ and /pa/, (b) forming **hypotheses** about which cues were critical for the particular speech feature by visually inspecting the spectrograms of these syllables, (c) using **speech synthesis** techniques to create syllables containing only the acoustic features hypothesized to be critical, and (d) **testing** the perception of the newly created syllables. These four steps — analyze, hypothesize, synthesize, test — still form the research plan for work in speech acoustics. The main difference is that each step in the early work was accomplished using fairly crude techniques. Speech was analyzed on a crude sound spectrograph rather than a digital computer. It was "synthesized" by literally painting (with acetate paint) on a device called the **Pattern Playback**, a machine invented for speech that converted the patterns drawn at various points on the frequency scale into a sound with corresponding frequency components. The test phase was accomplished by simply having the investigators stand around the machine and judge how the resulting synthesized syllable was identified, rather than by conducting a formal study.

The results of this early work, however, produced valuable descriptions of the acoustic events underlying phonetic perception. For example, early studies showed that the locations of the first two formants were sufficient to distinguish among the vowels, even though in natural speech four or more formants can often be identified. Figure 3–5 shows two-formant patterns painted on the Pattern Playback. When played, they reproduced eight of the most common English vowels. A comparison of Figure 3–3 and 3–5 shows that, although as many as four formants can be seen in the natural speech spectrograms, two formants are sufficient to distinguish the vowels.

The acoustic cues responsible for the perception of consonants were also identified. Studies showed that the perception of individual linguistic features, such as the **place of articulation** (the location in the mouth where the major constriction occurred) and the **manner of articulation** (whether the sound was voiced, nasalized, etc.), were governed by different aspects of the acoustic signal. Moreover, studies using computer-generated utterances showed that, even though naturally produced syllables contained many cues, single isolated cues were sufficient for indicating a particular feature value. For example, perception of the place of articulation in stop consonants indicating whether the major constriction occurred at the lips (/b/), alveolar ridge (/d/), or velum (/g/) depends primarily on the frequency content of the initial burst in energy at the beginning

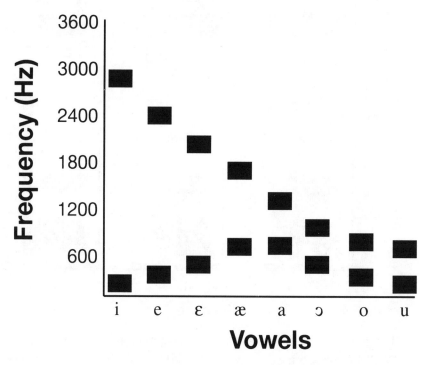

Figure 3-5. Two-formant patterns that are perceived as English vowels.

of the sound and the initial formant transitions. Studies using synthesized speech have shown that both cues are sufficient in isolation to distinguish the place feature. In Figure 3–6, the natural syllables /bae/, /dae/, and /gae/ are contrasted with their two-formant synthesized versions. Both sets of syllables can be identified as /bae/, /dae/, and /gae/, but the synthesized versions sound more machine-like.

Acoustic cues for the manner features, which indicate major distinctions in the ways sounds are produced, are generally associated with changes in the first formant. For example, the distinction between **voiced** and **voiceless** sounds produced at the same place

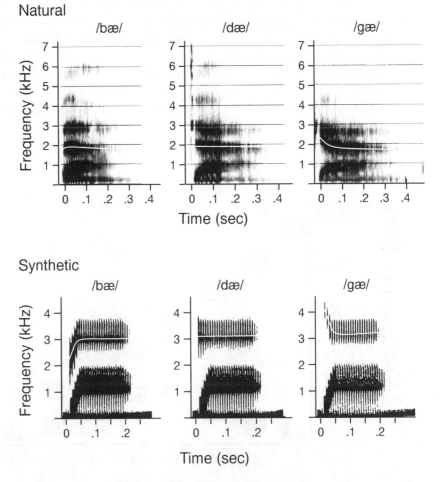

Figure 3–6. Naturally produced and computer-synthesized versions of the syllables /bae/, /dae/, and /gae/. Notice that the second formant transitions vary across syllables.

of articulation (e.g., /b/ vs. /p/) are related to an acoustic dimension called **voice-onset time (VOT)**. In English, voiced sounds are produced by simultaneously releasing the stop and instigating periodic laryngeal vibration (voicing); voiceless stops are produced by delaying the initiation of voicing in relation to the beginning of the syllable. Measurements of VOT indicate the difference (in msec) between the onset of the syllable (seen as a burst of frequency information that occurs when the stop is released) and the onset of voicing (seen in the first formant). This timing difference provides the critical cue used to identify whether a stop is voiced or voiceless. Voiced sounds typically have a VOT between 0 and +35 msec, depending on the place of articulation. Voiceless sounds have a VOT of between +30 and +150 msec.

In Figure 3–7, naturally produced /da/ and /ta/ syllables are contrasted with two-formant synthetic versions of the same syllables. The onset of voicing (V) and the onset of the burst (B) are marked for each syllable. Notice that the delay of voicing also produces a change in the first formant. The delay in voicing results in a "cutback" in the first-formant transition of voiceless sounds relative to their voiced counterparts.

Taken together, the spectrograms in Figures 3–6 and 3–7 illustrate two points. First acoustic cues that govern the perception of linguistic features have been identified. Second, the perception of linguistic features is controlled by what appear to be independent aspects of the acoustic signal.

To summarize, much has been learned about the acoustics of speech. We have learned that the physiologic gestures used during speech production give rise to specific dynamic acoustic events. For each speech feature a detailed set of acoustic events that are sufficient to govern perception have been described. However, as we will discuss in the next section, this did not completely solve the problem of speech perception. The same acoustic event was shown to be sufficient to govern perception of different phonetic segments, and quite diverse acoustic events were shown to be equivalent in their potential for indicating a particular phonetic value. These findings led to the idea that in order to account for the listener's ability to perceive the phonetic structure of language it was necessary to posit the existence of special perceptual mechanisms that evolved to analyze speech.

Acoustic Cues for Prosodic Features

In speech we perceive two distinct aspects of the sound, the phonetic identity of the sound units and the **prosody** of the utterance, its

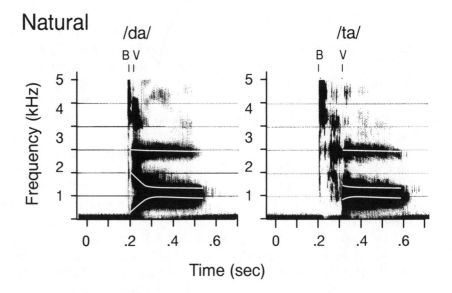

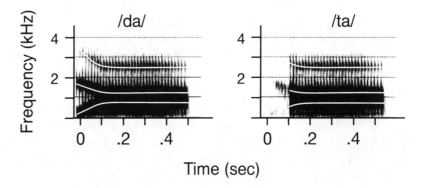

Figure 3–7. Naturally produced and computer-synthesized versions of the syllables /da/ and /ta/. The timing between the onset of the syllable (B) and the onset of laryngeal voicing (V) defines the voice onset time (VOT) of the syllable. The delay in the onset of laryngeal voicing in voiceless stops also causes a "cut-back" in the formant transitions.

pitch, rhythm, and tempo. As just reviewed, the identities of the phonetic units are determined by the pattern of formant frequencies over time. Prosody refers to the **stress** and **intonation pattern** of speech. The acoustic cues underlying the perception of prosody are also complex. The perception of stress is dictated by the relative values of three parameters — **duration, intensity**, and **fundamental frequency** — when compared across syllables. Stressed syllables are typically longer, louder, and higher in intonation. Figure 3–8 illus-

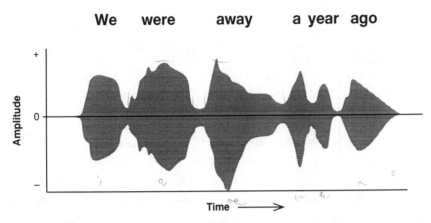

Figure 3–8. The amplitude envelope of the phrase "We were away a year ago," showing certain acoustic correlates of perceived stress (longer duration and higher amplitude). Higher stress occurs on the words "were" and "away."

trates the overall amplitude envelope of the phrase "We were away a year ago." The amplitude envelope provides information about the intensity and duration of the syllables contained in the phrase. As shown, each syllable produces an amplitude burst. The waveform envelope indicates that the second and third syllables in the phrase, "were" and "away," received primary stress. As shown, these syllables were more intense than those surrounding them and were also longer in duration.

Another prosodic characteristic of speech is its intonation (pitch) contour. A simple difference in intonation contour, as illustrated in Figure 3–9, differentiates sentences produced with a declarative (statement) as opposed to an interrogative (question) contour. The former is characterized by a rise-fall intonation contour, whereas the latter has a rising intonation contour. The perception of pitch contour is determined primarily by the fundamental frequency, that is, the frequency of glottal vibration. However, higher level linguistic variables can also play a role in its perception.

◆ ISSUES IN SPEECH PERCEPTION

The fact that the acoustic cues for speech sounds have been identified does not mean that humans' perception of speech is fully understood. There are two issues (at least) that complicate the story when running speech is perceived by a listener. Both problems have to do with how the consonants and vowels that make up words are recovered from the speech stream. The first is the issue of **speech seg-**

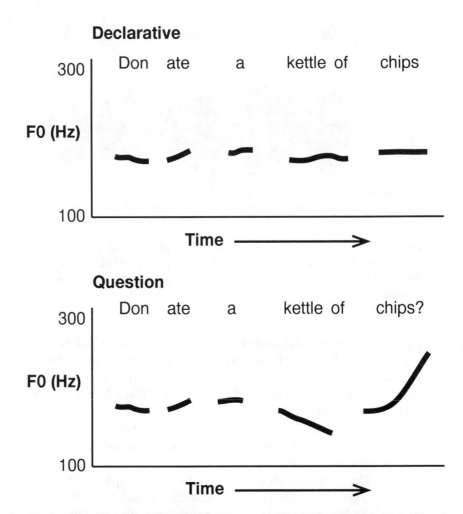

Figure 3–9. The fundamental frequency of the phrase "Don ate a kettle of chips," produced by the same speaker in a declarative (statement) and an interrogative (question) intonation contour.

mentation, the ability to break the spoken language signal down into segments that correspond to the consonants and vowels that make up words. The second is the issue of **speech variability**.

Speech Segmentation

Your perceptual system must track the formant frequencies in order to understand what was said. However, the tracking procedure is made difficult by the fact that the acoustic record does not segment the stream of speech into chunks that correspond with the consonants and vowels your perceptual system hears. For example, re-examine the spectrograph in Figure 3–4 which says, "Communication Sciences and Disorders." When you listen to someone produce these words, you hear the units of language. You hear four words, and can count the number of syllables quite easily (there are 12). You immediately grasp the meaning of the words.

How do we break a phrase down into units for analysis? A computer finds it very difficult to process speech because it cannot break phrases down into units. The computer cannot *segment* the stream. There are no silences between words or syllables to make segmentation easy. Silence often indicates a stop consonant rather than a break between words, and computers often make errors of this kind when attempting to segment speech.

One way to understand how difficult it is for a machine to segment spoken language is to try to segment printed words when the spaces between them have been removed, as in Figure 3–10. Without the spaces between words it is much more difficult to read the message. The letter string shown in Figure 3–10 can be broken down in different ways, and each is associated with a unique meaning. Segmentation is thus an important step in understanding a spoken message.

Another way to experience the segmentation problem, this time with spoken rather than written language, is to listen to a speaker of a foreign language. When we listen to a foreign speaker, we have the impression that the speaker is talking very fast. It does not sound like there are breaks between the words, and many of the individual sounds cannot be deciphered. Computers listening to speech are faced with a similar task. For a machine, analyzing speech is like reading words without spaces between them or listening to a foreign language.

Another problem with the analysis of spoken language is that speakers of the language do not always speak slowly and clearly.

THEREDONATEAKETTLEOFTENCHIPS

THE RED ON A TEA KETTLE OFTEN CHIPS

THERE, DON ATE A KETTLE OF TEN CHIPS

Figure 3–10. Segmenting printed letters into words is difficult when the spaces between words is eliminated. As shown, the string of letters can be segmented into two different series of words.

Speakers often do not articulate very well. Figure 3–11 shows two speech spectrograms of the same sentence: "Did you hit it to Tom?" The top record shows a spectrogram of a person saying each word very slowly and clearly. The bottom record shows a spectrogram of the same person speaking as we normally do, that is, quickly and easily.

Inspection of Figure 3–11 shows that the two records differ greatly. First, the well-articulated version is more than twice as long in duration when compared to the casually spoken version. Second, certain words and sounds virtually disappear. Words like "did you"

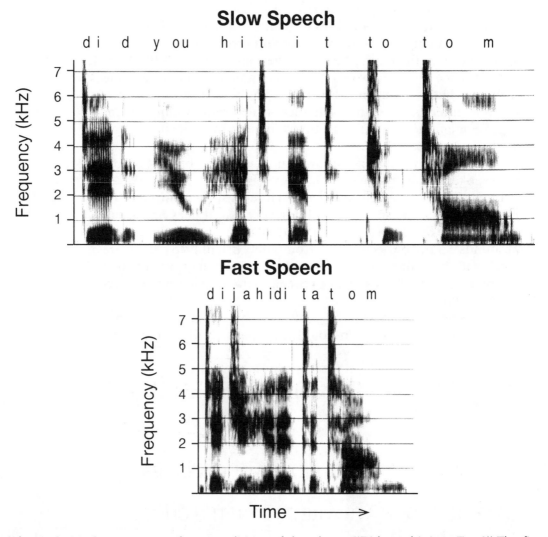

Figure 3–11. Spectrograms of two renditions of the phrase "Did you hit it to Tom?" The first phrase is produced slowly and clearly; the second is produced quickly and naturally. Both are perceived correctly by human listeners; however, machines cannot process the second version.

merge to become "dija." Words like "hit it to" merge to become "hidita." Items like "dija" and "hidita" are not real words and cannot be found in the brain's **mental lexicon**, its dictionary of words in the language. A computer could not find such words in its dictionary because they are not really words. This makes it difficult for a computer to decipher the message. It also makes our ability to understand speech all the more impressive and mysterious. As a listener, how do you segment the sounds and words you hear in order to understand the meaning or intent of the talker?

Variability in Speech

A second major issue has to be addressed when trying to explain speech perception. This problem is independent and would exist even if one could solve the segmentation problem. This problem is the extreme **variability** in speech. Variability makes it difficult to understand how we recognize a particular unit in speech, because the unit changes a great deal across different circumstances. There are three different sources of variability in speech: talker variability, context variability, and rate variability.

Talker variability refers to the fact that individual speakers produce speech differently. If one analyzes the speech of one speaker producing all of the English vowels, and plot the location of the first (F_1) and second (F_2) formant frequencies of each vowel in a two-formant coordinate plot, each vowel would have a particular location in the formant space (Figure 3–12A). If a computer analyzed these vowels, it would have no difficulty. Each vowel is specified by a particular set of coordinate values and has a unique location in the vowel space. Vowel categories do not overlap in the space. However, when a number of different talkers produce the same set of vowels, there is a great deal of overlap in the locations of individual vowels in the space (Figure 3–12B). It therefore becomes difficult to write a computer algorithm that correctly classifies the vowels.

Context variability is also a problem in speech perception. The information for a particular speech segment changes with the neighboring vowel. In other words, the acoustic information for the consonant changes with the vowel context in which it occurs. In the example shown in Figure 3–13, both natural and synthetic versions of the syllables /di/ and /du/ are shown. For the synthetic syllables the important acoustic information for /d/ is circled. In consists of the direction and extent of the **second formant transition** (see also Chapter 10 by Stevens). When the consonant /d/ occurs in the context of the vowel /i/, the second formant transition has to rise in order to hear /d/; however, in the context of the vowel /u/ the second for-

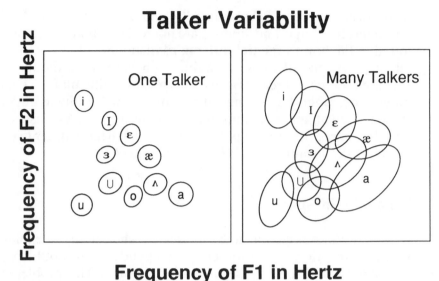

Figure 3–12. Schematic diagram showing the location of English vowels produced by a single talker as opposed to multiple talkers. The vowels of one talker are easily separated; however, when many talkers produce vowels, there is a great deal of overlap among categories.

mant transition has to fall in order to hear /d/. This is due to the fact that, at the level of spoken language, speech production involves **coarticulation**. When you plan to speak you adjust your articulators to prepare at least two or three units ahead, and this advance preparation alters the specific movement that is made when a given consonant occurs in different vowel contexts. This makes speech recognition more complicated because the recognition rules have to be specified for each context in which the unit might occur. Coarticulation in speech also raises the issue of the **basic unit of speech perception**. Many have argued that the basic unit of speech perception is probably larger than the phoneme, perhaps the syllable, because the acoustic cues to phonemes are so variable.

We learned earlier that some acoustic features are dynamic, that is, they change over time. For example, formant frequency transitions involve a change in formant frequency over time. We learned that these dynamic acoustic features are critical in speech perception, particularly for consonant sounds. Therefore, **rate variability** poses another problem for speech recognition. Rate of speech differs across speakers and also within a speaker over time. When a speaker adjusts his or her speaking rate, it alters the rate at which acoustic information occurs. This causes a problem because the critical value associated with a change from one phonetic unit to anoth-

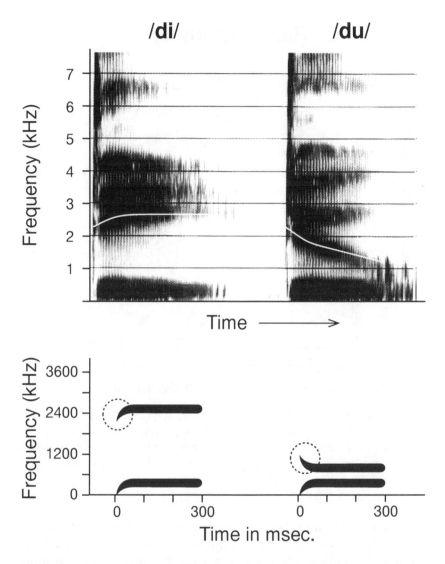

Figure 3–13. The acoustic cues for consonants change when a consonant occurs in different contexts, as shown here in both natural and synthetic versions of the consonant /d/. In front of the vowel /i/, the second formant transition rises in frequency; in front of the vowel /u/, the second-formant transitions falls in frequency.

er also changes. As shown in Figure 3–14, changing the rate of speech alters the transition duration that is necessary to produce a change in perception from one unit (such as the consonant /b/) to another (such as the consonant /w/). The important point is that one specific critical value (a particular transition duration) does not always indicate the consonant /b/; the exact transition duration that indi-

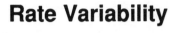

Rate Variability

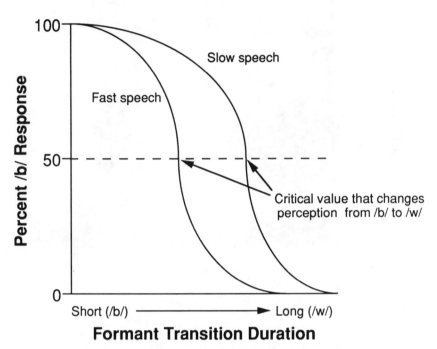

Formant Transition Duration

Figure 3–14. When the rate of speech changes from slow to fast, the acoustic cues that signal consonants such as /b/ and /w/ (the duration of the second formant transition) are altered. This means that two syllables each having the same formant transition duration can be perceived as either /b/or /w/, depending on the overall rate of speech.

cates /b/ (as opposed to /w/) changes with the rate of speech used by the talker. Once again, this complicates speech recognition by computer. This observation suggests that the listener must simultaneously analyze both the rate of speech and the phonemic content of the message.

To summarize the discussion thus far, three sources of variability have been the "bottlenecks" of speech recognition by computer. They are also the problems that make humans' processing of speech so mysterious and fascinating to speech scientists. In addition to variability, human listeners also have to contend with segmentation when trying to perceive speech. How do we so effortlessly understand speech when it is so difficult to segment it into units? How do we deal with the extreme variability in speech? After 40 years of research on humans' processing of speech, these topics still form the cornerstone of many research grants. Much progress has been made, but these issues continue to puzzle speech perception researchers. How is it that we perceive speech?

One clue to our effortless processing of spoken language is that we use other sources of information in addition to the acoustic analysis of the incoming message, as illustrated in Figure 3–15. When we process spoken language, we use two different types of information, "**bottom-up**" and "**top-down**." Bottom-up information refers to the on-line analysis of the speech information entering the auditory system. We assume that speech undergoes a series of transformations and that, at each successive stage, additional linguistic information is derived from the analyses.

For example, the first stages in bottom-up processing involve the conversion of the incoming auditory information into a neural signal. We assume that the auditory system converts the incoming acoustic signal into a kind of **neural spectrogram** that reveals the time-varying formant frequencies in speech. From this neural code the perceptual system has to derive the critical **phonetic features** contained in each segment of speech. **Phonological processing** consists of language-specific processing of the phonetic feature information. As described in the next section, different languages make use of different phonetic features in distinguishing between words. This stage in processing is posited to account for cross-language differences in speech perception.

Top-down processing refers to the use of **stored knowledge** that serves to constrain the number of plausible alternative messages one could be hearing. This stored information affects perception of the basic units of speech. For example, the **mental lexicon**, or list of all the words that you know, has a strong effect on your perception of words. If you hear a message produced in English, you automatically assume that it contains English words, and you attempt to listen to an incoming message with English words in mind. Studies show that if listeners are presented with real English words and words that follow the rules of English phonology but are not real words (such as the nonword "dreeb"), it takes a longer time and a louder signal to allow listeners to correctly identify the phonetic units contained in the nonword as opposed to the real word. Your mental lexicon affects perception by providing a list of candidate words for the listener to check incoming information against. If the incoming item has acoustic features that roughly match those contained in a word in your lexicon, your perceptual system assumes that you heard that word. If the incoming information does not match anything in your lexicon, your perceptual system remains uncertain until enough time has passed and the signal is loud enough to allow the listener to analyze each aspect of the incoming informa-

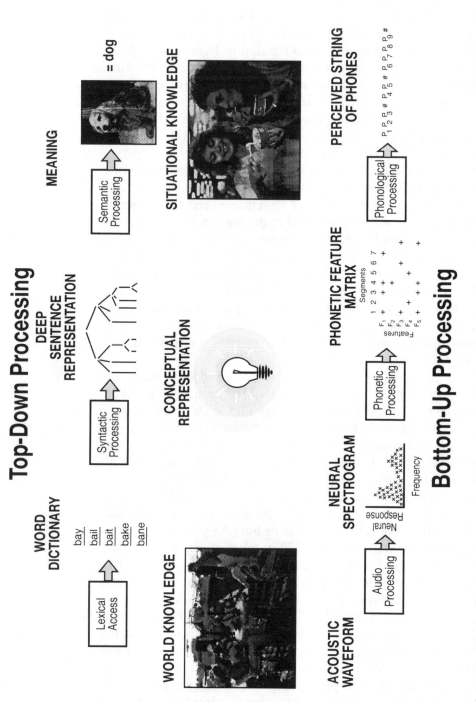

Figure 3–15. Spoken language processing involves both "bottom-up" and "top-down" processing. Bottom-up processing involves direct analysis of the incoming signal; top-down processing involves using stored sources of knowledge to form hypotheses about the message. Perception occurs when the interaction of these two kinds of analyses result in a single hypothesis about the message.

tion. Not having a mental lexicon would make perception much less efficient.

In addition to the mental lexicon, you have knowledge of the **rules of grammatical construction** in English and know that word order in English takes a certain form. This information also helps decipher the message. You also know the meanings of words and know that if a sentence contains the word "dog" it is likely that other words in the sentence have something to do with a dog. Other information is perhaps more subtle in nature. For example, you have **knowledge of the world** that specifies the content of typical sentences that might be uttered. When one is in a restaurant, it is likely that when the waiter comes to the table he or she will ask what you want to eat. **Situation-specific knowledge** specifies the context in which language occurs and that also serves as an aid to perception; if you're eating ice cream and you hear something that could either have been "ice cream" or "I scream," you would tend to perceive the first one because the situation suggests that this is the more likely of the two.

In summary, we not only analyze the incoming message using bottom-up tactics, we use stored knowledge about language and the world to constrain the possibilities. The two sources of information (bottom-up and top-down) *interact* during the perceptual processing of the incoming sound. Perception occurs when the bottom-up and top-down sources of information interact to sufficiently constrain the possible alternatives concerning what the speaker said, making only one alternative seem plausible to the listener. It is at this point that a listener *perceives* a specific message.

◆ A FOCUS ON PHONETIC PERCEPTION

One fact that has motivated research on the perception of the phonetic units of speech, the consonants and vowels that make up words, is that we know that bottom-up processes are very good even in the absence of top-down information. When someone introduces a new word completely out of context (such as the word "zabracon"), you perceive it. This is true despite the fact that "zabracon" is not listed in your mental lexicon and there is no contextual information to help you perceive the phonetic units it contains. Even in the absence of other contextual information, adult listeners recognize the consonants and vowels that make up words. Moreover, at the beginning of life, infants do not have any top-down sources of knowledge. Top-down sources of knowledge are acquired during development (see Chapter 4 by Bloom); they are not there to begin with. Infants must therefore come into the world prepared to process language from the bottom-up. Investigators have been interested in studying infant perception because it might provide the key to how bottom-up processing works in the absence of top-down information.

✦ INFANTS' PERCEPTION OF SPEECH

At birth, infants seem to be completely absorbed with the sound of the human voice and the sight of the human face. Evolution seems to have guaranteed infants' attentiveness to their own species' communicative signals. The infants of many animal species are specially sensitive to the vocal signals that are critical to their survival. Studies show that a diverse set of communicating animals — bats, birds, crickets, and frogs — are perceptually prepared at birth for the acquisition of species-typical vocal signals. They are very interested in them. This is also true of the human baby. Infants appear to be extraordinarily well prepared to respond to the human face and voice. Evidence supporting interest in the face comes from studies showing that young infants prefer to look at faces rather than at other visual configurations. More surprisingly, studies show that even newborns will imitate facial gestures presented to them by another person. In one study by Meltzoff and Moore (1983), it was demonstrated that infants as young as 42 minutes old can imitate gestures such as mouth opening and tongue protrusion.

My own work and that of others has demonstrated the human infant's exquisite sensitivity to human speech. For example, research has shown that, when given a choice, young infants prefer to listen to **Motherese**, a highly melodic speech signal adults use when addressing infants (Fernald, 1985). It is not the syntax or semantics of Motherese that holds infants' attention — it is the acoustic signal itself. When the syntax and semantics of Motherese are stripped away and only the melodic pitch component of Motherese remains, infants still demonstrate the preference (Fernald & Kuhl, 1987). Moreover, the prosodic features of Motherese, its **higher pitch, slower tempo**, and **expanded intonation contours**, appear to be universal across the world's languages (Grieser & Kuhl, 1988). We do not know what makes mothers (fathers too) speak to their infants in this way, but we do know that mothers in every language examined thus far produce this kind of speech, and that babies demonstrate a preference for it.

Infants' preference for human speech raises another question. Are infants interested in the sounds of human speech? And if so, are infants perceptually processing speech in a way that has any relevance to language acquisition? To answer these questions, studies have been conducted on very young infants.

Methods for Assessing Speech Perception in Infancy

How can one test very young infants to find out about their speech perception abilities? Two techniques have been used extensively: **high-amplitude sucking (HAS)** and **head-turn (HT)** (Jusczyk, 1985; Kuhl, 1985b). The HAS technique, shown in Figure 3–16, is used to test infants between 1 and 4 months of age. The technique works very well with infants this age, capitalizing on the young infant's willingness to suck on a pacifier. As the infant sucks on a nipple, which is

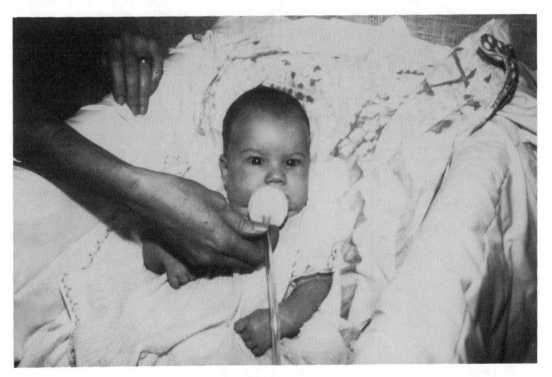

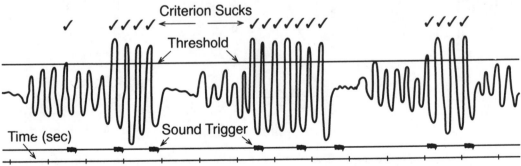

Figure 3–16. Young infant being tested using the high-amplitude sucking (HAS) technique. The infant sucks on a nonnutritive nipple and the pressure changes inside the nipple are recorded. Sucking responses that exceed a threshold result in the presentation of a speech sound.

connected to a pressure transducer, the infant's sucking responses produce pressure changes inside the nipple that are monitored by a computer. The resulting pressure waveforms are shown at the bottom of the figure. An amplitude criterion is set for each infant during a **no-sound baseline condition**.

After baseline is established, a speech sound is presented to infants when they produce a sucking response whose amplitude exceeds the preset criterion. The maximum rate of sound presentation to the infant is 1 sound per second. At this point, experimental infants are presented with a novel speech sound while control infants continue to be presented with the first sound.

Typical data from experimental and control infants are shown in Figure 3–17. The graph is labeled in minutes before and after the **shift point** (the point at which the sound is changed for experimental infants). During the first minute of contingent sound presentation, the number of responses typically decreases. Most infants appear mildly startled and stop sucking for a moment when the first sounds are presented, as suggested by the decrease in responses between the baseline minute and the first minute of sound presenta-

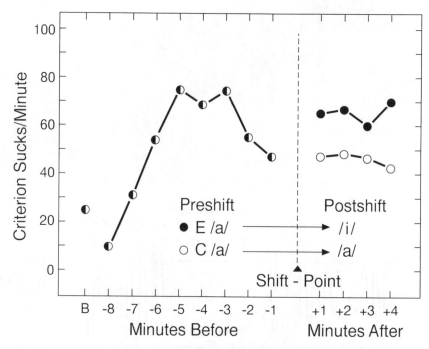

Figure 3–17. The number of sucking responses produced in each minute of the experiment by an experimental and control infant. The two infants are treated identically prior to the shift point; after the shift point, the experimental infant hears a new sound while the control infant continues to hear the first sound.

tion. Eventually, however, the number of responses increases and reaches the **maximum** as infants learn that sucking produces sound. The same speech sound is presented to the infant over and over. Eventually, the number of sucking responses occurring in a given minute drops below a **decrement criterion** (20% below the maximum for 2 consecutive minutes). The decline occurs when the infant tires of hearing the same sound presented over and over again. When this decrement criterion is met, infants in the experimental group are presented with a new sound while infants in the control group continue to hear the first sound. Both the experimental and the control infants are monitored for 4 minutes after the decrement criterion is met. Experimental infants typically increase their response rates when the speech sound is changed, whereas control infants either continue to decrease or do not change their response rates. Significant differences between the sucking rates shown by the two groups of infants are taken as evidence that infants of this age can discriminate between two speech sounds.

A second technique, **head-turn (HT) conditioning**, has also been used very successfully to test infants between 6 months and 1 year of age. In this procedure, infants are trained to make a **head-turn response** whenever a speech sound repeated once every second as a **background** stimulus, is changed to a **comparison** speech sound. A head turn that occurs during the presentation of the comparison stimulus is rewarded with a **visual stimulus**, for example, a toy monkey that claps cymbals when activated.

The test situation is shown in Figure 3–18. The infant is held by a parent so that he or she faces an assistant located to the infant's right side. The assistant maintains the infant's attention at midline or directly in front of the assistant by manipulating a variety of silent toys. A loudspeaker is located at a 90° angle to the assistant, and the **visual reinforcer** is placed directly on top of the loudspeaker. The visual reinforcer consists of a toy animal housed in a dark plexiglass box. The animal is not visible until the lights mounted inside the box are illuminated. The lights are illuminated when the infant produces a correct head-turn response at the point when the sound is changed from the background to the comparison. The experimenter is in an adjoining control room which also houses a computer that presents the stimuli and controls all of the contingencies delivered during the test.

Two types of trials, change and control, need to be used to make sure that infants' head turns are occurring only when the sound is changed. During a **change trial**, the stimulus is changed from one speech sound to another speech sound. During a **control trial**, the sound is not changed. For both types of trials, the head turns are scored. If a head turn occurs on a change trial, the trial is scored as

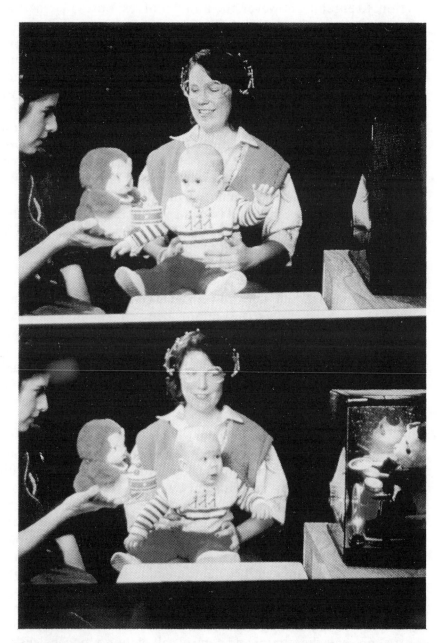

Figure 3–18. Infant at 6 months of age being tested in the head-turn (HT) technique. Infants sit on a parent's lap and are distracted by the toys held by an assistant. A background sound is presented from a loudspeaker located to the left of the infant. The infant is reinforced by the presentation of a toy animal (located in the black box above the loudspeaker) if the infant produces a head-turn when the sound changes from the background sound to a comparison sound.

correct, and the visual reinforcer is presented. If no head turn occurs during a change trial, the trial is scored as an *error*. During control trials, a head-turn is scored as an *error (false alarm)*; if no head turn occurs, the trial is scored as *correct*. Infants tested in this procedure seem to love the little game it involves and can be trained in about 20 trials (for an easy distinction such as /a/ versus /u/) to produce the head-turn response reliably.

These two behavioral techniques, the high-amplitude sucking (HAS) technique and the head-turn (HT) technique, have been widely used to study infants' perception of speech. HAS has been used with infants between 1 and 4 months of age; HT has been used with infants between 5.5 and 12 months of age.

Discrimination of Phonetic Contrasts and Prosodic Changes

One of the first questions one might ask about young infants' speech perception abilities is whether or not they can hear the differences between *syllables differing in a single phonetic feature* such as in the words "bat" and "pat." A large number of studies have shown that infants at the earliest ages tested are indeed capable of discriminating two syllables that differ with respect to a single phonetic feature. These tests have been done with both natural and with computer-generated syllables. For example, it has been shown that infants can hear the difference between syllables such as /ba/ and /pa/ or /da/ and /ga/. They can hear differences between quite similar consonants such as /sa/ and /za/. They can hear vowel distinctions as well, such as the difference between /a/ and /i/, or the more difficult vowel distinction between /a/ and /ae/. Virtually all the tests that have been done show that young infants have a keen sensitivity to the acoustic cues that distinguish the phonetic units of speech. This is very important to language learning. Without the ability to hear the fine distinctions that differentiate words, it would be very difficult for the infant to learn language.

Infants also have been tested on their ability to hear the difference between intonation contours, such as rising versus falling intonation contours. These tests show that infants have no trouble hearing these changes in intonation. Moreover, infants have been shown to discriminate the acoustic cues underlying adults' perception of stress when all three of the acoustic cues known to be related to stress perception by adults — increased fundamental frequency, intensity, and duration — are used.

Tests of infants' abilities to discriminate speech have used multi-syllabic contexts in an attempt to duplicate more natural (and more difficult) listening conditions. These tests revealed that infants discriminate two-syllable contrasts such as /daba/ versus /daga/ and /bada/ versus /gada/, /dawa/ versus /daga/, and /wada/ versus /gada/. These studies are important because they show infants' ability to discriminate in a more real-life context. This work also has shown that certain prosodic features can enhance the discrimination of a syllable embedded in a long string. For example, if a syllable in the midst of a sentence is produced with primary stress, with an elevated intonation contour, and at a higher intensity, it is easier to discriminate. That in fact is the way that mothers produce speech when they are talking to their infants.

Taken as a whole, these studies show that infants come into the world with the basic abilities to hear the distinctions important for language. The acoustic cues that differentiate phonetic units in the language are very subtle. It is considered very helpful that infants are born with the capacity to attend to and distinguish these acoustic cues.

Although these studies show that infants have a keen ability to hear speech-sound distinctions, they do not go so far as to say that infants are completely prepared to handle speech when they are born. When adults perceive speech, they do more than just discriminate differences between one sound and another. They **perceptually organize** speech into **phonetic categories**, ignoring some differences and listening to others. The question addressed in the next section is whether infants have an ability to perceptually organize speech sounds into phonetic categories.

◆ PERCEPTUAL ORGANIZATION FOR SPEECH

Categorical Perception in Adults and Infants

The first study published on speech perception by young infants addressed the question of infants' perceptual organization of speech. Published by Peter Eimas at Brown University (Eimas, Siqueland, Jusczyk, & Vigorito, 1971), the study demonstrated that infants exhibited a phenomenon called **categorical perception**. The study provided the first evidence that very young infants were perceptually organizing speech sounds in a linguistically relevant manner.

The phenomenon of categorical perception had been demonstrated in adults by Alvin Liberman and his colleagues at Haskins Laboratories in the 1960s. Tests of categorical perception used speech sounds created by a computer. The computer created a series of sounds that ranged from one syllable (such as /ba/) to a syllable that differed in only one phonetic feature (such as /pa/) by altering some acoustic variable in small steps. The acoustic variable manipulated to create a series that goes from /ba/ to /pa/ is voice-onset time. As illustrated in Figure 3–19, sounds on one end of the series are identified as the syllable /ba/; sounds on the other end of the series are identified as /pa/.

The test of categorical perception involved asking listeners to identify each one of the sounds in the series. Researchers expected that the sounds in the series would be perceived as changing gradually from /ba/ to /pa/, with many sounds in the middle of the series sounding ambiguous. But that is not what happened. Adults reported hearing a series of /ba/s that abruptly changed to a series of /pa/s. There was no in-between. And when researchers asked listeners if they could hear the difference between two adjacent /ba/s (or /pa/s) in the series, they could *not* do so, even though the two /ba/s (or /pa/s) were physically different. Listeners did not hear the gradual differences between adjacent stimuli in the series until they heard a big change — the change from /ba/ to /pa/. The fact that listeners' responses were "categorical" gave the phenomenon its name.

This phenomenon has been demonstrated for many phonetic features. Figure 3–20 shows the results of the **identification** and **discrimination** of sounds from a series that ranged from /ra/ to /la/ (Miyawaki et al., 1975). As shown in the top part of Figure 3–20, American listeners identified the sounds on the left end of the series as /ra/ whereas those on the right end of the series were identified as

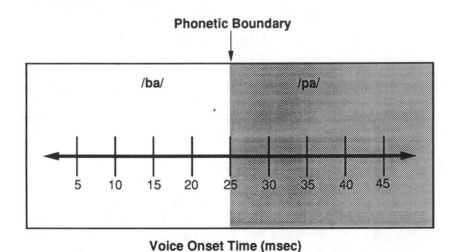

Figure 3–19. Categorical perception is tested using sounds from a series. The sounds vary in equal steps on some acoustic dimension. Tests show that the perception of stimuli in the series changes abruptly at the location of the phonetic boundary between the two categories.

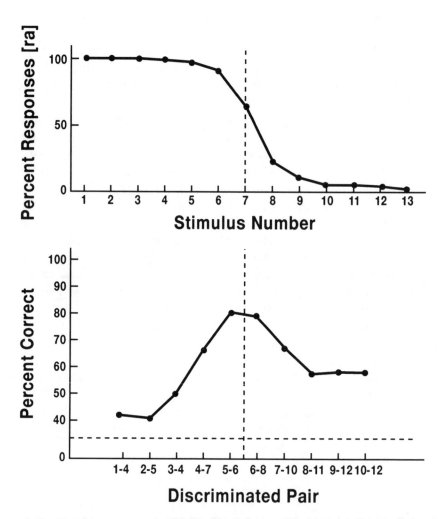

Figure 3–20. An example of categorical perception for the syllables /ra/and /la/. The ability to discriminate differences between sounds in the series (*bottom panel*) increases sharply at the location of the phonetic boundary on the identification function (*top panel*). Adapted from Miyawaki et al., 1975, with permission.

/la/. The bottom half of Figure 3–20 shows the discrimination results on American listeners. As predicted by the categorical perception phenomenon, discrimination performance improves at the boundary between the two phonetic categories. This means that when listeners hear two sounds (such as 5 and 8) in the series, one of which sounds like /ra/ and the other like /la/, they reliably discriminate between them. However, when they hear two sounds that are just as far apart and therefore just as different from an acoustic standpoint, such as the sounds 1 and 4, or 9 and 12, they fail to hear a difference between the two sounds.

Even more importantly, research on categorical perception in adults revealed that the phenomenon differed depending on the **linguistic experience** of the listener. It occurred only for sounds in an adult's native language. For example, when Japanese listeners were tested on the same series of /ra/ and /la/ sounds just discussed, they did not hear a sudden change at the **phonetic boundary** between /ra/ and /la/. They heard no change at all. The Japanese listeners showed a flat discrimination function, as shown in Figure 3–21, which compares the discrimination data of Japanese and American listeners. In other words, adults were shown to be very "culture-bound" in their discrimination of speech. These studies demonstrated that the perception of speech involved more than just the acoustic analysis of the signal; it involved some higher order process that took into account whether the distinction was meaningful (i.e., **phonemic**) in the person's language. In the Japanese language the distinction between /r/ and /l/ is not phonemic; it is not used to distinguish words, and Japanese adults did not produce categorical perception when tested with /r/ and /l/.

The finding that categorical perception was **language-specific** suggested that the phenomenon might be learned through exposure

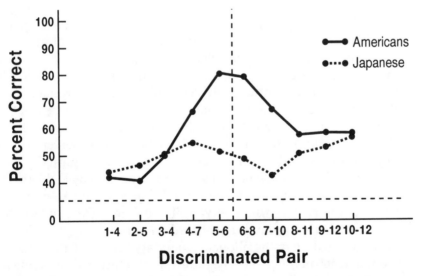

Figure 3–21. A comparison of the discrimination data obtained when American and Japanese listeners were tested with a series of stimuli that ranged from /ra/ to /la/. American listeners show the characteristic peak in discrimination shown in tests of categorical perception; Japanese listeners do not show the peak in discrimination.

to a specific language. This is what Eimas had set out to test in 1971. The question was: What would very young infants hear when presented with a series of /ba/s and /pa/s or /ra/s and /la/s? If hearing the sudden shift in the stimuli at the boundary between two categories was the result of experience with language (perhaps as a result of hearing their parents contrast words containing /b/ and /p/ — like "bat" and "pat") then young infants would not be expected to show it. Older infants, on the other hand, who had experienced language, might show the categorical perception phenomenon.

Infants' responses to the sounds were monitored using the HAS technique previously described. The results of the study revealed that infants' discrimination of /ba/ and /pa/ was categorical. They responded reliably to the change from /ba/ to /pa/ but not to an equal physical change when it occurred within the category /b/ or within the category /p/. Moreover, infants demonstrated categorical perception not only for the sounds of their native language, but also for sounds from foreign languages. In all cases, infants reacted to the sounds as though they heard a sudden shift in the series at the adult-defined boundary between the two phonetic categories. In contrast to adults, infants appeared to be born "citizens of the world." They responded to speech as though they heard all of the phonetic distinctions used in any language. What produced these multilingual abilities in infants? A special language acquisition device, or something else?

When the report from Eimas' lab was published, research was also being conducted on the cross-fostering of infant chimpanzees by human adults. It became clear from early work on cross-fostering that chimps could not learn to articulate human speech. Their vocal tracts and oral structures did not allow them to produce speech. Was it reasonable to assume that animals also would be unable to *perceive* human speech? Would nonhuman animals fail to demonstrate perceptual phenomena, such as categorical perception, that human adults and infants succeeded in demonstrating?

Tests of categorical perception were conducted by Kuhl and Miller in 1975 on animals such as chinchillas and monkeys, animals whose auditory systems are very similar to man's. The results of these tests showed that animals also heard an abrupt change in the stimuli at the location of the phonetic boundary between categories. Subsequent tests on other speech stimuli showed that this was true for a number of stimuli. In all cases, animals responded as though they heard a sudden change in the speech stimuli at the exact location where human adults perceived a shift from one phonetic category to another. On the basis of these findings, the authors speculated that phonetic boundaries were based on **natural auditory boundaries**. In the evolution of speech, the basic sensitivity of the auditory system must have played a strong role in defining the phonetic categories used in language.

These findings in animals affected our theories about the human infant and the nature of infants' initial predispositions with regard to language. Animals were not born with a language acquisition device, yet they performed in tests of categorical perception. The results on animals showing that the categorical perception of speech sounds was not unique to human beings suggested that we could not use the categorical perception phenomenon to support the idea that infants are born with an innate language acquisition device in place. Categorical perception could be accomplished in the absence of an innate module or mechanism dedicated to language.

Perceptual Constancy for Speech Categories

The studies on categorical perception tested infants' abilities to hear differences between sounds, and showed that their abilities were enhanced in the region of the phonetic boundary. This helps infants organize speech sounds into categories. However, perception of a phonetic category requires something else. In order to perceive a phonetic category, infants must be able to perceive a similarity among sounds that are obviously different. For example, as previously discussed, when different people (e.g., two adults, one male and one female) produce the same vowel sound (like the vowel /a/), you can hear the differences between them but you can also hear that they are similar. You perceive that the two people are producing the same vowel.

We know that computers are not good at this. Speech perception requires what cognitive psychologists call **categorization** — the ability to render discriminably different things equivalent — and computers are not good categorizers. Categorization is a phenomenon that characterizes all of perception. Because stimuli typically vary along many dimensions, categorization requires that we recognize similarities in the presence of considerable variance. Often the exact criteria used to categorize stimuli are not obvious. Consider the categories *cat* and *dog*. Describing what distinguishes them, and thus what uniquely categorizes them, is not simple. They both have two eyes, four legs, fur, a tail, and so on. Configurational properties of the face probably distinguish them, but trying to describe these features is difficult. Yet we would not expect an adult to mistakenly identify a cat as a dog, or vice versa. In the case of speech produced by different talkers, listeners must be able to categorize or "render equivalent" the sounds produced by different people, even though the sounds are very different acoustically.

The fact that computers fail to categorize speech produced by different talkers made infants' abilities all the more interesting. The question was asked: Do infants perceive similarity for speech produced by different talkers? Would infants outperform computers in the ability to "sort" speech into phonetic categories, to perceive a perceptual similarity — **constancy** — for the same vowel produced by different talkers?

The critical question for infants is whether they recognized that all /a/s are the same, regardless of the talker who produces them. It is of no small import to the child that such an ability exists early in life. It is critical to infants' acquisition of speech. Their vocal tracts cannot produce the frequencies produced by the adult's vocal tract, so they cannot mimic the exact frequencies that an adult produces. Infants must hear the similarity between the vowels they are capable of producing and those produced by adults in order to imitate them and learn speech.

In studies conducted by Kuhl (1979, 1983, 1985a), the head-turn procedure was used to test infants' abilities to hear a similarity between a vowel spoken by a diverse set of talkers. Infants were trained to produce a head-turn response when a single talker changed from producing one speech sound to producing another. After training, each infant was tested with the sounds produced by many different talkers to examine whether the training with one talker resulted in the generalization of the response to the speech of many other talkers. Generalization of the response from one talker to many different talkers would illustrate that the infant perceived speech produced by different talkers as similar.

Infants were first trained with the vowel sound /a/ produced by a male talker and the vowel /i/ produced by the same male talker. Once trained, the infant produced head-turning responses only when /i/ vowels occurred, and did not turn during the presentations of the vowel /a/. Control trials showed that infants turned their heads only when the vowel was changed. The experimental question was: What will infants do when they are presented with new instances of /a/ and /i/ vowels, instances clearly different from the /a/ and /i/ stimuli heard during training? If young infants can contend with talker variability — if they hear all /a/s (or all /i/s) as belonging to the same category — then their initial training to respond to a single /a/ and /i/ sounds produced by one talker should generalize to all members of the category, even those produced by different talkers. An infant trained to produce a head turn to one male's /i/ vowel, but not to his /a/ vowel, should produce head turns to all novel /i/s (produced by other males, females, and children), but not to equally novel /a/s.

The results demonstrated that infants have the ability to sort vowels by phonetic category. Infants responded correctly to novel vowels regardless of the talker producing the vowel. If the infant had been trained to turn to the male's /a/ vowel, then all novel /a/ vowels evoked the response, whereas very few of the novel /i/vowels evoked the response. Figure 3–22 shows the percent head-turn re-

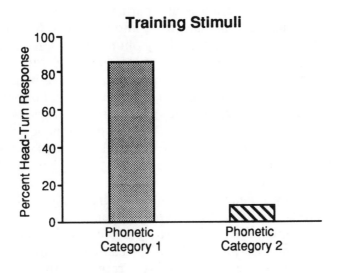

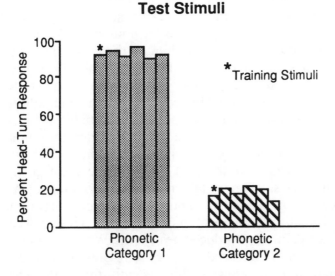

Figure 3–22. Categorization data from 6-month-old infants tested using the head-turn technique. Infants were trained to produce a head-turn response to one of two syllables (the vowel /a/ or /i/) spoken by a single talker (*top panel*). Then, infants were tested using /a/ and /i/ vowels produced by many talkers, including new male, female, and child talkers (*bottom panel*). Performance indicates that infants' responses generalized to novel instances from the two categories, indicating that infants can hear similarities between vowels spoken by different talkers.

sponses to all of the stimuli introduced in the experiment. In the *top panel*, infants' responses to the two stimuli used during the training phase are shown. In the *bottom panel*, infants' responses to the stimuli presented during the test phase of the experiment are shown. Each bar in the bottom panel of the graph represents the infants' responses to the utterances of a particular talker. Each talker produced one token from Category 1 and one token from Category 2.

Infants sorted the stimuli by phonetic class, regardless of the talker producing the sounds. Infants produced high numbers of head-turn responses to the novel stimuli that were members of the phonetic category they were initially trained to respond to (Category 1 stimuli). They produced very few head-turn responses to equally novel stimuli that were members of the second phonetic category (Category 2). An analysis of infants' first-trial responses showed that infants performed correctly on the very first trial. These results suggest that 6-month-old infants categorize all /a/s (and all /i/s) as the same — they appear to be capable of perceiving similarity among the sounds produced by different talkers.

In additional tests this issue was pursued further, making the experimental task more difficult by using many more talkers and close vowels — the /a/ in "pot" versus the /ae/ in "pat." This time the vowels were produced by 12 different men, women, and children. The vowels were produced naturally, rather than generated by a computer, as they had been in the previous study. We purposely chose voices that sounded very different so that extracting a constant vowel would be especially difficult. We used male talkers with deep voices, women with exceptionally high voices, even people with colds who sounded very nasal but could be understood. Adults could classify the sounds accurately. What about babies?

Figure 3–23 displays the infants' performance on both the two training stimuli (*top panel*) and the test stimuli (*bottom panel*). The results revealed two things. First, infants can categorize vowels by phonetic class when the talker is constantly changing. As shown, the percentage of head-turns to novel stimuli from the two categories differed greatly. When novel sounds from the reinforced category were presented, infants produced head-turns. When equally novel sounds from the nonreinforced category were presented, infants refrained from turning their heads. More recently, these results have been extended to even younger infants. In one study, newborns were shown to replicate this effect. The results thus confirm that, from birth, infants are capable of perceiving similarity for speech produced by different talkers — they demonstrate **perceptual constancy** for vowels across talkers. They sort speech into categories regardless of the talker producing the sound, something yet to be accomplished by a machine.

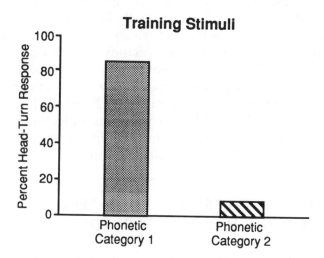

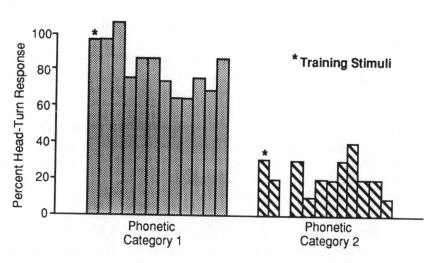

Figure 3–23. Categorization data from 6-month-old infants tested using head-turn technique on the vowels /a/ and /ae/. The top panel shows the training data for the vowels of a single talker. The bottom panel shows infant responses to the novel /a/ and /ae/ vowels spoken by 12 new talkers (men, women, and children). The data show that infants can perceptually sort vowels into phonetic categories regardless of the talker who produces the vowel.

And what of animals? Do they "categorize" speech across talkers? This question has not as yet been fully answered. Research shows that if the categories are sufficiently far apart so that they do not physically overlap, such as the categories /a/ versus /i/, animals can sort them into categories based on the phonetic identity of the vowel. However, there is insufficient data on animals for tests using categories such as /a/ versus /ae/, or /a/ versus /ɔ/, categories in which there is substantial physical overlap, to know whether animals will be able to sort the vowels into categories under these circumstances. Future research is needed to determine whether perceptual constancy across talkers is unique to humans.

✦ EFFECTS OF EXPERIENCE ON SPEECH PERCEPTION: WHAT IS LEARNED?

The results of tests on categorical perception revealed that infants are "multilingual" phonetic perceivers whereas adults are "culture-bound." This raises interesting questions about the developmental changes between infancy and adulthood. If we are all born with the general ability to hear the distinctions between all the sounds of all languages, when and by what process do we lose these abilities? When do our "language-general" speech perception abilities become "language-specific"?

Some information about *when* we lose the ability to discriminate foreign-language sounds was obtained by Janet Werker of the University of British Columbia (Werker & Tees, 1984). Her studies of infants showed that by 12 months infants failed to discriminate foreign contrasts they once showed an ability to discriminate. For example, when tested on a phonetic contrast used in the Hindi language but not in English, infants at 6 to 8 months of age showed the ability to discriminate the contrast; however, by 12 months of age the infants failed to discriminate the same contrast.

How does this change come about? What causes us to lose our abilities to perceive certain distinctions in speech? New work from my own laboratory suggests that infants' early listening experience alters their perception of speech in a way that explains this change in speech perception. These changes happen very early in life. In tests of speech perception conducted on 6-month-old infants in two countries, the United States and Sweden, it was shown that by 6 months infants already have begun to show a native-language pattern of phonetic perception (Kuhl, Williams, Lacerda, Stevens, & Lindblom, 1992). At 6 months of age, infants have not yet uttered a single meaningful word, nor do they understand a single word. We can conclude therefore that the initial change from a language-general pattern of phonetic perception to one that is language-specific does not depend on the acquisition of word meaning. In the next section I will describe these findings and a new theory on infants' development of speech perception.

The new studies focus on the perception of **phonetic prototypes**, which are exceptionally good examples of phonetic categories. **Prototypes** are the "best" members of a category, the ones most representative of the category as a whole.

There is good agreement among people as to the best members of many categories. Examples of birds and dogs are shown in Figure 3–24. Most people agree that a robin is a better (more typical)

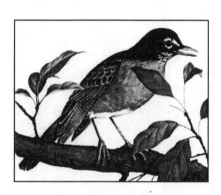
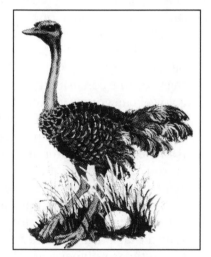
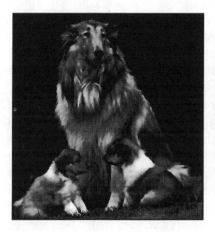
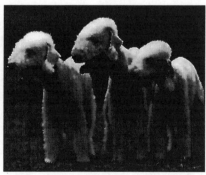

Figure 3–24. Prototypes are exceptionally good instances of categories. A robin is a prototype of the category bird; an ostrich is not. A collie is a prototype of the category dog; certain terriers are not.

member of the category bird than an ostrich is, and that a collie is a better (more typical) member of the category dog than a terrier is. The prototypes of categories appear to be easier to perceive than non-prototypes (atypical members) of the same categories. Prototypes often are processed more quickly, are more easily remembered, and frequently are preferred over nonprototypes. Our question was whether there were preferred instances (prototypes) for speech categories and, if so, whether those stimuli helped define speech categories.

To test the prototype hypothesis for speech, we computer generated many different instances of the vowel category /i/ — nearly a hundred (Kuhl, 1991). We then asked adults to judge the **category goodness** of each of the vowels using a scale from 1 to 7. A 7 indicated a particularly good exemplar — a perfect /i/. A 1 indicated an /i/, but a very poor one.

Adults ratings were very consistent. There was a certain location in the /i/ vowel space, a kind of **hotspot** that always resulted in better ratings. As you moved away from the hotspot for /i/, the ratings became consistently worse. It became clear that all members of a vowel category were not equivalent; some were better than others. Moreover, our studies showed that phonetic prototypes differed in speakers of different languages (Kuhl, 1992a). For example, Swedish listeners had different vowel prototypes than American listeners did. Even when both languages contained what ostensibly was the same sound, the vowel /i/, the listeners of the two languages differed with regard to which /i/ was the "best" in the two languages. Japanese listeners did not have prototypes for the sounds /r/ and /l/, but for a sound that was acoustically in between /r/ and /l/. In other words, phonetic prototypes were shown to be unique to a given language.

The discovery that there were phonetic prototypes and that they differed across different languages was important, but studies were needed to verify that the prototype made a difference in perception. Would listeners behave differently when listening to a prototype as opposed to a nonprototype of the category? The answer to this question was revealed by another set of studies.

Perceptual tests revealed that, when listening to a phonetic category prototype, a unique thing happened. Sounds that were close to a prototype could not be distinguished from the prototype, even though they were physically different. The prototype appeared to perceptually assimilate nearby sounds. This is conceptually illustrated in Figure 3–25. Imagine that the sphere in the middle of Figure 3–25A is a prototype, the "best" instance of a vowel category. The spheres around the prototype are other vowels from the same category. When listeners compare the prototype to the surrounding sounds, they find it difficult to hear any differences between the prototype and these other sounds. As illustrated in Figure 3–25B, the

A.

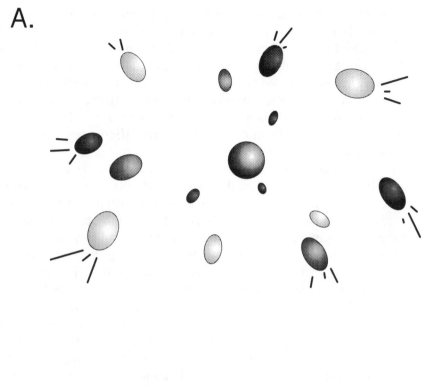

B.

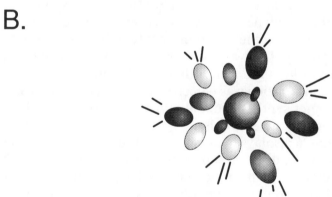

Figure 3–25. The perceptual magnet effect. When a variety of sounds in a category surround the category prototype (**A**), they are perceptually drawn toward the prototype (**B**). The prototype appears to function like a magnet for other stimuli in the category.

surrounding sounds are perceptually pulled toward the prototype. I named this effect the **perceptual magnet effect**, because the prototype appeared to act as a magnet for other sounds in the category.

The magnet effect is important because it offers an explanation for why adult speakers of a given language can no longer hear certain distinctions. A Japanese speaker's perception of the consonants /r/ and /l/ illustrate this point. The Japanese prototype is neither the American English /r/ or /l/, but something that is acoustically similar to these two sounds. When Japanese listeners listen to /r/ and /l/, they are assimilated to the Japanese prototype due to the perceptual magnet effect. Presumably, this is why a native speaker of Japanese has so much difficulty hearing the difference between the two sounds. American listeners can hear this difference because they have prototypes for both /r/ and /l/.

The question then becomes: How do prototypes form in the minds of people? One could speculate that there are two possibilities, two hypotheses about the origins of prototypes in people. One alternative is that infants are born with all of the prototypes of all languages registered in their brains. This view would argue that as language was learned prototypes that were never experienced by the language learner would disappear. A second possibility is that prototypes are not in the infants' mind at birth. This view would predict that prototypes develop as the infant learns language.

To test these two alternative hypotheses, experiments on young infants had to be conducted. I designed experiments in which 6-month-old infants were tested with prototypes and nonprototypes of the vowel category /i/ (Kuhl, 1991). To conduct the tests, two /i/ vowels were chosen from a large set that had been rated by adults. One was called the prototype because it had been given the highest good rating by adults. The other, the **nonprototype**, had been given a relatively poor rating. The two vowels were always identified by adults as /i/ vowels rather than some other vowel. Both were /i/s, but the one with the high rating was perceived to be a better instance of /i/. I then computer synthesized a number of variants of /i/ that surrounded both of these vowels.

Figure 3–26 displays the vowel sounds used in the experiment. Each circle on the diagram indicates an instance of a vowel. There are 32 stimuli around the prototype vowel, represented by open circles, and 32 around the nonprototype vowel, represented by closed circles. They form four rings around the center stimulus. An important factor about these rings is that the stimuli on them were physically scaled using the **mel scale** to equate the distance between the center stimuli and the surrounding stimuli for the two groups. The mel scale was invented by the famous psychophysicist S. S. Stevens in the 1950s to take into account the fact that equal changes in the frequency of a tone did not result in equal changes in the perceived pitch of the tone. The mel scale was used in an attempt to equate the physical changes represented in both sets of stimuli. Using the mel scale, stimuli on the first ring around the prototype were physically

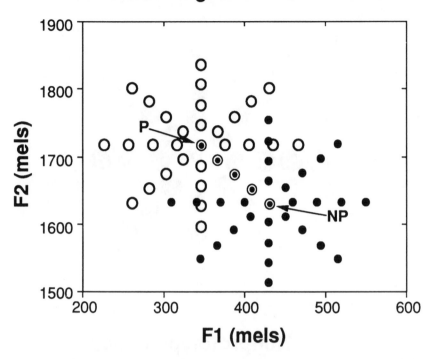

Figure 3–26. Vowel stimuli used in a test of phonetic prototypes. Each of two vowels, the prototype (P) and the nonprototype (NP), are surrounded by 32 vowel variants created by altering the formant values of the P and the NP vowels. The variants are scaled in mels to equate the distances between variants and the center vowel.

scaled to be just as far away from the prototype as the stimuli on the first ring around the nonprototype were from the nonprototype.

Two groups of 6-month-old infants were tested using the head-turn task previously described. Infants heard either the prototype or the nonprototype as the background sound during the experiment. During change trials, the stimuli surrounding that background sound were presented as the comparison stimuli to see which sounds the infant heard as different from the background sound. When infants heard a difference they produced a head turn.

Figure 3–27 shows the result of the experiment. Each solid circle on the diagram indicates that that particular vowel was indistinguishable from the center vowel. In the case of the prototype and its variations, the graph shows that infants could not hear a difference until they were three rings away from the prototype. In the case of the nonprototype, infants could hear differences as soon as they were

Prototype Group

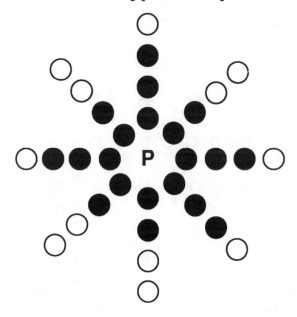

Nonprototype Group

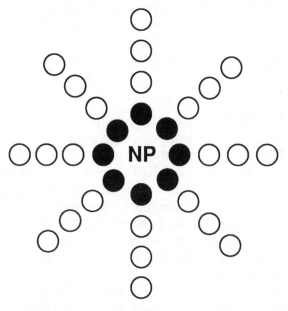

Figure 3–27. The results of vowel prototype tests on 6-month-old infants. The filled circles indicate stimuli infants equated to the P or the NP on over 60% of the trials. The data show that infants had to go much further away from the prototype than from the nonprototype to hear the difference, thus illustrating the perceptual magnet effect.

one ring away from the nonprototype. In other words, infants had to go much further away from the prototype to hear a change in the stimulus when compared to the nonprototype. Infants thus demonstrated the perceptual magnet effect.

The results of this 1991 experiment confirmed the fact that 6-month-old infants, growing up in America and listening to English, showed the perceptual magnet effect for American English vowels. What did this mean with regard to the **nature-nurture debate**? Did it indicate that infants were born with prototypes already specified? The data do not show that conclusively. Why? Because the infants tested in the experiment were 6 months old, and during the first 6 months of life infants are bathed in language. Perhaps the infants' responses to phonetic prototypes were dependent on the experience gained in listening to their parents speak. This question was not resolved by the 1991 experiment. What role did language experience play in the perceptual magnet effect?

To determine whether language experience played a role in the perceptual magnet effect, a **cross-language study** was conducted (Kuhl, Williams, Lacerda, Stevens, & Lindblom, 1992). Cross-language experiments typically involve testing listeners from two different languages on the same stimuli. This kind of experiment determines whether the two groups differ in their responses to the same stimuli, and therefore whether linguistic experience plays a role in the perception of those stimuli. Kuhl and an international team of colleagues tested infants from two different countries, the United States and Sweden, on vowel prototypes from two languages, English and Swedish. The stimuli used in the experiment are shown in Figure 3–28. The vowel prototypes of the two languages are very different, and adults from the two cultures rate the goodness of the same vowels differently. The /i/ vowel prototype is located in different places for American and Swedish adults; an English /i/ prototype is not perceived as a prototype to adult Swedes.

The experiment conducted in the two countries was identical. All aspects of the study were carefully controlled in the two settings. The testers, the stimuli, the equipment, the visual reinforcers, the toys used to distract the infants, even the table mothers sat at remained the same. The only variable that changed was the language experience of the 6-month-olds who were tested. The question was: Would the 6-month-old infants from the two countries resemble their adult counterparts, showing the prototype effect only for the vowels of their own language? Or would vowel prototypes be exhibited universally by infants from both cultures, in the absence of experience?

The results, shown in Figure 3–29, demonstrated that the perceptual magnet effect is strongly affected by exposure to a specific language. Both groups of infants demonstrated the perceptual mag-

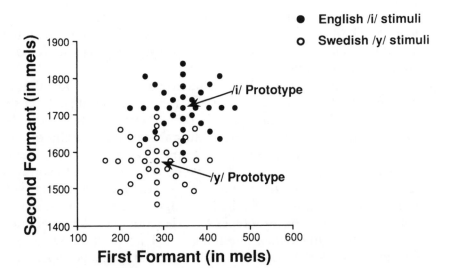

Figure 3–28. Stimuli used in a cross-language study of speech prototypes. Two vowel prototypes, American English /i/ and Swedish /y/, were used to test 6-month-old infants in the United States and Sweden. Each vowel prototype is surrounded by 32 vowel variants that were used in the test.

net effect only for their native-language sound. American infants showed a magnet effect only for the American English vowel. They did not show it for the Swedish vowel. Swedish infants showed the magnet effect only for the Swedish vowel. They did not show it for the American vowel. Thus, by 6 months of age, exposure to the ambient language alters infants' perception of the phonetic units of language. This is the earliest age at which linguistic experience has been found to affect perception of the building blocks of language.

The next question of interest was: How does language experience alter perception? What happens to infants in the first 6 months of life to make their perceptual systems change? As infants listen to speech, something is altered in their perceptual systems as a result of their listening experience. But what is it infants are listening to and how does it change their perception? Studies on infants' auditory preference show that they prefer listening to human speech more than any other auditory signal. Presumably, then, infants *are* listening to us speak. Infants are bathed in language from the time they are born (even before birth), and this early language experience affects infants. The findings highlight the importance of the speech parents address to infants.

Motherese, the special speech style used by caretakers when addressing infants, may make learning easier by producing better instances of speech sounds. As shown in Figure 3–30, Motherese has

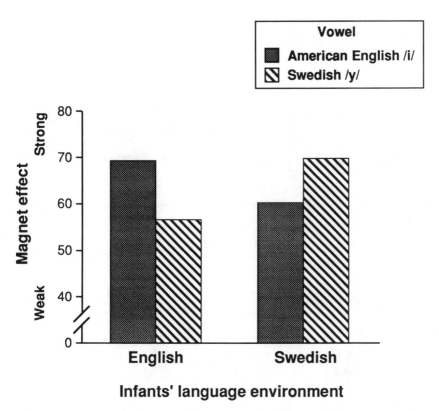

Figure 3–29. Results of a cross-language study on speech prototypes. Infants from both countries demonstrated a significantly larger perceptual magnet effect for the native-language vowel when compared to the foreign-language vowel.

a higher pitch, a slower tempo, and exaggerated intonation contours. It is a socially pleasing and attention-getting style of speech that mothers and fathers from all cultures use when speaking to their infants. Studies by Anne Fernald of Stanford University show that, when given a choice, infants prefer to listen to Motherese over speech that is directed toward other adults (Fernald, 1985). Motherese is like an acoustic "hook" that captures infant attention. Studies suggest that Motherese contains exaggerated acoustic cues for speech sounds. Motherese is also "vowel-drenched." Our studies show that mothers prolong vowels in the words used to address their infants, and moreover, that the vowels contained in Motherese words are rated as better instances when compared to the same words uttered by the same women when addressing adults (Kuhl, Gustafson, & Stevens, in preparation). These findings suggest that, in addition to its social-affective function, Motherese may serve to "tutor" infants on native-language speech sounds.

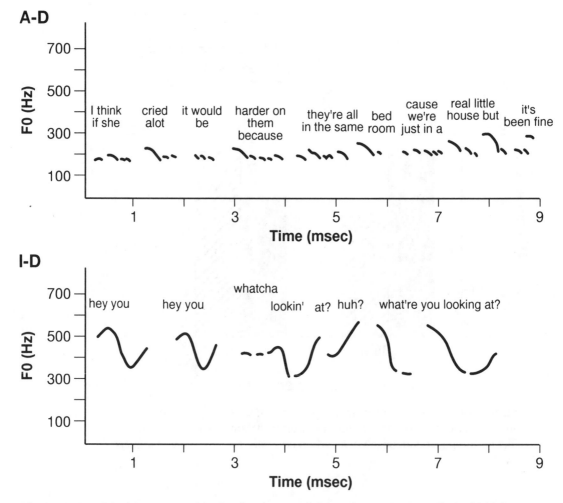

Figure 3–30. Displays contrasting the fundamental frequency pattern typical of Motherese, a form of infant-directed (I-D) speech used by adults when talking to their infants, with that used in adult-directed (A-D) speech. Motherese is higher in pitch, slower in tempo, and contains exaggerated intonation contours.

Given these findings on the impact of early language experience on the development of speech perception, it is also important to consider the possible effect of a hearing impairment in the early months of life on infants' language development. A hearing impairment would be expected to reduce the impact of the language environment on infants. This may account, in part, for the association between recurrent bouts of otitis media in infancy, an infection of the ear that produces a moderate, albeit temporary, impairment in hearing (see Chapters 14 by Berlin and 15 by Jerger and Stach), and language problems in later childhood.

There also are implications for bilingual exposure to language. We presume that when infants grow up listening to two languages, English and Spanish, for example, they form prototypes for the sounds of both languages. Only later do they sort them out and learn which prototypes belong to English and which to Spanish. Later in life we know that it is much harder to learn a foreign language because the prototypes of your native language can get in the way of new language learning. If you are a native-speaking Japanese adult, you have a prototype that is between English /r/and /l/. The English /r/and /l/ are perceptually drawn to the Japanese prototype because of the magnet effect, and this makes /r/and /l/ very difficult for Japanese adults to distinguish.

✦ CROSS-MODAL SPEECH PERCEPTION

Thus far the discussion of infants' perception of speech has been restricted to auditory events. We typically think of speech perception as an *exclusively auditory* phenomenon. Now the discussion will be extended to the auditory-visual (**cross-modal**) perception of speech, wherein our abilities to perceive speech go beyond those involving auditory perception.

Recent studies on adults show that the perception of speech is strongly influenced by information gleaned from watching the face of a talker. This raises profound problems for a theory of speech perception because it means that visual information, such as watching a talker's lips come together to produce the consonant /b/, is somehow equivalent to hearing acoustic information that auditorily signals the consonant /b/. One important question about such complex auditory-visual equivalences is how information as different as the sight of a person producing speech and the auditory speech event that is the result of production come to be related. To answer this, we decided to study the development of the ability to equate auditory and visual speech information.

Kuhl and Meltzoff (1982) designed an experiment to pose a **lip-reading** problem to infants. They asked whether infants could relate the sight of a person producing a speech sound to the auditory concomitant of that event. Figure 3–31 shows the procedure. Infants were shown two filmed faces, side by side, of a woman articulating two different vowel sounds. One face displayed productions of the vowel /a/, the other of the vowel /i/. While viewing the two faces, a single sound, either /a/ or /i/, was presented from a loudspeaker located midway between the two facial images. This eliminated any spatial cues as to which of the two faces produced the sound. The two facial images articulating the sounds moved in perfect synchro-

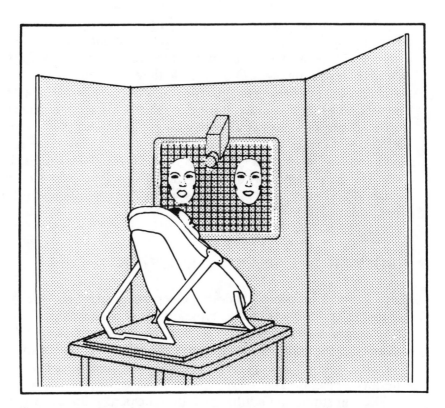

Figure 3–31. Technique used to test infants' cross-modal (auditory-visual) speech perception abilities. Infants watched two filmed faces, side-by-side, producing two different vowels, /a/ and /i/. At the same time they listened to a single vowel (either /a/ or /i/) presented from a loudspeaker located midway between the two faces. The results demonstrated that 18- to 20-week-old infants looked longer at the face that matched the vowel they heard.

ny with one another; the lips opened and closed at the exact same time, thus eliminating any temporal cues. The only way an infant could solve the problem was by recognizing a correspondence between the sound and the mouth shape that normally caused that sound. In other words, infants had to perceive a cross-modal match between the auditory and visual representations of speech.

The infants tested ranged in age from 18 to 20 weeks. They were placed in an infant seat facing a three-sided cubicle. The experiment had two phases, a *familiarization phase* and a *test phase*. During familiarization, infants saw each of the two faces for 10 seconds in the absence of sound. Following this both faces were presented side by side, and the sound was turned on. Infants were video- and audio-recorded. An observer who was uninformed about the stimulus conditions scored the videotaped infants' visual fixations to the right or left stimulus.

The hypothesis was that infants would prefer to look at the face that *matched* the sound. The results confirmed this prediction. Infants looked longer at the face that matched the vowel they heard. Infants presented with the auditory /a/ looked longer at the face articulating /a/. Those who heard /i/ looked longer at the face articulating /i/. The effect was very strong. Later studies produced the same results for the vowels /i/ and /u/.

These results demonstrated that 4-month-old infants perceive auditory-visual equivalents for speech. They recognize that /a/ sounds go with wide-open mouths, /i/ sounds with retracted lips, and /u/ sounds with pursed lips. What accounts for infants' cross-modal speech perception abilities? Have infants learned to associate an open mouth with the sound pattern /a/ and retracted lips with /i/ simply by watching talkers speak? Does some other kind of experience play a role in this ability? Future tests will need to be done to answer these questions.

We do know, however, that in adults auditory and visual speech information are very strongly linked. An experiment by Harry McGurk of England (McGurk & MacDonald, 1976; see also Green, Kuhl, Meltzoff, & Stevens, 1991) demonstrated that when adults listen to a simple syllable, such as /ba/, and watch a talker pronouncing some other syllable, such as /ga/, the observer combines the auditory and visual information and reports hearing the syllable /da/, a syllable that was not presented to either modality. This suggests that the brain integrates speech information entering the two modalities before phonetic perception occurs. Perception does not rely simply on auditory information. Apparently, there is more to speech than meets the ear.

◆ A THEORY OF INFANT SPEECH PERCEPTION

In this chapter we have explored speech perception and reviewed the results of many experiments on adults and infants. In this section I will integrate these studies by describing a **theory** of the development of speech perception.

Why do scientists create theories? Theories get invented for two reasons. First, there is a need to organize the large amount of data that result from experiments conducted in a particular field into a coherent framework. Theories provide a way of organizing the "facts" in a particular area of science. Often a theory points out areas in which there are holes, places where insufficient data have been collected to make the explanation complete. This is helpful because it suggests experiments that should be conducted.

The second purpose served by a theory is even more important. Theories offer explanations for the results of experiments, for the puzzles that data create. They provide answers to "Why" questions. For example, a theory of infant speech perception has to provide an answer to the question: Why can infants discriminate all phonetic contrasts at birth whereas later in life they can discriminate only a subset of these contrasts? Any theory of speech perception has to offer an explanation for these facts. It also has to explain how the change in infants' discrimination abilities is brought about.

In creating explanations for observed phenomena, a theory necessarily goes beyond the data and speculates about the *underlying causes* of behavior and the *agents of change*. A theory offers a sophisticated guess about how something, in this case, the mind, really works. Theories suggest new experiments to test the ideas put forward in the theory. This too is very helpful for the scientist who wants his or her next experiment to provide a critical test of the theory. Theories are thus helpful because they define the next best experiment to run, the one that will either provide strong support of the theory or prove the theory wrong and suggest an alternative theory. Science progresses toward the goal of providing answers to puzzles by offering theories and then testing them.

Returning to the issue of speech perception, a model of speech perception development has to account for infants' early speech perception abilities as well as the changes in those abilities that accompany language experience. What constitutes the infants' biological endowment for language at the phonetic level? What, on the other hand, is acquired in ontogeny?

The studies described in this chapter have led me to offer a new theory of the development of speech perception, called the **Native Language Magnet (NLM) theory** (Kuhl, 1992b, 1993, Kuhl & Meltzoff, 1994). The theory offers an explanation for the early period of speech perception, covering roughly the first year of life, prior to the time that infants acquire word meaning and contrastive phonology. The most important aspect of the theory is its claim that in the first year of life infants form **mental representations** of the speech information they hear. These representations constitute the beginnings of language-specific speech perception, account for infants' perception of both native- and foreign-language sounds, and serve as a blueprint which guides infants' initial attempts to produce speech.

I will first describe how the theory explains infants' initial speech perception abilities. NLM theory argues that what is "given by nature" is the ability to partition the world of sound into gross categories separated by natural boundaries. This is schematically illustrated in Figure 3–32 using an imaginary "vowel space" and lines to show the perceptual divisions. Any two sounds that are separated by a line are discriminable, according to the theory. These lines (perceptual boundaries) convey the fact that infants are born with a

Infants' Natural
Auditory Boundaries

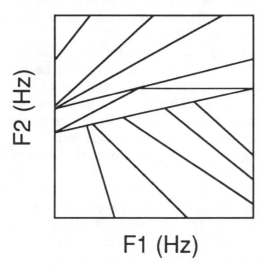

Figure 3-32. NLM Theory: At birth, infants perceptually partition the acoustic space underlying phonetic distinctions in a language-universal way. They are capable of discriminating all phonetically relevant differences in the world's languages.

capacity to resolve the acoustic differences between sounds that belong to different phonetic categories. In the tests of categorical perception reviewed earlier in the chapter, infants demonstrated that they are sensitive to the acoustic cues that underlie phonetic distinctions in language. Moreover, infants have shown that their abilities to discriminate speech sounds are particularly keen at the boundaries between phonetic categories. Recall that the studies on very young infants revealed their ability to discriminate sounds that straddled the boundaries between two phonetic categories, while failing to discriminate sounds that fall within a single phonetic category. As well, infants demonstrated this ability for sounds they had never heard. The theory argues, then, that infants are born with these abilities already in place. They do not have to experience speech sounds after birth in order to discriminate among them.

It is theoretically important to note, however, that the studies on animals demonstrated that the boundary effects associated with categorical perception are also shown by nonhuman animals. Taking the animal data into account, NLM theory claims that infants' abilities to hear the differences between phonetic units are innate;

however, the theory holds that the abilities are attributable to general auditory processing mechanisms. Infants' perceptual boundaries are not argued to be due to special processing mechanisms that evolved for language in humans. The theory holds that the phonetic distinctions used in the world's languages were selected on the basis of their acoustic distinctiveness and the abilities of early hominids to discern these differences.

To summarize the discussion thus far, NLM theory asserts that infants' initial abilities are perfectly suited to the task of speech perception. Infants can hear all of the distinctions used in the world's languages at birth. The theory holds, however, that these abilities stem from general mechanisms of perception rather than ones that evolved especially for language and speech.

The next question becomes: Given that infants' initial perceptual abilities result in the division of phonetic space into rough categories separated by natural boundaries, what is acquired in human ontogeny? Based on the data gathered in the studies on phonetic prototypes (the perceptual magnet studies discussed earlier), we can now say that by 6 months of age, infants have something more than the "basic boundaries" they were born with. By 6 months of age infants show evidence of language-specific magnet effects. The existence of magnet effects is illustrated in the plots shown in Figure 3–33. Schematically portrayed in the three panels of Figure 3–33 are the magnet effects that would be expected to be shown by 6-month-old infants being raised in Sweden, America, and Japan. The graphs convey, in conceptual terms, the idea that linguistic experience in the three different cultures has resulted in magnet effects that differ in number and location for infants growing up listening to the three different languages.

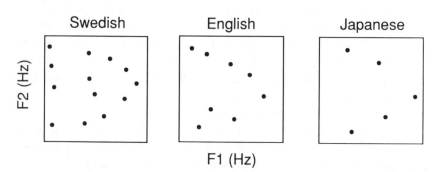

Figure 3–33. NLM Theory: By 6 months of age, infants reared in different linguistic environments show an effect of language experience. They exhibit language-specific magnet effects that result from listening to the ambient language.

NLM theory argues that the magnets shown in Figure 3–33 are acquired in ontogeny, that is, they are the result of infants' analysis of language input. Speakers of the three languages, Swedish, English, and Japanese, produce different numbers of vowels, with Swedish having approximately 16 vowels, while Japanese has only 5 vowels. Moreover, vowels of the three languages are located in different places in the vowel space. If the distributional properties of vowels produced by native speakers of the three languages were analyzed from samples of speech, the resulting data would show that vowels cluster at the points shown in Figure 3–33. What NLM theory argues is that infants analyze the distributional properties of the language spoken by their caretakers and mentally represent (commit to memory) that information in some form. The exact form in which the information is formed cannot as yet be described (it could be either a composite of all the items in the category experienced by the infant or many individual items that are remembered). The theory holds that, whatever form infants' representations take, these representations produce the perceptual magnet effect. It should be apparent that infants' perceptual boundaries assist in this process: The boundaries set limits on what infants' memory representations must organize.

Thus far we have discussed how infants' developing memory representations account for their perception of native-language sounds. What about infants' perception of foreign-language sounds? Recall that infants begin life with the ability to hear the differences between all sounds. Later, however, they fail to hear certain distinctions. The native-speaking Japanese adult, for example, cannot hear the difference between /r/ and /l/. How does NLM theory account for adults' and infants' eventual failure to discriminate foreign-language sounds?

The theory holds that the magnet effect reflects the formation of **perceptual maps** by the brain. These perceptual maps alter the perceived distance between sounds in phonetic space. Magnet effects alter perception by **warping** the acoustic space underlying phonetic distinctions. Recall Figure 3–25, which schematically illustrated the magnet effect. The perceptual space surrounding a category prototype is "shrunk" compared to the space around a nonprototype. In the region of the boundary between two categories, the perceived distance is "stretched." It takes a very large acoustic difference for a listener to hear a difference in the region of the prototype; however, a very small acoustic difference in the region of a nonprototype can easily be heard. This is the sense in which the perceptual space is "warped" by language experience. Around a native-language magnet, perceptual distinctions are "shrunk" (minimized);

near the boundaries between two magnets perceptual distinctions are "stretched" (maximized).

This warping of the perceptual space affects infants' abilities to hear certain distinctions in speech. Sounds that are close to a magnet are "pulled in" perceptually toward that magnet, and this can cause infants to fail to hear a distinction that is heard by infants from another culture. Consider the third panel of Figure 3–33, which shows the magnets formed by infants exposed to Japanese. The theory holds that Japanese infants would develop magnet effects in only five places in the vowel space. These five magnets will each pull in the sounds that surround them. Therefore, if Japanese infants listened to the vowels of a Swedish speaker, they would be expected to perform more poorly than Swedish infants listening to the same sounds. They might fail to hear the distinctions that speakers of Swedish hear. It is in this way that the magnet effect maximizes the perception of native-language distinctions while reducing the perception of foreign-language distinctions. The end result of the development of perceptual magnet effects on the boundaries that divide the underlying phonetic space is shown in the schematic diagrams of Figure 3–34. In essence, perceptual magnet effects cause certain boundaries to functionally "disappear," making it much more difficult to hear the distinctions made in a foreign language.

Research studies on adult listeners suggest that the boundaries do not literally disappear — that is, it is possible to increase performance on the discrimination of foreign-language contrasts if the training is very extensive, but training often does not generalize very well to new contexts or to new speakers. Training studies suggest that the alterations in perception that occur as a result of linguistic experience do not involve changes at a basic sensory level. Rather, the data suggest that the change occurs at a higher cognitive level, one

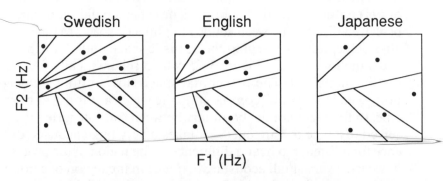

Figure 3–34. After language-specific magnet effects appear, certain phonetic boundaries "disappear"; magnet effects alter the perceived distance between stimuli, making certain distinctions more difficult to discriminate.

that involves memory and/or attention. The point made in Figure 3–34 is that exposure to a given language alters the underlying perceptual system, reducing the prominence of certain distinctions when compared to the language-general state of the perceptual system that existed prior to exposure to a specific language (Figure 3–32).

The theory thus explains adults' and infants' failure to discriminate certain foreign-language contrasts. Regarding infants, Janet Werker's studies discussed earlier suggested that infants aged 10–12 months fail to discriminate foreign-language sounds that they discriminated earlier. According to NLM theory, the developing magnet pulls sounds that were once discriminable toward a single magnet, making them no longer discriminable. According to this account, magnet effects occur first, before the failure to discriminate; they will developmentally precede and underlie the changes in infants' perception of foreign-language contrasts. NLM theory thus offers a causal explanation for the observed change in phonetic perception.

Regarding adults, NLM accounts for the results of studies showing their poor discrimination of foreign-language contrasts. Phonetic units from a foreign language that are similar to a category in the adult's native language have been shown to be very difficult for adults to perceive as different from the native-language sound. This includes the classic example of /r/ versus /l/ discrimination by native speakers of Japanese who have difficulty with the contrast even after considerable training. NLM takes the position that this is due to the fact that the prototype of the Japanese category is similar to both /r/ and /l/. The theory argues that the magnet effect of the Japanese prototype assimilates both /r/ and /l/, making the two sounds difficult for native-speaking Japanese people to discriminate.

Studies on **second language learning** conducted by James Flege of the University of Birmingham support the idea that the acquisition of a new language by adults poses difficulty at the level of phonology (Flege, 1987). In particular, it has been suggested that the native-language categories of the listener somehow interfere with the ability to perceive the phonetic distinctions in the new language. NLM theory argues that the magnet effect contributes to this difficulty. As described above, native-language magnets attract similar sounds, and this makes certain foreign-language distinctions, such as the segments /r/ and /l/ for native speakers of Japanese, difficult to perceive. The prediction that stems from the theory is that the difficulty posed by a given foreign-language unit will depend on its proximity to a native-language magnet. The nearer it is to a magnet the more it will be assimilated to the native-language category, making it indistinguishable from the native-language sound. The phonetic categories of the native language are analogous to a perceptual "sieve." The phonetic categories of the native language form holes in the sieve; the phonetic units of the newly acquired language must pass through the sieve, making some distinctions in the new language imperceptible.

The topic of second-language learning raises an interesting developmental issue, that of **bilingual exposure to language** early in life. Experiments have yet to be conducted on infants reared in a bilingual home in which the infant is regularly exposed to two different languages. It would be interesting to track the development of the perceptual magnet effect in infants reared in bilingual homes using the sounds of both languages as test stimuli. What outcomes would you predict? Would infants show magnet effects for the sounds of both languages?

One final point needs to be made about NLM theory. The results of experiments we reviewed on both adults and infants show that their knowledge of speech is not modality specific nor confined to perception. At a very young age, infants recognize the visual concomitants of an auditory speech signal. Moreover, we have data to suggest that infants have the capacity to vocally imitate speech very early in life; they hear speech and attempt to move their articulators to replicate what they hear. These kinds of data demonstrate that the speech representational system is **polymodally mapped** very early in life. This means that the memory representations formed by infants include not only auditory information but eventually visual information and the motor production rules necessary to produce speech.

NLM theory holds that speech representations initially are auditory but become polymodal as infants acquire information about the production of speech. Early listening experiences result in memory representations that are perceptual in nature. Infants' perceptual representations serve as **stored targets** for their acquisition of speech production gestures. Watching caretakers speak and the auditory information they hear is linked to the visual information that accompanies speech. When infants produce sounds themselves, they learn to relate the sounds they make with the speech gestures that caused those sounds. In this way, an **auditory-articulatory map**, which links speech sounds to speech gestures, is formed; eventually, speech representations become polymodal. This process of listening to language and committing the information to memory, which subsequently alters both speech perception and speech production, is the general framework suggested by NLM theory. The theory holds that a similar process occurs when infants first store in memory, and then attempt to produce, higher order linguistic units, such as intonation contours, stress patterns, and specific lexical items in the native language.

✦ SUMMARY AND CONCLUSIONS

Research on speech perception has shown that linguistic experience has an effect before infants utter or understand their first words. Infants' abilities to learn simply by listening to the ambient language suggest a powerful cognitive and linguistic representational system that, given proper input, responds automatically. At the level of speech, language acquisition is also guided, however, by nature's initial structuring of perception, in the form of natural auditory boundaries. These natural boundaries initially partition the perceptual space in a way that conforms to phonetic categories. Thus, nature provides the initial structuring of phonetic perception. When combined with the powerful role linguistic experience plays in warping perceptual space and thereby defining language-specific phonetic categories, we see that both nature and nurture play critical roles in the language acquisition process. The Native Language Magnet theory describes how infants' innate abilities interact with their early experiences with language to produce a language-specific and a species-specific pattern of speech perception. This theory accounts for the data in infant speech perception and serves as a model for the acquisition of higher order linguistic processes that presumably also rely on an interaction between innately given structure and primary linguistic data.

✦ REFERENCES

Eimas, P. D., Siqueland, E. R., Jusczyk, P., & Vigorito, J. (1971). Speech perception in infants. *Science, 171*, 303–306.

Fernald, A. (1985). Four-month-old infants prefer to listen to Motherese. *Infant Behavior and Development, 8*, 181–195.

Fernald, A., & Kuhl, P. (1987). Acoustic determinants of infant preference for Motherese speech. *Infant Behavior and Development, 10*, 279–293.

Flege, J. E. (1987). The production of "new" and "similar" phones in a foreign language: Evidence for the effect of equivalence classification. *Journal of Phonetics, 15*, 47–65.

Green, K. P., Kuhl, P. K., Meltzoff, A. N., & Stevens, E. B. (1991). Integrating speech information across talkers, gender, and sensory modality: Female faces and male voices in the McGurk effect. *Perception & Psychophysics, 50*, 524–536.

Grieser, D. L., & Kuhl, P. K. (1988). Maternal speech to infants in a tonal language: Support for universal prosodic features in Motherese. *Developmental Psychology, 24*, 14–20.

Jusczyk, P. W. (1985). The high-amplitude sucking technique as a methodological tool in speech perception research. In G. Gottlieb & N. A. Krasnegor (Eds.), *Measurement of audition and vision in the first year of* postnatal life: A methodological overview (pp. 195–222). Norwood, NJ: Ablex.

Kuhl, P. K. (1979). Speech perception in early infancy: Perceptual constancy for spectrally dissimilar vowel categories. *Journal of the Acoustical Society of America, 66*, 1668–1679.

Kuhl, P. K. (1983). Perception of auditory equivalence classes for speech in early infancy. *Infant Behavior & Development, 6*, 263–285.

Kuhl, P. K. (1985a). Categorization of speech by infants. In J. Mehler & R. Fox (Eds.), *Neonate cognition: Beyond the blooming and buzzing confusion* (pp. 231–262). Hillsdale, NJ: Erlbaum.

Kuhl, P. K. (1985b). Methods in the study of infant speech perception. In G. Gottlieb & N. Krasnegor (Eds.), *Measurement of audition and vision in the first year of postnatal life: A methodological overview* (pp. 223–251). Norwood, NJ: Ablex.

Kuhl, P. K. (1991). Human adults and human infants show a "perceptual magnet effect" for the prototypes of speech categories, monkeys do not. *Perception & Psychophysics, 50*, 93–107.

Kuhl, P. K. (1992a). Psychoacoustics and speech perception: Internal standards, perceptual anchors, and prototypes. In L. A. Werner & E. W. Rubel (Eds.), *Developmental psychoacoustics* (pp. 293–332). Washington, DC: American Psychological Association.

Kuhl, P. K. (1992b). Infants' perception and representation of speech: Development of a new theory. In J. J. Ohala, T. M. Nearey, B. L. Derwing, M. M. Hodge, & G. E. Wiebe (Eds.), *Proceedings of the International Conference on Spoken Language Processing* (pp. 449–456). Edmonton, Alberta: University of Alberta.

Kuhl, P. K. (1993). Innate predispositions and the effects of experience in speech perception: The native language magnet theory. In B. de Boysson-Bardies, S. de Schonen, P. Jusczyk, P. MacNeilage, & J. Morton (Eds.), *Developmental neurocognition: Speech and face processing in the first year of life* (pp. 259–274). Boston: Kluwer Academic Publishers.

Kuhl, P. K., Gustafson, K. T., & Stevens, E. B. (In preparation). The effect of Motherese versus adult-directed speech on goodness ratings of the vowel /i/.

Kuhl, P. K., & Meltzoff, A. N. (1982). The bimodal perception of speech in infancy. *Science, 218*, 1138–1141.

Kuhl, P. K., & Meltzoff, A. N. (1994). Evolution, nativism, and learning in the development of language and speech. In M. Gopnik (Ed.), *The genetics of language*. Oxford: Oxford University Press.

Kuhl, P. K., & Miller, J. D. (1975). Speech perception by the chinchilla: Voiced-voiceless distinctions in alveolar plosive consonants. *Science, 190*, 69–72.

Kuhl, P. K., Williams, K. A., Lacerda, F., Stevens, K. N., & Lindblom, B. (1992). Linguistic experience alters phonetic perception in infants by 6 months of age. *Science, 255*, 606–608.

McGurk, H., & MacDonald, J. (1976). Hearing lips and seeing voices. *Nature, 264*, 746–748.

Meltzoff, A. N., & Moore, M. K. (1983). Newborn infants imitate adult facial gestures. *Child Development, 54,* 702–709.

Miyawaki, K., Strange, W., Verbrugge, R., Liberman, A. M., Jenkins, J. J., & Fujimura, O. (1975). An effect of linguistic experience: The discrimination of [r] and [l] by native speakers of Japanese and English. *Perception & Psychophysics, 18,* 331–340.

Werker, J. F., & Tees, R. C. (1984). Cross-language speech perception: Evidence for perceptual reorganization during the first year of life. *Infant Behavior and Development, 7,* 49–63.

◆ RECOMMENDED READINGS

Aslin, R. N., Pisoni, D. B., & Jusczyk, P. W. (1983). Auditory development and speech perception in infancy. In M. M. Haith & J. J. Campos (Eds.), *Handbook of child psychology: Vol. 2. Infancy and developmental psychobiology* (pp. 573–687). New York: John Wiley.

Eimas, P. D., Miller, J. L., & Jusczyk, P. W. (1987). On infant speech perception and the acquisition of language. In S. Harnad (Ed.), *Categorical perception: The groundwork of cognition* (pp. 161–195). New York: Cambridge University Press.

Kuhl, P. K. (1987). Perception of speech and sound in early infancy. In P. Salapatek & L. Cohen (Eds.), *Handbook of infant perception: Vol. 2. From perception to cognition* (pp. 275–382). New York: Academic Press.

Werker, J. F., & Pegg, J. E. (1992). Infant speech perception and phonological acquisition. In C. A. Ferguson, L. Menn, & C. Stoel-Gammon (Eds.), *Phonological development: Models, research, implications* (pp. 285–311). Timonium, MD: York.

◆ GLOSSARY

Auditory-articulatory map: knowledge a speaker of a language learns early in life that links specific movements of the person's articulators to the specific sounds caused by those movements.

Basic unit of speech perception: the question about whether the unit analyzed by listeners in speech perception is the phonetic feature, the phoneme, the syllable, or the word; research suggests that the unit of perception may vary with the task, and that listeners analyze many different levels simultaneously during speech perception.

Bilingual exposure to language: simultaneous exposure to two different languages early in infancy or childhood.

Bottom-up analyses: the analysis of the incoming message that proceeds by attempting to analyze the signal to determine which acoustic and phonetic features are contained in the message. The information that results from these analyses interacts with that derived by top-down analysis of speech.

Brain mapping: the use of neuroscience techniques to identify the locations of major activity in the brain while the person is actively engaged in some form of mental activity.

Categorical perception: a situation in which the ability to discriminate speech sounds is limited to the ability to identify those sounds as different.

Categorization: the ability to group or sort items into categories based on common dimensions or features; requires more than simply the discrimination of two items from different classes; based on perceived similarity among discriminable items in a particular category.

Category goodness: the degree to which an item is judged to be representative of the category as a whole.

Coarticulation: the influence by neighboring sounds on the physical characteristics of a particular phonetic unit; it is caused by the fact that the speech motor system plans ahead and adjusts its motor movements depending on the next unit in the sequence.

Constancy: the perception of similarity among items that are discriminably different.

Context variability: when a phonetic unit is produced in different contexts, for example, when the phonetic unit /d/ occurs in the syllables /di/ as opposed to /du/, its physical characteristics vary a great deal, even though we hear the two /d/s as the same.

Critical periods: times in the development of an individual when he or she is particularly sensitive to the effects of experience.

Cross-language study: a study conducted with speakers of different languages.

Cross-modal perception: information from two different sensory modalities that is linked in some way by the perceptual system.

Cross-modal speech perception: the perception of speech through two modalities, such as audition and vision, as in lipreading.

Discrimination: the ability to hear a difference between two sounds.

Formants: particular frequency locations in speech in which the concentration of acoustic energy is particularly high.

Formant transition: rapid frequency changes in formants occurring over 50–100 msec.

Frequency/pitch: the frequency (periodicity) of a signal is determined by a physical measurement of the numbers of cycles per second that occur in that signal; its pitch is the perceptual correlate of that measure.

Fundamental frequency: the number of cycles per second of laryngeal vibration produced by the human voice.

Head-turn (HT) conditioning: a technique used to test infants' discrimination of speech sounds between the ages of 6 and 12 months of age. Infants sit on a parent's lap and watch an assistant located on their right play with silent toys. At the same time a loudspeaker located on the infant's left plays a background sound over and over. The infant is trained to produce a head-turn response when the background sound is changed to a comparison sound. If the infant does so when the sound changes, he or she is reinforced with a visual stimulus (a toy animal located in a black box is lighted and animated for a 6-sec period). Two kinds of trials are run: *Change trials* during which the sound is changed, the infant's head-turn responses are monitored, and a head-turn response results in the presentation of the visual reinforcer; and *control trials* during which the sound is not changed, but the infant's head-turn responses are still monitored, and head-turn responses that occur are scored as false alarms. If infants produce significantly more head-turns on *change trials* than *control trials*, they are assumed capable of discriminating the two sounds.

High-amplitude sucking (HAS): a technique used to test infants' discrimination of speech sounds between the ages of birth and 4 months. Infants suck on a pacifier and the strength of each sucking response is measured using a pressure transducer. A *baseline* is set in the absence of sound that results in a pressure threshold that allows about 25 sucking responses per minute to qualify as *criterion responses*. Once the baseline is established, a speech syllable is presented to the infants when a criterion sucking response occurs. Infants increase their criterion sucking responses under these conditions, eventually reaching a *maximum* number of sucking responses in a given minute. This continues until the infants' sucking responses meet a *decrement criterion*, which is defined as a 20% decrease from the maximum number that lasts for 2 minutes. At this *shift-point*, infants in the experimental group are presented with a new sound while infants in the control group continue to hear the original sound. After 4 minutes the experiment ends. A significant difference in the number of sucking responses that occur for the experimental versus control group after the shift point is taken as evidence that infants can hear the difference between the two sounds.

Hotspot: the acoustic location of the best instances of a phonetic category.

Hypothesis: a statement that specifies a conjectured relationship between two variables.

Identification: the labeling or naming of a stimulus.

Intensity/loudness: The amplitude of an auditory signal is determined by a physical measurement of its power; its loudness is the perceptual correlate of that measure.

Intonation contour: the perceived pattern of fundamental frequency change over time.

Knowledge of the world: Information about objects, people, and events experienced by the individual that is stored in the brain; human beings learn about the world by living and interacting in it; this knowledge plays an important role in all aspects of perception.

Language input: the spoken language produced by others that is experienced by an individual.

Language specific: listening and/or speaking in a way that is unique to a particular language.

Length/duration: The length of a signal is determined by a physical measurement of the span of time occupied by the signal; its duration is the perceptual correlate of that measure.

Linguistic experience: the total amount of exposure to a particular language that occurs for an individual.

Lip-reading: the phenomenon of perceiving speech information by watching talkers' articulatory movements.

Manner of articulation: a phonetic feature of speech sounds which specifies the overall manner in which the sound is produced; the manner feature specifies whether a sound was voiced or voiceless, nasal or nonnasal, and so on.

Mel scale: a frequency scale that equates for differences in the perceived pitch of a tone.

Mental lexicon: the dictionary of words and their meanings stored by the brain.

Mental representations: storage in memory of information about the items in a particular category; these representations could take many forms, ranging from some kind of composite image to a list of individual instances.

Motherese: the name given to speech that is directed by caretakers (men as well as women) to infants. When compared to the speech directed toward adults, Motherese has exaggerated intonation contours, a slower tempo, and a higher overall fundamental frequency.

Native Language Magnet (NLM) Theory: a theory of the development of speech perception in the first year of life that accounts for the change from a language-general mode of speech perception to one that is language-specific.

Natural auditory boundaries: enhanced abilities to discriminate between sounds that is present at birth in the absence of experience and is not attributable to special language-acquisition devices, but instead to the natural operation of the auditory perceptual mechanism.

Nature-nurture: Scientists are interested in the relative contribution to a given ability, such as intelligence, of a person's genetic endowment as opposed to what the person acquires by interacting in the world.

Neural spectrogram: The transformation of an incoming speech signal to a neural signal by the auditory system; the transformation is thought to produce a neural version of the frequency-over-time information that can be seen in a speech spectrogram.

Nonprototype: members of categories that are not good instances of the category.

Pattern Playback: a machine invented in the 1950s that allowed investigators to create the first versions of artificial speech by painting formants on an acetate belt which were then converted into sound.

Perceptual magnet effect: the finding that the best members of a category function like perceptual magnets for surrounding stimuli.

Perceptual maps: representations stored in memory that indicate the relationships among a variety of stimuli; specifically, their distances from one another.

Perceptual organization: the ability to group sounds into categories.

Phonemic: a phonetic change that is sufficient to change the meaning of a word in a particular language.

Phonetic boundary: the 50% point on an identification function; the point at which responses change from one category to another.

Phonetic categories: all speech sounds belonging to a particular class, such as all sounds composed of a certain set of defining features.

Phonetic features: the smallest building blocks of speech; phonetic units consist of bundles of phonetic features.

Phonetic prototypes: stimuli from a phonetic category that are judged by native speakers to be exceptionally good instances of the category.

Phonological processing: the language-specific aspects of phonetic perception; listeners of different languages learn which phonetic units are contrastive in the language and rules about how those units can be combined.

Place of articulation: a phonetic feature of speech sounds that specifies the location in the mouth where the point of major constriction occurred when the sound was produced; the place feature specifies whether a sound was produced with a bilabial closure, an alveolar closure, and so on.

Point vowels: the three vowels (/i/, /a/, and /u/) which are at the articulatory and acoustic extremes in vowel space.

Polymodally mapped: information that is stored in the brain in a way that is not specific to any one sensory modality.

Prosody: aspects of speech production involving the pattern of stress, rhythm, and intonation across syllables.

Prototypes: exceptionally good instances of a particular category.

Rate variability: When speech is produced at different rates, the physical characteristics of individual phonetic units vary and the phonetic boundary between two categories is shifted, making it impossible to specify an absolute physical value for a phonetic unit present in the signal regardless of the rate of speech.

Rules of grammatical structure: information stored in the brain about the way sentences are parsed in your native language.

Second language learning: learning of a second language by an adult who was previously exposed only to a single language.

Situation specific knowledge: People learn what to expect in certain situations by experiencing those situations repeatedly. This information helps us predict what is likely to happen next in an ongoing situation and this in turn aids perception.

Spectrogram: a physical display of speech that portrays changes in the formant frequencies over time.

Spectrograph: a machine used to create a frequency-over-time analysis of speech.

Spectrographic analysis: frequency-over-time analysis of the information in speech which is provided by a machine called the sound spectrograph.

Speech segmentation: the separation of speech into units (such as phonemes, syllables, or words) that can be analyzed, either perceptually or instrumentally.

Speech synthesis: the generation of artificial speech using a machine.

Speech variability: Individual units of speech (phonemes, words) are produced differently by different individuals, differently when produced in different phonetic contexts, and differently when produced at various rates of speech; each of these factors is responsible for the extreme acoustic variability observed in speech.

Stored auditory targets: auditory memories of sounds contained in the native language which guide speakers' attempts to produce articulatory movements that match those sounds.

Stored knowledge: the information contained in the human brain acquired during development. The information takes many different forms and includes both linguistic (the mental lexicon, word meaning, the rules of grammar) as well as cognitive (information about the world, information about specific situations) sources of knowledge.

Stress: the relative emphasis placed on individual syllables that occur in a multisyllabic string of speech.

Talker variability: When different talkers produce the same phonetic unit (such as /a/), its physical characteristics vary considerably; this is especially true when comparing male to female talkers or when comparing adult to child talkers. Nonetheless we hear the sounds as belonging to the same phonetic category.

Theory: an explanation of the facts and phenomena in a particular discipline; theories not only account for the experimental data that exist in a field but go beyond them to speculate about how and why particular phenomena exist; theories are educated guesses containing predictions that have to be tested in future experiments.

Top-down analyses: the analysis of an incoming message that proceeds by using sources of information stored in the brain to form hypotheses about the message; the hypotheses that are generated interact with the results of the bottom-up analysis of speech.

Voiced-voiceless: a phonetic feature of speech distinguished by voice onset time, an acoustic feature that describes the timing between two events in speech, the onset of laryngeal voicing and the onset of other acoustic events that mark the release of the sound; voiced sounds are produced when these two events occur nearly simultaneously; voiceless sounds when the release of the sound precedes voicing by over 40 msec.

Voice onset time (VOT): the measurement (in msec) of the time between the onset of the syllable and the onset of laryngeal voicing.

Warping of acoustic space: a change in the perceived distance between various phonetic stimuli that is brought about by exposure to a specific language.

Phonological Development and Disorders in Children

JUDITH R. STONE, Ph.D.
CAROL STOEL-GAMMON, Ph.D.

After reading this chapter, you should be able to:

✦ Define the terms **phonology** and **phonological system**, and give examples of how the phonological system works.

✦ Describe the different skills needed to learn phonology and how a young child gets experience with those skills.

✦ Describe how the phonological system develops from infancy to the school years.

✦ Give examples of the kinds of errors children make as they are learning to speak and discuss the reasons children make these errors.

✦ Describe what you might hear if you met a child with a **phonological disorder**, and discuss how the phonological disorder could affect your efforts to communicate with the child.

✦ Describe the responsibilities of a speech-language pathologist in working with children with phonological disorders.

✦ Describe the main differences between the **traditional approach** for remediating speech sound errors and current **phonological system approaches**.

Phonology is the component of language that relates to speech sounds and how they are used to form meaningful words. This chapter deals with normal phonological development as well as phonological disorders in children. Phonology develops during early childhood as a child learns which sounds are part of the language; how those sound combine into words; and how the sounds are produced by coordinating the lips, tongue, jaw, vocal folds, and breathing muscles. To learn phonology, a child must be able to discriminate sounds, learn and remember how speech sounds combine into words, and plan and execute the movements necessary for speech. Although children initially make many errors in speech production, they gradually become more accurate. By the elementary school years, children can produce all the speech sounds nearly perfectly. When a child does not develop sounds normally, a **phonological disorder** may be present. A phonological disorder often results in a child's speech being hard to understand, such that family, peers, and teachers have difficulty communicating with the child. Further, a child with a phonological disorder may feel embarrassed at sounding different and consequently become afraid to communicate. Phonological disorders may be severe, with many errors of pronunciation; they also may be mild, with just a few errors. In either case, a speech-language pathologist can help a child with a phonological disorder. The speech-language pathologist completes a **diagnosis** by identifying a disorder and assessing its nature and severity. A **treatment** program is then planned to help the child develop more normal ways of producing sounds so the child can extend that learning to new words. **Counseling** also can be provided to parents to help them understand phonological development and disorders and to support their communication with the child. The goals of treatment and counseling are to support the child's ability to be intelligible, communicate successfully, and maintain a positive sense of self as a speaker.

◆ WHAT IS THE STUDY OF THE PHONOLOGICAL SYSTEM ABOUT?

We take it for granted that when we speak other people will understand us. We do not think about how to pronounce words, or what speech sounds to use, or how to make our lips and tongue move in the way we want. We also take it for granted that we will understand others when they speak, that the sounds that come out of their mouths will form words we understand. In fact, when someone pronounces words in unusual ways or makes speech sounds poorly, we take notice; we may be irritated or confused, or we may think it sounds comical or even stupid.

The speech sounds that are used in our language form part of the **phonology** of the language, or the **phonological system**. The phonological system is more than just a collection of individual sounds, however. Just as our language is governed by rules of grammar, so is our speech sound system governed by rules. These rules are called **phonological rules**. They tell us which sounds are part of our language and which are not. For example, in American English, we make "r" sounds that are different from "l" sounds, so that the words "rip" and "lip" sound different to us and mean different things. But in Japanese, these sound differences do not exist. Because these differences are not part of the Japanese phonological system, a Japanese adult may not hear the difference between "r" and "l" and may have difficulty producing them when trying to speak English. As another example, consider some African languages. Their phonological systems include productions that are clicks of the tongue; these clicks are important sounds that combine with other sounds to make meaningful words. American speakers of English may use such clicks in play or when calling an animal; however, these clicks are not meaningful within words because they are not part of the English phonological system. Words of a language, therefore, have two components: They have specific meanings attached to them, and they use the sounds that are part of the language's phonological system.

Other phonological rules tell us the combination of sounds that can occur in a sequence within a word. Some speech sounds can occur in a sequence, but others cannot. For example, in English, we allow certain consonants to come together at the beginning of a word, which is called a consonant cluster. In the word "tree," "t" plus "r" form a consonant cluster; in the word "swim," "s" plus "w" form a consonant cluster. Other consonants cannot be combined in this way. Although "s" can combine with "t, p, k, w, l, m," and "n" sounds in a cluster, it cannot combine with "r" or "y." As a speaker of American English, you would not expect to say words like "srop" or "syop," even though you are familiar with the word "stop," which begins with "s" in a cluster. You know the rule about combining "s" with other sounds, even if you are not conscious of it (see box on the next page).

Another example of rules about how consonants can be used is that some consonants can only occur in certain positions of words. The consonant that is spelled by the letters "ng" can occur at the end of words ("bri*ng*, so*ng*") or in the middle ("si*ng*er, ba*ng*ing"); it cannot occur at the beginning of English words, however. We do

---

Consonant Clusters Beginning with "s"

Below are some of the forms that begin with "s" followed by one or two consonants. Some are *words* of English, some are *possible words,* that is, they are not words now, but could be selected as the name for a new product or a rock band; some would never be words of English. Look through the list and classify each form as one of the following: **RW** if it is a real word; **PW** if it is a possible word; **NPW** if it is not a possible word. It should be easy! The answers are provided at the end of the chapter.

1. scope RW
2. stroft PW
3. spring RW
4. smoog PW
5. slurn PW
6. sneak RW
7. smwill NPW
8. stlide NPW
9. splice RW
10. stwup NRW
11. swick PW
12. scrant PW

---

not have words like "*ng*o," even though this combination can occur in other languages, such as Vietnamese.

As described above, there are many phonological rules about speech sounds and their combinations. Although these phonological rules are important, they are not enough to make a person sound like a native speaker of a language. A whole other aspect of phonology is **prosody**. **Prosody** includes the following: (1) the intonation of speech productions (the rise and fall of our voices); (2) the stress patterns of multisyllabic words (some syllables are stressed; others are unstressed); and (3) the stress patterns of words in a sentence (the rhythm of the sentence, with some words louder and longer, and others quieter and shorter). Just as there are rules governing speech sounds, so there are rules governing these different aspects of prosody (see examples on opposite page).

Prosody is an important part of the phonological system. It makes our speech sound interesting and flowing, and it allows us to vary our speech patterns to ask questions, express different emotions, and emphasize important ideas. Different languages have different prosodic patterns; sometimes even when we do not understand a language, we can recognize some of the rhythmic or intonational patterns of the language as different from our own. Furthermore, even if we can produce the speech sounds of a language very well, we may sound like a foreign speaker if our prosody does not match the language. In movies and television shows, characters who are meant to be robots or aliens from outer space are often made to talk in a very altered prosody; for example, they speak with

---

Some Examples of Prosody

Use of intonation to indicate differences in meaning:
1. You're going? (Rising pitch indicates a question)
2. You're going! (Falling intonation indicating a statement)

Stress patterns of multisyllabic words (stressed syllables are indicated by capital letters)
1. MULtiply (but the stress is different in the word "multipliCAtion")
2. therMOmeter
3. uniVERsity

Use of stress to indicate different meanings:
1. BLACKboard (board written on with chalk, often green)
2. blackBOARD (a board that is black)

Use of stress in sentences:
1. Joe went to the STORE. (Answer to "Where did Joe go?")
2. JOE went to the store. (Answer to "Who went to the store?")

---

a flat tone and evenly spaced syllables and words. We can understand what such characters say because the sounds used are the sounds of the English language, but we recognize the speakers as non-native (and in these instances nonhuman) because of their unusual prosody.

✦ HOW DO WE STUDY THE PHONOLOGICAL SYSTEM?

Researchers have many vantage points from which to study the phonological system. Some researchers are interested in phonological development as it occurs in children developing normally during the early years of life (Menn & Stoel-Gammon, 1993). Other researchers are interested in children who do not develop as expected, or who exhibit **phonological delays** (or **phonological disorders**) (Shriberg, Kwiatkowski, Best, Hengst, & Terselic-Weber, 1986). By studying children, including those who are developing normally and those who are delayed, researchers can document what they observe happening as the speech sound system emerges. Several types of questions can be asked about phonological development. One type of question has to do with the *product* of development, that is, what sounds and sound sequences can be expected at different stages, and what prosodic patterns are observed? These questions attempt to describe what phonological development "looks like" in terms of speech output; therefore, in-depth descriptions of speech sounds and prosodic development are required. The descriptions can characterize both normal and delayed development and can increase our recognition of the similarities and differences across children.

A different type of question has to do with the *process* of development, that is, how do children learn the phonological system? What are the different factors that come together to allow for phonological learning, and how do children "figure out" the system? What factors are problematic for children with phonological delays, and how do these children ultimately succeed in learning the system? These questions do not focus on describing what happens but attempt to explain how and why phonological development occurs. As such, they require making inferences about how children think and learn based on what is observed, then testing hypotheses to confirm or disprove the explanations. Studying the process of development is always difficult because the mental activity involved in phonological development is covert; although we can observe the speech output, many different thinking processes are involved in the production of speech. Therefore, several explanations can exist for a certain kind of speech output.

Because a phonological delay can occur in association with other disorders, such as hearing loss and mental retardation, researchers must study children with varying histories. Some researchers focus on children who have a sensory, medical, or neurological problem that could be the cause of the phonological disorder; other researchers investigate children with phonological delays for which no known cause exists. Many children with phonological delays fall into the latter category; they clearly are learning more slowly or less well compared to other children, but there is no obvious explanation for their differences.

Because the phonological system develops over time during childhood, a key issue is the age of children studied. Some studies are longitudinal, following a few children intensively over time and documenting changes that occur. A longitudinal study might record the changes that occur in two children as they move from 12 months to 30 months of age. This kind of study is ideal for examining in detail subtle changes in phonological development and the ways children are unique in their development. Other studies, often of larger numbers of children, are cross-sectional, examining several groups of children, with each group at a different age. A cross-sectional study might examine separate groups of 12-month-olds, 18-month-olds, 24-month-olds, and 30-month-olds. Cross-sectional studies help us identify similarities across children, so that we can know what is most typical of a group of children. Longitudinal and cross-sectional studies are applicable to children with both normal development and phonological disorders.

Longitudinal and Cross-sectional Data

A **longitudinal** study of phonological development from 12 to 30 months involves the same subjects with data taken at different ages:

x x x x	x x x x	**x x x x**	**x x x x**
Joey Tom Sarah Amy	Joey Tom Sarah Amy	Joey Tom Sarah Amy	Joey Tom Sarah Amy
12 mos	18 mos	24 mos	30 mos

A **cross-sectional** study of phonological development from 12 to 30 months involves different subjects in each group:

x x x x	x x x x	**x x x x**	**x x x x**
Jake Bob Anna Kimi	Matt Tim Susan Judy	Peter Lars Mary Kate	Dan Sean Joan Ellen
12 mos	18 mos	24 mos	30 mos

A researcher studying phonological development or disorders faces numerous challenges in preparing and carrying out research. One of the first requirements is that speech must be sampled. Some of the decisions that must be made include what size sample (how many words and sentences), how often to sample, and the conditions of the sample (whether the child should be playing with toys, looking at a book, naming picture cards, or talking to a familiar adult). Once a speech sample is tape recorded, the researcher must listen to the tape and write down what the child has said. This may sound simple, but knowing what children say can be difficult, because child speech (especially disordered speech) is not as clear as adult speech. There are two steps involved in creating a record of what a child has said. First, the researcher writes the words he or she hears, without attempting to specify how the child has pronounced the words. This is called a *gloss* (illustrated on page 156).

Next, the examiner indicates the specific speech sounds used by the child in pronouncing (or mispronouncing) the words that are in the gloss. To focus on speech sounds, researchers use phonetic symbols in a process called *transcription.* Phonetic symbols represent the sound produced; they are different from the letters used to spell words. The alphabet of phonetic symbols is called the **International Phonetic Alphabet**, or **IPA**; the symbols used for transcription of English are shown in Table 4–1.

Glossing and Transcribing a Speech Sample

The gloss and phonetic transcription of 11 utterances (Utt) produced by a young child (J) as he plays with his mother are shown below:

Utt	Context	Gloss	Transcription
1	J holds play figure	"Daddy go store"	[dædi go sto]
2	J opens car door	"Daddy drive"	[dædi dwaiv]
3	Looks in car	"xxx"*	[xxx]
4	same	"Daddy go car"	[dædi go ka]
5	Turns to Mom	"Help me"	[hɛp mi]
(MOM: Help you? What do you want me to do?			
6	J points to car	"xxx* in here"	[xxx ɪn hɪr]
(MOM: What goes in there?)			
7	J holds up toy figure	"Him go"	[hɪm go]
(MOM helps J put figure in car)			
8	J looks at car	"There"	[dɛr]
9	Picks up another figure	"Baby go too"	[bebi go tu]
10	same	"Baby too"	[bebi tu]
11	J tries to put figure in car	"Him no fit"	[hɪm no fɪt]

*xxx denotes a word or phrase that is unintelligible and cannot be glossed.

TABLE 4–1. Symbols used for phonetic transcription

Symbol	Example	Symbol	Example	Symbol	Example
			Vowels		
[i]	heat	[ʌ]	hut	[ɔ]	caught
[ɪ]	hit	[ɝ]	hurt	[a]	hot
[e]	hate	[u]	hoot	[au]	house
[ɛ]	head	[ʊ]	put	[aɪ]	height
[æ]	hat	[o]	hope	[ɔɪ]	Hoyt
			Consonants		
[p]	pan	[θ]	thin	[dʒ]	jaw
[b]	ban	[ð]	than	[m]	met
[t]	tan	[s]	sun	[n]	net
[d]	Dan	[z]	zone	[ŋ]	ring
[k]	can	[ʃ]	shun	[l]	low
[g]	gun	[ʒ]	measure	[r]	row
[f]	fan	[h]	hand	[w]	wet
[v]	van	[tʃ]	chop	[j]	yet

For example, the first letter in the word "shoe" is "s," but the first *sound* that is pronounced is "sh." The phonetic symbol [ʃ] is used in transcription so that it cannot be confused with "s" (the phonetic symbol for the "s" in *see* is [s], just like the letter). In most papers dealing with phonology, writers use phonetic symbols to represent all speech sounds. In this chapter, we are representing speech sounds by writing letters in quotation marks because readers may be unfamiliar with the IPA.

Phonetic transcription is a skill that must be learned and practiced; even when people are skilled at transcription, they do not always agree on what they have heard. Making careful comparisons of transcriptions is an important part of phonological research. In the box on page 156, an example is given of transcription of a young child's speech. Included are the gloss, the transcription into IPA symbols, and a description of the context, or environment, in which the speech occurred.

Another decision that must be made in research is how to analyze the speech sample that is collected. There are different systems for looking at speech sounds and prosody; some systems look at each sound individually, whereas others look at patterns of sounds as they occur in words. Another system for analyzing a speech sample looks at *distinctive features* of sounds. *Distinctive features* are "pieces" of sounds relating to how a sound is perceived by the ear or how a sound is produced. For example, one group of speech sounds is called *fricatives*. Sounds in this group are all characterized by frication during production. Table 4–2 describes the consonants of English according to the *manner* and *place* of articulation. *Manner* of articulation refers to how consonants are produced; *place* of articulation refers to the **articulators** involved and where in the mouth the sounds are produced. In addition to manner and place, consonants are classified as *voiced* (produced with vocal fold vibration) and *unvoiced* (no vocal fold vibration). Classification systems of this sort are commonly used in both research and clinical work. Terms from this classification system are used throughout the remainder of this chapter. The reader is encouraged to refer back to Table 4–2 when these terms appear.

Some systems for analyzing distinctive features and prosody involve detecting acoustic changes that we cannot hear without special instrumentation. For example, we make some vowels longer and some shorter, depending on the final consonant in a word (the "a" in *cab* is longer that the "a" in *cap*) or where in a sentence a word falls (vowels are longer when the word is at the end of a phrase). In this case, research requires laboratory instrumentation and procedures that reveal more than the ear can reliably hear; transcription from a tape recorder is not sufficient. Researchers must decide

TABLE 4-2. Classification of consonants in English.

The consonants of English are grouped on the basis of *manner* and *place* of articulation as follows:

Stops: Stop consonants are characterized by a complete blockage of the airstream as it flows through the oral cavity. In English, the blockage is made by complete closure of (a) the lips, (b) the tongue tip against the alveolar ridge, or (c) the back of the tongue against the velum (back of the mouth). The *labial* stops (made with the lips) are [p] and [b]; the *alveolar* stops (tongue against the alveolar ridge) are [t] and [d]; and the *velar* stops (tongue and velum) are [k] and [g]. For each pair of consonants, the first is *voiceless* (no vocal fold vibration) and the second is *voiced* (with vocal fold vibration).

Nasals: Nasals are characterized by air flowing through the nasal cavity and a complete blockage of the airstream in the oral cavity. These consonants are produced at the same three places of articulation as the stops described above, giving us a *labial* nasal [m], an *alveolar* nasal [n], and a *velar* nasal [ŋ]. All nasal consonants are *voiced.*

Fricatives: Fricative consonants are characterized by a partial blockage of the airstream as it flows through the oral cavity; the articulators are positioned close to one another causing turbulence or frication. English has pairs of fricatives at four places of articulation (the first member of each pair is *voiceless,* the second is *voiced*): [f] and [v] are formed at the *labiodental* place of articulation (upper teeth touching lower lip); [θ] and [ð] have an *interdental* place of articulation formed with the tongue tip between the teeth; [s] and [z] are formed at the *alveolar* place of articulation (tongue against alveolar ridge); [ʃ] and [ʒ] are formed at the *alveopalatal* place of articulation (tongue contact beyond the alveolar ridge). The *voiceless* consonant [h] is produced with friction in the *glottis* (opening between vocal folds in the larynx).

Affricates: The affricates [tʃ] (*voiceless*) and [dʒ] (*voiced*) are consonants that begin like stops and end like fricatives. Both are *alveolar* in place of articulation.

Liquids and glides: Liquids [l] and [r] (both *alveolar*) and glides [j] (*palatal*) and [w] (*bilabial*) are *voiced* consonants produced by air passing through the oral cavity with little or no blockage. Glides have more rapid transitions to vowels than liquids do. (Note that you can produce a lengthened [r] in the word "ring," but if you lengthen the glide [w] of "wing," the onset sounds like [u] as in "*ooze*." Given the similarities between glides and vowels, [j] and [w] are sometimes refered to as *semivowels.*

what aspect of the phonological system they wish to study, and then they must develop methods appropriate to that part of the system.

Finally, even when data are collected, transcribed, and analyzed, there often is room for more than one interpretation of what the data mean. Part of the need for ongoing research is to keep testing and retesting hypotheses, when more than one interpretation is possible. As with many other areas of speech-language development and disorders, no one study can describe or explain all aspects of the phonological system. With any particular research project, one or more hypotheses can be tested that will help explain a phenomenon or event. The research will examine the problem from one perspective, controlling certain variables that may be important. It is possible that a different study, examining different hypotheses and controlling different variables, would yield conclusions different from those of the first study. Because of this, our understanding of a problem is best enhanced by many studies that address the problem from different perspectives. Over time, as results of different studies accrue, inaccurate conclusions can be ruled out, and evidence supporting specific hypotheses can be collected.

Speech-language pathologists work as clinicians to help people with **phonological disorders**. As clinicians, they may not be active in a big research program. However, they are involved in a similar process of investigation with each client who is seen. For each client, questions are raised about what the phonological system is for that child (i.e., the *product,* requiring description) and why the system is not developing properly (i.e., the *process,* requiring explanation). Clinical tasks associated with these questions are discussed in the final section of this chapter on the role of the speech-language pathologist in working with children with phonological disorders.

◆ HOW DOES THE PHONOLOGICAL SYSTEM DEVELOP?

The ability to produce the expected variety of speech sounds according to our phonological rules is one of the many abilities that develops during childhood. It proceeds in development along with many other skills that also require learning and practice. For example, early phonological development occurs at the same time as development of motor skills, such as walking and climbing stairs and using a crayon; play skills, such as pretend play and creating stories with toys; social skills, such as playing with other children and sharing toys; and self-help skills, such as eating with utensils and putting on one's clothing. In addition, the phonological system is only one part of the language system. Other aspects of language, such as grammar, are also developing at this time. (See chapter on language development by Bloom.)

Because phonological development occurs along with so many other skills, it is easy to forget how complicated it is. But many different abilities must come together for the phonological system to develop properly. These abilities involve listening to speech, recognizing differences according to the phonological rules of the language, storing information about words, and drawing on those stored words to produce words properly. We can depict these different abilities in a simple model, shown in Figure 4-1. As noted,

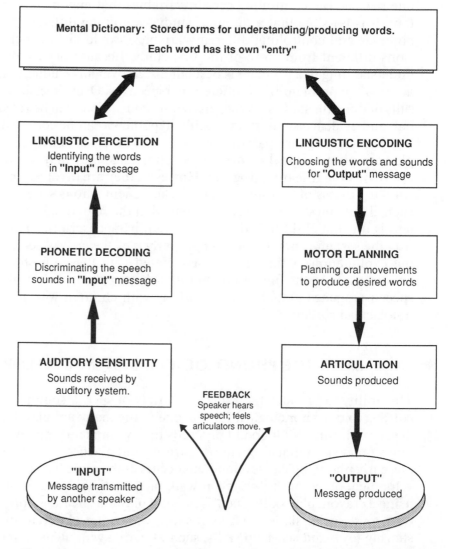

Figure 4-1. Processing model showing elements needed for comprehension and production of speech.

the left side of the model involves receiving and interpreting sound; the right side involves retrieving words from memory and producing words in speech. Different aspects of this model will be discussed as we consider normal development.

Some aspects of phonological development emerge during infancy, well before children produce sounds as meaningful words. For example, in listening to adults, infants are exposed to all the speech sounds of the language. Long before infants learn what words mean or how to produce words, they will start to hear differences among sounds in the language. From this experience, they begin to know which sounds belong in the language and which do not; in other words, they begin to learn some of the rules of phonology. Similarly, infants hear many different intonational and rhythmic patterns and begin to recognize these patterns; later on, these are the same patterns they produce as they learn to speak. For infants to learn which sounds and intonational patterns are part of the phonological system, they must be able to hear, and they must be able to **discriminate**, or hear differences among sound patterns. We know from research that infants are born ready to hear and discriminate certain basic phonological patterns; they must have experience, however, or they will not be able to build on these innate abilities that are so important for learning language.

Just as children need practice listening in order to learn which sounds are part of the phonological system, they also need practice producing sounds in order to combine them into words. Children begin producing sounds shortly after birth, although their earliest efforts do not sound like words and may even not sound like the phonological system of their native language. As young as a few months of age, infants begin "cooing" with sounds that are like vowels; later, they will begin using the lips and tongue to make consonant-like sounds that combine with those vowels, producing what we call **babbling** (Locke, 1983). Even though consonants and vowels are not made exactly the way adults make them, these babbled productions give infants practice in producing sequences of sounds and syllables. The most frequently occurring speech sounds in babbling are from the manner classes *stops, nasals,* and *glides* (see Table 4–2). Although infants produce a wide variety of speech sounds in the babbling period, the majority of sounds are similar to those that occur in the native language. Therefore, during babbling, infants are getting practice producing speech-like combinations that resemble the phonological system before the production of real words.

Infants with hearing impairment begin to vocalize in infancy, the way infants with normal hearing do; however, the vocalizations of these infants do not follow the same developmental patterns, indicating that some hearing is necessary for normal development.

Research has shown that a few infants with normal hearing also do not babble; they are at risk for delays later in the development of meaningful speech (Oller & Eilers, 1988). It is not clear why these infants do not babble; however, lack of babbling practice does seem to undermine their development of speech, with or without the complication of a hearing loss.

In addition to practicing speech sounds during the babbling period, infants practice the intonational patterns that are part of the language. Parents often talk about an infant "talking in sentences" because they hear long strings of speech sounds that sound like sentences or questions. These long strings are called *jargon*; they are children's opportunity to practice the prosody of the phonological system. Later, when learning words, children will use some of the same sound combinations and prosodic patterns they practiced earlier. For infants to produce the key elements of the phonological system, they must be able to coordinate different parts of the speech mechanism, including breathing, the start and stop of the voice, and the coordination of the lips, tongue, and jaw. Although many of these abilities are present in very rudimentary form at birth, much experience is needed for them to be refined into skills that can be used for meaningful speech.

Comprehension of words, or *receptive* language, develops before production of words, or *expressive* language. It is expected that children will comprehend many more words than they will produce, especially in the early stages of language development. Once children begin to produce meaningful words, a whole new stage of phonological development begins. This marks the beginning of the expressive **lexicon**, or expressive vocabulary. The lexicon is depicted in Figure 4–1 as the Mental Dictionary, at the top of the model. Just because children can hear some differences and can produce some babbled combinations does not mean they are ready to produce words accurately. For productions to be considered words, two criteria must be met: First, the children must have a production (sequences of sounds) that they can repeat relatively consistently. If children cannot produce sound combinations with some consistency, they will not be able to use a "word" more than once. Second, the production must have meaning attached. If meaning is not attached to the production, then the sound sequences are babble. Often, when an infant of 6 to 8 months babbles the sound combinations "mama" or "dada," parents think their child is talking in real words even though it is unlikely that meaning is attached to these syllable combinations. Parents, excited to be called by name, then encourage the infant to produce these forms over and over. There is nothing wrong with this; in fact, when parents encourage children to babble by smiling at them, repeating the babbled productions, and showing pleasure in face-to-face interactions, the children have a positive social interaction that is an important foundation for later communication. In trying to understand normal phonological development, however, we must recognize that such early productions are different from later words that are used meaningfully.

A child's first words usually are not pronounced exactly like adult words. In fact, first words are often merely approximations of what we recognize as the word (i.e., they may contain some of the sounds of the adult word or have the same number of syllables, but they have many differences). For example, a young child might say the word *blanket* as "bibi," *juice* as "du," and *cup* as "tuh." An adult who lives with the child is likely to understand most of what is being said, although a stranger might not be able to identify the intended words.

One important question is which sounds and sound combinations children are most likely to produce in early words. If we examine the words produced by young children who are learning how to speak, we find that there are certain similarities across children. The speech sounds produced tend to be the same sounds that predominated during babbling; specifically, the sounds are from the manner classes *stops, nasals,* and *glides* (see Table 4–2). The sounds are combined in simple syllables of consonants and vowels, as in babbling. Examples of consonants produced often by children who have small vocabularies of 10 to 50 words are "b, d, m, n, w," and "h." These sounds may be combined with vowels in single syllable words (e.g., "beh" for *bed,* or "moh" for *more*) and in syllable strings for multisyllabic words (e.g., "baba" for *bottle,* or "wawa" for *water*). Of course, children vary considerably in forms, and some children use a wider variety of sounds or combinations from the beginning (Stoel-Gammon & Dunn, 1985).

When children are first learning words and their lexicon is very small, some sound combinations stand for more than one word. For example, a child may use the word "da" to mean *down, dog, cat*; for this child, "da" is a *homonym,* one form that means several different things. Because children do not use many words and typically talk in familiar environments with familiar adults, the homonyms usually can be understood. As children grow older, however, the lexicon rapidly becomes much larger, and words are combined into sentences. In addition, children begin talking about different subjects, in different environments, with different people. Unless they can make differences between words that will be understood, communication will come to standstill. At this point, children must begin to expand the phonological system beyond the basic sounds and sound combinations used in their early words. To accomplish this expansion, they must learn to produce a great many more speech sounds. In addition, they must develop the **phonological rules** that govern how sounds can be combined.

We cannot see into a child's brain, and so we cannot really observe how the rules are learned. But we can listen to what the child produces and from that infer what kinds of rules the child is learning. Through studying children who are developing speech normally, researchers have learned that children learn phonological rules gradually (Ingram, 1986). Further, although children make errors in producing speech sounds, these errors often are systematic rather than random. People have called these systematic error patterns **phonological processes**. An example of a **phonological process** is the substitution of "w" for *liquids* "l" and "r"; this is called **gliding**, because the *glide* "w" is substituted for consonants from another manner class. Another example of a **phonological process** is the omission of consonants at the ends of words, such that *hat* is produced "ha" and *nose* is produced "no"; this is called **final consonant deletion**, because word-final consonants are deleted. Some common phonological processes are shown in the first box on the next page. Examples of another process are shown in the next box; see if you can figure out the error pattern.

The systematic error patterns children make give us clues about how much they have learned about the phonological system. Gradually, the error patterns become less frequent and children produce words in new ways; however, in the process of moving toward the adult production, children may change to a different error pattern. They may move from one incorrect rule to another, each time figuring out one piece of the phonological system. Or they may learn a phonological rule and apply it inappropriately in too many words. Finally, however, children put the pieces together and have the adult rule. Productions then match adult productions; that is, their productions sound correct to us.

At the same time children are figuring out the phonological rules of the language, they are becoming more skilled at controlling their **articulators**. This happens in part because of maturation of the neurological and physiological systems controlling movement (see Chapter 8 on the neuromotor system by Kent). For example, children become better able to use their tongues to make sounds in different parts of the mouth (e.g., back sounds, like "k," use a different part of the tongue than front sounds, like "t"). They also become more precise in the sounds they produce. Whereas children may initially produce *distortions* (i.e., imprecise sounds), gradually they are able to produce sounds more clearly and exactly. Finally, children become better able to control their articulators to produce more complex combinations, like consonant clusters or syllable combinations. People are used to hearing young children mis-

---

Examples of Common Phonological Processes

A brief definition and examples of some common phonological processes are shown below. See Table 4–2 for definitions of the terms marked with an asterisk (*).

Cluster Reduction

One consonant from a consonant cluster is deleted:

Target Word	Child's Production
spoon	"poon"
truck	"tuck"
play	"pay"

Unstressed Syllable Deletion

Unstressed, or "weak," syllables are deleted in a multisyllabic word:

Target Word	Child's Production
pajamas	"jamas"
elephant	"ephant"
tomato	"mato"

Stopping

A stop* consonant (p, t) is substituted for a fricative* consonant (f, s, sh, voiceless th):

Target Word	Child's Production
fan	"pan"
house	"haut"
ship	"tip"

Velar Fronting

An alveolar* consonant (t, d, n) is substituted for a velar* consonant (k, g, ng):

Target Word	Child's Production
gum	"dum"
kiss	"tiss"
singing	"sinin"

---

pronounce words like "spaghetti" or "aluminum"; we recognize that such words demand more skill in coordinating the articulators. Many children and adults enjoy the challenge of tongue twisters, where the movements required to produce the combination of sounds are particularly difficult, especially at rapid speech rates.

Speech sound development must occur fairly rapidly to keep pace with a child's vocabulary growth, sentence productions, and

---

Another Phonological Process

The child's pronunciation of each of the target words below contains errors in the consonants. These errors form a pattern that is common in early child speech. See if you can describe the pattern in terms of changes in *place, manner,* or *voicing* of the target consonants. The information on classification of consonants provided in Table 4–2 will be helpful in this exercise.

Target	Child's Form	Error
toe	"doe"	"d" for *t*
pat	"bat"	"b" for *p*
dug	"duk"	"k" for *g*
bad	"bat"	"t" for *d*
toot	"doot"	"d" for *t*
bag	"bak"	"b" for *p;* "k" for *g*
bib	"bip"	"p" for *b*
cake	"gake"	"g" for *k*
bed	"bet"	"t" for *d*

When an error occurs, does the *place* of articulation of the consonant change?

Does the *manner* of articulation of the consonant change?

Does the *voicing* of the consonant change?

Given the error patterns in the forms above, predict how the child would say

Bob _____ *top* _____ *get* _____ *pig* _____

---

social desires to communicate. One might wonder if there is a predictable sequence of sound development that all children go through in this period of great change. A set order of development would make sense, for example, with "easier" sounds learned early and "harder" sounds learned later. Many studies have examined speech sound development in groups of children from the ages of about 2½ to 9 years, examining at what ages children master different speech sounds (Smith, Hand, Freilinger, Bernthal, & Bird, 1990; Templin, 1957). Other studies have documented in detail how individual children develop sounds, following a few children's speech development over a long time (Smith, 1973). Results of these different types of studies have suggested that, although there are certain trends in children's sound development, there is no invariant order of speech sound acquisition. That is, different children master their sounds at different times. We cannot predict, for example, that all children will learn "f" before "s," or that all children will learn "l" before "t." We do know, however, that some sound classes like *liquids* ("l" and "r") and some of the fricatives (particularly "th" as in *these* and "v") may be mastered later by many children who are developing normally. Other sound classes, like *stops* ("p, b, t, d, k, g") and *nasals* ("m, n") typically are mastered relatively early. Therefore, normal development is not characterized by a specific order of phoneme acquisition, but rather by general trends in speech and sound acquisition, and the way children use sounds to communicate meaning.

Another difficulty with stating the exact order of phoneme acquisition is that children may produce a speech sound differently depending on a consonant's position in words. A child may appear to have acquired a speech sound relatively early, but then as more words are produced that use that sound, differences in pronunciation appear. One speech sound may start to appear sooner than another but may take longer to be produced correctly in a variety of word positions in the context of many other speech sounds. An example of an error pattern that is affected by the consonants' position in words is shown in the box below.

The Effects of Position in a Word

Note how the pronunciation of "s" is affected by its position within a word and by the adjacent sounds:

Target	Child's Form	Position of "s"	Pronunciation of "s"
soup	"toup"	initial, before a vowel	substituted by "t"
see	"tee"	initial, before a vowel	substituted by "t"
smoke	"moke"	initial, before a consonant	deleted
stop	"top"	initial, before a consonant	deleted
bus	"bus"	word final	correct
house	"house"	word final	correct

Clearly, the young child has a great deal to learn about the phonological system and needs considerable practice to produce accurate sound combinations. Not only is there a lot to learn, but many other areas of development are occurring simultaneously. It is no wonder that development occurs gradually; further, it should not be a surprise that there are many differences among children. Some children seem to be able to learn the phonological system rapidly and quite early, whereas others take a longer time to master the different elements. In general, however, by age 8 or 9 years, most children have established a phonological system that is the foundation for normal speech. They have mastered the variety of speech sounds and the basic rules for their combination, and they produce most words accurately, although they may still have difficulty with very complicated or unfamiliar words. They know the intonational and stress patterns of the language, and they sound like native speakers of the language. In all these ways, children in elementary school demonstrate their normal phonological development.

On entrance to elementary school, another aspect of development related to phonology becomes important. Children begin to take what they know about the phonological system and apply it to printed words for reading and writing. Reading and writing are both language tasks that rely on knowledge of the speech sound system; instead of the sounds being spoken out loud, they are translated into print form. Therefore, to read and write, a child must have a solid foundation in the speech sounds in the language, so the child can figure out how the auditory version of the sound (what is heard) relates to the printed sound (the letter). Even though phonological development for spoken sounds is largely complete by early elementary school years, phonological development continues as the child becomes more and more skilled at reading and writing. In addition, very subtle aspects of pronunciation, such as timing of complex movements, continue to develop until nearly adolescence.

◆ WHY DO CHILDREN MAKE SPEECH ERRORS?

One of the questions posed by researchers who study phonological development is: "Why do young children pronounce (or mispronounce) words the way they do? This section contains examples of some mispronunciations from a young child and a discussion of possible explanations for the underlying problems that lead to the mispronunciations. The same approach — examining errors and hypothesizing about the cause of the errors — also is important when speech-language pathologists work with children with phonological disorders. By attempting to understand the nature of the error, the speech-language pathologist can develop treatment that helps children master the specific abilities required. In this section, we will be referring back to the model shown in Figure 4–1; different explanations correspond to different components of the model.

Consider Rachel, age 3 years, 2 months, who consistently mispronounces the sound "v." In every word that has a "v," she substitutes a "b." Why does this error occur? We must begin by considering at least two possible explanations: (a) Rachel is unable to

discriminate between "v" and "b" (see Figure 4-1, left side of model) and (b) Rachel is unable to **articulate** "v" (see Figure 4-1, right side of model). We also must explain why she always uses "b" as the substitute for "v."

First, let us consider the possibility that Rachel cannot **discriminate** the two sounds. How can we determine whether Rachel can discriminate "v" from "b"? The most obvious way is to assess her discrimination abilities via a listening task. For example, we might set up some cards and ask Rachel to point to the letter V and the letter B. If she consistently points to the correct letter when we say the name of the letter, we can infer that she has perceived the difference between the two consonants. However, if she fails the task, there are at least two possible explanations. One is that she cannot hear the difference between "v" and "b"; the other is that she does not yet know the names of the letters of the alphabet. (Of course, a third possibility, always present with young children, is that Rachel was not interested in our task and so did not attempt to do what we were asking). Failure on the pointing task means that we need to ask more questions, such as "Can Rachel recognize the difference between the words *very* and *berry*? Between *vest* and *best*? Or *van* and *ban*?" In each case, accurate recognition of the words would indicate an ability to discriminate between the two consonants. On the other hand, failure to respond accurately might be attributed to a lack of understanding of the task or to the lack of words like *very* or *van* in her vocabulary. That is, when a child cannot complete a task, we must consider multiple explanations as to why she failed. By raising hypotheses about Rachel's problems and testing the hypotheses with different tasks (like "mini experiments"), we can draw more and more conclusions about her abilities.

If we conclude that Rachel can discriminate "v" and "b," we must move to tasks that will help us determine if Rachel can produce, or **articulate**, these different sounds. We might ask Rachel to do different movements with her lips to see if she can control where she places her lips to produce these sounds. We might ask Rachel to carry out movements that are not specific speech sounds to see if she controls her muscles well when not attempting to produce speech. We might ask Rachel to imitate syllables, such as "ba" and "va," to see if she can coordinate her lips for the consonant sounds in combination with movements for vowel sounds. Again, if she does not do the things we ask her, we must consider all the possible reasons, including lack of understanding of what we are asking her to do, disinterest, lack of experience with such strange activities, or inability to control the muscles.

A related question is why Rachel substitutes "b" for "v" — why not substitute "d" or "l"? The most reasonable explanation seems to lie in a combination of factors, related to both articulation and discrimination. The consonants "b" and "v" share many articulatory features: They are both produced by blockage of the airstream; the blockage involves the lips (for "v" the teeth also are involved); they are both produced with vocal cord vibration (see *voiced* versus *voiceless* sounds, Table 4–2). On the discrimination side, studies of speech perception of both adults and children have shown that "b" and "v" are more likely to be confused with one another than with other consonants. Therefore, substituting one for the other would be a likely outcome of perceptual confusion.

◆ WHAT HAPPENS WHEN PHONOLOGY DOES NOT DEVELOP AS EXPECTED?

In normal development, the phonological system develops gradually. As children grow older, they become able to produce words that sound more like adult words. They increase in this ability even as they are producing longer, more complex sentences and begin talking about more varied ideas and events. That is, phonological development keeps pace with other aspects of language development and allows children to communicate in the increasingly complicated ways that suit their growing social and intellectual development. Sometimes, however, a child does not develop phonology in expected ways. In this case, the child may become limited in what he or she can express or may be hard to understand. Lack of effective communication can cause frustration and limit the child's ability to participate in the world.

Children whose phonological systems do not develop as expected may be called **phonologically delayed** or **phonologically disordered**. (They also may be referred to as having disordered **articulation**, because of the role of the articulators in making speech sounds.) Phonological disorder is a very common communication disorder in childhood. Children may exhibit a phonological delay or disorder in many different ways. In some cases, a child speaks as a younger child would. For example, very young children often use repeated syllables (called *reduplication*) for complex words, producing "baba" for *bottle,* "wawa" for *water,* "kiki" for *kitten.* In normal development, these forms begin to change as the child's vocabulary grows, so that the child produces words that approximate adult forms more closely. A child who is phonologically delayed may continue to rely on reduplicated forms much longer than expected. Similarly, although children ages 2 to 3 years will often omit the "s" in words beginning with consonant clusters (*stop, spoon, sky* become "top, poon, ky"), a child with a phonological delay may continue to do this much longer, perhaps as late as 4 or 5 years of age. There-fore, the speech of some children with phonological delays has many characteristics of the speech of children who are younger.

In other cases, children who do not develop phonology nor-mally produce words in unusual or idiosyncratic ways that are not typical of younger children. They may omit consonants in the be-ginnings of words, producing *cup* as "up" and *baby* as "aby," which is something children rarely do in normal development. They may use sounds that are not part of the language they are learning. Al-though infants may normally babble sounds from other languages and may even produce some of them during the early development of the lexicon, they rarely continue to use those sounds. Children who are not developing typically may persist in using these sounds as if they are attempting to make them a part of the phonologi-cal system.

Finally, some children develop unusual error patterns that ap-pear to be their attempt to show what they know about words, even though their productions do not match adult productions. For ex-ample, a child may not have yet learned to produce consonants at the ends of words, such that words like *bed* and *bet* are potential homonyms (both would be produced as "beh"). To make a distinc-tion between these two words, the child may make the vowel in *bed* longer than the vowel in *bet*. This is similar to subtle vowel differen-ces in adult forms, but the child exaggerates the production to make the words sound very different. When a child does this, it is called **marking**; the child produces words differently, even though the forms are not correct. It is as if the child is attempting to say, "I know these words are different, but I cannot yet articulate them in the way you do." In the example in the next box, the child **marks** the different final consonants by making the preceding vowels different lengths. By paying attention to markings, we can learn more about what a child knows about the phonological system but cannot produce.

When a child has difficulty learning the phonological system, there may be many errors in production, and the child may be dif-ficult to understand. Problems with being understood, or **intelligi-bility** problems, are very serious because the child may not be able to express needs, ideas, and feelings, which in turn may lead to frus-tration. Even though children who are developing normally make some errors, they usually are understood by familiar adults, in part because they do not yet have complex enough language to make verbalizations long and complicated. Children with phonological delays may attempt to speak in longer sentences, but they become **unintelligible** quickly because of the lack of sound development, the confusing error patterns, and the complex sentences they are attempting to say. Although we do not have exact procedures to de-

---

Example of Marking

Some children use marking to avoid producing homonyms and thus make their speech more intelligible. Take, for example, the case of Jamie, age 3 years, 2 months. He was unable to produce "sh" (in words like *ship* or *fish*) accurately and substituted "s" for the "sh." Thus in his speech the word *ship* sounded quite a bit like *sip*. Jamie's parents, however, noted a difference between "s" and "sh" in their son's speech. When Jamie wanted to say a word with "sh," he would produce a lengthened "s" so that *fish* was "fis-s" and *shirt* was "s-sirt." By marking the difference between "s" and "sh" in this way, Jamie was able to distinguish between potential homonyms like *ship* (pronounced "s-sip") and *sip* ("sip").

---

termine how well a child "should" be understood at specific ages, we have guidelines for judging individual children's development. A child learning first words is not expected to be consistently intelligible to anyone but family and familiar adults, and even they may sometimes not recognize a word. By the time a child is 3 years old and talking in short sentences, strangers should be able to understand the child about 75% of the time and family members should be able to understand the child most of the time. By age 4 years and older, a child should be fully intelligible to strangers, even though speech production errors continue to occur. That is, errors should not be so frequent or so unusual as to prevent communication.

Some children have phonological delays but are not as hard to understand. The children may fail to learn some of the speech sounds that typically take most children longer to master. It is common for some school-age children to still have difficulty producing "r" or "s" correctly. When this is the only problem, the child is said to have a mild articulation problem, or a **residual error** (Bernthal & Bankson, 1993). A **residual error** is one that is "left over"; the child has developed fairly well but has one or two speech errors that are "left over" from early childhood. Examples of residual errors are a 7-year-old child who lisps an "s" sound or an 8-year-old child who produces a "w"-like sound for the "r" in words such as *road, hair*, and *carrot*. Although they may not interfere with communication as much as large numbers of errors, residual errors are still important because they make children sound different from their peers. If children still have speech errors in elementary school, they may be teased for "talking like a baby," or they may become self-conscious because they do not sound like their friends. Many of us have known someone who has had a residual speech error; often we remember that person in particular because of the speech error (e.g., "Susie was the girl with the lisp," or "Joseph could never say his 'r' sounds"). Some adults continue to have mild residual errors in their speech. A residual error can become a serious problem in someone's life, particularly if speaking is important to professional or personal goals.

◆ WHAT CAUSES A PHONOLOGICAL DISORDER?

When parents learn that their child is having difficulty learning to speak, they most frequently ask: "Why did this happen?" or "What caused this problem?" As much as speech-language pathologists want to address these questions, there are as yet no definitive answers.

As with many speech disorders, the causes of phonological disorders are not always known. Although certain congenital problems, such as hearing impairment and mental retardation, are associated with phonological disorder, many children with phonological disorders have no known deficit that would explain why they are having difficulty learning the speech sound system. In the past, such children were called *functional misarticulators.* The word *functional* meant there was no organic basis for the disorder. The word *misarticulator* described the fact that the children made errors of pronunciation. Although the word *functional* is still used, research is accruing that makes us question whether the disorders are really functional, or whether it is more accurate to say that we have not yet understood the many neurological and physiological factors that interact with the environment to influence development. Below we consider some of the possible causes of phonological disorders, based on what research has revealed thus far.

Middle Ear Infections

One of the key childhood problems that has been investigated as a possible cause of phonological disorders is middle ear infections, or *otitis media.* Young children often have ear infections, with accumulation of fluid in the middle ear. The fluid can block the transmission of sound, causing a temporary hearing loss. If these temporary hearing losses occur with regularity, they can interfere with children's ability to hear language and thus deprive them of the necessary stimulation for language learning. Children with chronic ear infections may not get enough experience to learn to discriminate among the sounds of the language, or they may misperceive sounds and store the wrong form of the word in the lexicon. If hearing acuity is reduced for a while, children may stop paying attention to speech, even when hearing returns to normal. Intuitively, it makes sense that hearing losses would interfere with learning the speech sound system; indeed, many children with phonological disorders have a history of otitis media.

In spite of the obvious importance of hearing, it is not so easy to conclude that otitis media causes phonological disorders. First, some children who have otitis media do not subsequently develop phonological disorders, while others who initially look delayed catch up quickly in speech development as soon as the otitis media is medically treated (Paden, Novak, & Beiter, 1987). Therefore, otitis media does not always lead to a phonological disorder. Further complicating the picture is that some children with a phonological disorder have no history of middle ear infections; therefore, it is possible to have a phonological disorder even if hearing has not been interrupted by ear infections. Some of the many factors not known at this point are (a) how frequently ear infections need to occur in order to influence development; (b) whether there are some periods of development where ear infections have a profound effect and other periods where they do not; and (c) whether some children are more vulnerable to developing phonological disorders from ear infections because of other, as yet unknown, causes. It is possible that some of the children who have a history of ear infections would have had difficulty with phonological development even if there had been no ear infections.

One reason we have trouble knowing the effects of otitis media on phonological development is that research on this condition is very difficult. Several factors complicate research efforts. One of the biggest research challenges is simply identifying the occurrence of otitis media. Knowing exactly when a child had otitis media, how long the episode lasted, and how severe the episode was can be difficult. If research is conducted on very young children, researchers may be able to track current medical care and thereby have documentation of episodes. However, much research has attempted to look back on children's development to judge the relation of otitis media to current phonological development. Such research, called *retrospective,* can be flawed by incomplete medical records and parents' imperfect memories, by the different kinds of medical treatment provided different children, and by the variety of educational or therapeutic opportunities that could affect children's development. It is very difficult to attribute the cause of phonological delay to otitis media when so many other factors (environmental, treatment, etc.) could be in play as well.

To counter the problems of retrospective studies, some researchers have begun doing *prospective* research. In prospective research, researchers follow the development of children from very early ages. In this way, careful documentation can be made of otitis media, medical treatment, and environment. These studies may improve our ability to understand the relationship of otitis media to phonological development and disorders. At present, we recognize the importance of immediate medical treatment for episodes of otitis media.

Control of the Speech Mechanism

Investigations of the cause of phonological disorders often have focused on children's abilities to control the speech mechanism. This is a logical area of inquiry, given the obvious importance of the speech mechanism to producing sounds. Possible problems with control of the speech mechanism have been noted in children with disorders ranging from very severe to mild. Several different types of speech mechanism control problems, and their possible causes, are discussed below.

Some children with a severe phonological disorder have unusual difficulty learning to coordinate their speech musculature for making speech sounds, despite the fact that there are no obvious impairments in their muscles. Although it is not clear that the only problem is muscular coordination (i.e., auditory perception and linguistic processing may also be difficult for these children), their difficulty telling their muscles what to do (sending signals from their brain to the muscles) stands out as a major barrier to learning to speak. In these cases, the children understand language well and want to communicate; often they will resort to complicated gestural systems because producing words is too difficult. The cause of this problem is unknown; it is different from a disorder such as cerebral palsy, where there is an identifiable disorder of muscle tone and control. People have labeled this problem **developmental apraxia of speech**, using terminology similar to an adult disorder caused by brain trauma from stroke or head injury (Hall, Jordan, & Robin, 1993) (see Chapter 9 on neurogenic speech and language disorders by LaPointe). Although research has not revealed neurological impairment in these children, future research may show neurophysiological deficits that can explain the extreme difficulty these children have learning to speak.

Another type of problem related to control of the speech mechanism occurs with **residual** articulation errors. As discussed earlier, residual errors are the few speech errors that remain in older children's speech when the phonological system should be mastered. Residual articulation errors may have different causes than more severe disorders where the child has multiple speech errors and is severely unintelligible. Residual articulation errors are often called *developmental* because the error types are characteristic of normal development. The presence of these errors at later ages may be due to habit, whereby a child continues to produce a sound as first learned.

Structural characteristics of the speech mechanism also can influence the development of speech errors. For example, a child with protruding front teeth may develop a tongue movement that moves forward to meet the teeth; the child may then lisp on certain sounds, such as "s" and "z." Once this pattern is learned, the child may habituate to it and not be able to resolve it independently, as in the habituation of residual errors. Similarly, children with a congenital cleft of the hard palate or inadequate tissue in the soft palate often attempt to compensate for the structural deficits by producing speech sounds unconventionally. Even if the structure of the speech mechanism is improved through surgery or the use of prostheses, the children may continue to produce the speech sounds as first learned.

Finally, there is a range of motor skills in young children. Just as some children are better at fine motor movements like arts and crafts or writing and drawing, so too are some children better at speech movements. Children who coordinate their muscles less well may be more prone to speech disorders, even of a mild variety. There are thus numerous ways that control of the speech mechanism can be related to phonological disorders, ranging from possible neurological impairment to structural abnormality, to habituation of mislearned movements.

Genetic Bases

More and more, research is showing us that disorders of speech and language run in families (Lewis, Ekelman, & Aram, 1989; Tomblin, 1989). When a parent has a history of a speech or language disorder, children in the family have a higher risk of a disorder as well. Some studies of several generations have shown clustering of disorders, with many individuals within one family having speech or language problems, often with multiple siblings having problems in later generations. A history of problems with reading also may show up in families where children have speech and language problems. As noted earlier, reading depends on knowledge of the speech sound system; therefore, problems in reading may be linked at times to problems in phonological development. Finally, boys are three to four times more likely to have a speech or language disorder than girls. This disparity between sexes also has been interpreted as genetically based.

Although there is strong research evidence that speech and language disorders run in families and are sex linked, we cannot conclude that all disorders are genetic. Similarities among family members can arise from environmental as well as genetic factors. The most recent research is consistent with the interpretation that the problems are inherited, but much work needs to be done before that conclusion can be drawn and generalized to the broad population of children with phonological disorders. At present, we can most accurately say that disorders often occur in more than one family member; that once a family has a member who has a speech and language problem, there is a higher risk for other members to also have a problem; and that boys are affected more often than girls. Again, some children have disorders even when no one else in the family has ever had a problem, and some children develop normally in families where other people have problems. Just as we cannot predict perfectly based on a history of ear infections, so too we cannot predict perfectly on the basis of family history.

We now return to the question posed earlier, "How do speech-language pathologists respond to a parent's question, 'Why did this happen?' " In light of the many possible causes of phonological disorders, and because conclusive answers are rarely available, speech-language pathologists are able to identify risk factors more easily than determine a specific cause. They look for a history of ear infections or other medical conditions that could influence development. They examine family history for other individuals with speech or language delays, persistent disorders, or reading or academic problems. In addition, they conduct a clinical evaluation that will help determine the child's ability to hear, to discriminate speech sounds, and to perform movements with the lips, tongue, and jaw, as necessary for speech. That is, they first obtain a history to consider possible medical, genetic, or environmental causes of speech problems. They then examine the child to evaluate the sensory, motoric, and linguistic systems necessary for learning the phonological system.

✦ WHAT DOES A SPEECH-LANGUAGE PATHOLOGIST DO TO HELP CHILDREN WITH PHONOLOGICAL DISORDERS?

Most of the time, we are not conscious of how we produce speech. Even when we stop and think about how we speak, we are not likely to be aware of the many things we do to produce clear, accurate speech sounds within a flow of sentences. It is difficult even for an adult to pay attention to speech and to make changes. What, then, can be done to help a child who is not developing speech normally? This is the challenge facing the speech-language pathologist who is working with a child with a phonological disorder.

Speech-language pathologists typically have responsibilities in at least three areas when working with individuals with communication disorders: **diagnosis**, **treatment**, and **counseling**. In working with children with atypical speech patterns, the speech-language pathologist first must conduct an examination to determine if there is a problem and, if so, the nature of the problem. This process of identifying who has a disorder is part of the **diagnosis**. The evaluation will reveal if the frequency and type of speech errors are outside of normal expectations; it also will help determine which underlying abilities the child has difficulty with, such as speech sound discrimination, memory for sound sequences, or motor control. As a result of the evaluation, the speech-language pathologist will make recommendations about whether **treatment** is needed. **Treatment** is a plan of remediation designed to help the child develop a more normal phonological system.

Along with providing treatment directly to the child, the speech-language pathologist may **counsel** the parents. **Counseling** includes information about expected development, ways the family can support the child's progress in therapy, and ways to maximize communication with the child even when speech remains hard to understand. Counseling also serves as support to parents in the form of listening, accepting the parents' concerns, and validating the parents' decisions to seek intervention. Counseling may be included in the child's treatment and may involve direct discussion of how the child feels about his speech, particularly with school-age children. Counseling also may occur indirectly by communicating to the child that he or she is valuable and capable; this can happen as the speech-language pathologist encourages the child to participate in treatment activities and supports the child in his efforts to communicate effectively.

Traditional Approach

Several different approaches have been developed to remediate phonological disorders; the approaches vary according to goals of treatment, methods for changing speech, and children for whom they are appropriate. One approach that has been used for a long time is designed to teach children specific speech sounds, like "r," "s," or "sh." In this approach, children are taught to move their lips, tongue, and jaw in new ways, then given lots of practice in making the new sounds. Children practice new sounds in syllables, then words, then sentences, until they can produce the new speech sound in everyday speech. This approach, which is called the "**traditional approach**," was developed by Van Riper, who was a major figure in the early days of speech pathology (Van Riper & Emerick, 1990). The **traditional approach** is still used widely with children, particularly school-age children with residual errors.

Phonological System Approaches

For children with more severe phonological disorders, for example, preschool children who make errors and are often unintelligible to listeners, a different approach is needed. These children make so many errors that teaching each sound in error takes too long. Further, it has been found that a sound-by-sound approach does not teach children what they need to learn about the phonological system as a rule-based system. Several researchers over the years have investigated ways of teaching children about the phonological system so that the children expand on what they are taught according to the rules of the system (Bernhardt, 1992; Gierut, 1989; Hodson & Paden, 1986). In this way, the children can be taught different "pieces" of the system (e.g., sound classes and syllable combinations) and can then begin spontaneously to learn other aspects of the system that they have not been taught directly. These approaches can be loosely called **phonological system approaches**. Although treatment can still take many months, the children can make great gains in intelligibility, far greater than if they were learning one sound at a time. An example of a remediation program based on the **phonological system approach** is described below.

Consider Elizabeth, age 4 years, who consistently deletes the final consonant in words, so that *talk* is "ta," *car* is "ca," and *fish* is "fi." Elizabeth's speech is hard to understand because words like *bee, bead, beet,* and *beach* sound alike when the final consonant is missing (they are homonyms, all pronounced as "be"). Although deletion of final consonants is a common error pattern, or **phonological process**, in the speech of 2-year-olds, most children produce some final consonants by age 2½, particularly as they begin to speak in sentences. Therefore, at age 4, Elizabeth is considerably behind expectations in her ability to produce final consonants. Intervention is appropriate to help her develop this important aspect of the phonological system.

A speech-language pathologist who sees Elizabeth will need first to evaluate Elizabeth's speech to determine which consonants

Elizabeth can produce accurately. Perhaps she can say "p" and "t" in words like *pie* and *two* but omits them in *cup* or *boat*. That is, Elizabeth may be capable of producing these speech sounds but may not know how to use them at the ends of words. In this case, therapy would focus on helping Elizabeth learn about speech sounds at the ends of words, rather than on producing individual sounds. The acquisition of a new *pattern* (consonants at the ends of words) would be more important than a production of a particular speech sound.

The speech-language pathologist would select several speech sounds to be the basis of practice in therapy sessions. Because the goal is for Elizabeth to learn the pattern, or the **phonological rule** about final consonants, it is important for more than one speech sound to be incorporated. Elizabeth might practice listening to and producing pairs of words, where the difference in meaning is illustrated by the presence or absence of the final consonant (e.g., *bee-beep, boo-boot*). She might learn to associate a concept to the pattern to be learned, for example, learning that words have "tails" like animals or "cabooses" like trains. Cues such as "remember the tail" or "put the caboose on the train" often are more meaningful and fun for children than abstract ideas about speech sounds. Examples of phonological processes, possible conceptual cues, and practice activities are shown in the box on the next page.

The advantage of this kind of therapy, as compared to the traditional approach, is that once Elizabeth knows the rule about using final consonants, she will begin to use the new word pattern with speech sounds that have not been practiced in therapy. When a child begins to extend what has been practiced to new examples, it is called **generalization**. The child **generalizes** based on rules that have been learned. As you can imagine, without generalization, a child with many sounds in error could spend years and years trying to learn each sound one at a time. Part of the speech-language pathologist's job is to plan a treatment program that will produce generalization, and to measure the child's progress over time to document that generalization is occurring.

In the present case, the speech-language pathologist would provide treatment until Elizabeth appears to have learned the rule well enough to continue developing it on her own. If Elizabeth has other error patterns, the speech-language pathologist would incorporate those patterns into treatment as well. The remediation program would be individualized to Elizabeth's needs, taking into account the number and type of error patterns she exhibits, their influence on her intelligibility, and her ability to participate in treatment. Family members could be involved by helping Elizabeth practice certain patterns at home, by encouraging Elizabeth, and

---

Treatment Targets, Concepts, and Activities

Targeted phonological process: Stopping (producing stops for fricatives)

Conceptual cues: "long sounds" (fricatives) versus "short sounds" (stops)

"noisy sounds" (fricatives) versus "popping sounds" (stops)

Activities: Moving a toy car while prolonging fricatives, then stopping the car when producing stops. Drawing continuous lines while prolonging fricatives, then drawing dots when producing stops. Sorting picture cards into one pile for the "noisy" sounds and one pile for the popping sounds.

Targeted phonological process: Unstressed syllable deletion

Conceptual cues: "Put in all the parts"

Activities: Putting big, cutout footsteps on the floor, then stepping on one footstep for each syllable in a word spoken (e.g., with the word "elephant," the child would step on three footsteps). Moving game pieces along a game board for each syllable in a multisyllabic word.

Targeted phonological process: Cluster reduction of words beginning with "s"

Conceptual cues: "Put the snake sound on first"

Activities: Sorting picture cards of minimal pairs, such as *sleep — leap, spot — pot, ski — key,* and talking about what makes the words sound different. Saying the word without the "s," then running a finger over a plastic snake while producing the cluster correctly. Pitching pennies onto cards on the floor and trying to make the pennies land on the minimal pairs, then saying the words on the cards.

---

by making communication enjoyable, even when Elizabeth is making errors. As noted above, part of the services provided by the speech-language pathologist would be **counseling** that helps the parents participate in these ways.

Treatment programs based on the **phonological system approach** vary according to the theory on which they are based, what specifically is taught during therapy, and the methods of teaching. However, they all have the goal of teaching children something about the phonological system as a whole to promote maximum gains incorporating rule-based learning. Some programs involve considerable drill work, where a child practices new phonological patterns in highly structured ways. Other programs involve more play and are particularly geared to the younger child. Listening practice often is incorporated to help children recognize differences among sounds and sound combinations; conceptual cues are used to help the child associate to the new speech pattern; and production practice is incorporated throughout.

Given the many individual differences among children, phonological disorders, and learning needs, no one treatment approach will be suitable for all children. Many speech-language pathologists combine teaching elements from different treatment approaches to meet the individual needs of children with phonological disorders. Some children require more training in discriminating sounds and recognizing which differences are important in the language; other children need more practice in producing new sounds and habituating the correct production. Part of the job of the speech-language pathologist is to pick the treatment approach that best matches the nature of the child's disorder and will bring about the greatest change in the shortest period of time.

The child as a whole, including the child's language abilities, social development, and emotional needs, must be considered in planning and implementing a remediation program. However important the phonological system is, it is but one piece of the communication system. A child is far more than a "phonological system." Our ultimate goal is to help children improve their intelligibility so they can feel successful and can be eager to communicate with others.

✦ SUMMARY AND CONCLUSION

In this chapter, you have read about phonological development in children and phonological disorders that can occur. You have considered how the phonological system is governed by rules, as are other aspects of the language system, and how the phonological rules are learned gradually during childhood. You have learned about the many capabilities that must come into play as a child learns the speech sound system, including listening skills, such as discrimination, and production skills, such as coordinating the articulators to produce meaningful combinations of sounds and syllables. You have studied different possible causes of phonological disorders, even while recognizing that in many cases specific causes are not known. You have been introduced to the responsibilities of a speech-language pathologist in diagnosing and treating children with phonological disorders.

The above paragraph simply summarizes the content covered in this chapter. It is hoped that the chapter provided a clear introduction to this topic and that it will be a solid foundation for your understanding of phonological development and disorders. Even more, however, it is hoped that the chapter has begun to stimulate you to ask questions about phonological development and disorders. Much remains to be learned about how the speech sound system develops and why some children have difficulty with this aspect of communication. In nearly every case of a child with a phonological disorder, whether in a research laboratory or in a clinic, what we do understand is shadowed by what remains a mystery. The route to better understanding of this complex topic is through asking questions in both research and clinical settings.

Think about what questions *you* would like to ask. Perhaps you find yourself asking about normal development; you might be interested in documenting phonological development in infants and children, to clarify and understand the characteristics of normal development. Perhaps you are curious about the medical or physiological/neurological conditions that influence development; you might wish to be involved with children who have organic or medical problems. Perhaps you are most drawn to methods of diagnosis and intervention, and how speech-language pathologists can produce the maximum development in children who have demonstrated phonological delays; you might be excited about a clinical setting and research on intervention.

In the study of phonological development and disorders, as well as in communication disorders in general, the magnitude of what remains to be learned is at once a source of frustration and excitement. Although we may find it difficult to face our incomplete understanding, particularly when dealing with children whose needs are immediate, we find it exhilarating to have so many choices for investigation and application. Whatever areas of interest have been awakened for you, there are questions to be asked and explorations to be conducted. We invite you into that process, confident that the opportunities will become increasingly vivid and exciting the more you deepen your involvement.

✦ ANSWERS TO BOXED QUESTIONS

Answers for Consonant Clusters Beginning with "s" (page 152)

RW (real words): 1, 3, 6, 9
PW (possible words): 2, 4, 5, 11, 12
NPW (not possible words): 7, 8, 10

Answers for Another Phonological Process (page 166)

There are no changes in *place* or *manner,* only in *voicing.* In word initial position, *voiceless* consonants "p, t," and "k" are substituted by their *voiced* counterparts; in word final position, *voiced* consonants are substituted by their *voiced* counterparts. These errors create a pattern whereby only voiced stops are produced in initial position and only voiceless stops occur at the ends of words.

✦ REFERENCES

Bernhardt, B. (1992). The application of nonlinear phonology to intervention with one phonologically disordered child. *Clinical Linguistics and Phonetics, 6,* 283–316.

Bernthal, J., & Bankson, B. (1993). *Articulation and phonological disorders* (3rd ed.). Englewood Cliffs, NJ: Prentice-Hall.

Gierut, J. A. (1989). Maximal opposition approach to phonological treatment. *Journal of Speech and Hearing Disorders, 54,* 9–19.

Hall, P. K., Jordan, L. S., & Robin, D. A. (1993). *Developmental apraxia of speech.* Austin, TX: Pro-Ed.

Hodson, B., & Paden, E. (1991). *Targeting intelligible speech: A phonological approach to remediation* (2nd ed.). Austin, TX: Pro-Ed.

Ingram, D. (1986). Phonological patterns in the speech of young children. In P. Fletcher & M. Garman (Eds.), *Language acquisition* (2nd ed.) (pp. 223–239). Cambridge: Cambridge University Press.

Lewis, B. A., Ekelman, B. L., & Aram, D. M. (1989). A familial study of severe phonological disorders. *Journal of Speech and Hearing Research, 32,* 713–724.

Locke, J. L. (1983). *Phonological acquisition and change.* New York: Academic Press.

Menn, L., & Stoel-Gammon, C. (1993). Phonological development: Learning sounds and sound patterns. In J. B. Gleason (Ed.), *Language development* (pp. 65–113). New York: Macmillan

Oller, D. K., & Eilers, R. E. (1988). The role of audition in infant babbling. *Child Development, 59,* 441–449.

Paden, E. P., Novak, M. A., & Beiter, A. L. (1987). Predictors of phonological inadequacy in young children prone to otitis media. *Journal of Speech and Hearing Disorders, 52,* 232–242.

Shriberg, L. D., Kwiatkowski, J., Best, S., Hengst, J., & Terselic-Weber, B. (1986). Characteristics of children with phonological disorders of unknown origin. *Journal of Speech and Hearing Disorders, 51,* 140–161.

Smit, A. B., Hand, L., Freilinger, J. J., Bernthal, J. E., & Bird, A. (1990). The

Iowa Articulation Norms Project and its Nebraska replication. *Journal of Speech and Hearing Disorders, 55,* 779–798.

Smith, N. V. (1975). *The acquisition of phonology.* Cambridge: Cambridge University Press.

Stoel-Gammon, C., & Cooper, J. A. (1984). Patterns of early lexical and phonological development. *Journal of Child Language, 11,* 247–271.

Stoel-Gammon, C., & Dunn, C. (1985). *Normal and disordered phonology in children.* Austin, TX: Pro-Ed.

Templin, M. C. (1957). *Certain language skills in children* (Monograph Series No. 26). Minneapolis: University of Minnesota, The Institute of Child Welfare.

Tomblin, J. B. (1989). Familial concentration of developmental language impairment. *Journal of Speech and Hearing Disorders, 54,* 587–595.

Van Riper, C., & Emerick, L. (1990). *An introduction to speech pathology and audiology* (8th ed.). Englewood Cliffs, NJ: Prentice-Hall.

◆ SUGGESTED READINGS

Aitchison, J. (1987). *Words in the mind: An introduction to the mental lexicon.* London: Basil Blackwell.

Bernthal, J., & Bankson, B. (1993). *Articulation and phonological disorders* (3rd ed.). Englewood Cliffs, NJ: Prentice-Hall.

Creaghead, N., Newman, P., & Secord, W. (1989). *Assessment and remediation of phonological disorders* (2nd ed.). Columbus, OH: Charles E. Merrill.

Ingram, D. (1986). Phonological patterns in the speech of young children. In P. Fletcher & M. Garman (Eds.), *Language acquisition* (2nd ed.) (pp. 223–239). Cambridge: Cambridge University Press.

Locke, J. L. (1983). *Phonological acquisition and change.* New York: Academic Press.

Menn, L., & Stoel-Gammon, C. (1993). Phonological development: Learning sounds and sound patterns. In J. B. Gleason (Ed.), *Language development* (pp. 65–113). New York: Macmillan.

Stoel-Gammon, C., & Dunn, C. (1985). *Normal and disordered phonology in children.* Austin, TX: Pro-Ed.

Van Riper, C., & Emerick, L. (1990). *An introduction to speech pathology and audiology* (8th ed.). Englewood Cliffs, NJ: Prentice-Hall.

◆ GLOSSARY

Articulation, to articulate: the formation of speech sounds by rapid, coordinated movement of the tongue, lips, jaw, and other structures (the **articulators**) (adj: **articulatory**).

Babbling: nonmeaningful sequences of consonants and vowels produced by infants.

Counseling: a process of educating and supporting clients and families through verbal discussion, exchange of information, and offering of emotional support.

Developmental apraxia of speech: a disorder of speech production in which a child is impaired in motor control for speech, specifically the voluntary planning and sequencing of speech movements, not attributable to muscle weakness or muscular neurological impairment.

Diagnosis: the act of identifying and classifying a disorder, and distinguishing it from other disorders in type and severity.

Discrimination, to discriminate: the ability to hear differences among different speech sounds; part of perception.

Final consonant deletion: an error pattern (see **phonological processes**) in which a child omits the consonant at the end of a word.

Generalization, to generalize: application of what has been learned in treatment to new words, more complex speech, new situations, and new communicative partners.

Gliding: an error pattern (see **phonological processes**) in which a child substitutes a "w" (a **glide**) for "l" or "r."

Intelligibility: the degree to which speech is understood by listeners; speech that cannot be understood is **unintelligible**.

International Phonetic Alphabet (IPA): the alphabet of phonetic symbols used for transcription of spoken language (shown in Table 4–1).

Lexicon: vocabulary used by a speaker; words stored in the mental dictionary.

Marking: producing a word with a subtle, unconventional error to make a distinction between it and another, similar sounding word (adj: **marked**).

Phonological delay, Phonological disorder: development of the phonological system that is slower than normal in accuracy or completeness, or follows an atypical pattern.

Phonological process: a systematic error pattern that affects a class of speech sounds, wherein one type of sound is substituted for another, or a class of sounds is deleted in certain word contexts.

Phonological system approach: any treatment approach for remediating speech errors that is based on the phonological system as a whole. It is designed to teach children new phonological rules so that systematic error patterns change and the child's phonological system becomes more adult-like.

Phonology, Phonological system: the speech sound system of a language, including all the elements and their rules (**phonological rules**) for combination.

Prosody: the part of the phonological system governing intonation and stress; these elements are also known as suprasegmentals.

Residual errors: referring to errors in children's or adults' speech that are left over from earlier development; usually referring to a small number of errors that were once developmentally typical.

Traditional approach: a treatment approach developed by Charles Van Riper for remediating articulation errors. It is based on discriminating and practicing new speech sounds in syllables, words, and sentences, in order to establish new production patterns for specific sounds.

Treatment: a plan to remediate or improve a communication disorder, as planned by a speech-language pathologist.

CHAPTER 5

Language Development

LOIS BLOOM, PH.D.

After completing this chapter, you should understand:

◆ How form, content, and use interact in language development.

◆ How developments in infancy, in particular, emotional expression and other aspects of cognition, are related to developments in language.

◆ That the single-word period in language development begins with a child's first tentative word sometime around the first birthday.

◆ That individual children differ in important ways in their language development.

◆ That children begin to acquire a grammar of simple sentences by learning different categories of verbs.

◆ How complex sentences begin between 2 and 3 years of age.

◆ How children learn to participate in conversations.

When children acquire a language, they acquire the power of expression — the ability to take something internal and private to themselves and make it external and public, so that other people can share it. Language expresses the beliefs, desires, and feelings we have as we relate to one another in everyday events. This means that language development is related to other aspects of cognitive development, as well as to emotional and social development. When something interferes with development, a child might learn language slowly or only with difficulty. To help the child with a language problem, we need to understand how language develops normally, without interference. Such understanding is the goal of this chapter. Development is described here in terms of the form, content, and use of language — as children acquire a vocabulary of words in the second year, simple and complex sentences in the third year, and learn to participate in conversations in this period of time.

The fundamental goal in development is to make sense of the world. The fundamental goal in acquiring a language is to know how the language and one's sense of the world fit together. Infants begin to work toward meeting these goals virtually from the moment of birth. In the first few hours of life, a human infant attends to sights, smells, and sounds and can make some sense of them. For instance, a newborn infant can tell the difference between its mother's voice and a female stranger's voice (DeCasper & Fifer, 1980). The infant will look into its father's face and, after wavering a bit, will settle on the eyes and stay there, intently gazing into another pair of eyes. Infants can appreciate that a moving object has boundaries and obeys certain physical laws when only a few months old (Baillargeon, 1992; Spelke, 1988, 1991), and they can tell the difference between speech sounds, such as the difference between the sound categories /pa/ and /ba/ (Eimas, Siqueland, Jusczyk, & Vigorito, 1971). All of these things and thousands more contribute to the development of an intentional being in the first year of life — a person, with thoughts and feelings about other persons and about objects and events in the world.

From the moment of birth, infants express something of what they are feeling through emotional displays — the frowns, cries, whimpers, and eventually smiles and coos that other persons interpret and respond to as meaningful. These displays of emotion in infancy are biologically determined — they are already a part of an infant's makeup at birth by virtue of human evolutionary history (Darwin, 1913). As the infant matures and develops in the first year, emotional expressions come under increasing control. By the end of the first year, infants are very adept at using such signals to let other persons know when they are delighted or distressed, interested, eager, or afraid, and their caregivers are very good at reading their meaning (Izard & Malatesta, 1987). Infant and caregiver are tuned into one another, and communication between them is well underway. This is because they are able to share something of what each is feeling and thinking through expressions of the face and the voice.

At the same time, infants are learning quite a lot about persons, objects, and events through their actions and interactions in the world. One result of this early cognitive development is the ability to think about things that are absent — things not there in the situation but represented instead in the mind as symbols (Piaget, 1954). Now the baby can think about mother, a bottle, something to eat, or the family dog even when these things aren't around. This is the symbolic capacity and learning language depends on it. Language itself consists of symbols: The word *dog* is a symbol because it stands for objects in the world that are dogs. But even more important, the word *dog* stands for the object we have in mind when we think about dogs; this mental object also is a symbol because it stands for what we know about dogs in the world. We use mental symbols when we think about things in their absence; we use language symbols — in words and sentences — to express mental symbols so that other persons can think about about them.

The symbolic capacity begins to develop in the first year and makes it possible for the 1-year-old to have thoughts and feeling about persons, events, and things that other persons cannot know. If what the infant has in mind is not also in the situation for others to see and hear, then it is discrepant from what others have in mind. This discrepancy between what two persons have in mind drives the development of language. This is because things that other persons cannot know about, because they are represented mentally in the child's mind, must be expressed if they are to be shared. Language makes it possible to express the contents of mind and to interpret what others have in mind. Saying "milk" or "I'm hungry" or "Where's the dog?" are expressions, and once they are said, they are out there for other persons to interpret and, therefore, know about.

Another result of cognitive development in the first year is that infants' thoughts and feelings become increasingly elaborate. They are able to hold in mind many more different sorts of things, and different relationships between things, because they now know more about the world. For example, in early infancy, babies cry simply because they are hungry; later they also know that milk or crackers will ease the hunger and that other persons can supply these things. But just whimpering or crying will not do; the 1-year-old will need to be more explicit than that and say the words. The increasingly elaborated and discrepant thoughts and feelings in the 1-year-old's mind can no longer be expressed by the displays of emotion that served the younger infant so well. If they are to be shared with others, the infant will have to learn a language to express them.

Languages are contrived by the persons in a society for sharing what cannot otherwise be known between them, and language needs to be learned. Language is learned to make what a child has in mind manifest — to give ideas, thoughts, and feelings an embodiment — so that other persons can know them (Danto, 1973; Taylor, 1979). Language makes it possible for individuals to share what they and others are thinking and feeling at a particular moment in time, through expression and interpretation. And language makes it possible for them to share the larger world view that holds the society and culture together across many moments of time — their customs, beliefs, and ways of living. But language does not take the place of those earlier emotional expressions from infancy. Children continue to express what they are feeling through their smiles, frowns, laughs, and cries as they are learning the language for expressing what those feelings are about and what to do about them (Bloom, Beckwith, Capatides, & Hafitz, 1988).

Acquiring the power of expression is the child's most important endeavor in the first few years of life, and language is the best medium of expression that we have. By saying words or making gestures, we are articulating the contents of mind and saying what they are, because the mental symbols we have in mind are embodied in the linguistic symbols — words and gestures — of the language. The purpose of this chapter is to describe how children acquire language and what it means to acquire a language for expression. Most of what is covered here will have to do with language as expression — what children actually say as they acquire language. We know that they acquire language through interpreting what they hear others around them say. However, the study of interpretation — how children learn to understand language — will not be stressed here, because children obviously are also learning to understand those aspects of language which are evident in their speech.

◆ A DEFINITION OF LANGUAGE

Language consists of three components: form, content, and use (Bloom & Lahey, 1978; Lahey, 1988). The shapes of words and sentences, the way the language sounds when it is spoken, or the way that it looks in sign languages and gestures, is language **form**. The forms of language consist of sounds, words, and sentence structures. The sounds of the language make up its phonology; the words of the language make up its dictionary or lexicon; and sentence structures are determined by the syntax of language.

What the words and sentences mean — what they are about — is the **content** of language. So, for example, the string of sounds /d-aw-g/ has meaning — it is the word *dog* — only if it connects with the mental symbol of an object dog. The content of the sentence "The dog chases the cat," for example, is the meaning of the individual words in the sentence plus the meaning relationships among the words *dog* and *chase* and *cat*. Meaning or the content of words and sentences is the semantics of language; the orderly arrangement of words in sentences is the syntax of language; and syntax and semantics together make up the grammar of the language.

The **use** of language is what we do with it to influence the thoughts and actions of other persons. We use language for different purposes — to get and give information, to get people to do things, to solve problems, read maps, organize events, and so forth. And we do these things differently in different sorts of circumstances: Saying "I'm thirsty," "I need a drink," "I'll have a glass of water, if you please," or "Gimme a Coke" would each serve the same purpose, but only if we take into account where we are and to whom we are talking. The purposes of language, and different ways of saying more or less the same thing to achieve a particular purpose, make up the pragmatics of language use.

Language is the integration of form, content, and use; these three components necessarily come together. Forms without meaning, like "dak" or "nef," are empty; randomly connected words, like "milk chase the" are gibberish; we do not say words and sentences just to talk, we have some reason or purpose in mind. Unless form, content, and use are integrated, we cannot use language for communication. It follows, therefore, that we need to understand how form, content, and use are integrated in order to help children and adults who have problems in communicating. And we need to understand how these things come together in normal language development in order to understand and be able to help children whose language is developing slowly or with difficulty.

◆ WAYS OF STUDYING LANGUAGE ACQUISITION

People who study language development make different kinds of assumptions about the child and about the language, and they bring different sorts of ideas to the research they do. For example, one such perspective takes its lead from linguistic theory and pursues the study of language acquisition from the viewpoint of the adult language-user. Beginning with a theory about the fully formed, adult language, one can ask how the structures and procedures of that language are acquired. The focus is on the end state — the language that needs to be learned — and evidence from children acquiring language is useful only if it can support or help to understand one or another linguistic theory (e.g., Baker, & McCarthy, 1981; Hyams, 1986; Pinker, 1984; Radford, 1990; Wexler & Culicover, 1980). And the emphasis typically is on the forms of language.

A second perspective takes its lead from anthropology and pursues the acquisition of language as the socialization of the child in a cultural context. Children acquiring language are always situated in relationships with other persons and learn a language through social interactions with other persons who already know the language. But a child does not just learn the language — by learning a language, the child is learning to participate in the "give and take of everyday life" (Schieffelin, 1990). Learning the language of a culture means acquiring the social practices and customs in the culture. Here the emphasis typically is on language use. For example, children need to learn when to talk and how to express themselves in different circumstances, taking into account such things as the relationships between the participants in a situation, their ages, relative experience, and the like. We talk differently to strangers than to persons we know well, differently at home than at school, and so forth. Here the focus is on the context — on how to use language for different purposes in different situations (e.g., Bates, 1976; Bruner, 1983; Ervin-Tripp, 1973; Ochs & Schieffelin, 1983; Schieffelin & Ochs, 1986).

Both of these emphases in studies of child language are important, but for different reasons. If one wants to understand the adult language more fully and, in particular, its grammar, then the option is to study how children's grammar either does or does not fit one or another theory of adult grammar. If, instead, one wants to understand how children are socialized to use language by the participants in different situations, then the option is to study children's language behaviors according to their cultural and social relevance.

A third theoretical perspective begins with the child and how what the child knows about the world influences how and what the child learns about the language. This is the **developmental perspective**. The organizing principle of development was articulated by Heinz Werner, one of the founders of developmental theory, as follows: Every behavior, whether it is an external bodily movement or an internal mental operation, gains significance from the part it plays in the overall functioning of the organism (Werner, 1948). In this view, language is just one among many aspects of human functioning. Both the external linguistic behaviors that we see and hear and the internal knowledge we have of words and procedures for sentences in memory gain their significance only in relation to other aspects of human functioning.

The 1-year-old child is not a language-learning machine — going through the steps of acquiring words and learning to say sentences according to a schedule or prescription — for the sake of the exercise. Instead, infants are thinking and feeling creatures who learn language in relation to everything else that they do and everything else they are learning. In this view, one cannot ignore what else is going on in a young child's life. In particular, one cannot ignore what the child knows about the world — the other aspects of a child's cognitive development that contribute to language. Neither can one ignore other aspects of expression, most notably a child's emotional expression, in seeking to learn how language is acquired for expression. And one cannot ignore the child's social context, because the driving force for acquiring a language is the need to share the contents of mind and thereby establish shared understandings with other persons.

The account of language development in this chapter is a developmental account. First, I will assume that those who are reading the chapter know little of how language is acquired. Accordingly, I will show the steps young children take in making the transition — in the first 3 years of life — from prespeech communication in infancy to the words and sentences of language. Second, true to the organizing developmental principle of Werner, I will show that these steps toward language are influenced by other developments going on at the same time — notably, developments in emotional expression, cognition, and social interaction.

What follows here is divided into five sections. The first is the transition from infancy to language, an account of developments in infancy that bring an infant to the threshold of word learning at the end of the first year. The second section is an account of word learning in the period between a child's first and second birthdays: from First Words to a Vocabulary Spurt toward the end of the second year. The third is an account of how children begin to combine words to form their first phrases and simple sentences sometime around the second birthday, often beginning at around 20 months. The next section is an account of complex sentences, which are sentences formed by combining the ideas and structures in a child's simple sentences. Complex sentences have their beginnings in the third year of life, with acquisition continuing well beyond the age of 3 years and into the early school years. The final section is a brief account of how children learn to participate in conversations with other persons.

These five sections add up to a developmental chronicle of language acqusition, but one with certain limitations that the reader should be aware of at the outset. The first is the space limitation in this chapter, and for this reason the chronicle necessarily will be selective. For example, we will be concerned with development through the first 3 years of life and will not go beyond what children typically have learned of language by the age of 3. However, everything else that happens later in acquisition builds on the knowledge of language a child acquires in the first 3 years. The second limitation comes from the fact that the author of a chronicle has the prerogative to stress certain things over other things deemed less interesting or important. Accordingly, certain important issues in the field will be covered while others will not. For example, I will not go into the issue of what is and what is not innately given about language, that is, what the child is born with that is specifically linguistic, such as principles of universal grammar. Instead, I will build on the fundamental and essentially noncontroversial assumption that certain basic and general cognitive abilities are present at birth, for example, the ability to form categories of things and categories of relationships between things. These general capacities are put in the service of acquiring a great deal of knowledge about the world, including the specifically linguistic knowledge that is language.

The guiding principles in the research to be covered here come from an explicitly psychological theory of language development, as opposed to one that derives from linguistic theory or the logical arguments in the philosophy of language (Bloom, 1991, 1993). Linguistic and philosophical theories are important, to be sure. But, for the child, the task of language acquisition is a psychological problem, not a logical problem, and the linguistic problems to be solved are always embedded in a personal and interpersonal — that is, a psychological — context.

We will begin with the infant in the last quarter of the first year, and the succession of child words and sentences shown here gives the reader some feeling for where the infant will be going in the next 2 years (and the pages to follow). These examples show the progress a child makes from saying only one word at a time, with words that cannot be readily interpreted out of context (as they are given here), to saying simple sentences and, eventually, complex sentences with meaning that is more or less transparent from the words and their arrangements.

Developments in Language: From Words to Sentences

CHILDREN PROGRESS FROM SAYING ONE WORD AT A TIME:
  "more" or "baby" or "uhoh"

TO SAYING A SERIES OF RELATED SINGLE-WORDS:
  "Mommy, juice"
  "button, open, button"

TO SAYING PHRASES AND SIMPLE SENTENCES:
  "no dirty soap"
  "this go there"
  "I writing circles"

TO SAYING MORE COMPLEX SENTENCES:
  "Mommy no play 'corder"
  "Where all the people go?"
  "Why don't like taste of of cheddar?"

TO SAYING INCREASINGLY COMPLEX SENTENCES:
  "Let's all take all the books out so we can read them"
  "I was crying because I didn't want to wake up because it was
    dark, so dark"

Adapted from Bloom, L., 1991. *Language development from two to three.*
New York: Cambridge University Press.

◆ THE TRANSITION FROM INFANCY TO LANGUAGE

The human infant is born to perceive, to interact, to learn. Certain
cognitive and social capacities that eventually serve speech and
language are already in place at birth, and others will evolve as the
result of experience in the first year. One of the tasks of development in the first year is to learn about a world of objects and become aware that the myriad sights and sounds that the baby sees
and hears have certain regularity and order. To that end, babies begin, very early, to attend to moving objects and salient noises. Gradually they begin to build memories, and those early memories provide the background against which they attend to new objects that
move and new noises that appear (Moscovitch, 1984). They also
discover that their bodies move and do things, and that the world of
objects and persons changes with the movements they make. Infants develop the capacities for learning language as they learn to
see, hear, and do.

  An infant, much less than an adult, could not possibly discriminate among all the visual and auditory input from the environment
at once. For this reason, the organization of the human nervous system has evolved over the history of generations so that certain stim-

uli in the environment stand out over others. Virtually from birth, infants select what they attend to and pay particular attention to patterns and to movement, because they find them interesting. In addition, infants enter a world in which persons, objects, and the kinds of things that happen to persons and objects are essentially orderly and consistent. Because events are orderly and consistent, they eventually are predictable. A major achievement in development is for infants to learn to predict the actions of persons and the effects such actions can have on objects and other persons. One particularly important effect of actions and movement is that objects change location, so that the infant comes to experience them anew in different places.

Certain knowledge about objects that is central to how adults view the world is already present in the first few months of infancy. A **theory of objects** clearly begins early in infancy, and experiments have shown its beginnings in infants' perceptions of objects that move in relation to a background (Baillargeon, 1992; Spelke, 1988, 1991). For example, infants appreciate that a moving object will continue to move unless it encounters another physical object; they have an early understanding of continuity and solidity. However, knowledge of gravity and inertia depend on having further experience with objects and so begin to develop somewhat later.

An infant's developing theory about objects is important for the infant's actions in learning to adapt and get around in the world. In the early months of life, infants act as though an object that is out of sight is also out of mind. When an object is hidden from view they do not look for it. But sometime toward the end of the first 6 months, they begin to understand that a whole object exists behind a cover when they can see only a part of it, and they will try to retrieve it. When children are able to search for objects that are hidden, we know they can think about absent objects. They no longer are limited to acting directly on the objects themselves. Instead, they construct a mental plan with symbols of the objects and act on the basis of the mental plan. This ability to think about absent objects and to act on the basis of those representations depends on the development of the symbolic capacity and marks the culmination of infant development. It is a gradual development in the first year-and-a-half that has its beginning in the first few months of life (Piaget, 1954).

An infant's early theories about objects have to do with objects in general: Behaviors like watching after a moving object, looking for hidden objects, and grouping objects together are things a child can do with many different sorts of objects. Babies learn to watch, search for, and find things as different from one another as bouncing balls, nursing bottles, and baby kittens. Such general, physical knowledge contributes to the process whereby babies begin to form concepts of individual objects according to their similarity or the functions they share. Thus, balls bounce, but baby kittens do not; kittens meow and scratch, have fur, and so on. By the end of the first year, in addition to a theory of objects in general, infants also have begun to form concepts of particular persons and objects that form basic categories, like balls, kittens, cars, and cookies. These concepts of persons and objects are embedded in a network of conceptual representations that also include **relational concepts** — such as disappearance and recurrence, which contribute to learning particular words like *gone* (for disappearance) and *more* (recurrence), for instance. Concepts of objects and relations are, in turn, embedded in the larger theories infants acquire — such as theories of causality, space, and movement (Keil, 1989, 1991; Murphy & Medin, 1985; Piaget, 1954, 1960). Concepts and theories about the world begin to develop before language and contribute to providing the content of language as it develops in the early childhood years (e.g., Bloom, 1973; Mervis, 1987; Nelson, 1974).

In particular, three basic theories about the world have begun to take shape at the beginning of the second year. They are the infant's emerging theories of objects, movement, and location, and they will be critically important for language. These theories will guide the 1-year-old's word learning, and they will provide the conceptual basis for the early sentences of the 2-year-old (Bloom, 1981, 1991). Ultimately, they determine the conceptual-semantic structure of the adult language (Jackendoff, 1983). Thus, the foundation for the semantic structure of language is in the theories of objects, movement, and location which begin to be formed in the first year of life.

We have already seen that the emergent infant on the threshold of language at the end of the first year is also an expressive infant. Cognitive developments bring the infant to the threshold of language only in conjunction with other developments in expression and social connectedness. At the same time an infant is learning about objects in the world, social developments and developments in expression are proceeding as well. Infants show us, in many ways, that they are biologically prepared for expression; virtually from birth, they have capacities that serve emotional expression and expression through speech or manual signs for language. An infant's cry in the first hours of life is an expression of discomfort and dismay and, at the same time, contains the rudiments out of which the sounds of speech will develop (Oller, 1980; Oller & Eilers, 1992; Stark, 1986). The ability to hear that categories of speech sounds are different, the tendency to gaze into another pair of eyes, the inclination to smile, and many other communication behaviors as well, are there to begin with — awaiting the caring, comforting, and coaction of responsive and responsible other persons. Hearing speech and seeing gestures, human infants cannot help but exploit their basic capacities to acquire the conventional forms of a language — if interpersonal and cognitive developments happening at the same time give them something to say and a reason to say it (Bloom, 1993).

The result is the emergence of an infant at around the 1st birthday who is ready to begin to meet the conventional requirements of language — ready for the first words. Development in infancy has been concerned with learning about the objective world of things and the subjective world of persons, both of which contribute to the representation of mental meanings that potentially are expressible in language. An infant's developing theories about the world and concepts in memory provide data for the construction of mental meanings for words to express. And the infant's social connectedness with other persons provides the interpersonal context within which the infant needs to share those mental meanings.

◆ EARLY VOCABULARIES: SAYING ONE WORD AT A TIME

First Words begin at about the first birthday, give or take a few months. First Words are tentative, imprecise, and fragile, and new words are acquired slowly in the several months after words begin to appear. Some time toward the end of the second year, things pick up and children begin to learn more and more different words, learn words more rapidly, and use their words more easily and readily. These are some well-known facts about early word learning. They were confirmed again in the results of a recently completed research project in which my students and I studied 14 children, every month, from 9 months to 2 years of age (Bloom, 1993). I will draw on that study in the following examples. Figure 5–1 is a summary of the children's progress in acquiring new words from one month to the next, beginning with their First Words (FW) in the playroom in which we studied their monthly progress in language development. They acquired words gradually over the next several months after FW, until a sharp increase in new words occurred, called a **Vocabulary Spurt** (VS). New words continued to increase in the month after VS (VS+1).

Individual Differences

Children differ greatly in when they begin to say words and how long it takes them to achieve a vocabulary spurt and, eventually, to

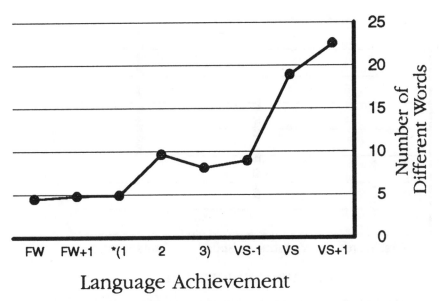

Language Achievement

Figure 5–1. Average number of different words learned each month. (*Each of the three data points in parentheses represents the average number of new words in one-third of the interval between FW+1 and VS−1.) (Bloom, L., Tinker, E., & Margulis, C., 1993. The words children learn: Evidence against a noun bias in early vocabularies. *Cognitive Development, 8,* 431–450, with permission).

begin saying sentences. Figure 5–2 shows the wide range in the ages at which the same 14 children reached these three landmarks in language development. Their average ages at First Words, the Vocabulary Spurt, and Simple Sentences were, respectively, about 14 months, 19 months, and 24 months. However, the range in the ages at which individual children reached these achievements was very wide, for example, from 10 to 17 months for FW and from 13 to 25 months for VS.

We do not know why children are so different in their onset and rate of word learning in the second year, but several reasons have been suggested. Certainly, exposure to words in the speech around them is an important factor. Children obviously have to hear words to learn them, and they are more likely to learn words when the words they hear are relevant to what they have in mind. This happens when caregivers talking to children say words that are about what a child is attending to, and we know that adults differ in their tendencies to do this. Children whose caregivers talk to them about what they are seeing and doing at the same time are more apt to acquire words earlier and have larger vocabularies (Masur, 1982; Tomasello & Farrar, 1986). Another factor often suggested to explain

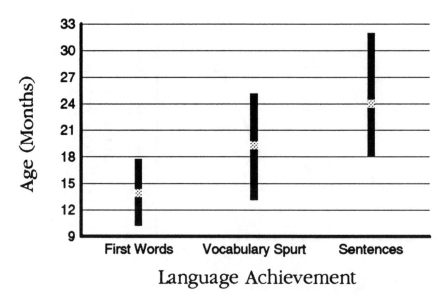

Language Achievement

Figure 5-2. Mean and range in age at the three language achievements: First Words, Vocabulary Spurt, and Sentences (Bloom, L., 1993. *The transition from infancy to language: Acquiring the power of expression.* New York: Cambridge University Press, with permission).

individual differences is social and economic background; poor children often are thought to be at risk for language acquisition. However, 4 children whose family incomes depended on public assistance were among the 14 children represented in Figures 5-1 and 5-2. Although one of them was the oldest child at VS and onset of sentences, the other three were not different from the others in the group; as is usually the case, differences within groups are typically greater than differences between them.

One thing that did differ among the children we studied was the frequency with which they expressed emotion. Infants who were more emotionally expressive tended to begin acquiring words somewhat later than those children who were more neutral in their expression (Bloom & Capatides, 1987a). We have interpreted this to mean that neutral expression supported states of attention needed for learning words; paying attention to the word and how it might be relevant to what a child has in mind requires cognitive effort. The thinking required for experiencing and expressing emotion — for evaluating a situation in relation to goals and plans — takes up the cognitive resources needed for learning words at the same time. We can see the difference between the two subgroups of earlier and later word learners in the same population of 14 children in Figure 5-3. The frequency of their emotional expressions is shown at the ages of 9, 13, 17, and 21 months. The earlier word learners, who began

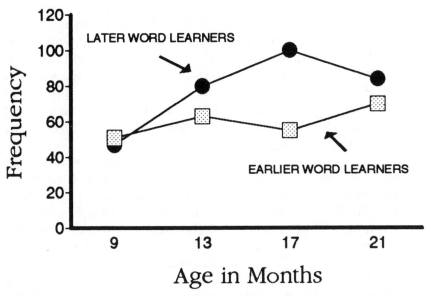

Figure 5–3. Mean frequency of emotional expression by earlier and later word learners (Bloom, L., 1993. *The transition from infancy to language: Acquiring the power of expression.* New York: Cambridge University Press, with permission).

saying words between 10 and 13 months, showed no change from 9 to 21 months in the frequency with which they expressed emotion. The later word learners increased in frequency of emotional expression from 9 to 17 months, instead of saying words **early**. Interestingly, when the later word learners made their move in language toward a vocabulary spurt, between 17 and 21 months, they decreased in how frequently they expressed emotion.

In addition to looking at expressing emotion and saying words separately, we also looked at how the two forms of expression came together in real time (Bloom & Beckwith, 1989). When they first started to say words, at FW, the children were more likely to be expressing neutral affect when they said words than to be expressing emotion at the same time. Again, we interpreted this to mean that the cognitive effort of emotional experience and expression was suspended in favor of the cognitive effort required for saying a word. However, by the time of the vocabulary spurt, they had gotten it together and were more likely to be saying words at the same time they expressed emotion than was expected by chance alone. They were learning words to express what their feelings were about. However, the words they said with emotional expression tended to be words they knew best and were, therefore, more automatic and easier to say. In addition, they said words with positive emotion more often than with negative emotional expression, and we know that positive emotional experience often requires less thinking. With positive emotion, a goal has been reached, and no new goals or plans are necessary. In contrast, negative emotion occurs when goals are blocked or a plan to reach a goal is not successful, meaning that a new goal or plan needs to be constructed (e.g., Oatley, 1992; Stein & Levine, 1989). These results show how emotional expression and cognitive factors collaborate in the effort of learning and saying words.

The conclusion in most descriptions of early word learning is that FW and VS mark the beginning and end of the single-word period in development. However, they usually are not sharp boundaries. In the beginning of word learning, infants grope to control phonetic and acoustic cues as they seek to grasp the connections between what they hear and what they see and know (Stone & Stoel-Gammon, Chapter 4). At some point a child is heard to say words that are somehow recognizable even though they may be incomplete and indistinct in sound and imprecise in meaning. Words are few and far between for a while, but the child eventually begins saying more different words, and using these words more readily and more frequently. And soon after a spurt in vocabulary, many children begin combining words for their first simple sentences, marking the end of the single-word period.

The Words Children Learn

Children learn a great many different kinds of words in the single-word period in the second year. However, one thing is clear: Children's early words cannot be classified according to their parts of speech in adult language: as nouns, verbs, adjectives, prepositions, and the like. These kinds of category assignments are valid only when children begin to combine words in sentences. When they are combined with one another in sentences, words can be defined on the basis of their distribution in relation to each other and by the semantic and syntactic functions they serve. Other classifications of children's words have been more successful when they are based on what a child's single-words appear to be expressing. Certain words name objects, like *ball, cookie,* and *car*; other words name relationships, like *more, gone,* and *up*. And still other words are parts of social exchanges and routines, like *hi, bye,* and *whee* (Bloom, 1973; Gopnik, 1988; Nelson, 1973). However, most accounts of early word learning have tended to emphasize the importance of object names among a child's words.

Again, going back to the early words of the 14 children already mentioned, we can look at the words they learned in the period between their First Words and continuing up to and including the month after their Vocabulary Spurt. Together, these children said a total of 11,404 words in this period in the playroom in which we studied them. However, many of these words were said very often; in fact, only 326 different words were included among the more than 11,000 words they said. Interestingly, the children tended not to be learning the same words. About three-fourths of the 326 different words were said by only one, two, or three children; only 49 different words (or 15% of the words) were said by seven or more children. And only 5 words appeared in the vocabularies of all the children; these words were *baby, ball, down, juice*, and *more*.

All the children played with the same toys in the playroom, in the same sequence, every month. However, one difference in the playroom context that obviously contributed to differences among the children was their mothers. In effect, the mothers represented the social and cultural experiences the children brought with them into the playroom each month. These experiences determined their word learning in the much larger contexts of their lives outside the playroom and contributed to the differences among them in their vocabularies.

Even though many people assume that object names are most frequent, object names do not, in fact, predominate in children's early vocabularies (Bates, Bretherton, & Snyder, 1988; Bloom, 1973; Bloom, Tinker, & Margulis, 1993; Gopnik, 1988; Hampson & Nelson, 1993; Nelson, 1973; Pine, 1992). Only about one-third of the different words learned by the 14 children we studied were names for things. When person names were included, the result was that little more than 40% of both word types and the more than 11,000 word tokens were names for persons and objects. The words learned by half or more of the children are shown in Figure 5–4, and the object names in the list are underlined. The diversity in young vocabularies is impressive, and words like *uhoh, hi, boom, on, this, moo*, and *yum* occurred in the vocabularies of seven or more children, along with object names like *box, ball, girl, bottle, cookie, juice*, and *spoon*.

Children's early words do not fall into neat, reliable categories according to either linguistic, conceptual, or pragmatic criteria. Even the common nouns children learn do not form a consistent class, because they name basic level objects like *shoe* but also include words like *lap, animal*, and *lunch* which are not names for basic objects (Nelson, Hampson, & Shaw, 1993). Evidently, children learn whatever words they hear that are relevant to the mental meanings they have in mind.

box							
choo-choo	**cookie**						
	door						
get	**eye**	**banana**					
girl	go	boom					
hammer	here	**bottle**	**apple**				
horse	moo	**cow**	**boy**				**baby**
in	no more	**daddy**	that			**mommy**	**ball**
out	on	**shoe**	this	**bead**	bye	no	down
sit	**truck**	**spoon**	uhoh	open	hi	oh	**juice**
two	woof	there	whee	yes	yum	up	more

| 7 | 8 | 9 | 10 | 11 | 12 | 13 | 14 |

Number of Children

Figure 5–4. The words learned by half (7) or more of the children in the Bloom (1993) studies; underlined words were names for things in the playroom (Bloom, L., 1993. *The transition from infancy to language: Acquiring the power of expression.* New York: Cambridge University Press, with permission).

What Are Early Words About?

The numbers and the kinds of words children learn are less important than the mental meanings a word can express. Certain words are specific to the concepts children acquire — words like *gone* or *more* or *up*. But those words probably were learned in the first place because they figured in events in which an infant's thinking and feelings were engaged — things that disappeared, recurred, or the like. One-year-old children learn to talk about the objects, causes, and circumstances of their beliefs, desires, and feelings with the words that say what these are — words like *Mama, uhoh, no, cow, cookie, more, gone*, and *up*. However, notably absent from these children's early vocabularies were the words that name the different emotions like *happy, angry, sad, scared*. Rather than telling their mothers what emotion they were feeling, they were telling them what their feelings were about and what they might do to change them — words for talking about the ways objects, and persons and objects, go together in everyday events.

If we look at the situation in which a child says words, we can attribute mental meanings that tell us what the child's words are about. When we did that with these 14 children, we found that they were far more likely to be expressing a desire to change the world than expressing a belief in the way the world appeared to be, to them. However, the desires they expressed were concerned primarily with themselves as the actors in events — the children were most likely to be talking about what they wanted to do or were about to do (Bloom, Beckwith, Capatides, & Hafitz, 1988). The finding that desires were about something the child wanted to do more often than what they wanted another person to do meant they were not learning words primarily to get other persons to do things. Thus **language as expression** was basic to their language learning, and more fundamental than learning language as a tool, for instrumental purposes. Language certainly is used to get people to do things, but that is only because it sets up a mental meaning in the hearer's mind that matches the mental meaning in the speaker's mind (Bloom, 1993).

Developments in mental meanings expressed in the single-word period pointed to the important changes taking place in the children's developing cognition. Two other aspects of the mental meanings these children expressed were noteworthy. First, the children were more likely to talk about what they anticipated in the situation — something that was about to happen in the context. The importance of this development is in what it tells us about the child's ability to construct a mental meaning cued by, but not given, in the context. Such anticipative meanings are private because they are represented mentally; they need to be made public, in an expression, if other persons are to know them.

Another development was an increase in expression of dynamic mental meanings involving actions. Talk about actions implied mental meanings with several elements, each having a different role and relationship to the others, depending on the participants in the action, for example, a child saying "cow," and moving to put the cow on top of a tower of blocks. Meanings with a focus on a single element, like holding out a spoon simply to show it to someone and saying "spoon," decreased as the children progressed from FW to VS. Thus, by the end of the period, the children were expressing more elaborate mental meanings: They were more likely to be talking about actions that they themselves were about to perform — their desires to do something. Such action expressions require that a child learn the verbs in a language and how verbs combine with other words the child might already know or learn. The increase in talk about actions, with the more elaborated mental meanings they entail, provides the impetus to learn the syntax of simple sentences.

✦ PHRASES AND SIMPLE SENTENCES

Combining words to form simple sentences is a great achievement. Children begin, tentatively at first, to put together words that they have already learned to say singly, for example, *more* and *juice* become *more juice*. They also might begin to repeat certain phrases that they've heard often, like *go byebye* and *all gone*, but these may well be learned as large whole phrases rather than combinations of the separate words. Certain of the meaning relations between words in children's earliest two- and three-word sentences are determined by particular words, for example, sentences with *no* mean nonexistence; sentences with *more* mean recurrence. Eventually, however, children begin to tap into the verb system of the language and to learn the structures and arrangements of words in sentences that are licensed by different verbs in the language. Most of the examples in the rest of this chapter come from the results of another investigation, by myself and my students, into the acquisition of simple and complex sentences by a different group of from 4 to 7 children as they acquired a grammar between 2 and 3 years of age (Bloom, 1991).

Most of the meaning relations in children's early sentences are determined by the verbs they learn; the development of verb relations — verbs combined with nouns or pronouns — is the foundation for their acquisition of grammar (e.g., Bloom, 1981; Bloom, Miller, & Hood, 1975; Tomasello, 1992). Children learn categories of verbs, and the different verbs determine sentence structures that are continuous with later syntax and the verb system of adult English. The three principal categories of verbs are action (e.g., *do, make, push, eat*), state (e.g., *be, have, want*), and locative action verbs (e.g., *go, put*). Sentences with action and locative verbs generally appear before sentences with state verbs. This finding confirms the importance of children's theories of objects, movement, and space, theories which had their beginnings in the cognitive development of early infancy.

Children also combine words with other meaning relations between them, for example, possession (*Mommy sock*), attribution (*big dog*), recurrence (*more milk*), negation (*no fit*), and so forth. With development, these separate relations are eventually embedded in verb relations to produce longer sentences. Examples are "Mommy drink more juice," "this lamb won't fit," and "I see boy's shoe."

Children differ, however, in whether they begin to combine verbs with nouns or pronouns in sentences (e.g., Bates, Bretherton,

& Snyder, 1988; Bloom, Lightbown, & Hood, 1975). Some children use nouns primarily and say things like "eat meat," "girl ride bike," "Mommy sock," "man making muffins." Other children tend to use more pronouns, with early sentences like "throw it," "my car," "I do it," "this go there." But regardless of how they start out — whether they are more likely to combine verbs with nouns or with pronouns — differences between children eventually diminish, and they become more similar to each other as they learn more about grammar and their sentences get longer. By the time the average length of children's sentences passes 2.5 words, they are no longer different in this respect. Regardless of how they start out, sentence subjects (*agents and actors*) become primarily pronominal and predicate objects (objects affected by the action named by a verb) are primarily nominal. Children also are able to switch between nouns and pronouns to mark differences in the situation or in interpersonal factors in conversations. For example, whether one says "the bus is coming" or "it's coming" depends on whether the hearer can know what *it* refers to. At the corner bus stop, "it's coming" will make sense, but in another context it might not.

Just as children differ in when they begin to say words and sentences, they also differ in how fast they progress in learning to say longer sentences with more complex structures. Figure 5–5 shows how differently four children increased in the average length of their sentences from their first tentative two- and three-word combinations just before 2 years of age until they were saying complex sentences at about age 3. Average length of sentences is frequently used to describe growth in language; the term used in the literature is **Mean Length of Utterance** or MLU. Progress in increasing MLU is shown here in relation to chronological age in months.

MLU is helpful for demonstrating individual differences, because it is an index of level of language development that can be used to compare children. Children of the same age can be very different in how much they know about language. We can talk about what the average 1-year-old or the average 2-year-old might know about language, but, in actuality, any group of 16-month-olds or 28-month-olds (or children of any age) will be very different from one another. For this reason, children are better equated on the basis of their language ability than on the basis of chronological age for research in language development and for assessment and intervention with children who have language problems.

However, MLU is only a superficial index of language development: It tells us how long a child's sentences tend to be, how fast a child is acquiring a grammar, and whether a child is similar to or different from other children of the same age. But MLU says nothing about what the child knows or is learning about the language,

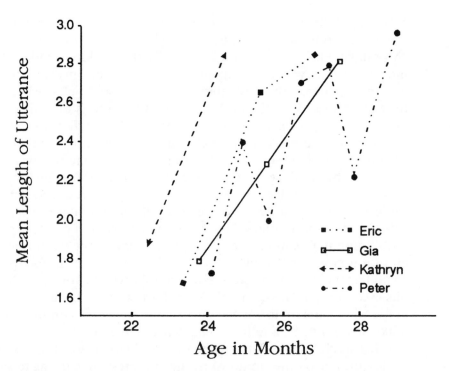

Figure 5–5. Increase in mean length of utterance (MLU) in relation to age by four children (Bloom, L., 1991. *Language development from two to three.* New York: Cambridge University Press, with permission).

aside from some very broad generalizations. An MLU between 1.3 and 2.0 usually means the child is limited to using single words and two-word or perhaps a few three-word phrases. Once MLU passes 2.0, utterance length increases when children begin to combine their two- and three-word phrases into longer sentences with negation, noun and verb inflections (endings like *-ing, -ed, -s*), asking questions, and the like. An MLU greater than 3.0 typically means a child has begun to learn something about complex sentences. These are the developments in language we will be concerned with in the rest of this chapter.

Negation in Simple Sentences

Negation is one of the earliest meanings in children's first word combinations, with phrases like "no fit," "no pocket in there," "no more cheese," and "milk all gone." Several things happen with the development of negation in simple sentences. First, there is development in content, with different meanings of negation in sentences; these meanings are, in general, nonexistence, rejection, and denial. The meanings nonexistence, rejection, and denial are quite general, and finer distinctions are possible: for example, nonoccurrence and disappearance in the nonexistence category; refusal and prohibition in the rejection category. Second, the forms of negation change from simple *no* or *no more* to more complex sentences with forms like *not, don't,* and *can't;* and the forms of sentences with different content become complex in different ways (Bloom, 1991).

The sequence in which children learn the different content categories of negation is based, first, on the order in which words and then sentences with these meanings appear over time. In the single-word period, 1-year-olds tend to express rejection most often, with the single word *no.* When they begin to combine words in phrases, however, they typically combine *no* or perhaps *all gone* or *no more* with other words to express nonexistence or disappearance. Thus, the first meaning of negation is rejection, with *no* as a single word, but early sentences tend to express nonexistence before rejection. This is because something that doesn't exist or that disappears needs to be expressed because it is simply not there; what the child has in mind (the absent object or event) is discrepant from what the listener has in mind and needs to be expressed. But rejection involves turning away from or pushing away something that is evident in the situation, and the single word "no" is enough. Thus, a child needs to say what it is that is nonexistent for someone else to know it, but when the child pushes away or turns away from something that can be seen in the context, the meaning is clear.

The number of sentences a child says with these different meanings changes over time; sentences expressing nonexistence are frequent at the same time that sentences expressing rejection and denial are infrequent. This development can be seen below in all the negative expressions over a period of about 7 hours by a child, Eric, when he was 22 months and his MLU was 1.42.

All Negative Words and Sentences Said by Eric at 22 months Expressing Nonexistence, Rejection, and Denial.

NONEXISTENCE	REJECTION	DENIAL
no more (8 times) no (2 times)	no (22 times)	
no more noise (13 times)	no train	no more birdie

(continued)

NONEXISTENCE	REJECTION	DENIAL
no more light (2 times)	no more dumpcar	no more blocks
no more car (2 times)	a want any shoes	
no more seal		
no more airplane		
no more round		
no more apple		
no more dumpcar		
a no more		
no go in		
no goes		
no ready go		
no fit		
no, it won't fit		

(Adapted from Bloom, L., 1991. *Language development from two to three.* New York: Cambridge University Press, p. 168).

The forms of sentences with different meanings also develop sequentially. Eric's earliest sentences expressed nonexistence with *no more* or *no* at the same time that the meaning of rejection was expressed most often with the single word *no*. When sentences began to express other meanings, first rejection and then denial, their structure was similar to the sentences learned earlier that expressed nonexistence, and the forms of sentences with different content were not different. Typically, they consisted of *no* or *no more* and another word, for example, "no more airplane" (nonexistence), "no more dumpcar" (rejection).

Thus, new content in sentences (first rejection and then denial) was learned originally with the old forms that had been first learned for expressing nonexistence. Later development consisted of learning new forms for expressing what was, by then, old content (Bloom, 1970). This developmental finding was consistent with a basic principle of development that Heinz Werner (Werner & Kaplan, 1963) had proposed years earlier: "Novel [content] is first executed through old, available forms; sooner or later, of course, there is pressure towards the development of new forms which are of a more [content] specific character, i.e., that will serve the new [content] better than the older forms" (p. 60).

Sentences expressing nonexistence developed and became more complex before sentences expressing rejection; rejection sentences became more complex before sentences that expressed denial. Eventually, different syntactic forms predominated to express the three different content categories of negation. We can see this development for Eric, almost 5 months later, with some examples of his many negative sentences when he was 26 months, 3 weeks old, and his MLU was 2.84 words.

Examples of Negative Sentences with Different Content and Form, Said by Eric almost 5 months later, at 26 months, 3 weeks and MLU = 2.84.

NONEXISTENCE	REJECTION	DENIAL
no more lollipop	no playing	that not lollipop
no choochoo train (4 times)	don't touch it	that's a not bridge
it doesn't go	dont' eat it	no, not a yellow
it doesn't fit	don't fall down	
I can't climb up	no, don't touch it	
		I can't find the bridge
		etc.
I couldn't see them		
	etc.	
etc.		
(TOTAL = 34)	(TOTAL = 13)	(TOTAL = 5)

(Adapted from Bloom, L., 1991. *Language development from two to three.* New York: Cambridge University Press, p. 195).

Development in the form of sentences was not simply a matter of adding more words or even of simply adding a negative word like *no, not, don't,* or *can't* to an otherwise positive sentence. The complexity of adding negation to a sentence had its cost, and this most often took the form of leaving out the sentence subject or some other part of the sentence. Thus, negative sentences often were shorter than affirmative sentences, even though or, more accurately, **because** they included the negation. This finding, among others, shows us how children struggle with learning the structures of grammar as different aspects of the language they are learning compete with one another. For example, sentences are also shorter when a child is using new words or responding to the demands of certain kinds of conversation (as we shall see in the last section). MLU indicates sentences increase in length with development, but children are not just adding words together to make their sentences longer.

Verb Inflections and Simple Sentences

One of the earliest developments in children's simple sentences is the addition of -s to nouns and inflections to verbs — the endings -ed, -ing, -s and the use of irregular verbs to indicate past tense, like *sang, ate,* and *did.* These additions to verbs are not automatically added to any or all of a child's verbs. Again, the verbs children learn determine how they learn the verb inflections, and they learn particular endings for different categories of verbs.

Certain verbs are very frequent in children's early speech, and they function like all purpose pro-verbs (similar to the way that pronouns can stand in for nouns). The most frequent of these are *do* and *go,* and they occur with all the inflections — children say *did, doing, gone, going* virtually from the beginning. However, other, more descriptive verbs, like *run, eat,* and *jump* take different inflections according to their inherent aspectual meaning. Aspectual meaning comes from the temporal shape of an event named by a verb: how long the event lasts and whether it has a clear end result, for example. Some verbs name events that last over time; they are durative, for example, *run, draw, try,* and *sit.* These verbs typically are the ones for which children learn the present, progressive ending -*ing,* for example, *running, drawing, trying, sitting.* Other verbs name events that are momentary and last a very short time, with a clear end result, for example, *jump, bite, touch, throw, break.* Momentary events with a completed end state like *jump* and *break* are most likely to occur with -*ed (jumped)* and irregular past *(broke)* than with -*ing.* Developmentally, then, aspect is a strong influence in guiding children in how they acquire verb inflections. The notion "aspect before tense" captures the general finding that aspectual distinctions — in particular, the duration of an event and whether it has an end state — are developmentally salient. Aspect leads the child in learning how to mark verbs for present and past tense.

Children's Early Questions

Children soon learn to turn their simple sentences with verbs into questions, using the familiar *Wh*-words: *What, Who, Where, Why, How, Which,* and *When.* The same simple sentence can be transformed into all of these different kinds of questions.

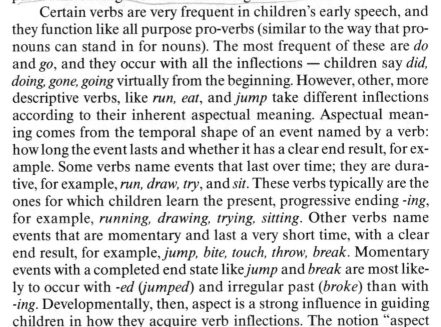

Taking, for example, the simple sentence "The girl rode her bike down the street," we could ask:

Who rode the bike?

What did the girl ride?

Where did the girl ride her bike?

Why did the girl ride her bike down the street?

When did the girl ride her bike?

Whose bike did the girl ride?

How did the girl ride the bike?

And so on.

Children learn both to ask these questions and to answer them, when they are asked by other persons, in a particular order. *What, where*, and *who* are learned before *why, how, which*, and *when*, and this sequence is shown in Figure 5-6 for a group of seven children who were studied between 2 and 3 years of age. Children learning different languages learn to ask questions in this same sequence. And children who learn a second language at a later age, for exam-

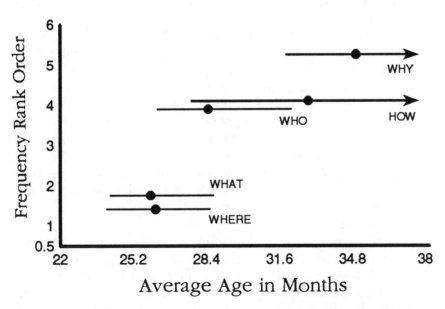

Figure 5-6. Sequence of development of *Wh*-questions, 7 children: Average age and ranges in age, in relation to average rank order of overall frequency (Adapted from Bloom, L., Merkin, W., & Wootten, J., 1982. *Wh*-questions: Linguistic factors that contribute to the sequence of acquisition. *Child Development, 53*, 1084–1092).

ple English-speaking children in Montreal who entered French-speaking schools at 5 or 6 years old, show the same sequence in learning the second language (Lightbown, 1978).

Several things contribute to this developmental sequence. One is that the question words themselves have different functions in the sentence. So, for example, in the sentence "The girl rode her bike down the street," *what, where, who* each ask about a particular part of the sentence, such as the subject (the girl is *who*) or object (the bike is *what*) or place (down the street is *where*). In contrast, *how, why*, and *when* ask about the entire event that the sentence is about: *How, Why, When* [did the girl ride her bike down the street?]

Learning to ask questions with the *Wh*-question words also depended on the difference between pro-verbs (all purpose verbs like *do* or *go* that can stand for other verbs) and descriptive verbs (like *run, jump, eat*, and *play*). The earliest questions, with *what, where*, and *who*, occurred with the copula (forms of *be*, for example, "Where is it?" or "What's that?") or with the small group of pro-verbs which were the children's most frequent verbs: *do, go*, and *happen*. Thus, just as the children first learned verb inflections with the pro-verbs, they also began to learn how to ask questions with the well-known and frequent *be*-forms and the pro-verbs. In contrast, the *Wh*-questions acquired later, *how, why, when*, were more likely to occur with descriptive verbs like *sing, jump*, and *break* which are more complex in their meaning content. The same group of seven children asked a total of 5,594 questions with these words, and the percentages of the different kinds of questions they asked with either pro-verbs or descriptive verbs can be seen in Figure 5–7.

Thus, two aspects of form and content contribute to the sequence in which children learn to ask questions with **Wh-question words**. One has to do with what the question word itself is asking for. And the other is the verbs children know. *What, where*, and *who*, the earlier learned questions, ask about one part of the sentence, with the frequent, familiar pro-verbs like *be, do, go*. *Why, how*, and *when* ask about the idea expressed in the whole sentence; they use more demanding descriptive verbs like *eat, ride*, and *throw*; and they are learned later.

Finally, questions also differ in how they are used by children in conversations. Overall, children are more likely to ask questions when they are introducing the topic of conversation; they are less likely, in general, to respond to what someone else says by asking a question. However, one question type — *Why* questions — is more likely than the others to be used in responding to what someone else says. And often, those *Why* questions have to do with some element of negation, for example:

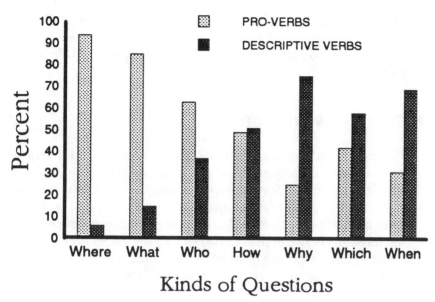

Figure 5–7. Use of different kinds of verbs in children's *Wh*-questions (Adapted from Bloom, L., Merkin, W., & Wootten, J., 1982. *Wh*-questions: Linguistic factors that contribute to the sequence of acquisition. *Child Development, 53*, 1084–1092).

David wants two pieces of bread;
His mother takes one piece and says

"I'll cut it so you'll have two."

And David says

"No, don't cut them.
Why you go an cut them?"

In sum, children learn to ask *Wh*-questions in a particular order, but in the context of learning the form and content of both the *Wh*-words and verbs, and their use in conversational discourse. Linguistic factors, together with other conceptual and pragmatic factors, contribute to the cognitive requirements for learning to ask questions.

The example just given, shows a child saying two sentences, one after the other; in this case, one was a simple sentence with negation ("No, don't cut them"), and the other was a simple sentence in the form of a question ("Why you go an cut them?"). Once children can say two simple sentences in a row like this, they can begin to learn how to combine two simple sentences to produce a complex sentence.

◆ COMPLEX SENTENCES

Having learned something about simple sentences, children between 2 and 3 years of age begin to combine the structures underlying their simple sentences to form complex sentences. One aspect of the development of complex sentences has to do with content: Children learn complex sentences in the first place to express particular meaning relations between the the two simple sentences they connect. At first, the only meaning is additive: two sentences are just added together, with no new meaning between them.

Additive Sentences

Adult: "Can you carry this for me very carefully?"

Kathryn: "Maybe you can carry that *and* I can carry this."

(Eric looking at a picture book)

Eric: "They're taking a vacuum cleaner *and* puppy dog's running."

Once children learn to simply add two sentences together without another meaning relation, they can begin to talk about more complex meanings, such as time and causality.

Temporal Sentences

(Kathryn pushing a toy car)

Kathryn: "I going this way to get the groceries *then* come back."

(Peter and adult looking for a lost toy)

> **Peter:** "You better look for it *when* you get back home."

Additive meaning is a part of temporal meaning; both things ("going this way" and "get the groceries") are happening. But a new meaning is added: the fact that the two things happen in a particular order (in the first example, you have to "go this way" **before** you can "get the groceries," and in the second example, you can "look for it" **after** "you get back home"). Both additive and temporal meanings also contribute to the third meaning of complex sentences, causality.

Causal Sentences

(Kathryn giving a little toy man to mother)

> **Kathryn:** "Maybe you can bend him *so* he can sit."

(Eric going towards a pile of toys)

> **Eric:** "Get them *cause* I want it."

In expressing **causality**, two things are necessarily added together ("bend him" and "he can sit"), and added together in a particular temporal order (first, it is necessary to bend the little toy man, **and then** he can sit). Here the element of causality is new: The little toy man can sit because he is bent; Eric goes to get the toys **because** he wants them. Thus, the meanings of complex sentences are cumulative: They build on one another. They also develop in a particular order. Children learn to express simple additivity with complex sentences before they learn to express temporal meaning relations, and they learn to express temporal meaning relations before they learn to express causality.

The second aspect of what children learn about complex sentences has to do with form. Children acquire the connecting words — like *and, because, so, then, but, if* — which connect two clauses to express these meanings. The first syntactic connective children acquire, in virtually all the languages of the world, is *and.* Because the earliest meaning of complex sentences is simple additive, that is not surprising: Children learn to add simple sentences and connect them with *and*. What is surprising is the fact that *and* also is used at first to express temporal and causal meanings. An example of a temporal sentence with *and* is "Jocelyn's going home *and* take her sweater off"; an example of causality with *and* is "She put a band aid on her shoe *and* it maked it feel better."

The other connectives are more specific in their meanings, and they are learned later with the different meanings of complex sentences, for example, *then* and *when* with temporal relations, *because* and *so* with causal relations. This is another instance of learning new forms (in this case, the different connective forms) to express old content (the meaning relations the children had already learned to express earlier with *and*).

Another aspect of form is that children acquire different structures for complex sentences. So far, we have been describing only one kind of complex sentences, those with the syntactic structure conjunction ("You carry this one and I carry that one" or "Maybe you can bend him so he can sit"). Another syntactic structure is complementation, where a particular verb in a simple sentence takes another simple sentence to complete (or complement) its meaning. The content of complementation sentences is determined by the meaning of the complement-taking verb. Certain of these verbs that children learn express their intention to do something: verbs like *want to, like to, have to, need to, try to*. Other verbs express their perceptions, what a child sees: verbs like *see, look (at), watch, show*. Still other verbs express an epistemic meaning which has to do with an aspect of the child's thinking: verbs like *think, know, forget, wonder, remember*.

Examples of Complementation in Complex Sentences

Intention Verbs:

"*Wanna* go playground."
"I *gonna* get it."
"I *want to* see Mommy."
"I *want* Mommy get balloon."

Perception Verbs:

"I *see* two bus come there."
"*Look* what my mommy got me."
"I'll *see* where it is."
"Let's *see* what's in the train."

Epistemic Verbs:

"I *think* the children go to bed."
"You *know* what's in this bag?"
"I *think* it's big enough.
"*Know* what's in here?"

(Adapted from Bloom, L., 1991. *Language development from two to three.* New York: Cambridge University Press.)

Again, as with other aspects of language development, the children we studied differed in how old they were when they acquired the different aspects of complex sentences. The children learned the content of complex sentences in the same order: the meanings additive before temporal before causal. However their ages were very different when they learned each of these. For example, they ranged in age from about 26.3 months to 31.5 months when they expressed temporal meaning in complex sentences, and from about 26.5 months to 31.3 months when they learned to express causality in complex sentences. The children were even more variable in when they learned the different syntactic connectives in complex sentences. The connective *and* was always learned first, and was learned at about the same time by the four different children in our studies: between 25 and 27 months of age. However, the other connectives were learned at very different ages; for example, the children differed by about 8 months in when they learned *because*, and by as much as 10 months in when they learned *so, then*, and *where* as connectives.

✦ EXPRESSION OF CAUSALITY

Finally, we will take one kind of complex sentence that children learn, causality, and describe it in more detail because it is particularly important to other aspects of a child's development. The notion of causality pervades just about all that we do and think about in the course of a day; things do not ordinarily happen just by chance. Instead, people do things that have a particular effect on how they and other persons think, feel, and do things. And most of the things that people do have reasons. Learning the language of causality is fundamental to the negotiations that are a part of the give and take of everyday life. Thus, acquisition of the form, content, and use of expressions of causality is important to many aspects of children's social and emotional development, as well as to their language development.

The famous Swiss scientist, Jean Piaget (1954), described how the concept of causality begins to develop in the first year of life: Very young infants soon learn to associate means with an end and to anticipate the consequences of their actions. However, Piaget, along with the other important developmental theorists, Heinz Werner and Lev Vygotsky, believed that true causal understanding develops slowly and is not in place until children are about 7 or 8 years old. They thought that younger children are aware of the temporal relations between events but cannot always appreciate the causal dependency between them.

However, we know from the development of complex sentences that 2-year-old children give every indication that they appreciate more than just the additive and temporal relations in causal connections. Earlier research had presented children with sequential actions using physical objects and asked them to talk about these events, which were external to their own beliefs, feelings, and desires. However, the causal sentences of 2-year-old children are most often about their causal intentions and motivations in everyday interactions. The children we studied clearly understood the causal connections between events and/or states and learned how to express causal content when it was relevant to the circumstances of their everyday lives.

With respect to both form and use, expressions of causality developed in a particular order (Hood & Bloom, 1979). The children learned to make causal statements, before they learned to respond appropriately when someone asked them a *Why* question. And they learned to respond to other person's *Why* questions, before they learned to ask *Why* questions themselves. Thus, children learn to respond appropriately to causal questions only after they express causality in their own statements and before they began to ask *Why* questions themselves. Statements, responses, and questions are fundamentally different kinds of events. Children are able to express their own semantic intention (in making a statement), before saying something that is influenced by what someone else said (in a response to someone else's question) which, in turn, is easier than asking about the intention of another (with a *Why* question). The children progressed from expressing their own intentions when making a causal statement to taking the listener's intentions into account when asking a *Why* question.

With respect to language content, children express both subjective and objective meanings in their causal statements, and these have to do with the reasons or results of actions (Bloom & Capatides, 1987b). But they expressed subjective meaning more frequently. Subjective causal meaning has to do with personal, emotional content, for example: "I was crying because I didn't want to wake up because it was dark, so dark." And subjective meaning was also concerned with social and cultural conventions, for example: "this [car] can't go . . . because that sign [traffic light] doesn't say go." Subjective causal connections are not fixed or self-evident in the physical world. Instead, they are social constructions and are learned largely from the language children hear. For example, waking up in the dark can be frightening, and children often cry when they awaken at night. In comforting them, parents provide the language of explanation that socializes the child's experience and expression of emotion (Kopp, 1987; Thompson, 1990). Eventually, this language is reflected in a child's own talk about the causes and circumstances of their feelings in events of the same kind.

SUBJECTIVE CAUSALITY has to do with Personal Reasons, for example:

"I'll help you if you have a little trouble."

or Emotional Reasons, for example:

"Wait my mommy comes . . . because I will be lonely."

or Social Reasons, for example:

Adult: "Why do you have him? (guinea pig) Did you take him home from school?"

> **Peter:** "Yeah, cause they don't belong in school."

OBJECTIVE CAUSALITY has to do with Consequences, for example:

"I don't have a Christmas tree . . . because throw it out."

or Relationships between Means and Ends, for example:

"I'm gonna pick this up so it can't step on the cord."

or Conditions, for example:

"You can't see it cause it's way inside."

Objective causal meaning has to do with action-based, means-end, and consequence relations. These were evident (perceptible or imaginable) and fixed in the physical order of things that result from actions in everyday events. Objective meanings are a continuity in language of the kinds of sensorimotor causality described in the actions of infancy (Piaget, 1954). For example, a child learns that a pull-toy will roll over a wire in its path from their actions with pull toys, leading the child to eventually learn to say "I'm gonna pick this up so it can't step on the cord."

Objective causal meanings were less frequent than subjective causal meanings. However, learning the syntactic connectives *and, because*, and *so* was associated, at first, with objective meanings. The children already knew something about objective causes and consequences in infancy. Thus, learning these forms was made easier with familiar and well-established content that was evident and verifiable in the physical context. This early association of connectives with objective meanings is another instance of learning new forms (syntactic connectives) with old content (the objective, perceptible means-end and consequence relations discovered in infancy). Learning to use the same connectives with subjective meanings later was, in turn, an instance of learning old forms with new content (see Bloom, 1970, regarding acquiring the forms and functions of negation).

In summary, the construction of a theory of causality begins in infancy with the early understanding of the relationship between change and the actions of oneself and others that bring about change. Before language, these actions are evident because they are perceptible; they are the child's only source of causal understanding and they later appear in complex sentences between 2 and 3 years of age in expression of objective causal meanings. As language is acquired, children can learn about other sorts of causal attributions from the language they hear the adults and older children around them using. As a result, they learn about social, personal, and culturally based causal connections and learn to talk about these in their subjective causal statements.

The maxim — new forms are learned with old content; new content is learned with old forms — has surfaced now in a number of places in this account of early language development. It has been observed in other contexts of language acquisition elsewhere and has even been given the status of a "basic operating principle" for language acquisition (Slobin, 1973, 1985). It means that children do not just add new aspects of language to their knowledge one at a time. Language development does not proceed in a straight line. Rather, the process of language development is synergistic, which means it requires cooperation and collaboration among the many aspects of language that are being learned. Think of how difficult it would be to learn something that is wholly new to you; learning is always helped by putting it into a familiar context. In the same way, children acquire the many aspects of language in relation to one another; this is why they learn new forms to express something they already know about and often learn to express new ideas using forms with which they are already familiar and comfortable.

old forms

◆ CHILDREN'S CONVERSATIONS

A major goal of language acquisition is for children to be able to take something from what an adult says and use it to form a related message. That is what converts simple turn-taking, before language, into conversational discourse, with language. Conversational discourse arguably is the most important use we make of language. We began this chapter by pointing out that infants acquire language to share what they and others have in mind. It should not be surprising, therefore, that sharing the topic of conversation is an important aspect of this development.

Conversations between adults and children ordinarily are studied by examining the form and content relationships between them when their messages share the same topic. We all know the tendency some children have to imitate what they hear others say. It turns out that repeating what an adult says is the earliest way in which children learn to share the topic in conversation. At first they simply repeat part or all of the adult's message. Soon, however, they repeat and also add something new. And, eventually, they repeat, add to, and also change something in the adult expression.

In our studies of discourse, child words and sentences were most often adjacent to — that is, they occurred immediately after — someone else had said something (Bloom, Margulis, Tinker, Rebello, & Fujita, 1993; Bloom, Rocissano, & Hood, 1976). This is not surprising, because we know that even when infants are only a few months old, they can take turns in vocalizing with an adult who is responding to them. However, once language begins, most child utterances that are adjacent to adult utterances do not share the same topic, for example:

Adult and child are looking out the window

Adult: "Where are the children?"

           Child: "want get down."
           (Climbing off the window ledge)

When adjacent child utterances begin to be contingent on adult utterances, they very often are imitations, sharing the same topic and form but not adding anything new, for example:

Adult: "She might pinch her fingers"

                    Child: "pinch her fingers."

An adjacent utterance is contingent when it shares the same topic and also adds new information to the preceding adult message, for example:

Adult: "I'm gonna build a high house"

                    Child: "I wanta build a high house too."

Development in the conversations of the children we have studied is shown in Figure 5–8, for the period from 21 months of age (Stage 1) to 36 months (Stage 3). Four categories of discourse are shown:

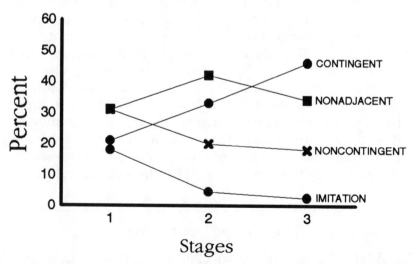

Figure 5–8. Developments in categories of discourse (Adapted from Bloom, L., Rocissano, L., & Hood, L., 1976. Adult-child discourse: Developmental interaction between information processing and linguistic knowledge. *Cognitive Psychology, 8,* 521–552).

nonadjacent speech, and three kinds of adjacent speech: contingent, noncontingent, and imitations. Nonadjacent (or adjacent) speech did not change. The major development was the increase in contingent speech; child responses that shared the topic of a previous message and added something new increased through the period. Adjacent speech that was not contingent and simple imitation, in which aspects of both form and content are shared but nothing new is added, decreased.

By the time children begin to say words at the end of the first year, they already know a basic rule of discourse: to say something after someone else says something. However, child utterances often are noncontingent until syntax is well underway. This means that, even though they engage in turn-taking, children are more apt to introduce a new topic or to change the topic. Between 2 and 3 years of age, contingent messages that share the topic of a prior utterance and add new information increase, as noncontingent messages and simple imitation decrease.

Developments in conversational discourse are a major aspect of language use, and they occur along with developments in other aspects of language. Children learn language form and content at the same time they are learning how to use language in conversation. We have already seen how learning one aspect of language often has a cognitive cost and influences other aspects. One example is leaving out sentence subjects in negative sentences. Another example is that children ordinarily do not ask topic-related questions for a long time. Although conversational contingency increases, and children also are asking many questions in this period of time, contingent responses generally are not questions. By the time the children we studied were 3 years old, contingent responses were more likely to be questions, particularly *Why* questions, but this was so less than 15% of the time.

The following dinner table exchange provides a good example of many of the things we've been talking about in this chapter.

At the Dinner Table:

        Child: "Do you perfer cheddar cheese?"

Mom: "no"

        Child: "Why don't you?"

Mom: "Because I like the taste of muenster better"

        Child: "Why don't like taste of of cheddar?"

This child was 2 years, 10 months old. Her question, "Do you perfer cheddar cheese?" began this conversational exchange. When she responded to her mother's answer, it was with a *Why* question. When she asked her mother "Why don't like taste of of cheddar?" her question was contingent, because it shared the same topic in her mother's sentence, and it also expressed negation. But it also showed some wear and tear, with omission of "you" and the dysfluency "of of." At the end of the period we have covered in this chapter, then, children are asking contingent questions, and even asking negative questions, but they are not asking them frequently or easily.

To participate in conversations, children must be able to take something they hear someone else say, use it as a cue to access something stored in memory, and create a mental meaning. They then have to hold that mental meaning in mind while they access the words and sentence procedures needed to express it. At the same time they are learning to do this, between 2 and 3 years of age, they also are acquiring the words and grammar of the language. It is not so easy, and children work hard at it. They take an active part in working at what and how they learn from the speech they hear. Language development is an active process, not a passive one, and a child doesn't just soak up words and sentences like a sponge. This chapter has been about the process of language development — about what and how children learn when they acquire the power of expression in the first few years of life. It is a process that will continue throughout the school years.

◆ SUMMARY

A great deal happens in the first year of life to make it possible for children to say their first tentative words, some time near the beginning of the second year. In the first few months of life, infants' cries and whimpers, coos and chortles, express something of what they are feeling and, at the same time, provide the groundwork out of which the sounds of speech will develop for the forms of language. By the time they reach their first birthday, infants also have learned a great deal about the world of persons and objects, and this knowledge contributes to what they learn about language content and use. Words are acquired slowly at first, but the pace picks up toward the end of the second year with a vocabulary spurt, when children suddenly learn a great many new words and use their words more easily. Soon, they begin to combine words to form phrases and simple sentences. This marks the beginning of a grammar. Acquiring the grammar of a language depends on learning verbs and the meanings and arrangements of verbs in relation to nouns and pronouns.

Simple sentences increase in complexity as children learn negation, inflectional endings on nouns and verbs, and how to ask questions. They soon learn to combine the structures underlying their simple sentences to learn complex sentences that express more complex meanings, like causality. And, at the same time that children are learning words and simple and complex sentences, they are learning how to participate in conversations by sharing the topic of what someone else has just said.

Several themes have been woven together in this story of language development. The first is that children learn language, in the first place, for sharing the contents of mind in acts of expression and interpretation. **Language as expression** is basic for language development. Language is the means of expression that a society has for taking the thoughts and feelings of individuals and making them public, so that other persons can know and share them. The second theme is the developmental principle: Children acquire language in relation to their social and emotional development and other aspects of their cognitive development; language is not learned for its own sake. And a third theme is that language development is an active process. Children work at learning language, because it does not happen easily or automatically. Language development requires collaboration among the several aspects of vocabulary, grammar, and conversational discourse; and these things are not just added together. And, finally, children are similar in many respects in their language development, but they also differ in important respects. Most importantly, children differ widely in age of onset and in how fast they progress in learning language. But barring any interfering internal or external factors, virtually all children acquire language. Students of communication disorders need to understand how that happens to be able to understand and help children for whom language learning is particularly slow or difficult. That has been the aim of this chapter.

◆ ACKNOWLEDGEMENT

Much of the material in this chapter has been drawn from my two recent books (Bloom, L., 1991, *Language development from two to three*, and Bloom, L., 1993, *The transition from infancy to language: Acquiring the power of expression*). I thank Margaret Lahey for her helpful, constructive comments after reading an early draft of this chapter.

◆ REFERENCES

Baillargeon, R. (1992). The object concept revisited: New directions in the investigation of infants' physical knowledge. In C. Granrud (Ed.),

Carnegie-Mellon Symposium on Cognition, Vol. 23. Visual perception and cognition in infancy (pp. 265–315). Hillsdale, NJ: Lawrence Erlbaum.

Baker, C., & McCarthy, J. (Eds.). (1981). *The logical problem of language acquisition.* Cambridge, MA: The MIT Press.

Bates, E. (1976). *Language in context.* New York: Academic Press.

Bates, E., Bretherton, I., & Snyder, L. (1988). *From first words to grammar.* Cambridge: Cambridge University Press.

Bloom, L. (1970). *Language development: Form and function in emerging grammars.* Cambridge, MA: The MIT Press. (Original doctoral dissertation, Teachers College, Columbia University, 1968).

Bloom, L. (1973). *One word at a time: The use of single-word utterances before syntax.* The Hague: Mouton.

Bloom, L. (1981). The importance of language for language development: Linguistic determinism in the 1980s. In H. Winitz (Ed.), *Native language and foreign language acquisition* (pp. 160–171). New York: The New York Academy of Sciences.

Bloom, L. (1991). *Language development from two to three.* New York: Cambridge University Press.

Bloom, L. (1993). *The transition from infancy to language: Acquiring the power of expression.* New York: Cambridge University Press.

Bloom, L., & Beckwith, R. (1989). Talking with feeling: Integrating affective and linguistic expression in early language development. *Cognition and Emotion, 3,* 313–342.

Bloom, L., Beckwith, R., Capatides, J., & Hafitz, J. (1988). Expression through affect and words in the transition from infancy to language. In P. Baltes, D. Featherman, & R. Lerner (Eds.), *Life-span development and behavior* (Vol. 8, pp. 99–127). Hillsdale, NJ: Lawrence Erlbaum.

Bloom, L., & Capatides, J. (1987a). Expression of affect and the emergence of language. *Child Development, 58,* 1513–1522.

Bloom, L., & Capatides, J. (1987b). Sources of meaning in complex syntax: The sample case of causality. *Journal of Experimental Child Psychology, 43,* 112–128.

Bloom, L., & Lahey, M. (1978). *Language development and language disorders.* New York: John Wiley.

Bloom, L., Lightbown, P., & Hood, L. (1975). Structure and variation in child language. *Monographs of the Society for Research in Child Development, 40* (Serial No. 160).

Bloom, L., Margulis, C., Tinker, E., Rebello, P., & Fujita, N. (1993). Contingencies between child and mother talk in the single-word period of language development. Manuscript.

Bloom, L., Merkin, W., & Wootten, J. (1982). *Wh*-questions: Linguistic factors that contribute to the sequence of acquisition. *Child Development, 53,* 1084–1092.

Bloom, L., Miller, P., & Hood, L. (1975). Variation and reduction as aspects of competence in language development. In A. Pick (Ed.), *Minnesota Symposia on Child Psychology*, (Vol. 9, pp. 3–55). Minneapolis, MN: University of Minnesota Press. Reprinted in L. Bloom (1991). *Language development from two to three* (pp. 86–142). New York: Cambridge University Press.

Bloom, L., Rispoli, M., Gartner, B., & Hafitz, J. (1989). Acquisition of complementation. *Journal of Child Language, 16,* 101–120.

Bloom, L., Rocissano, L., & Hood, L. (1976). Adult-child discourse: Developmental interaction between information processing and linguistic knowledge. *Cognitive Psychology, 8,* 521–552.

Bloom, L., Tinker, E., & Margulis, C. (1993) The words children learn: Evidence against a noun bias in early vocabularies. *Cognitive Development, 8,* 431–450.

Bruner, J. (1983). *Child's talk: Learning to use language.* New York: W. W. Norton.

Danto, A. (1973). *Analytical philosophy of action.* Cambridge: Cambridge University Press.

Darwin, C. (1892/1913). *The expression of the emotions in man and animals.* New York: Appleton.

DeCasper, A., & Fifer, W. (1980). Of human bonding: Newborns prefer their mothers' voices. *Science, 208,* 1174–1176.

Eimas, P., Siqueland, E., Jusczyk, P., & Vigorito, J. (1971). Speech perception in infants. *Science, 171,* 303–306.

Ervin-Tripp, S. (1973). *Language acquisition and communicative choice: Essays by Susan M. Ervin-Tripp.* Palo Alto, CA: Stanford University Press.

Gopnik, A. (1988). Three types of early word: The emergence of social words, names and cognitive-relational words in the one-word stage and their relation to cognitive development. *First Language, 8,* 49–70.

Hampson, J., & Nelson, K. (1993). The relation of maternal language to variation in rate and style of language acquisition. *Journal of Child Language, 20,* 313–342.

Hood, L., & Bloom, L. (1979). What, when, and how about why: A longitudinal study of early expressions of causality. *Monographs of the Society for Research in Child Development, 44,* No. 6.

Hyams, N. (1986). *Language acquisition and the theory of parameters.* Dordrecht: Reidel.

Izard, C., & Malatesta, C. (1987). Perspectives on emotional development. I. Differential emotions theory of early emotional development. In J. Osofsky (Ed.), *Handbook of infant development* (pp. 494–554). New York: John Wiley.

Jackendoff, R. (1983). *Semantics and cognition.* Cambridge, MA: MIT Press.

Keil, F. (1989). *Concepts, kinds, and cognitive development.* Cambridge, MA: MIT Press.

Keil, F. (1991). Theories, concepts, and the acquisition of word meaning. In S. Gelman & J. Byrnes (Eds.), *Perspectives on thought and language: Interrelations in development* (pp. 197–221). Cambridge: Cambridge University Press.

Kopp, C. (1987). The growth of self-regulation: Caregivers and children. In N. Eisenberg (Ed.), *Contemporary topics in developmental psychology* (pp. 34–55). New York: John Wiley.

Lahey, M. (1988). *Language disorders and language development.* New York: Macmillan.

Lightbown, P. (1978). Question form and question function in the speech of young French L$_2$ learners. In M. Paradis (Ed.), *Aspects of bilingualism* (pp. 22–43). Columbia, SC: Hornbeam.

Masur, E. (1982). Mothers' responses to infants' object-related gestures: Influences on lexical development. *Journal of Child Language, 9,* 23–30.

Mervis, C. (1987). Child-basic object categories and early lexical development. In U. Neisser (Ed.), *Concepts and conceptual development: Ecological and intellectual factors in categorization* (pp. 201–233). Cambridge: Cambridge University Press.

Moscovitch (Ed.) (1984). *Infant memory: Its relation to normal and pathological memory in humans and other animals.* New York: Plenum Press.

Murphy, D., & Medin, D. (1985). The role of theories in conceptual coherence. *Psychological Review, 92,* 289–316.

Nelson, K. (1973). Structure and strategy in learning to talk. *Monographs of the Society for Research in Child Development, 38,* No. 149.

Nelson, K. (1974). Concept, word and sentence: Interrelations in acquisition and development. *Psychological Review, 81,* 267–285.

Nelson, K., Hampson, J., & Shaw, L. (1993). Nouns in early lexicons: Evidence, explanations, and implications. *Journal of Child Language, 20,* 61–84

Oatley, K. (1992). *Best laid schemes: The psychology of emotions.* Cambridge: Cambridge University Press.

Ochs, E., & Schieffelin, B. (1983). *Acquiring conversational competence.* London: Routledge & Kegan Paul.

Oller, K. (1980). The emergence of the sounds of speech in infancy. In G. Yeni-Komshian, J. Kavanagh, & C. Ferguson (Eds.), *Child phonology. I: Production* (pp. 93–112). New York: Academic Press.

Oller, K., & Eilers, R. (1992). Development of vocal signaling in human infants: Toward a methodology for cross-species vocalization comparisons. In H. Papousek, U. Jurgens, & H. Papousek (Eds.), *Nonverbal vocal communication* (pp. 174–191). New York: Cambridge University Press.

Piaget, J. (1954). *The construction of reality in the child.* New York: Basic. (Original work published 1937; Ballantine Books edition published 1971)

Piaget, J. (1960). *The psychology of intelligence.* Paterson, NJ: Littlefield, Adams. (Original work published 1947)

Pine, J. (1992). How referential are "referential" children? Relationship between maternal report and observational measures of vocal composition and usage. *Journal of Child Language, 19,* 75–86.

Pinker, S. (1984). *Language learnability and language development.* Cambridge, MA: Harvard University.

Radford, A. (1990). *Syntactic theory and the acquisition of English syntax.* Oxford: Basil Blackwell.

Schieffelin, B. (1990). *The give and take of everyday life: Language socialization of Kaluli Children.* New York: Cambridge University Press.

Schieffelin, B., & Ochs, E. (Eds.). (1986). *Language socialization across cultures.* Cambridge: Cambridge University Press.

Slobin, D. (1973). Cognitive prerequisites for the development of grammar. In C. Ferguson & D. Slobin (Eds.), *Studies of child language development* (pp. 175–208). New York: Holt, Rinehart & Winston.

Slobin, D. (1985). Crosslinguistic evidence for the language-making capacity. In D. Slobin (Ed.), *The crosslinguistic study of language acquisition* (Vol. 2, pp. 1157–1256). Hillsdale, NJ: Lawrence Erlbaum.

Spelke, E. (1988). The origins of physical knowledge. In L. Weiskrantz (Ed.), *Thought without language* (pp. 168–184). Oxford: Clarendon Press.

Spelke, E. (1991). Physical knowledge in infancy: Reflections on Piaget's theory. In S. Carey & R. Gelman (Eds.), *The epigenesis of mind: Essays on biology and cognition* (pp. 133–169). Hillsdale, NJ: Lawrence Erlbaum.

Stark, R. (1986). Prespeech segmental feature development. In P. Fletcher & M. Garman (Eds.), *Language acquisition: Studies in first language development* (2nd ed., pp. 149–174). Cambridge: Cambridge University Press.

Stein, N., & Levine, L. (1989). The causal organization of emotional knowledge: A developmental study. *Cognition and Emotion, 3*, 343–378.

Taylor, C. (1979). Action as expression. In C. Diamond & J. Teichman (Eds.), *Intentions and intentionality, Essays in honor of G. E. M. Anscombe* (pp. 73–89). Ithaca, NY: Cornell University Press.

Thompson, R. (1990). Emotional self-regulation. In R. Thompson (Ed.), *Nebraska Symposium on Motivation, 1988*. Vol. 36. *Socioemotional development* (pp. 367–467). Lincoln: University of Nebraska Press.

Tomasello, M. (1992). The social bases of language acquisition. *Social Development, 1*, 67–87.

Tomasello, M., & Farrar, J. (1986). Joint attention and early language. *Child Development, 57*, 1454–1463.

Werner, H. (1948). *Comparative psychology of mental development*. New York: Science Editions.

Werner, H., & Kaplan, B. (1963). *Symbol formation*. New York: John Wiley.

Wexler, K., & Culicover, P. (1980). *Formal principles of language acquisition*. Cambridge, MA: The MIT Press.

◆ SUGGESTED READINGS

For an extensive list of readings in language acquisition, see:

Higginson, R., & MacWhinney, B. (1991). *CHILDES/BIB: An annotated bibliography of child language and language disorders*. Hillsdale, NJ: Lawrence Erlbaum.

The following list of suggested readings consists only of books published between 1983 and 1993 with two exceptions; one is the landmark book by M. M. Lewis, published in 1951, and the other, for the future serious student of language development, is the important four-volume study by Werner Leopold of his daughter's language development, 1939–1949.

Anisfeld, M. (1984). *Language development from birth to three.* Hillsdale, NJ: Lawrence Erlbaum.

Bates, E., Bretherton, I., & Snyder, L. (1988). *From first words to grammar: Individual differences and dissociable mechanisms.* Cambridge: Cambridge University Press

Bloom, L. (1991). *Language development from two to three.* New York: Cambridge University Press.

Bloom, L. (1993). *The transition from infancy to language: Acquiring the power of expression.* Cambridge: Cambridge University Press.

Bruner, J. (1983). *Child's talk, Learning to use language.* New York: W. W. Norton.

Fletcher, P., & Garman, M. (Eds.). (1986). *Language acquisition* (2nd ed.). Cambridge: Cambridge University Press.

Golinkoff, R. (Ed.). (1983). *The transition from prelinguistic to linguistic communication in infancy.* Hillsdale, NJ: Lawrence Erlbaum.

Ingram, D. (1989). *First language acquisition: Method, description, and explanation.* New York: Cambridge University Press.

Kuczaj, S., Barrett, M. (Eds.). (1986). *The development of word meaning.* New York: Springer.

Leopold, W. (1939–1949). *Speech development of a bilingual child* (4 Vols.). Evanston, IL: Northwestern University Press.

Lewis, M. M. (1951). *Infant speech, a study of the beginnings of language.* New York: Humanities Press.

MacWhinney, B. (Ed.). (1987). *Mechanisms of language acquisition.* Hillsdale, NJ: Lawrence Erlbaum.

Nelson, K. (1985). *Making sense: The acquisition of shared meaning.* New York: Academic Press.

Pinker, S. (1984). *Language learnability and language development.* Cambridge, MA: Harvard University.

Schieffelin, B., & Ochs, E. (Eds.). (1986). *Language socialization across cultures.* Cambridge: Cambridge University Press.

Slobin, D. (Ed.). (1985). *The crosslinguistic study of language acquisition* (2 Vols.). Hillsdale, NJ: Lawrence Erlbaum.

Smith, M., & Locke, J. (Eds.). (1988). *The emergent lexicon: The child's development of a linguistic vocabulary.* New York: Academic Press.

Wanner, E., & Gleitman, L. (Eds.). (1982). *Language acquisition: The state of the art.* Cambridge: Cambridge University Press.

✦ GLOSSARY

Content of language is the meaning expressed by words and sentences.

Conventional means that persons using a language share the same knowledge and agree on the elements of the language and the ways they can and cannot be combined with one another to express meaning.

A **developmental perspective** is the view that language is necessarily related to other developments happening at the same time in cognition, emotion, and social interaction.

First Words is the initial milestone in acquiring language and consists of the first use of a meaningful, conventional word at least two different times.

The **Form** of language is the inventory of elements — sounds and gestures — and the rules for combining them to form words and sentences.

Language is a conventional system of elements and the relationships between them for expressing ideas about the world for communication with other persons.

Mean Length of Utterance (MLU) is the average length of a sample of 50 to 100 child utterances. MLU is computed by dividing the total number of words in the utterances by the number of utterances.

Negation is the use of words like *no, not, can't, all gone*, and the like to express the opposite of something that would otherwise be affirmed or true.

Relational concepts consist of knowledge about how objects and events go together in the world.

A **theory of objects** is knowledge we have about objects in the world, their existence in time and space, and the relationships between them.

Use of language is the way language form and content are connected for different purposes according to the context.

A **Vocabulary Spurt** is the sharp increase in new words from one month to the next after a child has already acquired a small number of words in the second year.

Wh-question words are *who, what, where, when, how*, and *why*.

Language Disorders in Children

LINDA SWISHER, Ph.D.

After completing this chapter you will be able to:

◆ Define the term developmental language disorder.

◆ Describe some behavioral characteristics of specific language impairment, mental retardation, and autism.

◆ Describe the evaluation process and treatment approaches commonly utilized with language-disordered children.

◆ Appreciate the need to incorporate parents and professionals in the intervention process.

◆ Understand the legal rights of children with language disorders to receive appropriate attention in the public schools.

◆ In response to case presentations, answer the following questions:

Why is this child considered developmentally language disordered?

Which language components (form, content, or use) require attention?

What type of therapy approach is suitable for this child?

This chapter will introduce you to three different types of developmental language disorders. The model presented by Dr. Bloom in Chapter 5 describes language as a multidimensional skill involving form, content, and use. This model provides a framework for understanding the nature of the language disorders discussed in this chapter. After an overview of the evaluation and treatment of children with developmental language disorders, you will be introduced to the disorders of specific language impairment, mental retardation, and autism. Then you will be introduced to a child with each of these language disorders. Each child's case history, test results, and spontaneous language analysis are summarized for your consideration. Finally, based on the information presented in this chapter, you will be asked to discuss: Why we concluded that each of these children is language disordered, which language components (form, content, or use) require attention, and which treatment approaches would be appropriate for each of the children.

Brian: this the bell
David: this is the bell

Brian: the telephone do that too
David: the telephone does that too

Brian and David, who spoke the utterances transcribed above, are almost 5 years of age and from similar socio-linguistic backgrounds. David's use of complete sentences suggests his language acquisition is proceeding normally. In contrast, Brian's verbal output indicates he may have a developmental language disorder (DLD).

Unlike adults who acquire a language disorder such as aphasia (see Chapter 9) and lose normally developed, well-practiced language skills, in children with DLDs, the neuroanatomical substrate involved in language acquisition develops atypically before birth. Although child-parent language interactions may be adversely affected by the DLD, no evidence exists that poor parenting practices are the precipitating cause. During their preschool years, these children begin to face the social and educational disadvantages that result from DLDs. However, with therapy, some begin to function well within the normal range; others improve and avoid the frustrations of being labeled "dumb," "lazy," or "stubborn."

This chapter focuses on spoken language deficits that characterize children with a DLD during their preschool years. Dr. Bloom's model of language (Chapter 5) as a multidimensional skill involving form, content, and use is applied to the study of DLDs. After an overview of the evaluation and treatment of children with DLD, three categories of DLD will be described in greater detail: specific language impairment, mental retardation, and autism. Three individual case histories then will be summarized. Finally, based on the information presented in this chapter, you will be asked to discuss: why my colleague, Mrs. Vance, and I concluded that in each case study the child has a language disorder, which language components (form, content, or use) require attention, and which treatment approaches would be most appropriate for each of the children.

Although this chapter provides three case studies for consideration, I encourage you to observe and interact with local children in your area who have a DLD. Speech and language clinics typically welcome observers who understand the clients' need for confidentiality. Volunteer to help speech-language pathologists and audiologists employed in a variety of settings and, in the process, increase your knowledge of the far-reaching consequences of being born with less than the full capacity for relatively effortless language acquisition.

◆ EVALUATION

The age at which children are referred for a developmental evaluation varies from soon after birth to school age. Children determined to be at risk during the perinatal period typically are monitored by a team of professionals. This **interdisciplinary team** includes specialists from different disciplines (i.e., developmental psychology, pediatric neurology, audiology, speech-language pathology, occupational therapy, and physical therapy) who work together in an integrated plan of treatment to best accommodate the special needs of each child. In contrast, children who appear to have normal cognitive, motor, and sensory development usually do not concern their parents or pediatricians until they reach 2 or 3 years of age. At this point, referral directly to a speech-language pathologist usually occurs, and additional evaluations are recommended as necessary.

Still other children have language problems that parents and pediatricians do not notice during the preschool years. These children may be capable of adequately communicating their everyday needs with language and easily carry on a conversation. However, when they reach school age and the greater academic demands of learning to read and write challenge their language skills, academic problems may emerge. My colleagues and I call this phenomenon "growing into deficits" because the DLD does not surface until the child encounters the heavily language-laden tasks of learning to read and write.

For several important reasons, children who do not appear to be developing normally should be referred for evaluation as early as possible. Some will need considerable help to ensure that they enter kindergarten with as highly developed communication skills as possible. In addition, once the "red flag" of a DLD has been raised, periodic monitoring of the child's academic progress is warranted. Early identification and treatment followed by periodic monitoring encourages remediation of poor language skills as soon as they emerge. Early intervention, in turn, reduces the likelihood that the child will experience the frustration that accompanies social and academic failure.

Once referral occurs, the speech-language pathologist must first determine if the child has a language disorder and then further identify which language components (i.e., form, content, or use) require attention. To answer these questions, the clinician collects information from various sources including the child's primary caregivers (most often the parents), the child, and other specialists.

The speech-language pathologist follows several steps in the process of collecting information about the child. These include:

- ◆ obtaining a case history
- ◆ observing the child
- ◆ assessing the child's communication skills
- ◆ making referrals to other specialists.

Each of these steps will be discussed separately in the sections that follow. After completing the evaluation, the speech-language pathologist has the information necessary to develop an appropriate treatment program or to further monitor the child's prognosis at periodic intervals.

Case History

To obtain case history information, the clinician first administers a questionnaire designed to collect specific information regarding the child's development. Typically, parents complete the case history questionnaire at home where they have access to the child's baby records for reference. Some areas addressed and questions regularly asked on the questionnaire are presented in Table 6–1.

TABLE 6-1. Excerpts from a case history questionnaire.

Identifying Information

Child's Name:_____ Male___ Female___
    Age:_____ Date of Birth:_____

Statement of the Problem

Describe your child's problem:_____
When was the problem first noticed?_____
What changes in your child's speech and language have you noticed
    since then?_____
Do any relatives have problems with speech or language?_____

Speech, Language, and Hearing Development

Did your child babble and coo during the first 6 months?_____
At what age did your child say her/his first word?_____ What were her/his
    first words?_____
Does your child frequently use: sounds only_____ single words_____
    2-word sentences_____ 3-word sentences_____
    more than 3-word sentences_____

Developmental History

Were there any medical problems before this pregnancy?_____
    during this pregnancy?_____
When did your child first: sit unsupported_____ reach for an object_____
    crawl_____ walk unaided_____ run_____

Medical History

Has your child had middle-ear infections?_____
Did they occur frequently?_____ Describe the frequency:_____

After reviewing the completed questionnaire, the clinician forms
hypotheses about the nature of the child's problem and outlines an
interview to be conducted with at least one of the child's parents.
During the interview the clinician not only clarifies the reported
information but allows the parent(s) to expand on any items, encouraging them to voice their opinions about the nature and severity of their child's problem as well as what they hope to learn from
the evaluation. In addition, they are asked to provide specific information about the child's use of language in different situations.
Sample interview questions include:

How does your child tell you he wants a drink of water?

What are some words or sentences your child uses?

How well do strangers understand your child?

How do you react when you do not understand what your child wants or needs?

How does your child respond to this reaction?

As the evaluation proceeds, the clinician asks the parents whether the child's behavior in the clinic appears consistent with what they have observed at home. This question addresses the issue of representativeness, or how well what the clinician observes reflects what the child typically does. If, for example, the parents report that the child volunteers more complete sentences at home, observations of the child in the home environment or across additional sessions in the clinic might be required before appropriate recommendations can be made.

Behavioral Observations

Observations begin as soon as the child arrives for evaluation. At this time, the clinician makes a mental note of what the child does when greeted. What does the child say? Does the child make eye contact and acknowledge the greeting by waving or shaking hands without saying anything? Does the child act as though he did not hear what was said?

To help children and parents feel comfortable in the clinic environment, speech-language pathologists often begin an evaluation with the child and parent playing together. If an observation room with a two-way mirror is available, the clinician may choose to observe this interaction. Sample observations of the child's behavior might include:

Does the child typically use gestures, words, or sentences to communicate?

Does the child show signs of frustration when the parent does not understand what was communicated?

Does the child appear to understand what the parent says?

When the parent asks the child a question, how does the child respond?

Sample observations of the parent's behaviors might include:

Does the parent utilize a direct or conversational style of communication with the child?

Does the parent lead the activities or follow the child's lead?

Does the parent understand what the child wants and needs?

What does the parent do when unable to understand the child?

Finally, and perhaps most importantly, the clinician can begin to answer these questions: Does the interaction between parent and child appear positive and relaxed? Do they communicate successfully with one another?

Observation of the parent–child play interaction allows the clinician to obtain information that will guide the selection of appropriate activities and assessment procedures for the remainder of the evaluation. The tasks chosen will help the clinician determine whether a DLD exists and, if so, the nature and severity of the disorder.

Assessment of Language Skills

Assessment of the child's communication skills involves collecting two types of data that answer different questions. Norm-referenced measures, which allow the clinician to compare a child's performance to "peers" of the same age and socio-linguistic background, can be used to corroborate the impression of whether or not a language problem exists. Language sample analyses, which allow the clinician to study how the child uses language to communicate with others, help determine the nature of the problem or, more specifically, which language components (form, content, or use) require attention.

Norm-referenced Measures

The development of norm-referenced measures requires a great deal of expertise, time, and effort. Very briefly, the process includes the following steps:

◆ Outlining the skills thought to reflect language development

◆ Developing tasks that tap these skills

♦ Presenting these tasks to large numbers of normally developing children at different ages

♦ Documenting performance

♦ Analyzing the results in terms of describing performance standards for appropriate age levels.

The clinician must consider many variables when selecting norm-referenced measures for use with a particular child. For example, the test chosen must be appropriate for the child's age level and socio-linguistic background (see Chapter 2 by Orlando Taylor). Details in the test manual regarding the sample of children for whom the norms were determined form the basis for this important decision. Consider, for example, a Native American child whose parents speak both Navajo and English. If a vocabulary test normed on children whose parents speak only English is administered to this child, below-average performance may occur. However, this performance may not be indicative of a DLD. Instead, the child may have difficulty because Navajo rather than English words were acquired for certain objects and events. Likewise, the child may be unfamiliar with some of the tasks required by the test.

If the clinician believes that test performance accurately reflects the child's ability, and performance falls below that of the child's peers, corroborating evidence indicates a language problem exists. Prior to diagnosis however, most clinicians administer more than one standardized test and collect a spontaneous language sample. Results of such standardized testing and language sampling are compared to see if they appear consistent with the diagnosis.

Spontaneous Language Sampling

Language samples usually are collected in at least two situations — as the child plays with a parent and as the child plays with the clinician. When feasible, it also may be helpful to sample the child's utterances in interactions with siblings and peers because language may be used differently in these situations. In most cases, parents take the child to a clinic, school, or hospital for evaluation. In some instances, particularly with infants and toddlers, the clinician collects the language sample in the home.

The clinician must choose toys and other stimulus materials appropriate for the child's cognitive level, cultural background, interests, and perceptual and motor skills. Many clinicians ask the parent to bring a few of the child's favorite toys and books to the evaluation. Generally, toys found to elicit the most spontaneous language from preschool-age children include cooking and eating utensils; dolls; play sets such as a barn with animals, a gas station with cars, and a schoolhouse, airport, or castle with people and other manipulatives.

Clinicians frequently record language samples on audio and video tape for later analysis. This allows the clinician to play naturally with the child during the evaluation, knowing there will be a record of the entire interaction. After the language sample has been collected, the clinician chooses the portions that include the most talking from the child and transcribes the child's and adult's utterances, noting the contexts in which they occurred.

A **transcription** provides the clinician with a written record of what the child and adult(s) said and did as they played together. The sample then can be analyzed in several different ways depending on the child's level of development and what the clinician wants to learn from the analysis. For example, the language form analysis can determine if the child uses sentences as long and complex as those used by other children of the same age. Sample analyses include:

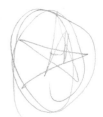

> Does the child use the plural ending ("s") when talking about more than one object?
>
> Does the child use the "ed" ending when talking about something that happened yesterday?
>
> Does the child use little words such as "is" and "am"?

Analysis of the content of the child's language occurs as well. The clinician determines the range and complexity of ideas expressed by the child. A sample analysis might include:

> Does the child express ideas such as ownership (e.g., "my doll")
>
> Does the child express disappearance ideas (e.g., "all gone")
>
> Does the child express location (e.g., "baby in")

Analysis of language samples of older children, who express more complex ideas, would include two events happening simultaneously (e.g., "Mom is going to the mall and Dad is taking us to the movies") or two events that oppose one another (e.g., "I want to go to the park, but mom said I have to stay home today").

Finally, the clinician analyzes the sample in terms of use. We use language for a variety of purposes such as commenting on objects and people in the environment (e.g., "That's a big dog"), regulating the actions of others (e.g., "I want you to take out the garbage now"), and requesting information (e.g., "What's that thing called?"). To accurately assess the child's use of language, the clinician must consider the interaction between the child and the adult or peer. Through analysis of this interaction, the clinician determines the range of purposes for which the child uses language and the child's success in accomplishing them. Sample analyses address: Does the child understand the back and forth nature of conversation? Does the child keep the conversation moving along by adding new information about a particular topic or by introducing new topics?

After the clinician has collected a case history, administered selected norm-referenced tests, and completed an appropriate language sample analysis, it is usually possible to determine: (1) whether the child is language disordered and, if so, (2) which language components require attention. In addition, based on informal observation of the child throughout the evaluation, the clinician can decide whether to refer the child to other professionals.

Referrals to Other Professionals

As discussed previously, many clinicians work with a team of professionals from related fields. When not part of a diagnostic team, speech-language pathologists may be the first professionals, besides the pediatrician, the parents contact regarding their child. If the clinician suspects the child's hearing is poor, or that cognitive, motor, or social-emotional development is delayed, referral to additional specialists becomes necessary.

✦ TREATMENT

In 1975, Congress enacted Public Law 94-142, The Education for All Handicapped Children Act. It mandates a free and appropriate education for all handicapped children ages 5 to 21. This was the first law that required public schools to provide speech-language therapy, occupational therapy, and physical therapy, as well as other special education services to all school-age children in need of them. In 1990 a second federal mandate, Public Law 99-457 (P.L. 99-457), extended the age range served by public schools. At the present time, public schools must also provide a free and appropriate education to all handicapped children between the ages of 3 and 5. P.L. 99-457 additionally provides each state with funds to establish evaluation and treatment programs for handicapped children ages birth through 2 years.

As you might imagine, P.L. 99-457 presents speech-language pathologists with new challenges. Providing services for many infants and toddlers involves focusing on the communication skills that precede the onset of speech and language (e.g., making eye contact, alerting to the sounds of language, and turn-taking). In addition, children identified as having communication problems before 2½ years of age typically exhibit other developmental disabilities that require a team approach to evaluation and treatment. As a member of the interdisciplinary team, the speech-language pathologist shares knowledge about speech and language development with parents and the other specialists involved. In return, the speech-language pathologist gains information from the other specialists, such as optimal physical positioning of the child during speech-language therapy.

Principles Guiding Clinical Practice

Now consider five components that reflect state-of-the-art services for preschool children with DLDs.

1. *An interdisciplinary approach to evaluation and treatment.* As previously mentioned, a team approach maximizes the probability that all of the child's needs will be met. In most programs, team members participate in both evaluation and intervention activities. Programs serving children ages birth through 2, conduct team evaluations in the home or at a clinic or agency. Treatment frequently occurs in the home where parents can assist specialists in enhancing the child's development across various skill areas. At the preschool level, team evaluations can be conducted at a school or agency, and classes often include "team teaching" instruction from early childhood educators, as well as speech-language pathologists and occupational or physical therapists.

2. *The provision of services in both group and individual formats.* A combination of therapy formats provides the necessary variety of contexts in which to practice communication skills. One-on-one and small group formats allow the clinician to focus on a child's individual needs. A large group or classroom format ensures opportunities for the child to use newly acquired language skills in a naturalistic situation and enhances the development of social skills. Individual or small-group therapy sessions can occur in a corner or special area of the classroom. Collaboration with the classroom teacher allows successful classroom-based therapy. For example, the speech-language pathologist may assist in planning the daily classroom activities or may present a daily or weekly language lesson that benefits all children in the classroom.

3. *Parent participation in the intervention process.* Parental participation greatly enhances the benefits of therapy. In programs serving children ages birth through 2, the parents rather than clinicians are regarded as the key members of the team, and are encouraged to participate in all aspects of the evaluation and treatment of their child. Parental responsibilities include observing therapy on a regular basis, and developing skills that will allow them to facilitate their child's language development. Clearly, the more parents understand about their child's needs, the better prepared they will be to enhance targeted language objectives at home.

4. *Mainstreaming.* Mainstreaming provides opportunities for children with a DLD to interact with normally developing children of the same age. For instance, some programs require children to attend a regular preschool on days they do not attend the program for children with language disorders. In this case, the speech-language pathologist works closely with the staff at the regular preschool to meet the child's communication needs. The clinician also provides special training to the preschool staff. Other programs use reverse mainstreaming to integrate normal children into the classroom for children with language disorders. Regardless of the implementation process, mainstreaming provides opportunities for children with DLDs to interact with normal peers who model age-appropriate language and social skills.

5. *The primary goal of intervention: Enhancement of functional communication skills in a naturalistic environment.* The primary goal of all intervention programs focuses on improving the child's ability to communicate with others in all situations of daily life. The components discussed above remain critical to the attainment of this goal.

Therapy Approaches

We will discuss approaches that fall at three points along a continuum of naturalness (Fey, 1986). As you can visualize, child-oriented approaches fall at the natural end of the continuum. These approaches are implemented by individuals familiar to the child (e.g., parents) who facilitate language development at home during everyday activities such as getting dressed and taking a bath. Trainer-oriented approaches, implemented by individuals less familiar to the child (e.g., clinicians) fall at the opposite end of the continuum. Hybrid approaches fall somewhere in the middle. Typically used in classroom situations, these approaches combine aspects of child- and trainer-oriented structures.

Child-Oriented Approaches

Child-oriented approaches do not directly attempt to change the child's speech-language behaviors. Instead, the clinician works with caregivers, teachers, and other significant adults in the child's life to modify their interactions with the child. In turn, modification of adult interactions enhances the child's speech-language development. Child-oriented procedures usually are implemented during the child's daily activities, both at home and at school.

Child-oriented approaches require adults to create an accepting, responsive communicative environment. The adult begins by following the child's lead. Thus, the adult observes the child and looks at, touches, or talks about the objects or events of interest to the child. During play, the adult attempts to facilitate the child's language development by simplifying language to a level just above the child's level. If the child uses predominately single words, the adult uses two- and three-word utterances (e.g., "Baby sleeping" or "Dog in wagon"). The adult also uses **self-talk** and **parallel talk** techniques. Whereas self-talk allows the adult to express personal observations, actions, and feelings, parallel talk requires the adult to comment on what the child is seeing, doing, and perhaps feeling. The adult can also use an **expansion,** which repeats the child's utterances in a longer and slightly more complex form. For example, if the child says, "baby sleep," the adult might expand the utterance by saying "Yes, the baby is sleeping." Child-oriented approaches never require the child to speak. However, when speech occurs, the parent, teacher, or clinician is immediately attentive.

In my experience, child-oriented approaches are most beneficial for very young children, those just beginning to talk, and those functioning at a low cognitive level. To achieve optimal results, these approaches require intensive parent training and consistent participation on the part of the child's parents and teachers. A child-oriented approach has the obvious benefits of facilitating language development across all daily activities.

Trainer-Oriented Approaches

As discussed earlier, trainer-oriented approaches fall at the less-natural end of Fey's continuum. If you stop and think for a moment, you can probably guess some characteristics of these approaches. The trainer-oriented approaches allow the speech-language pathologist to determine what the child will say, when he will say it, and what will constitute a correct or acceptable response. The clinician also selects the toys and materials the child will interact with, and determines when and where these materials will be presented. Implementation of these highly structured, trainer-oriented procedures typically occurs in a clinic or school environment.

Explore for a moment an example of trainer-oriented procedures. Consider a child learning to use "is" in statements to comment on what is happening in pictures. To initiate a response, the clinician might present a picture of a boy drinking juice and ask "What's happening?" If the child says, "The boy drinking," the clinician will consider this an incorrect response because "is" was omitted. At this point, the clinician will provide corrective feedback such as, "Tell me that again," or "The boy drinking?" These reactions from the clinician encourage the child to modify his response. If the child then provides a modified response ("The boy is drinking"), the clinician will provide positive feedback.

Trainer-oriented approaches have been documented to be very successful in establishing new language behaviors in the clinic environment. However, the extent to which these procedures facilitate the development of functional communication skills in naturalistic environments continues to be investigated. Although trainer-oriented approaches are effective in eliciting new language behaviors in children who produce sentences, I have not been satisfied with these procedures in isolation because of the limited transfer that occurs to natural communicative exchanges. For this reason, I use trainer-oriented approaches in the initial stages of teaching new skills, and then progress to more naturalistic approaches to facilitate the use of these new skills in naturalistic contexts.

Hybrid Approaches

Hybrid approaches fall somewhere near the middle of the "naturalness" continuum. These approaches, although most often implemented in the child's classroom or home, have been applied in clinical settings as well. Most hybrid approaches allow the child to take the lead, thereby determining when teaching will take place and what the consequences for communicating will be (e.g., obtaining a desired object). As with trainer-oriented approaches, the clinician has as least one language goal in mind while choosing the toys and materials for the therapy session. In addition, the clinician defines an acceptable response and provides the cues necessary for the child to produce this response.

Now consider the structure of a hybrid approach. Assume that a group of children is making peanut-butter crackers for snack. The clinician determines that during the task one child should work on using the negative form "can't" and another should practice a "where" question. Thus, the clinician places the peanut butter in view, but out of the child's reach and finds an accomplice to hide the knives. The clinician then asks the first child to pass the peanut butter, and the child replies "I can't." A prompt (e.g., "Say, I can't reach it") can be utilized if the clinician feels the child can produce a more complete response. If the child says "I can't reach it," the clinician responds, "Oh, you can't reach it. It's too high. I'll get it for you." At this point, the child has used the target structure in a meaningful, communicative exchange. Now in need of plastic knives, the clinician asks the other child to find them, initiating use of a "where" question, and the structure of the interaction occurs in the same format as described for the first child.

Hybrid approaches function optimally in group or classroom situations. In both individual and group therapy formats, the child can receive intensive practice on specified forms such as "can't" or other types of questions. These children additionally benefit from the opportunity to use forms in natural, communicative exchanges involving other children.

◆ SPECIFIC LANGUAGE IMPAIRMENT

> If you had a specific language impairment, the complexity of your language form would not match the complexity of your intellectual development. People who equate "intelligence" with spoken language skills would regard you as "dumb." Your thoughts and needs would outpace your means of expressing them. As a result, communication through words would often frustrate you. In the absence of appropriate help, you would either withdraw or act out. You would not look forward to starting school and would prefer to play alone rather than be ridiculed by your playmates.
>
> Now consider the alternative. Family members, preschool teachers, and a speech-language pathologist work together to improve
>
> *(continued)*

> your language skills so that your thoughts and needs can be expressed adequately. You are helped to avoid communication frustrations and start first grade confident and ready to learn. When you run into academic difficulty in the third grade, you immediately receive special help and therefore continue to keep pace with your classmates.

The term "specific language impairment" applies to preschool-age children with the following characteristics: normal intellectual development as assessed by a measure of nonverbal intelligence, poor language skills, and no other obvious handicapping conditions except in the area of speech. Terms that have been utilized in the past to refer to this type of DLD include "childhood aphasia," "delayed language," and even "delayed speech." Stevenson and Richman (1976) found that 5.7% of approximately 200 three-year-olds met standard criteria for specific language impairment.

The majority of these children have bilateral atypical development in the perisylvian areas of the brain that subserve language skills in adults (Plante, Swisher, Vance, & Rapcsak, 1991). Frequently, a family history of language disorders exists and speech skills vary from normal to profoundly impaired. In addition, co-occurring nonverbal cognitive deficits exist. For example, many of these children have difficulty rotating objects mentally to imagine the same object in a shifted position. The presence of hearing loss or mental retardation excludes a child from the category of specific language impairment.

Learning disability is defined in The Education of All Handicapped Children Act, P.L. 94-142, as "a disorder in one or more of the basic psychological processes involved in understanding or in using language, spoken or written, which may manifest itself in an imperfect ability to listen, think, speak, read, write, spell, or do mathematical calculations." Notice that a language disorder forms the core of the learning disability definition. In the research literature as well as clinical practice, children diagnosed as specifically language impaired during their preschool years are referred to as learning disabled during their grade school years. To qualify for services in the public schools, children with specific language impairment must be categorized as learning disabled, by federal law.

Children with this type of DLD characteristically come to the attention of a speech-language pathologist at about 2½ years of age. Although first words may have occurred when expected, the multiple-word utterances expected between 2 and 3 years of age do not emerge. In the great majority of cases, the expressive language form has poor grammatical structure with omissions of the "little" parts of language. Depending on the severity of this type of DLD, there may be an expressive vocabulary deficit and difficulty with language comprehension. As already mentioned, the behavioral constellation shifts over time to include written language deficits which become obvious during the child's school-age years.

The treatment for children with specific language impairment draws heavily on the knowledge you will gain as a speech-language pathologist in training. These children do not require simply more of what normally developing children require. Instead, they require intensive practice at their own "growing edge" of language. As with every child with a DLD, parents are encouraged to become part of the intervention team. In the case of a child with specific language impairment, parents should provide positive feedback for the use of newly emerging language forms during everyday activities.

A woman who observed the children with specific language impairment in therapy at the University of Arizona, Tucson Scottish Rite Center for Childhood Language Disorders, referred to them as "hurting where you can't see." Another observer referred to them as having an "invisible handicap." My colleagues and I have been drawn to children with specific language impairment primarily because of the likelihood that they can be helped to become full members of society: self-supporting and self-informing. With suitable help, they can advance academically and socially, and depending on the severity of the disorder, some even graduate from college.

✦ MENTAL RETARDATION

> If you were mentally retarded, you would not have the complexity of thought that characterizes most of your age-level peers. Because complexity of thought sets the pace of the development of language content, form, and use, all components of language acquisition would fall below age-level expectations. If your skill pattern included poor language skills relative to your nonverbal cognitive skills, you would be diagnosed with a DLD in addition to mental retardation. You might also have physical difficulties, for example, markedly poor motor coordination. The greater the level of retardation, the greater the difficulty you would experience with tasks easily performed by other children your age. Overall, the global nature of your dif-
> *(continued)*

ficulties would limit your choices in life remarkably. In short, you might look, act, and think differently from many other children your age. In addition, depending on the **etiology** of your mental retardation, (the cause of your condition), frequent bouts with conductive hearing loss might also occur.

The American Association on Mental Deficiency requires that individuals score at least two standard deviations below the average for their age group on a norm-referenced intelligence test and show significant impairment in adaptive behavior to be diagnosed as mentally retarded. In addition, these criteria must be met during childhood.

The prevalence of mental retardation currently is estimated to include 3% of the population. This figure has been broken down as follows (Schlanger, 1973):

Mildly retarded: IQ from 50 to 70
2.6% of the total population
85% of the mentally retarded population.

Moderately and severely retarded: IQ from 20 to 49
0.3% of the total population
11.5% of the mentally retarded population.

Profoundly retarded: IQ below 20
0.1% of the total population
3.5% of the mentally retarded population.

Considerable heterogeneity exists in the pattern and severity of strengths and weaknesses observed in children with mental retardation. As in all three categories of DLD discussed in this chapter, a relative disassociation between the form and content of language can be found. Sometimes the form is more developed than the content; sometimes the reverse appears to be true. For example, most children with Down syndrome appear to have particularly poor grammatical skills. In contrast, most children with Williams syndrome appear to have relatively strong grammatical skills (form) in the presence of poor language content.

Most known causes of mental retardation result from chromosomal abnormalities (e.g., fragile-X syndrome, Down syndrome), toxins present before birth (e.g., fetal alcohol syndrome and "crack" babies), and trauma to the brain before, during, or after birth. Many multiply handicapped babies are surviving whose developmental disabilities can be traced to parental use of crack, cocaine, alcohol, and prescribed drugs, to name a few of the substances that can adversely affect the neuroanatomical substrate of a child's cognitive skills. Frequently, parents report no family history of mental retardation.

At birth, multiply handicapped children are clearly at risk for mental retardation. Their atypical physical characteristics and mobility patterns draw attention to possible, co-occurring cognitive deficits. In contrast to most children with specific language impairment, but similar to some children with autism, first words do not emerge when expected. In fact, the development of children with mental retardation begins later than usual, proceeds more slowly, and reaches an overall lower level. With the help of therapy, the mildest form of this developmental disability does not exclude graduation from high school. However, the severest form requires caregiver assistance with the basic necessities of life, including toileting and eating, throughout the life span. The children most severely affected by mental retardation may not develop spoken language; others may speak only for food and relief from discomfort or pain.

The need to keep the focus of learning on the child's "growing edge" of language and to enhance learning in natural contexts through a team approach benefits children with mental retardation. Their slow process of learning new skills, limited success in transferring that learning to new contexts, and the probability of multiple handicaps makes priority setting especially important. Everyone who interacts with the child on a regular basis is encouraged to enhance the transfer of learning to new contexts. In addition, the team approach provides opportunities for the child to learn more than one type of skill simultaneously. For example, a speech-language pathologist may encourage an occupational therapist to include a word like "help" into a shoe-tying exercise to improve manual-dexterity skills.

As already mentioned, children with mental retardation have to work harder to accomplish less than their age-level peers. The majority can move into self-sufficiency, but some require parental support all of their lives. These children can make progress; however, the noteworthy gains achieved are best assessed in relation to their own individual skill level rather than in relation to age-level peers.

◆ AUTISM

If you saw the movie "Rain Man" starring Dustin Hoffman, you witnessed a remarkably accurate portrayal of an adult with
(continued)

autism functioning at a higher level than most. As a child with autism, a language disorder would be one of the most striking and long-lasting features of your developmental disability. For additional reasons not clearly understood, you would have proportionately more difficult encounters during your day than other children with roughly equivalent levels of intellectual ability. Your many weak areas of development would lead to frustrations that intermesh with those of your parents and teachers as they attempt to include you in everyday activities.

Autism is characterized by social development inappropriate for the child's intellectual level, language development delayed and/or deviant for the child's nonverbal intellectual level, and "insistence on sameness" as indicated by stereotyped play patterns, abnormal preoccupations, or resistance to change. In addition, these behaviors must be present before 30 months of age (Rutter, 1978). Other terms used to describe children with these characteristics have included "childhood schizophrenia," "atypical child," and even "psychotic child." Wing (1976) reviewed several epidemiological studies and concluded that the prevalence of autism is 4 to 5 in 1000 children. Of these, a small number function in the normal or mild to moderately retarded range with a much larger number functioning in the severely to profoundly retarded range.

Most children with autism have disabilities in three major areas of development: cognitive, linguistic, and social-emotional. Within this population of children, the degree of difficulty in understanding and reacting to the communication demands of everyday life ranges from mild to profound. Due to relatively well-developed, fine-motor skills, children with autism are less likely to be speech impaired than children with comparable levels of mental retardation. In addition, they are not at risk for hearing difficulties.

The great majority of children with autism lack the ideas expected for their age level as well as the range of intents to communicate expected for their degree of retardation. Because of the latter characteristic, difficulties in language use stand out as a major component of their DLD. Some children with autism, and some with mental retardation, produce language with a "superficial" form. Thus, the complexity of language form is at a higher level than their complexity of language content. These children often exhibit **echolalic** behavior, that is, they imitate words spoken by others. However, some children with autism speak infrequently and produce incomplete grammatical forms with paucity of content. Still others exhibit little or no verbal output.

The intellectual development of children with autism ranges from normal to profoundly retarded. For example, one high-functioning adult with autism became a successful entrepreneur. However, he considered himself lonely and did not know how to approach people for affection. Literal use of words and a muted social affect were the only features of his behavior that occasionally drew a minor degree of unfavorable attention. In contrast, many individuals with autism produce a range of nonverbal behaviors referred to as "stereotypic." Examples of these behaviors include hand flapping and a preoccupation with spinning objects. Stereotypic behaviors occur most frequently when an individual with autism confronts a difficult task or is left alone with little stimulation.

The search for the cause of autism has led to the following conclusions: Autism is a neurogenic disorder, the specific cause can rarely be identified for an individual child, and a variety of etiological agents may account for autism. Several years ago, autism was blamed on poor parenting practices, especially those of the mother. Since that time, abnormal brain development has been documented in some individuals with autism (e.g., Courchesne, Yeung-Courchesne, Press, Hesselink, & Jernigan, 1988) and numerous probable etiological agents have been proposed, for example, maternal rubella.

The possibility that a child is autistic surfaces early in life when a child appears to be either less social than expected or, in contrast, unusually clinging. After completing any pre-school-age child's evaluation, clinicians must strike a delicate balance between encouraging parents to hope for too much and deterring them from expecting too little. I recommend parents adopt a "one day at a time" approach until the child reaches 6 years of age. I also recommend that they remain open to many possible outcomes. Over time, the rate of change eventually becomes constant enough to discuss prognosis.

A slow process of learning new skills, limited transfer of learning to new situations, and limited motivation to communicate characterize many of these children. This constellation of differences presents noteworthy challenges to all who seek to enhance their development. In addition, the superficial form they produce makes it particularly difficult to find their "growing edge" — the level of language expression where form, content, and use interact normally but inconsistently. This challenge is met most successfully by well-prepared, persistent speech-language pathologists who analyze a carefully obtained language sample with attention to interactions among all three components of language: form, content, and use.

Intervention approaches for autistic and mentally retarded children overlap. For example, speech-language pathologists conduct language facilitation lessons in real-life situations that foster the back-and-forth, natural use of language. Two additional approaches successful with autistic children incorporate signing (language in another mode) as one speaks to help facilitate the reciprocal nature of language exchange and the use of parents as cotherapists. Parents evaluate their child's interests most accurately and can best determine what their child may be motivated to learn independently. In addition, they can aid the transfer of new skills across different situations.

Children with autism can learn. Many can also enjoy their accomplishments. Few will become fully independent members of society, but all can be helped to higher levels of proficiency and success. Their biological limitations are such that family members often have to plan for their long-term care and, while caring for them, seek respite from the constant attention their children with autism require.

◆ CASE STUDIES

Now you can apply what you have learned about children with DLDs. I will introduce you to three children. One child has specific language impairment, one is mentally retarded, and one has autism.

Ample evidence indicates (e.g., McCauley & Swisher, 1984) that "all tests are not created equal." Some are more useful for a given purpose than others. For this reason, when preparing an evaluation report, a clinician should always name the tests from which conclusions were drawn. In our case presentations, however, we have omitted the names of tests actually used during evaluations to emphasize that refinement of test batteries is an ongoing process.

After you read the background information and study the partial language samples for each child, answer the following questions:

Why do Mrs. Vance, the speech-language pathologist who initially prepared these case studies, and I regard this child as language disordered?

Which language components (form, content, or use) currently require immediate attention? Why?

What type of therapy approach might be suitable for this child? Why?

Brian

History

Brian is 4 years, 9 months of age. He is the youngest of three children. His two half-brothers are 12 and 15 years of age. One of his brothers was described as "dyslexic" or reading disordered.

Brian's birth history was unremarkable. He was born full term with no complications. His health history was also unremarkable with only one episode of **otitis media** (inflammation of the middle ear). Brian's motor developmental milestones were within normal limits: He sat alone at 6 months and walked unsupported at 13 months. Parental report of his independent decision-making skills indicated no referral for assessment of his "general" intellectual status was warranted.

Brian's speech-language development was slow in comparison to his motor development. He used his first word at 9 months, but did not begin combining words until the age of 3 years. At age 3, he used approximately 20 words and was "difficult to understand." Brian was referred for a speech-language evaluation at the age of 3 years, 1 month. Results of norm-referenced tests and a spontaneous language sample indicated that Brian's understanding of language was "borderline normal" and his ability to express himself was significantly delayed. His articulation skills were also found to be disordered. Therapy was recommended and initiated.

Prior to the initial evaluation, Brian underwent a pure-tone audiological screening and a tympanogram. Results indicated that his hearing sensitivity and middle-ear function were within normal limits in both ears.

Results of Norm-referenced Tests

A battery of tests that assessed both language and speech skills was administered when Brian was 4 years, 9 months of age to determine whether he still qualified as language disordered. The receptive language tests revealed that Brian's understanding of language was within the average range for his age. In contrast, the expressive tests revealed that his ability to use grammatically correct sentences to express ideas was well below the range expected for his age. Finally, an articulation test indicated significant difficulty in pronouncing sounds correctly.

Results of the Language Sample Analysis

A spontaneous language sample was collected as Brian played with his mother and with the clinician. A portion of the sample appears in the box below. The language sample was used to analyze the form, content, and use of Brian's spontaneous language.

Brian's Language Sample

Brian is playing with his mother at the clinic. They are playing with a fire station, cars, and people.

(Mom lines up toy men on the roof of the fire station)

B1: **no, put him down here**

(Brian moves the men to the table)

M: Oh, you don't want them up there?

B2: **(unintelligible response)**

M: Well.

(Brian plays with the bell on the fire station)

B3: **this the bell**

M: That's the bell? Does the bell ring when there's an emergency?

B4: **no the bell it has _____ some _____ _____ when the cars come out**

M: When what?

B5: **when the kaws, the cars come out**

M: When the cars come out the bell rings? I thought the bell rang when there was an emergency.

B6: **the telephone do that too**

M: What?

B7: **oh no!**

B8: **the doors**

B9: **the doors close Mom**

M: What?

B10:   **that doors close on the, that fireperson**

M: The fire what? The fire department?

B11:   **that close**

M: That's closed.

(Brian opens the fire station door)

M: Now it's open. What is this?

B12:   **that the door**

M: That's the door, right

(Brian makes a siren noise)

M: When the door is down can the cars come out?

B13:   **huh?**

M: When the door is down can the cars come out?

B14:   **no**

M: Nope. They're locked in there right?

B15:   **yes**

B16:   **and the door it open up and the cars go**

M: Right! They're released. They come out. There's no door in the back It's open. Did you see the back end of the fire station?

(Brian moves the station so he can see the back)

B17:   **I see in there**

First, review the sample with language form in mind. You will probably notice almost immediately that Brian leaves out little words like "is" in utterances B3 and B12. Although he uses the plural marker in utterance B5 (. . . the cars), he fails to use the present tense marker in utterance B16 (and the door it open [for opens] up . . .). He makes another error in utterance B6 ("The telephone *do* [for does] that too.") Also notice several blank lines that indicate words the transcriber (in this case the clinician) did not understand. In many instances, Brian's mother did not understand what he was saying either. Reduced intelligibility is the result of Brian's difficulty in pronouncing speech sounds correctly. Further analysis of Brian's form indicated that this aspect of his language was well below the range for his age.

Now consider the content or meaning expressed in Brian's utterances. He talks about what is happening in the immediate environment (utterances B1, B3, B12, and B17). In addition, he talks about things not present in the environment, but related to the topic of conversation. Consider utterance B6. After his mother says that the fire bell rings when there is an emergency, Brian says the telephone rings too. In utterance B16, Brian talks about what will happen when the door opens. In this case, he is talking about what will happen even though the event is not actually taking place. The ability to reflect on future events requires abstract thought. Further analysis of the content of Brian's language revealed that he expressed a wide variety of both concrete and abstract thoughts despite significant limitations in form.

The final language component that we must consider is that of use. Recall that use refers to what we wish to accomplish when we talk and how well what we say relates to what our communication partner is saying. To analyze use, then, we must look not only at what Brian says, but at what his mother says to him. Begin by analyzing Brian's responses to questions. When his mother asks a question, Brian almost always responds. Sometimes, his response is simply "yes" (B15) or "no" (B16), and sometimes it involves a complete sentence (B12) or an explanation (B4). When Brian's mother asks him to clarify what he has said (usually because she did not understand him), he tries to provide the information she needs. This is clear in utterances B5 and B10. Brian also adds information to the conversation with utterances such as B6 and B9. So far, the analysis of use indicates that Brian follows many of the rules of conversation. Now consider what Brian accomplishes when he talks. With utterance B1, Brian regulates his mother's behavior by telling her that he wants the people on the table, not on the roof. Utterance B3 informs Brian's mother that he has found a bell and draws her attention to the bell. With utterance B13, Brian acknowledges that his mother asked a question, but communicates that he did not hear or understand the question. Note that his mother repeats the question, then he answers it. Further analysis of this component of Brian's language indicated that he expresses a variety of communicative functions.

Questions

Now you have the information you need to answer the questions posed at the beginning of this section. See if you can answer them yourself and discuss the answers with your classmates and instructor before reading the answers provided.

Q: Why do Mrs. Vance and I regard Brian as language disordered?

A: Brian's score on the nonverbal cognitive test was well within the normal range for his age level. Although norm-referenced language tests revealed age-appropriate understanding of language, Brian's ability to express himself in grammatically correct sentences was well below the range expected for his age. This difficulty was also apparent in the language sample. Based on these results, we can conclude that Brian has a language disorder.

Because Brian's nonverbal cognitive abilities appear to be age appropriate, and because he has normal hearing and social-emotional development, we can further conclude that he qualifies as specifically language impaired.

Q: Which language components (form, content, or use) currently require attention?

A: The language sample analysis indicated that Brian has difficulty with form. He omits many of the "little words" and makes errors in verb tense. Language content and use were relatively well developed, but should be monitored as therapy progresses.

Q: What type of therapy approach might be suitable for this child?

A: Because Brian is not retarded and because he needs to learn the "little" parts of language, a combination of trainer-oriented and hybrid approaches would be suitable in his case. Trainer-oriented approaches would provide the structure and repetition necessary for learning new language forms. Hybrid approaches would provide him with opportunities to use newly learned language forms in naturalistic environments. Brian's parents should be involved in the therapy process so they can reinforce target structures at home.

Claire

History

Claire is 6 years, 3 months of age. She is the youngest of two children; her sister is 13 years of age. There is no family history of speech or language problems.

When Claire was born, she was diagnosed with Down syndrome. As an infant, she suffered from several upper respiratory infections. In addition, she has had repeated middle-ear infections throughout her childhood. Her motor developmental milestones were delayed: She sat alone at 11 months and walked unaided at 22 months.

Claire's speech-language development was slow as well. She used her first word at 20 months and reportedly was slow to acquire new words after that time. Claire began combining words into short phrases and sentences at approximately 50 months of age. Claire's mother reported that she and her husband understand most of what Claire says.

Claire and her family have received special services through a state-funded agency since she was an infant. A team of specialists including a pediatrician, speech-language pathologist, audiologist, physical therapist, occupational therapist, psychologist, and social worker have worked together to provide the family with information and a wide range of intervention services.

Results of Norm-referenced Tests

Although Claire has undergone periodic team evaluations, this discussion will focus on the results of cognitive and speech-language testing only. In addition, the discussion will center on the results of the most recent evaluation.

At the age of 5 years, 7 months, tests that assessed both nonverbal cognitive abilities and language skills were administered. A clinical psychologist assessed her cognitive status; and a speech-language pathologist assessed her language skills. Results indicated that Claire's nonverbal cognitive abilities were significantly below the range expected for her age. Receptive language tests revealed that her understanding of language was also well below the range expected for her age. A comparison of results from these measures indicated Claire's receptive language skills were commensurate with her nonverbal cognitive development.

The expressive tests indicated Claire's ability to communicate ideas verbally was well below age-level expectations. Comparison of scores across all tests revealed that her expressive language skills were even lower than expected given her level of nonverbal cognitive development and receptive language abilities. In summary, Claire's profile indicates the presence of a DLD that affects expressive skills more than receptive skills.

Results of the Language Sample Analyses

A spontaneous language sample was collected as Claire played with her mother at home. A portion of this sample appears in the box below. The sample was used to analyze the form, content, and use of Claire's language.

Claire's Language Sample

Claire is playing with her mother at home. They have a bag filled with toys. As Claire pulls toys out, they talk about them.

(Mom takes out playdough and a knife)

M: I found a knife too, look.

C1:   knife, yuck

(Claire is blowing bubbles)

M: Why don't you show Mom how you can cut?

(Claire continues to blow bubbles)

M: You're making big bubbles now.

C2:   little bubbles

(Claire catches a bubble on her wand)

C3:   Mom, I did it.

(Mom points to the playdough)

M: Does this look like a birthday cake?

C4:   yep

M: Should we cut it?

C5:   yes

M: Why don't you cut it for me? Can you cut it?

C6:   I can't

(Mom puts Claire's bubbles aside. Claire tries to cut the "cake.")

M: Oh isn't that nice.

C7:   to eat with

M: Yes, we eat it.

C8:   at eight thirty

M: Eight thirty?

(continued)

C9:	**yeah**
M:	Eight thirty is bedtime.
C10:	**look**
C11:	**＿＿＿ ＿＿＿ ＿＿＿** (unintelligible utterance)
C12:	**the middle**
M:	Cut all the way down. Just a little bit more. Then we can have some.
C13:	**look, I make it**
M:	How many pieces do we have? One for you and one for me.
(Mom hands Claire a piece of playdough cake)	
M:	Here you are.
C14:	**yuck!**
M:	Yuck?
(Mom starts to play with playdough)	
M:	I'm going to play with mine.
(Claire picks up some grapes and hands them to Mom)	
C15:	**Mom, you like some?**
M:	Sure, I'd like some. Do you want some?
C16:	**no**
M:	Don't you like grapes?
C17:	**yeah**
M:	Then have a grape — just pretend.
C18:	**I play bubble**

First begin with a discussion of language form. As you read through the transcript, you may be struck by the fact that Claire's utterances are very short and simple. Indeed, analysis of 100 utterances indicated that Claire's sentences were an average of two words in length. You may also notice that she makes some grammatical errors. For instance, in utterance C13, Claire says "look I make it" when she means I made it or I'm making it. This is an example of a tense error. In utterance C18, she fails to use the plural marker on bubbles, even though she used the plural correctly in utterance C2. Inconsistencies such as these are common in the speech of children with a DLD. Further analysis of utterance C18 indicates that Claire has left out some important words. We as adults would probably say "I want to play with the bubbles" or "I'm gonna play with the bubbles" if we were engaged in this communicative exchange. Finally, Claire used some words that were not intelligible to the transcriber. This is common in children with Down syndrome because they often have motor difficulties that affect speech skills. Clearly, the form of Claire's language is well below the level we would expect for a 6-year-old child.

Now review the transcript with content in mind. As you may have noticed, the vast majority of Claire's utterances refer to what is happening in the immediate environment. When she refers to past events, they are those that have just happened (utterances C3 and C13). Utterance C3 is interesting for another reason. Without knowing the context, you would not know what "I did it" means. She did not say something specific such as "I caught the bubble." In fact "I did it" is an utterance that Claire uses repeatedly to refer to many different events. This may indicate limitations in vocabulary development that result in the overuse of generic or all-purpose utterances such as "I did it." In utterance C7, Claire says "to eat with" to mean that cake is something to eat (at least this is her mother's interpretation). Utterance C8 is interesting because Claire makes reference to time ("at eight thirty"). This is one of the few instances where she talks about something not immediately present. Unfortunately, her mother fails to understand what she means. Further analysis of Claire's language revealed that she could name most of the objects in the bag. However, her ability to talk about how these objects were used or how they related to her own toys or experiences was extremely limited. In addition, Claire rarely talked about objects or events that were not present in the immediate environment.

Review the sample once again and this time think about Claire's use of language. Remember to consider what both partners in the communicative exchange are saying. Begin by looking at Claire's response to questions and her ability to move the topic of conversation forward. For the most part, she responds when her mother asks her a question (C4, C5, C6 and C16). In addition, she asks her mother if she would like some grapes (C15). These behaviors indicate that Claire, like Brian, understands some of the "tacit" rules of conversation. In contrast to Brian, however, Claire usually responds to questions with yes or no. Consider utterances

C8 and C9. After Claire says "at eight thirty," her mother asks for clarification or additional information about what she means. Claire's response is a simple "yeah" which provides no additional information to her mother. Claire's inability to elaborate on her original thought is most likely due to limited development of language content and form. There are a few instances in which Claire adds to the topic of conversation. Utterance C2 informs her mother that she's making little bubbles, not big ones. Utterances C8–C12 add new information about cutting the cake. Again, these behaviors show that Claire understands some of the basic rules of conversation.

Now examine what Claire accomplishes when she talks. With utterance C3, she calls attention to herself and informs her mother that she has caught a bubble. Utterances C1 and C14, although limited in form, clearly communicate that she does not like what is being shown or offered to her. With utterance C15, Claire politely asks her mother if she would like some grapes. Finally, utterance C18 communicates that Claire would like to play with bubbles instead of pretending to eat a grape. Overall, Claire used her language to accomplish a variety of communicative functions.

Questions

At this point, you should be able to answer some key questions about Claire. As I suggested before, discuss these questions with your classmates and instructor before reading the answers provided.

Q: Why do Mrs. Vance and I regard Claire as language disordered?

A: The results of norm-referenced tests indicated that, although Claire's receptive language skills were commensurate with her nonverbal cognitive skills, her expressive skills were reduced relative to nonverbal cognitive and receptive language functioning. The language sample also showed significantly delayed expressive language abilities. Based on these results, we can conclude that Claire has a language disorder.

Q: Which language components (form, content, or use) currently require attention?

A: The language sample indicated that Claire has difficulty with language form and content. She has a tendency to use all-purpose utterances to talk about various objects and events. Improving Claire's ability to use a greater number of vocabulary items and language forms to express these ideas would enhance her ability to communicate. Some attention to the structure or form of utterances may also be necessary to help Claire communicate more effectively. Finally, although her use of language appears relatively well developed at this time, it is important that this aspect of language be carefully monitored.

Q: What type of therapy approach might be suitable for this child? Why?

A: Claire's therapy should focus on helping her develop new ways to talk about the objects and events in her environment. In addition, she may need assistance in learning to talk about objects and events not immediately present. Although she makes some grammatical errors, improving language form would not be the priority at this time. Because child-oriented and hybrid approaches provide opportunities to talk about objects, people, and events throughout the child's daily routine, both would be utilized with Claire. Her parents and teachers could be trained to model a variety of three- to five-word utterances when interacting with her. Hybrid approaches could be used in the classroom to stimulate and reinforce production of novel utterances throughout the course of the day. Collaboration between clinician, teacher, and parent could help Claire learn to tell her parents what happened at school and vice versa. This could be an important step in helping Claire talk about people, objects, and events not present in the immediate environment.

Ken

History

Ken is 6 years, 4 months of age. He is an only child who lives at home with his parents. He attends a special education class in the public schools five days per week.

Ken's birth history was unremarkable. He was born full term with no complications. His health history was also unremarkable. Ken's motor developmental milestones were within normal limits: He sat alone at 6 months and walked unaided at 12 months.

Ken's parents reported normal speech and language development until the age of 20 months, followed by a regression in verbal expression and the emergence of stereotypic hand movements, high-pitched screaming, social withdrawal, hand biting, and irregular sleep patterns. At 31 months of age, Ken was evaluated by a pediatrician who reported a marked delay in his emotional development. Physical and neurological development were found to be within normal limits.

At age 31 months, the diagnosis of autism was assigned by a clinical psychologist who noted delays in Ken's play behavior. Ken's nonverbal IQ was assessed and was found to be within the normal range.

At age 33 months, Ken's language skills were assessed by a speech-language pathologist. At that time, his receptive and expressive language skills were at the 14-month level. Ken communicated mainly through gestures and leading his parents to desired objects. A general development scale indicated that his motor skills were at the 32-month level and his nonverbal problem solving abilities were at the 34-month level.

Shortly after he was diagnosed with autism, a team of specialists began providing services to Ken and his family. Initially, the team worked with the family at home, and later Ken was placed in a special needs classroom at a local agency. At the age of 5, he began receiving services through the public schools.

Results of Norm-referenced Tests

Ken has undergone various assessments since the age of 3. This discussion will focus on the results of the most recent speech and language testing only. As was reported in the history, a clinical psychologist found Ken's nonverbal cognitive skills to be within the normal range for his age.

When Ken was 5 years, 10 months of age, his speech and language skills were reassessed. When norm-referenced tests designed for children Ken's age were administered, his responses were often judged to be unreliable, presumably because the test items were too difficult.

Only one of the language tests administered yielded valid, scorable results. This test assessed Ken's understanding of single words (receptive vocabulary). Results placed his receptive vocabulary skills well below the range expected for his age. A language test designed for younger children was also administered. Because norms for 5-year-old children were not available, a score could not be obtained, and results could only be used to describe Ken's language skills. During administration of this test, Ken named familiar objects and repeated words on request. He did not comment on immediate experiences and did not ask or answer questions. Receptively, Ken pointed to body parts and to familiar objects and people. He also demonstrated understanding of simple requests involving action (e.g., "Sit down"), number (e.g., "Put one spoon in the box"), function (e.g., "Show me what you read"), and size, shape, and color attributes (e.g., "Point to the green block"). Ken responded correctly to commands involving the words "on," "under," and "beside" and to commands requiring him to follow two or more steps (e.g., "Give me the dog and put the shoe on the floor"). An articulation test revealed that Ken's ability to pronounce speech sounds was below the range expected for a child his age.

Results of the Language Sample Analyses

A language sample was collected as Ken played with his mother at home. A portion of the sample appears in the box below. The language sample was used to analyze the form, content, and use of Ken's spontaneous language.

Ken's Language Sample

Ken and his mother are playing together at home. They have crayons, coloring books, legos, cars and trucks.

(Mom has made a plane from legos. She puts a pilot in the plane. Ken makes the plane fly and turns it upside down)

K1: **no, no, no**

M: Oh no, he's gonna fall out of the plane. He's hanging on by   a string (in a high-pitched voice). He's falling out of the   plane.

K2: **oh no, oh no, oh no**

(Mom puts the pilot back on top of the plane)

M: He's standing on top of the plane.

(Ken turns the plane over and the pilot falls off)

M: Oh no, He's all broken. His leg is broken, his arm is broken.

(Ken laughs. He picks up the pilot and looks at it)

K3: **leg is broken**

M: His leg is broken. He fell out of the plane.

(Mom looks at the airplane)

M: The wing is broken.

(continued)

K4:   wing is broken

M: The wing on the airplane is broken.

(Ken picks up the pilot. Mom runs the airplane into the pilot)

M: Oh no.

(Ken laughs)

K5:   oh no

(Mom looks through the legos)

M: I'm gonna build a car. What do you want?

(Mom works on her car. Ken drinks some lemonade)

K6:   lemonade please

K7:   drink

M: How about a car with two wheels? Oh no. I need
        some more   wheels.

(Mom finishes the car and moves it toward Ken)

K8:   oh no, oh no, oh no, oh no, oh no

(Mom picks up the car to adjust something. Ken drinks all
of his lemonade and holds his cup out to Mom)

K9:   lemonade

K10:   give me some lemonade (Ken uses a high-pitched voice)

M: What do you want?

K11:   can I have some lemonade, please (Ken uses an
        appropriate pitch)

M: Sure.

(Mom pushes the car)

M: Look, over the bumpy road.

(Mom gets up to get more lemonade)

(Ken pushes the car toward the edge of the table)

K12:   oh no, oh no

(Mom comes back with the juice and holds it in front of Ken)

K13:   juice

(Ken laughs. He reaches for the lemonade and his microphone falls off)

M: Oh, you lost your microphone. Here it is — we need to put it   back.

K14:   six

M: What?

M: I know what you're looking for. You want that car that goes   all by itself. Want mama to get it?

K15:   red

M: Huh?

K16:   red bus

M: Red bus? The red bus is right there.

(Mom and Ken play with the bus)

As you read through the sample the first time, you may notice that the conversation between Ken and his mother lacks the smooth back and forth flow that we observed in the other samples. Ken's mother takes on most of the responsibility for keeping the interaction going. She supplies the words to describe Ken's actions as well as her own. Also notice that, at times, Ken repeats all or part of what his mother says (utterances K3, K4, and K5). You may recall from the introduction to autism that this behavior is called echolalia. Ken's mother asks few questions, especially those that require him to provide new information (e.g. "What do you want to do now?"). Throughout the sample (50 utterances), Ken responded to only half of the questions his mother asked. Of these responses, only half were considered appropriate or related to the question. Similarly, Ken often produces utterances that seem unrelated to the topic of conversation. Examples include K14 and K15. Children with autism often say things that seem unrelated to what their communication partner has said. These observations indicate that Ken's understanding of the conversation rules is less well developed in comparison to the other children discussed.

Now consider what Ken accomplishes when he talks. With utterance K1, he calls his mother's attention to what he is doing. Utterances K2 and K12 appear to be comments about what is happening in the immediate environment. With utterances K3 and K4,

Ken acknowledges what his mother has said by echoing her, but he does not extend the topic in any way. Finally, he asks for lemonade with utterances K6, K10, K11, and K13. In summary, Ken accomplishes some communicative functions with his language. The variety of forms he uses to express these functions, however, is extremely limited. We will discuss this finding in a moment.

The content of Ken's language is interesting and further sets him apart from Brian and Claire. As with Claire, Ken rarely talks about objects and events not present in the immediate environment. In addition, analysis of the complete sample indicated that the vast majority of Ken's utterances made reference to the color or size of objects (e.g., "It's blue" or "A hair's brown") or to ownership of the object (e.g., "That's mine"). Recall that both Brian and Claire talked more frequently about what was happening around them. In Ken's case, most comments about ongoing action appeared limited to "oh no, oh no" (see utterances K2, K5, K8, and K12). In fact, Ken used verbs to describe different actions in only 4 of 50 utterances. Overall, the ideas Ken expresses are extremely limited. He talks about attributes such as color, size, and number, and about ownership. He asks for things using memorized phrases such as "Can I have _____, please?" Finally, in addition to difficulty talking about past and future events, Ken has great difficulty talking about what is happening in the immediate environment.

Now consider the form or structure of Ken's language. Due to his limited expressive output, and the paucity of sentences, it is difficult to gain a good understanding of this language component. In utterances K3 and K4, Ken uses the word "is," a form which Brian usually omitted. Caution must be used when analyzing utterances such as these, however, because Ken was imitating his mother. Utterances K10 and K11 were grammatically correct. Analysis of 50 utterances indicated that Ken made few grammatical errors. Some of the utterances he used spontaneously included "This is mine" and "It's carnation pink." Language that appears to be intact grammatically is common in children with autism. Language form appears well developed relative to content and use.

Questions

Once again, answer the three important questions. Think about the answers and discuss them with your classmates and instructor before reading the answers provided.

Q: Why do Mrs. Vance and I regard Ken as language disordered?

A: Ken clearly has a language disorder. His extremely limited ability to communicate effectively with others, even his mother, contrasts with that of the other children we have discussed. He appears to lack the ability to carry on a meaningful conversation with another individual.

Q: Which language components (form, content, or use) currently require attention?

A: Ken's limited ability to communicate relates to difficulties in the areas of language use and content. Ken's understanding of the conversation rules is limited. He needs help in developing the skills necessary to initiate and respond appropriately in a conversational exchange. In addition, he needs assistance in developing a variety of forms to accomplish his communicative needs. For example, helping Ken develop a variety of ways to ask for things would make his language sound more natural. In addition to language use, Ken needs assistance in developing language content. He needs to learn to talk about ongoing actions, locations of objects and people, feelings or emotions, and, eventually, about objects and events not present in the immediate environment.

Q: What type of therapy approach might be suitable for this child? Why?

A: Because Ken needs help in learning to participate in a conversational exchange, and because he needs practice in talking about the objects, people, and actions in the immediate environment, a child-oriented approach would be suitable at this time.

It is difficult to maintain a normal conversational exchange with a child with autism. If Ken's mother can be trained to modify her interactions with Ken, his language skills might be improved indirectly. Ken's mother needs to learn to follow his lead and to "tune in" to what Ken says and does. Instead of guessing what he wants, (see Mom's utterances) she should be encouraged to let him tell her what he wants and needs. At times, Ken's mother expands his utterances (see Mom's utterances following K3 and K4), an excellent way to facilitate language development. If Ken were producing more utterances relevant to the context, his mother could do more expansions. In addition, she should be encouraged to talk about what Ken is seeing, doing, and feeling using a variety of action words. Ken's father and teachers should also be trained to use child-oriented procedures with him so that improved language skills can be facilitated across daily activities.

◆ SUMMARY AND CONCLUSIONS

Children with DLDs differ from one another in many ways. Those with specific language impairment have their major difficulty with language form. In contrast, children with mental retardation have diminished complexity of thought accompanied by language content, form, and use levels lower than expected for their age. Children with autism are disinclined to communicate, have difficulty with language use, and exhibit deficits in form and content ranging from mild to profound.

During the evaluation process, a speech-language pathologist addresses three major questions: Is the child language disordered? If so, which language components require attention? And which treatment approach is suitable for the child? To answer these questions accurately, the clinician must understand the appropriate use of norm-referenced measures, how to analyze a spontaneous language sample, and how to interpret case history information and observations collected during the evaluation process. In many cases, more than one treatment strategy, and especially in the cases of autistic or mental retarded children, more than one specialist is required to serve the child well.

◆ ACKNOWLEDGMENT

Mrs. Rebecca Vance, who directs the clinic of the University of Arizona, Tucson Scottish Rite Center for Childhood Language Disorders, helped prepare the initial draft of this chapter. Her insights and advocacy regarding children with DLDs are invaluable to those fortunate enough to benefit from her attention. Together, Mrs. Vance and I thank the Tucson Scottish Rite Charitable Foundation for the unwavering support that has made it possible for us to serve and study children with specific language impairment in one facility. I also thank Janette Ressue for serving as an associate editor and student reader during the final drafts of this chapter. She, like many of you, is in the process of becoming a speech-language pathologist. We dedicate our work on this chapter to our friend, the late Lyle Coolidge, 33°, and his beloved wife, Ethel, without whom there may well have been no Center.

Endnote: I recommend you check out the video "Rain Man" and have a class party. (If that is a success, check out "Wild Child" and compare and contrast the intervention methods used with those mentioned in this chapter.) Get your instructor to spring for the popcorn.

◆ REFERENCES

Courchesne, E., Yeung-Courchesne, R., Press, G., Hesselink J. R., & Jernigan, T. L. (1988). Hypoplasia of the cerebellar vermal lobes VI and VII in infantile autism. *New England Journal of Medicine, 318,* 1349–1354.

Fey, M. (1986). *Language intervention with young children.* Boston: College-Hill Press.

McCauley, R. J., & Swisher, L. (1984). Psychometric review of language and articulation tests for preschool children. *Journal of Speech and Hearing Disorders, 49,* 34–42.

Plante, E., Swisher, L., Vance, R., & Rapcsak, S. (1991). MRI findings in boys with specific language impairment. *Brain and Language, 41,* 52–66.

Rutter, M. (1978). Language disorder and infantile autism. In M. Rutter & E. Schopler (Eds.), *Autism: A reappraisal of concepts and treatment.* New York: Plenum Press.

Schlanger, B. (1973). *Mental retardation.* Indianapolis: Bobbs-Merrill.

Stevenson, J., & Richman, M. (1976). The prevalence of language delay in a population of three-year-old children and its association with general retardation. *Developmental Medicine and Child Neurology, 18,* 431–441.

Wing, L. (1976). *Early childhood autism.* Oxford: Pergamon Press.

◆ GLOSSARY

Echolalia: repetition of the words spoken by another person.

Etiology: the cause of a disease/disorder.

Expansion: the repetition of a child's utterance in a longer and slightly more complex form.

Interdisciplinary team: a group of representatives from different disciplines who work together within an integrated plan of treatment.

Mainstreaming: providing the opportunity for handicapped children to interact with normally developing peers in a regular classroom.

Otitis media: inflammation of the middle ear.

Parallel talk: a language facilitation technique in which an adult talks about what the child is doing.

Self talk: a language facilitation technique in which an adult talks about what the adult is doing at the moment.

Transcript: a written record of the utterances spoken by a child and another individual. Frequently, a description of the physical environment is included.

Human Communication Disorders in Context and Environment

JAMES R. ANDREWS, PH.D.

When you have completed this chapter, you should be able to:

✦ Define a linear paradigm and a systemic paradigm and discuss treatment models for which they form a basis.

✦ Describe the concepts of (1) defining the treatment system, (2) the role of the clinician, and (3) counseling as they are used in the individual treatment model and in treatment in context.

✦ Discuss systemic principles and their application to contextual treatment in speech, language, and hearing disorders.

✦ Discuss issues related to speech, language, and hearing treatment of clients in the context of interactive systems.

New service delivery models are emerging in speech-language pathology and audiology. In addition to the individual, one-on-one, approach in which treatment is offered in the clinician's office, treatment is now being offered in the environment or context of the client. Specialists in communication disorders are learning to use the resources of others, such as family members, teachers, and other habilitative specialists, to extend their influence far beyond the traditional therapy room. This expansion of treatment options requires new ways of thinking. In this chapter, you will learn about communication disorders in context through a discussion of issues and through case illustrations selected from the writer's clinical experience.

It is the clinical practice of the profession that captures the interest and imagination of most speech-language pathologists and audiologists. Intervening to improve the quality of life for clients by enhancing their ability to communicate is both satisfying and challenging to most clinicians. The search for ever more effective treatment methods has become especially active and interesting over the past several years. New models for serving people with speech, language, and hearing problems are emerging that require expanded clinical skills and new ways of thinking. As these models are perfected by innovative clinicians, the clinicians themselves will be in the best position to test their effectiveness. In other words, the clinicians who master the techniques and knowledge that new service delivery models require will be in the best position to add to the clinical knowledge of the discipline of communication sciences and disorders.

Speech-language pathologists traditionally have provided treatment services to clients on an individual basis with the clinician meeting alone with the client in the clinician's office. However, new forms of professional practice are emerging in which clinicians use a variety of approaches to change a client's behavior. These may result in clinicians including clients' entire families in treatment and working with their assistance; providing services in the classroom with teachers; consulting with teachers to help *them* make interventions in the classroom; and sharing knowledge with groups of other professionals on treatment teams. The purpose of this chapter is to introduce the beginning student to these varied approaches to clinical treatment and to the rationales behind them.

At the outset we must appreciate that making one's knowledge usable by family members, teachers, and persons from related disciplines such as physical therapy, occupational therapy, and medicine requires special skills and knowledge in addition to those used to provide services directly to clients in a one-on-one situation. First, let's define what is meant by "treatment in context." When a clinician provides services in which interventions are integrated into family interactions, interactions in the classroom, or interactions that take place while another service is being provided (e.g., physical or occupational therapy) it is said that the speech, language, or hearing treatment is occurring "in context." That is, interventions are occurring in real life situations, outside of the clinician's office and in the context or presence of family members, classmates, teachers, and/or other habilitative specialists.

These additions to to the individual service delivery model have resulted in an expansion of our focus of attention. Besides focusing on the communicative characteristics of individuals, we also are beginning to attend to communicative interactions between clients and others in their environments. We pay attention, then, not only to what and how clients communicate, but also to the responses of listeners. This double description (Keeney, 1983), this attention to both sides of natural interactive sequences, opens new possibilities for intervening in the context of everyday communication.

Thinking about treatment in context also has led us to think more about how a communicative disorder may manifest itself in social situations, about who may be affected by a client's communicative disorder, and who might be involved in the process of change. As you will learn later in this chapter, the underlying assumptions that form the basis for traditional one-on-one individual treatment seem insufficient to support treatment in contextual situations. It is well known that the way we think determines what we do. More broadly, our view of the world serves to direct our attention and influence our perceptions of reality. The changes that are occurring in the way we provide clinical treatment for speech, language, and hearing disorders are so profound that they are understood most completely when we make a shift in some of our most basic ways of thinking.

The remainder of this chapter will be a discussion about two types of thinking, that is, two world views, and how each influences our understanding of communicative disorders and the manner in which change is elicited. The connection between thinking and clinical practice will be discussed and described. Several clinical examples will be used to demonstrate the use of treatment provided in context.

◆ TWO WORLD VIEWS

In this section we will discuss two **paradigms**, or world views. Most of us are so familiar with a **linear** cause-effect view of the world that it is difficult to imagine any other. This view assumes that one event is caused by another and that a correct interpretation of the cause can be identified. A second paradigm, less familiar to most of us, is called a **systemic** world view. This view assumes that each event is unique to the context in which it occurs and that interpretations of an event are likely to differ. Although the field of communicative disorders traditionally has been based on the former view, it now seems likely that clinical services are most effective when the practitioner integrates these views and uses elements of *both* perspectives. Clearly, the manner in which a speech-language pathologist or audiologist provides clinical services is dependent on how that person thinks about relationships, communication, communicative disorders, and the clinical process. It is not an exaggeration to say that the professional's view of the world determines how he or she will provide clinical services to persons with communicative disorders.

The Linear Paradigm

Most of us have learned to view the world from a linear cause-effect perspective. This type of thinking is typical in western culture and has facilitated the development of many important scientific advances. Certain bacterial organisms, for example, *cause* illness in humans; heating food to a particular temperature *causes* the bacteria to be killed. Linear thinking can be envisioned as "in a line." It is characterized by a search for causal relationships, by orderliness, and by reducing complex reality or phenomena into a number of smaller, simpler parts. It is anti-contextual in that phenomena are studied outside of their natural environments (i.e., in the laboratory) and atomistic, meaning that a phenomenon may be divided into small parts that may be studied independently of the whole. This implies that there is little or no interaction between the parts and that nothing is lost when a small unit of the whole is studied outside of its relationship to the other parts that comprise the phenomenon. The practice of medicine in Western culture is based on a linear perspective. In fact, the practice of medicine in our part of the world is so tied to a linear perspective that some use the term "medical model" as being nearly synonymous with linear perspective. The medical model, in fact, provides us with such a good example of the application of a linear perspective that we will analyze its characteristics to help us understand how specialists in communicative disorders (speech-language pathologists and audiologists) traditionally have conducted their professional practices.

The medical model assumes that (1) there is one correct truth; (2) the view of the expert (the physician) is paramount; (3) the physician should seek the cause of the patient's illness; (4) the physician should decide the course of action that is to be taken, based on the cause of the problem; (5) the unit of treatment is the individual who is ill; (6) the patient should comply with the physician's recommendations; and (7) anything that interferes with the physician's treatment of the patient is intrusive and to be avoided.

Consider the individual with a persistent headache who seeks medical treatment. The physician first attempts to determine the cause of the headache. The treatment of a headache due to a brain tumor obviously is different than treatment for a headache related to tension. It is the physician's opinion that is important; he or she will determine the "truth" about the patient's headaches. The patient's friends and family members may have other views about the cause of the problem, but their views are not likely to be sought or used by the attending physician who, alone, will determine the course of treatment. The individual with the headache is the unit of treatment (i.e., the patient) and will be expected to comply with the physician's request to come for further tests, take a particular medication, make a change in life style, and so on. The fact that the patient is busy and finds it difficult to make time for further testing or to purchase medication is irrelevant and unlikely to be part of the physician-patient conversation.

This perspective, applied to communication disorders, leads the speech-language pathologist to assess the potential communication disorder and search for its cause; provide treatment for the communication disorder that is independent of the context in which the client is seen (i.e., the treatment is the same whether the person is seen in a hospital, school, clinic, or at home); view the client as the unit of treatment and attend to change as it occurs in the client, presumably, as a result of treatment; determine the course and frequency of treatment services; and make prescriptive recommendations for others to follow (typically homework assignments to practice a new skill or understanding).

To illustrate, Mark is 8 years old and in the third grade. Mark's teacher noticed that his speech is difficult to understand and she referred him to the school's speech-language pathologist. The speech-language pathologist asked Mark to come to her office where she listened to him speak and administered an articulation test (a set of pictures or words designed to elicit all of the sounds of American English). In addition to determining Mark's

(continued)

speech-language characteristics, the clinician searched for causes of the problem. She screened his hearing and checked his school records for any indication that he had ever failed the standard hearing test administered to all children in the school. While she had his file, she also read it for any indication of a learning disability, any notes about poor motor coordination, and any information about general intellectual functioning. As she interacted with Mark, the clinician watched how he used his tongue and lips to form sounds, looked at his teeth to rule out the possibility that poor alignment of teeth or missing teeth might be the cause of any of his articulation errors, and asked him to engage in a set of predetermined movements of his tongue and lips. The speech-language pathologist found that Mark had many articulation errors. A missing tooth might be responsible for his distortion of the /s/ sound, but could not account for most of his other misarticulations. Although his hearing sensitivity was within normal limits, his records indicated that he had many recurring ear infections and, likely, mild to moderate hearing losses between the ages of 2 and 5. This, the clinician speculated, might account for a good part of his present difficulty with speech. The pattern of Mark's speech sound errors was such that the clinician decided to analyze them using an additional and more elaborate procedure that would allow her to determine underlying "rules" that Mark might be using to select articulatory gestures and, therefore, speech sounds. She found, for example, that he often omitted the final sounds of words and that he tended to use his tongue tip to produce sounds that ordinarily are produced with the back of the tongue. As a result of this evaluation, the speech-language pathologist determined that Mark did have a significant speech articulation problem, that Mark would be unlikely to improve his speech on his own, and that his problem likely is related to frequent temporary reductions of hearing sensitivity that occurred when Mark was younger. The clinician recommended that she work with Mark in her office for 30 minutes, two times each week. She will see Mark alone during that time. Mark's mother indicated that she appreciated the attention that Mark was getting, and the clinician informed her that, at a later time, she would be sending work home with Mark that she hoped would be completed.

The Systemic Paradigm

A systemic world view is characterized by attention to interaction, relationship, wholeness, and context. In this perspective, reality is viewed as being based on one's perception and is the result of the interaction between an event and an individual's interpretation of the event. An individual's perception of truth is acknowledged as valid. Rather than seeking the one correct truth, or perspective, each person's perspective is accepted as truth as it exists for that individual. Systemic thinking can be envisioned in the form of a circle, rather than a line.

Interactive problems, rather than disease, provide the best example of use of a systemic paradigm. Rather than a physician, then, consider a family therapist as the expert. In a systemic therapeutic approach: (1) each person's perspective of truth, or reality, is viewed as valid; (2) the perspective of the expert (the therapist) is one of several views, each of which is important; (3) the cause of the problem may be impossible or difficult to determine and/or may be irrelevant to treatment; (4) the therapist guides the course of action that is to be taken based on everyone's view of the problem; (5) the unit of treatment is the group of individuals who compose the relevant interactive system (i.e., a family); (6) the therapist talks about the situation in a manner that is based on the views of everyone involved and makes suggestions that are reasonable reframes of these perspectives; and (7) extraneous factors that are part of the family's situation are sought out and accommodated in suggestions for change.

Consider the young married couple who find themselves arguing so much that they seek help from a family therapist. The therapist first determines each person's view of the problem. The wife may, for example, report that her husband withdraws from her and seems unwilling to interact with her in the close, personal way that she believes should typify a good marriage. The husband's perspective, on the other hand, may be that his wife is forever asking him questions and probing into his life in an intrusive, inappropriate, and irritating manner. His view of a good marriage is that a couple enjoys one another, but that each maintains a certain amount of privacy. There is no one correct truth in this situation; there are two truths. The therapist's perspective may add a third truth. Neither the wife nor the husband is the cause of the problem, although each may blame the other. The cause of the problem would be difficult to determine and will not be the focus of the therapist's attention. Rather, the clinician will use techniques that take into account each of their perspectives on their situation. The therapist will attempt to learn
(continued)

about the couple's life style and values as well as significant influences currently on them to frame suggestions in a manner that each will accept. Change will be expected to occur in the context of the couple's everyday interactions, not in the therapist's office.

The systemic perspective, applied to communicative disorders, leads the speech-language pathologist to define a group of people who have influence on the person with the speech-language problem; determine the perspective each of these persons has about the problem, what each has done to help the person with the problem, and what each believes has been successful in helping the person; assess the disorder to search for a likely cause; and provide treatment that uses the resources of everyone in the defined interactive system of involved people. Much of the treatment will occur in interactions between these people and the person with the communicative disorder. In other words, treatment will occur in the context of conversations and everyday interactions. The unit of treatment includes not only the person with the speech-language problem, but those who make up the group referred to as the "interactive system." The speech-language pathologist will attend both to changes in the client (the person with the problem) and to changes in interactions that occur in the interactive system. Suggestions will be given that are based on each person's perspective. The types of interactions that are believed by those involved to have been helpful, and that the clinician also believes will be helpful, are expanded on to become a significant part of the clinician's suggestions.

Using Mark as the illustration, recall that he is 8 years old and in the third grade. His teacher found his speech difficult to understand and referred him to the school's speech-language pathologist. This time, let us assume that the speech-language pathologist provides treatment services based on a combination of a linear paradigm and a systemic paradigm. Consequently, the speech-language pathologist asked Mark's teacher to describe what she had noticed about Mark's speech and what she does that she believes is most helpful to Mark. She also asked his teacher: (1) if she thought Mark had a hearing loss; (2) if she thought Mark's academic learning might be negatively affected by his speech problem; and (3) if she (the speech-language pathologist) might observe Mark in the classroom. The teacher believed that

Mark's hearing was normal but was concerned that his speech was causing him difficulty in learning to read. The teacher suggested that the speech-language pathologist come to the classroom during the time reading was being taught. The speech-language pathologist subsequently visited Mark's classroom and found his speech to be characterized by many imprecisions and difficult to understand. Later, she met briefly with the teacher and told her that she concurred with her observations. She also pointed out that the teacher's technique of letting Mark watch her face as she repeated some of the words from the reading book was a good idea. The speech-language pathologist called Mark's mother and told her that she had observed Mark in his classroom and asked if she or Mark's father had concerns about Mark's speech. Mark's mother said that everyone in their family could understand him and that they had not considered his speech to be a problem. The speech-language pathologist told her that Mark's teacher was having difficulty understanding him and that both his teacher and she were concerned about this and the possibility that his speech patterns might interfere with his learning to read. Would his parents, she asked, be willing to help Mark with his speech to help his teacher and other people at school understand him better? Mark's mother agreed to speak with Mark's father and suggested that they would both be willing to participate in any way possible to help the teachers.

The speech-language pathologist indicated that she would like to administer an articulation test to Mark and asked if there was a time that both Mark's mother and father could come and participate in that session. As it turned out, neither parent was available. The clinician searched Mark's school records for any indication that he had ever failed a hearing test or any indication of a learning disability, notes about motor coordination, information about Mark's intellectual ability, or any information that might help her better understand Mark' speech-language situation. The clinician then talked to Mark about his teacher's concern and discussed, with him, his awareness of his speech difficulties in the classroom. Mark agreed that it would be a good idea to improve his speech so that his teacher and friends could understand him more easily. The clinician administered the articulation test and, at the same time, watched how he used his tongue and lips to form sounds, and looked at his teeth to rule out the possibility that poor alignment of teeth or missing teeth might be the cause of any of his articulation errors. She also asked him

(continued)

to engage in the set of predetermined movements of his tongue and lips. The speech-language pathologist noted that Mark's front teeth might account for his distortion of the /s/ sound, but not for most of his other misarticulations. Although his hearing sensitivity currently was within normal limits, his records showed that he had experienced many recurring ear infections when he was younger. The clinician speculated that this might account, in part, for Mark's present difficulty with speech. The pattern of Mark's speech sound errors was such that the clinician analyzed them using a more elaborate procedure designed to uncover underlying "rules" that Mark might be using to select articulatory gestures and the resulting speech sounds. Mark, she found, often omitted the final sounds of words and tended to use his tongue tip to produce sounds that ordinarily are produced with the back of the tongue.

At this point, the speech-language pathologist had informally defined a treatment system as consisting of Mark's teacher, his father and mother, Mark, and herself. This group consisted of the primary set of people who could be used to help Mark improve his speech. Her task now was to determine what each of these people might do to help Mark and when they could do it. To elicit their cooperation, the clinician spoke again with Mark's teacher and described the testing she had done. She asked the teacher if she could continue to repeat some of the words that Mark said during reading and have him look at her face in the way she had done during the first classroom visit. The teacher said that this came very naturally to her and that she could easily do this. The speech-language pathologist added that if she could exaggerate the final sounds of some of the words as she did this it would be especially helpful. The teacher agreed and asked the speech-language pathologist to visit the classroom another time just to be sure that she was following her suggestions accurately. The speech-language pathologist concurred and also arranged to see Mark herself, on an individual basis, one time per week. Mark's parents were pleased with this arrangement. The speech-language pathologist inquired about family activities and times that Mark's parents typically interacted with him. His mother reported that she read a book to Mark nearly every evening and that Mark's father liked to roughhouse with him. Mark's mother was asked if she could exaggerate the final sounds of some words as she read to Mark and she agreed to do so. Mark's mother also suggested that Mark's father might be able to do the same thing as he wrestled with Mark. The speech-language pathologist reminded Mark's mother to keep these activities enjoyable for both Mark and his parents and, for now, to merely let Mark listen rather than ask him to repeat words. The clinician asked Mark to pay attention to times when his friends understood him the best. Finally, the speech-language pathologist invited Mark's parents to visit during the time she worked with him and indicated that she would be calling in another week or so to see how her suggestions were going.

✦ LINEAR AND SYSTEMIC VIEWS IN CLINICAL PRACTICE

The manner in which the profession is practiced depends on the clinician's treatment paradigm and the treatment situation. Three specific and important ways in which clinical practice varies with the clinician's paradigm are: (1) definition of the treatment system, (2) the role of the clinician, and (3) the use of counseling techniques.

Definition of the Treatment System

In the individual direct services delivery model, which is based on a **linear paradigm**, the interactive system is assumed to be the client and the clinician. In this model, the clinician's attention and primary intervention is directed toward the client. Change is expected and attended to only in that person (the client). Further, the primary change in communicative ability is expected to occur during the treatment sessions with the clinician. Toward this end, parents of children with special needs typically argue for more time for their children to be served by clinicians. For many years, the linear paradigm for clinical service provision was not questioned. It seemed obvious that the clinician would work solely with the person who had the problem. Another model of clinical service delivery could hardly be imagined.

More recently, other models of service delivery have emerged. For example, definition of the **treatment system** becomes an issue for the clinician whose treatment services are based on a **systemic paradigm**. In this model, one of the first steps in treatment is to determine who will be involved. The treatment system is defined as the client and a group of people who interact with the client, have influence on the client, and are concerned about the client's problem. A client's family typically would meet this definition even if the family was not the traditional two-parent, married, birth mother and father. The definition also could be met by counselors in a residential setting or selected staff in a school, hospital, or nursing home. Friends of a client, including selected children in a school, also may be included within the system.

Change is expected in the client, but changes also are expected to occur in the interactions of the family or other persons making up the system. The clinician's primary intervention is with the client and the people in the treatment system. Treatment often is indirect and suggestions are given to be used by members of the system as they interact with the client. In other words, treatment typically occurs in the client's context whether it be the home, school, hospital, or nursing home.

Role of the Clinician

In the individual direct services model, the clinician learns about the client's speech-language problem from the clinician's perspective. The views of others are not attended to and are considered unimportant. Typically, the views of others are not sought. Once the clinician has learned about the problem, he or she begins to use techniques with the client designed to improve the client's ability to communicate.

In contrast, the clinician using a systemic service delivery model learns about the client's problem from everyone in the defined system. The clinician learns what each person has done about the problem and the successes he or she has had. The clinician also develops his or her own view of the problem and conducts a clinical assessment of the client. After everyone's perspective is known, the clinician develops a way of talking about the problem (i.e., a language for talking about it) that makes sense to everyone participating in the treatment system and talks with them about it in that way. Further, the clinician determines how and when other people in the system can be involved in creating communicative change in the client. In other words, the clinician determines the kind of interactive differences that will promote change. Changes are expected to occur in both the client and the system. For example, the process of family members hearing one another's views, in and of itself, sometimes causes family members not only to begin to view the situation somewhat differently, but also to interact differently with the client. As the clinician listens and learns, he or she notices points of agreement and disagreement between people; attends to spontaneous communication patterns within the system, particularly those involving the client; and looks for behavioral sequences in which the problem may be embedded. Typically, some interactions that tend to promote change are seen as well as interactions that may perpetuate the problem. These issues are addressed during the process of treatment.

Use of Counseling Techniques

Clinicians using an individual direct services model of treatment tend to view counseling as providing the client and the client's family with educational information about the problem. For example, verbal explanations, brochures, and information about support groups that may be helpful to the client may be provided.

In a systemic model, the clinician must have good counseling skills for treatment to be successful. These skills are used for a variety of purposes: to interview and learn the different perspectives of those making up the treatment system; to respond to differences in points of view; to enlist cooperation and participation in treatment; to respond to emotions; to problem solve with the group; and to present unwelcome information.

✦ FOUR SYSTEMIC PRINCIPLES

In what follows, four systemic principles that relate to professional practice in context are described. They may be easiest to link with your experience when they are viewed as applied to the interactive system of a family. They can also, however, be applied to other systems, including classrooms and professional teams.

Principle 1

One part of a system cannot be understood in isolation from the rest of the system.

Applying this principle to a human interactive system such as a family, the principle may be restated to read that one member of a family cannot be understood in isolation from the rest of the family (Epstein & Bishop, 1981). Behaviors of an individual are understood more completely when they are viewed in relation to, or in the context of, the interactions of the individual's family members than when they are observed apart from that context. As Trout and Foley (1989) stated, "we do not know a child unless we know his or her family" (p. 59). This principle is particularly significant for speech-language pathologists because communication is an interactive event. Each family has its own values, communication style, family vocabulary, mutually shared jokes and memories, and its own manner of relating meaning to events. It is difficult, if not impossible, to understand one member of the culture of a particular family by learning about that person individually, separate from the other members of that culture. Parents, for example, are able to explain many of their child's behaviors that may be uninterpretable to an outsider; siblings commonly are able to understand the speech of their unintelligible brother or sister; nonverbal behaviors of clients often are understood by family members; and parents know their children's tolerances, moods, frustration levels, imminent illnesses, energy levels, and so on. Family members typically can communicate with one another in a combination of verbal and nonverbal manners that conveys far more information to one another than to those outside of the family system. Finally, children are apt to talk and interact more in the presence of family members than they are when alone in the presence of a stranger — even if the stranger is a skilled specialist in communication sciences and disorders.

An example of this principle in clinical practice is the case of a 4-year-old child whose parents reported that he stuttered. Timmy lived with his mother, father, and 7-year-old brother. Early in the session, it became apparent that Timmy's mother was the family spokesperson and did most of the talking for the family. Timmy's father was rather quiet and spoke with a slight hesitancy that, itself, resembled stuttering. Timmy's older brother monitored the conversation that was occurring between his parents and the speech-language pathologist and, seemingly, corrected it for accuracy. As the parents reported factual data (e.g., about dates, family activities, interactions with friends and neighbors, etc.), the older brother made corrections. His parents acknowledged that he was nearly always accurate about these details. Further, while Timmy was described as being of average intelligence, his older brother was "at the top of his class." When all four family members were engaged in conversation with the speech-language pathologist, the mother and older brother did nearly all the talking. Questions addressed to the father or to Timmy were readily answered, simultaneously, by the mother and older brother. When the speech-language pathologist looked directly at Timmy and moved closer to him to talk with him, mother and older brother were essentially "on the edge of their seats" ready to answer, and frequently did.

Timmy's communicative environment seemed to be a clear factor in his problem. The speech-language pathologist, in response to the frenzied talking by two of the four family members, asked permission to play a game of checkers with Timmy. Timmy's mother said that Timmy and his brother frequently played checkers together and that Timmy knew how to play and would enjoy doing so with the clinician. The speech-language pathologist used the opportunity to create a different communicative environment by saying very little and talking in a quiet voice in short sentences when he did talk. At the end of the game Timmy's parents expressed amazement! It had, they said, not occurred to them that it would be possible to play with Timmy and not talk through the entire game. They went on to describe how they interrupted one another and suggested that this probably did not create an environment that was conducive to fluency. This insight by Timmy's parents provided the content of conversation for the next several sessions and was a significant factor in family-initiated change in communication style among family members. This change, in the clinician's view, was the basis for a resolution of Timmy's stuttering.

Timmy's stuttering could not possibly have been understood in the manner it was if he had not been seen in the context of his family. This is not to say that his stuttering might not have been resolved by a speech-language pathologist using a more individual perspective. Clearly, however, seeing Timmy in the context of his family gave the speech-language pathologist a "different look" at him and his situation than would have been derived by seeing him alone or with only one parent present.

Principle 2

Change in one part of the system creates change in other parts of the system (Epstein & Bishop, 1981).

When one member of a family has a hearing loss or a speech-language problem, every other member of the family reacts in some way. The exact type and variety of responses that are typical have not yet been identified because specialists in communication sciences and disorders are only beginning to realize the power and potential that lies within interactive systems. It is apparent from clinical observations, however, that some of the responses of family members may be used to promote change whereas others are likely to perpetuate the problem. Family members, themselves, have written more about the impact of disability on the family than professional specialists. Family members' accounts of the powerful influence of head injury (Demichelis, 1989), cleft palate (Seibel, 1987), hearing loss (Luterman, 1991), and other disabilities (Buscaglia, 1983) exist in the literature. Other, even more personal, descriptions of the profound influence of hearing loss and communication disorders likely sit on the desk of many practitioners in the form of letters from clients.

If there is truth in this principle, it follows that the responses of family members of our clients have a powerful influence on the success or failure of the communicative change we seek to make. Family members may, then, enhance or diminish the influence that speech-language pathologists and audiologists have on their clients. Clinicians who understand the power of the family and have the ability to use the resources of the family to promote communicative change are likely to be more effective than their counterparts who continue to attend solely to the individual with the disorder. Further, as more is learned about the specifics of family responses and influences, it is important that this becomes public knowledge. Clinical researchers, practitioners who have the ability to make astute observations as they practice the profession, and the skills to gather clinical data, are in a position to make substantial changes in the way we practice the profession and interpret the profession to the public. Although we have been slow to educate society about communication sciences and disorders, the current level of understanding among parents of children receiving services seems to be that 90 minutes of direct services with a speech-language pathologist is better than 60 minutes. Although this may be true, skillful use of the resources of everyone in the child's interactive system is, to this writer, far and away more powerful than 60 or 90 minutes of individual therapy. This conclusion has not been objectively proven! It is but one example of the type of information related to interactive systems that lies ready to be uncovered by creative practitioners-researchers.

One description of the application of this principle relates to changes in family members that occur *after* a communication disorder has improved (Andrews & Andrews, 1986).

In this case study, "T" is described as a 5-year-old child who lived with his parents, two older brothers, and an older sister. T's speech intelligibility was not a problem to his family; they reported that they could understand everything he said. His teacher and other children at school, however, had considerable difficulty understanding T's speech. T's family agreed to participate in sessions with the speech-language pathologist. They would all come to 1-hour sessions held approximately every other week, and carry out mutually agreed-on activities at home. These activities would be as "natural" as possible, in that they would be activities that could be done in the context of everyday interactions with T. Both parents and siblings agreed to help. Initially, it seemed that surgery might be necessary to improve the separation between T's mouth and nose at the point where his soft palate approximated the back wall of his throat. This proved to be unnecessary, however, when the precision of his speech began to improve. As this occurred, however, several additional and unexpected changes were reported by T's family. T's personality seemed to change. he became more verbally aggressive with his siblings who now described him as "mean" and as someone who said "dirty words." T's parents viewed this change as positive. Now that their young son could talk better, they said, he was able to stand up for himself and protect his toys, just as his siblings did with theirs. They also reported that T was less physically aggressive than before. This case study is a clinical example of how changes in T's ability to communicate influenced the way he was reacted to by others in his family (change in one part of the system resulted in changes in other parts of the system). Further, unexpected changes also occurred in T that seemed to be linked to his improved communicative ability. He brought a friend home from school for the first time; his teacher reported that he was dressed better and was more kempt; and a social worker reported that his parents were keeping dental appointments on a regular basis, for the first time. This is only one example of the richness of the family system and its influence and reaction to communication disorders and change. The foregoing example is only the beginning — there is much more to be learned about this process.

Principle 3

Transactional patterns of the family determine the behavior of family members (Epstein & Bishop, 1981).

The style and content of interactions among family members determines the behavior of its members. We all have seen examples of this; some are superficial, others are not. A particular mannerism may be used, for example, by both a parent and a child. This might be as simple as a way of sitting or a particular vocal inflection that is characteristic of members of the same family. On a deeper level, it may relate to values held by family members. Often, these values seem to be ones that run so deep that, more than being the subject of family discussions, they form the basis of decisions, assumptions, and life style in an unspoken manner. Everyone has attitudes about money, work, education, success, other people, and so forth. These attitudes tend to be passed from generation to generation. The manner or form in which values are expressed by children may be different than those of the parents. However, underlying assumptions usually persist.

Specialists in communication sciences and disorders are only beginning to apply this principle to treatment of communicative disorders. Current thinking tends to focus on the manner in which family members can be involved in effecting communicative change in a member with a speech-language or hearing problem. Following, is an example of a family with a 2-year-old child who does not talk.

Matt lives with his parents and baby sister. He has said a few words from time to time, but says no words on a consistent basis. In fact, attempts to encourage him to do so usually result in his walking away from the adult. When more pressure is put on Matt to imitate a sound or word, he becomes particularly resistive by fussing or, eventually crying. In spite of the fact that he says no words, Matt communicates. He uses a rather elaborate system of gestures combined with facial movements, head nods, and phonation to ask for things, express his desire to do things, respond to comments made by his parents, initiate and terminate "conversations," and greet people. Hearing loss was ruled out through audiological testing. Matt shows that he comprehends by carrying out complex commands and pointing to pictures, although sometimes he ignores an adult's attempt to engage in these activities, just like he fusses when asked to repeat words and sounds. Matt's mother believes that he will talk when he is "ready." Matt's father believes that Matt can talk, but is stubborn and is refusing to do so. The speech-language pathologist believes that Matt has great difficulty talking due to a defect in the automatic function of connecting oral-motor movements with the words Matt wants to say.

As each person's perspective about Matt's situation was learned, it became apparent that there was truth in each. Matt does refuse to try to imitate and to try to say words. He sometimes even refuses to carry out commands to demonstrate his understanding. He does seem "stubborn" some of the time. Matt communicates well without using words. He has developed an elaborate system to interact with his parents. It is possible that, when he is "ready" to talk, he will do this just as he decided to communicate through gestures. Finally, it does seem that oral speech is particularly difficult for Matt. He seems to know that he is more successful with the communication system he developed than he could be with speech. The characteristics of (1) being able to say words occasionally but not being able to repeat them or say them again, (2) being unsuccessful in imitating words on the rare occasions that he will try, (3) comprehending seemingly within normal limits, and (4) communicating readily, all make it seem as if Matt is unable to use his oral mechanism to speak in a reliable and normal manner. In other words, it does seem that Matt cannot rely on talking to communicate. All three perspectives contain truth; so what should be done?

At the first session, Matt's parents suggested that they would like to pretend not to understand his communicative attempts to create a "need" to talk and to respond to his "refusal" to talk. Because transactional patterns of the family influence the behavior of family members, this decision about how to interact with Matt was very important. The speech-language pathologist (SLP) pursued the parent's suggestion by asking questions and responding to their imagined descriptions of the likely outcome of such actions. In this way, they were able to develop visual and auditory images of interactions with Matt. "How will this work?" "What will you do?" "What will Matt do?" What will you do in response?" A script of the conversation went something like this:

SLP: All right. So if you pretend you don't understand Matt, what will happen?

Mom: Well, for one thing, he won't eat because, so far at least, he won't say the word for what he wants.

SLP: Yes. He communicates what he wants through gestures, but not through words. So if he won't say the words, you won't give him the food.

Dad: Exactly. He'll just have to go hungry.

Mom: But, he won't go hungry. He'll climb up and get the cereal. He'll just eat cereal all the time.

(continued)

SLP: Okay. You'll let him get the food that he can reach, but you won't give him anything unless he says the word.

Dad: Right.

Mom: He'll probably cry all the time. He knows I can understand his gestures. He won't really think I don't understand him. He'll think I'm being mean.

Dad: He might think we don't like him.

SLP: And, of course, you do like him. You love him!

Dad: Right! . . . I'm not sure we can do this. Maybe it's not a good idea.

Mom: We don't want to create another problem. He already can't talk; now he'll be emotionally disturbed, too!

Dad: Maybe there's something else we could do.

SLP: I think so. In fact, I think we should make an even greater effort to understand his gestures and encourage him to use these as much as possible.

Dad: Sounds good to me! I don't think we can pretend not to understand him after all the time we've spent trying to figure out his gestures.

Mom: Yes, he'd be a mess and so would we!

SLP: Okay. Let's encourage his desire to communicate. Let's try to connect with him in any way we can. Rather than pretending not to understand him, let's try to understand him even more. How would it be if, this week, you pay particular attention to his gestures and begin to keep a list of the things he communicates?

Mom: Okay. It's going to be a long list. He tells me a lot.

Dad: Yeah! He just doesn't say the words; he has lots of things to tell us.

This conversation was very important. It is likely that the parents, initially, really believed that the best way to help Matt would be to pretend not to understand his gestures. The first half of the session, in fact, was riddled with this implication as they described Matt. That theme was so predominant that the speech-language pathologist had the impression that the parents felt guilty for being so good at figuring out Matt's communicative intentions. It seemed clear that they could not be talked out of their belief that, in the long run, it would be helpful to Matt to refuse to comprehend his gestures. Had that occurred, Matt's refusal to talk would have been matched by his parent's refusal to accept anything other than "talk." There is little or no research data to guide the speech-language pathologist in this situation, but it seemed that other efforts to use transactional patterns of Matt's family members in helpful ways would be best based on positive communicative interactions. Further, one of the truths about Matt is that speaking is difficult for him. Forcing him to rely on a potentially defective speech-language neurological system for all of his communication with those who were most significant in his life did not seem to be a solid base on which to build further interventions.

At the present time, Matt's family is involved in his treatment. Their interactions with him include responding with pleasure to any syllables or words they hear Matt say, imitating sounds Matt says, singing songs and saying rhymes with Matt, and encouraging him to practice vowels and syllables he is able to say perfectly. These transactional patterns, along with encouraging Matt to communicate in other ways, provide the basis for using family transactional patterns to promote change in Matt's ability to speak.

Principle 4

A family's structure, organization, and developmental stage are important factors in determining the behavior of family members (Epstein & Bishop, 1981).

This principle is similar to the one just discussed, but rather than emphasizing interactive patterns, it focuses on the hierarchical structure of the family, the roles/relationships of those who make up the family system, and the family's developmental stage. Traditionally, families were organized around two birth parents and their children. Occasionally, a grandparent also lived in the home. Today, there is a variety of family structures. These include traditional families, solo parent families, three- and four-generation families, foster families, homosexual families, and grandparent-headed families. In most cases, a parenting team of two caregiving adults can be identified. In some cases, the parenting team consists of family friends or relatives, foster parents or even counselors from a residential facility. The concept of "family" is then enlarged to include related and unrelated people who are concerned about the well-being of the child. The point is that the structure of the family is one variable that determines the definition of the term "family" and, therefore, the parenting team that may be convened by the speech-language pathologist.

Family members also assume different roles and families organize themselves around the functions that different family members assume in these roles. Examples of roles include breadwinner, family spokesperson, caregiver, housecleaner, disciplinarian, shopper, and cook. Further, family members assume more subtle roles that affect their style of parenting; their manner of communicating; and the extent to which they reinforce, listen to, play with, and respond to their children.

Another variable that determines the behavior of family members is the family's developmental stage (Carter & McGoldrick, 1980). Just as individuals develop and change, so do families. The family with preschool children is different from the family in the process of launching children into adulthood or a family that is retired. Specifics of speech-language or hearing services vary with the developmental stage of the family.

When speech-language services are provided in the context of family members, it is considered important to give family members suggestions that are consistent with their roles in the family and their particular style of interacting with other family members. In other words, assignments should be congruent with the family members' roles in the family and their style of interacting. Elise and her family provide a good example.

Elise is 27 months old and lives with her foster parents and three other children ranging in age from 18 months to 18 years. Speech-language services are offered in the foster parent's home when both parents can be present. Elise's comprehension of language and her use of language are below that of most other children her age. In addition to her slow communication development, she has microcephaly, may have been exposed to cocaine in utero, and takes medication to control seizures. Elise's hearing is within normal limits, and she imitates words when looking at books with an adult and when playing with an adult. Her spontaneous speech is limited to less than 50, one-word, utterances.

Elise's foster mother, Mrs. Briggs, seemed to enjoy participating with the speech-language pathologist in the assessment of Elise's speech-language. Prior to the first session with the speech-language pathologist, she had already written down words she had heard Elise use and had other notes about Elise's medical history and developmental accomplishments. When asked questions about Elise's comprehension and use of language, Mrs. Briggs had ready answers and was able to elaborate on many of the details about Elise's behavior. When asked if she would show the speech-language pathologist how she looked at books or played with Elise, Mrs. Briggs became obviously uncomfortable. Mr. Briggs, who had sat quietly thus far, got out of his chair and sat down on the floor and began to play with Elise. As he did so, he followed Elise's lead and talked about the objects she was looking at. When Elise phonated, he imitated her. When Elise looked at him, he smiled and encouraged her to do the same.

Clearly, both Mr. and Mrs. Briggs have ready resources that the speech-language pathologist can tap to help Elise. The clinician continued to observe these resources as she watched interactions between Elise and each of her foster parents at the second session. Toward the end of the session, the speech language pathologist held a conversation with the Briggs' and asked each of them what they enjoyed doing with Elise. Mrs. Briggs indicated that she had a background in medical record keeping and enjoyed maintaining written accounts of Elise's behaviors and accomplishments and reading books about some of Elise's medical problems. Mr. Briggs, on the other hand, was quick to point out that he was happy to turn those functions over to his wife. He liked to play with children, and Elise was no exception. He enjoyed rolling a ball back and forth to her, playing with her toys with her, and reading books to her. The speech-language pathologist expressed appreciation for the importance of the roles that each parent found natural and indicated that both roles were important and could be used to help Elise. The strengths of each parent, then, were used as the clinician and foster parents worked as a team to help Elise. The speech-language pathologist was sensitive to the principle that behaviors of family members vary with the structure, organization, and developmental stage of families and elaborated on the idiosyncratic resources of both Mr. and Mrs. Briggs in a manner that allowed each to participate fully in Elise's treatment process.

◆ PROFESSIONAL PRACTICE ISSUES IN COMMUNICATION DISORDERS

For many years, the linear medical model provided a sufficient set of assumptions for the clinical practice of speech-language pathology and audiology. The small size of the therapy rooms in most university speech and hearing clinics provides vivid evidence for the extent to which the individual approach has been part and parcel of the profession. The mindset of future practitioners and future university teachers, alike, was influenced not only by the coursework and clinical supervision they received, but by the unspoken assumptions present in every corner (literally) of the educational program. Even now, the medical model provides an adequate framework for the clinician who works with clients on an individual basis and assumes responsibility for providing services directly to the client without the assistance of significant persons in the client's life.

Speech-language and hearing treatment that attends to interactions between the client and others and utilizes the resources of influential persons in the client's environment has been called **contextual therapy**. Several emerging forms of clinical practice illustrate the meaning of the term contextual therapy. These approaches include (1) the involvement of family members in the assessment and treatment process, (2) the provision of speech-language services in school classrooms, and (3) participation of speech-language pathologists and audiologists on interdisciplinary treatment teams. Each of these approaches involves making the speech-language pathologist's or audiologist's knowledge usable by others and using resources beyond those of the lone professional. *Each is more appropriately based on a combined linear-systemic paradigm than on a linear paradigm alone.* The clinician must draw on many of the same concepts and skills whether he or she is working with clients in the context of families, collaboratively with personnel in the context of a school, or with other professionals on interdisciplinary teams. Some of these concepts and skills are discussed in the sections that follow. The clinician who is able to use these concepts is not only in a good position to provide contextual therapy, but also to elaborate on them and add to our understanding of their use.

Appreciating Difference and Diversity

Differences in culture, life style, values, perception, and professional orientation become apparent when one works contextually. In 1986, for example, Public Law 99-457 provided start-up funds for states to provide services to children with disabilities between the ages of birth and 3 years. By law, these services must be **family-centered**, meaning that (1) professionals work to promote family competence, (2) treatment is under the control of the family, and (3) professionals are viewed as the agents of families. Frequently, services are offered in the family's home. This one feature of services, meeting with the family in their home, is significantly different from meeting the family at one's office. The idiosyncratic style of each family is more readily apparent in the home than in the clinic or in the professional's office. The professional who can respect family differences and work within their structure is likely to be more effective than the professional who makes negative judgments, even when the judgments are subtle and unspoken. Imagine a professional person coming to your home. What would make you want to cooperate with the service that he or she provides? Likely, you would want someone who was respectful of your family's life style and of you as a person, and who was positively curious about how you interact as a family.

We already have indicated that one assumption of a systemic paradigm is that there are many truths as opposed to one correct view. The clinician who is skillful enough to respectfully learn about a family and then to use this understanding to make his or her knowledge usable to the family is likely to be successful in offering contextual therapy. Similarly, the professional who listens to the views of fellow professionals on an interdisciplinary treatment team will be in a position to explain his or her points of view and treatment suggestions more effectively than the professional who is critical of other person's perspectives.

deShazer (1985) uses the term "polyocular view" to describe a perspective that takes into account many views of the same situation. Each is accepted as valid for the person holding the view. In clinical situations, the practitioner listens to the different views held by others and accepts each as truth for the person expressing it. This listening and acceptance creates a situation in which each person is freed to become effectively involved in the process of communication change.

Joining

Joining is a term used in the family therapy to refer to behaviors that result in the therapist being accepted into the interactive system of a family (Minuchin, 1974). When working contextually, this term seems more appropriate than the term "rapport," which professionals in our field have used for many years to refer to a positive relationship between a clinician and a client. Rapport is an important concept for clinicians who use an individual approach. The situation of the clinician working contextually, however, is more accurately described by the word, joining.

It has been suggested that joining is promoted by using language that invites participation by other members of the treatment system (Andrews & Andrews, 1990). The clinician may say, for example: "Let's work on this together" or "Let's think about this and see what we believe will work best," "What do you think of this idea?" or "I really need your input on this." Other ways that clinicians join with others are by interacting respectfully, acknowledging the expertise of others, and assuming a cooperative interactive style. Although this concept is simple, its importance should not be diminished. The speech-language pathologist or audiologist who cannot interact in a style that allows him or her to join successfully with those who make up the treatment system will not be effective in working contextually. The relationship that develops between members of the treatment system is a critical component in the success of interventions, as we will see next.

Co-evolution and Family Fit

Contextual therapy involves joining of individuals and groups of people, whether it is the speech-language pathologist or audiologist with a family, with teachers and other personnel in a school, or with an interdisciplinary team of other professional persons. In each case, the joined individuals create a treatment system whose members develop assumptions and a unique style that is idiosyncratic to their newly formed system. Like other interactive systems, the treatment team cannot help but evolve or change over time as the participants interact and respond to one another.

Consider a group of specialists including speech-language pathologist, physician, nurse, physical therapist, and occupational therapist working within the context of a family having a 22-year-old son with a traumatic brain injury. The treatment team, that is, the defined system, includes the family members and the professionals. The characteristics of the interactive system formed by the family and the group of professionals are significant because they will determine the nature of the services provided and the eventual outcome for the son with a disability. As family members and professionals become better acquainted and more fully joined, each influences the others. Together, they co-create a unique family-professional relationship. Another way of describing this changing, mutually influenced situation is to say that the treatment system "co-evolves" over time (Hoffman, 1982).

The concept of **co-evolution** deserves attention as a subjective means of evaluating clinical services. Clinical researchers who choose to investigate this area will find it rich in depth of information and usefulness to the field. Most clinicians have a sense of the family-professional relationship and the degree to which the system is evolving in a positive direction. Ideally, the expertise of the professional vis-a-vis the family being served improves as the system evolves and as more is learned about the family's capabilities, needs, and desires. The clinician's ability to make his or her knowledge usable to the family and to make effective interventions improves as family members gradually reveal more about themselves and their member with a communicative disorder. In addition, the ability of the family to respond to mutually created ideas and suggestions also improves over time. Family competencies are sharpened, and new competencies are uncovered. Another way of saying this is that the **fit** between the professional's expertise and the family's resources becomes increasingly more comfortable. A good fit, according to Campbell, Draper, and Crutchley (1991), means that the family can allow the professional to explore its meaning system (i.e., its unique characteristics as a system), and the professional is able to use feedback from the family in a way that both respects and challenges the family. In other words, the clinician improves in his or her ability to help the family meet the needs of their member, and the family improves in its ability to respond to the professional.

Viewing the change process interactively and as co-evolving, we can conceive, then, of both professionals and family members becoming more competent in using their areas of expertise. The interactive process that takes place between professionals and family members, in this case, is the core of teamwork, utilizing and promoting the resources of everyone involved in a nonhierarchical manner.

The same concept can be applied to a speech-language pathologist working together with a fourth grade child, the teachers the child encounters (e.g., a classroom teacher, a learning disabilities resource teacher, and a teacher's aide), and the child's parents. The speech-language pathologist or audiologist may consult with the members of this treatment system to develop interventions that can be carried out by each as he or she interacts with the child. The relationship between participants of the group can be expected to change over the course of time. The fit between the expertise of the speech-language pathologist and the expertise of all others in the group may improve in such a way that the ability of each to respond to mutually created interventions improves. Consequently, services to the child become increasingly effective.

Encouraging Participation of All Members of a System

It may seem odd to address the issue of participation of members who comprise the treatment system. Consider, however, the clinician working with a family consisting of a mother, mother's friend, and two children. In some situations, a child's mother may be reluctant to disclose that a friend shares the home with her and her children. Yet, this friend is likely to be an integral and important part of the children's family system. When this is so, and we always assume it is, it is important to include that person as well as the mother and both children. Even in families composed of two birth parents, it is not uncommon for mothers to assume that they can represent the family in the absence of the father. Fathers play important roles in families, as do other children. To develop effective interventions, the clinician working contextually needs access to all family members. It is necessary to know the perspective of each family member if the clinician is to have an accurate understanding of how to use this system to promote change in its member with a communicative disorder. A fruitful topic for further investigation is the influence that fathers have on the treatment system. It seems, for example, that their very presence positively influences change in the involved family member.

Similarly, the influence and expertise of each member of the professional team is very important. When one person's contribution is weak or missing, that member's ideas are not accessible and the treatment process is weakened. Team participation is an area that is being explored by some speech-language pathologists and deserves the attention of researchers with knowledge about contextual therapy (Briggs, 1991).

Use of Counseling Techniques

Second only to a thorough knowledge about normal processes and the various disorders of communication, effective contextual intervention requires skill in using counseling techniques. These are used to elicit participation and cooperation, to explore the views of the client's problem as experienced by other members of the system, to find points of accommodation for differing views, and to know when it is appropriate — and when it is not — to respond to emotions expressed, to arrive at and deliver effective interventions, and so on.

The distinction between using counseling techniques and providing counseling is an important one. From the above description, it should be apparent that it is not counseling that is being done. Rather, the clinician is using the techniques of counseling to enhance the contextual treatment process.

Common counseling techniques useful for the contextual clinician include **attending, restating, reflecting, tracking, neutral questioning, summarizing, amplifying**, and **reframing** (Andrews, 1986; Luterman, 1991). These form a basic set of techniques that are used by speech-language pathologists and audiologists who work contextually. These techniques are likely to become part of the professional preparation of speech-language pathologists and audiologists as leaders in our field come to recognize their importance. The manner in which each of these techniques is used and the effect it has varies, of course, with the particular situation. Treatment of communication disorders in context is a rapidly growing practice. The field could benefit from research into these techniques and how they may be used most effectively by speech-language pathologists and audiologists.

Isomorphic Interventions

Clinical experience indicates that our interventive suggestions to others within the treatment system are most effective when they are consistent with interactive behaviors already practiced by the listener and when they are described in relation to the listener's perspective about the communication disorder. This is a subtle, but large, departure from the more common practice of suggesting standard intervention techniques used by speech-language pathologists and audiologists, which are independent of (1) the usual manner in which the person interacts with the client, (2) the normal activities and life style of the person, and (3) the person's view of the communicative disorder.

Isomorphism is a concept that refers to equality of form and may be described most simply as a pattern that persists throughout the subsystems of a larger system. One way to think about this is in terms of the different generations within a family. Parts of the attitudes and habits that were characteristic of grandparents may be seen in their children and grandchildren. Optimism, as a rule of life, for example, may be repeated in different forms as one learns about preceding, current, and subsequent generations of a family. Another example is the repeated pattern of respect for others within an institutional structure. For example, when owners respect managers, managers respect supervisors, supervisors respect workers, and workers respect customers.

Applied to clinical practice, interventions suggested to family members, to other professionals of a treatment team, or to teachers using facilitative techniques in a classroom are likely to be most effective when the suggestions are consistent with the activities and interactions already used by individuals. Further, the manner in which interventions are presented to others seems to determine their success. Specifically, when a suggestion for an intervention is explained in words consistent with the way a person understands the problem, the intervention is more likely to be implemented and be successful than when the person's perspective is ignored.

◆ SUMMARY AND CONCLUSIONS

You have learned about the manner in which two world views influence the treatment services that speech-language pathologists and audiologists provide. Although a linear, cause-effect paradigm is adequate for direct individual services, contextual treatment flows best from an integration of the linear and systemic paradigms. Case illustrations were used to show the importance of systemic principles in contextual treatment. Issues such as appreciating difference/diversity, adopting a perspective that includes the perceived truths of everyone involved, co-evolution of the family-professional relationship, joining, encouraging participation of all persons in the treatment system, use of counseling techniques, and interventions tailored to family life styles and interactive patterns were discussed. These concepts, when appropriately applied, can enhance the quality of clinical services provided and the success of such services.

◆ REFERENCES

Andrews, J. & Andrews, M. (1986). A short-term family systems approach to speech-language treatment as a supplement to school-based services. *Seminars in Speech and Language, 7*, 407–414.

Andrews, J., & Andrews, M. (1990). *Family based treatment in communicative disorders: A systemic approach.* Sandwich, IL: Janelle Publications.

Andrews, M. (1986). Application of family therapy techniques to the treatment of language disorders. *Seminars in Speech and Language, 7*, 347–358.

Briggs, M. H. (1991). Team development: Decision-making for early intervention. *Infant-Toddler Intervention: The Transdisciplinary Journal, 1*(1), 1–9.

Buscaglia, L. (1983). *The disabled and their parents.* Thorofare, NJ: Slack.

Campbell, D., Draper, R., & Crutchley, E. (1991). The Milan systemic approach to family therapy. In A. S. Gurman & D. P. Kniskern (Eds.), *Handbook of family therapy* (pp. 325–362). New York: Brunner/Mazel.

Carter, E. A., & McGoldrick, M. (1980). The family life cycle and family therapy: An overview. In E. A. Carter & M. McGoldrick (Eds.), *The family life cycle: A framework for family therapy* (pp. 3–20). New York: Gardner Press.

Demichelis, A. (1989). Never the same. *Asha, 31*, 87–88.

deShazer, S. (1985). *Keys to solution in brief therapy.* New York: W. W. Norton.

Epstein, N., & Bishop, D. (1981). Problem centered systems therapy of the family. In A. S. Gurman & D. P. Kniskern (Eds.), *Handbook of family therapy* (pp. 444–482). New York: Brunner/Mazel.

Hoffman, L. (1982). A co-evolutionary framework for systemic family therapy. *Australian Journal of Family Therapy, 4*, 9–21.

Keeney, B. P. (1983). *The aesthetics of change.* New York: Guilford Press.

Luterman, D. (1991). *Counseling the communicatively disordered and their families.* Austin, TX: Pro-Ed.

Minuchin, S. (1974). *Families and family therapy.* Cambridge, MA: Harvard University Press.

Rogers, C. (1965). *Client centered therapy.* Boston: Houghton Mifflin.

Seibel, N. (1987). A parent's perspective. *The ACPA/CPF newsletter* (pp. 1–2). American Cleft Palate Association, Pittsburgh, PA.

Trout, M., & Foley, G. (1989). Working with families of handicapped infants and toddlers. *Topics in Language Disorders, 10*, 57–67.

◆ RECOMMENDED READINGS

Andrews, M., & Andrews, J. (1991). Family based treatment: A system model for involving families. In A. Halper, L. Cherney, & T. Miller (Eds.), *Clinical management of communication problems in adults with traumatic brain injuries* (pp. 147–159). Gaithersburg, MD: Aspen.

Andrews, M., & Andrews, J. (1993). Family centered techniques: Integrating enablement into the IFSP process. *Journal of Childhood Communication Disorders, 15*, 41–46.

Donahue-Kilburg, G. (1992). *Family-centered early intervention for communication disorders.* Gaithersburg, MD: Aspen.

Ferguson, M. L. (Ed.). (1992). Clinical forum: Implementing collaborative consultation. *Language, Speech, and Hearing Services in Schools, 23*, 361–372.

Frassinelli, L., Superior, K., & Myers, J. (1983). A consultation model for speech and language services. *Asha, 25*, 25–30.

Manolson, A. (1991). *It takes two to talk: A Hanen early language parent guide book.* Toronto: Hanen Early Language Resource Centre.

McGonigel, M. J., Kaufman, R. K., & Johnson, B. H. (Eds.). (1991). *Guidelines and recommended practices for the individualized family service plan.* Bethesda, MD: Association for the Care of Children's Health.

Miller, L. (1989). Classroom-based language intervention. *Language, Speech, and Hearing Services in Schools, 20*, 153–169.

◆ GLOSSARY

Amplifying: identifying a resource for change, describing the resource, and discussing it in a manner that helps the people involved assume ownership of it.

Co-evolution: this term refers to the concept that systems influence one another and change, or evolve, together, over time. Therapists have applied the concept to the changing relationship between family and therapist in which each affects the other.

Contextual therapy: therapy that occurs in the natural environment of the client, that attends to interactions between the client and others, and that uses the resources of others who have influence on the client.

Family-centered: refers to attitudes and actions that support the family, enhance family members' competencies, and keep families in charge of decision-making. Usually used in reference to the treatment model; required by federal law to be used when providing services to infants and toddlers with disabilities and their families.

Isomorphism: a mathematical concept used by therapists to refer to behavioral patterns that are repeated in subsystems of a larger system, such as generations of a family. More practically, the term also is used to refer to similar elements of different views of a situation as distinguished from elements that are dissimilar. When making suggestions for change, these are thought to be most effective when they are related to the family's existing life style and activities (i.e., they are isomorphic to the family), and when they also result in a new interpretation for elements that are different.

Joining: therapists use this term to refer to their attempts to form a partnership or alliance with the members of a family so that the therapist is accepted into the interactive system of the family.

Linear: specifically, used to refer to a sequence of causal events that do not return to the original point of origin. Feedback processes are not involved and relationships are not, therefore, circular in nature. We use this word to refer to a world view that is cause-effect oriented; that seeks the one, correct truth about each situation; and that treats complexity by reducing it into small parts.

Neutral questioning: questions asked from a nonjudgmental position of curiosity with the intent of understanding clients' concerns, exploring interactive patterns, and identifying resources to facilitate change.

Paradigm: we use this word to refer to the internal map or world view that provides a broad conceptual framework for thought and action.

Professional-family fit: this term refers to the relative degree to which the therapist's suggestions match the family's ability to respond to them. This is expected to improve over time as each uses feedback from the other during the process of constant change. When the fit is good, interventions are uniquely appropriate and effective.

Reductionism: a style of thinking that understands and studies complex phenomena by breaking them down into smaller and simpler parts.

Reflecting: a technique originally described by Rogers (1965) in which a therapist, from a position of unconditional positive regard, restates the feelings and content that a person is expressing.

Reframing: a discussion of a situation that results in a change in meaning or value attributed to the situation even though the facts remain the same. This change in thinking is expected to result in subsequent changes in behavior related to the situation.

System: used here to refer to a group of people who interact, behave, have influence, and respond in such a manner that the group becomes qualitatively different than the totality of each individual person's behavior, influence, and response. Thus, the whole is greater than the sum of its parts.

Systemic: a term used to refer to a system's use of feedback to transform events in ways that cannot be predicted by traditional cause-effect analysis. We use this word to refer to a world view that recognizes differing perceptions of reality, focuses attention on interactive patterns, is more solution- than problem-focused, and seeks system transformations more than cause-effect changes.

Tracking: the use of observation and/or questioning to develop an understanding of sequences of events that occur between people.

Neurological Bases of Communication Disorders

RAY D. KENT, Ph.D.

After completing this chapter, you will be able to:

◆ Describe the Neuron, the Microscopic Unit of the Nervous System.

◆ Identify the major parts of the Human Nervous System, including the Central Nervous System (cerebral hemispheres, thalamus and related structures; basal nuclei; brain stem; cerebellum; limbic system; and spinal cord) and the Peripheral Nervous System (especially the cranial nerves).

◆ Discuss the primary methods of brain imaging.

◆ Answer the following questions about language and the brain: Why is it often said that the left hemisphere is dominant for language? What are the language areas within the left hemisphere? What are some contemporary theories of language representation within the brain? How does the brain control the production of speech? What are the primary neural structures involved in understanding and producing language?

◆ Describe some major changes in the brain during development and aging.

The understanding of many communicative disorders is closely link-ed to an understanding of the human brain. This chapter is an intro-duction to basic neuroanatomy for speech and language. The pri-mary objective is to identify the parts of the brain that are considered to be most directly involved in human communication, and to con-sider how these structures participate in the comprehension and pro-duction of language.

"This human brain . . . is without any qualification the most highly organized and most complexly organized matter in the universe"
(J.C. Eccles, *The Understanding of the Brain*, 1973, p. 1).

For good reason, the human brain has been called the most com-plex system in the known universe. The complexity results first from the tremendously large number of basic anatomical units that make up the brain. These basic units are neurons, or nerve cells. The number of neurons has been estimated to be in the range of 20–100 billion, and some scientists believe that the number may be closer to a trillion. Neurons are so numerous that counting them is tedious and inexact. The complexity of the brain arises as well from the fact that the neurons are multiply interconnected. A single neuron in the brain may have connections with more than 1,000 other neurons. The number of possible connections is enormous and greatly increases the challenge of studying the brain. One could spend several lifetimes trying to discover the individual con-nections among the neurons that make up just a few parts of the brain.

Alternatively, one can try to understand the nervous system in terms of major components, each of which contains millions of neurons. This is the approach taken in this chapter, which will de-scribe the basic organization of the nervous system relevant to speech and language. An understanding of this basic organization is requisite to an understanding of communication disorders asso-ciated with neurological disease or damage.

◆ THE NEURON, THE MICROSCOPIC UNIT OF THE NERVOUS SYSTEM

The neuron is the basic anatomic unit of the nervous system. One of the most famous scientists in the study of the nervous system,

Ramon y Cajal, described each neuron as an independent living cell. He recognized that each neuron is a genetic, anatomical, and functional unit. But even though the neurons are individual units, they function collectively by means of connections among them. The basic structure of a neuron is shown in Figure 8–1. The major divisions are the **cell body** (which contains the nucleus with its genetic material) and two major types of processes, **dendrites** and **axons**. Dendrites carry information toward the cell body and axons carry information away from the cell body. The information is in the form of electrical impulses that travel along the axon or dendrite. A burning fuse is a good analogy of the neural impulse, which

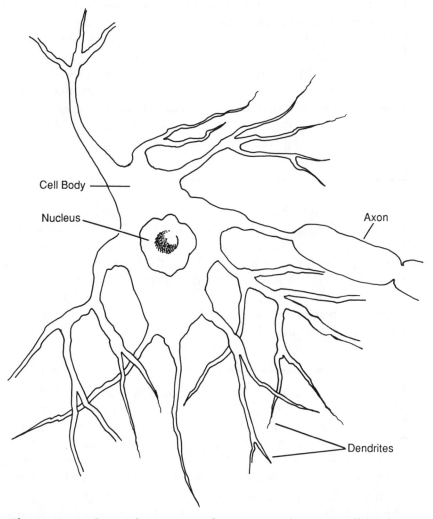

Cell Body

Nucleus

Axon

Dendrites

Figure 8–1. General structure of a neuron, showing cell body, nucleus, dendrites, and axon.

moves in one direction along the axonic or dendritic process. Figure 8–1 shows only a few dendrites, but an actual microscopic view of a neuron may reveal hundreds of dendrites. These processes enable the neuron to receive information from hundreds of other neurons. The connections between different neurons are made at **synapses**, which are like communication terminals that connect one neuron with another. The communication is chemical in nature, involving specialized substances called **neurotransmitters**. The neurotransmitter substance is released into the microscopic space, the **synaptic cleft**, between one neuron and its neighbor.

Neurotransmitters are the chemical messengers in the nervous system. Different parts of the brain are linked in chemical watersheds in which a particular neurotransmitter is the primary messenger. Many neurological and psychiatric disorders are now being understood and treated in terms of deficiencies or excesses of particular neurotransmitters. Some neuroscientists think of the brain as a gland, in recognition of its important chemical activities. Some of the chemical messengers found in the brain are also found in other parts of the body, which obscures the brain-body division.

Imagine now that neurons like the one illustrated in Figure 8–1 are collected in groups of thousands or even millions to form the various structures of the brain. Collectives of neurons often serve a particular function, so an examination of function usually is described in terms of large groups of neurons. Neurons typically are arranged in the nervous system such that their cell bodies cluster together in **nuclei** and such that their axons run together in bundles called **tracts** or **fascicles**.

Notice the dual use of the word "nucleus." First, it can refer to the nucleus of a cell, that is, the part of a cell that contains the genetic material. Second, it can refer to a collection of neuron cell bodies. Therefore, a neuron, which contains a cell component called a *nucleus,* can be grouped with other neurons into a neural structure called a *nucleus.* This dual usage can be confusing, but it is unfortunately just one example of many terminologic hazards in the study of the nervous system. Although this chapter will attempt to avoid these potential confusions, it will be necessary on occasion to admit that confusing terminology is a fact of life in the study of the nervous system.

When many axons run together in the nervous system to form nerves or tracts, they often are wrapped within a white fatty substance called **myelin**. The myelin coating is rather like the insulation around an electrical wire. It keeps neural messages intact and speeds their transmission. Diseases that cause **demyelination**, or loss of myelin, impair the reliable transmission of neural impulses. Multiple sclerosis is one of these diseases.

✦ THE HUMAN NERVOUS SYSTEM

The human nervous system consists of the brain, the spinal cord, and the nerves by which the various parts of the body are connected to the brain or spinal cord. This system will be discussed according to the organization given in Table 8–1.

The **central nervous system** (CNS) is made up of the brain and spinal cord. The major structures of the CNS are shown in Figure 8–2, which is analogous to a gross anatomical dissection in which the major parts of the CNS have been isolated. The **peripheral nervous system** (PNS) includes 12 pairs of cranial nerves that emerge from the base of the brain and 31 pairs of spinal nerves that emerge from the spinal cord. The PNS essentially connects the CNS with the receptors (eyes, ears, and so on), muscles, and glands of the body.

TABLE 8–1. The major divisions of the nervous system.

Central Nervous System (CNS)
Cerebral hemispheres
Thalamus and associated structures
Basal nuclei
Brain stem
Cerebellum
Limbic system
Spinal cord
Peripheral Nervous System
Cranial nerves (12 pairs)
Spinal nerves (31 pairs)

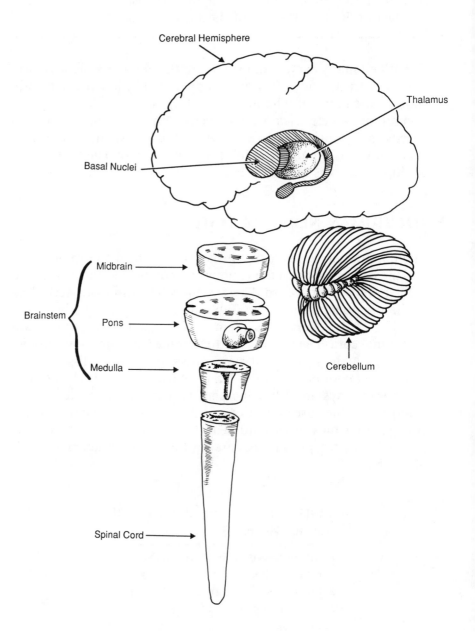

Figure 8-2. A graphically dissected central nervous system, showing the following major parts: cerebrum (cerebral hemisphere), thalamus, basal nuclei, midbrain, pons, medulla, cerebellum, and spinal cord.

Central Nervous System

Cerebral Hemispheres

The **cerebral hemispheres** are often what we think of when we visualize the brain. These are two large structures divided by a large fissure that runs from front to back. Fissures are also called **sulci** (singular form is **sulcus**) and folds of brain tissue are also called **gyri** (singular form is **gyrus**). The cerebral hemispheres are the largest part of the brain (about 80% of the brain by weight, averaging about 3–4 lbs) and they dominate the visual appearance of the brain when it is removed from the skull (Figure 8–3). The two cerebral hemispheres are connected by tracts of nerves so that neural messages can be exchanged between them. One of the most important of these tracts is the **corpus callosum** (Figure 8–4), a large bundle of fibers that connects the left and right hemispheres. Major connections within each hemisphere are the **fasciculi**, shown in Figure 8–4.

The cerebrum (the cerebral hemispheres) is the largest part of the brain, weighing about 3–4 pounds. The entire brain is only about 2% of total body weight but it demands about 25% of the blood from the heart.

Models and illustrations of the brain often give the misleading impression that the brain is a kind of solid or semi-solid organ that retains its general shape when removed from its bony case. In fact, brain tissue has the consistency of jelly. Unless the brain is fixed with chemicals before it is removed from the cranium, it slumps and oozes into a puddle. The living brain is held in shape by the bones of the cranium and three sacklike tissues called the meninges. The meninges are three layers of tissue that lie under the skull and over the brain. The skull and meninges give shape to the brain and protect it from injury.

The cerebral hemispheres as shown in Figure 8–3 are divided into four major **lobes**. The **frontal lobe** is the part that lies anterior (toward to the front) of the central fissure. The **parietal lobe** is the upper part of the hemisphere that lies behind the central fissure. The **temporal lobe** is situated beneath the lateral fissure. The **occipital lobe** is located toward the back. The lobes can be associated with major functions as follows:

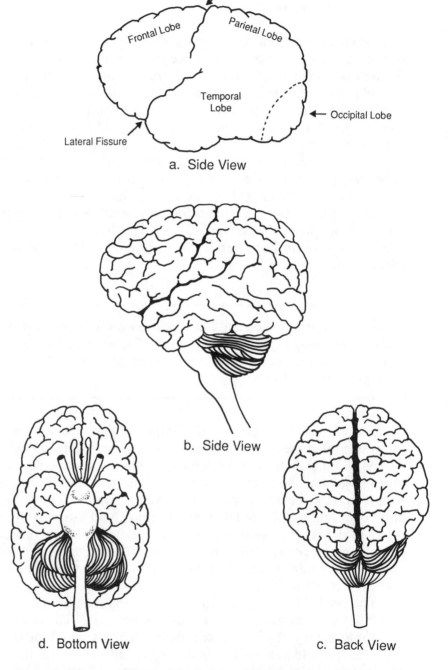

Figure 8-3. Various views of the brain and spinal cord: **a.** side view of brain showing major fissures and lobes; **b.** side view of brain and spinal cord; **c.** back view of brain and spinal cord; and **d.** bottom view of brain.

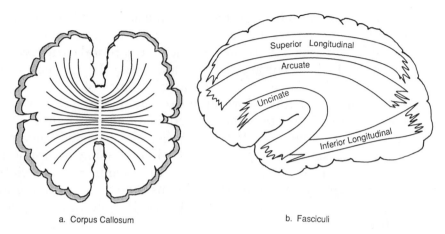

a. Corpus Callosum   b. Fasciculi

Figure 8-4. Major fiber tracts of the cerebral hemispheres: **a.** the corpus callosum, which connects the two hemispheres (seen from above, with part of the brain removed); and **b.** the tracts within the same hemisphere (seen in a side view).

Frontal lobe — thinking, planning and social judgment. This lobe is sometimes called the "executive" of the brain.

Parietal lobe — reception and interpretation of external and internal stimuli, and storage of information.

Temporal lobe — processing of auditory information, memory, and emotion.

Occipital lobe — processing of visual information.

(One other lobe, the **limbic lobe**, lies more internally and will be discussed later as we look inside the brain.)

Casual observation of the cerebral hemispheres does not reveal many distinctive landmarks except the wrinkles of the surface. The pattern of wrinkling varies somewhat from brain to brain, but it is regular enough that names have been given to the major fissures. Figure 8-3 shows two major fissues that will be important landmarks throughout this chaper. One fissure is the **central fissure** (also called the Fissure of Rolando), and the other is **lateral fissure** (also called the Fissure of Sylvius). The wrinkling of the brain's surface permits the organ to accommodate a much larger number of neurons than if it were perfectly smooth. The brain tissue appears to be essentially the same everywhere. In this respect, the cerebral hemispheres are rather like the liver, which, on superficial examination, looks everywhere about the same. However, microscopic study of the cells of the cerebral hemispheres reveals regional differences. As a first step in understanding these regional variations, we must first recognize that the neuron cell bodies of the cerebral hemispheres are contained in a thin layer or bark that is about 2–3 mm thick. This bark is called the **cerebral cortex** (cortex means bark). The neuron cell bodies are arranged in six microscopic layers within the bark. Shortly after the turn of the century, a famous neuroscientist, Korbinian Brodmann, studied the neuronal structure of the brain and divided the brain into a kind of mosaic based on structural differences from region to region. The Brodmann areas shown in Figure 8–5 are still used today in describing brain structure and function. Only the Brodmann areas associated with language will be emphasized in this chapter. Many important language areas — 22, 41, 42, 39, 40, and 44 — lie near the lateral fissure.

To many people, the word "cortical" is nearly synonymous with higher level processes, such as thinking, language, and plan-

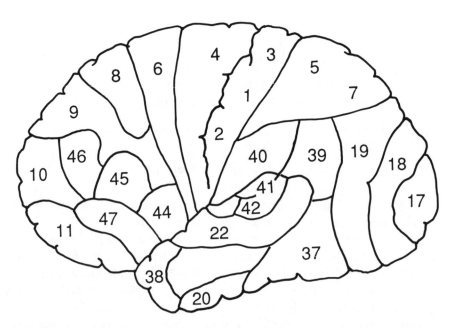

Figure 8–5. Brodmann areas of the cerebral cortex. The Brodmann areas are a quiltwork of fields that cover the surface of the cortex. The ones shown in bold outline are most important to speech and language. General functions typically ascribed to selected Brodmann areas are as follows: **1, 2, 3** — "sensory strip" for body sensation; **4** — "motor strip" for control of voluntary movement; **6** — premotor area for motor planning; **9, 10** — planning, judgment, foresight; **5, 7** — general sensory associations; **17, 18** — vision; **41** — audition; **22, 42** (Wernicke's area) — auditory association; **39, 40** — language processing; **44** (Broca's area) — expressive language.

ning. This view has been reinforced by popularized maps of the brain that link a particular function such as language or thought with a limited region on a cerebral hemisphere. However, this conceptualization is not supported by recent discoveries about the nervous system, and there is reason to be skeptical about simplified schemes that assign complex functions to small regions of the cortex isolated from other neural systems. This chapter will have a good deal to say about the cerebral cortex, but it will not be the exclusive subject by any means. Keeping this caution in mind, consider Figure 8–5 as a tentative map of cortical function. The labels indicate the presumed function of localized regions of the brain. This is an example of **localization**, or the attempt to define the functions of specific areas of the brain. A strict localizationist believes that the brain can be subdivided into functional areas. An anti-localizationist believes that the brain operates through the participation of many different parts. Much of the controversy in the history of brain research can be discussed with respect to these polar views of brain function. Figure 8–5 has a definite clinical usefulness. Indeed, much of the evidence for the functional assignments in Figure 8–5 comes from clinical data in which damage to the brain is associated with particular dysfunctions.

Although the cerebral hemispheres are the most conspicuous parts of the brain when it is viewed in isolation, there is much more to the brain. To visualize the remaining structures, it is necessary to remove the cerebral hemispheres, as has been done diagrammatically in Figure 8–6. Lying within the cerebral hemispheres are important structures including the thalamus, the basal nuclei, and the limbic system. These islands of gray matter are often called **subcortical** structures, meaning that they are located "beneath" the cortex. These parts of the brain cooperate with the cortex in the neural regulation of behavior, including speech. These structures have been neglected in many discussions of how the brain controls speech and language, but mounting evidence confirms that they play very important roles indeed. To understand these roles, it is helpful to take a look at the general roles of these brain structures in human behavior.

Thalamus and Associated Structures

The **thalamus** is a spherical object about the size of a small egg — actually two small eggs, because the thalamus, like many brain structures, is paired, with one thalamus on either side of the midline. It is divided into a number of different nuclei, or clusters of

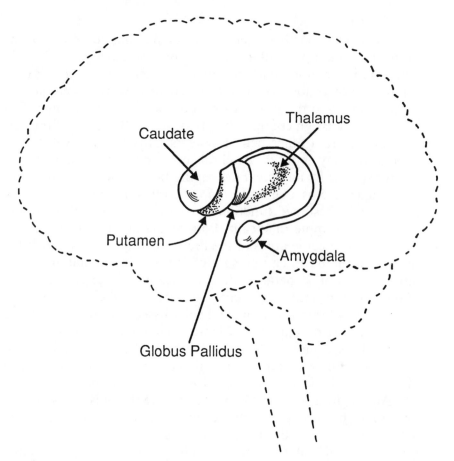

Figure 8–6. Basal nuclei seen within a side view of the brain.

neuron cell bodies. Recall that in the cerebral cortex the cell bodies are arranged in a sheet or bark. The thalamus is an example of another common geometry of cell body clusters, spherical mass. The word "thalamus" means chamber, and this derivation can be helpful in understanding the role of the thalamus. We might think of the thalamus as kind of grand chamber in which neural information converges and is then sent to other brain structures. The information can be of several types, including instructions sent to the muscles (**motor** impulses) and information received from sensory organs such as the eyes, ears, nose, and skin (**sensory** impulses). Sometimes the thalamus is likened to a major relay station in which neural messages are received and transmitted to other structures. The thalamus has ample connections with other parts of the brain, and there is good evidence that the thalamus may set the "tone" of other structures. It alerts other parts of the brain to prepare them to receive and act on neural information.

Cell bodies of neurons within the CNS are collected together in three major ways — a thin bark (as in the cerebral cortex), rounded masses (as in the basal nuclei), or in long columns (as in the spinal cord). Therefore, gray matter in the brain often appears in one of these forms.

Basal Nuclei

As noted earlier, the word nucleus can refer to collections of neuron cell bodies. The **basal nuclei** are such collections. Before further discussion, a few words of caution are in order. First, although basal nuclei is the preferred term, many books and articles use the term "basal ganglia." Ganglia means "nerve knots," and although the word ganglia should be reserved for cell body aggregates in the peripheral nervous system, the term "basal ganglia" is frequently encountered. Second, writers on neuroanatomy disagree on exactly which structures should be included in the basal nuclei. However, all of them probably would agree that the basal nuclei include the **caudate** (meaning "tail"), **globus pallidus** ("pale globe"), and **putamen** ("stone"). These structures are located in roughly the same area of the brain and are especially important in regulating motor functions. Damage to these structures often results in muscle control problems, as will be discussed later.

Brain Stem

The **brain stem** includes a number of important nuclei that regulate functions such as respiration, swallowing, and chewing. The major structures of the brain stem are the midbrain, pons, and medulla.

Cerebellum

The **cerebellum** literally means "little brain" and this may be an appropriate name for it. The cerebellum, like the cerebrum, has two hemispheres. The cerebellum is richly connected with other parts of the brain and these connections allow the cerebellum to possess privileged information on both motor and sensory functions. One conception of the cerebellum's role is that it provides for the smooth coordinated control of muscle activities. In doing so, the cerebellum appears to monitor the instructions that the cerebral cortex issues to the muscles and revises these instructions as needed to insure that the muscles are activated to produce accurate movements. However, the cerebellum probably does more than insure that movements are precise. For example, it has been observed that some individuals with autism have abnormally small cerebellums. Perhaps the cerebellum is somehow involved in autism but the exact nature of the involvement is not known.

Limbic System

Limbic means "border." Some of the structures that comprise the **limbic system** are illustrated in Figure 8–7. These structures also are called the **limbic lobe**. The limbic system lies deep within the brain and was only quite recently described as a functional system. It is thought that the limbic system is involved in emotion and memory. The role of one limbic structure, the **hippocampus** ("sea horse") was discovered inadvertently in neurological surgery for epilepsy. When

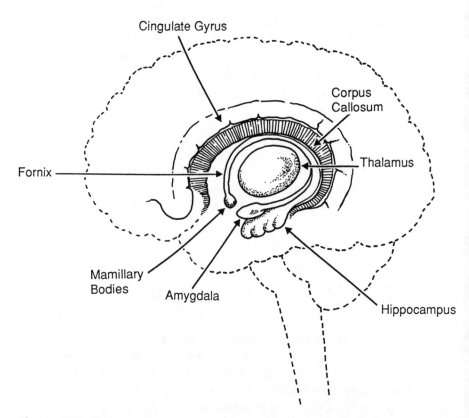

Figure 8–7. Limbic system seen within a side view of the brain.

epileptic seizures cannot be controlled by medications, neurosurgeons sometimes will remove neural tissue that is thought to be the trigger zone for seizures. In one surgery of this type, a patient called H.M. had his hippocampus removed on each side of the brain (the hippocampus is a paired structure). The result of this surgery was a profound memory impairment (**amnesia**). H.M. simply could not form new memories. He could read the same magazine over and over again, always finding it to contain new information. This surgical experience pointed to the importance of the hippocampus as a part of the brain's memory circuit. This is just one of many examples of how the study of individuals with damage to the brain has yielded important information on how the brain works. The limbic structures have many connections with the frontal lobe of the cerebrum and these two parts of the brain form an important circuit for emotion.

Spinal Cord

The **spinal cord** is the portion of the central nervous system that is located within the spinal column. As shown in Figure 8–8, the spinal cord is a pencil-thin cable of nervous tissue in which a H-shaped central core of neuron cell bodies (gray matter) is enclosed by a white wrapping of myelinated fibers. We saw in earlier sections that neuronal cell bodies could be aggregated in a thin bark (cerebral cortex) or rounded masses (basal nuclei or thalamus). In the spinal cord, the cell bodies are arranged in long columns. The spinal cord gives rise to 31 pairs of peripheral nerves that (a) transmit messages from the CNS to muscles and glands and (b) receive sensory messages from the body. These spinal nerves constitute part of the peripheral nervous system and are described in the next section along with the cranial nerves.

The Peripheral Nervous System

The peripheral nervous system (PNS) lies outside the CNS and consists of 12 pairs of **cranial nerves** and 31 pairs of **spinal nerves**. These nerves are the means by which the CNS communicates with the rest of the body. The peripheral nerves are commonly divided into motor and sensory parts. **Motor nerves** innervate muscles or glands. **Sensory nerves** transmit sensory information on qualities such as vision, hearing, touch, movement, and pain to the CNS. Table 8–2 shows the major functions of the 12 pairs of cranial nerves. These nerves emerge from the base of the brain and then reach to the structures they innervate. Note that the nerves identified by the

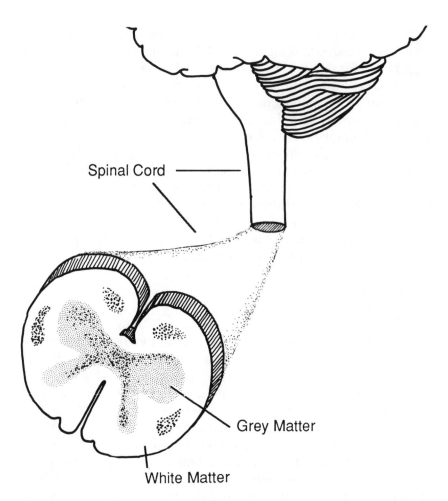

Spinal Cord

Grey Matter

White Matter

Figure 8–8. Cross section of spinal cord, showing gray and white matter.

Roman numerals V, VII, VIII, IX, X, XI, and XII are especially important for speech production.

Brain Imaging

Modern **brain imaging** is giving new insights into the structure and function of the living human brain. Brain imaging is the process of revealing brain structure or physiology. The major types of brain imaging systems are summarized in Table 8–3. Some of these techniques are capable of yielding detailed information on the brain's structure. Other techniques can be used to study function, such as metabolism or blood flow to various regions of the brain. Although the brain imaging methods differ considerably in how they work

Table 8–2. The twelve cranial nerves, identified by Roman numeral and by name, and their major functions.

Number	Name	Function
I	Olfactory	Smells
II	Optic	Sees
III	Oculomotor	Moves eyeball and constricts pupil
IV	Trochlear	Moves eyeball
V	Trigeminal	Somatosensation to front half of head; motor to chewing
VI	Abducens	Moves eyeball
VII	Facial	Moves face, tears, tastes, and salivates
VIII	Statoacoustic	Balances and hears
IX	Glossopharyngeal	Tastes, salivates, and swallows
X	Vagus	Tastes, swallows, lifts soft palate, and phonates; sensorimotor to the viscera of the thorax and abdomen
XI	Spinal accessory	Turns head and shrugs shoulders
XII	Hypoglossal	Moves tongue

Table 8–3. Some methods of brain imaging and the brain characteristics they reveal.

Method	Brain Feature Examined
Computerized tomography (CT)	Physical structure
Magnetic resonance imaging (MRI)	Physical structure
Positron emission tomography (PET)	Brain metabolism, such as oxygen or glucose uptake
Electroencephalography (EEG)	Electrical activity
Magnetoencephalography (MEG)	Magnetic fields

and what they can reveal about the brain, they can be understood in terms of the logical sequence explained below.

1. Brain structure refers to the physical composition of the brain. Magnetic resonance imaging (MRI) is one of the newest and most powerful tools to examine the detailed structure of the nervous system (or other parts of the body). A more conventional x-ray technique, called computerized tomography (CT) is also used to make pictures of brain structure.

2. Brain chemistry or **metabolism** pertains to the way in which chemicals are used in functions of the brain. The brain is a chemical engine in which oxygen and glucose are the basic fuels. One way of studying brain function, then, is to trace these chemicals as they are used in the brain's metabolic processes. Positron emission tomography (PET) uses radioactive markers (labels) that are "attached" to chemicals that are taken up by the brain. Chemical activity can be determined by following the distribution of the radioactively labeled chemicals. Unlike conventional x-ray methods, in which the source of x-rays is *outside* the body, PET works by getting the source of x-rays *inside* the body, usually by injecting them into the blood stream or by mixing them in air that is breathed in. Monitoring regional blood flow is another way of studying brain function. Regions of the brain that are most active demand more blood, so that increased blood flow usually indicates increased brain activity. A new tool under development is Functional Magnetic Resonance Imaging (FMRI), in which magnetic resonance imaging is used to study blood flow.

3. Electrophysiology is the study of electrical activity in living tissues. Functions of the brain can be monitored by recording the electrical activity generated within it. The magnitude of this electrical activity is very small but can be recorded with electrodes attached to the scalp and then amplified. This procedure is called **electroencephalography** (electro- = electrical; encephalo- = brain; -graphy = recording; hence, literally, recordings of brain electricity). Computers are used to sum up the electrical activity recorded from different regions of the brain and to display the resulting patterns in multicolored "maps."

4. Magnetic fields are generated by the brain's electrical activity. It should be possible to record these very weak magnetic fields and display the results as an indication of brain function. This process is called **magnetoencephalography** and is one of the newest, and most experimental, methods of brain imaging.

With the increased application of imaging systems, the understanding of the brain may change dramatically. Accordingly, it is imortant to recognize the impact of these technologies of neuroscience.

✦ LANGUAGE IN THE BRAIN

If language is a function of the brain, then can language be assigned to particular parts of the brain? This question is one of localization, or the attempt to relate particular functions or behaviors to local regions of nervous tissue. But it is not necessarily the case that the brain is divided into distinct regions that serve discrete functions. Rather, it may be that some, if not all, functions, are carried out by a concerted action of many different regions of the brain. The extreme version of this perspective is called **mass action** which holds that the brain functions essentially as a whole to carry out a given function or behavior.

Can language be localized? Figure 8–9 schematizes a search for an answer to this question. As a first step, one might ask: Do the

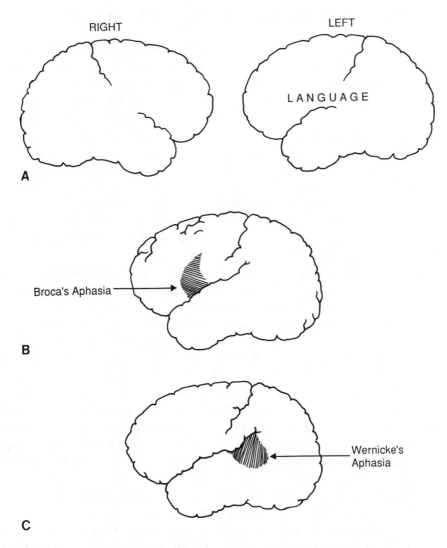

Figure 8-9. Major aspects of localization within the brain. **A.** hemispheric asymmetry — left hemisphere is typically dominant for language in right-handed individuals. **B.** Broca's area is hypothesized to be involved in speech output. **C.** Wernicke's area is hypothesized to be involved in the auditory comprehension of speech.

two cerebral hemispheres participate equally in language? The human body has many paired structures, such as kidneys, lungs, ovaries, or testicles, and usually the two members of a pair perform very similar functions. For this reason, a person can lose one lung or one kidney and still function in an apparently normal way. Is the same true of the brain? Can a person lose one cerebral hemisphere and still have apparently normal language?

Cerebral Asymmetry of the Brain for Language

Reports on a number of types of brain damage have led to a very important conclusion: language is located primarily in the left cerebral hemisphere, at least in right-handed individuals. When language functions were examined in individuals who suffered **strokes** (disturbances to the blood supply of the brain) or brain **trauma** (physical injury, as from a blow to the head), the preponderance of persons who suffered language impairment were those with damage to the left hemisphere. In fact, the evidence that language is based in the left hemisphere is so strong that language is often cited as the best example of **cerebral asymmetry**, or the idea that the two cerebral hemispheres are not equal in their control of a given behavior. Some writers took the position that language is lateralized to the left hemisphere. However, that position is too extreme, for it appears that the right hemisphere does have some language capability. For example, when certain drugs are used to incapacitate the left hemisphere, the subjects who received the drug do not lose language altogether. Rather, they demonstrate a reduced ability to use language, functioning more like a young child than an adult.

The body of evidence points to the conclusion that the left hemisphere (in right-handers) is generally dominant for language. Therefore, damage to the left hemisphere is a particular jeopardy to language. Some exceptions to this general rule should be noted. First, some left-handed persons demonstrate language dominance of the right hemisphere. Second, some children who suffer severe damage to the left hemisphere develop a right-hemisphere dominance for language. Third, there are some reports indicating that some individuals with speech disorders such as stuttering may differ from the usual pattern of left-hemisphere dominance for spoken language. One theory of stuttering holds that people who stutter have anomalous (atypical) asymmetries of cortical function (see Chapter 13 by Prins). As mentioned earlier, the two hemispheres are connected by a large bundle of fibers called the corpus callosum, which is a major pathway for communication between the two hemispheres. A type of surgery called **commissurotomy** severs this major pathway and leaves the two hemispheres relatively independent. Studies of persons who have this brain surgery (sometimes called "split brain") have yielded important information about the relative capabilities of the left and right sides of the brain.

The two hemispheres also participate differently in the perception of sounds. Generally, for right-handed persons, the left hemisphere seems better able to process the information for brief or rapidly changing events, such as the consonants in the words *top, dog,* or *lock.* The right hemisphere, in contrast, seems better suited to process information of longer duration or information with a slowly changing time pattern, such as the overall rhythm of speech. These differences between the hemispheres are evident within a few weeks after birth, and probably emerge during fetal development.

Language Areas Within the Left Hemisphere

As shown in Figure 8–9, our inquiry to this point has indicated an incomplete lateralization of language, meaning that language functions are strongest in the left hemisphere but not completely absent from the right. The next step is to ask if language can be localized *within* the left hemisphere. To answer this question, it is helpful to introduce the term **aphasia**, which refers to an impairment of language use as the result of damage to the brain. Much of the knowledge about how language is represented in the brain has come from clinical studies of persons with aphasia. This chapter will consider the subject of aphasia only briefly, as a way of showing where language may be located in the brain. The topic of aphasia is discussed more thoroughly in Chapter 9.

There are various classifications of aphasia, but for present purposes it is sufficient to consider two types of aphasia that have been particularly important in the history of research on this language impairment. One type is called **Broca's aphasia**, which is characterized by difficulty in producing spoken language. The other type is called **Wernicke's aphasia**, which involves a primary difficulty in understanding spoken language. Each of these types of aphasia was named for an 18th century neurologist who described patients with aphasia. Paul Broca described a patient named Tan (the name was given to him because this was the only word the patient could say). Tan had an impairment of language expression, and Broca deduced that Tan's primary area of brain damage was the region shown in Figure 8–9B (Tan actually had a much larger area of damage but Broca concluded that one isolated region was of primary importance in explaining the language disorder). Carl Wernicke reported on another person with aphasia, but in his case the language impairment affected primarily the comprehension of spoken language. Wernicke's patient had brain damage like that shown in Figure 8–9C.

These clinical reports were highly influential in the understanding of aphasia. Even today, many clinicians diagnose forms of aphasia called Broca's or Wernicke's. But for present purposes, the issue is what these aphasias might tell us about the localization of language in the brain. One interpretation of these two types of aphasia is that the brain has one center that controls the expression of language as speech. This center is known as Broca's area and is located as shown in Figure 8–9B. Another center controls the comprehension of heard speech and is located in a region called Wernicke's area (Figure 8–9C). The idea thus emerges that different language functions might be assigned to different parts of the brain. Broca's and Wernicke's areas are two important centers, but not necessarily the only ones. The conceptualization that emerges from this kind of thinking is that language functions of the brain should be understood in terms of interconnected centers, located principally in the area around the lateral fissure and in the parietal lobe. As we will see in a following section, this is a popular perspective but it has been challenged by other points of view.

Theories of Language Representation Within the Brain

As new information is gathered, new theories of language representation in the brain, or at least revisions of older theories, are likely to appear. To be sure, still other theories could be mentioned, but two theories in particular have been selected for discussion here to give some idea of the range of possibilities without making the chapter excessively long.

The **Centers and Pathways Model** was an outgrowth of the pioneering work of Broca and Wernicke. The basic idea of this model formulated by Lichtheim, is that language is represented in a small number of centers which are connected by pathways, as illustrated in Figure 8–10. The centers are responsible for a particular function, such as motor expression (Broca's area) or auditory comprehension (Wernicke's area). The connecting pathways transmit information between centers. Damage to either the centers or pathways can result in a language disturbance. By analogy, a telephone system serving a large community could be interrupted either by damage to its central office or to the transmission lines that connect the central office with the switchboard of an office building. An appealing feature of the Centers and Pathways Model is that it

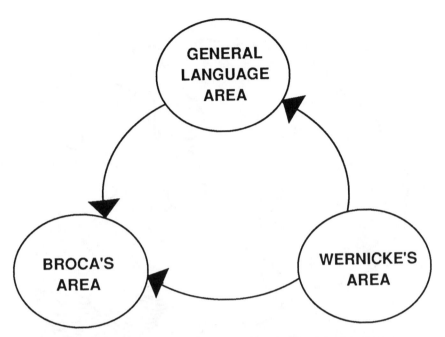

Figure 8–10. Diagram of the Centers and Pathways Model of Language: The centers are a General Language area, Broca's area, and Wernicke's area. The connecting lines are the pathways.

clearly relates location of damage to type of aphasia. However, this model has failed to account for some types of brain damage and the resulting aphasia. Aphasia sometimes results from damage to parts of the brain that were not expected to serve a language function.

The **Convergence Zone Model** is a more recent conceptualization developed by a neurologist, Antonio Damasio. This model holds that language is processed in a number of regions of the brain and that the different types of information are gathered and interpreted in a convergence zone. This model is shown schematically in Figure 8–11. Various types of information on an object are funneled to the convergence zone where a language function, such as naming, is finally performed. Many of the objects and events that we name are associated with a variety of types of information which may be represented in different parts of the brain. Naming a single piece of clothing such as a hat may involve the integration of information about fabric (texture), color, size, shape and even function (e.g., a rain hat versus a sun bonnet). This model allows that large regions of the brain may be active in speech and language functions, such as recognizing a word, producing a word, or formulating a sentence.

The **Modular Model**, variants of which have been described by a number of scientists, is based on the idea that brain functions

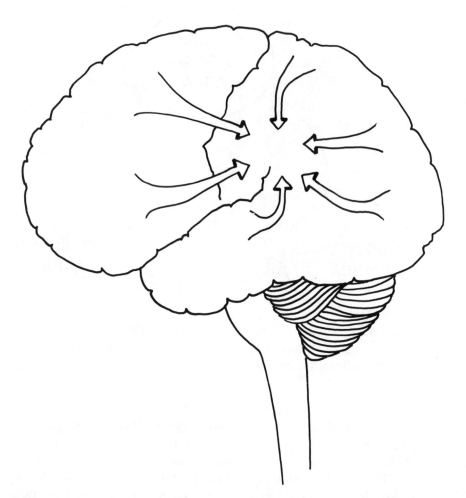

Figure 8–11. Diagram of the Convergence Zone Model of Language: Information from various parts of the brain is integrated and interpreted in a field of converging inputs.

are modularized, or subdivided into separate components. A rough analogy is a computer that has several different circuit boards, one to control graphic displays, one for an input device such as a mouse, another for sound output, and so on. A modular model of the brain holds that the brain is organized so that various functions are represented in independent or semi-independent neural circuits. Because the modules can operate simultaneously and in parallel, complex behaviors such as language can be accomplished with great speed and flexibility.

Neural Control of Speech

Once a language message is formulated, it must be expressed if any one other than its originator is to know about it. The message can be transmitted through writing, speech, manual signs, or gestures. Each of these output systems has its own musculature and control problems. If the message is to be written, the muscles of the arm and hand must be regulated to produce legible writing. Similarly, if the message is to be spoken, the muscles of the speech production system must be regulated to produce an intelligible utterance. This issue brings up the general problem of motor control. Every language message, from the most banal to the most profound, ultimately relies on motor coordination for its expression. Because speech is movement, specifically movement of structures such as the lips, tongue, jaw, vocal folds, and respiratory organs, one way to understand speech is to understand movement.

> Sperry (1952) spoke to the significance of movement when he wrote, "The entire output of our thinking machine consists of nothing but patterns of motor coordination" (p. 297).

Active movement is the result of muscular action. To move, we send neural impulses from the brain to selected muscles. These impulses, or instructions, tell the muscles when, how much, and how long to contract. The brain structures and pathways involved in movement control are schematized in Figure 8–12. The neural control of voluntary movement is complicated and involves a number of different structures that are connected by various loops. Figure 8–12 is a simplified representation of the neural control system but it conveys the essential components for an introductory description. The classic description is in terms of two systems — **pyramidal** and **extrapyramidal**. In fact, these two systems cooperate very closely in the control of movement. The distinction between them at least simplifies the description of this complex system and that reason alone may justify their separate discussion. The pyramidal system is discussed first.

The pyramidal system, or pathway, of motor control is usually described as the primary system of voluntary motor control. The basic neural plan is relatively simple, as shown in Figure 8–13. The pathway originates in the cortex, primarily in a strip of cortex commonly known as the **motor cortex** (corresponding to area 4 in Figure 8–5). Classically, this strip was thought to be quite narrow (about

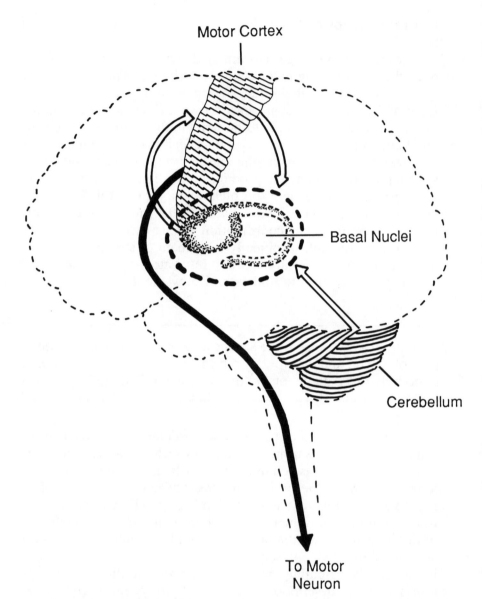

Figure 8-12. Diagram of the major brain structures involved in motor control.

1 cm wide) and readily distinct from the **sensory cortex** (corresponding to areas 1, 2, and 3 in Figure 8–5). But newer information suggests that the strip may be as wide as 4 cm and that the motor and sensory cortices overlap. Different parts of the body can be mapped along the motor cortex, as shown in the inset of Figure 8–13. Thus, one part of the cortex represents movement of the arm, another part movement of the tongue, and so on. But the mapping of movement on brain is not a simple one-to-one pattern; recent ex-

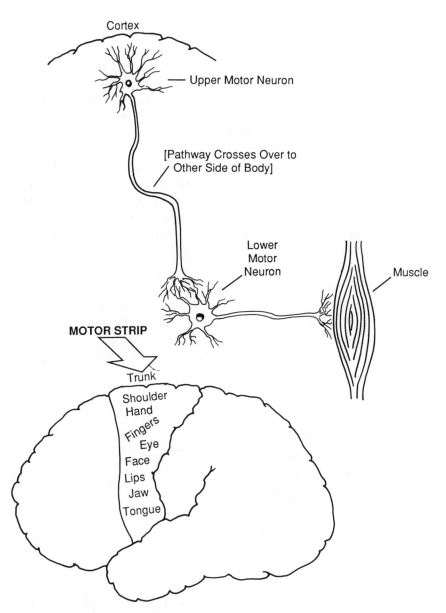

Figure 8–13. Schematic of pyramidal motor pathway, showing upper motor neuron and lower motor neuron. Inset shows representation of body on the motor strip (Brodmann area 4).

periments have shown that a given muscle or movement can be multiply represented in the motor cortex. The axons of the neurons in the motor cortex descend through subcortical structures, crossing from one side to the other at the level of the medulla. This crossing over is highly important in neurology because it means that **one**

side of the brain controls motor function on the opposite side of the body. That is, motor control is primarily **contralateral** (contra = opposite; lateral = side). After crossing, the neuron then synapses (connects with) another neuron that in turn directly innervates muscle. This basic two-neuron plan of an upper-motor neuron and a lower-motor neuron constitutes the pyramidal pathway.

But the pyramidal pathway does not work alone. Rather it cooperates with another system, the extrapyramidal pathway, to control movement. The extrapyramidal pathway is shown in a highly simplified form in Figure 8–14. Many of the structures should be familiar at least by name, for they were introduced earlier, for example, under the heading of basal nuclei. In fact, the structures of the basal nuclei, together with the thalamus, are major participants in the extrapyramidal pathway. It should be emphasized that Figure 8–14 is a simplified and incomplete representation of this complex system, but it suffices for purposes of introduction.

A division between the pyramidal and extrapyramidal pathways is somewhat artificial because they control movements together. However, one reason to maintain the distinction is because of the effects of various neurological diseases. One example of an

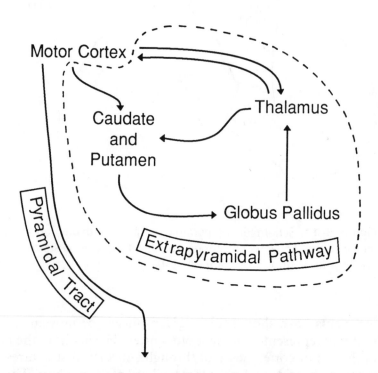

Figure 8–14. Combined system of pyramidal and extrapyramidal pathways of motor control.

extrapyramidal disease is Parkinson disease, which typically involves the symptoms of rigidity (stiffness), tremor (an involuntary rhythmic shaking), and slowness of movement. Many people with Parkinson disease have rigid muscles (and therefore a masklike, almost unblinking facial expression), a shaking of the limbs or fingers, and a difficulty initiating movement. This disease is linked with loss of cells in a particular part of the brain within the extrapyramidal motor system. As these cells die, the brain suffers a kind of chemical malnutrition, in which one particular neurotransmitter is in short supply. Drug therapy for Parkinson disease aims to correct for this deficiency in a chemical messenger. Another way to treat the disease is to replace the dysfunctional tissue through transplants of similar tissue from the same person, or from another person. Transplants of neural tissue are one of the newest and most controversial forms of therapy for neurological diseases.

Speech disorders that result from damage to the parts of the nervous system that control movement are called **dysarthrias**. The damage can occur at several different levels, including the motor cortex, the structures of the extrapyramidal system, the lower motor neuron, or even the junction between the lower motor neuron and the muscle itself. Although the various forms of dysarthria tend to have some characteristics in common (such as slow rate of speaking and abnormal voice quality), an experienced clinician can distinguish them with a high degree of accuracy.

◆ A SUMMARY OF NEURAL STRUCTURES INVOLVED IN UNDERSTANDING AND PRODUCING LANGUAGE

Figure 8–15 is a summary illustration which shows some of the most important structures thought to be involved in (a) producing speech in response to a spoken message, and (b) reading aloud a written word. These illustrations simplify the process considerably but they give some idea about the major parts of the brain that are involved in listening to speech, reading, and producing speech.

Figure 8–15A shows the basic neural pathways involved in listening to speech and then producing a verbal response. The auditory signal is first received at the cortex in a region of the temporal lobe called the **primary auditory area** which accomplishes an initial processing of sound patterns. By the time auditory information reaches this area, it already has been processed by many neural centers along a complex pathway that leads from the ear to the cortex. Information from the **primary auditory area** is then transmitted for additional processing in Wernicke's area and in the **auditory association area**. Wernicke's area is linked to the **supramar-**

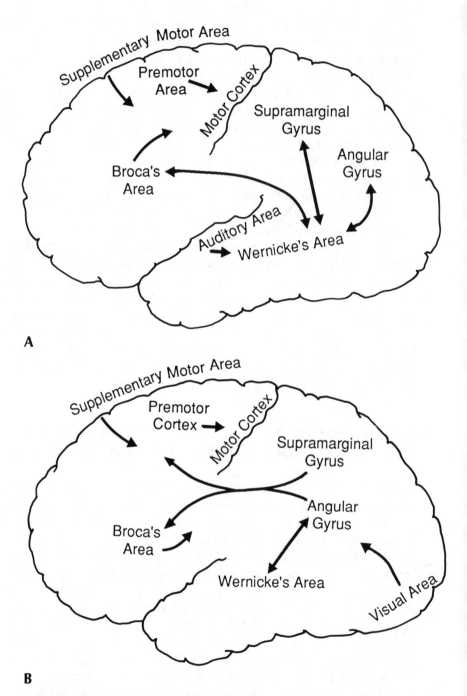

Figure 8–15. General pathways of brain activity: **A.** Hearing and repeating a spoken word. **B.** Reading a printed word.

ginal gyrus and the **angular gyrus**, which assist in the linguistic interpretation of the message. Communication between the posterior areas of the cortex discussed so far with the more frontal regions is accomplished largely via an important tract called the **arcuate fasciculus** (shown in Figure 8–4). Broca's area plays a role in the preparation of a motor response (i.e., the act of speaking). Broca's area transmits information to the motor cortex (especially the orofacial and laryngeal areas of the motor strip). However, as shown in the diagram, several other structures participate in motor control of speech. These include other cortical regions such as the **supplementary motor area**, **premotor cortex** (some authors regard the supplementary motor area and premotor area as the same), and **somatosensory cortex** (the sensory strip). In addition, speech production is regulated by subcortical structures including the basal nuclei, thalamus, and cerebellum. Obviously, many different parts of the brain participate in listening to speech and responding in kind. But many other relevant structures have been omitted in the interest of simplicity. For example, no mention has been made of the right hemisphere, but it too is involved in processing the speech message. Also neglected are the various nuclei and ganglia of the limbic system, pons, cranial nerves and spinal nerves.

Figure 8–15B depicts the major pathways involved in seeing a printed word and reading it aloud. The sense of vision projects to the occipital lobe, which contains both the **primary visual area** and **visual association area**. Information from these areas is then transmitted to the angular gyrus, which in turn projects to areas of the frontal lobe that regulate the process of speaking, as described in connection with Figure 8–15B.

◆ A BRIEF LOOK AT THE DEVELOPMENT AND AGING OF THE BRAIN

The brain undergoes many lifespan changes. Of course, the periods before birth, infancy, and childhood are primarily years of formation. The years of adulthood, especially after the age of about 40 years, are conspicuous periods of loss — loss of brain weight and loss of neurons. But the loss of neurons begins much earlier — in infancy. We are born with as many neurons as we will ever have. Many neurons fail to make functional connections and are shed from the developing brain. It appears that brain development is largely a selective carving of a huge neuronal population into functional ensembles. As one scientist put it, nature is "profligate" and neurons are wasted in large numbers during the developmental process. In some sense, our mental selves are what is left after masses of our neurons die.

Table 8–4 is a timetable of some major events in brain development from shortly before birth until about 6 years. Also listed are some corresponding events in the development of spoken language. Notice, for example, that the age at which corticocortical connections (meaning connections between different areas of the cortex, as shown in Figure 8–4) are established matches up against the age at which the infant demonstrates initial word comprehension, such as understanding "No!" or "bye-bye." The table also describes changes in dendritic density in the language areas of the cortex. Dendritic density is the degree of branching of a neuron's dendrites. Dendritic branching is the means by which neurons are connected with other neurons. The greater the branching, the greater is the connectivity among neurons. Recent research indicates that dendritic branching initially is greater in the right hemisphere than the left, and in the oral motor area of the cortex than in Broca's area. But the pattern changes during development so that eventually the left hemisphere has a greater branching than the right, and Broca's area has a greater branching than the oral motor area. Development of the nervous system continues until the age of 18–21 years, by which time myelination is complete and the brain's activity patterns have reached maturity. Recent findings indicate that the frontal lobe (the "executive" of the brain) is the last to mature.

At about the age of 40 years, neuronal loss accelerates and metabolic waste products accumulate in the nervous tissues. The loss is not uniform. Some areas, such as the temporal lobe, lose neurons at a faster rate than other parts of the brain. Among the brain areas with the fastest losses of neurons are structures that serve memory (parts of the limbic system, shown in Figure 8–7). Some disease conditions, such as Alzheimer's disease, result in extremely high rates of neuronal death. Persons with Alzheimer's disease gradually lose memory and the capacity to live independently. In the advanced stages of the disease, there may be severe personality changes and loss of speech. Aging and many diseases common in the elderly also are associated with changes in the availability of neurotransmitters, the brain's chemical messengers. A major direction of research on the aging brain is to explore the possibility of replacing neurotransmitters by drug therapy or surgical implants.

> Would it be possible to distinguish geniuses from people of normal intellect by studying their brains? Perhaps so, but the differ-
> *(continued)*

Table 8–4. Some events in brain maturation related to language.

5 MONTHS GESTATIONAL AGE: By this time the full complement of neurons is established, meaning that the brain has as many neurons as it will ever have.

BIRTH: Neuronal cell formation is complete and the neurons have completed their migration to their target sites. Migration is a process in which neurons relocate from the embryonic sites to the sites they will have in the mature brain.

3 MONTHS: At this age, the dendritic density (amount of branching in dendrites) is greater in the right hemisphere than in the left, and the density is greater in the oral motor area of the cortex than in Broca's area.

6 MONTHS: There is a peak in development of inner layers of cortex in the brain's language areas. The cortex has six layers of neurons with the inner three devoted largely to receiving input from other parts of the brain. The early development of the inner three layers is therefore a possible preparation for input.

8–9 MONTHS: Corticocortical connections are being established, and an adult-like metabolic activity is observed across regions. Corticocortical refers to connections across different regions of the cortex. It is at about this time that a child first demonstrates comprehension of a spoken word.

15 MONTHS: Hippocampus is fully mature, giving the infant an important neural system for memory. There is also a rapid acceleration in the number of cortical synapses, so that more and more neurons are in functional contact.

24 MONTHS: Dendritic density increases in Broca's area to catch up with the density in the oral motor cortex. Dendritic density in the left hemisphere is also catching up with that in the right. The age of 2 years is for many children the beginning of an explosive stage of language learning.

48 MONTHS: There are peaks in the overall level of brain metabolism, and in the development of the outer three layers of language cortex (perhaps reflecting increased output potential).

72 MONTHS: Dendritic density of Broca's area is now greater than that in oral motor cortex.

ences are not easily detected. A study of Albert Einstein's brain showed one difference in the inferior part of the parietal lobe, a part of the brain that seems to be involved in the processing of information from different senses. Perhaps one factor in Einstein's genius was that he had an unusual ability to integrate information from different senses.

◆ CONCLUSION

This chapter has been a short guided tour through the most complicated system in the known universe — the human brain. The tour was necessarily selective, leaving many interesting and important features unexplored. But for those who choose to learn more about the human nervous system, the fundamental concepts introduced in this chapter should serve as a basic outline. One of the human brain's most remarkable accomplishments is language. Some scientists believe that language is the faculty that most clearly distinguishes humans from other species. This chapter has discussed some major ideas about how language is represented in the brain, including lateralization to the left hemisphere in right-handers, and possible localization of language within this hemisphere.

But without a means of motor output, language has no communicative value. A person without some capability of motor output cannot communicate. Speech is the most common form of language expression throughout the world and is usually the first to be learned. The motor control of speech is accomplished by the interaction of many parts of the nervous system, reaching from the cerebral cortex, through the basal nuclei, thalamus, and cerebellum, to the cranial and spinal nerves that innervate the muscles of speech production.

Many of the disorders discussed in this book are associated with impairments of the nervous system. Therefore, a fundamental knowledge of the nervous system is needed to understand the origin, assessment, and management of these communication disorders.

◆ REFERENCES

Eccles, J. C. (1973). *The understanding of the brain.* New York: McGraw-Hill.
Klivington, K. (1989). *The science of mind.* Cambridge, MA: MIT Press.
Sperry, R. W. (1952). Neurology and the mind-brain problem. *American Scientist, 40,* 291–312.

✦ RECOMMENDED READINGS

Most of these books were written for a general audience, and some of them are highly entertaining as well as informative.

Calvin, W. H., & Ojemann, G. A. (1980). *Inside the brain.* New York: New American Library. The authors discuss neuroscience from a neurologist's perspective. Much of the book is based on dialog concerned with persons who have neurological disorders.

Ewing, S. A., & Pfalzgraf, B. (1990). *Pathways: Moving beyond stroke and aphasia.* Detroit, MI: Wayne State University Press. The authors, who are speech-language pathologists, describe and follow six individuals and their families as they contend with stroke and aphasia.

Gazzaniga, M. (1988). *Mind matters.* New York: Houghton Mifflin. This book reports on brain research, especially the supposed functions of various parts of the brain. The author offers a neuroscientist's view of pain, love, dreams, and memory, and presents a theory of the brain based on a modular-interpreter organization.

Klawans, H. L. (1989). *Toscanini's tumble and other tales of clinical neurology.* New York: Bantam Books. A neurologist describes a number of patients and what he learned from them about neurological disorders and the people who contend with them. Klawans and Oliver Sacks are prominent contributors to a genre in which specialists recall their most interesting clinical encounters.

Klawans, Harold L. (1990). *Newton's madness.* New York: Harper & Row. Continuing very much in the vein of *Toscanini's Tumble and Other Tales of Clinical Neurology,* Klawans describes patients with a variety of neurological disorders.

Knox, D. (1985). *Portrait of aphasia.* Detroit, MI: Wayne State University Press. The author's wife suffered a stroke that left her with aphasia. Much of the book describes the recovery process and its accompanying emotions.

Martin, R. (1986). *Matters gray and white: A neurologist, his patients and the mysteries of the brain.* New York: Henry Holt. The title effectively summarizes the book. The author uses his clinical experiences to tell about the practice of neurology, about how neurological disorders affect people, and about what these disorders reveal about the brain.

Noonan, D. (1989). *Neuro– (Life on the frontlines of brain surgery and neurological medicine).* New York: Simon & Schuster. The author accompanies a neurologist as he diagnoses and treats a variety of disorders. Noonan tells the story from the point of view of both the doctors and patients. The book offers personal insights and a fair amount of information on diagnosis and treatment of neurological disorders.

Restak, R. (1979). *The brain: The last frontier.* New York: Warner Books. Restak discusses at length a number of discoveries about the human brain. A little outdated but still a good and broad introduction to the topic.

Sacks, O. (1970). *The man who mistook his wife for a hat and other clinical tales.* New York: Summit Books. Sacks describes his experiences with a variety of patients. Written with wonderment and affection, the book also teaches about the practice of neurology and neurological disorders.

Sacks, O. (1990). *Awakenings.* New York: Harper Perennial. Sacks describes the results of L-Dopa medication given to a number of people afflicted with parkinsonism resulting from encephalitis lethargica (a kind of sleeping sickness). This book was the basis for a movie, called *Awakenings*, which starred Robert De Niro and Robin Williams.

Smith, A. (1984). *The mind.* New York: Viking Press. A wide-ranging book that presents many facts in masterful prose. Not a single illustration, but Smith makes his words work quite well, as he writes on topics ranging from anatomy to disorder to exceptional accomplishment.

Sylvester, E. J. (1993). *The healing blade.* New York: Simon & Schuster. Subtitled *A Tale of Neurosurgery*, this book is mostly about a neurological institute in Phoenix and a neurosurgeon named Dr. Robert Spetzler. The author, who spent hundreds of days and nights at the Institute, describes surgical procedures and the surgeons who perform them. Reads rather like a journalistic novel.

Wulf, H. H. (1973). *Aphasia, my world alone.* Detroit, MI: Wayne State University Press. Wulf describes her recovery from aphasia, giving a vivid account of her frustrations and victories. Speech-language therapy figures prominently in her recovery.

◆ GLOSSARY

Amnesia: an impairment of memory resulting from damage to the brain.

Aphasia: an impairment of language resulting from damage to the brain. Several types of aphasia are recognized.

Axon: the process of a neuron that carries information away from the neuron's cell body. Axons tend to have few branches and can vary greatly in length.

Basal nuclei: (also called **basal ganglia**); Specialized subcortical structures that help to regulate movement and integrate sensory information.

Brain imaging: any method used to show the structure or function of the intact brain.

Brain stem: the part of the brain consisting of the midbrain, pons, and medulla.

Cell body: the part of a neuron that contains the nucleus and its genetic material.

Central Nervous System (CNS): the part of the nervous system that is contained within the bony cavities of the skull and spinal column; it consists of the brain and spinal cord.

Cerebellum: the "little brain," or the structure located behind and beneath the cerebral hemispheres. The cerebellum is involved in the control of coordinated movement.

Cerebrum: the major portion of the brain, consisting of the cerebral hemispheres.

Cerebral asymmetry: the idea that the two cerebral hemispheres are not equal in size or function.

Cerebral cortex: literally the "bark" of the cerebral hemispheres. It consists of six layers of neurons that form a rind of gray matter around the cerebrum.

Corpus callosum: the thick band of axons that connect the two cerebral hemispheres. The corpus callosum is one example of a commissure, or band of fibers that connects the hemispheres.

Cranial nerves: the 12 paired nerves that emerge from the base of the brain to innervate various structures of the head, neck, thorax, and abdomen. The cranial nerves, together with the spinal nerves, constitute the Peripheral Nervous System.

Dendrite: the process of a neuron that carries information toward the neuron's cell body. Dendrites tend to be short and highly branched.

Dysarthria: an impairment of speech production as a result of damage to the nervous system.

Extrapyramidal motor system: a brain system that participates in the regulation of movement. It is considered to be parallel to, and relating with, the pyramidal system of motor control. The extrapyramidal system consists principally of the basal nuclei.

Gyrus (plural form is **gyri**): an outfolding or ridge on the cerebral hemispheres.

Limbic system: a set of brain structures thought to regulate emotions, memory, and some aspects of attention. Some limbic structures are the cingulate gyrus, septal region, fornix, mammillary bodies, hippocampus, and amygdala.

Lobe: one of the five major divisions of the cerebral hemispheres. The lobes are called frontal, parietal, temporal, occipital, and limbic.

Localization: the principle that focal regions of the brain can be associated with particular functions or behaviors.

Myelin: the fatty, white tissue that surrounds large axons to provide an insulating coating. The so-called white matter of the brain takes its color from myelin.

Neuron: the nerve cell, or basic unit of the nervous system. It is composed of a cell body and processes called axons and dendrites.

Neurotransmitter: a chemical messenger in the nervous system.

Nucleus: (1) the part of the cell body that contains genetic material; or (2) a collection of cell bodies in the Central Nervous System (also called "gray matter").

Peripheral Nervous System (PNS): the major division of the nervous system that lies largely outside the bony protection of the skull and spinal column; it consists of the cranial and spinal nerves.

Pyramidal motor system: along with the extrapyramidal motor system, a system for the control of voluntary movement. The pyramidal system arises primarily from Brodmann Area 4 (motor strip), Brodmann Area 6, and the parietal lobe. It was classically regarded as the primary system of voluntary motor control, but it is now thought to work closely with the extrapyramidal system and to include sensory as well as motor fibers.

Spinal cord: the part of the Central Nervous System that extends through the spinal column. It gives rise to the spinal nerves.

Spinal nerves: the nerves of the Peripheral Nervous System that emerge from the spinal cord.

Stroke: a focal neurologic deficit with a sudden or rapid onset caused by a cerebrovascular disease (the deficit usually lasts longer than 24 hours).

Sulcus (plural form is **sulci**): a fissure in the surface of the cerebral hemispheres.

Synapse: the juncture or functional connection between neurons.

CHAPTER 9

Neurogenic Disorders of Communication

LEONARD L. LaPOINTE, Ph.D.

After reading this chapter, you should be able to:

◆ Understand the history of the study of brain damage and communication disorders.

◆ List some of the causes of nervous system damage that result in impaired communication.

◆ List the principle types of neurogenic disorders of communication.

◆ Understand the nature and characteristics of aphasia, right hemisphere impairment, traumatic brain injury, dementia, and neuromotor speech disorders.

◆ Appreciate general principles and strategies of evaluation and treatment of these disorders.

◆ Recognize that clinical intervention can aid in the restoration of improved quality of life for people who have experienced neurogenic communication disorders.

In this chapter you will be introduced to the disorders of speech, language, movement, and thinking that result from damage to the brain and related parts of the nervous system. The roots and origins of these disorders will be outlined as will the variety of diseases, traumas, and conditions that create them. Most of the chapter will be devoted to explanation and description of the disorders themselves. Case vignettes and examples of disrupted communication drawn from the experience of working with hundreds of individuals with these disorders will illustrate the aphasias, right hemisphere syndrome, traumatic brain injury, dementia, and the neuromotor speech disorders. All of this will be set against the backdrop of the role of the professional in communication disorders and the responsibilities, challenges, and rewards of working with people with these conditions.

Word soup. Word salad. "I'd like some twink . . . quankit. No camorrit, dammit." Every time Albert tried to put a sentence together, about the only thing that came out was a mish-mash of words — or swear words that he couldn't seem to control. He called the cigarette lighter an "appleholtent." Who knows where that came from? The knife and spoon were "Nighfolt" and "Cuffolt." He tried to retrieve the name for a picture of chocolate cake. "I know that one. Fred Cake. Goddamn. Jesus H. Pwell. Is that right?" He couldn't understand a lot of what people said either. It sounded like they were using words that he never learned or weren't in the dictionary. It was like trying to understand Bulgarian or Lithuanian. Word soup. Word salad. What a mess. I never knew a stroke could create such a disaster. Aphasia, huh? Sounds like language that's been put in a Cuisenart.

"Sorry, Beth . . . it's a brain tumor." Two of the most feared words in the English language. She broke it to me as gently as she could. Brain tumor. Unwanted growth. It wasn't malignant, and they said it probably wouldn't grow back. But they had to do surgery and take it out. Good break, she said. It was pretty much confined to the right hemisphere of the brain. The surgery was a success, though they had to destroy some healthy brain tissue to get all of the "neoplasm," their term for the unwelcome, infiltrating little growth that tried to ruin my 32-year-old life. Except that I still have trouble with my left arm and leg. I'm worried about whether or not I'll be able to take care of my baby. And this "Right Hemisphere Syndrome." I get lost easier. I can't find my way around the hospital halls. Seems like I can't pay attention. I don't seem to be able to get the big picture. They keep telling me I don't finish the food on my hospital tray. I thought I finished it. No wonder I'm always hungry. I feel less emotional, kind of flat most of the time. I don't seem to get the punch line in some jokes; though I still like the Three Stooges. I love it when that horseshoe hits Curly on the head. Oh, a wise guy, huh? I still have some trouble recognizing faces. I even had trouble with Matthew when they brought him to me. Sometimes I wonder whether that person was really my cousin who stopped in to see me. I have the faint impression it was someone pretending to be my cousin. I wonder if this will ever get better? I guess I can kiss off my plans for graduate school, at least for now. Maybe I'll get better. Maybe this rehab stuff will work. I wish I had all of my right hemisphere back. Dah, ta daht ta da tah dadaah . . . . If only I had a brain . . . What was that Wizard of Oz song?

My name is Bennett. My Hopi name is much longer. It would be difficult for you to say. It is difficult for me to say now. I am a silversmith and make intricate village scenes on silver bracelets. Little pueblos with tiny detailed kachinas. I don't like people to tell me what to do. I used to feel that it was a violation of my civil rights for anyone to prescribe that I wear a helmet. I've changed my mind. Ha. No pun intended. I wish I would have had one on when my Harley twisted sideways and threw me on that stretch of gravel going up the Third Mesa. I wish it could be like in our legends. Spider Woman and the Twins. The First People suffered no illness, no injury. I wasn't so lucky. I suffered deep cortical and brain stem damage and the path of rehabilitation has not been easy. The people in Phoenix helped me a lot. In a way, there has been some good fortune in my cloud house, since I still have the use of my arms and hands and can use my Macintosh Powerbook and communicate this way. But my attempts at talking are still not very successful. I have trouble controlling my breathing for speech. My tongue movements are

(continued)

very slow, and most of the words I try to say are dragged out and not very clear. I still have some trouble swallowing, too. The speech-language pathologist told me I have a condition called Flaccid Dysarthria. Sounds pretty exotic. I never heard of it before. Apparently, there's a lot of it caused by traumatic brain injury from motorcycle accidents. Maybe when I get a little further along, I'll join that group that's lobbying the legislature to try to get a mandatory helmet law passed. Maybe it would prevent a few of these. A lot of the accident victims I've met will need help the rest of their lives. And most of them ran out of insurance long ago. A violation of civil rights. Restriction of personal choice. Yah, right. It's been rough. Sometimes I feel like Cha'-kwaina, the kachina called One Who Cries. I'll keep trying, though. I can still create beauty from silver. I won't lose my spirit. We have a rich tradition of persistence. Maybe by the Hawk Moon I'll be doing better.

This chapter is about the disorders of speech and communication that are caused by damage to the brain and nervous system. This territory of fascination and heartbreak is mapped and introduced by Kent in Chapter 8. As the stories above illustrate, there is a human side to all of this. A person is the nucleus around which each story revolves. These disorders can be counted, analyzed, interpreted, researched, and described but none can be divorced from the person. Each happens to an individual and each creature exists within the little constellation of a family. The human side is the most compelling side. Although the study of the workings of the brain and what happens when things go wrong is mesmerizing, the contemplation of the puzzling catalog of communication disorders that are created out of disease or damage to the nervous system is even more alluring. The person who chooses to specialize in neurogenic communication disorders must be part detective, counselor, laborer, monk, confessor, artist, teacher, and friend. Study of the brain has been called one of the last frontiers of science, so immediately that means that there will be many unanswered questions. People we work with will be desperate and frustrated as they seek solutions and demand answers that may not exist. We will not be able to satisfy them always. Many times, the inadequacy of the state of the clinical science will result in professional identity and competency crises that create sleepless nights for us with sheets hopelessly twisted around our ankles. But there is a balance to all of this. And the balance will be the small steps of accomplishment that add up to even greater gains — the retrieved word; the improved comprehension; the step toward independence and acceptance. All of these can ripen into a sense of wellness and improved quality of life. This is no small reward. These benefits can make for a sense of fulfillment and accomplishment and an infusion of good reasons to get up in the morning. These are not tiny harvests.

In this chapter we will learn about these disruptions of talking and writing and reading and thinking and communicating that are the result of brain damage. To appreciate this, it will be necessary to learn our way around the warps and woofs of the enchanted loom of the brain, and be surprised by the parade of diseases and conditions that disrupt this delicate tapestry. We will be introduced to the relatively recent history of interest in these disorders. We will learn about the disorders; the nature and characteristics of them; and how they can drastically change so many facets of human living, loving, and learning. We will learn as well what efforts are being made to deal with them and to help restore some balance to the lives of the players who must put up with them. First, some history.

◆ ORIGINS: THE MURKINESS OF THE PAST

"A prisoner with a very visible Organ of Tune turned out . . . to be passionately fond of music but 'spent his youth in debauchery' [and] was in jail because of an unnatural crime."

"An infanticide in whom Love of Offspring was 'absolutely flattened' but the Organ of Murder was very largely developed."

"A thief with a large Organ of Acquisitiveness who also had large but somewhat smaller Organs of Murder and Compassion robbed a woman and strangled her. He later returned to his victim to untie the cord he had used."

Franz Joseph Gall, *On the Functions of the Brain and Each of Its Parts* (1835, cited in Mac Millan, 1992)

Criminal behavior can be related to bumps on the head. So thought Dr. Franz Joseph Gall and his followers. In fact a lot of other emotions, personality traits, attributes, and "powers," as they were called by Dr. Gall, could be localized simply by feeling the bumps and prominences on the skull. For years, in the middle part of the 19th century the "science" of brain and behavior was advocated and advanced by Gall, the German anatomist and founder of "Phrenology." **Phrenology** was the science or pseudoscience of determining a person's character or attributes by noting the pattern of skull bumps. Gall claimed to have discovered his principles of phrenology by observing people and animals with marked character traits and then noticing that they had distinctive skull shapes or "bumps" that could be felt with the fingers. Figure 9–1 is a reproduction of one of the many "Phrenology Charts" that were popularly used to read the character of clients. These readings were conducted in physicians' offices, in the tents of road shows, and in "Phrenology Parlors" of the cities of Europe and North America.

In addition to the qualities of Murder and Tune, such traits as Wonder, Vanity, Wit, Adhesiveness, and Language (associated with bulging or protruding eyes) could be readily discerned from the head and facial features of individuals.

Phrenology was immensely popular in the 1800s, until it was discredited by advances in science and by its failures in predicting or deducing saints and geniuses from sinners. Eventually, it became the target of satire and lampoon in verse and on the stage, and one can imagine it becoming an easy target for the Saturday Night Live troupes of the 1900s. While this pseudoscience took things quite a bit too far, in it can be seen the seeds of many contemporary ideas and approaches to our understanding of the brain and behavior.

The picture of the brain and its association with speech and language came into much sharper focus in the 19th century. At the very least, Gall was no doubt responsible for fanning the debates on the relationships between skull size and intelligence and on the localization of language in the brain that flared intensely at this time in the European professional societies. From these debates came the case studies of the 1860s that tried to provide evidence of a connection between the frontal lobes of the brain and language.

The French physician, Ernest Auburtin, presented a remarkable case study of a failed suicide, in which the man had torn off part of his skull with a revolver shot that left a large portion of his brain exposed but not damaged. Auburtin described how he had treated the man for his wound and decided to conduct an experiment in nature by pressing a pancake turner against the conscious man's exposed brain while the patient was talking. As Auburtin (Wertz, LaPointe, & Rosenbek, 1991) described it:

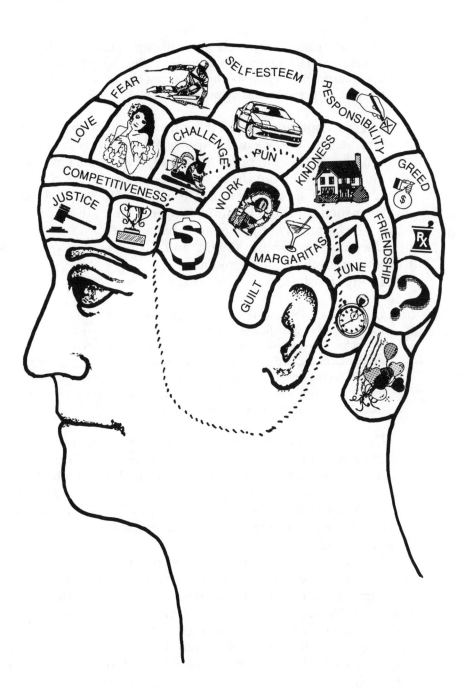

Figure 9–1. Phrenology. Bumps and areas on the skull that phrenologists thought corresponded to human traits and characteristics.

> While the patient was interrogated the flat surface of a large
> spatula was lightly applied; on gentle pressure speech was sud-
> denly suspended; a word begun was cut in two. Speech returned
> as soon as pressure was removed. (p. 8)

This description provided the impetus for perhaps one of the
most eminent milestones in the history of brain and language. For
in the audience was the prominent French anatomist, physician,
and anthropologist, Paul Broca. This description of the role of the
frontal lobes in speech prompted him to be on the lookout for
further evidence on the location of speech and language in the
brain. The biography of this remarkable and versatile scholar has
been detailed by Schiller (1992), and in it one can appreciate
Broca's contribution to neuroscience.

In the translated words of Broca:

> On April 11, 1861, a fifty-one-year old man named LeBorgne
> suffering from a diffuse gangrenous inflammation of the entire
> buttocks, was admitted as a surgical patient to the general infir-
> mary of the Bicetre [hospital]. When I questioned him the next
> day about the onset of his illness his only response was the mon-
> osyllable, "Tan", repeated twice in succession, and accompa-
> nied by a movement of the left hand. (p. 9)

One week later LeBorgne died. Broca performed an autopsy
and the fresh brain specimen was shown to the Anthropological
Society of Paris a few hours after it was taken. With this classic case
study, Broca described the damage to be confined to the second
and third convolutions of the superior part of the left frontal lobe
and thereby implicated this region of the brain as the "seat of articulate language."

This area of the brain was subsequently labeled "Broca's
Area," and has been associated with the processes of speech and
language ever since. Kent illustrates and discusses the area in
Chapter 8. This confluence of interest and case study activity in the
middle and late 19th century marked an unprecedented period of
discovery about the brain and about neurogenic communication
disorders. Only the Great Wars (World War I and World War II)
with their tragic contributions of hundreds of brain-damaged sol-
diers would contribute more to our understanding of the effects of
brain damage on behavior. Today, we have built on these early
musings and have a much deeper appreciation of brain function
and its relation to the assorted varieties of speech, language, and
other disturbances that are invoked by brain damage. The causes of
brain damage are numerous.

✦ NEUROPATHOLOGY: DISEASE AND DAMAGE

Strokes, knife wounds, drive-by shootings, brain infections and abscesses, deadly microbes and viruses, shrapnel, AIDS/HIV, tumors, dashboard rebounds, bathtub tumbles, baseball bats, Harley-Davidson skids, Alzheimer's disease, chemical abuse, multiple sclerosis, lightning, chopstick penetration, hang-glider crashes, rock slides, foul balls, Huntington's disease, cerebral palsy, puff adder bites, drunken roof dives into shallow pools, carbon monoxide poisoning — all of these and dozens more can damage the nervous system.

Neuropathology is the study of the diseases and injuries that can affect the nervous system. The bad things that can happen to good people. While the brain enjoys a reasonable amount of protection, because it is encircled by the bony helmet of the skull and rests in the shock-absorber liquid of cerebrospinal fluid, it is certainly not impervious to insult. Brain disorders include over 650 different conditions — ranging from the small explosions of stroke or cerebrovascular accident (CVA) (bleeding or blockage of brain blood vessels), head or traumatic brain injury (physical damage to the brain or nervous system caused by laceration or bruising), to Alzheimer's disease (slow, degenerative damage to large areas of the brain), or Parkinson's disease (damage to select motor centers caused by neurochemical abnormality). Some of these disorders can be killers, such as brain tumors (out-of-control growth of cells) and multiple sclerosis (loss of myelin around nerves) or amyotrophic lateral sclerosis (Lou Gehrig's disease) (widespread, rapid deterioration of movement control).

Brain disorders are one of the leading categories of disease that cause death in the United States. Others are more subtle, and while they are not killers, they greatly change the quality of life that children and adults enjoy. Brain disorders do not respect social position, status, money, age, or gender. They strike priests, prime ministers, orange-pickers, telephone linemen, politicians, jockeys, clowns, proctologists, blues guitarists, babies, teenagers, and grandmothers. No one is safe from the devastation that can be created by brain damage and an estimated 50 million people in the United States are touched in some way by diseases of the nervous system. Approximately 1 out of every 70 people will have some form of diagnosed nervous system disease, but if such things as learning disabilities, sleep disorders, schizophrenia, alcoholism, and drug addiction are counted (and these conditions are intimately related to nervous system pathology) as many as 1 in 5 people are affected (*Scientific American,* 1992, p. BR3).

The toll of these brain disorders can never be fully measured in terms of the suffering of people afflicted and their families, but the economic cost is enormous. The National Foundation for Brain Research (NFBR) recently estimated the economic impact of brain disorders to be as much as $401.1 billion. This includes not only the direct charges of medicines, hospitalization, rehabilitation, and overall health care, but the indirect costs of lost wages, lost taxes, family caregiver expenditures, and other hidden societal expenses of the conditions (*Scientific American,* 1992, p. BR3).

Not all of these diseases and conditions affect the areas of the brain necessary for communication or cognition, but many do. In Chapter 8, the neurological bases of communication are presented lucidly. While it is obvious that damage could occur in parts of the brain that allow speech and thought to escape unscathed, there exist special regions and special systems that are vital to the functions necessary for these processes. Much of the cerebral cortex in both the left and right hemispheres is involved in language, memory, thought, attention, and speech movements.

The areas of the brain that appear to be involved frequently in language use include those areas of the left cerebral hemisphere nourished by the left middle cerebral artery. This *perisylvian area,* so-named because it is "around the Sylvian fissure," appears to be the crucial zone of aphasia, and damage within this region almost inevitably results in aphasia. The perisylvian area includes three smaller zones that have been associated with language loss, including areas first cited by Paul Broca in the frontal lobe (Broca's area); an area in the temporal lobe (Wernicke's area); and a region encompassing the borderlines of the parietal, temporal, and occipital lobes referred to as the **PTO cortex**. Figure 9–2 shows the zone of aphasia and the perisylvian area of the left cerebral hemisphere. Certainly, these are not the *only* areas involved in speech and language, but they appear to be primary.

Although over 650 conditions or diseases can damage the brain, by far the greatest contributor to neuropathology is cerebrovascular accident (CVA) or stroke. This condition remains the third leading killer in the United States, particularly of adults over 45. It is the result of interruption of the vital blood supply to the brain and can take the form of hemorrhage (excessive bleeding) or thromboembolic events (either stationary or moving blood clots). If the blood supply to the brain is interrupted for longer than about 4½ minutes, permanent damage may be caused and the brain cells (neurons) can suffer death (necrosis). The National Stroke Association (1991) has emphasized some key facts about stroke, as listed in Table 9–1.

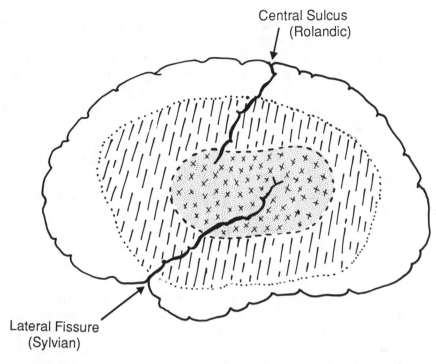

Figure 9-2. Areas of the left cerebral hemisphere important for language functions.

TABLE 9-1. The scope of stroke.

STROKE affects 500,000 Americans every year

STROKE is a major cause of death of American women, claiming more than 90,000 female lives a year

3 million U.S. STROKE survivors exist and nearly one-third are permanently disabled

About 72% of STROKES occur to persons over 65

STROKE results in need for nursing home care for about 180,000 older persons per year

STROKE is the second most common cause of dementia after Alzheimer's

Source: National Stroke Association. *Clinical Updates.* January, 1990 (p. 1).

Although stroke is the *leading* cause of brain damage (about 70% of all neuropathology), another significant type of neuropathology is brain injury, most frequently referred to as **traumatic brain injury (TBI)**. Some experts disagree on the exact label for this disorder and suggest that the "T" in TBI be dropped because "traumatic" sometimes confuses the issue by mixing the disorder in with emotional or psychiatric conditions. Traumatic brain injury seems to be the most frequently used term in the literature, however. It has been called the "Silent Epidemic," because not much public or even professional awareness has been stirred up over the hundreds and hundreds of cases of head and brain injury reported every year. Falls and vehicular accidents, especially automobile and motorcycle crashes, take their toll primarily on the younger population. TBI strikes the 15- to 24-year-old segment of the population especially, and the number of lives lost or devastated is enormous. From 30,000 to 50,000 young people in this age group suffer TBI every year to the extent that it prevents them from returning to their normal life style.

Dementia, too, is a significant type of brain disorder. It arises from many causes, not just Alzheimer's disease, and may affect the memory, thinking, language, and other cognitive functions of as much as 20% of the older population in the United States.

These are the sources of neuropathology. They are abundant, and they are formidable, and most of them can create the assortment of neurogenic communication disorders to which we will turn now. What must not be lost during the emphasis on diseases, damage, and havoc surrounding these disorders is the fact that they can be understood and treated, and in many cases the great reward of working with people with these conditions is that they can regain skills that have been lost, or they can find ways to compensate or adjust so that an acceptable quality of life can be enjoyed. The struggles can be arduous, but the rewards of rehabilitation can be equally intense. We turn now to the specific disorders.

◆ THE DISORDERS

Aphasia

Perhaps the most dramatic and certainly one of the most puzzling of all of the neurogenic communication disorders is **aphasia**. About 300 people become newly aphasic every day in the United States. Each will awaken, if he or she has been laid unconscious by the stroke or other cause, into a twisted-language Wonderland in which the words people are saying to them sound like a strange, unfamiliar mix of sound combinations that carry little meaning, almost as if they have been transported to a foreign language environment, where no one uses words that have meaning. During attempts to speak, the newly aphasic person will struggle to find correct words and put them in the right order.

As Betty, one of the first individuals with aphasia I evaluated, remarked after recovering and reflecting on her dawning experience with aphasia:

> I thought they had cut my tongue out. I had gone in for surgery on my wisdom teeth; they had put me under general anesthesia; and I developed a stroke during the surgical procedure. When I awoke and struggled to find words, I thought for sure I had lost my tongue. But it was far worse than that, as I was to find out. My tongue was fine but I couldn't come up with the right words or put them in the right order. And then when I tried to write or read, I had the same trouble. And it sounded like everyone was speaking a language I didn't know. Talk about terrifying!

Aphasia means "without language" or "loss of language." In some parts of the world people use the term *dysphasia.* Language purists insist that the term with the prefix *a-* (aphasia) means total loss of language, and to be more precise, the term *dys-* should be used (*dys*phasia), because it more accurately refers to partial loss of language. These distinctions have little clinical reality since even the most severely involved people have some residual language, and these days the term *aphasia* is commonly accepted in the literature and in the jargon of the professional communities to mean all gradients of language loss caused by brain damage. In fact, *aphasiology* is the term that is used increasingly to refer to the study and research of this disorder in all of its variants of severity and type.

The language functions that are affected in aphasia are related primarily to the use of word meaning and use of the *grammar* or rules of putting words together. To linguists, these processes traditionally are referred to as *lexical-semantic* and *syntactic.* The lexicon can be thought of as the little Golden Dictionary of about 50,000 words that we carry around in our heads at all times. We gain experience with language and layer and store new word meanings at an early age ("mama, doggy, nano, pee-pee") and continue to add to this seemingly ever-expanding semantic storehouse ("Fax, microchip, cyberpunk"). So *semantics* refers to the study of meanings; of words, thoughts, concepts, and their relationships to referents or things. **Lexical-semantic processes**, then, are those language processes that deal with storage and use of word meanings.

Syntax refers to the way in which words are arranged to show relationships of meaning within and between sentences. It relates to the rules of language use, and in fact the term comes from the Greek word *syntaxis,* for "arrangement."

Disturbances of lexical-semantic or of syntactic aspects of language can cross the modalities of language use, and therefore the aphasia that results might be apparent in reading, writing, speaking, or understanding. Related areas of symbol use such as arithmetic, telling time, counting money, producing and understanding gestures, or even appreciating auditory signals that have meaning (such as the siren of a fire truck), can be part of aphasic impairment as well as the more traditional types of communication. By far the most obvious signs and symptoms of aphasia are revealed in attempts at spoken language. What does aphasia sound like? The hallmark is variety and variability. Trying to characterize all of aphasia is a little like trying to answer the question, "What is an animal like?" The examples in Table 9–2 give a flavor to the variety of verbal behaviors characteristic of aphasia. These examples are representative, and taken from actual dialogues with individuals who were aphasic. Certainly, the possible examples of types of verbal impairment are as diverse as the number of speakers who are aphasic. It must be remembered that, while the broken verbal language of aphasia is the most apparent and well-known, much of aphasic impairment is somewhat veiled and not as obvious. The second major category of aphasic deficit is in auditory comprehension or understanding spoken speech. This has nothing to do with reduced hearing ability or problems in hearing acuity. The basic problem is in interpreting and making sense of the incoming spoken messages. Reading and writing also are frequently affected, and the same types of errors in word retrieval, substitution, and syntax heard in spoken aphasic speech are apparent in the reading and writing of people with aphasia.

In addition to the vast differences across individuals with aphasia (and within any given person over the course of time) in the qualitative aspects of the disorder, a wide range of severity can exist as well. Some of the most severely involved language users may be limited to a few unintelligible, relatively undifferentiated words or responses. On the other hand, many who suffer aphasia have a difficulty that is hardly noticeable on the standardized tests used to measure the disorder, but their language problems are confined to subtle, high-level linguistic processes, such as the ability to generate word synonyms or semantic alternatives with as much linguistic agility as they could before the cerebral insult. One former patient complained about how much difficulty he had with poetry writing, with organizing and giving classroom lectures, and with reading technical articles. These deficits were interpreted by him not to be "mild," but to be significant influences on the quality of his life, and he was desperately motivated to do all he could to improve his linguistic skill. The relative severity or "mildness" of aphasic impairment must indeed be compared to the value system and beliefs of the person experiencing the disorder. Severity level is

TABLE 9–2. Examples of aphasic verbal deficit.

Deficit Description	Example
Vocabulary reduction	"I can't think of the names of those things . . . let's see . . . uh . . . they're lost . . ."
Verbal paraphasia (use of nonintended words)	"I took the train . . . cab, no, bus. I took bus. Leave the damn driving to them."
Agrammatism (omission of function words, telegraphic speech)	"Drove store. Shop. Wife. Find Spam. Good. Have supper. Nap. Great cook."
Neologistic jargon (new words)	"Oh, that's a boy . . . a meoy. He's flinder. He's flample. Fall. Cookies. His peenchers. A hog . . . a hoss . . . a dog. A hayveness. Is that right?"
Recurrent, stereotypic utterances	"Boy, oh boy, oh boy, oh boy." "Anything else but . . . anything else but . . ." "Sumbitch. No. Sumbitch. No, no. Smitch . . . sumbitch. No. Oh, sumbitch."
Delay, abnormal silent time	"I'm . . . . nearly . . . . ready . . . . to . . . ."
Reduced output (decreased words per minute; decreased phrase length)	"By the time . . . I get a Kleenex . . . she'll be risin' . . . Me, too . . ."
Abnormal, hyperfluent output	"The works, words come in, I can't, come in but it won't seem to come right, hear it, hear o.k. right, with right coming to understand, but won't work words coming near right time to hear . . ."
Circumlocution	"It's a raft . . . graft . . . no, big, yellow, long-necked animal. Long necker. Spots. Skinny legs, eat from trees. I know it. Africa. Wobbly, long neck. Giraffe. That's it. That big sucker."
Morphosyntactic errors (number, tense, gender, possessives)	"He's of, on, on it. She's on 'er. She've was, were, weren't. He won't. He did."
Repetition impairment	Clinician: "Say Oh." Client: "I can't say that. I know. I don't happen to say it. No. On. Nope. No way . . ."

related to many differences across medical and behavioral variables of people with aphasia, but perhaps the most relevant are related to cause of the disorder and location and size of the brain lesion.

Types of Aphasia

The variability of aphasia is not so great that the study of the disorder is in chaos. Some patterns and rules and order have emerged over the years to present levels of understanding to the aphasiologist that, if not comforting, at least indicate trends of explanation as well as directions of remediation. One of these trends has been the observation that clusters of aphasic behaviors occur regularly enough to create syndromes or patterns of impairment. These types of aphasia will be discussed in the following section.

Aphasiologists have had a difficult time coming to agreement on classification and types of aphasia. Some experts feel that it is inappropriate to categorize aphasic characteristics into groups or syndromes. They feel that aphasia should be viewed and studied "without adjectives" that refer to specific type. One of the bits of evidence cited by those who choose a more holistic view of aphasia is that the aphasia test batteries that have been designed and used to attempt to categorize patients with aphasia into syndromes or groups are not always successful. In fact, about 15 to 40% of the aphasic patients tested cannot be classified unambiguously (Brookshire, 1992). Others have argued that the classical approaches to classifying aphasia do not sit well with what we have learned about normal cognitive processes. Others suggest that the emerging evidence from viewing neural activity during speech by functional brain imaging methods such as Positron Emission Tomography (PET) or Single Photon Emission Computed Tomography (SPECT) has shown much more widespread activation of brain areas during speech and language tasks than originally understood. (See Chapter 8 for illustrations.)

While the relationships between specific aphasic behaviors and the location of brain damage associated with them is less than perfect, there is no doubt about the predictability of certain more global speech/language functions and their association with regions of the brain. For example, areas of the temporal lobe (Wernicke's area) are undoubtedly related to auditory comprehension and the storage and retrieval of auditory word images and word meaning. This area also seems important for the knowledge and use of certain syntactic linguistic rules. Broca's area, in the frontal lobe, appears to be important for speech fluency (the rate, rhythm, and amount of verbal output), as well as in the use of certain "functor" words such as articles, conjunctions, and prepositions. Despite the drift in belief by many contemporary aphasiologists away from a strict "connectionist" or "localizationist" view of areas of the brain damage and associated syndromes of aphasia and the modification of the view of aphasia more toward a "Convergence Model" (see Kent's discussion in Chapter 8), many believe that there are enough regularities in the signs and symptoms of the disorder to permit predictions about location of brain damage in aphasia.

A lot of schemes of classification exist. This may be one of the most confusing aspects of studying this disorder. In fact, it was alleged that one instructor at the University of Florida Medical School warned his neurology students, "Read only *one* book on aphasia. If you read two you'll become too confused with the classification terms and labels."

Although this may be an exaggeration, it reflects a long-standing frustration with the literature on aphasia that is replete with inconsistency in the use of terms, labels, and systems of classification. At the very least, dividing aphasia types into **Nonfluent** and **Fluent** appears to be useful both for understanding and clinical usefulness (see Table 9–3). Further the Nonfluent and Fluent categories can be further subdivided into some of the more commonly used syndrome categories of aphasia. While evidence these days suggests that there may be both "cortical" and "subcortical" types of ahasia (depending on where the suspected or confirmed brain damage is located), for our purposes the most commonly agreed-on types of cortical aphasia are found in Table 9–3.

Although not all people with aphasia can be classified into these categories, many can, and the following speech/language attributes have been associated with each language type.

Nonfluent Aphasias

BROCA'S APHASIA. This syndrome is associated mostly with damage to the anterior or forward parts of the left cerebral hemisphere.

TABLE 9–3. Classification of aphasia syndromes or types.

Nonfluent Aphasia	Fluent Aphasia
Broca's Aphasia	Wernicke's Aphasia
Transcortical Motor Aphasia	Transcortical Sensory Aphasia
Global Aphasia	Anomic Aphasia
	Conduction Aphasia

Usually larger lesions, that include more than just the area traditionally known as Broca's area, are necessary to create the syndrome of characteristics called Broca's aphasia. In this condition, the most apparent components are agrammatism (telegraphic speech) and nonfluent speech production. Phrase length is short; naming ability and repetition ability (imitative speech) may range from mildly to severely impaired; and the agrammatism is depicted by reduced use of auxiliaries (e.g., *have, be, may, can, shall,* etc.), copulas (linking verbs), articles (e.g., *a, an, the*), prepositions (e.g., *in, by, with, for, to,* etc.), and inflectional and derivational endings (word ending changes that signal differences in tense, number, gender, etc.)

"Small words. Small words. Can't do small words. Large words fine. Small words no good" is a common expression of frustration by a person with Broca's aphasia. Usually auditory comprehension is relatively intact, although it is frequently not normal and careful testing can reveal deficits in understanding. Verbal output sounds slow, strained, and labored; and frequently phonological or articulation errors, along with attempts at revision and self-correction, are evident.

TRANSCORTICAL MOTOR APHASIA. The damage that creates this remarkable condition is often around the top and anterior border zones of the perisylvian region, although some have suggested that the damage may be deep below the brain surface in these frontal regions. Nonfluent, severely impaired spontaneous speech is characteristic of this type. But an unexpected finding tips off the transcortical aphasias. Despite meager attempts at conversation or discourse and very nonfluent, impaired production when speech is produced, the hallmark of this condition is "remarkably well preserved repetition ability." It is surprising to evaluate a person with very nonfluent, impaired ability to initiate and maintain conversation, and then find that he or she can repeat words, phrases, and even sentences, sometimes flawlessly. Naming is usually superior to spontaneous attempts at speech and auditory comprehension is only mildly to moderately impaired. A typical dialogue might be:

Clinician:	Tell me about your problems with speech.
Client:	. . . (long pause) . . . Stroke. Talk. Arm, leg bad.
Clinician:	Try to say these things after me. Cup.
Client:	Cup.
Clinician:	Cup of coffee.
Client:	Cup of coffee.
Clinician:	Sandwich.
Client:	Sandwich.

Clinician:	I'd like a turkey sandwich and a cup of coffee.
Client:	I'd like a turkey sandwich and a cup of coffee.
Clincian:	Wow. You really do a good job repeating things.
Client:	. . . . (long pause). . . No good alone. Talk. Now, hungry.

GLOBAL APHASIA. As the name implies, the condition of global aphasia may reflect a level of severity rather than a distinctive quality of disturbance. Profoundly impaired language abilities across all of the modalities of speaking, understanding, reading, and writing are apparent. Oral expression is very nonfluent and may be limited to just a few words, emotional utterances, or a little bit of verbal ability on serial or overlearned utterances (i.e., *"NO." "Oh boy." "one, two, three . . ."*). Repetition and imitative speech as well as naming ability are severely impaired. Auditory comprehension is very limited, usually correct only for single words or short phrases that are surrounded by contextual clues to understanding. Reading and writing are usually just as impaired as speech and understanding. The lesion is usually large and deep, and may cover the entire perisylvian region. Two separate cortical lesions, one anterior and one posterior, create global aphasia. Sometimes a global aphasic syndrome can be created by a relatively small, but critically placed lesion in the subcortical, deep brain regions. This has been called *"global capsular/putaminal aphasia"* after the deep brain structures that may be damaged (Helm-Estabrooks & Albert, 1991).

Fluent Aphasias

The fluent aphasia syndromes are many times the most startling, dramatic, and unusual types since they are seasoned with much word substitution, neologistic jargon (*"fracker . . ." "trabnoll" "fireman's hafner, helmet"*), and copious, verbose verbal output. The primary fluent syndromes are:

WERNICKE'S APHASIA. Very fluent, often hyperfluent, speech and impaired auditory comprehension are hallmarks of this type. Speech is often peppered with verbal paraphasias (use of nonintended words). Word substitutions may or may not be semantically related to the intended word (*"I rode on a horse, a hearse, a bus, I mean a bus."*), or may be neologistic jargon. The jargon may be truly neologistic (new word) or may be strings of genuine English words that are inappropriate or out-of-context (*"A knife, a spoofolt, and a fork . . . a settin' forth." "Perhaps there was a possibility that they would* *reach or have been asked or gotten to level the degree of yes, no, or maybe." "Whew, my hands. They just got jummed up and they lump on the 'leventh or the seventh.")*

Conversational speech is marked by what some have called "press of speech," that hyperfluent, rapid expulsion of strings of sentences with hardly a pause or an acknowledgment that conversation requires turn-taking by both speaker and listener. This monologue type of discourse production has led some to suggest that fluent aphasic speakers may well have a disturbance in **pragmatics**, or the rules that govern and regulate language use, especially in conversational discourse. Auditory comprehension may be disturbed, not only evidenced by special tests of understanding, but also by the apparent lack of self-monitoring or error-awareness during speech production. Naming may be mildly or severely affected, as may be repetition or imitative speech. For the most part, the damage in Wernicke's aphasia is in the posterior or back parts of the left cerebral hemisphere, around the auditory association areas in the temporal lobe.

TRANSCORTICAL SENSORY APHASIA. This is the fluent counterpart of transcortical motor aphasia. Again, the hallmark of this transcortical aphasia is remarkably preserved ability to repeat or imitate words. Conversation and spontaneous speech are fluent, somewhat like that of the speech in Wernicke's aphasia, but are full of paraphasias or word substitutions and lacking in nouns. In fact, naming is usually severely to moderately impaired. Auditory comprehension is impaired, usually much more profoundly than in transcortical motor aphasia, but the cardinal characteristic remains the intact ability to parrot or repeat words, phrases, and sentences. The damage that creates transcortical sensory aphasia may be around the edges of the posterior portions of the perisylvian area, especially around the PTO cortex.

CONDUCTION APHASIA. This is another type of fluent aphasia. Conversation is abundant and fluent. Phrase length, syntax, and prosody of language is good. Naming deficits may be present and range from mild to severe. Auditory comprehension is impaired, but in some cases may be only mildly impaired. The hallmark of this type of aphasia is in repetition or imitative speech performance. Repetition is extremely poor, and some have suggested that selective deficit in repetition is the distinguishing feature of conduction aphasia (Goodglass, 1980). One area of damage that has been implicated in conduction aphasia is the arcuate fasciculus, a band of fibers just below the cortical surface that connects Wernicke's and Broca's areas. (See Kent, Chapter 8, for an illustration of the arcuate fasciculus.)

ANOMIC APHASIA. Anomia, characterized by misnaming and word retrieval problems, is an aphasic feature that is scattered across all types of the disorder, and has been called the most ubiquitous characteristic of aphasia. Anomic aphasia, on the other hand, as a type of aphasia as opposed to a feature of all aphasias, has received a mixed reception. Some experts feel it is rare, some believe it is most common. Those who accept it as a separate type of aphasia suggest that spontaneous speech is fluent, auditory comprehension and repetition are only moderately to mildly involved, but that a specific disturbance in using labels and names of objects, pictures, and other referents is the prime feature of the disorder. Pictures cannot be named, or they are misnamed with either semantically related or unrelated responses (*"Yes. That has four legs, a tail that wags, and is woman's best friend. It's a ... frog. No. A cow. Wait a minute. Did I say cow? A seeing-eye cow? Jeez. No ... a ... a ... you know, I have one at home. Mickey. No, Skippy. A ... dog. Dog. That's it. Jeez. I couldn't fetch that word up"*).

While damage to many locations within the "zone of aphasia" in the perisylvian region can result in word retrieval and naming problems, the areas specifically around the **PTO cortex** seem to be important for these processes.

OTHER TYPES. While the aphasia types listed above seem to constitute the most frequently seen categories, atypical or "pure" aphasias are reported occasionally in clinical reports or in the aphasia literature. There is some question as to whether or not these atypical patterns should be classified as aphasia syndromes. Some of these are conditions that affect reading primarily, with or without concomitant writing impairment. These atypical syndromes include **Alexia without Agraphia** (reading impairment with no accompanying writing disorder); **Alexia with Agraphia** (reading and writing impairment without significant deficit in oral expression or auditory comprehension); **Pure Word Deafness** (totally absent auditory comprehension with error-free spontaneous speech, naming, reading, and writing); **Pure Agraphia** (severe writing disorders with other aspects of language usage intact); and **Crossed Aphasia** (aphasia in right-handed individuals who have suffered right hemisphere damage).

The tempest of controversy over aphasia classification and aphasia types, no doubt, will roll on for years to come; as with all scholarly or clinical debate, the elements of compromise and acceptance of some features of both positions is often the most prudent course. Some of the storm has weakened to occasional gusts of wind these days, and even some of the most staunch champions of aphasia syndromes have had the insight and courage to revise and soften their earlier views on the matter. More and more, it appears that the vast majority of individuals with aphasia who are seen and treated in clinics and hospitals present a mixture and variety of aphasic communication disorders that include disruption across all or most of the language modalities and are intertwined in nearly double-helix fashion with deficits in such cognitive processes as working memory, attention, resource allocation, and information processing. This does not negate the existence or the clinical and theoretic importance of predominant aphasia types or syndromes. It only suggests that clinicians may expect to see mostly a mixed bag of aphasia; but regularly some unique hybrids or peculiar variants will happen along. Good clinicians learn early in their careers that, if unambiguous classification or typing does not seem possible, careful observation and operationally based description of specific aspects of communication impairment and intactness not only will aid understanding of the nature of the disorder but also can serve as a springboard for enlightened clinical intervention.

Right Hemisphere Syndrome

Right hemisphere syndrome or **right hemisphere impairment (RHI)** refers to a group of performance deficits that are the result of damage to the "nondominant" (usually right) hemisphere of the cortex of the brain. A profuse collection of sensory, perceptual, linguistic, and other unusual and sometimes strange behaviors can result from right hemisphere damage. Many of these deficits are readily or subtly apparent during communication or during attempts to interact with others. The role of the right hemisphere in communication is appreciated far more today than in earlier times. It will become increasingly apparent that the right hemisphere is no longer regarded as the poor second cousin of the left, as a "minor" hemisphere or a sort of spare tire, nice to have around in case the left hemisphere blows out. Significant behavioral change can emanate from diseases and lesions to the right hemisphere, and as the experts have become increasingly sophisticated at observation and testing, the catalog of these disorders has thickened.

Very little information exists about the incidence or prevalence of right hemisphere impairment, and even less is known about the relative distribution of behavior deficits created by RHI. Some data suggest that among stroke patients counted in a national study over

3 years about half (51%) were found to have left side of the body (right hemisphere) involvement. With about 500,000 people each year having a new stroke in the United States, this means slightly more than 250,000 people per year will have right hemisphere damage (Granger, 1990). Although this gives us at least a glimmer of an idea of how many people suffer right hemisphere damage from stroke, it says nothing about all of the other causes of brain damage that exist. Tumors, diseases, accidents, and the wicked salad bar of other etiologies also contribute their strife and compromise the right hemisphere.

SIGNS AND SYMPTOMS. Disturbances that result in RHI are not as obvious as those from the left himisphere.

As Russell, a person with RHI, described it:

> It's weird. I *cannot* read a road map. I used to drive a truck, and I was good at maps and things. In fact I won a merit badge in the Boy Scouts for it, and I even played around in Orienteering . . . you know, that competitive sport that started in Sweden where you test your skill of finding checkpoints with just a compass and a topographical map. Man, I could no more Orienteer now than I could put toothpaste back in the tube. I couldn't even find my way home. I get lost around the park across the street from my house. My reading is a little messed up, too. Maybe it's my eyes. 'Cause they told me I had neglect or something, and I didn't notice the food on the left side of my hospital tray. Also, I can't play Chess worth a Tinker's damn anymore. I can't seem to figure out the moves or strategies. When I do get a few moves in, I play like a man with a paper head. I guess Chess is out. I used to play like a Russian. Now I play like a cushion. And there's something wrong with my earholes, too. Especially in long conversations. Seems like I can't . . . Sheez, . . . follow everything. I just lose track of the gist or the main idea during long discussions. Maybe I just don't pay attention. Seems like I drift. My wife tells me that I seem kind of flat. Like I'm kinda just inside lookin' out and observing everything, but not really getting involved in things. I used to be pretty emotional. I'd argue or let out a thigh-slappin' laugh at the drop of a hat. Now, nothing seems very funny. I really am flat. Except the other day one of those real heavy nurses slipped on a piece of lettuce in the canteen and fell on her butt, and I cracked up. Now that was funny. What the hell is goin' on with me anyway? Is this all due to that stroke in the right side of my brain? It's spooky, isn't it? Can you help me with any of this?

The strange variety of perceptions and behaviors described by Russell capture many, but not all, in the constellation of altered behaviors in RHI. Since 1980 much more clinical and research attention has been directed to RHI and the picture is beginning to come into clearer focus. Myers (1983) has suggested that the most frequently seen or reported deficits in RHI include:

1. Neglect of left half of space

2. Denial of illness or of limb involvement.

3. Impaired judgment and self-monitoring

4. Reduced motivation

Further, classification of RHI, along with specific examples in each category can be appreciated from Table 9–4.

Disturbances of RHI are often very subtle, but nevertheless they can have a profound effect on the quality of life. It takes some real detective work and ingenious assessment to uncover these disturbances. One intriguing, if rare, complication of RHI is called "Capgras Syndrome," in which the person with right hemisphere damage not only fails to recognize the faces of his friends and family, but is convinced that some of these people may be "doubles" or impostors (Bienemann, 1989).

Certainly one of the most apparent effects of the so-called "inference" failure of RHI is the tendency for people with this disorder to fail to go beyond the face value of a communicative message. This leads to a literal interpretation or meaning and affects such subtle aspects of language as *metaphor, humor, idioms, indirect requests,* and *aspects of discourse of general conversation.*

Thus, a person with RHI might err in the interpretation of such bits of language as:

"What does it mean when I say, 'They were just sitting around shooting the bull?' "

"I don't know. A bunch of ranchers or hunters killed a bull with a rifle?"

"If you saw smoke coming out of the upstairs window and a fire truck came roaring up and stopped outside your neighbor's house on Bayview Drive, what do you think would be going on?"

"How should I know? I just saw the truck pull up. They didn't tell me. I don't know what's happening."

TABLE 9-4. Right hemisphere impairment.

Visual-spatial Deficits
 Visual discrimination and integration
 Impaired facial recognition ("prosopagnosia")
 Geographic, topographic confusion
 Poor scanning and tracking
 Visual-constructive deficits ("constructional apraxia")

Affect and Prosody
 Apathy; indifference
 Impaired sensitivity to emotional tone
 Impaired comprehension, production of emotional language

Linguistic Deficits
 Poor word discrimination
 Poor auditory understanding of long, complex material
 Reduced verbal fluency for categories
 Impaired visual word recognition
 Poor word-picture matching
 Poor body part identification
 Poor reading comprehension for paragraphs

Higher Order Communication Deficits
 Poor ability to organize information meaningfully, efficiently
 Production of impulsive, tangential, unnecessary details
 Poor judgment of what is important and what is not
 Overpersonalization
 Literal interpretation of figurative language
 Poor use of contextual cues
 Poor sensitivity to pragmatic, paralinguistic, or body language cues
   in communication

"What does it mean when I say 'It's raining cats and dogs,' or, 'Go jump in the lake?' "

"You better have a strong umbrella." "I don't feel like swimming."

These and other figures of speech and subtleties of language are lost or impaired to the person with RHI. Because humor is so dependent on unexpected twists or incongruities and on double meanings, the person with RHI has a great deal of trouble with certain aspects of humor, especially with puns or other punch lines that are dependent on delicate differences of meanings. On the other hand, it is frequently reported that a characteristic of RHI is "gallows humor" or a heightened jocularity at situations depicting injury or the misfortunes of others. So elements of classical slapstick humor, such as tumbling down stairs, slipping on a banana peel, skidding off a roof, and all of the other typical Three Stooges maneuvers of eye-gouging, nose-twisting, and baseball bat clubbing seem to tickle the person with RHI disproportionately to other types of humor.

As with all of the conditions described in this chapter, the damage that creates the communicative and cognitive impairments also can create a variety of other physical and psychosocial problems. The most common related physical condition is weakness or paralysis of the arm or leg on one side of the body. This **hemiparesis** (one-sided weakness) or **hemiplegia** (one-sided paralysis) can prevent the person with RHI from walking or using the affected arm. **Hemisensory impairment** is another accompanying condition. This is a one-sided loss of the ability to perceive or feel things. Common complaints include numbness, or tingling sensations, or the reduced ability to feel pain, touch, vibration, or even hot and cold. Sometimes loss of sensation or movement in the face and mouth region affects ability to chew or swallow, and this may be accompanied by drooling, taste alteration, or droopy facial appearance. If the brain damage is widespread or deep, or affects crucial deep brain structures, such basic functions as bowel or bladder control can be altered.

Another physical or medical condition that may be a part of the brain damage is a seizure disorder, or epilepsy. This is a factor in about 20% of strokes or CVAs, and it occurs often enough to suggest that clinicians who deal with brain-damaged individuals should be aware of the possibility of seizures. In most cases the seizure disorder is well controlled by medication.

The psychosocial disturbances that accompany RHI are abundant. Alterations in mood, including apathy, indifference, and denial appear more frequently with RHI than many other disorders. Families report changed personality, and the distinctive alterations in cognitive, perceptual, and emotional functions, along with poorer self-evaluative capabilities, altered discrimination of emotional aspects of facial expression, and an inability to tune-in to the gist of things, contribute to the common perception that "this is not the same person." Mood disorders, especially depression, also may be a part of the symptom complex of RHI, although some experts report that it is more common in left than in right hemisphere lesions. Many of these physical and psychosocial concomitants are not unique to RHI but can accompany damage to either hemisphere and are frequently seen in aphasia as well.

All of these differences and unique alterations in communication and behavior are part of the RHI package surely suggest that this hemisphere can no longer be regarded as "minor" or as just a spare. Increasingly, speech-language pathologists are being called on to deal with people who have these exotic and debilitating behaviors, and the more both professionals and the general public are informed about these conditions, the more likely it will be that RHI will be clinically managed instead of ignored.

Traumatic Brain Injury

As indicated earlier, **traumatic brain injury (TBI),** sometimes referred to as just "brain injury," is known as the "silent epidemic." Considering its impact on the society, it is amazing that the disorder is characterized as "silent." But it is ill recognized by both the public and by professionals. In the United States, about once every 16 seconds someone suffers a head injury and incurs a TBI. (In the literature, "traumatic brain injury" [TBI] is increasingly used as the term of choice, but the labels "head injury" and "closed head injury" [CHI], are used quite frequently. Recently, some have suggested dropping the qualifier "traumatic" and simply referring to the disorder as "brain injury." Time and usage will clarify the evolution of the label.) About 400,000 new cases are admitted to hospitals in the U.S. each year with this condition. Although many of these people recover, and just undergo the effects of concussion or "post-concussive syndrome," from 30,000 to 50,000 sustain a head injury so severe that they can never return to a normal life style.

Most of these injuries occur in the teenage and early adulthood years, from ages 15 to 24; but the pediatric population from birth to 5 is another segment of the population susceptible to head injury. What causes these substantial numbers of injuries? Mostly, the proliferation in the use of motor vehicles has resulted in steadily increasing rates of head injury from vehicular accidents. Cars and trucks are the principle culprits (or rather the drivers or circumstances that create the accident), but increasingly motorcycles and off-road vehicles are implicated in head injury. For the infant-toddler age group, and for the elderly, falls, especially around the home, are the leading causes. With pediatric TBI, another significant cause is child abuse, particularly violent shaking of an infant or toddler. Among adolescents and adults, homicide attempts and firearm accidents are a soaring factor in head injury, especially in economically depressed neighborhoods of metropolitan areas. Guns, cars, motorcycles, and young adults equal increasing numbers of traumatic brain injuries. Other causes include the many ways other than by motor vehicular accidents, falls, or shootings that the head can be struck, crushed, or accidentally traumatized. Males comprise as much as 70% of the persons hospitalized with the diagnosis of traumatic brain injury. For some reason, and that reason is probably linked to the well-documented risk-taking and aggressive behavior of males, traumatic brain injury remains predominantly a masculine phenomenon. Although the demographics and the numbers of traumatic brain injury are impressive and shocking, they do not even begin to capture the amount of human suffering involved.

I was alone in a freakish one-vehicle automobile accident. It happened at about 2:25 a.m., not too long after my girlfriend's high school semi-formal dance. The newspaper articles all said how I jumped the median and went down a highway's wrong lanes for a distance. I went up an embankment and slid sideways, slamming into a tree with the full impact on the driver's door. I had four bruised ribs, a collapsed left lung, and a severe concussion that left me comatose for thirteen days. I was on thirteen life-support systems . . . Once my blood pressure and other vital signs started showing them that I was going to pull through after all, they advised my family to expect not much more than "a vegetable." . . . in the middle of May, the memory of the night that changed my entire life finally came back. I had a car crash because I was driving drunk. I had learned how to barely walk with a walker, and I got discharged on May 28th. . . . At Heinz I had Psychological Services, Cognitive Therapy, and Social Skills Therapy, plus Speech, Occupational and Physical Therapy. I feel committed and obligated to preventing EVERYONE from driving under the influence. Please don't take a chance. . . Appreciate life, and remember that I am part of your world and you're part of mine.

(Richards, 1991, p. 8)

The day is lawn-mowing, hiking, bar-b-que, and fireworks. Walking back to the car, I opt for a short-cut that my niece and nephew decline. Dark and steep, the slope reminds me of skiing. I lean forward and reach for the overhead branches. But the terrain is surprising — grasses instead of tundra. As my feet slip out from under me, my hip and shoulder strike a concrete piling, invisible in the dark, tall grasses. In slow motion, my head snaps back onto a steel spike set in the concrete. The world goes black. My life changes forever.

> . . . (Now) I look fine on the outside. Tan, rested, working, playing. People expect I am my old self. And I try to be. But I'm not the same. I don't have a scar or cast to show the damage. But there is physical damage that I and the doctors are unaware of. And I am working hard to overcome the emotional damage. I don't know it yet, but the next three years will prove just as challenging as the first eight months. I will continue to struggle and grow. And I will survive.   *(Bauer, 1992, p. 10)*

As can be appreciated from the true stories above, the events surrounding traumatic brain injury can be life-twisting. And because the areas of brain damage can be widespread and involve many regions, the signs and symptoms of TBI can be profound. The damage from strokes and some types of trauma are frequently focal and pick off only selected areas, but the damage from a serious fall or vehicular accident can be diffuse and related to rotational and twisting forces of the brain slamming against the inside of the skull. Not only is damage related to the sites of direct impact, but a *contre coup* area of damage is not unusual to the areas of the brain directly opposite the point of direct impact. Also, certain bony prominences inside the skull contribute to shearing and lacerating forces that particularly affect the underside of the brain.

CHARACTERISTICS AND DEFICITS. Generally the results of traumatic brain damage are grouped into the focal lesion effects that create speech, voice, language, or swallowing disturbances and the disruptions of cognitive processes of memory, attention, information processing, and higher level disruptions of problem-solving or reasoning caused by more diffuse damage. In addition, it is not uncommon to see a variety of behavioral deficits in TBI that include impulsivity, lack of social judgment, poor insight, planning, and organization (sometimes called disruptions in "executive function"), and occasionally aggressiveness or combativeness. Personality changes and psychosocial problems are legion with serious TBI and a perusal of the literature reveals many such changes. Table 9–5 lists some of these changes that have been reported in studies of brain injury.

Physical problems frequent with TBI include problems walking and with use of the arms and hands, and changes in vision or hearing. Two hallmarks of TBI that have been used in attempts to classify severity or type of TBI are **altered levels of consciousness** and **post-traumatic amnesia (PTA)**. The most common type of al-

TABLE 9–5. Personality and emotional changes reported after brain injury.

Agitation
Aggressiveness
Increased Anger
Anxiety
Apathy
Changed Affect
Denial of Illness
Depression
Changed Self-Awareness
Disinhibition
Facetiousness
Helplessness
Impatience
Impulsivity
Indifference
Emotional Lability (crying or laughing)
Phobias
Changed Sexual Interest (increased or decreased)
Socially Inappropriate Comments
Suspiciousness
Withdrawal

Source: From M. D. Lezak and K. P. O'Brien, Chronic emotional, social, and physical changes after brain injury. In E. D. Bigler, *Tramatic brain injury* (pp. 365–380), 1990. Austin, TX: Pro-Ed.

tered consciousness is *coma,* the state of deep or prolonged unconsciousness. However, altered consciousness does not always mean deep sleep or total unresponsiveness, and in fact milder levels of altered consciousness include states of stupor or lethargy. Not all people who suffer TBI lapse into a coma, and many never lose consciousness; but coma is a familiar accompaniment to head injury.

The *Glasgow Coma Scale (GCS)* is a measure developed in the 1970s to rate states of wakefulness or consciousness (Teasdale & Jennett, 1974). With this scale the examiner rates the stimulation required to induce eye opening, motor responses, and verbal responses. A numeric scale is used with a score of 3 (on a 15-point scale) indicating the deepest level of coma with no eye opening to any stimulation, including pain, no movement, and no verbal utterances. Scores on the *Glasgow Coma Scale* at the time of hospital admission are a reliable and fairly accurate prediction of the level and degree of severity of the brain damage as well as the prognosis or prediction for recovery.

Post-traumatic amnesia (PTA) also has been used as a predictor of severity of TBI. Memory loss, or amnesia, is a common result of brain injury, and people with head injury have difficulty retaining new information and laying down new memories as well as remembering the events surrounding the trauma. The length of PTA has been used to predict severity and eventual outcome, although these predictions are not always perfect.

COMMUNICATION DEFICITS. The nature of the impairment in communication that accompanies TBI has been discussed and dissected for years. Many feel that some of the same reading, writing, talking, and understanding problems seen in aphasia are part of the disorder. Others emphasize the interwoven aspects of speech, language, and deficient cognitive processes. Evaluation and treatment surely must consider all of these factors. People with TBI have been said to "talk better than they communicate" (Holland, 1982). Certainly the tests usually given to assess the communication of people with aphasia do not capture all of the problems of TBI communication, and lately many have suggested that the rambling ineffective communication of the person with TBI is due to disturbances in **pragmatics** or language discourse and use. Communication deficits revealed by looking at aspects of language pragmatics include such things as poor affect or emotional language, poor topic selection, poor topic maintenance, and poor turn-taking during conversations. Some of the rambling nature of TBI communication may be due to difficulty with such subtle aspects of conversational discourse as *cohesive ties* and *coherence,* those processes by which aspects of narratives and conversations are melded together. Neuromotor speech disorders, which will be discussed in a following section, as well as muscle or nerve impairment that alters moving the mouth, chewing, and swallowing, also may be part of the picture.

Dementia

One of the myths and stereotypes surrounding the aging process is that if we live long enough all of us will lose our intellectual edge; we will become intellectually slower and the joys and gifts of youth will be eroded. This contribution to the stereotypes of aging and indeed to another rampant "-ism" in our society ("ageism" joins racism, sexism, and a host of other distorted societal perceptions about groups of people) is perpetrated by the thousands of advertising, commercial, and media messages that inundate us every day with the idea that "youth is good/old is bad." We are cajoled to invest in products and services, including major surgical alteration of offending body parts, that camouflage, cover, hide, recolor, blot out, disguise, conceal, darken, veil, or in other ways obliterate the signs of the natural aging process. This is a stark revelation of societal values. Not all societies fall into this trap. Some revere the wisdom and experience of the elderly. Certain indigenous peoples in North and South America and several Asian societies and other world subcultures hold "old" as precious. Accumulated wisdom is called upon and revered; and the visible signs of aging are badges of accomplishment. Perhaps with a growing realization of the inevitability of the process and with the increasing numbers of people who enter the cohort of the elderly, the destructive nature of these societal values will change.

Although intellectual decline is not an inevitable part of aging, there is no denying that certain physiological and behavioral changes occur. Hearing, vision, and certain motor skills (the ability to hit a curve ball is affected fairly early) are skills and processes that change with age. Another truism is that certain medical conditions and syndromes are more likely to be present in the elderly. The occurrence of cancer, stroke, and other pathologies of the body are age-related. **Dementia**, too, is a condition associated with aging. Dementia is an acquired syndrome characterized by persistent intellectual decline which is due to neurogenic causes. The most common sign associated with dementia is impairment in memory. This may or may not be accompanied by certain changes in reasoning or judgment, disturbed cognitive processes of attention, or changes in personality. Problems of communication can be associated with dementia also, and only in the past few decades have clinicians and researchers begun to sort these out.

Dementia springs from many causes, but it is important to understand that diseases, conditions, and abnormal changes in the nervous system create dementia, and it is not merely a by-product of the natural aging process. The nature and eventuality of the dementia depend on the cause; and although most are progressive and foretell a slow decline, some are static. Another group of the dementias mercifully are treatable, and as many as 10 or 20% have been reported as the result of reversible causes (Shekim, 1990). Contrary to the widely held myth that nearly everyone over 65 has some form of dementia, studies have found that only 1 to 15% of the elderly have a true dementia. Diseases, infections, or strokes are the most frequent causes with the most common cause being Alzheimer's disease, sometimes referred to as dementia of the Alzheimer's type (DAT). Alzheimer's disease accounts for over 50% of all those with dementia, and vascular problems related to a series of strokes (called multi-infarct dementia) are the cause of another 20%. Other conditions include varieties of exotic diseases usually named after the physician or researcher who first described it such as Pick's disease, Parkinson's disease, or Creutzfeldt-Jacob disease. Another cause is Huntington's disease, the genetic degenerative combination of dementia and movement disorder that claimed the great American song-writer/poet, activist, and balladeer, Woody Guthrie:

> This land is your land . . . This land is my land . . . From California . . . to the New York Island;

> The crops are all in and the peaches are rotting . . . The oranges are piled in their creosote dumps . . . ;

> Your waters have turned . . . the darkness to dawn . . . so roll on, Columbia, roll on . . . ;

and over 1000 more.

These days, much research effort is being expended on finding out more about dementia, particularly Alzheimer's disease, and the underlying culprit that creates the problem has been hypothesized to be due to genetic causes, aluminum and other intoxications, and viral infections. Time will sort out the real transgressors, and no doubt the blame will be laid on a gang of causes rather than a singular explanation.

STAGES OF DEMENTIA. Some writers have characterized distinctive stages of the progression of the disorder. Mostly these stages are temporal from time of diagnosis, such as "early," "middle," and "late" dementia. Behaviors characteristic of these stages range from moderate cognitive and mental decline such as disorientation in the early stage (Question: *What year is it?* Answer: *1939. The year of Gone with the Wind and the pregnancy of Mickey Mouse.* Question: *Where are you right now?* Answer: *Government substation number 2. Or the Lake Panasoffkee dump.*) to the severe cognitive and communication decline of late dementia where the individual may be perseverative, echolalic, or virtually mute.

COMMUNICATION AND DEMENTIA. The precise nature of the communication deficit in dementia is not crystal clear, though more agreement is emerging as continued study results accumulate. The semantic system of the language such as naming and word retrieval seems much more vulnerable to the dementing process than does the speech sound system or the grammatical rules of language. The classic features of language breakdown are anomia (*"Bike, no, trike, no, car. Car."*); reduced efficiency in verbal formulation (*"I ah . . . ah . . . I had toast. Toast or bagel. Bagel. And some . . . ah . . . some oat meal . . . some oat meal. I mean oat bran. Lot's of oat bran. Maybe a* *little too much... Excuse me a minute."*); or circumlocution (*"We went to the... ah... the place where the seats rock and you eat the popcorn... the movie place... the movie... the screen house... the little projector guy place... you know... the movie house."*).

Discourse or connected speech can reveal many of these communication deficits, and they are amplified by the disjointed nature of conversation when memory loss increases. Conversations lack cohesion, do not seem to be tied together, and may be filled with incomplete phrases, phrase repetitions, stereotypic sayings (*"Don't ya jist know. Don't ya jist know."*); irrelevant intrusions (*"So we went to the bank and made out a withdrawal... Sic 'em Spotty, bit the hell out of all of 'em. We withdrew some money and bought the Jacuzzi."*); and an increase in jargon or nonsense words (Shekim & LaPointe, 1984).

Evaluation of the communication deficits of dementia has been accomplished by the administration of a variety of standarized batteries traditionally used to evaluate aphasia. Recently, the publication of the *Arizona Battery for Communicative Disorders in Dementia* has addressed the specific receptive, expressive, orientation, and memory deficits seen in the disorder (Bayles & Kazniak, 1987). An array of language and communication assessment measures for use with individuals with dementia is suggested in a chapter on language and communication in dementia by Ripich (1991). In addition to recommended measures for language comprehension, semantics, syntax, and phonology, several approaches are given for appraisal of pragmatics and discourse (such as evaluating turn-taking, topic management, conversational repair, and paralinguistic features).

Dementia is a disorder that can easily overwhelm caregivers, family, and friends. The progression and decline in irreversible dementia is as inevitable as the passage of time, and it is easy to understand that some would feel little can be done about this downhill march. But creative health care providers and clinicians have suggested ways of stemming the tide or even improving communication so that acceptable quality of life can be sustained. The focus of treatment comes from many professionals, and may well be on the people and environment surrounding the person with dementia. Adjusting environmental factors such as talking about the present, reducing sources of conflict and distraction, cutting down the number of conversational participants, as well as adjusting complexity, rate of speech, and using both written and verbal instructions can enhance the probability of communication success (Shekim, 1990).

Trying to maintain viable communication and the merit of life in the face of dementia is not easy. These are some of the most challenging and frustrating experiences for everyone involved. But we are well past the societal attitude where people with these disorders are warehoused or abandoned. The increase in basic and clinical research, along with the patience and devotion of families and creative clinicians, will unfold new and effective ways of making the communicative lives of these individuals not only tolerable but positive. These are the challenges that will tax and reward all of us who choose to face them.

Neuromotor Speech Disorders

Motor means movement. It does not refer to the popular conception of what is under the hood of a Honda. Medical dictionaries define *motor* as "moving or causing movement." It applies to a nerve or a group of nerve cells through which, or from which, impulses travel that excite activity. Neuromotor speech disorders are disturbances of movement of the speech production system that result in someone being imperfectly understood or creating the impression that something is unusual or bizarre about his or her speech pattern. The two major types of neuromotor speech disorders are the **dysarthrias** and **apraxia of speech**. In the neuromotor speech disorders, so long as they do not co-exist with language or cognitive impairment, the linguistic processes involved in the use of semantics and the use of syntax are not affected. Usually, the most apparent results are in clear and precise production of speech segments (sounds) and suprasegments (rate, stress, intonation).

All of the same neuropathologies that can cause the other neurogenic communication disorders also can create neuromotor impairment, although the damage must be at selected levels or sites of the nervous system that are involved in speech movement. That means that strokes, diseases, accidents, poisons, and other bandits that rob neural integrity also can affect speech movement, if they strike the right locations.

A few astute specialists in speech production have suggested that the motor speech system can be conceptualized on a simple basis by viewing it as a system comprised of a couple of bags of air that produce energy (the lungs and respiratory system) and a series of valves that act on that air stream. At the level of the larynx and vocal folds, phonation or voice may or may not be added; at the level of the velopharyngeal port (the valve comprised of the velum and the posterior pharyngeal wall), resonance options can be selected; and other valving choices can be exercised by tongue, lips, and jaw movements. Figure 9–3 depicts these levels of the speech production system.

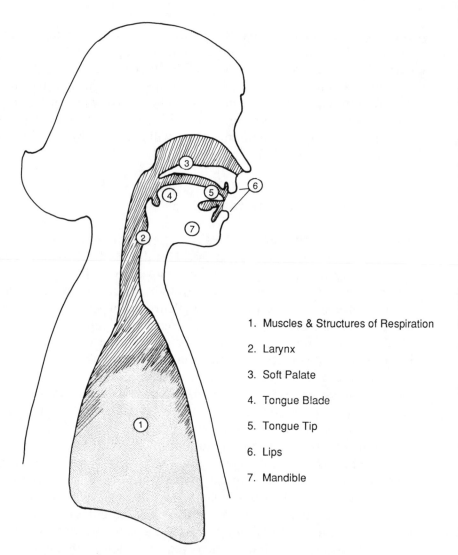

1. Muscles & Structures of Respiration

2. Larynx

3. Soft Palate

4. Tongue Blade

5. Tongue Tip

6. Lips

7. Mandible

Figure 9–3. The speech production system. Important functional components of the motor speech system.

All of this results in molding and modification of the air or sound stream that results in the creation of patterns of sounds and silence that impart familiarity and meaning to the ideas we have created and selected to express. These speech movements must be carefully programmed and synchronized if they are to result in speech sounds that fall within recognizable limits, and some speech science accountants have suggested that over 100 muscles must be involved in this speech movement symphony. The brain and relevant portions of the central and peripheral nervous system (including cranial and spinal nerves) must conduct and orchestrate this speech harmony. But sometimes the music is sour. Dissynchrony of speech movements can create dis-harmony of the speech signal.

DYSARTHRIAS. The most frequently occurring disturbances of motor speech production are the dysarthrias. In the old days, the term was singularized as "dysarthria," and it was thought that the disorder was one that primarily affected the articulation of speech. Now it has been pointed out repeatedly that *types* of the disorders exist and can be differentiated from one another, and that not only articulation but all of the speech production process can be impaired. Thus, damage to the neuromuscular control of speech can affect respiration, phonation, resonance, articulation, and prosodic aspects of speech. These contemporary refinements in the conceptualization and definition of motor speech disorders is largely the result of milestone research emanating from the Mayo Clinic in Rochester, Minnesota in the early 1970s (Darley, Aronson, & Brown, 1975).

In fact, some of the early Mayo Clinic research in the dysarthrias associated neurological conditions and damage to certain levels of the nervous system with identifiable types of dysarthrias. Although clinicians these days recognize that many of the people they see who present a dysarthria might be difficult to clearly pigeonhole and end up with a speech diagnosis of a "mixed" dysarthria, some speech patterns are clearly different and relate to the disease or condition that caused it. Table 9–6 presents some of the recognizable dysarthria types along with the neurological conditions or level of brain damage associated with them.

DYSPHAGIA. Swallowing problems (frequently referred to as **dysphagia**) are related to neuromotor speech disorders in that they frequently, though not necessarily, accompany disturbances of speech movement. Some estimates have placed the incidence of swallowing problems as high as 13 to 14% of all hospitalized patients and from 40 to 50% of all residents of nursing homes or extended care facilities (Logemann, 1993). Increasingly, caseloads of speech-language pathologists who work in a medical environment reflect the need for services for individuals who have difficulty swallowing and eating. Although dealing with the evaluation and treatment of swallowing disorders requires careful collaboration and teamwork among several health care professionals, the speech-language pathologist many times coordinates these efforts.

Normal swallowing is a quick and easy thing. It is a safe and efficient process and it takes less than 2 minutes to move a mouthful of pasta primavera or a gulp of strawberry shake from the

TABLE 9–6. Types of dysarthrias.

Dysarthria Type	Neurogenic Condition or Level of Damage	Speech Deviations
Flaccid	Brain stem, lower motor neuron	Hypernasality, breathiness, poor articulation
Spastic	Bilateral motor strip	Strained-strangled voice, low pitch, very poor articulation
Ataxic	Cerebellum	Irregular speech and syllable repetition
Hypokinetic	Basal ganglia, Parkinsonism	Reduced loudness, rushes of speech
Hyperkinetic	Many levels of extra-pyramidal motor system	Unsteady rate, pitch loudness; sudden or slow variations in speech or voice; stoppages; tics; grunts

mouth, through the pharynx, and into the esophagus, that elastic tube that conveys food to the stomach. During this 2-minute process, the airway is protected so we don't breathe food into the lungs and get pneumonia, and the glob of Twinkie or swig of Snapple is propelled under pressure from the mouth to the back of the throat into the esophagus.

Most of the time this process is a cinch and no problems with swallowing occur. Sometimes, if we try to talk or take a breath while eating, we choke a bit and "get something down the wrong pipe," but mostly it is safe and nearly automatic. But the brain and nervous system disorders (stroke, disease, brain injury) that create neuromotor speech disorders can cause lasting problems with swallowing as well. When this occurs the distress can be serious and even life-threatening. It is more than just an inconvenience, and more and more speech-language pathologists are rewarded by being able to play a major role in the identification and treatment of dysphagia. For the person who cannot eat or swallow normally, improvement in these vital life functions can mean a drastic change in quality of life.

The signs and symptoms of dysphagia are several, and frequently very obvious. Some people cough and choke when the bad swallow alarm goes off and the reflexive reactions take over to try to expel food from the airway. Others simply cannot clear the food from the mouth, and residuals of breakfast or lunch can be observed in the mouth and pharynx. Frequently, the problems in eating and swallowing result in dehydration, nutritional deficiency, weight loss, or pneumonia; and patients with dysphagia are frequently medically managed and even may require surgery for tube feeding.

The multidisciplinary approach is as evident in the evaluation and treatment of dysphagia as it is in any of the disorders. The speech-language pathologist frequently coordinates these efforts and may be referred to as the "swallowing therapist" on the team. In some settings, the occupational or physical therapist, a dietitian, or a nurse may perform the duties of the swallowing therapist. Other professionals involved include the attending physician, as well as perhaps a neurologist, otolaryngologist, or gastroenterologist. For the evaluation, a radiologist usually works closely with the swallowing therapist. Other members of the team may include a respiration therapist or a specialist in maxillofacial prosthetic appliances.

The swallowing therapist usually coordinates both the evaluation and treatment of dysphagia, and the assessment in the acute care setting or hospital typically involves a **bedside evaluation** so that determinations can be made of cognitive status, language abilities, mentation, and other behavioral or medical variables that might influence readiness to eat or swallow (Logemann, 1993). After these determinations are completed, the most frequent evaluation of swallowing function involves the swallowing therapist and a radiologist who conduct a **modified barium swallow** to allow motion picture X-rays to be taken of the oral and pharyngeal regions. During this procedure, the person is required to assume an eating position and swallow predetermined amounts of liquid or food. The food may be of varying consistencies such as pudding, puree, or chewed portions of a cookie. The swallowing therapist and the radiologist, in consultation with other team members, then try to pinpoint what is wrong with the swallowing process and recommend treatment procedures or procedures that improve efficient swallowing, eliminate aspiration (food or foreign substances in the lungs), and prescribe a diet that helps to ensure adequate nutrition and hydration (Logemann, 1983).

APRAXIA OF SPEECH. A second major category of neuromotor speech disorders is the problem seen in people who have trouble programming and sequencing the sounds of speech in a normal and coordinated manner. Typically, these individuals have no difficulty knowing what they want to say (unless, of course, they have a co-existing aphasia), but the motor speech problem reveals itself by struggle in getting the sounds out in a well-timed and synchronized fashion (*"I know what I want to say, but I can't say it right."*).

Many labels and terms have been used for this motor speech problem including *verbal apraxia, aphasic phonological disorder, phonetic disintegration, apraxic dysarthria, phonemic paraphasia, aphemia,* and many others. The terminological confusion resulted in great debates about the best name for the disturbance, and even whether or not it existed. These days, however, usage has leaned to the term **apraxia of speech**, although not everyone agrees with the label or that the disorder is separate from that seen in types of phonological involvement in aphasia.

Most experts agree on the characteristics of it, though. It primarily affects the speech process of articulation and the prosodic elements of rate, speech rhythm, and stress. Speech sounds get misplaced, distorted, and substituted, and the initiation of words or sentences may be characterized by silent groping and posturing of the speech articulators (tongue, lips, jaw), by audible verbal groping with speech sound intrusions or overflow, and by syllable and word repetitions or restarts (*"I'd like a bigaret, . . . ah . . . snigaret, tigaret . . . What the heck's the matter with me. I want a . . . stig . . . stig . . . stigaret. Not a stigaret. I want to smoke a cigaret and I can't even ask for one. . . . A sinkaret. Gimme a damn Marlboro . . . I can't say that word."*).

The late 1960s and the 1970s were marked by social and political turmoil, disruption, and change along several national and international fronts, and this time span corresponded to tumult and significant productivity in the area of neuromotor speech disorders as well. Several important doctoral dissertations on the topic of apraxia of speech, as well as clinical research from hospitals and the increasingly sophisticated *speech motor control laboratories,* contributed to our understanding of the disorder.

A dozen or so speech and nonspeech characteristics have been advanced as typical of apraxia of speech, and a series of descriptive and experimental studies of the behavior, acoustics, and physiology of the disorder formed the foundation for contemporary thought about it (Wertz, LaPointe, & Rosenbek, 1991). Although universal agreement has not been reached, some clinicians feel that the most fruitful differentiating characteristics or cardinal features of apraxia of speech are those listed in Table 9–7.

Although some experts would argue with the selection and priority of these characteristics, and perhaps select personal favorites, these features with accompanying examples capture much of the essence of apraxia of speech. Once the disorder is heard a few times from several individuals, the distinctive nature of the speech impairment becomes firmly entrenched, and the clinical utility of these features as differentiators from the other neurogenic disorders becomes apparent.

TABLE 9-7. Cardinal features of apraxia of speech.

1. **Numerous speech sound substitutions (including additive substitutions); some speech sound distortions; few speech sound omissions.**

   "He's on the tel... tel... tef... telfalone... He's on the twelfalone. He's talking on the felaphone. I mean the telephone. That's it. Felaphone."

2. **Groping, posturing, speech initiation problems.**

   "She's in the... Camelback Terrace complex... the... partments... ah... pahpartments... the... Ca... Cam... Tamel... Tuh... Ca... aaahhh... Tambleback... Caaa... (visible mouth and tongue movements) *Camelparts... Camelparts? I just said Camelparts. I don't know any Camelparts. Ahhhh... Ca...* (more visible mouth posturing, groping, searching behavior of tongue) *Camel... back... Terrace... a... part... ments. That's where she lives."*

3. **Inconsistency. Changes in errors or speech production on repeated trials.**

   "Gingerbread. Gingerbread. Gingergread. Gringerjed. Grinjer. Brinjer-jed. Ginger. Gringe. Ahgin. Aginger. Gingerbed. Gingerbread. There. Gingerbread. I got it now. Gingerbread. Whew!"

Although the specific sites of damage in the brain are open to some question, clearly the portions of the nervous system responsible for planning, programming, and sequencing the complicated muscular events needed for linking speech sounds into meaning are responsible. Most people believe that these responsibilities are conducted in the motor association areas of the cerebral cortex, but widespread cortical and even subcortical areas might be participants.

Apraxia as a concept referring to disturbances of programming movements has been around since the turn of the century. Liepmann (Wertz, LaPointe, & Rosenbek, 1991) was one of the first to describe in detail patients who demonstrated disturbed volitional nonspeech movements of the mouth (oral apraxia) or of the arm (limb apraxia). One of Liepmann's patients could not use a toothbrush properly with his right hand but demonstrated its use perfectly when it was presented to his left hand. Sometimes he used the toothbrush as if it were a spoon, shoveled with it, or put the handle in his mouth. He also had great difficulty demonstrating the use of musical instruments (even though he was a musician) and could not successfully show Liepmann how to produce sound from a trumpet or harmonica. The patient attempted to pound with or comb his hair with the harmonica, while sometimes recognizing with great embarrassment that he could not plan and execute the appropriate movement sequences. According to Liepmann's description, the general condition of apraxia was an inability to act or move the movable parts of the body in a purposeful manner, even though motility was preserved and paralysis or weakness was not responsible.

When this disrupted programming of movement affects the movable parts of the speech production system such as the tongue, lips, or jaw, the result is jumbled speech with the characteristics described above. Fortunately, and depending on severity, this disorder lends itself to a degree of correction with strategies of compensation and other means of intervention. The outcome for people with apraxia of speech can be quite favorable with appropriate diagnosis and treatment. That leads to another important issue, the matter of recovery and therapy.

◆ RESTORATION, RECOVERY

Study of the neurogenic disorders of communication necessitates dwelling on diseases, disasters, abnormal conditions, and heartbreak. Bad things happen to good people and change the lives of good families. Students of pathology and disaster become discouraged and pessimistic with the necessity of having to tread water in this seeming swamp of misfortune. But it is extremely important to recognize the positive end of choosing to get involved with the hardships of others. The dark clouds, the struggle, the adversity, the challenge, the frustration, the disappointment that accompany those struck with disorders of communication can be balanced with equally sanguine notions. For every wreck there is a raft. Recovery. Restoration. Relearning. Overcoming obstacles. Adjustment. Acceptance (LaPointe, 1990). All of these are good reasons to get up in the morning and provide solace not only to the individuals who choose to expend the effort to face unique challenges, but provide as well the balance and satisfaction necessary for the professionals who choose a life of helping others get on the raft and look for shore. Said a prospective graduate student in communication disorders at Arizona State University, "I know this isn't for everybody, and we all have to match our own values and personality traits with how to spend our days, but for myself, I would rather live a life trying to help people instead of trying to con them."

Not all of those we work with will make the gains we would hope for, but all have the potential to take steps toward adjustment or acceptance with an enhanced quality of life. The professional in neurogenic communication disorders must learn the brain, must learn the fundamentals and science of human communication, must learn the disorders, must learn the tests and appraisal instruments, must keep on the cutting edge of treatment and intervention principles and strategies. But most of all he or she must learn, adopt, and inculcate into the spirit and self the values of humanity and respect for the individual. We work with people. We work with families.

The challenges are plenty but the rewards are legion. John Fowles (1970) has reminded us of the ancient Greek concept of *Aristos,* striving for and assisting others in their search for the best in a given situation. The gale of disaster that inevitably accompanies a shattered nervous system and loss of communication can be followed by the faint and then brighter rainbow of recovery, restoration, and *aristos.*

◆ SUMMARY AND CONCLUSIONS

This chapter introduced and described the disorders of communication, cognition, and movement that can accompany damage or disease to the brain and other relevant parts of the nervous system. In addition to a brief outline of the history and origins of the clinical study of this topic, a description and scope of neuropathology — the diseases, traumas, conditions, and other causes of these impairments — was presented. The principal disorders were explained, described, and illustrated with quotations and case studies. These disorders included several types of aphasia, right hemisphere syndrome, traumatic brain injury, dementia, the neuromotor speech disorders (dysarthrias and apraxia of speech), and dysphagia. Throughout the presentation of the disturbances that can be created by a shattered nervous system, the role of the professional in assessing, treating, counseling, and guiding the clinical management process in a humane and individualistic manner was stressed.

◆ REFERENCES

Bauer, C. (1992). From the patient's point of view. *Cognitive Rehabilitation, 10*(2), 8–11.

Bayles, K., & Kazniak, A. (1987). *Communication and cognition in normal aging and dementia.* Boston: Little, Brown.

Bienemann, K. L. (1989). Psychological implications of right hemisphere injury. In P. A. Pimental & N. A. Kingsbury (Eds.), *Neuropsychological aspects of right brain injury* (pp. 65–72). Austin, TX: Pro-Ed.

Brookshire, R. H. (1992). *An introduction to neurogenic communication disorders* (4th ed.). St. Louis: Mosby Year Book.

Darley, F., Aronson, A., & Brown, J. (1975). *Motor speech disorders.* Philadelphia: W. B. Saunders.

Fowles, J. (1970). *The aristos.* Boston: Little, Brown.

Gall, F. J. (1835). On the functions of the brain and each of its parts. In Mac Millan, M. (1992). Inhibition and the control of behavior: From Gall to Freud via Phineas Gage and the frontal lobes. *Brain and Cognition, 19,* 72–104.

Goodglass, H. (1980). Disorders of naming following brain injury. *American Scientist, 68,* 648–655.

Helm-Esterbrooks, N., & Albert, M. C. (1991). *Manual of aphasia therapy.* Austin, TX: Pro-Ed.

Holland, A. (1982). When is aphasia aphasia? The problem of closed head injury. In R. H. Brookshire (Ed.), *Clinical aphasiology: Conference proceedings 1982* (pp. 345–349). Minneapolis: BRK Publishers.

LaPointe, L. L. (Ed.). (1990). *Aphasia and related neurogenic language disorders.* New York: Thieme Medical Publishers.

Lezak, M. D., & O'Brien, K. P. (1990). Chronic emotional, social, and physical changes after traumatic brain injury. In E. D. Bigler (Ed.), *Traumatic brain injury* (pp. 365–380). Austin, TX: Pro-Ed.

Logemann, J. (1983). *Evaluation and treatment of swallowing disorders.* Austin, TX: Pro-Ed.

Logemann, J. (1993). *A professional's guide to swallowing disorders.* Rockville, MD: American Speech-Language-Hearing Association.

Myers, P. S. (1983). Treatment of right hemisphere communication disorders. In. W. H. Perkins (Ed.), *Current therapy in communication disorders* (Vol. 3, pp. 57–67). New York: Thieme-Stratton.

National Stroke Association. (1991). The scope of stroke. *Clinical Updates, 1*(3), 1–3.

Richards, W. (1991). From the patient's point of view. *Cognitive Rehabilitation, 9*(5), 8.

Ripich, D. (1991). *Handbook of geriatric communication disorders.* Austin, TX: Pro-Ed.

Rosenbek, J., LaPointe, L. L., & Wertz, R. T. (1989). *Aphasia: A clinical approach.* Austin, TX: Pro-Ed.

Schiller, F. (1992). *Paul Broca: Explorer of the brain.* Oxford: Oxford University Press.

Scientific American. (1992, September). Decade of the brain, pp. BR3.

Shekim, L. (1990). Dementia. In L. L. LaPointe (Ed.), *Aphasia and related neurogenic language disorders* (pp. 210–220). New York: Thieme Medical Publishers.

Shekim, L., & LaPointe, L. L. (1984, February). *Production of discourse in patients with Alzheimer's dementia.* Paper presented at the International Neuropsychology Society meeting, Houston.

Teasdale, G., & Jennett, W. B. (1974). Assessment of coma and impaired consciousness. *Lancet, 2,* 81.

Wertz, R., LaPointe, L. L., & Rosenbek, J. C. (1991). *Apraxia of speech in adults: The disorder and its management.* San Diego: Singular Publishing Group.

◆ SUGGESTED READINGS

Bayles, K., & Kazniak, A. (1987). *Communication and cognition in normal aging and dementia.* Boston: Little, Brown.

Brookshire, R. H. (1992). *An introduction to neurogenic communication disorders* (4th ed.). St. Louis: Mosby Year Book.

Chapey, R. (1994). *Language intervention strategies in adult aphasia.* Baltimore: Williams & Wilkins.

Helm-Esterbrooks, N., & Albert, M. C. (1991). *Manual of aphasia therapy.* Austin, TX: Pro-Ed.

LaPointe, L. L. (Ed.). (1990). *Aphasia and related neurogenic communication disorders.* New York: Thieme Medical Publishers.

LaPointe, L. L., & Katz, R. C. (1994). Neurogenic disorders of speech. In G. Shames, E. Wiig, & W. Secord (Eds.), *Human communication disorders: An introduction* (pp. 480–518). New York: Macmillan.

Ripich, D. (1991). *Handbook of geriatric communication disorders.* Austin, TX: Pro-Ed.

Rosenbek, J. C., LaPointe, L. L., & Wertz, R. T. (1989). *Aphasia: A clinical approach.* Austin, TX: Pro-Ed.

Wertz, R. T., LaPointe, L. L., & Rosenbek, J. C. (1991). *Apraxia of speech in adults: The disorder and its management.* San Diego: Singular Publishing Group.

◆ GLOSSARY

Agraphia: impaired writing usually associated with brain damage. Characterized by spelling errors, reversals, impaired word order, and other manifestations of faulty written language use. Sometimes called **dysgraphia**.

Agrammatism: a characteristic of aphasia marked by omission of language function words (prepositions, articles, etc.). Telegraphic speech.

Alexia: impairment in reading the printed word. May be acquired or developmental. Acquired alexia is a reading impairment that accompanies or is a part of aphasia. Frequently called **dyslexia**.

Aphasia: impairment in the comprehension and production of language symbol systems that results from fairly localized damage to the brain. Usually accompanies focal areas of damage to the left cerebral hemisphere. Affects reading, writing, speaking, understanding, gestures, and other symbol systems used in communication.

Apraxia of speech: one of the major types of neuromotor speech disorders caused by brain damage that results in faulty planning, programming, or sequencing of the sounds of speech.

Cerebrovascular accident (CVA): damage or injury to the blood vessels of the brain or nervous system. Most frequent types of CVA are thromboembolic (either stationary or moving blood clots) or hemorrhage (excessive bleeding). A popular term for CVA is **stroke**.

Dementia: abnormal reduction in memory, thinking, language, and other cognitive functions that results from diffuse brain damage from a variety of diseases and conditions.

Dysarthria(s): a group of neuromotor speech disorders caused by impaired movements of the speech production system as a result of damage to the brain or nervous system. May affect respiration, sound production, resonance, or speech prosody.

Dysphagia: disturbance in swallowing or the oral preparation and movement of food from the mouth, through the pharynx, and into the esophagus.

Hemiparesis: weakness or partial paralysis of one side of the body after brain damage. Usually involves the lower and upper extremities (leg and arm) on one side.

Hemiplegia: paralysis on one side of the body after brain damage. Usually involves the lower and upper extremities.

Hemisensory impairment: reduction or loss of sensory functions on one side of the body. May result in reduced appreciation of touch, hot and cold, or pain sensation.

Lexical-semantic processes: language processes that deal with storage and use of word meanings.

Neologistic jargon: language use in aphasia marked by nonsensical, new words. Words not found in the dictionary such as *hayveness* or *appleholtent*.

Neuropathology: the study of diseases and injuries that can affect the nervous system. The causes of brain or nervous system damage.

Phrenology: the science or pseudoscience of the 19th century that attempted to determine a person's character or personality attributes by noting patterns of bumps and protuberances on the skull.

Post-traumatic amnesia (PTA): a period of memory loss characteristic of the span of time after an incident of traumatic brain injury.

Pragmatics: study or implementation of language systems in a real-life context. The elements and practice of language use.

Right hemisphere impairment (RHI): a constellation of linguistic and extralinguistic deficits created by damage to the right cerebral hemisphere. May include impaired perception, visual field neglect, alterations in certain emotions, and reduced ability at tasks that require synthesis or inference.

Syntax: the rules governing the arrangement, grammar, and ordering of language units.

Traumatic brain injury (TBI): also called **closed head injury** or just **brain injury**. Refers to the physical damage to the brain or nervous system caused by bruises, lacerations, penetrations, or shearing as a result of such causes as motor vehicular accidents, falls, or skull-penetrating missiles.

Scientific Substrates of Speech Production

KENNETH N. STEVENS, Ph.D.

After reading this chapter, you should be able to:

◆ Describe an utterance as a sequence of words, and describe the words as sequences of phonetic units.

◆ Interpret the production of a speech sound in terms of the generation of sound sources and the shaping or filtering of these sources.

◆ Recognize that a sound can be described as a waveform that changes with time or as a spectrum that represents the sound as a sum of sinusoidal waveforms.

◆ Describe how sound is generated by vibration of the vocal folds.

◆ Describe how sound is generated by turbulence in the flow of air at an obstacle or constriction in the airway.

◆ Interpret vowel sounds in terms of vocal tract shapes and acoustic characteristics.

◆ Classify consonant sounds in terms of how they are produced in the vocal tract and in terms of their acoustic properties.

A theory of speech production is reviewed, with emphasis on the mechanisms of sound generation in the vocal tract. The sound that emerges from the lips is the result of a two-step process: the generation of sound sources that are the result of modulation of airflow through a constricted part of the airway between the larynx and the lips and the filtering of these sources by the acoustic cavities of the vocal tract. The acoustic properties of a number of different classes of sounds are described, including influences on the sounds when they occur in sequences of words and in casual speech.

As an initial step in the generation of an utterance, a speaker must generate a thought, select a set of words to be produced, and organize these words into a proper sequence. Once this sequence of words has been laid out or planned, instructions are given to the **articulators** (movable structures within the vocal tract or airway extending from the larynx to the mouth opening) and to the respiratory system to perform an appropriate sequence of movements. In his or her memory, the speaker has access to a list of words or a lexicon. Each word in this lexicon contains a set of instructions that specify how the various articulators are to be maneuvered to produce that word. These instructions for each word can be organized to produce a sequence of sounds or **segments**. This pattern of organization provides specific instructions for moving the articulators that are crucial to the production of each of the component sounds. The movements of the articulatory structures specified by the lexicon result in the generation of sound that is radiated from the mouth, nose, and neck surfaces of the speaker.

The primary articulators that are active in producing different speech sounds are shown in Figure 10–1. This figure is a section through the midline of the head, and it shows the trachea or windpipe, the **larynx** located above the trachea, and the structures that shape the airway above the larynx. During speech production, the primary function of the respiratory system below the trachea is to provide a supply of air that is converted to sound in the vicinity of the larynx or in the airway downstream (toward the mouth opening) from the larynx. The articulators that can be manipulated to produce different sound patterns during speech include the vocal folds, which are located within the larynx, structures in the pharyngeal region, the soft palate, the tongue body, the tongue blade, and the lips. The function of each of these structures in producing different sounds will be discussed in the following sections.

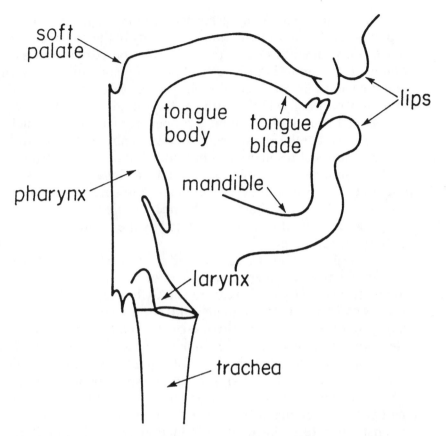

Figure 10–1. Sketch of the shape of the human vocal tract in the midline. The various parts of the system that are active in speech production are identified.

◆ SOUND SOURCES AND SOUND FILTERS IN SPEECH PRODUCTION

The generation of most sounds, including the sounds of speech, can be described in terms of two processes: (1) generation of a **source** of sound energy and (2) a **filtering** or shaping of this source. This distinction between a sound source and a filter can be illustrated by examining the sound generated by a drum beat. The source in this case is the sound produced by the initial tap of the drumstick on the drumhead. This source sets the stretched drumhead in motion, and the character of the sound that emerges depends on the shape and tension of this surface. The drumhead acts to filter the initial brief pulse of sound energy imparted by the drum beat.

As another example, a brief sound source is generated when a guitar string is plucked. In this case, the filtering is dependent on the tension and mass of the string, where along its length the string is plucked, and the configuration of the body of the guitar. For some musical instruments, such as the violin, the source of sound is continuous rather than impulsive. The bow is passed over the string, and the sound from this continuous source is filtered by the string and the violin body. The filtering of the sound source in these examples is the result of mechanical properties of a structure (such as the drumhead or the guitar string), but it can also be an acoustic filtering by tubes or resonators, as in woodwind or brass instruments.

A familiar example of a sound produced by an acoustic source and filter is the sound that is generated by blowing over the top of a pop bottle. The flow of air over the neck of the bottle produces a sound source, and this source is filtered by the resonance of the air column in the bottle.

In the production of speech, sound sources are generated by narrowing the airway, either at the larynx or at some location downstream from the larynx, and causing air to flow rapidly through this narrow constriction. When there is little or no narrowing of the airway, as in quiet breathing, the passage of air causes little or no audible sound to be generated. If the narrowing is produced by placing the vocal folds close together, the folds may be set into vibration, and the modulated flow of air through the space between the vocal folds (the glottis) forms the acoustic source. A source also can be generated by creating turbulence in the flow of air in the vicinity of a constriction (e.g., during the production of an /s/ sound). Such sound sources are much like the sound that is produced at the outlet of an air conditioner. This sound source for an /s/ sound has a noisy character that is quite different from the sound that is generated by vocal fold vibration.

The filtering of these sound sources is achieved by shaping the airway between the glottis and the lips. The adjustment of the source-generating constrictions as well as the shaping of the airways for acoustic filtering is accomplished by manipulating the positions and shapes of the various articulators, as discussed above.

✦ CHARACTERIZATION OF WAVEFORMS, SOURCES, AND FILTERS

One way of describing a sound at a point in space is in terms of the time variation of the pressure fluctuations in the air. This variation in pressure can be depicted as a graph of sound pressure versus time. This graph is called a **waveform**. An example of such a graph for a sound in which the pressure variation with time is sinusoidal is shown in Figure 10–2A. The pattern of sound pressure is repeti-

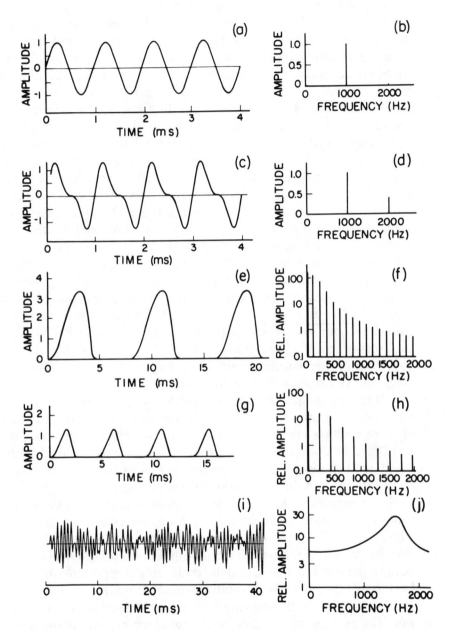

Figure 10-2. Examples of several different waveforms (right panels). The top panels A and B show a sinusoidal waveform, which has just one component in the spectrum, depicted by the vertical line at 1000 Hz. The waveforms in the next three panels C, E and G are periodic, and their spectra D, F and H have several components with equal spacing between the components. The bottom panel I shows a noise waveform for which the spectrum J is continuous.

tive or **periodic** (repeats itself in the same amount of time), and the number of complete cycles per second is the **frequency**. In this example, the frequency is 1000 Hertz (or cycles per second) and the period is 1 millisecond. (This means the waveform repeats itself 1000 times per second.) An alternative way of depicting such a sinusoidal waveform is given in Figure 10–2B. In this representation, the horizontal axis indicates the frequency of the sinusoidal waveform, and the vertical axis indicates the amplitude of the waveform, which in this case is unity. The vertical line at 1000 Hz (abbreviation for Hertz) gives the frequency and amplitude of the sinusoid. This second representation is called the **spectrum** of the waveform. The two representations are equivalent. The time waveform shows a sinusoidal variation with a particular amplitude and frequency. The spectrum is a somewhat more compact representation, which shows the frequency by the placement of the vertical line along the horizontal axis and the amplitude by the vertical length of the line.

Figure 10–2C shows a waveform constructed by adding two sine waves — one at a frequency of 1000 Hz and an amplitude of 1 unit, and the other at a frequency of 2000 Hz and an amplitude of 0.5 unit. This complex waveform (nonsinusoidal) repeats itself every 1 millisecond, and hence is periodic with a frequency of 1000 Hz. The spectrum of this waveform, shown in Figure 10–2D, has two components, as depicted by the two vertical lines.

It turns out that any **complex periodic waveform** can be constructed by adding a set (two or more) of sinusoids whose frequencies are multiples of the frequency of the waveform. The waveform in Figure 10–2C is an example with just two components. Figures 10–2E to H show two more examples. As before, the waveform is given at the left, and the corresponding spectrum is on the right. Each of these waveforms has a number of components, with the amplitudes of the components being smaller as the frequency increases. The sinusoidal component whose frequency is equal to the repetition frequency of the waveform is called the **fundamental** component or the first harmonic, and the remaining components are called **harmonics** (whole number multiples of the fundamental). Note that in these examples the amplitude scales for the spectra are logarithmic. The examples in Figures 10–2E and G have different fundamental frequencies, and hence different spacing between the harmonics. The sounds from many musical instruments are rich in harmonics, and these sounds can also be represented by spectra like those in Figures 10–2F and H.

Some speech waveforms such as the fricative sound shown in Figure 10–2I are not periodic. Such waveforms are called **aperiodic** because they do not repeat themselves. These waveforms also can be represented by spectra, but these spectra have a very large number of closely spaced components. It is convenient to represent the spectra of such sounds by a continuous curve, as in Figure 10–2J. This curve gives the relative amplitudes of the closely spaced frequency components at each frequency.

The fundamental frequency F (in Hz) is inversely related to the amount of time (the period P in seconds) needed to complete one cycle of the waveform. The equation $F = \frac{1}{P}$ describes this relation. For example, if the waveform repeats itself once every 0.005 sec, then the frequency is

$$F = \frac{1}{0.005} = 200 \text{ Hz, or cycles per second.}$$

There are at least two motivations for representing sounds such as speech in terms of spectra. One motivation is that the ear processes sounds to give an approximate spectral representation of sounds in the neural pathways from the ear to the brain. Thus, when sounds of the type shown in Figure 10–2 impinge on the ear, there is a representation of these sounds inside the ear that is similar to spectral patterns like those shown at the right of the figures.

A second motivation for characterizing waveforms in terms of sums of sinusoidal components comes from the special characteristics of certain "filters," such as the human vocal tract, amplifiers, loudspeakers, organ pipes, and so on. When an input signal is applied to these devices, there is an output signal in response. The special characteristic of these systems is that if the input signal is a sinusoid with a particular amplitude and frequency, then the output is a sinusoid with the same frequency but with a different amplitude. The situation is depicted schematically in Figure 10–3A, B, and C.

Figure 10–3A is an example of a filter characteristic. If the input to the filter is a sinusoid with a particular frequency, the curve in Figure 10–3A gives the amount by which to multiply the amplitude of the sinusoid at that frequency to obtain the amplitude of the output sinusoid. For example, if the input is a sinusoid with a frequency of 1000 Hz, as shown in the spectrum in Figure 10–3B, then the filter characteristic in Figure 10–3A indicates that the amplitude of that sinusoid is multiplied by 3 to obtain the amplitude of the output. Because the amplitude of the input is 1, the output amplitude is 3, as in the spectrum in Figure 10–3C. In general, the amount by which the filter changes the amplitude of the input sinusoid depends on the frequency of the sinusoid. Suppose, for example, that the input signal is periodic but with several frequency components,

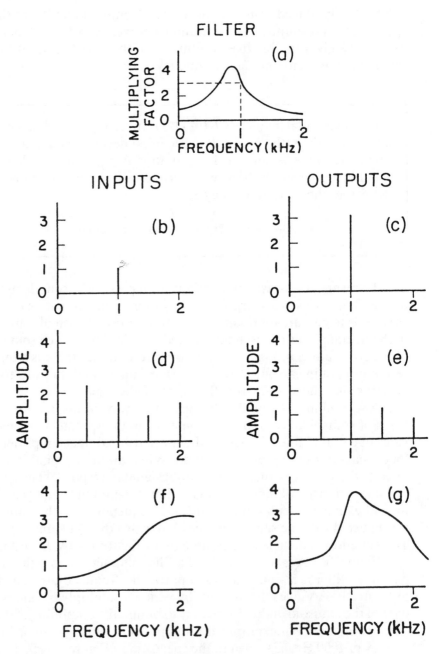

Figure 10-3. Illustration of the filtering of different waveforms. The filter characteristic, shown in A, indicates the factor by which the amplitude of each frequency component of the input is multiplied to obtain the output amplitude of that component. Panels B, D and F show the spectra of three different input signals, and panels C, E and G show the spectra of these signals after they have been passed through the filter.

as in the spectrum shown in Figure 10–3D. Each sinusoid in this spectrum is multiplied by a different factor as it passes through the filter. After passing through the filter, the spectrum of the signal has the form shown in Figure 10–3E. In this example, some of the harmonics in the output signal are larger than those in the input signal, and some are smaller.

If the spectrum of the input signal is continuous, like the spectrum shown in Figure 10–3F, then the output of the filter also has a continuous spectrum, as illustrated in Figure 10–3G. At each frequency, the output spectrum is equal to the input spectrum multiplied by the filter characteristic.

When we consider how different sound sources are generated in the **vocal tract** and how the vocal tract filters these sources, we generally describe the sources in terms of their spectra. We will examine how these sources are filtered by the vocal tract to give the spectrum of the output sound pressure.

✦ VOCAL-FOLD VIBRATION

The source of sound that is used for the generation of vowels and some other speech sounds is produced by setting the **vocal folds** into vibration. The vocal folds are located in the larynx, which is positioned at the upper end of the trachea or windpipe. The position of the vocal folds is shown in Figure 10–4, with their front ends attached to a structure called the thyroid cartilage, and their back ends attached to small cartilages called arytenoid cartilages. The vocal folds are about 1 cm long for an adult female and about 1½ cm for an adult male. Viewed from above, the vocal folds appear as two bands of tissue, about 2–3 millimeters thick, as shown in Figure 10–4.

During normal quiet breathing the vocal folds are set rather far apart, as in Figure 10–4A. The vocal processes of the arytenoid cartilages are rotated toward the side of the airway. This causes a large opening between the vocal folds (glottis). Under this condition very little sound is produced by the gentle inward and outward flow of air. When the vocal folds are positioned close together during exhalation of air from the lungs (as in Figure 10–4B), pressure is built up in the trachea, and the vocal folds are set into vibration.

The series of pictures in Figure 10–5 demonstrates how this vibration occurs. These pictures show how the middle of the vocal folds would appear if they were observed in a coronal cross section (from the front). The series of pictures indicates what would be observed if a rapid series of photographs of the vocal folds were taken during 1 cycle of vibration. At the time of the first frame, the upper edges of the folds remain closed, and the air pressure in the trachea exerts a

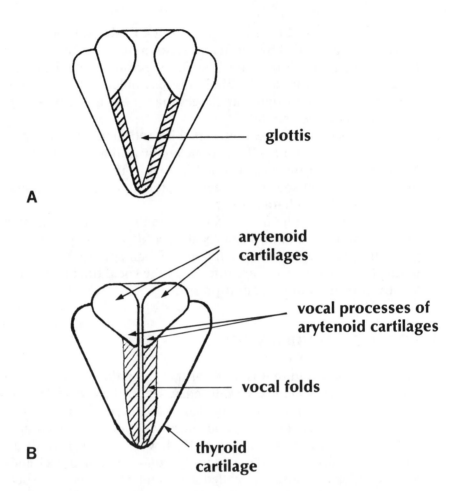

Figure 10–4. Schematized representation of the vocal folds and surrounding structures as seen from above. **A.** Configuration of these structures during quiet breathing. **B.** Configuration when the structures are in a position that leads to vocal fold vibration.

force on the lower parts of the folds, as shown by the arrows. This force pushes the lower surfaces apart (frame 2), until the upper edges open at frame 3. At this time, air begins to flow through the channel between the vocal folds, called the **glottis**. The upper edges of the folds continue to move outwards (frame 4), but because of the flow, the pressure in the space between the folds decreases. Due to the elasticity of the vocal folds, and the rate of airflow through the glottis, the folds spring back together (frame 5), first touching at the bottom and then at the top. The flow of air is cut off and the cycle repeats itself.

As a consequence of this vocal fold vibration, brief pulses of air flow through the glottis (see volume velocity graph in bottom

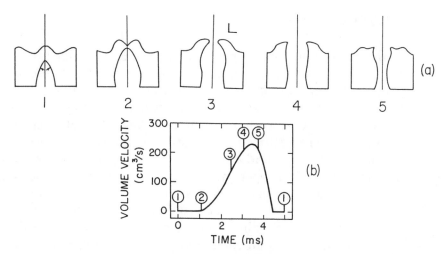

Figure 10-5. A. Schematized coronal sections (i.e., as viewed in a plane perpendicular to the vocal folds) showing the configuration of the vocal folds at various instants of time during a cycle of vibration (adapted from Baer, 1975). Successive times are labeled 1–5, with the **glottis** (the opening between the vocal folds) being closed at 1 and 2, and open at 3, 4, and 5. The cycle is repeated after 5. The arrows in panel 1 show the outward force of air pressure caused by the subglottal pressure. The vertical lines depict the midline of the glottis. The horizontal and vertical lines above panel 3 indicate dimensions of 1 mm. **B.** Schematized representation of the glottal airflow during a cycle of vibration. The points on the waveform correspond roughly to the times in the various panels in A. The values of volume velocity and time are appropriate for female vocal folds with a subglottal pressure of about 8 cm H_2O.

panel of Figure 10–5). These pulses constitute the acoustic source for vowels and many other speech sounds. The velocity of the flow of air through the glottis looks something like the periodic waveforms that have already been shown in Figures 10–2E and G. The frequency of vibration of the folds, and hence the frequency of the pulses of air, depends on the thickness, mass, and tension of the vocal folds. For adult female speakers, this frequency is usually in the range 150–300 Hz (e.g., as in Figure 10–2G), whereas for adult males, this range is about 90–180 Hz (as in Figure 10–2E). The frequency is somewhat higher for children than for adult females.

The waveform and spectrum of the air pulses through the glottis may vary from one individual to another. Normally the pattern is regular and produces a complex periodic waveform like those in Figure 10–2E and G. Sometimes the vocal folds do not function correctly, and the pattern of pulses emerging from the glottis is irregular and noisy. That is the case with certain voice disorders.

◆ VOWELS

During the production of a phrase or sentence, the various articulators above the larynx are moved around to change the shape of the airway between the glottis and the lips. This tortuously shaped airway is called the **vocal tract**. The sequence of articulatory movements tends to alternate between times when this airway is relatively open and times when a narrowing or constriction is formed by one of the articulators. **Vowel sounds** are produced during the times when the vocal tract is relatively open, whereas consonants are generated during the constricted intervals. We look first at the vowel sounds, for which, as we have seen, the acoustic source is at the glottis.

For vowels, the shaping of the airway by the articulators determines how the sound source at the glottis is filtered. Figure 10–6 shows a sagittal cross section (from the side) of the shape of the airway for four different vowels. This shape is the outline of the surfaces of the vocal tract in the midline, and does not show the dimensions in a lateral direction (away from midline, toward the side). Nevertheless, the midsagittal shapes in Figure 10–6 show how the positions of the tongue body and the lips can be manipulated to produce very different configurations for the airway. The sound from the glottal source is filtered differently for each of these shapes. The filtering is determined by the variation of the cross-sectional area of the airway along its length from the glottis to the lips. For the vowels /i/ (as in *beat*) and /u/ as in *boot*), the tongue body is raised up in the mouth, leaving only a narrow passage between the tongue surface and the palate. The tongue body is displaced farther back in the mouth for /u/ than for /i/, and the lips are more protruded and form a relatively narrow opening at the front of the vocal tract. In the case of the vowel /ɑ/ (as in *father*), the tongue body is low in the mouth, and the mandible or jaw is lower than for /i/ and /u/. The tongue body is displaced back to form a rather narrow opening in the pharyngeal region during the production of /ɑ/. In the case of the vowel /ə/ (as in the first vowel in *about*), the cross-sectional area is approximately the same along the length of the airway.

The filtering produced by the vocal tract for the uniform configuration represented by /ə/ is shown in Figure 10–7. This filter characteristic gives the amount by which each frequency component of the pulses of airflow at the glottis is multiplied to give the amplitude of this component of the velocity of back-and-forth fluctuations of the air at the lips. There are several peaks in the filter characteristic in Figure 10–7, and these peaks are approximately uniformly spaced. At the frequencies of the peaks, the source spectrum is multiplied or amplified by a factor of 5–10, whereas at the valleys

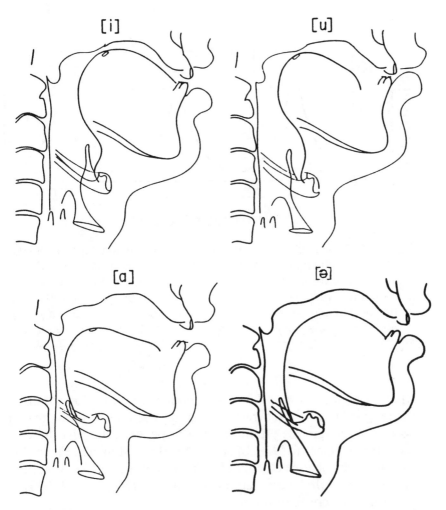

Figure 10–6. Sketches of the outline of the vocal tract at the midline when four different vowels are being produced: /i/ as in *beat*, /u/ as in *boot*, [ɑ] as in *father*, and /ə/ as in the first vowel in *about*. The figures are adapted from illustrations in Perkell (1969).

the multiplication factor is close to unity. The peaks in the filtering are evidence of **resonances** of the vocal tract, called **formants**. The frequencies of the formants depend on the speed of sound and on the overall length of the vocal tract along a path from the glottis to the lips. For this example of a uniform airway with a length *l*, the formants are located at frequencies of

$$\frac{c}{4l}, \frac{3c}{4l}, \frac{5c}{4l}, \text{ and so on,}$$

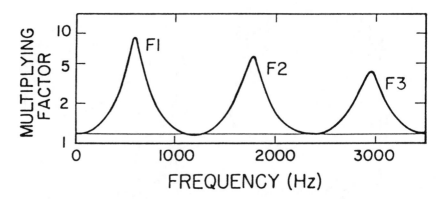

Figure 10–7. Filter characteristic of the vocal tract when it is in a configuration for which the cross-sectional area is uniform along its length. The filter characteristic gives the factor by which the spectrum of the acoustic source at the glottis is multiplied to obtain the acoustic output at the lips. The length of the vocal tract is taken to be 15 cm, corresponding to the average length for an adult female. The peaks corresponding to the first three formants are identified.

where c = speed of sound = 35400 cm/second. Thus, for example, if the length l is 15 cm (corresponding approximately to the average vocal-tract length for an adult female speaker), the first three formant frequencies are 590, 1770, and 2950 Hz, as shown in Figure 10–7. The average vocal-tract length for an adult male speaker is about 17 cm, leading to formant frequencies of 520, 1560, and 2600 Hz for this uniform configuration.

As we have observed, the result of filtering the spectrum of the glottal pulses by the filter characteristic in Figure 10–7 is the spectrum of the velocity fluctuations at the lips. There is some additional modification of these frequency components at the lips to account for radiation of the sound, leading to the spectrum of the sound pressure at a distance from the speaker's mouth. The steps in the production of the sound, from the glottal source to the sound pressure at a specific distance from the lips, are summarized in Figure 10–8. At the initial step, both the waveform $U_s(t)$ and the spectrum $U_s(f)$ of the source are shown. This source is filtered by the vocal tract and by the radiation, and the result is the waveform $p(t)$ and spectrum $P(f)$ of the sound pressure, as displayed at the right of the figure.

When the shape of the vocal tract is not uniform (e.g., for the vowels /i/, /u/, and /ɑ/ in Figure 10–6), the filtering component of this process in Figure 10–8 is modified. The filter still shows evi-

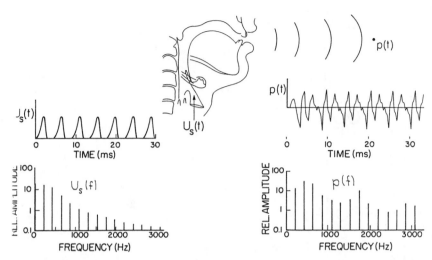

Figure 10–8. Showing how the acoustic source $U_s(f)$ at the glottis is modified by the vocal tract and by radiation from the lips to obtain the sound pressure $p(t)$ at some distance from the lips. At the left of the figure both the source waveform and its spectrum are shown. The waveform and spectrum of the sound pressure at a specified distance outside of the mouth are given at the right.

dence of prominences or formants, but these formants no longer have uniform spacing. The first two formants in particular are displaced to higher or lower frequencies depending on how the airway is shaped by the tongue body and the lips. For example, when the tongue body is raised (as for /i/ and /u/ in Figure 10–6), the frequency of the first formant moves downward from its value for a uniform configuration, and when the tongue body is lowered (as for /ɑ/) it moves upward. Lowering of the tongue body usually is accompanied by lowering of the jaw or mandible, leading to a vocal tract shape that is more open in the front. On the other hand, forward and backward movements of the tongue body in the mouth displace the frequency of the second formant toward a higher and lower frequency, respectively.

The frequencies of the first and second formants for several different vowels are plotted in the chart in Figure 10–9. The vowels represented in this chart are the four vowels whose vocal-tract shapes are displayed in Figure 10–6, together with the vowel /æ/ as in the word *bat*. The chart is arranged so that the vowels produced with a high tongue-body position (and a low first-formant frequency) are at the top, and those produced with a low tongue-body position (high first-formant frequency) are at the bottom. Front vowels are at the right and back vowels at the left.

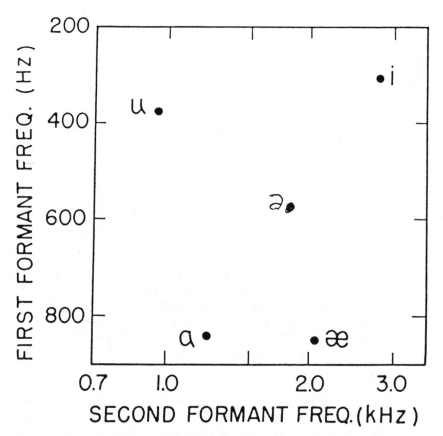

Figure 10–9. The frequency of the first formant is plotted against the frequency of the second formant for five different vowels of American English. These are average values for adult female speakers.

In English, there are several vowels in addition to those shown in Figures 10–6 and 10–9. The first two formant frequencies for these vowels generally lie on or within the contour joining the four outer vowels in Figure 10–9. Several of the vowels in English are produced with a vocal tract shape that changes with time, so that the frequencies of the formants are moving through the duration of the vowel. These vowels are called **diphthongs** (vocalic glides within a single syllable). Examples of diphthongs are the vowels in the words *bide, shout*, and *void*.

Changes in the spectrum of speech sounds over time are often displayed in the form of a spectrogram, as illustrated in Figure 10–10. A **spectrogram** is a plot of frequency versus time, with spectrum amplitude represented as degree of blackness of the pattern. The vowel formants are evident as dark bars on the spectrogram. These bars are relatively horizontal or fixed in frequency for vowels that

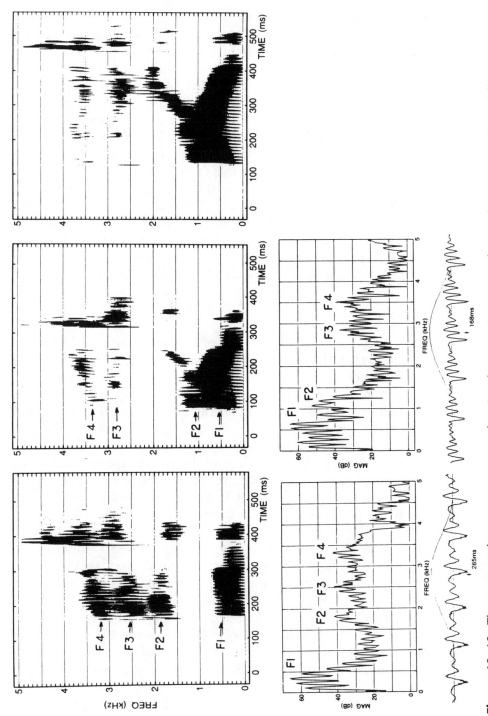

Figure 10–10. The top panels are spectrograms showing the acoustic patterns for words containing three different vowels: *bid* (left), *bud* (middle), and *bide* (right). The vowel in the right panel is a diphthong. The spectra below the first two spectrograms are measured in the middle of the vowels [I] and [ʌ]. A section of the vowel waveform is shown below each spectrum. The formant frequencies are identified in the spectra and spectrograms of [I] and [ʌ].

are not diphthongs, but show substantial movement for diphthongs. Vowels of both kinds are displayed in Figure 10–10. For the type of spectrogram shown in Figure 10–10, the regular vertical striations are evidence of the individual glottal pulses that occur when the vocal folds are vibrating. For example, in the spectrogram of the word *bid*, these pulses are spaced about 8 milliseconds apart near the middle of the vowel produced by a male talker, indicating that the frequency of vocal fold vibration is 125 Hz at this point.

Also shown in Figure 10–10 are spectra measured around the middle of the vowels in the words *bid* and *bud*. The individual harmonics are evident in these spectra, and the effects of the formants are observed at frequencies where there are peaks in the spectrum envelope drawn through the tips of the harmonics. The amplitude scale for displaying these spectra (as well as the spectra in later figures) are logarithmic, similar to the amplitude scales used for plotting spectra in Figure 10–8. The vertical axis for these spectra is in decibels (or dB). If a particular spectral component has an amplitude **A**, then its amplitude expressed in decibels is

$$20\log_{10}A \ \text{dB}$$

Thus if *A* is multiplied by a factor of 10, the increase on the vertical scale of Figure 10–8 is 20 dB, whereas for a multiplying factor of 100, the increase is 40 dB.

Figure 10–8 depicts vowel production as the generation of a periodic source at the glottis and the filtering of this source by a vocal tract that has well-defined resonances. These resonances lead to several peaks in the filter characteristic of the vocal tract. This simple picture is sometimes modified, depending on the speaker and on the influence of other sounds that are produced adjacent to the vowel. For example, there may be irregularities in the glottal source, so that the glottal pulses are not completely periodic, or the pulses are accompanied by noise, leading to a voice that sounds rough or breathy. Or, the filtering by the vocal tract may be modified by lowering the soft palate (**velum**). The opening to the nasal cavity that is created by this movement (called the **velopharyngeal opening**) introduces extra prominences into the filter characteristic. (Recall those shown in Figures 10–7 and 10–8.) In English, a velopharyngeal opening is created in a vowel when that vowel is followed by a nasal consonant such as /m/ or /n/. The acoustic effect of this velopharyngeal opening can be seen if we compare the spectrograms and spectra in Figures 10–10 and 10–11. The vowel in the word *bin* in Figure 10–11 shows evidence of the opening to the nasal cavity, whereas there is no such evidence in *bid* in Figure 10–10. For the vowel in *bin*, there is an extra peak in the spectrum at around 1000 Hz.

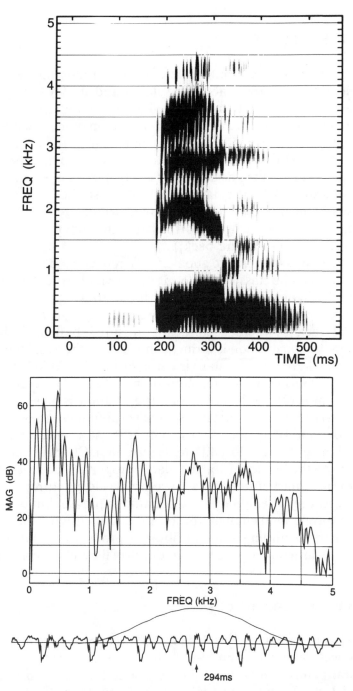

Figure 10–11. The spectrogram at the top is an utterance of the word *bin*. The spectrum in the lower panel is sampled in the vowel of this word. Comparison of this spectrum with that of the vowel [ɪ] in the word *bid* in Figure 10–10 shows some differences, particularly in the frequency range around 1 kHz. The extra peak and valley in the spectrum of the vowel in *bin* is evidence that a velopharyngeal opening has been created in anticipation of the nasal consonant at the end of the word.

✦ CONSONANTS

When vowels are generated, there is only a minor narrowing or constriction in the airway above the glottis, and air flows freely through the vocal tract. **Consonants**, on the other hand, are produced by creating a major constriction in some region of the vocal tract. This constriction is formed by moving one of the articulators (usually the lips, the tongue blade, or the tongue body) so that there is complete closure of the vocal tract, or a very narrow opening in the airway between that articulator and the outer surface of the vocal tract (usually the upper lip or incisors, the **hard palate** [bony roof of the front of the mouth], or the **soft palate** [muscular portion of the roof of the mouth — in the back]).

In English there are about 25 different consonants. These consonants can be classified in terms of: (1) which articulator is used to form the constriction; (2) whether the narrowing produced by this articulator forms a complete closure or only a partial closure of the vocal tract; (3) whether significant pressure is built up in the mouth when the constriction is formed; and (4) how the vocal folds are adjusted when the consonant is being produced. For example, these different properties for the consonant /b/ are: (1) the lips form the articulator, (2) the closure is complete, (3) there is pressure build-up, and (4) the glottis is adjusted so that vocal fold vibration is facilitated. By modifying one of these properties at a time, the consonant /b/ can be changed to a different consonant. Changing the articulator from the lips to the tongue blade (property 1) changes /b/ to /d/; forming a partial rather than a complete closure (property 2) gives /v/; creating a velopharyngeal opening to prevent build-up of pressure (property 3) changes /b/ to /m/; and modifying the glottal adjustment to inhibit vocal fold vibration produces /p/ rather than /b/.

We turn now to a discussion of each of these classes of consonants.

Sonorant Consonants

Consonants that are produced with a narrowing in the vocal tract but with no pressure build-up behind this narrowing are called **sonorant consonants**. The source of sound for these consonants is at the glottis. Because there is no impediment to the flow of air above the glottis, the vocal folds vibrate in much the same way as they do for vowels. Examples of spectrograms of several sonorant consonants as they occur in intervocalic position are shown in Figure 10–12. For all of these consonants, the continuing vertical striations provide evidence of vocal-fold vibration throughout the interval.

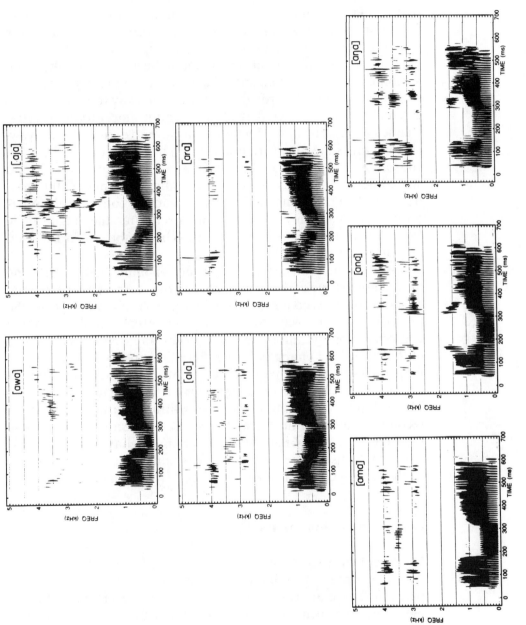

Figure 10–12. Spectrograms of several sonorant consonants in the phonetic environment [ɑ-ɑ].

Sonorant consonants differ from vowels in at least two ways. One is that the filtering that occurs in the vocal tract while the tract is constricted has characteristics different from those for vowels. Additional resonances may appear in the spectrum, or some resonances may be suppressed (as in the nasal consonants in Figure 10–12) or two resonances may come close together, merging into a single spectral peak (as in /w/ and /j/ in Figure 10–12). (The symbol /j/ represents the initial consonant in the word *yacht*.) A second attribute of sonorant consonants is that they are always produced with movement of the articulators toward or away from a constricted configuration; hence they always exhibit time-varying spectral characteristics. The movement is usually toward or away from a vowel. Sometimes the time variation is rapid or abrupt (as for the nasal consonants /m, n, ŋ/ or the consonant /l/ in Figure 10–12) and sometimes it is slow (as in /w, j, r/). The abrupt changes in the spectrum for the nasal consonants occur because a complete closure is formed by one of the articulators: the lips for /m/, the tongue blade for /n/, and the tongue body for /ŋ/. (The symbol /ŋ/ is the final consonant in the word *sing*.)

Immediately preceding the closure or immediately following the release for one of these nasal consonants, there is a time interval of about 50 milliseconds in which the vocal tract is moving from the preceding vowel toward the consonant configuration or from the consonant configuration toward the following vowel. As the shape of the vocal tract changes during these time intervals, the formant frequencies move in ways that indicate which of the three articulators (lips, tongue blade, or tongue body) is forming the constriction. These differences in the **formant transitions**, particularly for the second and third formants, can be seen in the spectrograms for these three consonants in Figure 10–12. Experiments have shown that listeners make use of these formant transitions in determining which of the three consonants was produced by a speaker.

Obstruent Consonants

Obstruent consonants are produced when the consonantal constriction causes pressure to build up in the vocal tract behind the constriction. There are two acoustic consequences of this build-up of pressure in the vocal tract. As the pressure in the vocal tract increases, the difference between the pressure in the trachea below the glottis and the pressure in the vocal tract above the glottis decreases. This decreased pressure across the glottis results in a reduced amplitude of the glottal air pulses, and with a sufficient increase in the pressure in the vocal tract, the vocal folds may stop vibrating altogether. A second consequence of the increased pressure in the vocal tract behind a constriction is that a rapid flow of air can occur through the constriction. This airflow can become turbulent, and result in the generation of noise in the vicinity of the constriction. Familiar examples are the hissing sound when the consonant /s/ is produced or the short burst of noise that is generated when the lips are opened at the beginning of a word like *pat*. The **turbulence noise source** has a continuous spectrum of the type illustrated in Figure 10–2J. The source is filtered as the sound passes through the vocal tract that is downstream from the constriction. There is a greater variety of obstruent consonants than sonorant consonants in English and in most languages. As noted earlier, these consonants can be produced with different articulators (different places of constriction), with different voicing characteristics, and with complete or partial closure at the constriction. Spectrograms of a number of obstruent consonants as they occur in intervocalic position are shown in Figures 10–13, 10–15, and 10–16.

The consonants in Figure 10–13 are **stop consonants**, for which the articulator forms a complete closure. These consonants are produced by forming the closure with the lips (/b/), the tongue blade (/d/), and the tongue body (/g/). The shape of the vocal tract in the midline when the closure is formed for each of these consonants is shown in Figure 10–14. In the case of the voiced stop consonants, the vocal folds continue to vibrate through all or most of the time interval when there is a closure. This vocal fold vibration can be seen as vertical striations near the bottom of the spectrograms in Figure 10–13 in the interval between the two vowels. Immediately following the time when these stop consonants are released (closure ceases as articulators move toward positions required for the following vowel sound), there is a rapid flow of air through the rapidly increasing opening. This flow of air creates a brief burst of noise, which acts as a source of sound. This source is filtered by the airway downstream from the constriction. The burst of sound that is radiated from the lips, therefore, has a different spectrum depending on the place in the mouth where the constriction is formed.

Spectra of the bursts for the three consonants /b, d, g/ are shown at the right side of Figure 10–13. The spectrum of the burst for /g/ has a prominence at a frequency of about 1750 Hz, reflecting the resonance of the portion of the vocal tract in front of the constriction formed by the raised tongue body. For the consonant /d/, there is a spectral prominence at a much higher frequency (about 4000 Hz), because the cavity in front of the constriction is relatively short (1.5–2 cm), as shown in Figure 10–14. There is no significant prominence in the spectrum of the burst for the labial consonant /b/, because there is no cavity in front of the constriction to filter the source.

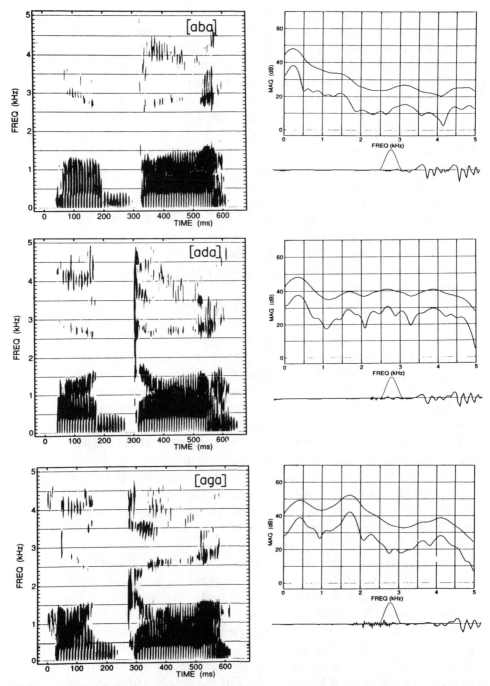

Figure 10–13. The left panels show spectrograms of three voiced stop consonants in the phonetic environment [ɑ-ɑ]. The spectra in the right panels (*lower lines*) are sampled on the release bursts of the consonants, with the waveforms displayed below the spectra. The upper line in each panel is a smoothed version of the spectra. The different spectrum shapes reflect the different positions of the articulators at the time they are released to generate the bursts.

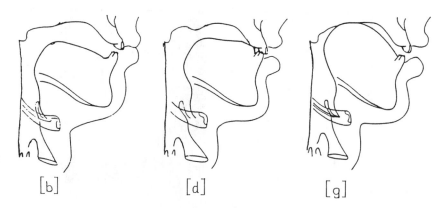

[b]   [d]   [g]

Figure 10-14. Sketches of the outline of the vocal tract in the midline when the closure is formed for three different stop consonants: /b/ (*left*), /d/ (*middle*), and /g/ (*right*). (From Perkell, 1969.)

As with the nasal consonants discussed above, the pattern of change of the formant frequencies (particularly the transitions of the second and third formants) immediately preceding or following the closure interval for the stop consonant provides information to a listener as to whether the consonant was produced with the lips, the tongue blade, or the tongue body. The different movements of the second and third formants just before the consonant closure and just after consonant release are evident in the spectrograms for the three stop consonants in Figure 10-13. This information supplements the information available in the properties of the burst.

For the stop consonants /b, d, g/, the noise burst at the consonant release is relatively short (5–20 ms), and vocal fold vibration occurs immediately after the burst. The vocal folds are already in a configuration such that they begin to vibrate as soon as pressure in the mouth is released and air begins to flow through the glottis. In the case of the voiceless stop consonants /p, t, k/, the vocal folds are spread apart at the time the consonant is released. A spectrogram of the consonant /t/ as it occurs between vowels is shown in Figure 10-15. When air begins to flow through the glottis after the consonant is released, the vocal folds are sufficiently far apart that vibration is not initiated immediately. Around the time of release, the speaker begins to bring the vocal folds together so that they are in a configuration that permits vibration to occur. This movement of the vocal folds takes about 50 milliseconds, and as a consequence, there is a delay of about 50 milliseconds from the time of release to the onset of vocal fold vibration. (This is called the **voice onset time**, or VOT.) During this time interval, turbulence noise is generated, first in the vicinity of the constriction formed by the lips, tongue blade, or tongue

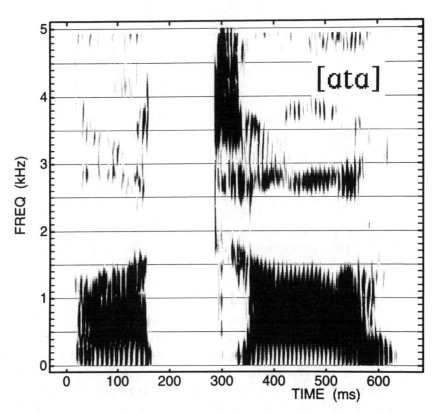

Figure 10–15. Spectrogram of the voiceless stop consonant [t] in the phonetic environment [ɑtɑ].

body (burst), and then in the vicinity of the glottis (**aspiration**). As was true of the voiced stop consonants /b, d, g/, the spectra of the noise bursts and aspirations reflect the places of articulation for /p, t, k/, namely at the lips, tongue blade, or tongue body. This delay time with noise can be seen in the spectrograms in Figure 10–15. The beginning of the noise (at a time of 270 ms on the spectrogram) occurs well in advance of the onset of vocal fold vibration at about 320 milliseconds.

The spectrograms in Figure 10–16 show examples of the **fricative consonants** /s/ and /z/ in intervocalic position. For these consonants, a narrow constriction is formed by the tongue blade, which is grooved at the midline and placed against the front part of the hard palate. The rapid airflow through the narrow air channel at the constriction creates a turbulence noise source which is shaped or filtered by the short cavity in front of the constriction. This filtering enhances the high frequencies for these consonants, as the spectrograms show. During the time interval in which the noise is generated, there is no vocal fold vibration for /s/. Glottal vibration contin-

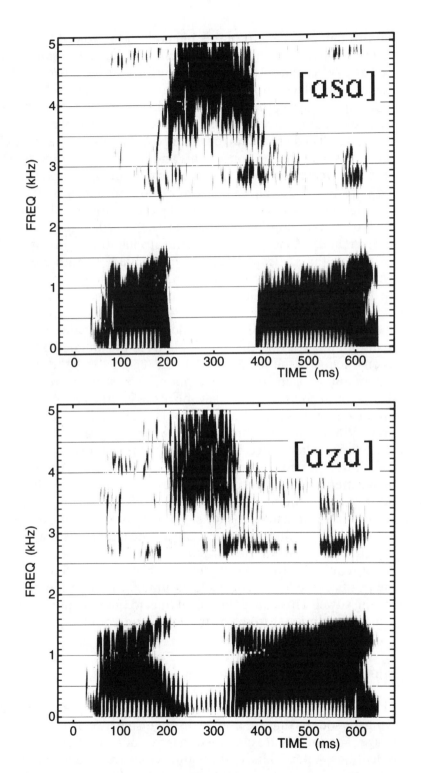

Figure 10–16. Spectrograms of the voiceless and voiced fricatives [s] and [z] in the phonetic environment [ɑ-ɑ].

ues through at least part of this interval for the voiced fricative /z/. Other fricative consonants (/ʃ/ as in *shoe*, /ʒ/ as in *measure*, /f/ as in *face*, and /v/ as in *vase*) are produced by forming the narrow constriction at other places along the front part of the vocal tract. As can be observed by saying these words aloud, each fricative pair has cognate voiced and voiceless consonants at each place of constriction.

In English there are two obstruent consonants that have the characteristics of both stop consonants and fricative consonants. These are the **affricate consonants** /tʃ/ and /dʒ/, as in the words *church* and *judge*, respectively. These consonants are produced by forming a complete closure of the airway by placing the tongue blade against the hard palate, similar to the closure achieved on the stop consonants /t/ and /d/. However, during the production of affricates, when the tongue tip is released, the part of the blade behind the tip continues to form a narrow constriction, and turbulence noise is generated for a time immediately following the release. This latter phase of the affricate release is similar to a fricative consonant.

All of the consonant sounds described above are produced by manipulating the lips, the tongue blade, or the tongue body to form a constriction in the vocal tract in some region above the glottis. The consonant /h/ as in *hat* is an exception, because no narrow constriction is formed in the vocal tract above the glottis. This consonant is produced by spreading the vocal folds apart so that they do not vibrate. When air flows through this relatively spread glottis, turbulence noise is generated in the vicinity of the glottis, and this noise constitutes the acoustic excitation for the vocal tract. A spectrogram of the utterance /ɑhɑ/, shown in Figure 10–17, illustrates the kind of noise that is generated for this /h/ sound. In contrast to fricative consonants or noise bursts for stop consonants, /h/ shows spectral peaks corresponding to several of the vocal tract resonances, and therefore has some of the attributes of a vowel. Because the tongue is not required for the production of /h/, talkers tend to anticipate the position the tongue needs to assume for production of the following vowel. This causes the vocal tract to filter the noise source in a manner similar to that of the following vowel.

Summary of Classification of Consonants

Linguists have developed a framework and terminology for classifying the sounds that are used to distinguish between words in a language. The sounds are classified in terms of a number of properties or features. A partial list of the features that are used to classify consonants is given in the first column of Table 10–1. The remaining columns indicate, for each of a number of different consonants, wheth-

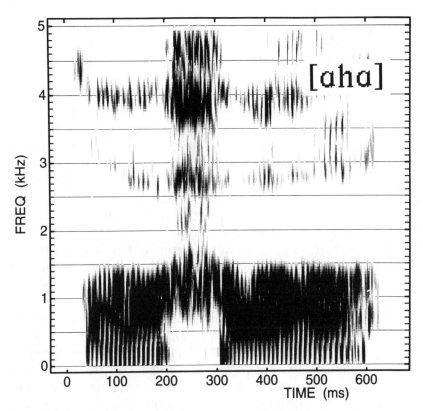

Figure 10-17. Spectrogram of the consonant [h] in the phonetic environment [ɑhɑ].

Table 10-1. A partial listing of feature values for some of the consonants
in English.

Feature	p	t	k	b	d	g	f	s	v	z	m	n	ŋ
Lips	+	−	−	+	−	−	+	−	+	−	+	−	−
Tongue blade	−	+	−	−	+	−	−	+	−	+	−	+	−
Tongue body	−	−	+	−	−	+	−	−	−	−	−	−	+
Voice	−	−	−	+	+	+	−	−	+	+	+	+	+
Continuant	−	−	−	−	−	−	+	+	+	+	−	−	−
Sonorant	−	−	−	−	−	−	−	−	−	−	+	+	+

er the various features are present or absent in the sound. This list
of six features must be expanded to about 15–20 features to permit
classification of all the vowels and additional consonants that can
occur in language. See Chapter 3 by Stoel-Gammon and Stone for
a more complete list.

The first three features in Table 10–1 specify which of the three articulators is active in forming the constriction in the vocal tract. The feature [**voice**] indicates whether or not the laryngeal structures are adjusted to permit continued vocal fold vibration during the consonant, [**continuant**] indicates whether the articulator forms a complete closure (i.e., [−continuant]) or just a partial closure in the airway, and [sonorant] specifies whether or not pressure builds up in the mouth behind the constriction when the consonant is produced. Pressure build-up occurs for a [−sonorant] consonant. Table 10–1 shows, for example, that the consonant /b/and /p/ share all features except [voice]. On the other hand, for the consonants /n/ and /s/ the features specifying the articulator are the same but the remaining features are different.

Classification of sounds in terms of features also provides an efficient way of describing the constraints on sound sequences that occur in different languages. For example, in English the plural for a noun is formed by appending /s/ to the ends of words like *back* and *laugh*, and by appending /z/ for words like *bed* and *cave*. That is, the [−voice] consonant /s/ is appended if the final consonant of the word is [−voice], and the [+voice] consonant /z/ is appended if the final consonant is [+voice]. Another constraint in English applies when a word ends in an obstruent consonant that is preceded by a nasal consonant, as in *send, lymph*, and *think*. The constraint here is that the nasal segment takes on the same feature [lips], [tongue blade], or [tongue body] that characterizes the final obstruent consonant. A word such as *semt* is not possible in English because it violates this constraint.

◆ SPEECH SOUNDS IN SENTENCES

When phrases and sentences are produced, some of the properties of the sounds that form the words in the sentences may undergo modification, relative to the properties that have been illustrated for the simpler utterances in Figures 10–10 to 10–16. The kinds of modifications depend the speaking style and the context in which the sounds occur. Examples of these influences of context can be seen in the spectrogram of the sentence in Figure 10–18. The sentence is "He will list some words in that book," and there are several places in the sentence where the sounds do not have the form that would be observed if the individual words were spoken clearly. For example, in the sequence *list some*, there is a long fricative interval between 520 and 720 ms, but no evidence that a closure occurred for the stop consonant /t/. Or, in the word *that*, the initial consonant /ð/ (occurring at around 1300 ms) is produced as a nasal consonant rather

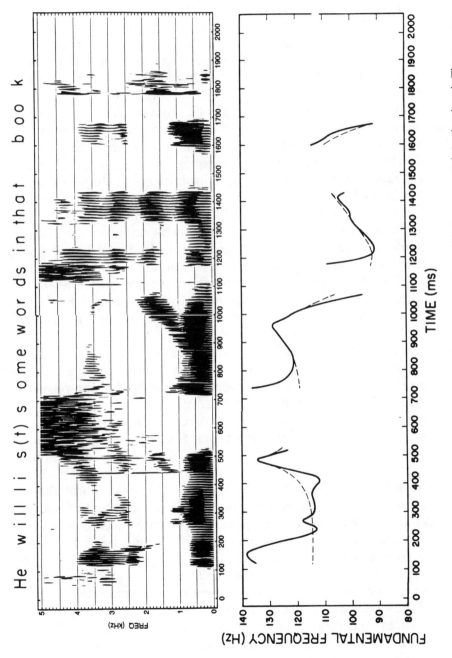

Figure 10–18. The upper panel is a spectrogram of the sentence: *He will list some words in that book*. The spectrogram illustrates some modifications of speech sounds when words are spoken in a sentence context. The solid line in the lower panel gives the contour of fundamental frequency versus time for the same sentence. The dashed line is an estimate of the shape of the fundamental frequency contour if local perturbations due to individual vowels and consonants were removed from the original contour. This dashed contour is intended to show which words in the sentence are produced with prominence and to mark the boundaries of the utterance. See text.

than as the expected voiced fricative consonant. The kinds of modifications that can occur in running speech are constrained in particular ways, and native listeners appear to take these modifications into account without much difficulty.

The spectrogram in Figure 10–18 also illustrates the range of durations of phonetic units that can occur between speech sounds, especially when the sounds occur in longer utterances. For example, some syllables have greatly reduced prominence, and the durations of the vowels in these syllables are considerably shorter than the durations of vowels in syllables with greater prominence. In Figure 10–18, the vowels in *some* (740 ms) and *in* (1200 ms) undergo this kind of reduction. Other vowels receive special prominence in the sentence (i.e., the vowel in *words*), and consequently have a greater duration. Linguists refer to these changes in prominence as changes in syllable **stress**. In addition to the influence of the prominence of a syllable, several other factors contribute to the durations of the vowels and consonants. For example, some vowels are intrinsically longer than other vowels, and vowels at the end of a phrase or a sentence tend to be longer than vowels in the middle of the utterance.

The durations of vowels, then, as well as the durations of consonant units, provide information to a listener as to which syllables are more prominent than other syllables and also help to delineate the boundaries of phrases or sentences.

A speaker also marks prominences and boundaries by causing variations in the frequency of vocal fold vibration during the vowels in an utterance. The **fundamental frequency** (F_0) for a vowel can also undergo changes due to modifications of the vowel quality and to attributes of the consonant that precedes the vowel. The F_0 contour for the sentence "He will list some words in that book" is shown below the spectrogram in Figure 10–18. Some of the fluctuations in F_0 are a consequence of local effects of individual vowels and consonants. For example, the high F_0 on the first vowel is probably because the vowel /i/ is known to raise F_0 relative to its value for a vowel with a lower tongue-body position. Likewise, certain consonants that are adjacent to vowels can cause a local increase or decrease in the fundamental frequency near the vowel boundaries. An example is the increased F_0 at the beginning of the word *some* (at about 730 ms), caused by the voiceless consonant /s/. The main variations in F_0, however, are a consequence of the speaker's plan to place prominences on certain syllables, as well as to mark the boundaries of the utterance. In this example, the dashed line gives an estimate of the component of the fundamental frequency that is intended to mark the prominences and boundaries, with local effects due to particular vowels and consonants subtracted out. There are prominences on the words *list, words,* and *book,* with the final fall in fundamental frequency indicating the end of the utterance.

◆ SPEAKER DIFFERENCES AND SPEECH STYLES

We have focused up to now on the acoustic properties that distinguish one speech sound from another. It is well known, however, that the speech of a particular talker has individual characteristics that distinguish him or her from other speakers independent of the attributes that identify which sounds and words were spoken. We have seen, for example, that the frequency of vocal fold vibration for adult female speakers is higher, on the average, than it is for adult male speakers, and the formant frequencies for vowels spoken by women are, on the average, higher than for vowels produced by men. Speakers can differ from each other, however, in many other ways that are reflected in the acoustic patterns of their utterances. For example, people have different voice qualities, either because their laryngeal structures are different or because they choose to adjust the configuration of their vocal folds in different ways. These different voice qualities can be a consequence of different waveforms of glottal vibration, turbulence noise generation at the glottis, or irregular vibration of the vocal folds. Different talkers also can produce certain sounds or sequences of sounds, such as nasal consonants or particular types of vowels, in unique ways.

The acoustic characteristics of a particular speaker also may vary depending on the speaker's emotional state or the speaking situation. For example, the range of fundamental frequency, the glottal waveform, and the temporal pattern of the speech can be influenced by the talker's emotional or physiological state. There are a variety of disorders of speech production that can have a marked influence on the speech patterns of a talker.

To illustrate the kinds of differences that can occur between speakers, we show in Figure 10–19 spectra of the same vowel (in the word *but*) produced by two different female speakers. The first formant frequency is about the same for the two speakers (approximately 900 Hz), and the second formant frequencies are slightly different. Substantial differences between the speakers can be seen in the amplitudes of the first two harmonics (both of which are below 500 Hz) in relation to the amplitude of the first formant peak around 900 Hz. Also the first formant peak is much more prominent for speaker 2 (in the right panel) than for speaker 1. The spectrum for speaker 1 shows regularly spaced harmonics only up to about 1500 Hz, with an irregular spectrum shape at higher frequencies indicat-

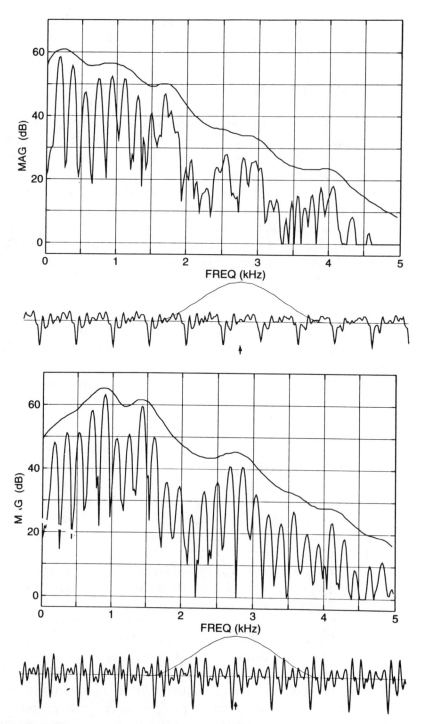

Figure 10–19. Spectra of the vowel in the word *but* produced by two adult female speakers. The spectra illustrate the differences that can occur between speakers. See text.

ing the presence of turbulence noise. For speaker 2, on the other hand, there are uniformly spaced harmonics throughout the frequency range up to 5000 Hz. Listeners hear the words with these two vowels as the same word *but*, but one voice (speaker 1) is clearly judged to be more breathy than the other. These differences are related to differences in the glottal sound source.

Figure 10–20 illustrates a more severe individual difference: a comparison of spectrograms of the production of the word *knot* by a normal speaker and by a speaker with a disorder in the control and coordination of the muscles used in speaking, known as dysarthria. One obvious difference is in the duration of the utterance, with the vowel and the final consonant closure being much longer for the dysarthric speaker. More detailed examination of the spectrograms shows that the dysarthric speaker exhibits some instability in the vowel and has difficulties in forming the final consonant. These kinds of quantitative acoustic analyses can have considerable value in diagnosing deviations from normal speech patterns, and in prescribing measures that might be taken for remediation of speech disorders. The differences seen in Figure 10–20 reflect temporal and spatial adjustments in the deployment of articulators in the vocal tract. These adjustments in the acoustic filter change the acoustic output of the vocal tract.

✦ SUMMARY AND CONCLUSIONS

The words that make up an utterance are represented in a speaker's memory as sequences of sounds or segments. Each of these seg-

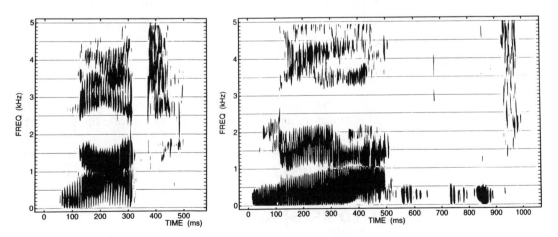

Figure 10–20. Spectrograms of the word *knot* produced by a normal speaker (*left panel*) and by a speaker with a disorder of muscle control (*right panel*).

ments contains instructions that specify how to move and to shape various articulators to produce the appropriate sound pattern. Movements of the articulators must be coordinated to perform two functions. One function is to generate sources of sound by modulating the flow of air in the vocal tract, either at the vocal folds or at a place in the upper airway where a constriction gives rise to turbulence in the airflow. The second function is to adjust the shape of the airway to filter the sources. Taken together, these two functions form the basis for the **source-filter theory of speech production**.

Descriptions of this acoustic process are most conveniently formulated in terms of source spectra and filtering mechanisms that modify these spectra. Speech sounds can be classified according to the kinds of sources that are used to generate the sounds and the nature of the filtering of these sources. A basic classification is in terms of vowels and consonants. Other categories are based on which articulator is used to form a constriction, how this articulator is positioned, and how the larynx is adjusted.

When an utterance consisting of a sequence of words is produced, a speaker can manipulate the durations of speech sounds and the frequency of vocal fold vibration to mark certain syllables as more prominent than others and to indicate boundaries between groups of words (e.g., at phrase and sentence boundaries). In casual speech, certain attributes of some speech sounds may be modified relative to their properties when they are produced slowly and clearly.

Speakers have particular characteristics that distinguish their speech from that of other speakers. Certain acoustic attributes of the speech of a given individual may vary depending on the emotional state of the speaker or the speech style that the speaker chooses to use in a particular situation. Acoustic analysis can also be used to interpret deviations from normal speech production.

◆ REFERENCES

Baer, T. (1975). *Investigation of phonation using excised larynxes.* Unpublished doctoral dissertation, Massachusetts Institute of Technology, Cambridge, MA.

Perkell, J. S. (1969). *Physiology of speech production: Results and implications of a quantitative cineradiographic study.* Cambridge, MA: MIT Press.

◆ SUGGESTED READINGS

Clark, J., & Yallop, C. (1990). *An introduction to phonetics and phonology.* Cambridge, MA: Blackwell.

Denes, P., & Pinson, E. (1973). *The speech chain.* Garden City, NY: Anchor Books.

Fant, G. (1960). *Acoustic theory of speech production.* The Hague: Mouton.

Flanagan, J. L. (1972). *Speech analysis, synthesis, and perception.* Berlin: Springer-Verlag.

Kent, R. D., & Read, C. (1992). *The acoustic analysis of speech.* San Diego: Singular Publishing Group.

Kent, R. D., Atal, B. S., & Miller, J. L. (Eds.). (1991). *Papers in speech communication: Speech production.* Woodbury, NY: Acoustical Society of America.

Ladefoged, P. (1982). *A course in phonetics.* New York: Harcourt Brace Jovanovich.

Pickett, J. M. (1980). *The sounds of speech communication.* Baltimore: University Park Press.

Rosen, S., & Howell, P. (1991). *Signals and systems for speech and hearing.* San Diego: Academic Press.

✦ GLOSSARY

Affricate consonants: obstruent consonants produced with characteristics of both stop consonants and fricative consonants. Examples are the first and last sounds in the words *church* and *judge.*

Aperiodic: waveforms that are nonrepetitive. Waveforms that are not periodic.

Articulators: movable structures within the vocal tract or airway extending from the larynx to the mouth opening.

Aspiration: noise generated in the vicinity of the glottis.

Complex periodic waveform: a waveform constructed of two or more sinusoids whose frequencies are multiples of the frequency of the waveform.

Consonants: speech sounds produced by creating a major constriction in some region of the vocal tract.

Continuant: a consonant produced without complete closure of the vocal tract.

Diphthong: a vocalic glide within a single syllable (as in *bide* or *shout*).

Filtering: frequency-selective modifications of a sound source resulting from the resonating characteristics of the vocal tract.

Formants: peaks in the acoustic spectrum resulting from resonances within the vocal tract during speech production.

Formant transitions: time varying changes in resonant frequencies resulting from changing positions of articulators within the vocal tract during speech production.

Frequency: the number of complete cycles of a waveform per second. Frequency is measured in Hertz (Hz).

Fricative consonant: a continuant consonant produced by creating a narrow constriction within the vocal tract and supplying sufficient air flow to cause a continuing turbulence noise source.

Fundamental: the sinusoidal component of a complex wave whose frequency is equal to the repetition frequency of the waveform. The fundamental frequency is sometimes called the first harmonic.

Fundamental frequency: frequency of vocal fold vibration.

Glottis: the air channel opening between the vocal folds (in the larynx) through which air escapes during voice production, and through which air passes during normal respiration.

Hard palate: bony roof of the front of the mouth. Located anterior to the soft palate, which forms the back portion of the roof of the mouth.

Harmonics: whole number multiples of the fundamental frequency.

Larynx: the cartilaginous structure, located above the trachea and below the pharynx, that houses the vocal folds. The larynx is used to generate voiced sound and whisper during speech production.

Obstruent consonant: a consonant produced with a narrowing of the vocal tract that causes pressure to be built up behind the constriction.

Periodic: a pattern of sound pressure that is repetitive (repeats itself in the same amount of time).

Resonance: peaks in the transfer function of the vocal tract during acoustic filtering of the sound source. Resonance peaks are related to the speed of sound and the dimensions of the vocal tract.

Segment: an identifiable sound within a sequence of sounds that form a word.

Soft palate: the muscular portion of the roof of the mouth (also called the velum). Located posterior to the hard palate; forms the back portion of the roof of the mouth.

Sonorant consonant: a consonant produced with a narrowing of the vocal tract, but with no pressure build-up behind the narrowing.

Sound source: the generation of sound energy somewhere within the vocal tract, usually by narrowing of the airway.

Sound spectrum: a graph displaying frequency on the horizontal axis and amplitude on the vertical axis.

Source-filter theory of speech production: theory that describes the production of speech sounds as the generation of sound sources and the filtering of these sources by the vocal tract.

Spectrogram: a three-dimensional graph displaying frequency versus time, with spectrum amplitude represented by the degree of blackness in the pattern.

Stop consonant: a consonant sound produced as a result of a complete closure formed by an articulator in the vocal tract.

Stress: changes in the prominence of a syllable as a result of changes in fundamental frequency, intensity, and duration of the syllable.

Turbulence noise source: sound produced with a continuous spectrum. Turbulence noise sources result from the random variation of air pressure created when air particles pass through a narrow constriction at high velocity.

Velopharyngeal opening: the opening between the posterior portion of the oral cavity (actually oro-pharynx) and the nasal cavity.

Velum: soft palate, the back portion of the roof of the mouth.

Vocal folds: muscles and connective tissue located within the larynx that are used to produce voice (through vocal fold vibration). The two vocal folds are attached anteriorly to the thyroid cartilage and posteriorly to the arytenoid cartilages.

Vocal tract: the tortuously shaped airway extending from the larynx to the lips. The vocal tract can include the nasal airway during the production of nasal sounds.

Voice: sound produced by the larynx, usually through vibration of the vocal folds.

Voice onset time: the time interval between the release of pressure, built up as a result of vocal tract constriction during stop consonant production, and the onset of vocal fold vibration (voicing).

Vowel sounds: sounds produced when the vocal tract is relatively open (unconstricted).

Waveform: a graph of sound pressure versus time.

Genetics, Syndrome Delineation, and Communicative Impairment

ROBERT J. SHPRINTZEN, Ph.D.

After completing this chapter, you should be able to:

◆ Understand basic principles of human inheritance.

◆ Understand how syndromes are delineated.

◆ Know the difference between a syndrome and isolated anomalies.

◆ Know when to be suspicious of a possible syndromic diagnosis in a child.

◆ Interact with colleagues in the fields of genetics and dysmorphology.

◆ Contribute meaningfully in the full description of a child with multiple anomalies.

Congenital anomalies occur in at least 14% of the general population, often as part of multiple anomaly disorders known as syndromes. There are thousands of syndromes which have anomalies that result in abnormal speech, language, cognition, and hearing. The most recent advances in molecular genetics have led to the identification of the mechanisms by which many human anomalies occur. This chapter will discuss how to identify children with multiple anomaly syndromes and the importance of reaching a correct diagnosis. The direct impact of syndrome identification on patient care will be illustrated. The future of how molecular genetics will interface with the communicative sciences will also be discussed.

There is little question that the most exciting area of activity in the biomedical sciences is genetics. An intimate coordination between basic laboratory science and clinical practice has occurred over the past several years and has opened up bright promise for more effective treatment and even eradication of many human diseases. Specialists practicing in the area of communication disorders have been somewhat slow to respond to the progress taking place in human genetics. Undergraduate and graduate curricula have not focused on congenital anomalies and the manner in which they cause communicative impairment. Few speech-language pathologists and audiologists have developed significant expertise in the area of human genetics so that their contributions to the scientific literature relating to congenital anomalies have been sparse.

This chapter provides a basic introduction to the disciplines of dysmorphology, syndromology, human genetics, and molecular genetics (described below). The root causes of many types of communicative impairment will be discussed and related to basic biological mechanisms that result in human malformation.

◆ SYNDROME IDENTIFICATION

What Is a Syndrome and Why Study It?

The study of human anomalies is known as **dysmorphology**, but may be variously referred to as **syndromology**, **medical genetics**, and **clinical genetics**. Although the term **genetics** is used to describe the study of individuals with anomalies, not all abnormalities are caused by genetic factors; but the term *genetics* typically is used to describe the study of what was previously known as *birth defects*. The term *birth defects* is not typically used any more; **anomaly** is the preferred term. An **anomaly** may be defined as any deviation from normal structure, form, or function in an individual. The reason for the preference of the term *anomaly* over *birth defect* is that not all anomalies are present or detectable at birth. This is particularly true of communicative disorders. You will note that the definition of *anomaly* is not limited to structural deviations. Disorders of function also are considered to be anomalies which would include mental retardation, language impairment, certain articulation impairments, and voice disorders if they can be shown to be related to a problem of dysmorphogenesis (abnormal embryonic and fetal development). Because speech or language disorders cannot be present or detected at birth, the term *birth defect* is inappropriate, but because these communicative impairments can result from dysmorphogenetic influences (such as brain malformations, cleft palate, or clefts of the larynx), they must be considered to be anomalies.

Syndrome is a term commonly used in human disease. The word *syndrome* is derived from the Greek roots, *syn* (together) and *dramein* (to run), so that an appropriate definition of syndrome is "things which run together." *Syndrome* typically is used to imply a symptom pattern which has been seen before and recognized to be a pattern of disorders that occurs frequently enough so that the co-occurrence of the symptoms cannot be attributed to chance. *Syndrome* is used frequently in the biomedical sciences, as in AIDS (*A*uto*I*mmune *D*eficiency *S*yndrome), Munchausen-syndrome-by-proxy (a psychological disorder), and Pickwickian syndrome (a sleep disorder characterized by obstructive apnea in obese middle-aged males).

In dysmorphology, *syndrome* has a more specific meaning. A syndrome may be defined as the presence of multiple anomalies in a single individual with all of those anomalies having a common cause. In other words, it is unrealistic to think that someone who has a congenital heart anomaly, short stature, and an inguinal hernia in association with severely hypernasal speech, language impairment, and severe articulation disorder has all of these findings occurring together strictly by chance, even though each of these anomalies occurs with frequency in the general population (see case study 1). One might ask why it is so unlikely for several common anomalies to occur in a single individual strictly by chance? One needs to invoke nothing more complicated than simple mathematics to answer this question. Incidence statistics have been computed for most anomalies detected at birth, such as cleft palate, inguinal hernia, and congenital heart anomalies. For example, congenital heart disease occurs with a frequency of at least 1:400 live births. Cleft palate (without cleft lip) has a frequency of approximately 1:2,500 live births. What is the probability that one child will be born with both a cleft palate and a congenital heart lesion such as a ventriculoseptal defect? The odds would be 1:1,000,000 (see case report). At this rate, only one or two children per year would be born in the United States with the combination of cleft palate and heart anomalies. Is this truly the prevalence of children with this combination? Not at all. In fact, well over 5% of children with cleft palate have heart anomalies. If one were to add inguinal hernia and small stature as additional findings in the same child, the probability of this association would be less than one per billion. However, the association of cleft palate, heart anomalies, inguinal hernias, and small stature is seen in at least 1:5,000 live births. The association of these anomalies at frequencies far higher than would be expected by chance indicates that the association is not caused by random assortment, but rather as a recurring pattern of anomalies, or a syndrome.

The study of genetics has become increasingly sophisticated with the advent of new biochemical tests for the study of DNA, the substance which serves as the basis for human heredity. The study of human genetics currently consists of two branches which of necessity overlap to establish the correct diagnosis: clinical genetics and molecular genetics. **Clinical genetics** refers to the process of physical examination and direct patient contact, including the process of genetic counseling. The information derived from the physical examination results in the patient's **phenotype** which is the sum total of all clinical findings, including both physical and functional characteristics. Although physical findings such as the height, weight, head circumference, number and shape of the fingers and toes, and heart characteristics such as congenital heart anomalies are all a part of the phenotype, so are functional and behavioral features such as intellect, language, articulation, hearing, and psychological aspects.

Molecular genetics is the newer field of study and refers to the application of biochemical tests to study the actual mechanisms of heredity. By utilizing new techniques of DNA analysis, it is now possible to locate specific genes and trace their effects. The genetic makeup of the individual is the person's **genotype**. Clinical genetics and molecular genetics interface in matching the phenotype to the genotype, thereby allowing the assessment of an abnormal gene's effect. To properly study genotype, clinical geneticists must first identify the correct phenotype so that molecular analysis can be applied to the correct diagnosis.

Etiologies of Syndromes

Syndromes, and anomalies in general, may be caused by four different categories of etiologies: chromosomal, genetic, teratogenic, and mechanical. To date, thousands of syndromes with known causes have been identified. Several excellent source books are listed at the end of this chapter, as well as several computer programs which may prove to be informative. Identifying the type of cause (chromosomal, genetic, teratogenic, or mechanically induced) often assists the clinician in understanding the potential outcome for the affected child, but the primary importance of identifying the type of cause is the ability to counsel parents regarding their reproductive future, including the risks they may be facing. Identifying the etiology allows parents to make informed reproductive decisions guided by the knowledge of their recurrence risk.

Chromosomal Syndromes

Children with chromosomally induced syndromes are usually small of stature, mentally retarded, and may be severely malformed. **Chromosomes** are long strands made of DNA and protein which carry the genetic material that guides the formation of the developing embryo (see Figure 11-1). Each human cell contains 46 chromosomes. Forty-four of these chromosomes contain the majority of genetic information that guides human formation and function and are called **autosomes**. These chromosomes are paired with each member of the pair being identical in appearance to its partner and are identified by number from 1 through 22. The remaining pair of chromosomes are called the **sex chromosomes** because their primary purpose is to determine the sex of the organism. These two chromosomes are labeled by the letters X or Y. The X chromosome is larger than the Y chromosome. Males have an X and a Y chromosome, females

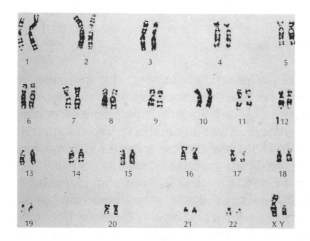

Figure 11-1. An example of a karyotype with banding of a normal male.

have two X chromosomes. It is apparent that the purpose of the Y chromosome is to produce male individuals. The X chromosome carries a number of genes which have functions unrelated to producing a sex phenotype. Chromosomes are large enough to be seen under a microscope during cell division. A chromosome analysis, or **karyotype**, is performed by observing human cells (usually white blood cells) during cell division, applying stains which define small sections of the chromosome with alternating dark and light bands (hence the term "banding"), photographing the chromosomes, and carefully examining the photographs for the integrity and size of the chromosomes. The bands are measured to determine if very small pieces of chromosome might be missing. Deletions of whole chromosomes or pieces of chromosomes, extra chromosome material, abnormal breakages of chromosomes, or abnormal configurations of chromosomes are noted. If abnormalities are found in the structure or amount of chromosomal material, it is of major significance because even small pieces of microscopically visible chromosome contain many genes and the abnormalities resulting from chromosome alterations would represent the effect of many errors in gene action. A karyotype should be suggested when a child presents with multiple anomalies, especially if they include small stature, mental retardation, major limb anomalies, major brain anomalies, and major heart anomalies. A karyotype would not be suggested if the pattern of anomalies seen in the child fits a pattern known to be consistent with a recognized genetic, teratogenic, or mechanically induced syndrome. A positive karyotype yields a firm diagnosis which will explain all of the anomalies seen in the child. Because most chromosomal syndromes result in a broad spectrum of major anomalies and often include brain and craniofacial anomalies, disorders of speech, language, cognition, and hearing are very common.

Genetic Syndromes

Syndromes of genetic etiology are not the same as chromosomal syndromes because the amount of abnormal genetic material is much smaller, usually amounting to a single gene. Genes are the basic units of human heredity and actually represent small segments of the large DNA molecules that comprise the chromosomes. DNA molecules consist of two strands of intertwined sugar and phosphate molecules connected by pairs of amino acids called **base pairs** (see Figure 11–2). Genes vary in size according to the number of base pairs necessary to perform a particular function. If an error occurs in the sequencing or structure of the base pairs, the gene's function will be

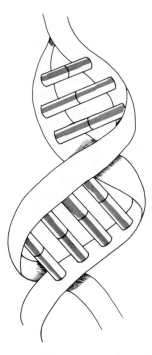

Figure 11–2. Drawing of a portion of a DNA molecule.

altered. An alteration in the gene is referred to as a **mutation**. Genes also can be deleted which also would result in an error in the process of embryonic development. The 22 pairs of autosomes contain strings of genes, approximately 100,000, placed in specific order along each chromosome. The sequencing of the genes along the chromosome is the set of instructions which causes development of the organism. This set of instructions encoded by the genes is known as the **genome**. The approximately 100,000 genes making up the human genome is made of 3 billion base pairs. It therefore is obvious that deciphering the human genome code is a monumental task, yet it is proceeding nonetheless.

Each gene on the autosomes has a corresponding partner in the same location on the matching chromosome. The genes on the X chromosome do not have corresponding partners on the Y chromosome in males, but do have counterparts on the matching X chromosome in females. Abnormal traits caused by single mutant genes can be inherited in the following manner:

1. Autosomal dominant

2. Autosomal recessive

3. X-linked

It is not the purpose of this chapter to teach the principles of elementary Mendelian inheritance. This information is easily obtained by reading any elementary biology text. However, suffice it to say that in **autosomal dominant inheritance**, the mutant gene is located on one of the 44 autosomes and its effect is expressed in the individual even though its partner gene is normal. Because offspring inherit half of their chromosomes from each of their parents (they inherit one chromosome from each pair from each parent), the risk of inheriting a single mutant gene is 50% (see Figure 11–3). In **autosomal recessive inheritance**, both members of the gene pair must be mutant for the trait to be expressed. Parents who give birth to children with autosomal recessive disorders do not show the trait because they have only one half of the genetic complement necessary to express the trait (see Figure 11–3). The recurrence risk is 25% because that is the chance that an offspring will inherit both mutant genes from the parents, each of whom has one normal gene and one abnormal gene.

In **X-linked recessive disorders**, the mutant gene is carried on the X chromosome. It is rare for females to express X-linked traits. In order to do so, they would need to inherit an abnormal X chromosome gene from both parents. Usually, the mother's X chromosome, if abnormal, will be counteracted by the father's normal X chromosome (thus making the child female). Males express X-linked traits because their Y chromosome has no normal gene to counteract the mutant X chromosome gene (see Figure 11–3). There also may be X-linked dominant traits, but these are very rare and do not comprise any of the common conditions associated with speech, language, or hearing disorders.

There are two other types of genetic causes of traits: polygenic (or multifactorial) and contiguous gene syndromes. **Multifactorial** disorders are those caused by an interaction of several (or many) genes and environmental influences. For many years, cleft lip and cleft palate were thought to be multifactorially caused traits because they did not follow simple patterns of dominant, recessive, or X-linked inheritance (Fraser, 1970). Today, the majority of clinicians and researchers understand that clefting has many causes, and only a small percentage of cases are inherited multifactorially.

Contiguous gene disorders are a newly recognized group of diseases caused by deletions of small portions of DNA which contains several genes occupying a continuous segment of chromosome. Each DNA molecule contains a series of genes. A deletion or mutation of a large DNA molecule will cause the alteration or deletion of a number of genes that are spatially connected in a chain on the chromosome and therefore called contiguous. Some syndromes that have a large number of anomalies, which would be difficult to at-

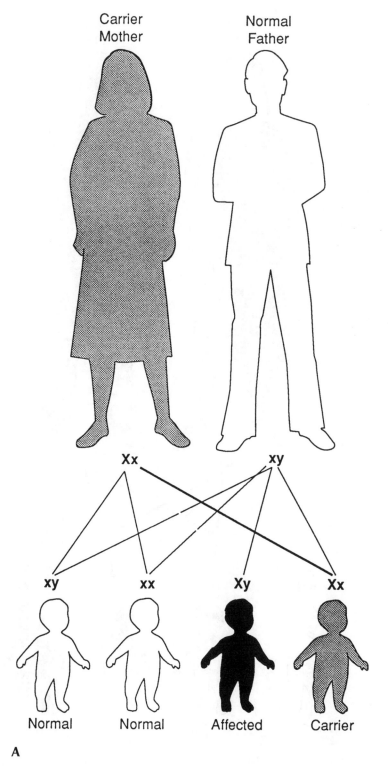

Figure 11-3. Diagramatic representation of the patterns of inheritance.

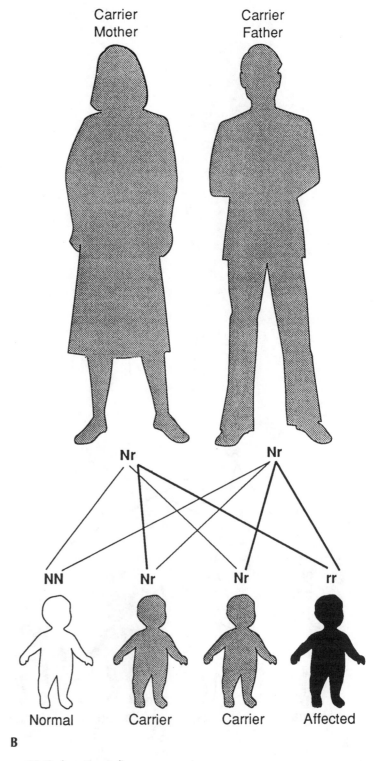

B

Figure 11-3 *(continued)*

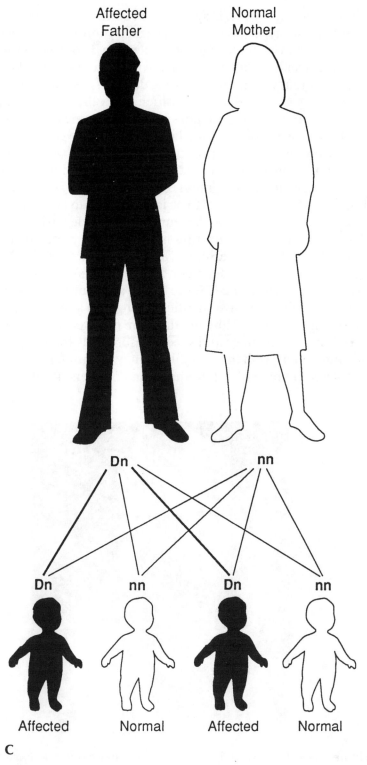

C

Figure 11-3 *(continued)*

tribute to a single gene, may represent contiguous gene syndromes. There are two types of contiguous gene syndromes: those with and those without visible chromosome deletions. Those with visible chromosome deletions can be detected with high resolution karyotypes. Those without visible chromosome deletions require the use of new molecular genetics techniques which allow the analysis of individual genes and DNA sequences on chromosomes and have found deletions of areas of DNA too large to be a single gene, yet too small to be seen under the microscope. For example, velo-cardio-facial syndrome, a disorder inherited in an autosomal dominant manner, has been located to a segment of the long arm of chromosome 22. The deleted region appears to be large enough to encompass at least several genes, which may account for the wide variety of anomalies in this syndrome affecting multiple body parts, including the palate, brain, heart, face, hands, abdomen, and genitals. Other contiguous gene syndromes include Prader-Willi syndrome, Beckwith-Wiedemann syndrome (Figure 11–4), and Rubinstein-Taybi syndrome, all of which have significant language and speech disorders as common features. Although these are relatively rare disorders, the prevalence of language and speech disorders is frequent enough so that individuals with these problems may be seen fairly often by specialists in the field of communication disorders. Prader-Willi syn-

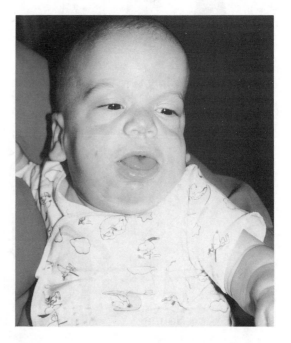

Figure 11–4. Child with Beckwith-Wiedemann syndrome. Note the large lower jaw and large tongue.

drome is an interesting disorder because it is characterized by severe obesity, hypotonia (poor muscle tone), developmental delay, and compulsive overeating. Language disorders also may be accompanied by severely hypernasal speech during early childhood. However, with advancing age, the hypernasality tends to resolve spontaneously (Sadewitz & Shprintzen, 1987), probably because the hypotonia diminishes with age. Beckwith-Wiedemann syndrome is a disorder with the key findings of an omphalocele (a herniation of the abdominal organs through a defect in the umbilical region), macroglossia (an abnormally large tongue), developmental delay, hypotonia, overgrowth, and creases in the ear lobes. Cleft palate also may be found. The enlarged tongue, hypotonia, and developmental delay nearly ensures the presence of speech and language disorders in this syndrome. Rubinstein-Taybi syndrome is characterized by small stature, mental retardation, a characteristic facial appearance including a beaked nose, and broad thumbs and big toes.

Teratogenic Syndromes

Teratogens, literally translated, are things that produce "monsters" (from the Greek *teratos*). In essence, a **teratogen** is an agent in the embryonic environment that interferes with the normal embryologic process, resulting in anomalies. The most publicized teratogens have been alcohol and thalidomide (a drug used for morning sickness during pregnancy which was popular in Europe in the 1950s and 1960s). Thalidomide is used infrequently today, but fetal alcohol syndrome (Figure 11–5) probably is one of the most common of all multiple anomaly disorders and is clearly under-reported. There are five basic types of teratogens: viruses and bacteria, medicinal drugs, illegal drugs (i.e., "street drugs"), naturally occurring or common environmental substances, and maternal exposure to external energy sources. The effects of viruses are best known in association with rubella (the "German measles" virus), but other viruses also are potent teratogens, including cytomegalovirus (a virus that causes cellular enlargement), herpes simplex (the class of viruses that cause cold sores and genital herpes), and varicella zoster (the chicken pox virus), all of which cause eye anomalies, **microcephaly** (reduced head circumference, usually related to small brain size), and mental retardation. Teratogenic medicinal drugs include many of the anticonvulsants (antiseizure medications), especially phenytoins and hydantoins (which result in craniofacial anomalies, limb anomalies, growth deficiency, and cognitive disorders); anticoagulants such as coumarin and warfarin (which result in craniofacial anomalies, growth deficiency, and cognitive disorders); retinoids

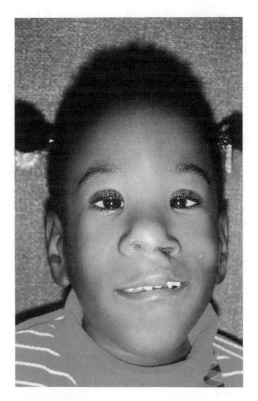

Figure 11–5. Child with fetal alcohol syndrome. Note the small eyes and epicanthal folds.

such as vitamin A and vitamin A congeners (which result in heart, craniofacial, ear, and central nervous system anomalies); antibiotics such as tetracyclines (which cause tooth discoloration and thinning of the enamel), streptomycin, kanamycine, and chloroquine (which cause sensory hearing loss); psychotropics such as benzodiazepines (which cause cleft palate) and lithium (which causes Ebstein anomaly); and chemotherapy drugs (which cause a wide range of anomalies including growth deficiency, mental retardation, cleft palate, limb anomalies, and genitourinary malformations). It is probable that many if not most psychoactive illegal drugs, including cocaine, are teratogens. Naturally occurring substances that cause anomalies include mercury, toluene (commonly found in house paint), and PCBs (polychlorinated biphenyls). Malformations caused by radiation exposure and excessive heat have linked maternal exposure to energy emitting sources to teratogenic effects. Exposure to ionizing radiation has been linked to genetic mutation, neoplasms, and central nervous system anomalies. Exposure to heat could be from an external source, such as a sauna or hot tub, or from a high maternal fever, resulting in maternal hyperthermia which also raises the temperature in the uterus and has been linked to central nervous system anomalies.

Teratogenic anomalies show some variability of expression because the action is not directly on the developing baby, but is mediated through the maternal anatomy and physiology; and there is a time- and dose-dependent effect. Therefore, the effects on the embryo of maternal exposure to alcohol rely on the amount consumed, the period of time over which it was consumed, the stage of development of the embryo (different structures and functions will be susceptible to malformation at specific stages of development), and the mother's ability to metabolize alcohol which in turn is dependent on maternal liver size and function, vascular function, basal metabolism rate, and the manner of consumption of alcohol (with versus without food). Some women may be able to metabolize several ounces of alcohol with none of it reaching the embryo via the maternal bloodstream, while in other circumstances, nearly all of the alcohol will circulate through the embryo.

Mechanically Induced Syndromes

Mechanical factors that cause anomalies are of two types: those that impinge on the embryo and cause a redirection or inhibition of growth called **deformations** and those that tear or mutilate the embryo called **disruptions**. In the majority of deformations and disruptions, the assumption is that the embryo or fetus is intrinsically normal and anomalies would not have occurred if an external mechanical factor had not interrupted normal development. An example of a deformation would be head molding caused by the descent through the birth canal or by prolonged placement in a breech position. A variety of anomalies can be caused by mechanical compression of the developing baby, including micrognathia, club foot, facial asymmetry, craniosynostosis (premature fusion of the skull bones), and arthrogryposis (congenital joint contractures).

The most common form of disruption is the amnion rupture sequence, sometimes known as ADAM sequence (ADAM being an acronym for amniotic deformities, adhesions, and mutilations). Estimated to occur with a frequency of 1:8,500 live births, the anomalies are caused by tears in the amnion. As the amnion heals, bands of fibrous tissue form and may adhere to, or wrap around, portions of the developing embryo or fetus. That portion of the developing anatomy may then develop ringlike constrictions, amputations, or be mutilated by the amniotic band (see Figure 11–6). The craniofacial complex and limbs are particularly susceptible to amniotic ad-

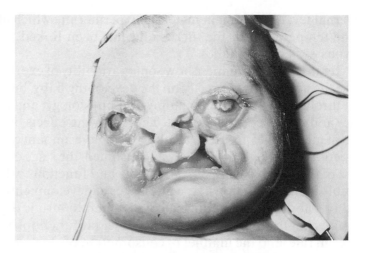

Figure 11–6. Patient with amnion rupture sequence.

hesions, resulting in cleft lip, facial clefts, and anencephaly. These bands may even be "swallowed" by the fetus or adhere to the bucco-pharyngeal membrane resulting in clefts of the palate.

In some cases, deformations can occur secondary to anomalies in the developing baby. For example, the majority of amniotic fluid is derived from fetal urination. If the fetus cannot swallow, or if the fetus has renal agenesis (absent kidneys), a deficiency of amniotic fluid results, a condition known as oligohydramnios. The lack of amniotic fluid can cause compression of the developing fetus, resulting in deformation of the compressed body parts, such as the jaw, face, skull, or limbs.

Sequences

Not all children with multiple anomalies have syndromes (as defined earlier). It is appropriate here to define the term *sequence*. **Sequence** is defined as multiple anomalies derived from a single known or presumed structural anomaly or mechanical factor. Therefore a single malformation, deformation, or disruption can secondarily cause other anomalies. However, the primary anomaly which causes the other anomalies may itself have many possible causes (i.e., not a single etiology), unlike syndromes in which there is a single pathogenesis.

The best known and most recognizable sequence is the Robin sequence. Originally labeled the Pierre Robin syndrome, it is now recognized that this common disorder is not a syndrome, but rather a sequence with etiologic heterogeneity. "Pierre Robin syndrome" was regarded to be the triad of findings of micrognathia (a small lower jaw), a wide U-shaped cleft palate, and upper airway obstruction secondary to glossoptosis (the tongue falling into the airway). The pathogenesis of Robin sequence is as follows. **Micrognathia** is the primary anomaly which secondarily causes both the cleft palate and airway obstruction. At approximately the seventh week postfertilization, the tongue rests against the skull base and the small palatal shelves (the embryonic structures that will form the palate) are located on either side of the tongue, vertically oriented (see Figure 11–7). Normally, as the mandible (the lower jaw) continues to grow, room is made in the oral cavity for the tongue to descend away from the skull base so that the palatal shelves can flip into a horizontal orientation above the tongue and begin growing towards the midline for eventual fusion at approximately the tenth gestational week (Figure 11–7). If, however, the mandible is abnormally small or retropositioned, the oral cavity will remain small and the tongue will not be able to descend from between the palatal shelves. The growth potential in the palatal shelves must be greater than the rapid lateral expansion of the skull so that the medial growth of two halves of the palate will exceed the laterally expanding oral cavity. If physically obstructed from growing medially, the lateral expansion of the oral space will be greater than the medial narrowing of the palate.

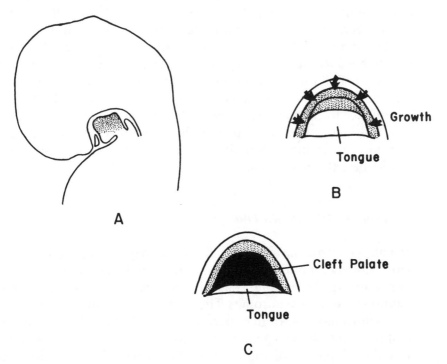

Figure 11-7. Drawing of the pathogenesis of Robin sequence.

Eventually (after 11 weeks), the growth potential in the palatal shelves is lost and a palatal cleft results. Therefore, because the micrognathia ultimately results in the impeding of the palatal shelves, the cleft occurs only because of the micrognathia. At birth, newborns are obligate nose breathers and reflexively keep their mouths closed. In Robin sequence, the micrognathia persists at birth. With the mouth closed, the tongue becomes entrapped in a more posterior position, thus obstructing the airway (Shprintzen, 1988). It also has been found that infants with Robin sequence have a short lingual attachment in the floor of the mouth (a short genioglossus muscle) which also acts to keep the tongue from moving forward to open the airway (Argamaso, 1992).

Although micrognathia can cause secondary anomalies, a small lower jaw may have many possible causes. Many chromosomal, genetic, teratogenic, and mechanically induced syndromes have micrognathia as a clinical feature. For example, Stickler syndrome is an autosomal dominant genetic syndrome related to a mutation of a gene on chromosome 12 which regulates the formation of collagen II, a basic component of connective tissue and cartilage. Stickler syndrome has a variety of clinical features including micrognathia, epiphyseal dysplasia, and congenital myopia which can progress to retinal detachment in adult life. Stickler syndrome is one of the most common syndromes of clefting, accounting for just under 5% of all children with cleft palate (Shprintzen, Siegel-Sadewitz, Amato, & Goldberg, 1985). Because micrognathia is a common feature of Stickler syndrome (as is cleft palate), many infants with Stickler syndrome have Robin sequence, and vice versa. In fact, approximately one third of all infants with Robin sequence have Stickler syndrome. It should therefore be obvious that it is possible for a syndrome and a sequence to co-exist, the sequence being a secondary effect of the syndrome. It is, however, unlikely that one individual would have two syndromes, the odds of that occurrence by random assortment would be extremely high.

Syndromes of Unknown Etiology

Not all syndromes have an identifiable etiology. In some cases a common etiology for multiple anomalies in a single individual can only be presumed. Cohen (1982) has labeled these types of syndromes as **unknown genesis** syndromes. There are two types of unknown genesis syndromes: recurrent pattern and provisionally unique. Recurrent pattern unknown genesis syndromes are those where the individual has a pattern of anomalies that has been seen before in other unrelated individuals. No etiology for the pattern has been identified; karyotypes have been negative, there is no history of teratoge-nesis, and there are no familial occurrences. In other words, all cases are sporadic, but the pattern is a familiar one. Williams syndrome is a good example of a recurrent pattern unknown genesis syndrome. The phenotype of Williams syndrome is familiar, including a dis-tinctive facial appearance, cognitive impairment, and a characteristic personality. Language usage in Williams syndrome is very sophisti-cated, especially considering the presence of mental retardation in the majority of cases. To date, no one has been able to identify the etiology of Williams syndrome. Chromosome analysis has proven normal and teratogens are not implicated. No one with Williams syndrome has had a child with the syndrome. Although no cause has been identified, the pattern of anomalies still is considered to be a syndrome because it has been seen repeatedly and it is not pos-sible that this pattern is a random assortment of anomalies in so many individuals. It is probable that the etiology of this fairly com-mon disorder will be identified as molecular genetics continues to progress as a science as has already happened with other syndromes which previously had no known etiology, such as Prader-Willi syn-drome and de Lange syndrome.

Provisionally unique syndromes refer to individuals who have multiple anomalies of unknown etiology, but the pattern has not been seen or reported before. As far as the diagnostician is aware, the pattern of anomalies in this individual is unique, but it must represent a syndrome because it is unlikely that multiple anomalies will occur together by chance assortment. The term *provisionally* is added to "unique" because, at some point in time, another patient may be seen with the same pattern of anomalies, a cause may be found, or the individual may reproduce and have a child with the same pattern of anomalies.

✦ THE IMPORTANCE OF SYNDROME IDENTIFICATION

Why is it important to determine whether a child has a syndrome? Be-cause accurate diagnosis leads to better patient care. There are literal-ly thousands of possible syndromic diagnoses, perhaps the majori-ty of which will cross the paths of specialists in the communicative disorders. Many of these conditions are extremely rare, occurring with frequencies of 1:30,000 live births. Although the most common syndromes may be seen frequently by experienced clinicians, most are unknown to the lay public. When parents are presented with their child who has multiple anomalies, it is natural for them to ask, "why?"

Behind this question is the parent's desire for the clinicians man-aging the care of their child to know what the problem is so they can manage it correctly. Also, having a name for the condition provides significantly more comfort than an "I don't know." But even more important, behind every diagnosis, three factors become known to both the clinicians and parents: the phenotypic spectrum, the natural history, and the prognosis.

Phenotypic Spectrum

Phenotypic spectrum refers to all of the anomalies associated with a syndrome. The phenotypic spectrum is compiled from the clinician's observations plus all reports in the scientific literature that have described the syndrome. By knowing the phenotypic spectrum of a syndrome, if the clinician is suspicious of the diagnosis in a patient, he or she would know what to look for in the process of evaluation. This would include not only visible or easily studied anomalies, like cleft palate, microtia (a malformed external ear), or abnormal fingers, but also suspected problems (based on previous descriptions) that might require specialized diagnostic tests.

Two examples of the importance of knowing the phenotypic spectrum will be provided for syndromes with communicative impairment as common clinical findings. An excellent example of the way in which knowing the phenotypic spectrum will lead to better patient care is illustrated by Stickler syndrome (also known as hereditary arthro-ophthalmopathy) which is, as mentioned earlier, an autosomal dominant genetic disease caused by a mutation of a single gene on chromosome 12. Imagine that an infant has been born with the provisional diagnosis of Robin sequence based on the presence of micrognathia, cleft palate, and upper airway obstruction. As an astute clinician, you are aware that the majority of Robin cases are syndromic and there may be an underlying primary diagnosis. Being as astute as you are, you also remember that at least a third of all Robin cases represent Stickler syndrome. You go to the literature and find that the common anomalies associated with Stickler syndrome include congenital myopia (nearsightedness), a 15% likelihood of sensorineural hearing loss (hearing loss caused by abnormalities of the inner ear), conductive hearing impairment (abnormalities in the conduction of sound to the inner ear) secondary to the chronic otitis media (ear infection) which often accompanies cleft palate, epiphyseal dysplasia (abnormalities of the growth plates of the long bones such as the legs), and both maxillary (upper jaw) and mandibular hypoplasia (deficiency) with a characteristic antegonial (concave) notching of the body of the mandible (see Figure 11–8). The nose is usually short, the nostrils are anteverted, the bridge of the nose is usually flat or "saddle" shaped, there can be slight bulg-

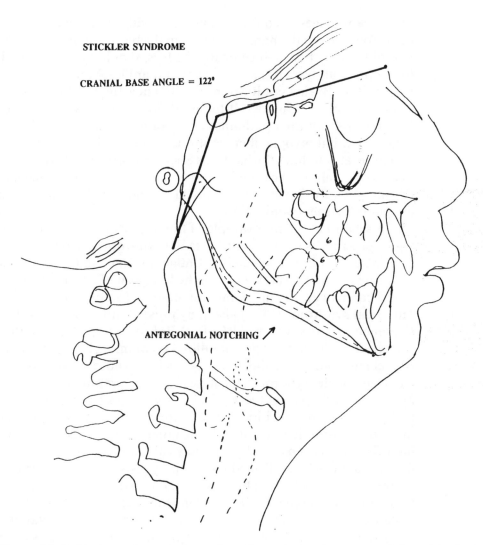

Figure 11-8. Tracings of a cephalometric radiograph showing antegonial notching in the mandible of a patient with Stickler syndrome.

ing of the eyes, and the joints may be hyperextensible. You examine the baby, immediately feeling the body of the mandible for the characteristic shape. Although this type of antegonial notching can be found in other syndromes with facial abnormality, such as Treacher Collins syndrome and Nager syndrome (which also may be associated with Robin sequence), you do not find other anomalies consistent with those diagnoses. You do find a depressed nasal root, anteverted nostrils and a long philtrum which is often indicative of a short nose. Your suspicions of Stickler syndrome continue to be strong. Based on the known phenotypic spectrum of Stickler syndrome, you suggest an ophthalmologic consultation to look for myopia. You also tell the parents that when the baby is a little older, X-rays of the long bones, specifically the legs, should be done to look for epiphyseal dysplasia at the knees and ankles. You also request an Auditory Brainstem Response (ABR) hearing test to check for sensorineural hearing loss. If the ABR does not show evidence of hearing loss, but the ophthalmologic examination reveals significant congenital myopia, there is strong enough evidence to tell the parents that you think the baby has Stickler syndrome. It is unlikely that an ophthalmologic examination would have been requested had not the phenotypic spectrum of Stickler syndrome been used as a template for the examination.

A second excellent example of the importance of the phenotypic spectrum is the velo-cardio-facial syndrome (also known as Shprintzen syndrome) which is a contiguous gene syndrome caused by the deletion of several genes on the long arm of chromosome 22 inherited in an autosomal dominant manner. Infants with velo-cardio-facial syndrome (VCF) also may present initially with Robin sequence (approximately 11% of all Robin cases). Retrognathia (posterior positioning of the mandible) is common, but without the typical antegonial notching found in Stickler syndrome. Also different from Stickler syndrome, the nose is usually prominent and long. Myopia is not a part of the VCF phenotypic spectrum, but abnormally tortuous retinal blood vessels are common, so an ophthalmic examination is warranted. Congenital heart disease is a common finding, as is hypocalcemia (low calcium levels). All of these features are easily confirmed by specialty tests, but if not suspected, they might not be sought. However, it is extremely important to locate these anomalies both for diagnostic accuracy and for immediate treatment of potentially life-threatening heart or metabolic disorders. Also a part of the phenotypic spectrum of VCF is both generalized hypotonia and hypotonia specific to the pharynx (throat) which may present an early problem for both feeding and possible upper airway obstruction. Being alert to this problem will allow clinicians to be especially attentive to early feeding and respiration problems which can prevent the baby from deteriorating to the point of "failure to thrive," thus preventing unnecessary crisis situations and allaying parental anxiety.

Natural History

The natural history of a syndrome refers to the course of the clinical findings over time. Understanding the natural history is critically important to knowing when to apply necessary treatments or when to look for anomalies that may not be evident until later in life. In the previous example of Stickler syndrome, it was mentioned that epiphyseal dysplasia may become evident radiographically later in infancy. However, most important is the progressive nature of the eye impairment. Congenital myopia often progresses to vitreous and retinal degeneration and possible retinal detachment. It has been reported that over 70% of adults with Stickler syndrome develop areas of retinal detachment, as well as other eye problems including astigmatism, glaucoma, strabismus (eye muscle problems), and cataracts (Gorlin, Cohen, & Levin, 1990). With proper ophthalmologic care, blindness is preventable, but timely treatment following the detection of a retinal detachment is essential. Therefore, understanding the natural history of Stickler syndrome allows the clinician to schedule frequent eye examinations and intercept serious problems. Another aspect of the natural history of Stickler syndrome is the development of joint pains in childhood which could be misdiagnosed as juvenile arthritis. These joint pains tend to be minor and related to minor skeletal anomalies. Parents should be counseled as to the benign nature of these complaints and advised that, unlike arthritis, they are not progressive or symptomatic of an underlying disease. Understanding the natural history of Stickler syndrome can prevent unnecessary parental worry, and expensive diagnostic tests for diseases that are not present, and allow the timely delivery of necessary treatment while avoiding the delivery of unnecessary treatment.

Velo-cardio-facial syndrome also provides an important example of the natural history of a common syndrome associated with communicative impairment. Speech and language development often is delayed. Nearly all cases reported to date (over 120) with overt or **submucous clefts** (see Glossary) of the palate have developed severely disordered articulation, including abnormal **glottal stop** substitutions (see Glossary) for nearly all consonant productions (Golding-Kushner, 1991). Early intellectual development often is perceived to be normal, but by age 7 years as school work involves more abstraction and conceptualization, learning disabilities in mathematics and reading comprehension become obvious (Goldberg, Motzkin, Marion, Scambler, & Shprintzen, 1993; Golding-Kushner, Weller, & Shprintzen, 1985). At this same time, in part because of the change in the intelligence tests from rote tasks to more abstract ones, IQ scores often deteriorate. A characteristic personality has been described in association with the various cognitive disorders in VCF, and this personality pattern seems to be a predictor of more serious problems which have come from a study of the natural history of VCF (Goldberg et al., 1993; Shprintzen et al., 1992). It has been found that at least 20% of individuals with VCF develop psychosis as adolescents or adults, although it is probable that the actual frequency of severe personality disorders is higher (Shprintzen, Goldberg, Golding-Kushner, & Marion, 1992). This aspect of the natural history of VCF was totally unexpected when the syndrome was initially described in a series of young children (Shprintzen et al., 1978), which stresses the need to observe individuals with a particular disorder longitudinally in order to fully determine the effects of the syndrome. In both of the examples presented above, the advantages of understanding the natural history of the syndrome are obvious.

Prognosis

The prognosis is the expected outcome of the syndrome, both in terms of the naturally determined longevity, intellect, general health and function, and the expected outcomes of treatments which have been applied. Longitudinal observation of a syndrome also allows professionals to determine the long-term prognosis. The phenotypic spectrum guides the clinician in the evaluation and treatment process, the natural history provides the timing for the application of diagnostics and treatments, and the prognosis predicts the effectiveness of treatments.

The majority of syndromes have prognoses that are sufficiently positive to make treatments worthwhile. Children with Stickler syndrome can lead perfectly normal lives, especially if needed treatments are applied in a timely manner. The prognosis for velo-cardio-facial syndrome is somewhat more guarded, but it has been demonstrated that speech disorders can be successfully resolved, cardiac anomalies repaired, and learning disabilities managed with limited success. Even psychotic disorders such as schizophrenia can be treated effectively with a variety of psychopharmaceuticals. There are several syndromes, however, where the prognosis is so poor that one must question the wisdom of applying treatments which are unlikely to have any positive benefit. There are syndromes with progressive degeneration of the central nervous system, such as Cockayne syndrome, Refsum syndrome, ataxia-telangiectasia syndrome, Hurler syndrome, Tay-Sachs syndrome, and Huntington syndrome. To date, there are no effective treatments to counteract the neurologic, metabolic, and deteriorating aspects of these genetic disorders, although it is possible that once gene effect (what the gene does) is isolated, treatments may become available. At this point in time, however, clinicians must question the wisdom of applying treatments that will have no advantage for the patient.

◆ SYNDROMIC EFFECTS ON COMMUNICATION

Human communication can be impaired in many ways, none mutually exclusive. Hearing, language, articulation, phonation, and resonance may be impaired singly or in combination because of syndromic anomalies that directly affect anatomy or function. The full scope of communicative disorders associated with multiple anomaly syndromes is not known because, as mentioned at the outset of this chapter, few scientists from the communicative sciences have become involved in the process of syndrome delineation. It is imperative that the process of contributing to syndrome delineation begin in earnest so that speech-language pathologists, audiologists, and deaf educators can add to the phenotypic spectrum, natural history, and prognosis for the thousands of conditions that result in congenital anomalies. The areas of investigation are many.

Syndromes of Hearing Impairment

Hearing may be impaired by many syndromic features, not all of which necessarily directly involve the ears. Certainly the most familiar syndromes will be those which do directly involve ear anomalies of the external, middle, or inner ear (see Chapter 14 by Berlin and Chapter 15 by Jerger and Stach).

Ear Anomalies

External ear anomalies occur as frequent features of all types of syndromes with known causes (i.e., chromosomal, genetic, teratogenic, and mechanically induced). It is unusual to find external ear anomalies without associated middle ear anomalies unless the external ear anomaly is minor, such as the small ears associated with Down syndrome (trisomy 21).

Minor ear anomalies, such as ear tags (extra pieces of tissue, usually comprised of cartilage and skin which are usually found somewhere between the ear canal and outer corner of the mouth) or preauricular pits (small openings also found between the ear canal and outer corner of the mouth) are very common anomalies that may appear as isolated minor malformations. However, they frequently are associated with multiple anomaly syndromes, many of which have middle ear anomalies and conductive hearing loss as common findings. Ear tags and pits also may be associated with varying degrees of facial asymmetry, facial paresis (weakness), and the possible presence of extra pieces of tissue (choristomas) elsewhere on the body, particularly in or near the eyes.

External ear anomalies are not often associated with inner ear malformations or sensorineural hearing loss, but on rare occasions, inner ear malformations may be found. The presence of any external ear anomaly should certainly lead the observant clinician to recommend a thorough audiometric assessment, even for minor malformations such as ear tags which would not by their physical nature seem to result in a conductive hearing loss.

Microtias (incompletely formed external ears) are almost always related to middle ear anomalies, including ossicular anomalies (abnormalities of the small bones in the middle ear), reduced size of the middle ear space, and most frequently, fixation of the footplate of the stapes (the smallest bone of the middle ear), all of which lead to conductive hearing loss. An abnormal course of the facial nerve (Cranial Nerve VII) through the middle ear (often right through the footplate of the stapes) is frequently found in association with microtia, particularly in syndromes where microtia is a common anomaly, such as Treacher Collins syndrome (Figure 11–9), oculo-auriculo-vertebral dysplasia (also known as hemifacial microsomia and, on occasion, Goldenhar syndrome), and Nager syn-

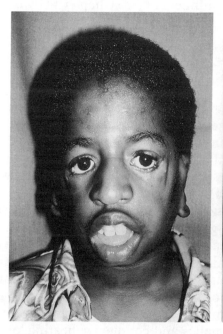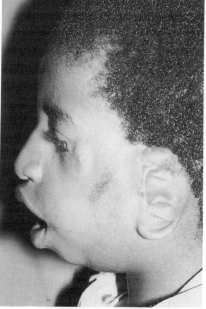

A   **B**

Figure 11–9. Patient with Treacher Collins syndrome in full face and profile. Note the projection of hair onto the cheek and the downslanting eyes.

drome. Knowing that the facial nerve may be abnormally placed is important because surgery to the middle ear could inadvertently sever the nerve and cause facial paralysis.

Inner ear anomalies may involve abnormalities of the membranes (common in syndromes involving connective tissue dysplasia), the structure of the cochlea, and hair cell anomalies. Inner ear anomalies, particularly those associated with organ of Corti disorders, often are accompanied by pigmentary anomalies elsewhere in the body, such as unusual hair color or streaks of hair color, eye color, or patches of unusual skin color (including vitiligo), the best known of these disorders being Waardenburg syndrome (both types I and II).

True neural hearing loss can be caused by syndromes that have neoplasias (growths or tumors) as common findings, especially those which appear on the acoustic nerve. The best known of these disorders is neurofibromatosis type II (NF II), which is an autosomal dominant genetic condition resulting in tumors called neurofibromas, abnormally colored patches of skin, and brain abnormalities. The gene for neurofibromatosis type II has been mapped to chromosome 22, with acoustic neuromas (tumors growing on the acoustic nerve), usually bilateral, as the presenting feature.

As mentioned earlier, hearing loss also may be caused by anomalies unrelated to the ears. Neural hearing loss can be caused by damage to the acoustic nerve caused by physical compression secondary to abnormal bone growth in the skull. A number of syndromes present in this manner later in life (another reason to pay attention to the natural history), including craniometaphyseal dysplasia, craniodiaphyseal dysplasia, frontometaphyseal dysplasia, Van Buchem disease, and sclerosteosis, all of which are syndromes characterized by severe overgrowth of bone throughout the skull.

Syndromes of Language Impairment

It should be obvious to the reader that syndromes associated with hearing loss will have significant effects on language development. However, language impairment also should be expected to occur in association with syndromes that have any type of central nervous system impairment, learning disabilities, or mental retardation as possible findings. Syndromes with these types of impairments are too numerous to list, and language impairment can be caused directly or indirectly (i.e., as a sequence in a secondary manner) by chromosomal, genetic, teratogenic, and mechanically induced causes. Language is a brain-mediated function, and the brain is unique in organ development in that it develops its structure initially in the first trimester, but grows actively throughout the third trimester. As a result, the brain is particularly susceptible to malformation because of its extremely long developmental stage. The brain also is very susceptible to metabolic disturbance and teratogenic influence.

In disorders where there are structural malformations of the speech mechanism without central nervous anomalies, language impairment would not be expected to occur. In cases where cleft palate is associated with a language disorder, the clinician should not mistakenly associate the language impairment with the patient's difficulty with intelligibility because of a resonance or articulation disorder. Isolated cleft palate (in the absence of other anomalies) does not cause language impairment. Therefore, in cases where cleft palate is associated with language impairment, the clinician should be highly suspicious of a possible syndromic relationship.

Syndromic Contributions to Articulation Disorders

Articulation disorders should be anticipated in disorders that have oral anomalies including dental abnormalities, jaw malformations, cleft lip and/or cleft palate, tongue aberrations, neurologic impairment, and abnormal innervation or sensation of the mouth. The articulation impairment associated with dental and jaw abnormalities should be obvious and are not syndrome specific. The type of articulatory impairment tends to be related to the specific anatomical defect. These have been described in more detail elsewhere (Bloomer, 1971; LeBlanc & Shprintzen, 1993; Witzel, 1983; Witzel, Ross, & Munro, 1980).

Similarly, articulation problems associated with cleft lip and palate have been described in detail elsewhere and are related to the presence of dental anomalies, maxillary abnormalities, and resonance imbalance secondary to **velopharyngeal insufficiency** (an inability to separate the nasal cavity from the oral cavity during speech). Of particular importance are the unusual articulation substitution patterns often observed in individuals with clefts, including glottal stops, pharyngeal fricatives, mid-dorsal lingual contacts, pharyngeal stops, and laryngeal stops (Hoch, Golding-Kushner, Sadewitz, & Shprintzen, 1986; Trost, 1981). It does appear, however, that certain syndromes have a higher prevalence of abnormal articulatory substitutions than others. Golding-Kushner (1991) found that glottal stops and other "compensatory" articulation substitutions occurred in nearly all patients with velo-cardio-facial syndrome, but were found relatively infrequently in patients with Stickler syndrome and van der Woude syndrome (a genetic disorder characterized by small pits or openings in the lower lip in association with cleft palate or cleft lip and palate). It should be noted that neither Stickler nor van der Woude syndrome has hypotonia or cognitive dysfunction as features, whereas VCF has significant hypotonia during the speech learning stage and subsequent cognitive impairment.

Articulation also may be impaired by neurologic or neuromuscular dysfunction. Many genetic syndromes of neuromuscular disease, such as myotonic dystrophy (Steinert syndrome) and facio-scapulo-humoral muscular dystrophy include abnormal muscle response as well as secondary malocclusions caused by abnormal facial muscular forces. Neurologic impairments can occur with any syndrome that has central nervous system anomalies or any of the metabolic diseases (such as Hunter syndrome and the other lysosomal storage diseases) that cause brain abnormality secondary to the storage of cellular waste products. Lysosomal storage diseases, such as Hunter syndrome, are genetic disorders which result in the inability of the body to rid itself of cellular waste products which become stored in the body's tissues. The storage of these waste products causes physical distortion and cellular dysfunction and, in certain cases, may result in early death. Oral tissues also become thickened causing abnormal articulatory contacts and difficulty in navigating the tongue around the oral cavity.

Syndromic Contributions to Voice Disorders

Laryngeal anomalies that lead to phonatory disorders are relatively unusual, but do occur in a number of syndromes. Cleft larynx (in Opitz syndrome), vocal chord atrophy (in Werner syndrome), loose mucosa in the glottis (in cutis laxa syndrome), lack of mucosal lubrication in the glottis (in hypohidrotic forms of ectodermal dysplasia), and a small glottis with short vocal cords (in many forms of dwarfism) are some of the possible causes of voice problems. Unilateral vocal cord paresis may also occur, as in oculo-auriculo-vertebral dysplasia (hemifacial microsomia). Short neck, an abnormality found in a number of syndromes (including syndromes of short stature and syndromes with spinal anomalies) also may cause an abnormal voice, although the problem may really be due more to an aberrant resonance pattern in the supraglottic area.

In determining if an unusual voice is a syndromic feature versus the typical vocal abuse common to many children, a careful history is invaluable. Besides a history of hyperfunctional vocal usage (previously referred to as *voice abuse*) which could confirm a behavioral component to a hoarse voice, the clinician should specifically seek out responses to questions regarding histories of upper airway obstruction, difficulties with feeding, chronic coughing, and chronic vomiting.

Resonance Disorders in Syndromes

Syndromic anomalies can cause hypernasal resonance, hyponasal resonance, and unusual patterns of oral resonance. These disorders are quite common in syndromes with craniofacial malformations.

Hypernasal Resonance

Any syndrome that has cleft palate as a clinical feature may have hypernasal speech as a secondary anomaly. This includes over 400 syndromes which have been delineated to date that have either cleft palate or cleft lip and palate as a possible finding. However, some syndromes are more likely to have velopharyngeal insufficiency and hypernasality resulting from the cleft than others (Golding-Kushner, 1991; Shprintzen, 1982). Variation in the prevalence of hypernasality in various syndromes is related to a number of factors including cognition, general muscle tone, adenoid size, and the overall size of the nasopharynx which is, in large part, related to the angle of flexion of the skull base (Arvystas & Shprintzen, 1984; Gereau & Shprintzen, 1988; Shprintzen, 1982). The skull base in Stickler syndrome tends to be more acute in flexion which reduces the volume of the nasopharynx; whereas in velo-cardio-facial syndrome, the skull base tends to be more obtuse which increases the volume of the nasopharynx. As the volume of the nasopharynx increases, increased movement in the velopharyngeal mechanism is needed to overcome the enlargement (see Figure 11–10). In other words, cleft palate by itself does not necessarily lead to hypernasal speech because other structures are contained in the velopharyngeal valve and influence its function. Craniofacial morphology is highly variable from syndrome to syndrome so that the prevalence of velopharyngeal insufficiency after palate repair will not be uniform for each condition.

Although to many clinicians cleft palate is the most obvious cause of hypernasal resonance, it is probable that at least an equal number of individuals have hypernasal speech for reasons unrelated to clefting (although there are no available data to substantiate this clinical impression). Even if head trauma and other sources of brain and peripheral injury are eliminated from the population of individuals with hypernasal speech, there remain many conditions with central and peripheral nervous system anomalies that precipi-

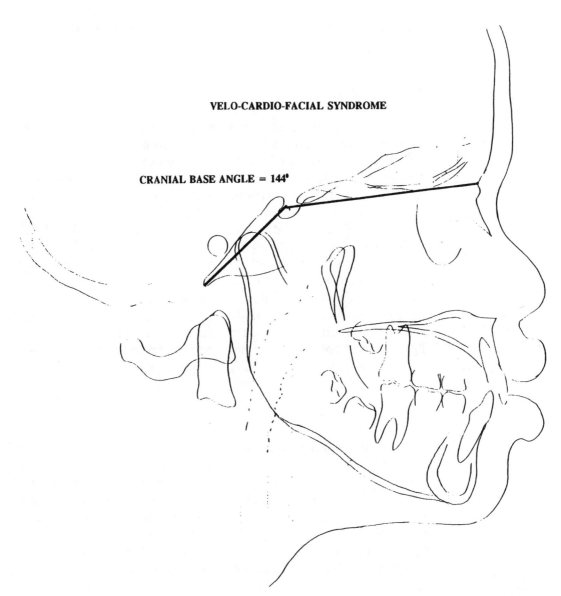

VELO-CARDIO-FACIAL SYNDROME

CRANIAL BASE ANGLE = 144°

Figure 11–10. Tracings of cephalometric radiographs showing cranial base angles for Stickler syndrome and velo-cardio-facial syndrome.

tate velopharyngeal dysfunction. They include nearly all forms of genetic neuromuscular disease, various myopathies (muscle disease or degeneration), many syndromes which have central nervous system anomalies, and syndromes which have central or peripheral hypotonia (weakness) as features. They include syndromes such as Down syndrome, myotonic dystrophy, Moebius sequence, Dubowitz syndrome, Rubinstein-Taybi syndrome, velo-cardio-facial syndrome (secondary to pharyngeal hypotonia), Prader-Willi syndrome, and Weaver syndrome.

Hyponasal Resonance

Hyponasal speech (speech with too little nasal resonance) can result from both a small nasopharynx and from a small nasal cavity, including the choanae (the entrance from the nasal cavity into the pharynx above the palate). Syndromes that include acute flexion of the skull base are likely to result in reduced nasal airflow, both during respiration and during speech. In fact, in many of these syndromes, children often are chronic mouth breathers. Besides Stickler syndrome, as mentioned above, other syndromes with reduced nasopharyngeal volume include Treacher Collins syndrome, Crouzon syndrome, Apert syndrome, Pfeiffer syndrome, and Nager syndrome. These syndromes also tend to have very short anterior cranial bases. The anterior cranial base comprises the roof of the nasal cavity so that reduction in size of the anterior cranial base will reduce the total volume of the nasal airway. In such cases, the choanae are often small, stenosed (narrowed), or even atretic (absent).

Abnormal Oral Resonance

Abnormalities in the shape, size, and configuration of the pharynx can alter oral resonance during speech. Micrognathia, short neck, macroglossia (large tongue), a long palate, enlarged tonsils, and other head and neck anomalies all can cause a muffled oral resonance quality. This type of problem is common in Robin sequence, Treacher Collins syndrome, Nager syndrome, Crouzon syndrome, Apert syndrome, Noonan syndrome, Klippel-Fiel anomaly, fronto-metaphyseal dysplasia, and craniometaphyseal dysplasia.

✦ WHEN TO BE SUSPICIOUS

Although this chapter is meant to be a broad introduction to the process and logic behind syndrome delineation, it should be apparent that syndrome diagnosis is not always instantaneous and may involve referral to several specialists before a proper diagnosis can be reached. Therefore, the first step is to be suspicious. The specialist in communicative disorders should follow the following steps in developing this suspicion:

1. Know how to obtain a careful and accurate history. Ask specifically about diagnoses which might have been rendered by other professionals. A history of anomalies in relatives (especially first degree relatives) is of particular importance. Questions should be leading because factors the clinician might consider important may not be considered important by the historian. Family histories of anomalies, especially those similar to the presenting problems of the patient, should prompt referral for further study.

2. If the patient presents with two or more major anomalies or three or more minor anomalies, it is probable that there is a syndromic diagnosis. A major anomaly can be defined as one that requires immediate or eventual medical management or which, if untreatable, will adversely affect the quality or quantity of life. Examples of major anomalies include cleft palate, coarctation of the aorta (an abnormality of the aortic arch), anophthalmia (an absent eye), or mental retardation. Minor anomalies are those that are easily recognizable, but have no major impact on the quantity or quality of life. Examples of minor anomalies would be a missing finger nail, a supernumerary tooth, absent eye lashes, or a small umbilical hernia.

3. If the patient has multiple problems that would not be expected to occur together by chance because the odds of coexisting problems would be too great.

When the clinician's suspicion is aroused, appropriate referral sources should be identified and referrals made. Referral sources can be identified by contacting the American Society of Human Genetics, the National Society of Genetic Counselors, or the American Board of Human Genetics.

It also is recommended that the clinician have one or more compendiums which describe syndromes available. Excellent text sources include, but are not limited, to the following books: *Smith's Recognizable Patterns of Human Malformation* (Jones, 1991), *Syndromes of the Head and Neck* (Gorlin et al., 1990), *The Birth Defects Encyclopedia* (Buyse, 1991), and *Mendelian Inheritance in Man* (McKusick, 1992). Several computer data bases also are available which allow interaction with the clinician for the purpose of assisting the diagnostic process. Two of these data bases are *POSSUM* and *The London Data Base*.

Case Report

Tim had caused his parents enormous concern since birth. As soon as he was born, his color caused his Apgar score to be low and a pediatric cardiologist was called to examine him. The thrill
(continued)

and joy of a new birth were replaced by the anxiety and concern of a major heart anomaly. Tim's breathing was also labored and his muscle tone was very poor. Doctors kept referring to him as a "floppy baby." The heart disorder was obviously serious. His parents were told that Tim had a right-sided aortic arch (it is normally on the left), a hole in the upper chambers of the heart called a ventriculoseptal defect (VSD), another heart abnormality called a patent ductus arteriosus (PDA), abnormalities of some of the large cardiac blood vessels, absence of the thymus gland which is important to normal immunologic function, and hypocalcemia (insufficient calcium levels) which could cause seizures. The doctors said that this set of abnormalities often occurred together in a group. The cardiologists said that surgery would be necessary to ligate (close) the PDA and repair the VSD or Tim could die. They also said that the hypocalcemia could be handled with supplements and that Tim would probably outgrow it shortly. The floppiness, or hypotonia, that Tim had might be caused by his serious cardiac anomalies.

Surgery was an ordeal because it was a life and death decision Tim's parents needed to endure. Fortunately, all went well. Tim remained hypotonic in the months following his surgery, but the doctors said that this was not unusual for a child undergoing such a traumatic event and prolonged hospitalization. Tim's suck was weak and his feedings needed to be handled with a nasogastric tube, often called gavage feeding. His parents had enormous difficulty getting him to feed normally, and when he was finally able to take food orally, some came out of his nose. The doctors said that Tim's weakened condition was responsible for these problems.

After the cardiac surgery, an inguinal hernia (a hernia near the groin) was noticed, as was an anomaly of the genitals known as a hypospadias. These problems also required surgery. Tim's parents wondered why one little baby had so many different problems. One doctor tried to calm their fears by saying that each of these problems was very common and it would not be so rare to see them all happening in one child.

Finally, with Tim's heart condition stable and his other anomalies repaired, his parents felt as if Tim had been through the worst and life could get back to normal. However, Tim was frequently ill with colds, ear infections, bronchitis, and even had several bouts of pneumonia which required hospitalizations. He was treated with antibiotics and recovered. The pediatrician said that these illnesses were not unexpected in very sickly children who were more susceptible to these types of upper respiratory infections. These additional problems were discouraging, but fortunately treatable.

As Tim grew older, he remained small, but the pediatrician assured the parents that this was to be expected because of the serious cardiac lesion and the long period of hospitalization and feeding difficulties. Tim's motor milestones were also mildly delayed, but even Tim's parents expected this under the circumstances. Tim walked at 15 months and he was still small, but growing. However, Tim's parents were concerned about his lack of intelligible speech development. He had said his first words at about the time he started walking. Tim had said "ma-ma" at 15 months and "no" at 16 months, but little intelligible speech followed. It did seem, however, that he was trying to say words. His parents described his speech as "nasal" and lacking in consonant production. The pediatrician offered them platitudes, saying that some children developed speech much later than others, especially those who had histories of prolonged illness or hospitalizations. He added that Tim's problem with ear infections and the mild hearing loss which accompanies it often result in speech and language impairment. The parents accepted the explanation, grasping at hope and not wanting anything else to be wrong with their baby.

Tim continued to grow and develop motor milestones. Although the parents realized that Tim was not exactly like other children, they were happy that he was "catching up" to other children and that he did not appear to be severely impaired. They were, however, still concerned about his speech delay and lack of intelligibility at his third birthday. Finally, the pediatrician agreed that the speech problem was pathologic and required assessment. Tim was referred to a speech pathologist who diagnosed something called "velopharyngeal insufficiency" and "hypernasality" with severe articulatory impairment characteristic of a child with a cleft palate. An oral examination showed the presence of a submucous cleft palate. The speech pathologist explained that a submucous cleft palate was a separation or cleft of muscles in the palate, but the skin covering of the palate remains intact (see Figure 11–11). The effect on speech could be the same as in a cleft palate where the skin was cleft, as well. The speech pathologist thought Tim should be seen at a place called a Craniofacial Center which was located at a large teaching hospital in nearby large city.

(continued)

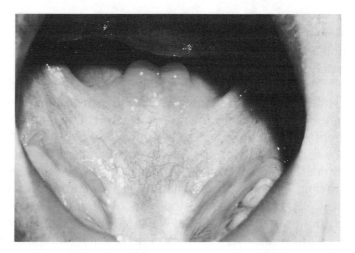

Figure 11–11. Oral view of a submucous cleft palate showing a bifid uvula, zona pellucida (the translucent area in the midline), and a notch in the posterior border of the hard palate.

At the center, the family was greeted by a genetic counselor who took an extensive history and asked many questions about abnormalities in other family members. There were none. It was explained that Tim would be examined by a clinical geneticist. When they asked why, Tim's parents were told that it was unreasonable to think that all of Tim's problems were unrelated. Tim's mother repeated what she had been told by many of Tim's previous doctors, that Tim was having problems with his growth, development, speech, and language because of his illnesses, hospitalizations, operations, and poor feeding and that all of his abnormalities were high frequency birth defects so that Tim was just "unlucky." The geneticist replied that Tim's problems probably were all related to a single cause and that she and her colleagues had seen many patients with the same combination of anomalies.

The clinical geneticist, who was also a pediatrician, examined Tim carefully, took many measurements of his head, face, hands, and ears. She pointed out Tim's small ears with their thickened folds and missing lobules, something Tim's mom had always noticed but had never been mentioned by other doctors. She noted his inguinal hernias and hypospadias, palate abnormality, almost anticipating that they would be there, as if she knew where to look. Tim's parents began to realize that this doctor knew what she was doing.

After the examination, Tim's parents received genetic counseling while their son played in the waiting room. They were anxious to hear what the geneticist had to say, especially because
of the confidence they had in her after watching the methodical manner in which Tim was examined.

"Your son has a condition we have seen frequently which
almost always results in the kind of speech disorders Tim displays. It is called velo-cardio-facial syndrome, and it is also responsible for all of the other abnormalities Tim has. As the name
implies, there are heart abnormalities and a typical facial appearance. The "velo" refers to velum which is a medical term for soft
palate. Over 40 abnormalities are known to be features of this
syndrome. We even know what the cause is, and to confirm the
diagnosis, we would like to draw some blood from Tim's arm for
a chromosome and DNA analysis."

Tim's mother asked, "You mean this is genetic?"

"Yes. It is caused by the deletion of a small piece of genetic
material from chromosome 22."

The geneticist then went into a long explanation of what
genes and chromosomes do, how abnormalities can cause congenital anomalies, and then showed them a diagram of chromosome 22 and the region where the genetic material known
as DNA was missing. The geneticist further explained that neither parent seemed to have the same problem, but that an analysis of their DNA would be able to confirm that the problem began anew in Tim.

"But everyone told us that because all of Tim's problems
were such common birth defects, it might be that Tim had them
all together by chance. Isn't that true?" asked Tim's mother, still
trying to comprehend the enormity of the diagnosis and how it
contradicted years of misconception. The explanation she received was astoundingly simple.

"I'll give you an example," said the geneticist. "Cleft palate
without cleft lip happens in 1 of every 2,500 live births. Congenital heart disease in 1 per 400 live births. The odds of those happening together, as they did in Tim, are as follows. You have a
barrel at your right hand with 2,500 ping pong balls in it, one of
them painted red. At your left is a barrel with 400 ping pong balls,
one painted red. What is the probability that you will stick one
hand in the left barrel and the other hand in the right barrel and
pick out the two red balls simultaneously? If you pick a red one
in the right hand, you don't hold on to it and keep picking with

(continued)

the other hand. You throw it back in and shake them all up each time. The odds of getting the two red balls together is 400 times 2500, or 1 in a million. Now, add to that the inguinal hernia, hypospadias, and all of the other abnormalities, and the odds of these things being together by chance are astronomically high. Therefore, when we see one child with a number of abnormalities, we always think it is a syndrome."

◆ REFERENCES

Argamaso, R. V. (1992). Glossopexy for upper airway obstruction in Robin sequence. *Cleft Palate Journal, 29,* 232–238.

Arvystas, M., & Shprintzen, R. J. (1984). Craniofacial morphology in the velo-cardio-facial syndrome. *Journal of Craniofacial Genetics and Developmental Biology, 4,* 39–45.

Bloomer, H. H. (1971). Speech defects associated with dental malocclusion and related anomalies. In L. E. Travis (Ed.), *Handbook of speech pathology* (pp. 715–767). New York: Appleton-Century-Crofts.

Buyse, M. L. (1990). *Birth defects encyclopedia.* Cambridge, MA: Blackwell Scientific.

Cohen, M. M., Jr. (1982). *The child with multiple birth defects.* New York: Raven Press.

Fraser, F. C. (1970). The genetics of cleft lip and cleft palate. *American Journal of Human Genetics, 22,* 336–352.

Gereau, S. A., & Shprintzen, R. J. (1988). The role of adenoids in the development of normal speech following palate repair. *Laryngoscope, 98,* 99–103.

Goldberg, R., Motzkin, B., Marion, R., Scambler, P. J., & Shprintzen, R. J. (1993). Velo-cardio-facial syndrome: A review of 120 cases. *American Journal of Medical Genetics 45,* 313–319.

Golding-Kushner, K. J. (1991). *Craniofacial morphology and velopharyngeal physiology in four syndromes of clefting.* Unpublished doctoral dissertation, City University of New York.

Golding-Kushner, K. J., Weller, G., & Shprintzen, R. J. (1985). Velo-cardio-facial syndrome: Language and psychological profiles. *Journal of Craniofacial Genetics and Developmental Biology, 5,* 259–266.

Gorlin, R. J., Cohen, M. M., Jr., & Levin, L. S. (1990). *Syndromes of the head and neck* (3rd ed). New York: Oxford University Press.

Hoch, L., Golding-Kushner, K., Sadewitz, V. L., & Shprintzen, R. J. (1986). Speech therapy. *Seminars in Speech and Language, 7,* 311–323.

Jones, K. L. (1988). *Smith's recognizable patterns of human malformation* (4th ed). Philadelphia: W. B. Saunders.

LeBlanc, E. M., & Shprintzen, R. J. (1994). Speech and the maxillofacial complex: A structural-functional perspective for diagnosis and management. *Oral and Maxillofacial Surgery Clinics of North America, 6*(1), 113–120.

McKusick, V. A. (1990). *Mendelian inheritance in man* (9th ed). Baltimore: Johns Hopkins University Press.

Randall, P., Krogman, W. M., & Jahina, S. (1965). Pierre Robin and the syndrome that bears his name. *Cleft Palate Journal, 2*, 237–244.

Sadewitz, V. L., & Shprintzen R. J. (1987). Communication impairment in children with multiple anomaly syndromes. [Video tape]. White Plains, NY: March of Dimes Birth Defects Foundation, 1987.

Shprintzen, R. J. (1982). Palatal and pharyngeal anomalies in craniofacial syndromes. *Birth Defects, 18*(1), 53–78.

Shprintzen, R. J. (1988). Pierre Robin, micrognathia, and airway obstruction: The dependency of treatment on accurate diagnosis. *International Anesthesiology Clinics, 26*, 84–91.

Shprintzen, R. J., Goldberg, R., Golding-Kushner, K. J., & Marion, R. (1992). Late-onset psychosis in the velo-cardio-facial syndrome. *American Journal of Medical Genetics, 42*, 141–142.

Shprintzen, R. J., Goldberg, R. B., Lewin, M. L., Sidoti, E. J., Berkman, M. D., Argamaso, R. V., & Young, D. (1978). A new syndrome involving cleft palate, cardiac anomalies, typical facies, and learning disabilities: Velo-cardio-facial syndrome. *Cleft Palate Journal, 15*, 56–62.

Shprintzen, R. J., Siegel-Sadewitz, V. L., Amato, J., & Goldberg, R. B. (1985). Anomalies associated with cleft lip, cleft palate, or both. *American Journal of Medical Genetics, 20*, 585–596.

Trost, J. E. (1981). Articulatory additions to the classical description of the speech of persons with cleft palate. *Cleft Palate Journal, 18*, 193–203.

Witzel, M. A. (1983). Speech problems in craniofacial anomalies. *Communicative Disorders, 8*, 45–59.

Witzel, M. A., Ross, R. B., & Munro, I. R. (1980). Articulation before and after facial osteotomy. *Journal of Oral and Maxillofacial Surgery, 8*, 195–202.

✦ SUGGESTED READINGS

Cohen, M. M., Jr. (1982). *The child with multiple birth defects.* New York: Raven Press.

Fraser, F. C. (1970). The genetics of cleft lip and cleft palate. *American Journal of Human Genetics, 22*, 336–352.

Siegel-Sadewitz, V. L., & Shprintzen, R. J. (1982). The relationship of communication disorders to syndrome identification. *Journal of Speech and Hearing Disorders, 47*, 338–354.

✦ GLOSSARY

Anomaly: any deviation from normal structure, form, or function in an individual.

Base pair: pairs of amino acids which connect two strands of intertwined sugar and phosphate molecules to comprise DNA.

Chromosome: long strands made of DNA and protein which carry the genetic material (genes) which guides the formation of the developing embryo. Humans have 46 chromosomes, or 23 pairs, each member of the pair resembling the other with the exception of the male sex chromosomes (see below).

> **Autosome:** 22 pairs of the chromosomes are called autosomes which carry the majority of human genetic information and do not play a role in sex determination.

> **Sex chromosome:** a single pair of chromosomes which are responsible for sex determination. Females have two X chromosomes which are identical to each other in structure and do carry a number of genes, whereas males have an X and Y chromosome, which do not resemble each other. The Y chromosome's purpose is to produce the male phenotype.

Cleft palate: an opening in the palate (which forms the roof of the mouth) caused by a failure of the embryonic elements of the palate to fuse.

> **Submucous cleft palate:** a separation of the muscle fibers in the soft palate and on occasion a separation of the palatal bone with an intact skin covering. The uvula is cleft (split), called a *bifid uvula*.

> **Occult submucous cleft palate:** a separation of the muscle fibers in the soft palate with an intact skin covering, but without a cleft uvula so that on oral examination, the palate appears normal.

Congenital: present at birth.

Deformation: mechanical factors which cause anomalies by impinging on the embryo and cause a redirection or inhibition of growth.

Disruption: mechanical factors which cause anomalies by tearing or mutilating the embryo or fetus.

Dysmorphology: the study of congenital anomalies.

Embryo: the developing baby in the mother's uterus during the first three months of gestation (the first trimester).

Fetus: the developing baby in the mother's uterus during the last six months of gestation (the last two trimesters).

Gene: a unit comprised of DNA responsible for determining human structure and function and accountable for human heredity.

Genetics: the study of heredity.

> **Clinical genetics:** the science of studying human beings and diagnosing genetic disease.

> **Molecular genetics:** the science of studying the structure and function of genes to determine how human disease is caused and how genes function.

Genetic counseling: the delivery of information to an individual or family regarding a genetic trait or abnormality.

Genome: the human genetic code.

Genotype: an individual's genetic make-up.

Glottal stop: an abnormality of articulation where consonants are produced by hard contact of the vocal cords causing a stoppage of air and sudden release. This articulatory error is common in individuals with cleft palate.

Hypoplasia: an abnormally small or incompletely formed body part.

Hypotonia: weakness, usually generalized to the entire body.

Karyotype: chromosome analysis.

Laryngeal web: an abnormal piece of skin stretching across the larynx which can cause breathing problems or an abnormal production of voice.

Mandible: the lower jaw.

Maxilla: the upper jaw.

Microcephaly: abnormally small head size.

Micrognathia: an abnormally small lower jaw.

Microtia: an abnormally formed external ear (i.e., hypoplastic).

Mode of inheritance: the pattern with which a trait is inherited in a family.

> **Autosomal dominant:** a 50% risk of inheriting an abnormal trait because of the presence of an abnormal (mutant) gene on one of the autosomes from one parent.

> **Autosomal recessive:** a 25% risk of inheriting an abnormal trait because of the presence of an abnormal (mutant) gene on one of the autosomes in both parents.

> **X-linked:** a 50% chance for males to inherit an abnormal trait because of the presence of a mutant gene on one of the mother's X chromosomes. Also known as *sex-linked*.

Multifactorial: expression of an abnormal trait caused by several or many genes plus environmental influences.

Mutation: a change in a gene causing it to produce an abnormal trait.

Neoplasia: literally "new growth," usually referring to a tumor.

Phenotype: the physical and behavioral characteristics of an individual.

Sequence: multiple anomalies derived from a single known or presumed structural anomaly or mechanical factor. Therefore a single malformation, deformation, or disruption can secondarily cause other anomalies. However, the primary anomaly which causes the other anomalies may itself have many possible causes (i.e., not a single etiology), unlike syndromes where there is a single pathogenesis.

Syndrome: the presence of multiple anomalies in a single individual with all of those anomalies having a common cause.

Teratogen: an agent in the embryonic environment which interferes with the normal embryologic process resulting in anomalies.

Velopharyngeal insufficiency: an inability to separate the oral cavity from the nasal cavity during speech, usually resulting in speech with excessive nasality.

Voice Disorders

LORRAINE OLSON RAMIG, PH.D.

After completing this chapter, you should be able to:

◆ Describe how you produce your voice.

◆ Explain how you change the pitch, loudness, and quality of your voice.

◆ Describe why your voice sounds low in pitch, soft and breathy when you have a cold or allergies.

◆ Describe how voice is evaluated.

◆ List three categories of voice disorders.

◆ Explain the basic principles for improving disordered voice.

◆ List eight vocally abusive habits.

◆ Explain how to keep your voice healthy.

Voice production or phonation is the foundation of oral communication. This chapter will enhance your awareness of the critical role of the voice in effective communication as well as its role as a window to physical and emotional condition. The anatomical and physiological bases of normal and disordered voice production will be described in relation to the voice characteristics of pitch, loudness, and quality and their acoustic correlates. Voice disorders of use/misuse, psychogenic/stress, and medical/physical origins together with their multidisciplinary assessment and treatment will be discussed. Techniques for maintaining a healthy voice will be presented.

Take a deep breath and say "oh" for as long as you can. Listen to the pitch, the loudness, the quality of that "oh." **Now say "oh" with surprise, now say it with fear, now say it with sadness.** Listen to the pitch, loudness, and quality of your voice and how your voice changed to reflect each of these emotions.

- ✦ **Think of how your voice sounds when you have a cold or allergies.**
- ✦ **Think of how your voice sounds the day after you have cheered at a sporting event.**
- ✦ **Consider your ability to "hear" good or bad news in the voice of your best friend within the first 2 seconds of his or her phone call.**
- ✦ **Think of the sound of a baby's cry, a child's laugh, a teenager's shriek, and a grandma's whisper.**
- ✦ **Think of your favorite singers and how their music makes you feel.**

These examples demonstrate that voice has a great impact on communication, both in conveying meaning as well as in revealing information about the age, physical health, and emotional intent of the speaker.

Voice, or **phonation**, is the foundation for the production of oral communication. The understanding of phonation is a multidisciplinary endeavor. It involves knowledge from such disciplines as anatomy, physiology, acoustics, aerodynamics, engineering, perception, as well as the professions of otolaryngology, neurology, psychology, and vocal performance. The speech pathologist blends knowledge from these basic sciences and professions to improve the effectiveness of vocal communication.

✦ HOW DO YOU CREATE YOUR VOICE?

Look at Figure 12–1 on page 484. This is your speech mechanism. Your respiratory system includes your lungs surrounded by your rib cage and intercostal muscles on the sides and your diaphragm and abdomen on the bottom. **Put your hands on your rib cage and inhale and exhale; now put your hands on your abdomen and inhale and exhale.** As your rib cage and abdomen move out during inhalation, you are filling your lungs with more air. This is the air supply you use to produce voice.

Your respiratory air supply (the air in your lungs) causes the vocal folds in your larynx to vibrate during voice production. Look again at Figure 12–1 on page 484. The larynx sits on top of the trachea (windpipe) which is the airway from the lungs. **Take in a breath, put your hand on your "Adam's Apple" and say "ah."** After you inhale, your vocal folds come together (adduction) and valve the air stream to produce the vibration you feel in your neck. This vibration creates the acoustic voice source. The vibration of your vocal folds occurs approximately 200 times per second if you are a female and 125 times per second if you are a male. The number of vocal fold vibrations per second is the fundamental frequency of your voice. The fundamental frequency, intensity (acoustic power), and regularity of this acoustic voice source are related respectively to the *pitch, loudness*, and *quality* you perceive in your voice.

To produce speech, this acoustic voice source is filtered in your vocal tract (mouth and throat) by the movement and position of your articulators — tongue, lips, jaw, and velopharynx. **Take in a breath and say "ah," "ee," and "oh."** Notice the movement of your lips, tongue, and jaw as they change position to generate these different speech sounds. The sound of your voice as it is heard by listeners is related to the characteristics (frequency, intensity, and regularity) of the acoustic voice source (at your larynx) as filtered by the vocal tract (your mouth and throat).

How Does Your Larynx Work?

To understand how voice is produced, it is necessary to review basic *laryngeal anatomy and physiology*. The **larynx** or "voice box" is composed of muscles and cartilages pictured in Figure 12–2. Their function is to change the position and shape of the vocal folds. The vocal folds move apart (abduct) to allow air to flow into the lungs,

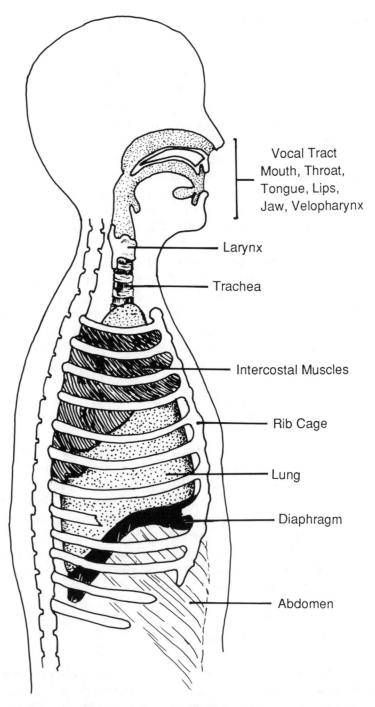

Figure 12–1. Functional components of the speaking mechanism. The respiratory system includes the lungs surrounded by your rib cage and intercostal muscles on the sides and your diaphragm and abdomen on the bottom. The larynx sits on top of the trachea. The vocal tract includes your mouth, throat, tongue, lips, jaw, and velopharynx.

move together (adduct) to produce voice, and they are stretched and thinned to change pitch. Five pairs of laryngeal muscles are used in voice production (Figure 12–2**A**): the thyroarytenoids (or vocalis muscles located within the vocal folds), cricothyroids, lateral cricoarytenoids, interarytenoids, and posterior cricoarytenoids.

The intrinsic laryngeal muscles have attachments to cartilages within the larynx. There are three primary laryngeal cartilages (Figure 12–2**B**); the thyroid is the largest. **Put your finger on your Adam's apple (thyroid notch) and swallow.** You have just felt your thyroid cartilage move. Below the thyroid cartilage and above the trachea is the cricoid cartilage, a ring-shaped cartilage. The arytenoid

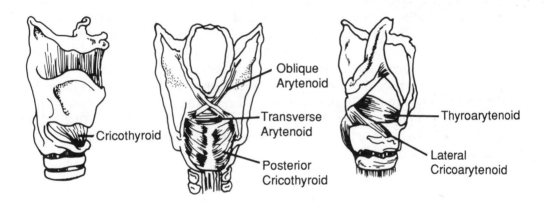

View A Muscles

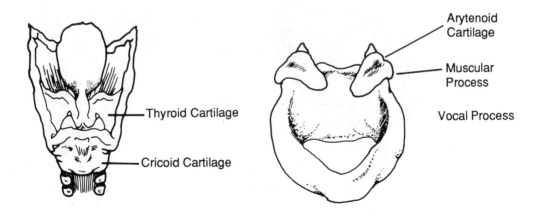

View B Cartilage

Figure 12–2. The intrinsic laryngeal muscles (**A**) including the thyroarytenoids (vocalis), cricothyroids, lateral cricoarytenoids, transverse and posterior cricoarytenoids shown in lateral and posterior views. The laryngeal cartilages (**B**) including the thyroid, cricoid, and arytenoids.

cartilage pair is positioned on the top of the posterior portion of the cricoid cartilage. The arytenoid cartilages are shaped like pyramids and have two processes or points for muscular attachment: the vocal processes and the muscular processes.

The vocal folds attach anteriorly to the thyroid cartilage and posteriorly to the vocal processes of the arytenoid cartilages (Figure 12–2**B**). **Sing up the scale.** You have just used your cricothyroid muscle to stretch and thin your vocal folds to make them vibrate faster and produce a higher pitch. **Say "oh-oh-oh."** You have just used your lateral cricoarytenoid and interarytenoids to close (adduct) your vocal folds to produce each "oh." **Say "oh-oh-oh" again and take a breath between each "oh."** You have just used your posterior cricothyroid muscles to open your vocal folds for each breath.

The **vocal folds** themselves are composed of five layers as pictured in Figure 12–3. the epithelium is on the edge of the vocal fold. The next three layers are within the lamina propria: superficial, intermediate, and deep. The thyroarytenoid (or vocalis) muscle comprises the "body" of the vocal fold. The superficial layer of lamina propria (Reinke's space) vibrates the most during phonation. The glottis is the air space between the open vocal folds through which air flows to and from the lungs. The **false vocal folds** or ventricu-

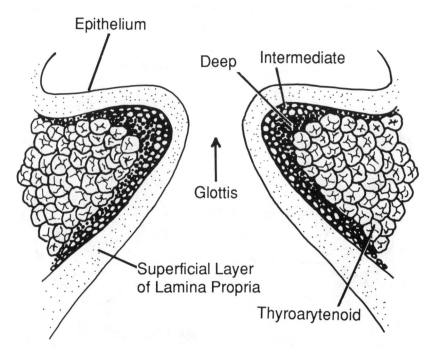

Figure 12-3. The five layers of the vocal folds: the epithelium, the superficial, intermediate, and deep layers of the lamina propria, and the thyroarytenoid (or vocalis) muscle.

lar folds (see Figure 12–4) are located above the true vocal folds, and they may vibrate during disordered phonation. **Sing down the scale as low in pitch as possible until your voice makes a low "fry rumble" sound; in many cases you may be vibrating your false vocal folds.**

The nervous system controls the larynx (Figure 12–5) through bilateral cortical and subcortical connections to the nucleus ambiguus of the vagus (or 10th) cranial nerve as described in Chapter 8. Because this control is bilateral, unilateral damage to the brain does not affect voice production significantly. Muscles in the larynx are controlled (innervated) by two branches of the vagus nerve. The superior laryngeal nerve branch of the vagus innervates the cricothyroid muscle pair. All other intrinsic laryngeal muscles are innervated by the recurrent laryngeal nerve branch of the vagus. Given the exquisite sensitivity of the larynx to emotions such as fear, anger, and joy, it is not surprising that autonomic and limbic sys-

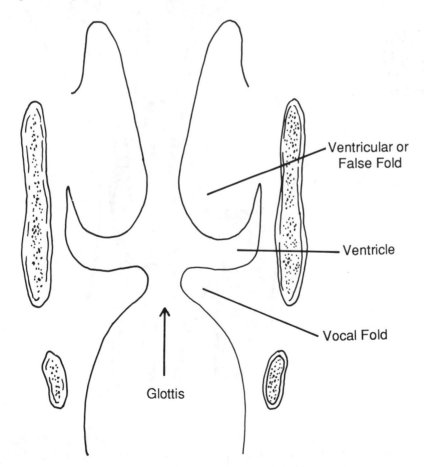

Figure 12–4. The location of the false (ventricular) folds and the true vocal folds on coronal section.

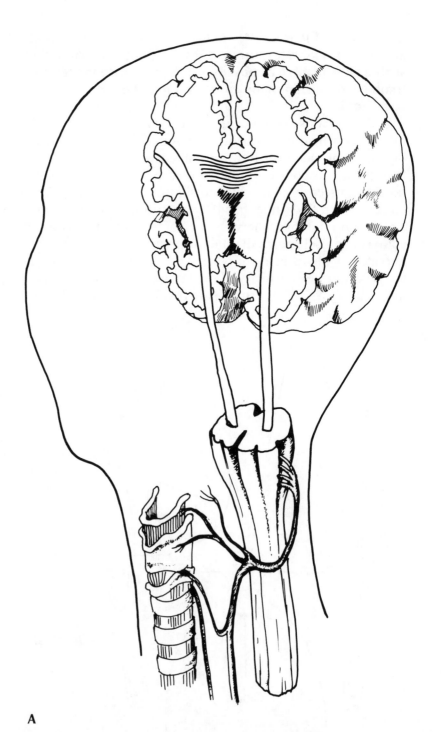

A

Figure 12–5. (**A**) Cortical and subcortical connections to the nucleus ambiguus of the vagus (tenth) cranial nerve. (**B**) Superior and recurrent laryngeal nerve branches of the vagus innervate laryngeal muscles.

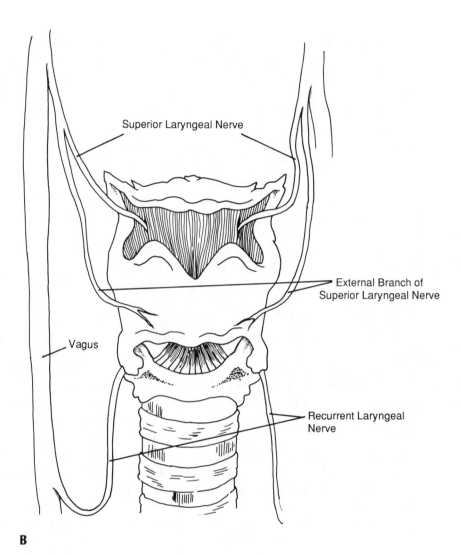

B

Figure 12-5 *(continued)*

tems (discussed in Chapter 8) play an important role in control of phonation as well. **Remember how your voice sounded when you made your first speech to a large audience?** Your autonomic and limbic systems were affecting your voice. The nervous system control of your larynx is discussed in more detail in Chapter 8.

◆ HOW DO YOU EVALUATE THE CHARACTERISTICS OF THE VOICE?

A goal in the assessment of voice and its disorders is to establish a relationship between how the voice sounds (the perceptual characteristics) and what the speech mechanism — the larynx in particular — is doing to create that sound (the physiological characteristics). Knowledge of that relationship contributes to diagnosis of a voice disorder and to its treatment. We may reasonably refer to sound produced within the larynx as the sound source (technically, the voice source). Therapy improves the sound of the voice by modifying (through behavioral, surgical, or pharmacological methods) how the larynx is creating voice. The speech pathologist evaluates the perceptual features of *pitch, loudness,* and *quality* together with their *acoustic* (physical sound) *correlates* to gain insight into the physiologic bases of a disordered voice and consequently insight for treatment. Acoustic information is useful because it permits objective quantification of voice characteristics. The speech pathologist and the otolaryngologist (ENT) also view the vocal folds through *endoscopy* and evaluate anatomical and physiological characteristics that contribute to voice production (Figure 12–6). Integrating the information gained through physiologic, aerodynamic, acoustic, and perceptual evaluations is critical in understanding and treating the voice.

Pitch is the psychological sensation resulting from perception of the **fundamental frequency** (the number of vocal fold vibrations per second) from the acoustic voice signal. Fundamental frequency is determined by the length and tension of the vocal folds. When there is more tension in the vocal folds, the vibratory rate is higher and the fundamental frequency and pitch are higher. **Sing up the scale and think of your vocal folds stretching and thinning like a rubber band as your pitch goes up.** As your vocal folds stretch and thin, they have more tension and so they vibrate at a higher frequency. As a result your voice has a higher pitch. When you are nervous or anxious, your vocal folds may have more tension, and your voice frequently reflects this tension through faster vocal fold vibration and a higher pitch.

Loudness is measured from the acoustic voice signal as *sound pressure level* and is associated with the degree of adduction of the vocal folds in combination with air pressure beneath the vocal folds (subglottal pressure). **Say the word "Hello" very softly** — you did not fully adduct your vocal folds and your voice was reduced in loudness. **Now shout the word "Hello"** — notice how you took in a deeper breath, adducted your vocal folds with greater force, and impounded more air pressure below the vocal folds to produce a louder voice.

The relationships between perceptual dimensions of **vocal quality** such as breathiness, hoarseness, tremor, and their acoustic and physiologic correlates are not straightforward. Vocal quality has been associated with dimensions of both vocal fold **vibratory insta-**

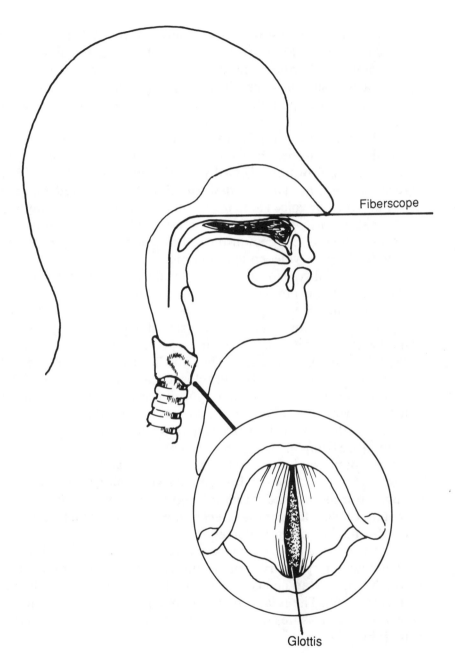

Fiberscope

Glottis

Figure 12–6. Visualization of the larynx through fiberoptic examination.

bility and **adduction**. In addition, vocal quality has been associated with vocal tract characteristics.

Vibratory instability has been thought of as "long-term," such
as vocal tremor, and "short-term," such as hoarseness. **Produce "oh"
with a shaky voice.** This is **vocal tremor** or, if you did this with an

artistic flair, **vocal vibrato**. Vocal tremor is produced at about 5 to 6 times per second. **Now produce "oh" with a hoarse voice.** This is an example of short-term instability which may be reflected in acoustic measures such as jitter (cycle-to-cycle differences in time, sometimes called pitch perturbations), shimmer (cycle-to-cycle differences in amplitude), and spectral noise.

Another way to think of voice quality is on the continuum of breathy-normal-pressed as related to amount of vocal fold closure (adduction). **Produce a breathy "oh," now a normal "oh," then really squeeze out an "oh" that sounds tight or pressed.** You have just moved your voice along the breathy-normal-pressed continuum of vocal quality by changing the amount of vocal fold adduction (closure). Figure 12–7 demonstrates the breathy-normal-pressed continuum through videoendoscopic pictures of vocal folds.

Vocal quality also can be associated with characteristics of the vocal tract. For example, the passage from the pharynx to the nasal cavity is called the velopharyngeal port. If this passage is open during non-nasal sounds, speech may sound hypernasal. By contrast, if there is too little nasal resonance, speech may be called hyponasal (the sound of your speech when you have a stuffed nose). Speakers with normal velopharyngeal closure can alter the shape of their mouth (vocal tract) through tongue and jaw movements. This affects the perceived quality of the sounds produced by changing the acoustic filtering of the voice source by changing the vocal tract shape. (See Chapter 10 for a more complete discussion.) **Keep your tongue bunched in the back of your mouth and your jaw closed and sustain "ah." Now while you are sustaining "ah," gradually open your mouth and let your tongue relax on the floor of your mouth. Could you hear the effect of the different vocal tract shapes on the quality of your voice?**

The optimally healthy voice is created through a combination of adequate respiratory support and easy onset vocal fold valving which generate an acoustic signal that is enhanced through vocal tract filtering. The relationships among perceptual, acoustic, and physiologic measures related to laryngeal function are summarized in Table 12–1.

◆ WHY DO VOICE PITCH, LOUDNESS, AND QUALITY CHANGE WITH AGE?

When you talk to a stranger on the telephone you often are able to estimate his or her age. You can tell whether you are talking to a child, a teenager, an adult, or an elderly person by the characteristics of their voices. People at different ages have different character-

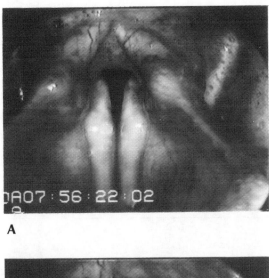

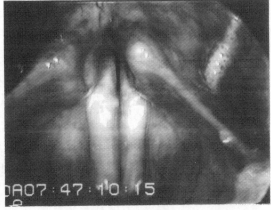

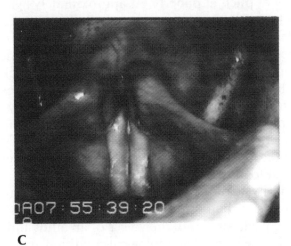

Figure 12–7. Vocal fold configuration during production of a breathy voice (**A**), a normal voice (**B**), and a pressed voice (**C**).

TABLE 12–1. Perceptual features of voice and their acoustic and physiologic correlates.

Perceptual	Acoustic	Physiologic
Pitch	Frequency	Vocal fold mass and elasticity
Loudness	Intensity	Subglottal air pressure, vocal fold adduction, vocal tract shape
Quality	Waveform regularities and spectral features	Vocal fold vibratory regularity and vocal fold adduction

istics of the pitch, loudness, and quality of their voices. These characteristics change because the speech mechanism and larynx grow, change, and then deteriorate with age.

Imitate the voice of a 4-year-old child saying "Hello, how are you?" Now repeat that sentence using the voice of a 70-year-old. How did you change the pitch, loudness, and quality of your voice to create those perceptions of age?

The voice of a baby is high in pitch — think of the sound of an infant crying. This sound reflects the very small vocal folds and short vocal tract of an infant. As a baby grows into a child, the size of the larynx and vocal folds increase and the fundamental frequency decreases. Into the teenage years, the larynx of the male grows considerably, and this growth is associated with the nearly one octave lowering of pitch at puberty. At approximately age 18, the voice is adult-like and remains consistent until approximately age 60 when age-related deterioration begins. Male voices go up in pitch after age 60, reflecting atrophied (shrinking) vocal folds. Some female voices go down in pitch with advanced age, reflecting thickening of vocal folds related to hormonal changes; other female voices go up in pitch, reflecting atrophy of the vocal folds. Voices also may become hoarse and tremorous with age, reflecting both muscle atrophy and age-related deterioration in neurological control of the larynx. It is important to note that the progression of age-related changes in voice may be related to an individual's physical condition; older individuals in good physical condition may have fewer age-related changes in their voices than those in poor physical condition. Figure 12–8 shows acoustic signals of the voices of an adult and two elderly individuals, one in good physiological condition and one in poor physiological condition.

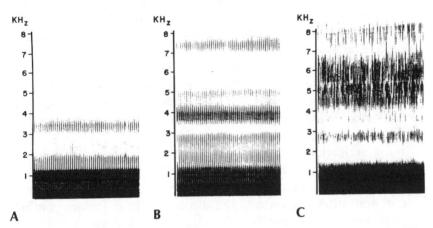

Figure 12–8. Wide band (300 Hz) sonograms of the vowel /a/ produced by males of different chronological ages and physiological conditions; young in good condition (**A**), old in good condition (**B**), and old in poor condition (**C**). A sonogram is a three dimensional representation of acoustic spectra. Time is represented on the abscissa (horizontal dimension), frequency in KHz is represented on the ordinate (vertical dimension), and intensity is reflected by the darkness of the pattern. Each sonogram represents approximately 300 ms of sustained phonation sampled from the mid-section of each vowel.

◆ WHAT CAN GO WRONG WITH THE VOICE?

Voice disorders can affect individuals of all ages. Approximately 5% of children and 3% of adults have disordered voices. The continuum of voice disorders (dysphonia) is broad. It can range from the professional voice user having a subtle breakdown in voice, which reduces the effectiveness of vocal performance but does not affect speech effectiveness or intelligibility, to a disorder of the voice such as a vocal nodule which results in a hoarse voice, reducing both speech effectiveness and intelligibility, to surgical removal of the larynx which eliminates the voice source and requires an alternative mode of voice production. The degree of *communication impairment resulting from a voice disorder* relates to both the severity of the disorder and its impact on the voice user. It is generally true that voice disorders are among the most successfully treated of all disorders seen by a speech pathologist.

Perceptual signs of a voice disorder can include problems with *pitch, loudness,* and *vocal quality.* For example, pitch may be too high for a person's age, sex, and body size and may distract the listener. Loudness may be too soft and prevent the listener from understanding the speaker. Voice quality may be hoarse, too breathy, or tremorous. Any of these conditions can distract the listener and reduce the degree to which the speaker will be understood. These disordered perceptual characteristics will have acoustic and physiological correlates.

The *etiologies* or causes of voice disorders are varied and frequently there are many contributing causes for one voice disorder. Three major categories of etiology include: (1) *misuse/abuse*, (2) *psychological/stress*, and (3) *medical/physical*. As illustrated in the diagram in Figure 12–9, these categories overlap, and in many cases a number of etiological factors contribute to one voice disorder. There may be a *primary etiological factor* which is the basis for the disorder and then subsequent *secondary factors* which relate to the patient's compensatory response to the disorder. These factors combine to generate the characteristics of the disordered voice.

For example, a medical or physical condition can affect the production of voice and generate corresponding stress and misuse/abuse behaviors. **Think of how your voice sounds when you have laryngitis accompanying a cold or allergies.** When you have a cold, your pitch is frequently lower, your voice is softer, and it has more of

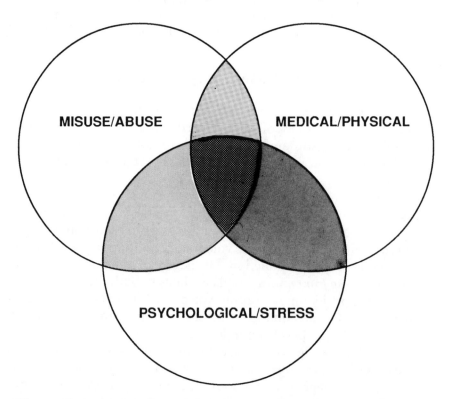

Figure 12–9. Model of voice disorder etiologies: use and misuse, medical and physical condition, and stress and psychological factors and their interactions.

a hoarse quality than your normal voice. This happens because your vocal folds become swollen (edematous) and they vibrate at a lower frequency, generating a lower pitch. Because your vocal folds are swollen, they cannot close (adduct) normally; therefore you cannot easily project your voice, thus reducing loudness. Also when the vocal folds are swollen (edema), they may vibrate irregularly, causing your voice to sound hoarse. Thus when you have a cold, you often have a low-pitched, weak, hoarse voice. When this happens, you notice that people misunderstand you, and you are unable to get their attention easily. You are unable to control your voice precisely to express emotions. This annoys you and you may "work harder" to create an understandable voice. You work harder by hyperadducting (tightly closing) your vocal folds, which only makes the problem worse. You feel stressed because you can't express yourself, and this makes the laryngeal muscles tighter. When you try harder, your voice sounds strained. In these circumstances, rather than working your voice harder, you should rest your voice (reduce the amount of talking) so that the edema and irritation subside. Fortunately, voice disorders associated with colds usually are temporary. In most cases your cold will go away and your voice will return to normal within a few days. However, for people with more significant voice disorders, their voices sound continuously disordered, and they feel this frustration every day. If you have a hoarse voice for over 10 days, you should see an otolaryngologist.

Although the preceding example demonstrates how etiologic factors may overlap, each of the three general categories of voice disorder etiologies are discussed independently in the following sections.

Misuse/Abuse

Many times the *vocal habits* (e.g., throat clearing, coughing) of a speaker, together with the manner or style in which a speaker produces his or her voice when talking, contribute to the development of a voice disorder. A speaker also may have life-style habits that damage the vocal folds. Smoking cigarettes and drinking alcohol can irritate the vocal folds. Any activity that causes the vocal folds to close with excessive force can be characterized as vocal misuse/abuse. **Clear your throat, now cough.** These activities forcefully adduct your vocal folds and are called hard glottal attacks. Chronic throat clearing, coughing, screaming, or loud talking for a long period of time can cause damage to your vocal folds. **Think of how your voice sounds and feels after you have cheered loudly throughout a sporting event.** As many as three out of five cheerleaders have a laryngeal pathology, usually directly related to vocal misuse/abuse.

The *manner or style in which you produce voice* when you speak can also lead to a voice disorder. **Produce the phrase "My voice is tight" with a pressed or tight sounding voice. Now produce the phrase "My voice is relaxed" with a breathy voice.** When voice is chronically produced with too much tension in the laryngeal muscles — when your voice sounds pressed and tight — it is called vocal hyperfunction. *Vocal nodules, vocal polyps,* and *contact ulcers* are examples of voice disorders associated with vocal misuse/abuse and vocal hyperfunction.

Initially, the symptoms of vocal misuse/abuse and hyperfunction may be mild hoarseness and vocal fatigue. Later, after prolonged periods of vocal misuse/abuse, **vocal nodules** (sometimes called singer's or screamer's nodes), which are like calluses, may form on the vocal folds at the point of maximum vocal fold adduction. The nodules may add mass to the vocal folds so the pitch of the voice may be lower. The nodules prevent complete adduction, so air escapes and the voice may be breathy and reduced in loudness. Nodules may prevent the vocal folds from vibrating regularly so the quality of the voice may be hoarse, husky, and have breaks in pitch. Lower pitch, reduced loudness, pitch breaks, and husky voice quality are the classic characteristics associated with vocal nodules. Vocal nodules are the most common voice disorder in children and, in some cases, have been associated with aggressive vocalization secondary to a psychological etiology. In adults, vocal nodules have been associated with habits of vocal misuse and hyperfunction and are frequently observed in individuals who spend much of their day talking. Vocal nodules are pictured in Figure 12–10**B**. Vocal nodules can be managed effectively by behavioral voice therapy designed to identify and reduce habits of vocal misuse/abuse, reduce vocal hyperfunction, and teach an easy, healthy manner of voice production. Habits of vocal misuse/abuse and healthy voice use are summarized in Table 12–2.

TABLE 12–2. Habits of vocal misuse/abuse and healthy voice habits.

Vocal Misuse/Abuse	Healthy Voice Habits
Throat clearing	Reduce or eliminate habits of misuse/abuse
Excessive coughing	
Screaming or yelling	Use relaxed voice onset
Loud talking for extended periods of time	Use adequate respiratory support
Habitual speaking with tight, pressed voice	
Hard glottal attacks	Drink 8 glasses of water each day
Smoking	
Drinking alcohol in excess	

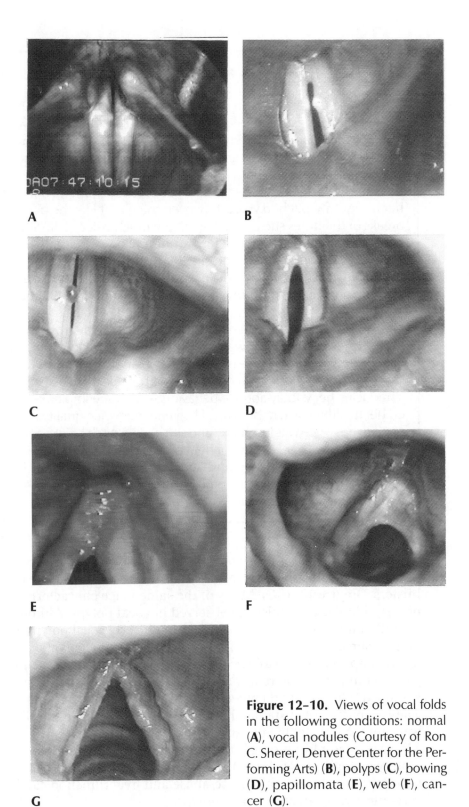

Figure 12–10. Views of vocal folds in the following conditions: normal (**A**), vocal nodules (Courtesy of Ron C. Sherer, Denver Center for the Performing Arts) (**B**), polyps (**C**), bowing (**D**), papillomata (**E**), web (**F**), cancer (**G**).

Case Study

Mary Jo was a sophomore in college. She was referred to our University Clinic because of bilateral vocal nodules. The interview revealed that Mary Jo was very socially active with a vocally gregarious personality. She did a great deal of highly animated talking, cheering at sporting events, and talking over loud background noise in smoky rooms. She admitted that she actually didn't mind her husky, low-pitched voice; however, she didn't like the pitch breaks or the times she couldn't generate much voice at all. She had come to the clinic primarily at the urging of her father.

Therapy consisted of educating Mary Jo about how voice is produced and how voice is misused, identifying vocal misuse/abuse in her daily living (through vocal diaries), and suggesting alternative activities (e.g., when talking at a party over loud background noise, suggest the conversation move away from the noise). She was taught how to produce a well-supported voice which allowed her to "take the load off the larynx." Mary Jo was successful in increasing her awareness of her vocal misuse and in reducing her vocally abusive behaviors. When she implemented her healthy voice habits (vocal hygiene) her voice quality improved; her voice was less husky and she had no pitch breaks. She was pleased with the sound of her voice and understood clearly the relationship between how she used her voice and how it sounded. The report from the otolaryngologist after three months was that the nodules were gone.

Vocal misuse/abuse also may be associated with polyps on the vocal folds. **Vocal polyps** are more pliable than nodules and are like blisters. (Figure 12–10**C**). Many of the same voice characteristics observed in vocal nodules are observed in vocal polyps. Although voice therapy may be useful in patients with early vocal polyps, laryngeal surgery sometimes is necessary to remove the polyp(s). Figure 12–11 presents a histological example of a vocal polyp, the surgical technique used to remove the polyp, and the acoustic signal of sustained "ah" phonation pre- and post-surgical removal of a polyp. The polyp disrupted stable phonation before surgery; phonation was much more stable after surgical removal of the polyp (Figure 12–11**D**). A combination of surgical removal of the polyp by the otolaryngologist (ENT doctor) and voice therapy (by the speech pathologist) to reduce vocal misuse/abuse and hyperfunction can be very effective in treating vocal polyps.

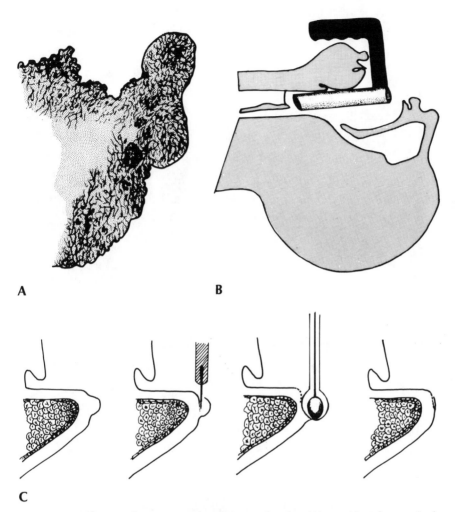

A   **B**

C

Figure 12–11. Histological picture of a vocal polyp (**A**), position for surgical procedure (**B**), surgical removal of vocal polyp (**C**), and examples of sustained "ah" phonation pre- and post-surgical removal of polyp (**D**) (overleaf).

Another vocal misuse/abuse disorder is **contact ulcers**. These are ulcerations in the mucosa of the tips of the vocal processes of the arytenoid cartilages (Figure 12–10**D**). Contact ulcers have been associated with low-pitched phonation characterized by a quality that sounds throaty and pressed, with many hard glottal attacks. Contact ulcers are most often observed in middle-aged males who speak with excessive force. They also have been associated with gastroesophageal reflux, a condition that occurs when digestive juices come in contact with the vocal folds. Gastroesophageal reflux is associated with heartburn, burping, and acidic taste in the mouth. Clients with contact ulcers may complain of vocal fatigue and radi-

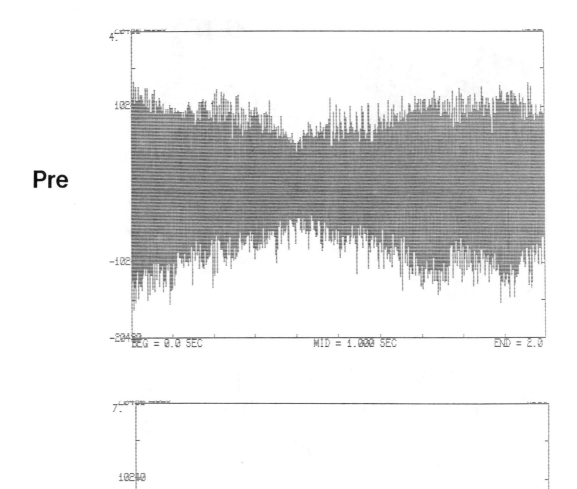

Pre

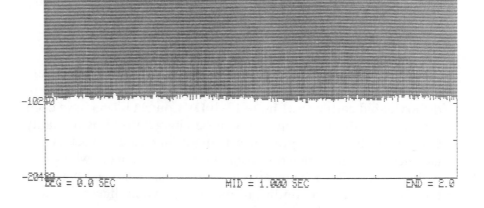

Post

D

Figure 12–11 *(continued)*

ating pain in the throat or a lump in the throat. Treatment may include the identification and reduction of vocal misuse/abuse; teaching relaxed, easy-onset voice production; and medically managing the gastroesophageal reflux.

In general, misuse/abuse disorders can be successfully treated by a speech pathologist through behavioral treatment which helps patients reduce habits of vocal misuse/abuse and hyperfunction and teaches principles of healthy voice production. Certain cases require a combination of medical and surgical intervention preceded and followed by behavioral management.

Psychogenic Voice Disorders

Voice characteristics reflect the emotions of the speaker. **Think of your voice when you had an argument with a good friend, when you told a lie, when you told someone you loved them for the first time.** You expressed yourself through your words and your voice.

It is clear that voice characteristics enhance communication when they reflect the speaker's emotion. However, when the voice becomes disordered as a result of disordered emotions, a psychogenic voice disorder is said to exist. Extreme states of anxiety or depression can affect the voice and result in characteristics ranging from mild hoarseness to complete voice loss (aphonia). Although the larynx can function normally in these patients during automatic, vegetative tasks such as coughing and throat clearing, typically during speech production the voice sounds disordered without a corresponding laryngeal pathology. In most cases, the larynx is capable of producing a normal voice, but the emotions of the speaker prevent this from happening. Musculoskeletal tension disorder, conversion dysphonia and aphonia, and mutational falsetto are examples of psychogenic voice disorders.

Musculoskeletal tension disorders occur when laryngeal muscles hyperfunction in response to stress. Intrinsic laryngeal muscles (both attachments in the larynx) and extrinsic laryngeal muscles (one attachment in the larynx, one out of the larynx) may be affected by excessive tension. **Put your fingers on your thyroid cartilage and move it gently from side to side. Say "ah" while you do this.** Your larynx should move easily without pain and the "ah" should not sound tight or pressed. **Now tighten the muscles in your neck. Try to move your larynx side to side while you say "ah."** Notice how tight and pressed the "ah" sounds and how difficult it is to move your larynx. This is how a musculoskeletal tension disorder would feel. Imagine talking all day with these tight laryngeal muscles. Prolonged periods of musculoskeletal tension dysphonia may result in laryngeal pathologies such as nodules or contact ulcers. Treatment of a musculoskeletal tension disorder may involve both direct laryngeal massage to reduce tension in laryngeal muscles and voice therapy to facilitate healthy (nonhyperfunctional) voice production as well as counseling to address the origin of the stress.

The mechanism of a *conversion voice disorder* is loss of voluntary control over voice production due to stress or conflict. The voice may be disordered (conversion dysphonia) or there may be no ability to voluntarily generate voice and the client whispers (conversion aphonia). In either case, the laryngeal pathology is minor, the client believes the problem is organic and the disordered or absent voice allows the client to avoid an emotionally painful situation. Because the larynx is normal, the treatment for this disorder is to get the voice back through a very brief period of various vocal fold adduction activities such as yawning, sighing, coughing, throat clearing, or gliding into a sustained "ah." Once the voice has returned, the underlying psychological etiology for the voice loss should be addressed through counseling.

Case Example

Jane, a 45-year-old woman, came to our clinic because of a consistently hoarse voice. She had seen an otolaryngologist who told her that her vocal folds were normal. During our interview when she was asked to describe any stress in her life, she stated that due to financial reasons, approximately 3 months ago, she had moved in with her relatives. In exchange, she worked in their jewelry store. She said that this was very difficult both at work and at home, because she felt that her relatives treated her poorly. She reported that they were always criticizing her at work in the presence of customers and barely spoke to her at home. Because her current state of living was dependent on her relatives, however, she felt as though she could not complain to them or speak up for herself. Stimulation to briefly cough and clear her throat and prolong "ah" resulted in a clear voice after a number of trials. It was apparent that Jane could produce a voice of normal quality. However, her inability to confront her relatives and her repressed anger had affected her voice in the form of a conversion dysphonia. Jane discussed her anger regarding her relatives while simultaneously working on mechanisms to allow her to move out of the living and working situations. Her dysphonia improved. Within 2 months, Jane was able to move out of state and she wrote back to report to us that she had a new job and a clear voice.

Mutational falsetto (puberphonia) is an example of a psychogenic voice disorder associated with puberty. When the voice does not change at puberty despite the growth of the larynx, the disorder is called mutational falsetto or puberphonia. **Say "Hello, how are you?" in your normal pitch and loudness. Now, using a pitch twice as high, say the sentence again.** This high-pitched sentence is an example of the sound of a voice with mutational falsetto. The psychologic etiology proposed for this disorder is that the client is resisting the transition to adulthood and so maintains the child-like voice. Because the larynx is of normal size, with the potential to generate a normal pitch, the focus of treatment is to elicit the pitch that is representative of the size of the larynx. In addition, psychological etiological issues are addressed through counseling.

In general, a speech pathologist can elicit an improved voice from patients with psychogenic voice disorders and will establish the need and make the referral for additional counseling on a case by case basis.

Voice Disorders Produced by Medical or Physical Conditions

A variety of medical or physical conditions affect the production of the voice. In these cases, voice disorders occur because either the actual physical characteristics of the vocal folds are changed through a disease or trauma or the nervous system's ability to control the larynx is affected.

Neurological Disorders

As discussed in Chapters 8 and 9, many disorders of the nervous system affect movements necessary for speech production. Some of these *neurological disorders*, or *movement disorders* may also affect the larynx and respiratory system and be reflected in a disordered voice. In certain cases, specific neurological disorders are associated with specific vocal symptoms. Figure 12–12 shows examples of acoustic characteristics of voice in different neurological diseases. Voice disorders may be the first, or an early, sign of a neurological disease, and voice may deteriorate as a disease progresses. This means that analysis of voice may contribute to diagnosis and the documentation of disease progression. Figure 12–13 shows an example of voice in a patient with Lou Gehrig's disease (amyotrophic lateral sclerosis) over a 6-month time span as the voice becomes more unstable.

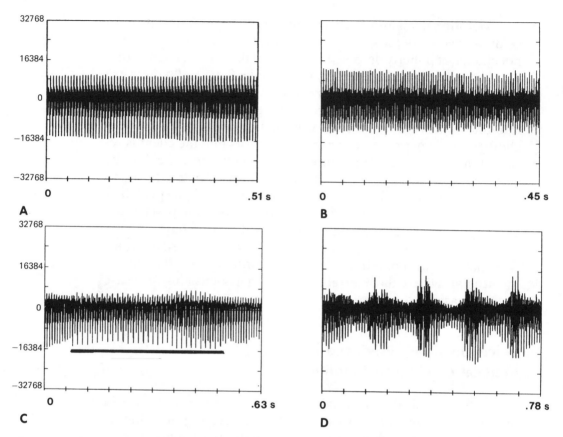

Figure 12–12. Acoustic waveform examples (microphone recordings) of less than one second of sustained vowel phonation from a normal male speaker (**A**), a patient with myotonic muscular dystrophy (**B**), a patient with Huntington's disease (**C**), and a patient with Parkinson's disease (**D**).

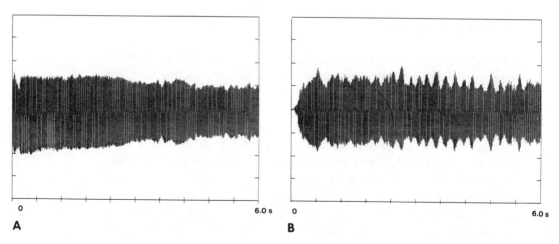

Figure 12–13. Acoustic waveform examples (microphone recordings) of sustained vowel phonation from a patient with Lou Gehrig's disease (amyotrophic lateral sclerosis) over a six month time frame as his disease progressed.

Neurologically based voice disorders historically have been considered within the framework of the movement (motor speech) disorders or dysarthrias. As discussed in Chapter 9, these classifications have been related to the site of neurological damage and referred to as flaccid, spastic, ataxic, hypokinetic, hyperkinetic, and mixed dysarthria. Another approach to neurological voice disorders is to consider them in relation to the laryngeal disorders of hypoadduction (reduced adduction), hyperadduction (increased adduction), and instability (unsteady voice). This approach may have particular relevance to the design of treatment for these voice disorders and is the approach we will take here.

Hypoadduction occurs in many neurological disorders of phonation. Flaccid (lower motor neuron) and hypokinetic (Parkinson's disease) neurological disorders are two examples where reduced vocal fold adduction results in a disordered voice. As discussed in Chapter 8, lower motor neuron dysarthria can involve damage to one of the components of the motor unit: nucleus, nerve, myoneural junction, or muscle. Laryngeal nerve paralysis is one of the most common neurological voice disorders. It may result from isolated trauma to branches of the vagus nerve resulting from an accident during thyroidectomy, chest, or neck surgery. It may be characterized by reduced vocal fold closure and a breathy voice that is reduced in loudness (hypoadduction). **Say "Hello, how are you?" in a breathy, whisper-like voice. Imagine the rest of your life with that voice. How would your life change?** If nerve regeneration and improved function is not observed within 6 months, surgical treatment may be necessary to facilitate vocal fold closure. In these cases behavioral voice therapy is designed primarily to improve vocal fold closure and increase vocal loudness.

Other lower motor neuron disorders that result in vocal fold hypoadduction include myasthenia gravis (disease of the myoneural junction) and myotonic dystrophy (disease of the muscle). These lower motor neuron disorders may affect other aspects of speech production such as articulation and resonance as well as phonation. The diagnosis and treatment of these disorders are designed within the context of the entire motor speech disorder (dysarthria).

Another neurological disease which typically results in vocal fold hypoadduction is Parkinson's disease. As discussed in Chapter 9, Parkinson's disease, a hypokinetic dysarthria, is a disease of the extrapyramidal system. The majority of Parkinson's disease patients are diagnosed after age 50 and receive neuropharmacological (drug) treatment for their symptoms. Although neuropharmacological treatments have positive effects on limb movement, speech and voice disorders are not consistently improved. Imprecise articulation and disordered rate are observed in patients with Parkinson's disease, and 90% of patients have disordered voice. Reduced loudness, monotone, and hoarse voice quality have been related to bowed vocal folds (see Figure 12–10**E**) and rigidity and hypokinesia in the muscles of the larynx. Intensive (daily) voice treatment focusing on increased phonatory effort and vocal fold adduction has been successful in improving patients' vocal loudness and speech intelligibility.

Case Example

Eugene was a 68-year-old male diagnosed with Parkinson's disease 6 years ago. His voice was reduced in loudness, breathy, hoarse, and monotone. Consequently, he had a difficult time being understood, especially by his aged hard-of-hearing friends. His pretreatment laryngeal examination revealed moderate vocal fold bowing. He enrolled in a program of intensive voice therapy focusing on increased phonatory effort and vocal fold adduction. He attended therapy daily for 16 sessions. The intensity of his speech increased 10 decibels after therapy. His posttreatment laryngeal examination revealed reduced bowing and increased vocal fold adduction. He reported that after therapy, he "talked a lot more" because people could now understand him.

Hyperadduction occurs in many neurological disorders of phonation. Spastic pseudobulbar palsy and hyperkinetic dysarthria are two examples of neurological disorders where hyperadduction of the vocal folds results in a disordered voice. When there is *bilateral upper motor neuron damage, spastic pseudobulbar palsy* occurs. Because the larynx is bilaterally innervated, unilateral upper motor neuron damage does not significantly affect voice production. Bilateral strokes and spastic cerebral palsy are the most common causes of this disorder. The classic voice characteristic of spastic pseudobulbar palsy is a strain-strangled voice quality (hyperadduction). As discussed in Chapters 8 and 9, this voice disorder typically occurs in the context of disorders of articulation (dysarthria) and in some cases language (aphasia). The effectiveness of treatment is variable and may focus on generating a consistent voice source.

Hyperadduction also is observed in various forms of *hyperkinetic dysarthria* such as dystonia, chorea, and tics. As described in Chapter 9, these are motor speech, or movement, disorders characterized by increased movements. When these movement disorders affect laryngeal muscles, a randomly hyperadducted voice may occur.

Dystonia is characterized by abnormal, involuntary action-induced movements. Sustained muscle contractions cause twisting and repetitive movements or abnormal postures that may be sustained or intermittent. When these movements affect laryngeal muscles, they are associated with the voice disorder *spasmodic dysphonia*. The adductor form of spasmodic dysphonia is characterized by choked, strain-strangled phonation and, in some cases, vocal tremor; the abductor form is characterized by a breathy effortful voice quality.

Clench tightly the muscles in your hand to make a fist ten times rapidly. Now clench the muscles in your larynx 10 times rapidly. While you are rapidly clenching and unclenching your laryngeal muscles, try to produce "ah" for 10 seconds. Imagine talking all day with a voice like this.

Vocal hyperadduction may be observed in another hyperkinetic disorder called *chorea*. As described in Chapter 11, chorea is characterized by involuntary, purposeless, nonrhythmic, abrupt, rapid, unsustained movements that flow from one body part to another. The movements have been reported to be "dance-like," hence use of the Greek word *chorea* meaning "dance." Choreiform movements are most frequently associated with Huntington's disease, an autosomal dominant (hereditary) movement disorder. When these choreic movements affect the larynx, the voice is strained and characterized by voice breaks (both adductory and abductory).

Tics are most frequently associated with the disorder Gilles de la Tourette syndrome. This syndrome develops in childhood and is associated with grimacing, twitching tics of the face and eyes. The most notable characteristic is the generation of noises, barks, and outbursts of profanity. Drug treatment has been successful in reducing the symptoms of this disorder.

The efficacy of behavioral voice therapy for the *hyperkinetic* patient population has not been established.

Phonatory instability is observed in many neurological disorders of voice. One primary example is the unstable voice observed in the patient with vocal tremor. *Tremor* is associated with many movement disorders such as Parkinson's disease, essential tremor, and cerebellar ataxia. When the muscles of the respiratory or laryngeal systems are affected, vocal tremor results.

Shake your hand at the rate of about 5 times per second. Imagine the muscles in your larynx shaking at that rate. Produce an "ah" with a voice that shakes at about 5 times per second. Imagine the rest of your life with a vocal tremor.

Most vocal tremor has been reported in the range of 4–8 times per second (Hz). Faster rates of tremor (10–13 Hz) have been reported in patients with amyotrophic lateral sclerosis or Lou Gehrig's disease and referred to as "flutter." Neuropharmacological treatment is the primary form of treatment and has been successful in reducing vocal tremor in some patients.

The majority of neurological voice disorders are observed in the context of disorders of the entire nervous system. Therefore, the focus of their assessment and treatment must include consideration of the characteristics and etiology of the neurological disorder as well as the role of the voice disorder in reducing overall speech intelligibility. Although the efficacy of behavioral treatment for neurological voice disorders is not well-established, the classifications of disorders of hypoadduction, hyperadduction, and instability provide direction for treatment planning. The basic interdisciplinary team involved in the treatment of neurological voice disorders includes the speech pathologist, otolaryngologist, and neurologist.

Other Medical or Physical Conditions

Other physical conditions that may affect laryngeal function and result in a voice disorder include *trauma, viruses, congenital conditions, endocrine disorders*, and *cancer. Trauma* to the larynx may damage the nervous system and then be classified as a neurological voice disorder or it may cause structural damage to laryngeal cartilages. Fracture of cartilages may require laryngeal reconstruction surgery. Two examples of trauma that can occur during surgical intubation and result in voice disorders are: (1) a vocal fold granuloma (granulated sac) and (2) hemangioma (blood-filled sac). Both of these conditions interfere with vocal fold vibration and must be surgically removed.

Viruses may affect the physical characteristics of the vocal folds. One example is papillomata, a benign, tumor-like condition that may recur throughout childhood (Figure 12–10**F**). It must be removed surgically because the primary danger of this condition is occlusion of the airway.

Some disordered physical conditions of the larynx occur at birth. One example is *congenital laryngeal web* (Figure 12–10**G**). This is a webbing between the anterior vocal folds, which may interfere with breathing. Webbing also can occur when two sides of the vocal folds are affected as a result of trauma or bilateral removal of lesions and results in a high-pitched, hoarse voice. This condition must be treated surgically.

Endocrine disorders such as hypothyroidism (insufficient thyroxin output by thyroid glands) may result in a hoarse, coarse, gravelly voice due to increased mass of the vocal folds.

Laryngeal cancer (Figure 12–10**H**), which has been linked to cigarette smoking and alcohol use, occurs most often between 50 and

70 years of age. Squamous cell carcinoma is the most common type observed in the larynx. Hoarseness may be the only initial symptom. Because early diagnosis is important for survival, hoarseness occurring for over 10 days (in the absence of a cold or allergies) should not be overlooked. Hoarseness is a primary sign of cancer.

The spread of cancer is the major cause of removal of the larynx in these patients. If total laryngeal removal (laryngectomy) is necessary, the patient will require an alternative mode of voicing. The surgical procedure basically removes the larynx and pulls the trachea to the neck to form a stoma through which the patient now breathes (Figure 12–14). One mode of voicing used by many speakers without a larynx (alaryngeal speakers) is esophageal speech. In this case, another muscle in the vocal tract, the cricopharyngeus (or pharyngoesophageal segment), is used as pseudo-vocal folds to valve the airstream from the esophagus and generate voice. The esophagus (rather than the lungs) is used as the source of air (Figure 12–14). It is frequently said that esophageal speakers speak on "burps." Because the vibratory source for production of voice has changed to the cricopharyngeus, the pitch, loudness, and quality of the esophageal speaker's voice will reflect that new vibratory source. Typically, the esophageal voice is softer, lower in pitch, and rough.

Not all laryngectomees are able to produce functional esophageal speech, and a number of prostheses have been designed to assist the alaryngeal speaker. One alternative mode of voice production is through the use of a tracheo-esophageal shunt which shunts air from the trachea into the esophagus, thus allowing the speaker to use respiratory air to produce voice. (Figure 12–14**C**). This method is considered the easiest and most successful method for alaryngeal speakers to produce voice. Another alternative approach is through use of the electro-larynx, a battery-operated device that generates a sustained sound. The sound of the electro-larynx produces an alternative source of voice and is placed against the neck as the speaker articulates.

◆ ASSESSMENT AND TREATMENT OF VOICE DISORDERS

Assessment and treatment of voice disorders is multidisciplinary. The speech clinician and otolaryngologist work together to evaluate and optimize the patient's voice. Additional team members may include a psychologist, neurologist, oncologist (cancer specialist), pediatrician, vocal coach, and singing teacher. Some voice disorders can be managed by behavioral voice treatment only; other voice disorders require surgical intervention preceded or followed by voice

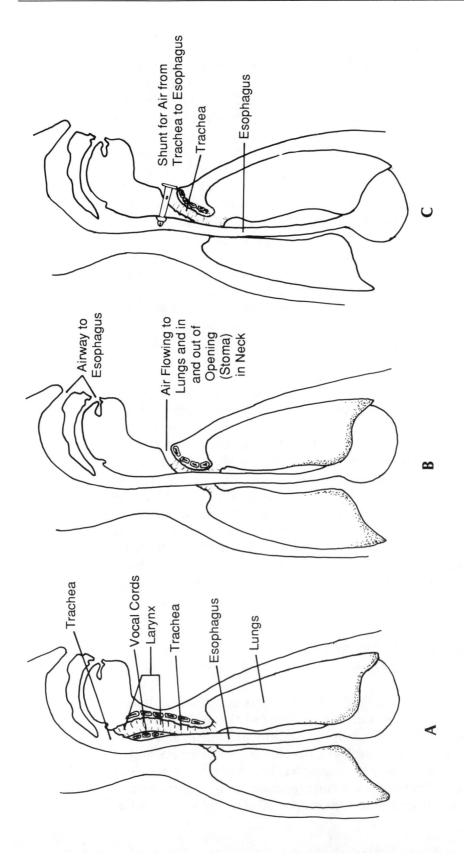

Figure 12–14. Before (**A**), after (**B**) total laryngectomy, and with tracheoesophageal shunt in place (**C**). Notice after the laryngectomy the patient breathes through a stoma. Sound is generated by vibration of the pharyngoesophageal segment.

therapy. And some voice disorders, such as vocal tremor, may respond well to pharmacological intervention.

Assessment of a voice disorder always includes an assessment of the *history* of the disorder and the client's impression of the disorder and its effect on his or her daily living. The voice is evaluated on a *perceptual* level to describe its pitch, loudness, and quality and to assess the impact of the voice disorder on speech intelligibility and communication effectiveness. Various tasks such as sustained "ah" phonation, reading, conversational speech, and phonation range (highest and lowest pitches) are routinely included in such an assessment. Measures of *acoustic* characteristics of voice such as the average fundamental frequency, intensity and residual noise (and the variability of these measures) frequently are obtained to provide objective data for comparison with normative data and to establish a baseline of behavior for pre- to post-treatment comparisons. An evaluation of the *physical condition* of the larynx is essential to assess the relationship between the sound of the voice and the physical condition of the larynx and to determine if there are any disorders which require medical treatment. A speech pathologist and/or an otolaryngologist may view the physical condition of the larynx. This may be done in many ways including a mirror examination, nasal fiberoscopy (fiberoptic bundle inserted through the nose), or oral endoscopy (endoscope rod inserted into the mouth). Often, these examinations are videotaped for later use in describing the physical condition of the larynx. In some cases a stroboscopic light source is used to allow cycle-by-cycle viewing of the details of vocal fold vibration. If additional information regarding the *aerodynamic support for voice production* (air pressures and flows generated by the respiratory system and valved during speech production) is desired, measures of respiratory system function, such as vital capacity (maximum air supply) and subglottal air pressure (air beneath the vocal folds) may be obtained. If neurophysiological information about laryngeal function is desired, *electromyographic recordings* (electrical activity in the muscles) may be carried out by a neurologist or otolaryngologist. The various types of information gathered by a speech pathologist, otolaryngologist, and any other professionals are combined to establish the medical diagnosis of the patient and to develop a treatment plan.

Voice Treatment

Treatment for disordered voice can involve behavioral voice therapy, surgical or pharmacological treatment, psychological counseling, or a combination of these treatments. Decisions for treatment approaches are based on the established efficacy of the treatment together with the specific needs of each patient.

Behavioral voice treatment plays an important role in the management of most voice disorders. The primary goal is to maximize vocal effectiveness and speech intelligibility by teaching techniques of healthy voice use in relation to the existing vocal mechanism and vocal needs of the individual.

In cases of **misuse/abuse**, the primary focus of treatment is to identify and eliminate vocal misuse habits (e.g., coughing, throat clearing) and teach principles of healthy voice production. Treatment focuses on helping the client manage his or her environment, activities, and habits to improve the health of the larynx. In the case of children with voice disorders, family members and teachers may play an important role in treatment.

Healthy voice production frequently includes maximizing respiratory and vocal tract support to reduce hard voice onset and "take the load off the larynx." Voice production should be easy and effortless. In some cases, treatment techniques using biofeedback-enhanced relaxation procedures to reduce overall body tension may be useful. It has been said that voice is so sensitive to body tension that "if your shoes pinch, you'll hear it in your voice."

Say "ah" with a pressed sounding voice. Now yawn and sigh when you say "ah." Did you observe the difference in sound and feel of your voice?

In many cases of vocal misuse/abuse, voice therapy will work very well to improve the voice. Voice therapy can reduce and eliminate vocal nodules, polyps, and contact ulcers. In certain cases, when nodules and polyps must be removed surgically, voice therapy is essential to teach habits of healthy voice use so that the nodules or polyps do not return.

In cases of voice disorders of *psychological origin*, the goal of behavioral treatment is to elicit the best voice possible and provide counseling to address the psychological problem. Because the larynx is virtually normal in most cases, eliciting phonation may involve a brief period of vegetative activities such as yawn-sigh, coughing, and throat clearing with focus on producing voice. In certain cases, treatment is provided in combination with a counselor or psychologist.

The primary focus for treatment of voice disorders accompanying *medical or physical conditions* centers on compensation. Given the condition of the phonatory mechanism and its neurological control, treatment should be directed toward generation of the best voice possible within the physical limitations. In certain cases, surgical treatment followed by voice treatment will be indicated.

Surgical and pharmacological voice treatment is required for many medical or physical problems. The speech pathologist works closely with the medical personnel during these treatments to maximize the resulting laryngeal function.

Surgical treatment of the vocal folds (phonosurgery) may be needed to remove tissue, such as nodules, polyps, cysts, granuloma, and cancer, from the vocal folds. Surgery may be needed to change the position of the vocal folds. For example, when the vocal folds are paralyzed, various surgical procedures to increase adduction may be carried out such as injection of a substance (teflon, silicone, collagen, human fat) to add mass to the vocal fold or to push the fold inward (thyroplasty) (Figure 12–15).

Surgical and *pharmacological treatment* have been used to eliminate neural input to the laryngeal muscles through recurrent laryngeal nerve section and injection of botulinum toxin to reduce symptoms of spasmodic dysphonia.

Psychological treatment may be necessary in certain voice disorders. Because the voice is a sensitive indicator of emotion, it is not surprising that voice disorders can arise from psychological causes. In addition, it is not surprising that a disordered voice can generate an emotional response on the part of the speaker. So whether emotions played a role in the etiology of the voice disorder or were the result of the disordered voice, it is reasonable to consider the psychological dimensions of all voice disorders. In some cases, the speech pathologist is able to provide the necessary counseling. In other cases, it will be necessary to make a referral to a counselor, psychologist, or psychiatrist.

◆ WHAT CAN "GO RIGHT" WITH THE VOICE?

A well-trained voice can be a beautiful musical instrument which conveys meaning through speech and song. Eloquent speakers (e.g., actors, ministers, politicians) and singers (opera, rock, jazz, country western) can move audiences through well-trained use of the human vocal instrument and have developed careers based on their vocal skill.

This power of the voice extends to others as well. **Remember teachers you have had who have influenced you significantly and recall their voices. Think of people you admire and think of their voices.** The salesperson with the sincere, confident voice probably sold you something you would not have purchased from the salesperson with the hesitant or annoying voice. Consider the role of the lawyer's voice when she reached the hearts of the jury in her final argument.

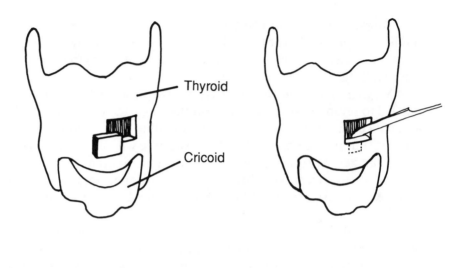

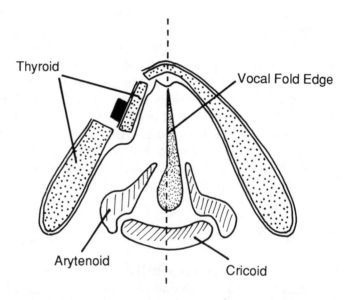

Figure 12–15. Thyroplasty surgical procedure to improve vocal fold adduction.

Various professionals contribute to the development and maintenance of the "maximally effective" voice, including speech pathologists, otolaryngologists, singing teachers, and vocal coaches. These individuals form a team with knowledge of techniques to facilitate a maximally effective voice.

Your voice is a powerful tool. The right words paired with the right voice can be a critical element in maximizing your communication effectiveness.

Do you like your voice? Does it reflect your personality? Do you feel you could be a more effective speaker? Would you like to develop your singing voice? One powerful way to learn about voice is to take singing or speaking lessons. Write to the Voice Foundation, 1721 Pine Street, Philadelphia, Pennsylvania, 19103, for the name of a speech pathologist, singing teacher, or vocal coach in your area.

◆ SUMMARY AND CONCLUSIONS

This chapter introduced you to normal and disordered voice production and its significant role in oral communication. You learned about laryngeal and vocal tract anatomy and physiology underlying the generation of your voice. You learned how pitch, loudness, and quality are controlled by the larynx and how they are measured acoustically (fundamental frequency, intensity, and regularity). You learned "what can go wrong" in the larynx because of etiological factors of: misuse/abuse, psychogenic/stress, and medical/physical conditions. You learned how voice disorders are evaluated and the basic principles of voice treatment for each etiology. You learned "what can go right" in the larynx and the significance of keeping your own voice healthy to maximize your vocal effectiveness.

◆ ACKNOWLEDGMENTS

This work was supported in part by NIH-NIDCD Grants No. R01 DC01150 and No. P60 DC00976.

◆ SUGGESTED READINGS

Andrews, M. L. (1991). *Voice therapy for children.* San Diego: Singular Publishing Group.

Aronson, A. E. (1990). *Clinical voice disorders.* New York: Thieme Medical Publishers.

Baken, R. J. (1987). *Clinical measurement of speech and voice.* Boston: College-Hill Press.

Bless, D., & Hirano, M. (1993). *Videostroboscopic examination of the larynx.* San Diego: Singular Publishing Group.

Blitzer, A., Brin, M. F., Sasaki, C. T., Fahn, S., & Harris, K. S. (1992). *Neurologic disorders of the larynx.* New York: Thieme Medical Publishers.

Boone, D. R., & McFarland, S. (1988). *The voice and voice therapy.* Englewood Cliffs, NJ: Prentice-Hall.

Colton, R., & Casper, J. (1990). *Understanding voice problems.* Baltimore: Williams & Wilkins.

Gould, W. J., Rubin, J. S., Korovin, G., & Sataloff, R. T. (in press). *Diagnosis and treatment of voice disorders.* Tokyo: Igaku-Shoin.

Hirano, M. (1981). *The clinical examination of the voice.* Vienna: Springer-Verlag.

Hixon, T. J. (1987). *Respiratory function in speech and song.* San Diego, CA: College-Hill Press.

Keith, R. L., & Darley, F. L. (1986). *Laryngectomee rehabilitation.* Austin, TX: Pro-Ed.

Sataloff, R. T. (1992, December). The human voice. *Scientific American*, pp. 108–115.

Stemple, J. (1993). *Voice therapy: Clinical studies.* Chicago: Mosby Yearbook.

Sundberg, J. (1987). *The science of the singing voice.* DeKalb, IL: Northern Illinois University Press.

Titze, I. R. (in press). *The principles of voice production.* Englewood Cliffs, NJ: Prentice-Hall.

Wilson, F. (1967). *Voice disorders in children.* Baltimore: Williams & Wilkins.

✦ GLOSSARY

Contact ulcers: ulcerations in the mucosal linings of the airway at the tips of the vocal processes of the arytenoid cartilages.

False vocal folds: folds of tissue above the true vocal folds in the larynx. Sometimes used in the production of "vocal fry" sound.

Falsetto voice: vocal sounds produced with taut and thinned vocal folds. Falsetto voice has relatively few harmonics compared to vocal sound produced with normal voice (in modal the register).

Fundamental frequency (F_0): the number of complete cycles of vocal fold vibration per second. Fundamental frequency is measured in Hertz (Hz).

Hyperadduction of vocal folds: overly strong adduction of muscles which causes the vocal folds to be pressed at midline.

Hypoadduction of vocal folds: reduced vocal fold adduction resulting in disordered voice (flaccid or hypokinetic). Usually of neurological origin.

Intensity: the amplitude of sound (a physical measure).

Larynx: the cartilaginous structure that houses the vocal folds. It is located above the trachea (windpipe) and below the pharynx. The larynx is used to generate voiced sound and whisper during speech production.

Loudness: the psychological perception of the amplitude of sound.

Misuse/abuse: life style habits that damage the vocal folds or contribute to a voice disorder.

Musculoskeletal tension disorder: disorders that occur when laryngeal muscles hyperfunction in response to stress.

Mutational falsetto: a psychogenic voice disorder associated with puberty in which the patient uses a falsetto voice; also called puberphonia.

Normal voice: sound produced with normal vibration of the vocal folds.

Phonation: voiced sound production.

Pitch: the psychological perception of the fundamental frequency of the voice.

Vibratory instability: irregular vocal fold vibration.

Vocal fold abduction: the vocal folds are positioned near the side of the airway in the trachea; the vocal folds are open.

Vocal fold adduction: the vocal folds are positioned near midline in the trachea; the vocal folds are closed.

Vocal folds: muscle and connective tissue located within the larynx that are used to produce voice (through vocal fold vibration). The two vocal folds are attached anteriorly to the thyroid cartilage and posteriorly to the arytenoid cartilages.

Vocal fry: a "rumble-crackling" of sound resulting from abnormal vibration of the vocal folds, or a low-frequency vibration of the false vocal folds.

Vocal nodules: small growths (that resemble calluses) that form on the vocal folds at the point of maximum vocal fold adduction.

Vocal polyps: small blister-like growths that form on the vocal fold.

Vocal tremor: low-frequency (4–6 Hz) shaking of the voice that is observed in some neurological disorders.

Vocal vibrato: low-frequency (5–6 Hz) musical ornament used in singing.

Voice: sound produced at the larynx, usually through vibration of the vocal folds.

Voice disorder: an abnormal voice quality resulting from anatomic, physiologic, or psychogenic causes.

Voice quality: perceptual characteristics of the vocal tone (normal, breathy, harsh, hoarse).

Fluency and Stuttering

DAVID PRINS, PH.D.

After reading this chapter, you should know:

◆ How speech that is stuttered compares with fluent speech.

◆ How to define the problem of stuttering as event and as disorder.

◆ How the severity of stuttering is described in terms of speech characteristics and their effects on personal adjustment.

◆ How stuttering severity can vary under different speaking conditions.

◆ When stuttering begins and how it develops in the individual.

◆ How stuttering varies within and across societies.

◆ How five pivotal ideas have come to shape our thinking about the nature of stuttering.

Fluent speech is a dazzling human achievement that we usually take for granted. But when it falters and the problem of stuttering emerges, we begin to realize how fragile, yet essential, the fluency of speech really is. This chapter portrays stuttering as both a *speech event* and as a *disorder of human communication.* The onset and development of the problem are traced from its beginnings in early childhood. Its occurrence and variability are described in individuals and societies. Five pivotal ideas concerning the nature of stuttering are examined for their impact on research and treatment and the way we think about this complex problem today.

"I am a stutterer. I am not like other people. I must think differently, act differently, live differently — because I stutter. Like other stutterers, like other exiles, I have known all my life a great sorrow and a great hope together, and they have made me the kind of person I am. An awkward tongue has molded my life."
(from the autobiography of Wendell Johnson, 1930, p. 1)

Try to imagine what it would be like if, day-by-day, you could not control the flow of your speech; if suddenly, often unexpectedly, your speech movements would seem to freeze in place, only to be followed by seemingly uncontrollable repetition or prolongation of the sound you just uttered, or no sound at all, as you struggled to continue. If you spoke like that, how would you feel? What levels of dread and panic would accompany speaking situations? How would your life be affected, the way you think about and interact with people, the kind of person you are?

Some recent reactions of one of my students may help you to answer these questions. As a part of her preparation to become a clinician, she took the role of a person who stutters while making a purchase in a local drug store. Here is what she said about that experience: "I felt so very young — like a little girl who lost her mother. My hands grew cold and my stomach was tight with fear. Until then, I hadn't thought how many trips down an aisle a stutterer might need before simply asking for hand cream. I hadn't imagined the urgency I would feel to get through my sentence, or how stupid and young and conspicuous I would sound. Nor had I thought I'd be angry at the quizzical stares of customers and clerks, silently saying, 'What is wrong with her?'"

In this chapter, you will learn about the problem of stuttering. Many have said it is the most baffling of all speech disorders. This chapter portrays a problem that:

◆ has apparently existed since the recorded history of human kind;

◆ usually begins in early childhood, but at its onset has no absolutely distinctive speech characteristic;

◆ after early, intermittent signs may last for months or even years, may vanish completely with no identifiable reason;

◆ occurs inconsistently, so persons who stutter chronically can, on some occasions, speak with effortless fluency but cannot explain why or how they do so;

◆ when it persists into adulthood, often seems impossible to eliminate completely.

First, we will try to get a picture of stuttered speech: what it sounds and looks like, and how it varies under different conditions. Then, we will consider when and how it begins in individuals and how its prevalence varies in societies. Finally, we will journey through modern history to see how principal ideas have unfolded to explain the nature of the disorder and what we understand about it today.

◆ FLUENT VERSUS STUTTERED SPEECH

What does it mean when we refer to stuttering as a disorder of *fluency*? To appreciate the answer, you need to know something about the characteristics of fluently uttered speech. Let's start with a simple phrase, "just all living things." It contains 4 words, 5 syllables, and 14 speech sounds. As spoken aloud, it looks like this when transcribed into the International Phonetic Alphabet (IPA): /dʒʌstɔlɪvɪŋθɪŋz/. Each *sound* is represented by a different letter symbol, and the phrase is written as one continuous "word," because, as uttered, it contains no perceptible pauses. Spoken at a comfortable rate by an adult with normally fluent speech, it requires less than 1 second when uttered at the beginning of a sentence (.91 second, to be exact). Imagine it, to utter speech at the stunning rate of more than 14 sounds per second, effortlessly, and in a continuous stream! Just as amazing — this coded signal is immediately understood by the listener.

When you consider what the speaker has to achieve *before* the sounds are created, the rate and continuity, or fluency, of speech is all the more incredible. First, there are what we call the "psycholinguistic" processes by which words are retrieved from memory, according to their meaning and according to their sounds, and then encoded with other words into a pronounceable "program." This program is then translated into motor commands and executed as movements which, in turn, become the audible speech sounds. It boggles the mind to conceive of doing all these things so quickly and synchronously. Yet, you do them over and over each day and pay no heed to the miracle. In fact, if you are a typical speaker, you have been uttering speech more-or-less like this since you were about 3 or 4 years old, although your current rate is perhaps twice as fast as it was at that time.

Although seemingly impossible, the rate and continuity of human speech is nonetheless *necessary* for normal, efficient speech communication as we know it. For example, if you were to utter the phrase, "just all living things," *discontinuously* at about two separate sounds per second, it would not only take much more effort, but you would likely lose track of the intended message while your listener would not comprehend it at all. (You might experiment by uttering the phrase, one sound at a time with brief, distinct pauses between each sound.)

Nonspeech sounds do not share this fluency characteristic. When they are presented at rates above seven to nine per second, only half the rate of typical adult speech, they cannot even be recognized by listeners! Likewise, a skilled transcriber of Morse code completely loses track of the message at speeds that are a mere five sounds per second.

It is, then, the *fluency* of speech that makes it most distinctive as a communication system, not simply the fact that we produce sounds to convey meaning. In fact, speech has evolved so that its fluency is imperative if speakers and listeners are to communicate normally.

But, what happens if this imperative is not achievable? Let's look again at our phrase, "just all living things," this time spoken by a 15-year-old boy who stutters. As before, it is transcribed in the IPA, each speech sound represented by a different symbol.

/wʌʌ-wʌʌʌ-w-w-wʌ__dʒ-hhh__dʒʌstɔlɪvɪŋ_____hhh-n-n-n__θɪŋz/

Typically spoken in less than 1 second, the phrase required 9 seconds for him to utter! But the slow rate did not result from simple prolongations of continuously uttered sounds. Rather, it resulted from what seems like chaos: extraneous sounds, repeated and prolonged sounds, and unexpected silent gaps (shown by the lines between sounds).

Imagine what it would be like to speak this way on a daily basis; to take almost 10 times longer to say a simple phrase than the average speaker, not to mention the degree of effort required. You would be robbed of the opportunity to interact normally with others in the way that is most uniquely human. And so it is with the person who stutters as severely as this 15-year-old boy. He is denied that part of being alive that we have come to take for granted: effortless, fluent speech.

But I'm getting ahead of our story, thinking about the *effect* of stuttered speech on the speaker before we've had a chance to study the speech itself and consider a working definition of the problem.

◆ DEFINING THE PROBLEM

Core Features

Let's return once more to our sample phrase as spoken by the young man who stutters. It abounds with sound prolongations, unexpected speech gaps, and sound repetitions. These "elemental" prolongations of sound and silence, along with sound repetitions, are the central features in the following definition of stuttering: "Speech events that characterize stuttering can be specified succinctly as silent or audible elemental repetitions and prolongations" (Wingate, 1964, p. 488). This definition is often used as a standard because it specifies the so-called core disfluencies necessary to mark the occurrence of stutter events, whether they occur in the speech of persons who stutter or who are normally fluent. In other words, when these fluency errors occur in *anybody's* speech, the speaker may be said to have "stuttered" on those occasions. In fact, persons with normal speech sometimes display such episodes of stuttering as you may have observed.

Accessory Features

After viewing a video tape of the 15-year-old boy who stutters, 20 adults with normally fluent speech were asked to describe how his speech sounded and looked. Nineteen said it *sounded* "strained, effortful, forced or strangled." Nine mentioned "gasping, breathy sounds"; and five emphasized "popping and clicking" noises. Eighteen said his speech also *looked* "tense or strained," while 10 described excessive "jerky, groping, tick-like movements or spasms."

Three listeners gave this analogy: "His speech looks like a machine running out of control." Another listener, comparing the speech to walking, said it was as if "his legs were jerked abruptly backward while he was in mid-stride." These characteristics are often called **accessory features** of stuttering. They usually accompany the core disfluencies, particularly in older children and adults who stutter. Sometimes accessory features can become quite elaborate and ritualistic.

Frank was a teenager who used to have long silent episodes of stuttering during which he pressed his lips together and uttered no sound. While doing this, he would often shudder and repeatedly flick his right index finger along the side seam of his trousers. I asked him why he flicked his finger that way. Frank smiled rather sheepishly and said, "to help me get the word out." Clearly, Frank could identify the reason for his actions, however irrational. Unfortunately, he had been caught in the accident of sequential events (a flick of the finger and the utterance of a word), and had interpreted them as having a cause-effect relationship. This interpretation, perhaps resulting from a one-time occurrence, then served to sustain the reflexive ritual even though he realized how ridiculous it was.

Together, these core and accessory features identify what we have come to call the stutter event. It is generally believed to consist of two principal components: (1) an interruption of fluency, perceived by the speaker as a loss of control and (2) the speaker's coping reactions (Bloodstein, 1987; Prins, 1991; Rosenfield & Nudleman, 1987; Van Riper, 1971; Wingate, 1976). Apparently, behavior that we, as listeners, observe and identify as stuttering is associated mainly with the second component. This includes the excessive effort and tensing of muscles that lead to multiple sound repetitions, long periods of silence or sound prolongations, facial grimaces, extraneous head and bodily movements, and the like. Concerning the first component, much disagreement exists about possible source factors that could interrupt fluency and thereby *set the occasion* for observable stutter events. There is, however, substantial agreement about the nature of the reactive behavior that constitutes the second component. It appears to be defensive in nature; what persons who stutter do to contend with a perceived emergency, the instant when the flow of speech is interrupted.

Associated Features

Core and accessory features characterize the events, or *disability*, of stuttering, but there is more to the *disorder* than the description of stuttered speech. Sometimes, the most damaging features of stuttering are its *handicapping effects*: how it shapes the person's life. When extreme, the extent of handicap may affect all aspects of the individual's personal, social, educational, and occupational adjustment.

> Pat had come to a time in her life when she wanted to go back to school to study early childhood education. As she contemplated this change, she began to evaluate the effects of stuttering on her life. Rarely did she answer the telephone, and she would initiate a telephone call only in the most dire circumstances. In stores, she merely muttered answers if spoken to. Others ordered for her in restaurants. She never initiated speech in groups, and would usually decline to answer questions in such situations. Pat justified her silent life by saying, "I really don't have anything important to say." Her stuttering disability was an obstacle, but the handicap she had allowed it to become was much worse.

✦ PROBLEM SEVERITY

This brings us to the matter of stuttering severity and how to judge it — by no means a simple matter. Generally speaking, severity is described in terms of the speech disability: the frequency of stuttering episodes, their duration, and the extent of visible and audible accessory features. Depending on speaking circumstances, these dimensions vary enormously among, and even within, adults who stutter. For example, *frequency* of stuttering may range from 1% of words uttered (very mild) to more than 25% (very severe). Similarly, the *duration* of stutter events may be fleeting (less than 1 second) or more than 5 seconds which is generally regarded as quite severe. The *visible and audible accessory features* also vary, from barely noticeable to painful appearing.

In the spontaneous speech sample from which the phrase, "just all living things," was taken, our 15-year-old stuttered on 44% of words uttered, some stuttering episodes lasted more than 5 seconds, and our listeners judged the visible/audible accessory features to be "painful and upsetting." There is no doubt; he stutters very severely.

Although we use these more-or-less objective dimensions to describe severity of the speech disability, they do not necessarily reflect the *handicapping potential* of the disorder. For example, individuals with quite mild speech characteristics of stuttering sometimes reveal very high degrees of handicap.

Rick had a stuttering problem but rarely displayed any overt stuttering episodes. In fact, as a casual acquaintance you probably would not know that he stuttered at all. He used a lot of tricks and subterfuge to avoid stuttering. When he answered the telephone, he draped a handkerchief from the corner of his mouth because he believed he could then speak fluently. One day he explained that he had recently met a girl in a bar. When she asked him where he was from, he replied, "Oh, over on the Eastern seaboard;" a curious answer, particularly since he was from Montana! He simply could not accept the fact of his stuttering or run the risk that his problem might be revealed. The very idea of stuttering was repugnant to him — a serious threat to his self image. His disability was mild, but his handicap was severe.

◆ INTERMITTENCY

You are quite perceptive if you have begun to wonder whether the speech of persons who stutter is more-or-less the same on all occasions. In fact, it is not. People who stutter will do so very little, or not at all, when they: (1) speak or read aloud in chorus with other speakers, whether or not those speakers are stutterers; (2) utter syllables or words to the beat of a metronome; (3) speak while hearing their own speech after it is delayed a fraction of a second (delayed auditory feedback); (4) speak while hearing noise that is loud enough to mask the sound of their own voice. For persons who stutter, these are commonly called **fluency inducing conditions,** and they are almost universally effective in reducing or eliminating stuttering, no matter how severe it is. This is particularly true of speaking in chorus or to a metronome beat.

Many explanations have been given to account for these effects. Included among them are that fluency inducing conditions: (1) simplify or impose a timing mechanism for the coordinated execution of speech movements; (2) reduce demands upon speech programming processes; (3) alter auditory feedback which, in turn, masks the stutterer's voice or changes his manner of producing speech; (4) reduce communicative responsibility. Individually or in combination, these explanations suggest possible source factors that could serve to interrupt speech fluency and thereby underlie the occurrence of stutter events.

Other circumstances that often lead to a reduction in stuttering include: whispering, singing, speaking at a slow rate by prolonging sounds, talking to oneself or to young children or animals, and counting or uttering other "automatic" speech sequences.

On dozens of occasions during treatment sessions I have seen the following sequence: A client begins to speak, and immediately triggers an episode of stuttering that he can't seem to terminate. The clinician finally interrupts, "What word are you trying to say?" "Baseball," (or some other word) comes the fluent reply. The clinician responds, "Okay, go ahead and say it," at which time the speaker returns to his stuttering routine in a futile attempt to utter the word.

The intermittency of stuttering is one of the problem's most perplexing, if not frustrating, characteristics. How is it possible that persons who stutter can speak with seemingly effortless fluency under one condition, only to return to stuttered speech when that condition is terminated? The apparent ease with which fluency is attainable tantalizes adults who stutter and their clinicians alike, imploring them to devise techniques that will allow the *effortless* fluency to endure. That seldom happens, however, in adults who have stuttered chronically since early childhood.

◆ ONSET OF STUTTERING

Typically, stuttering does not emerge full-blown. It most often develops slowly with first signs when children are between 2½ and 5 years of age. In fact, it has been estimated that 75% of those who stutter as adults began before age 6 (Bloodstein, 1987).

Stuttering usually emerges when speech and language development are at a period of greatest acceleration: when children are moving from short, one-and two-word utterances to the production of sentence-long responses that emulate the fluency of adult speech. Disfluencies of all types abound during this period; for example, repetitions of phrases, words, syllables, and sounds; sound prolongations; unexpected pauses; revisions, and interjections. They often occur on 5 to 10% of words uttered, three-to-five times the frequency found in adult speech. In particular, repetitions stand out, especially of whole, monosyllabic words at the beginnings of sentences or clauses. These often involve the repetition of pronouns ("I-I-I-I," "you-you-you") or of conjunctions ("but-but-but," "and-and-and-and").

Distinguishing the Child Who Has a Stuttering Problem

A great puzzle about the onset of stuttering concerns how to distinguish between a child who is *normally disfluent* and one who is *stuttering*. We can begin by asserting that there is no absolute behavioral criterion, the single occurrence of which will identify a preschool child as having a stuttering problem. In other words, all types of disfluencies found in the speech of children who are believed to show early signs of stuttering are also found to some extent in most normally disfluent children. This is referred to as the **Overlap Phenomenon** (Bloodstein, 1987), and it should remind us of something very important: **The onset of stuttering appears to reflect a special condition of breakdown in fluent speech which, to some extent, is experienced by most preschool children.**

If no single type of disfluency distinguishes the child who is beginning to have a problem with stuttering, how can the distinction be made? Usually, it is done by combining the amount with the type of disfluency. On average, the speech of preschool children who are considered to be problem stutterers tends to be more disfluent overall. Even more important, it usually contains substantially higher percentages of part-word repetitions and sound prolongations, the so-called core features of stuttering identified earlier. This characteristic has been reported over a period of decades.

Along with the high percentage of part-word repetitions and sound prolongations (e.g., "Ca-Caa-Caaaa-Caaaaa-Caaaaa-Caaaaa-Can I go too?"), preschoolers who are believed to have a problem with stuttering also tend to have a higher number of repeated speech elements per instance of repetition than normally disfluent children. Sometimes as many 10, or more, repetitions occur before a word is uttered. Audible signs of tension in vocal pitch and volume changes and visible signs of effort in facial and neck muscles are also frequent.

✦ DEVELOPMENT OF STUTTERING

In a child whose speech and language are otherwise developing normally, it is not uncommon for quite severe characteristics of early stuttering to appear over a period of several days, sometimes almost overnight. In such cases a child may repeat partial words or initial sounds of words over and over at the beginning of nearly every utterance, perhaps never completing the sentence, or even the word. These children sometimes become upset, ask "Why can't I talk?," cover their mouths, or even pull on their tongues. This behavior may last for days or weeks and then, without warning or any apparent explanation, vanish just as quickly.

Episodes of "stuttering" may continue in a preschool child for months, or even years, before going away completely or becoming a chronic condition. In fact, the *episodic character* of early "stuttering" has become its hallmark (Bloodstein, 1987) and one of the most difficult features to explain. It should tell us, however, **that to understand the nature of the disorder, it may be just as important to determine why it persists in a few youngsters as to explain why it occurs at all.**

Sometimes, periods of "stuttering" can be associated with periods of unusual excitement and uncertainty in the family, for example, birthdays, holidays, moving to a new home or community, visits by relatives, birth of a sibling, and the like. But, just as often, stuttering can seem to have a life of its own, quite apart from what appears to be going on in the observable life of the child.

In a relatively small fraction of children who show early signs of stuttering, perhaps 20%, the problem becomes *chronic.* When this happens, they enter what Bloodstein (1987) calls a second phase. During this phase, the core features of their stuttering (elemental repetitions and prolongations) tend to occur more on principal parts of speech and throughout an utterance, as well as on initial words. Stuttering also is particularly noticeable when these children become excited and try to speak rapidly. Later, in what Bloodstein calls a third phase, accessory features become more severe, and tension more evident; yet, these cases remain willing talkers, showing little fear or embarrassment about speaking. In a fourth phase, which some never reach, Bloodstein describes the emergence of fearful anticipation of speaking, speech avoidance, and extreme sensitivity to the problem.

Although this sequential development is typical and often takes 10 to 15, or more, years from onset to full-blown disorder, Bloodstein is quick to point out that these phases can be substantially compressed.

A 3½-year-old boy, who stuttered on 60% of the words he uttered in spontaneous speech, was referred to our clinic. Stuttering episodes lasted up to several seconds during which time severe signs of tension were evident in his neck and in the pitch and volume changes of his voice which frequently sounded almost strangled. For all intents and purposes, at age three(!) the speech characteristics of his stuttering were those of a very severe, chronic adult stutterer.

After a study of detailed case records, Van Riper (1971) reported a somewhat different pattern to account for the onset and development of stuttering, one of disorder *subgroups*. About 50% of his cases seemed to follow a sequence similar to the one reported by Bloodstein, but the remainder were different. About 25% constituted a subgroup with retarded speech development. These children began to stutter almost with the onset of multiple-word utterances, and they showed no episodic periods of normal fluency. About 10% of his cases constituted another subgroup whose problems began later, typically between the ages of 5 and 9. The onset was sudden and usually coincided with a traumatic event. Finally, Van Riper described an additional 10% of cases whose "stuttering" began latest of all and whose speech was characterized by lengthy, stereotyped repetitions of words and phrases.

The reports by Bloodstein and Van Riper clearly indicate that there is no single pattern of onset and development for all persons who stutter. It is not clear, however, whether the various patterns reflect different source factors that interrupt fluency in unique ways, or whether the patterns reflect unique reactions of individuals to common sources of fluency interruption, or both.

After stuttering has become a chronic condition, it does not always persist throughout life. It is fairly common to hear reports that stuttering has gradually subsided without the aid of direct therapy in persons who have stuttered for as many as 20, or more, years. This occurs most often, however, when the severity of stuttering is relatively mild.

◆ SOCIETAL OCCURRENCE

Universality

We have looked at the occurrence of stuttering in individuals. Now, to get a broader picture of the disorder, we need to observe its occurrence in societies. References to stuttering have appeared since the recorded history of civilization. An Egyptian hieroglyph is believed to represent the problem. Moses is thought to have stuttered, and there are many references to stuttering in ancient Greek literature. In more contemporary times, we also find stuttering among celebrated figures: for example, Charles Darwin, Winston Churchill, King Edward VI; and even more recently, country-western singer Mel Tillis, actress Marilyn Monroe, and professional basketball player Bob Love.

In research reported over the past 100 years, the prevalence of stuttering in various cultures has been remarkably constant. Among studies of school children in the United States, a figure somewhat less than 1% is most commonly reported (Bloodstein, 1987). Surveys of Japanese school children have reported similar results (Van Riper, 1982), whereas the percentage appears to be somewhat higher in Europe (Bloodstein, 1987).

You should understand the difference between *prevalence* and *incidence* of stuttering as a disorder. When we speak of prevalence, we mean the number of existing cases at a given point in time. Incidence, on the other hand, refers to the number of cases that have ever occurred, taking into account that an individual may begin, but not continue, to stutter. Principally because many preschool children who show early signs of stuttering do not become chronic stutterers, incidence is generally reported to be substantially higher than prevalence. There is evidence to suggest that incidence may be as high as 4 to 5% in populations where the prevalence is about 1% (Bloodstein, 1987).

Variability

Cultural Differences

Stuttering does not occur with the same frequency in all societies. Some years ago, it was reported to be less frequent in certain American Indian tribes (e.g., the Bannock and Shoshone) as well as in some primitive cultures throughout the world (e.g., in New Guinea and Borneo). These societies were also characterized as being relatively noncompetitive, placing little premium on speaking ability, and having permissive child rearing practices. But there are other primitive cultures, for example the Ibo of West Africa, where the problem is reported to occur at more than double the typical 1% figure. Among the Ibo, ability to speak is much admired and there is substantial ridicule of youngsters who stutter or otherwise speak poorly.

Sex Ratio

Studies spanning almost a century report consistently that stuttering is more prevalent among males than females. The ratio is usually 3:1, or somewhat higher, depending on the age range of the study. Many suggestions have been given to explain this phenomenon, including a sex-linked genetic factor, child rearing practices that place greater demands on male children, generally slower speech and language development among males than females, and a lower capacity in males to generate timing programs.

Familial Patterns

Experts and casual observers alike have been fascinated by the tendency for stuttering to recur among generations of the same family. To put it another way, a person who stutters is much more apt to have a near-relative who stutterers than is a person who is normally fluent. Andrews et al. (1983) have estimated that first-degree relatives of stutterers (parents and siblings) are over three times more apt to stutter than are such relatives of normally fluent speakers.

Geneticists have tried to account for the familial pattern, often as they would human traits that run in families: The genetic influence is a predisposing factor, and the disorder occurs when this factor coincides with the necessary environmental conditions. New developments in the techniques of gene isolation could, however, bring about a much more specific identification of genetic linkages to stuttering. In the 1940s and 1950s, it was more popular to blame environmental influences for the familial pattern. Today, however, these speculations are less in tune with recent advances in science and therefore appear less credible.

Twinning

The occurrence of stuttering in twins has intrigued researchers for many years. A particularly interesting question concerns the appearance of stuttering in both members of a twin set. If stuttering were *always* to occur in both *identical* twins, but to occur in fraternal twins at only the normal expectancy for siblings, then a genetic link would be sufficient to explain the disorder's occurrence. As it turns out, this is not the case. Although stuttering more often appears in both twins when they are identical, its occurrence in only one identical twin is not uncommon when twins are reared apart.

We have defined stuttering, described certain features of stuttered speech, considered onset and development of the disorder, and reviewed some unique characteristics about its occurrence in individuals and societies. To complete our picture, we need now to consider how people have tried to explain this perplexing problem.

◆ THE CAUSES OF STUTTERING

What causes stuttering? Before we can answer that question, we must answer another: "What is it about stuttering that we are trying to find a cause for?" Well, in relation to *stutter events* we need at least to consider causes of the two components: (1) the interruption in fluency and (2) the speaker's reaction thereto. Most "theories of stuttering," although not always making the distinction clear, have tried to explain one, or both, of these components.

You would not believe the number of explanations that have been advanced to account for stuttering. Within the scope of this chapter, it would be impossible to mention, let alone describe, all of them. Yet, **it is important for you to become aware of what I will call pivotal ideas that, during their ascendancy, dominated thinking, research, and treatment of stuttering.** We will consider ideas that have emerged during the so-called modern era which began in about 1930 when the first truly academic program in speech pathology was established at the University of Iowa.

The ideas will be classified into three categories, depending on their point of view concerning the principal source factors that underlie stutter events: (1) speech motor control, (2) learning, and (3) personality. From the start, you should understand that these categories are not mutually exclusive. For example, a viewpoint that emphasizes speech motor control does not, or should not, exclude the role of learning and vice versa. Both points of view are necessary to any complete explanation of stutter events, as we shall see.

Figure 13–1 shows the pivotal ideas in each category. Their periods of ascendancy sometimes overlap; however, we will take up each idea in the order in which it became popular, then consider its basic concepts, impact on research and treatment, and status. Be patient as you go along. At first, some of the concepts may seem a little difficult to understand.

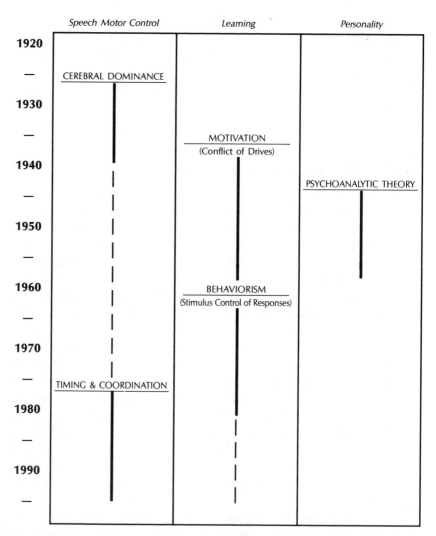

Figure 13–1. Nature of Stuttering: Pivotal ideas and their periods of ascendancy in the Modern era.

Cerebral Dominance

Basic Concepts

For some time the general idea had been around that people who stutter may lack the cerebral (brain) dominance required for controlling speech movements. Beginning with what we are calling the modern era, however, Orton (1927) and Travis (1931) were the first to popularize this theory. Travis captured its essence with these words: "The symptoms of stuttering are then mainly the peripheral signs of rivalry between the two sides of the brain" (Travis, 1978, p. 277). He and Orton reasoned that because the muscles of speech structures receive nerve impulses from *both* the left and right hemispheres of the brain, one hemisphere would have to be dominant over the other in order for speech movements to be synchronized.

Clearly, they were trying to account for an impairment source factor that would predispose persons to fluency interruptions: a central nervous system that had not matured sufficiently to achieve hemispheric dominance over speech movements. Orton and Travis allowed that the maturational failure could result from hereditary influences, disease, or injury. Travis also made clear that factors such as emotional arousal and fatigue might be involved, or even necessary, to destabilize speech movements in persons who suffered from marginal dominance.

Research

Considering the few people working in the speech disorders field at the time, the number of published studies concerned with the dominance theory was enormous during the period from 1929 to 1940. There were **four principal areas of focus in these studies: (1) muscle contraction patterns from the left and right sides; (2) patterns of electrical discharge from the brain; (3) handedness; and (4) innate dominance.**

Early findings appeared to support the theory. For example, people who stuttered seemed to have a greater tendency than normally fluent speakers to be left-handed and to have *less* innate dominance of the cerebral hemispheres. Eventually, however, as more information was collected, stutterers appeared to show about the same amount of right- handedness, and the same latent tendency toward ambidexterity, as nonstutterers. Also, no *consistent* differences were found in muscle contraction patterns from the two sides' speech structures or in patterns of electrical discharge from the two sides of the brain.

Although never failing altogether, interest in the question of cerebral dominance waned during the 1940s and 1950s. However, beginning in the 1960s, more sophisticated questions, techniques of measurement, and experimental procedures began to attract new interest. **The question shifted somewhat from concern about conflict between the hemispheres to interest in left hemisphere control of speech functions.** In contrast to what was known in the 1930s, it was now well established that the left cerebral hemisphere is especially adapted for controlling speech processes. Researchers began therefore to question whether persons who stuttered would show the typical pattern of left hemisphere control. Results of the more recent work suggest that there could be a tendency for some persons who stutter to make more use of the right hemisphere for speech processing than do normally fluent speakers.

Treatment

Early on, the **Cerebral Dominance Theory** had a profound impact on treatment. Clients were given batteries of diagnostic tests to determine their handedness and innate dominance. They were made to shift handedness if it differed from what the tests found to be innate. At its most extreme, treatment might involve putting a cast on the nondominant arm so the other one would be used exclusively for extended periods. The right arm was often subjected to this treatment because many stutterers were judged to be innately left-handed. At lesser extremes, all kinds of unilateral activities, such as writing, throwing, racket sports, and so on, were emphasized using the native side. To train dominance for speech control, simultaneous writing and talking activities became particularly popular. The first letters of words were written with deliberate emphasis and timed to the onsets of words as they were spoken aloud.

> Van Riper (1958) reported that in 1936 his clients were required to perform simultaneous writing and talking with such vengeance that they produced no fewer than 15 pages per day of writing/talking exercises!

Although these approaches often were accompanied by improved speech fluency, the effect did not last. More than anyone else, Van Riper, himself a stutterer, led the movement away from these methods. He believed they had only a temporary effect because they were "repressive," having as their objective the avoidance, rather than the acceptance and modification, of stuttering (Van Riper, 1957).

Current Status

The idea remains alive that fluency could be interrupted and stuttering could begin, and even be sustained, in some individuals because of difficulties with hemispheric dominance in speech motor control (Moore, 1990). New techniques for imaging the brain undoubtedly will be useful in shedding more light on this subject. As the research continues, you should recognize some of its past, and even current, limitations:

1. Most of the work describes characteristics of groups of subjects. It does not test for cause-effect relationships between the occurrence of stuttering and some other variable.

2. Most studies involve adults who stutter, and their hemispheric dominance for speech may reflect the effects, rather than a cause, of the disorder.

3. Over the years, it has been difficult to replicate findings. Although there may be many reasons, this strongly suggests that subject selection has a major effect on outcome. In other words, persons who stutter probably differ substantially from each other with respect to factors that contribute to the onset and perpetuation of their disorders.

4. Even when differences are found between groups of stutterers and nonstutterers in a given study, there is virtually always overlap in individual subject performance. That is, there are invariably stutterers who perform within the range of nonstutterers, and vice versa. This means that one-to-one cause-effect relationships probably will not fully account for the occurrence and perpetuation of stuttering.

As we shall see, **these limitations do not apply only to the work in cerebral dominance. They apply to much of the research in other pivotal areas as well.**

Motivation: The Conflict of Drives

Basic Concepts

In the mid-1930s, one of Travis' students led a revolt, of sorts, against the ideas of his teacher. His name was Wendell Johnson, and he was destined to become world renowned for his writings about stuttering. He introduced the concept of the *stuttering moment* (what we now call the stutter event). To Johnson, himself a stutterer, it was the window to understanding the nature of the disorder and its treatment (Johnson, 1933). As a result of his own, his student's, and his colleagues' extraordinary program of research, Johnson came to regard stuttering as an intermittent, yet consistent and predictable, "response made to identifiable stimuli or cues." (Johnson, 1955b, p. 16). In other words, he came to regard stuttering as a *learned behavior.* **In contrast to Travis, Johnson denied any underlying impairment to account for fluency interruptions. To him, the critical factor in stuttering was to be found in the reactive component — how the speaker responded to what otherwise were normal interruptions in fluency.**

Johnson's definition of the moment, rather than describing its speech characteristics, captured his ideas concerning the *reason* for its occurrence: "Stuttering is an anticipatory, apprehensive, hypertonic, *avoidance* reaction." (Johnson, et al., 1956, p. 261). To Johnson, stuttering was what persons who stuttered did to keep from stuttering.

But how did they get this way? Johnson believed that the problem originated in the "ear of the listener." There then followed a series of interactions involving adult listeners, the child, and his speech (Johnson, 1938, 1959). The first interaction began with adults (usually parents) reacting to the child's normal disfluencies as if they were episodes of stuttering. By doing this, they labeled and isolated the behavior. They did so, according to Johnson, because the word, "stuttering," meant something abnormal that they believed the child was doing.

As Johnson explained it, this first interaction was crucial to onset of the problem. However, **for stuttering to develop, the child had to interact by internalizing the parent's negative beliefs and, in turn, trying to avoid his own disfluencies.** Although Johnson thought it unlikely, he granted that a child might be sufficiently sensitive to disfluencies in his speech, or that they might occur with such frequency, that stuttering (i.e., avoidance reactions) could develop without the need for parent labeling.

Johnson relied heavily on the concepts and language of general semantics in developing his theory (Johnson, 1946). It remained for two others, George Wischner and Joseph Sheehan, to apply learning and conflict theory more specifically to Johnson's ideas. Wischner explained how stuttering moments began, stopped, and were reinforced due to the speaker's *anxiety motivation* (Wischner, 1950, 1952). Somewhat later, using principles derived from laboratory experiments with animals, Sheehan (1953) described stuttering moments as *approach-avoidance acts,* the kinds of ambivalent behavior that result when our responses have had a history of both rewarding and punishing consequences.

Research

Johnson's ideas, coupled with his energy and enthusiasm, dominated the thinking and research concerning stuttering from the mid-1930s until a few years before his death in 1965. No other person before or since has inspired or motivated research in such quantity over such an extended period. Most notably, this work dealt with the onset of stuttering, its distribution in ongoing speech, and its variability under different speaking conditions.

Johnson's early work concerning onset provided, and the work that followed upheld, the discovery of the **Overlap Phenomenon** between disfluencies that occur in the speech of normally fluent children and children who are regarded as having a problem with stuttering. (Recall, no type of disfluency absolutely distinguishes children who stutter from those who do not.) Even in his own studies, however, Johnson chose to overlook what may have been a very important finding: **Children diagnosed as stutterers had far more part-word repetitions in their speech than did children who were normally disfluent.** (You will remember that part-word repetitions are the very behavior that defines a core feature of stuttering.)

Johnson and his colleagues also found that **stuttering moments were not distributed randomly in the speech sequence and that, under certain conditions, their frequency varied predictably.** Today, it is hard to imagine the excitement caused by these findings! Until this point, stuttering had been regarded as a "random disintegration" of speech movements. Now, research demonstrated that stuttering tended to occur at word onsets, on the first three words of sentences, on words beginning with consonants more than vowels, on principal parts of speech, and on stressed syllables in polysyllabic words. Other studies showed that when stutterers re-read the same passage aloud, there was a tendency for stutter events to decline about 50% in frequency from the first to the fifth reading. If these same speakers were brought back to read later in the day, their stuttering frequency returned to its original level! The decline in frequency was called stuttering *adaptation* and its return was called *spontaneous recovery.* Adaptation did not occur for all who stuttered, but for groups the pattern has remained consistent in dozens of studies. Along with these findings, Johnson and others reported a consistency effect, the tendency for stuttering to occur on the same words when a passage is re-read aloud. They also found that people could predict when they would stutter with more than a chance degree of accuracy (Johnson, 1955b).

Johnson interpreted these results as supporting his theory of onset and the moment of stuttering. To him, stuttering occurred on words that were prominent and called attention to themselves, and it varied according to stimuli with which it had occurred in the past. It was permanently sustained in the speaker's repertoire by motivation to avoid its occurrence. **As we shall see later, Johnson could not have anticipated that the very studies concerning location and variability of stuttering that he used to support his ideas would provide the basis for a totally different kind of explanation for the problem.**

Treatment

In the late 1930s, Johnson wrote a paper describing two essential principles of treatment for the adult who stutters: (1) the *descriptional principle* and (2) the *principle of static analysis* (Johnson, 1955a). By the former, he meant that stutterers needed to replace such statements as, "The word is stuck in my throat," with statements like, "I tensed and pushed my tongue to the roof of my mouth." Johnson believed that by talking this way, stutterers would also begin to think this way. They would come to accept responsibility for what they did when they stuttered and what they needed to do to speak normally, rather than to view stuttering as something that happened to them and that they were almost helpless to change.

In the principle of static analysis, Johnson essentially provided a technique to achieve the descriptional principle's objectives. Stutterers were, at a given signal, to freeze their position during a stuttering moment; then study in detail what they were doing and thinking, the levels of tension, the postures, and so on. By doing so, they would come to identify the irrationality of their behavior.

It was Van Riper, however, the second of Travis' students to become a world-recognized authority on stuttering, who was to make "the moment" the essential target of treatment. With a zeal matched by no other, Van Riper developed a systematic program for helping persons who stutter to modify their behavior *during* stuttering moments. His basic approaches emphasized nonavoidance; teaching the person who stutters to stutter in a new, easy, acceptable manner (Van Riper, 1957). Over the years, Van Riper evaluated and honed his procedures and techniques and described their nature and evolution in copious detail (Van Riper, 1958, 1973).

Current Status

Several studies directly controverted Johnson's notion that parental diagnosis in some form was essential to the *onset* of stuttering.

These, and another study that we will take up shortly, made suspect Johnson's specific idea about the effect of parent labeling. As a result, it became irrational to believe that such an act by parents was a necessary or sufficient condition to cause the onset of stuttering. And clearly it was possible for persons who stutter to do so without engaging in avoidance acts, as such (Bloodstein, 1987).

Unfortunately, along with his ideas about onset, Johnson's important concepts about *the moment* of stuttering also tended to be discarded. These were that: (1) cues in the environment, and in the chronic stutterer's speech movements themselves, could have special meaning for the expectation of stuttering and thereby trigger the reactions that make up the second component of stutter events; and (2) the thoughts and beliefs that persons who stutter retain about their speech may be crucial to sustaining the disorder.

These ideas, wrapped by Johnson and his colleagues in the language of semantics and motivational learning, actually form the basis for applying contemporary social cognitive theory to understanding stutter events. According to social cognitive concepts, most of our reactions to environmental stimuli are not evoked "automatically." Rather, they are *self-activated* based upon our learned *expectations* which are retained in memory.

What I call the "Crystal Goblet Phenomenon" may help you understand stutter events in light of cognitive learning theory. This phenomenon occurs when, seated at the dinner table, you heedlessly touch . . . then in panic, retract . . . your hand from a liquid-filled goblet. The cue of the moist glass has a unique **meaning** because of what it **predicts.** Although your reflexive retraction is instantaneous, it is sustained because the touch of the glass evokes stored images of cascading liquid, people leaping to their feet, verbal rebukes, and other mortifying consequences.

Underlying Personality Disorder

Basic Concepts

Could it be that stuttering is a neurotic symptom; that is, the expression of an underlying personality disorder? During and immediately following the time of Freud, there was substantial speculation that this might be the case.

By neurotic symptom, we mean an action performed to relieve internal personality conflict. The conflict usually results from a strong need of unconscious origin that the individual cannot accept or express directly. The symptom partially satisfies the need but also blocks its full expression. The symptom is therefore an act that for the individual is both rewarding and punishing at the same time.

Regarding stuttering, the question concerns the source of underlying conflict and why it would be expressed in a breakdown of speech fluency. Three principal psychoanalytic theories became popular. Each implicated a different period in the early life of the child as being the source. Two theories stated that persons who stutter experienced trauma during the period of early nursing. As a consequence, they sustained a strong unconscious need to be gratified by modes of behavior related to that period. Later, the *movements* of speech, or its *content,* awakened the overpowering need. Another theory said the source of conflict originated during the so-called anal period of socialization. For stutterers, speaking resurrected a need to express aggressive "soiling" type feelings that had their origin in the period just before and during toilet training. In all of these theories, it is the intensity and character of unconscious needs that make them unacceptable. As a result, the speaker cannot express them directly, and the consequence is a blocked or repetitive speech pattern. In this way, **the psychoanalytic theories tried to account for both the source of fluency interruptions as well as the speaker's reactions.**

Research

Although they never had the impact of Johnson's ideas, the psychoanalytic theories launched a period of quite concentrated research in stuttering that began in the 1940s and reached its height during the 1950s. Sheehan (1970) provides a nice review of this work. In general, most studies compared a group of subjects who stuttered with a normally fluent group using personality trait inventories or projective tests. The results were inconsistent. Overall, persons who stuttered were not found to be abnormal in relation to fluent speakers or to have, in common, personality profiles suggested by the theories.

Due to the negative outcomes of this work, later studies changed the focus from personality as a *cause,* to personality as an *effect,* of stuttering. The results remained obscure, however, finding no common maladjustment pattern among persons who stutter and no clearly identifiable relationships between personality and treatment outcome.

Treatment

Purely psychoanalytic treatments of stuttering were never widely practiced although they prospered more during the period of the 1940s and 1950s than they have since. One problem was that talking was sufficiently disabled for some who stuttered that it was impossible for the therapist to cover much ground during the psychoanalytic hour. To offset this problem, hypnosis was sometimes used to facilitate fluency. Its positive long-term effects, however, were never substantiated. Gradually, it became clear that (1) personality abnormalities did not underlie the onset of stuttering and (2) whatever their personality characteristics, people who stutter chronically need direct help with the mechanics of speaking.

Current Status

The failure to turn up consistent relationships between personality and stuttering led to a substantial decline of work in this area. Today, it is almost universally accepted **that stuttering is not a symptom of underlying personality disturbance.** Further, it is widely held that **the role of personality in stuttering is probably individualistic in nature, unlikely to be revealed by studies that compare a group of subjects who stutter with a group of subjects who do not.**

Stimulus Control of Responses

Basic Concepts

A study published in 1958 shook the world of stuttering. Its title was, "Operant Stuttering: The Control of Stuttering Behavior through Response-Contingent Consequences" (Flanagan, Goldiamond, & Azrin, 1958). It not only challenged conventional dogma about the nature and treatment of stuttering, it launched a 20-year period during which "behaviorism" dominated research and treatment.

For three subjects, the study demonstrated clearly that a loud, 1-second blast of noise, contingent upon (i.e., occurring soon after) stuttering episodes was accompanied by a *decrease* in their frequency. Following a subsequent study of disfluencies in nonstutterers, Flanagan and his colleagues concluded that, "breaks, pauses, repetitions and other nonfluencies can be considered operant responses;" they can be "controlled by ensuing consequences" (Flanagan, Goldiamond, & Azrin, 1959, p. 979). If true, this meant that stutter events were explainable simply as behavior that is shaped and controlled by environmental occurrences! In other words, there need not be any unique source factor(s) of fluency interruption.

At first, you might think this study supported Johnson's ideas about onset. But, in actuality, it did the opposite, and many clinicians and theorists were stunned. To them, the results seemed unbelievable. Since the time of Johnson, it had been generally accepted that aversive (punishing) consequences for stuttering would increase avoidance motivation and thereby *increase* the severity of stuttering. In fact, at least two earlier studies (Frick, 1951; Van Riper, 1937) had reported that an *increase* in stuttering did follow the *threat* of shock.

But now a new experimental procedure had been used, the actual *presentation* (not the threat) of an aversive stimulus, and a different outcome had resulted. Enter the age of behaviorism, the experimental period. **Within the operant model of behavior, if stuttering could be brought under stimulus control, that would be sufficient to define not only its nature, but effective treatment procedures as well.** In the aftermath, literally dozens of studies were undertaken to determine whether the early results would be replicable and under what conditions.

Research

In the early 1960s, the most concentrated and the best of the experimental work of this era was begun at the University of Minnesota under the direction of Richard Martin and Gerald Siegel (see Prins & Hubbard, 1988). The basic research designs changed from describing characteristics of different *groups* of subjects to studying the effects of stimuli on stuttering responses in *individuals.*

In an early study, electrical shock not only reduced the frequency of stuttering in one subject, but in two others had a more specific effect on reducing nose wrinkling and tongue protrusion during moments of stuttering (Martin & Siegel, 1966). The results were nothing short of sensational, and they clearly supported the earlier findings of Flanagan, Goldiamond, and Azrin.

Martin and Siegel, and others elsewhere, continued studying various types of response contingent stimuli (RCS), ranging from different noises and tones to verbal rebukes and praise, time out from speaking, and even money. As so often has been the case in the stuttering literature, the results (with one exception we will take up later) became inconsistent. This led Martin to state, some 10 years after his initial studies, that **"results ... yield only very**

equivocal support to the notion that stuttering is an operant response class" (Martin, St. Louis, Haroldson, & Hasbrouck, 1975, p. 489). Somewhat later, Ingham distanced this research completely from the operant model: **"The RCS studies never had a necessary connection with operant conditioning or to the concept of stuttering as an operant"** (Ingham, 1984, p. 235).

Among the many stimuli studied during this period, however, there was one that stood out from all the rest: *response contingent time-out from speaking (RCTO)*. This condition required subjects to stop speaking for several seconds each time a moment of stuttering occurred. The effect was a reduction, or sometimes complete elimination, of stuttering, and it was consistent in more than 15 published studies (Prins & Hubbard, 1988). This outcome occurred not only in the laboratory, but in the clinic as well.

How could the time-out effect be explained? Some held to the operant model and simply concluded that RCTO served as a "punisher" more consistently than other stimuli. But others ventured that time-out makes subjects more aware of what they are doing. Thereby, it may cause them to take control and do what is necessary within their ability to speak more fluently (James, Ricciardelli, Rogers, & Hunter, 1989). If this is true, then time-out would not bring stuttering under stimulus control, per se, but under the control of the speaker! As we shall see in a moment, other studies reinforced this interpretation.

Research questions turned more and more to evaluating clinical effects. For example, Martin reported that when stutterers provided *their own* time-out following stuttering episodes, the effects lasted longer and generalized more to another speaking situation than if the *experimenter* administered the time-out (Martin & Haroldson, 1982). Ingham (1982) showed that when stutterers were taught to *self-evaluate* their stuttering, it improved the long-term effects of treatment. **These outcomes added strength to the suggestion provided by the earlier time-out studies: that speech change may be determined not by the occurrence of consequential events alone, but rather by what these events mean to the speaker.**

Treatment

Behaviorism in the laboratory ushered in the age of accountability in treatment: Treatment procedures became more carefully described and defined; baseline measures were collected on stuttering severity so that progress and outcome could be evaluated; client progress in treatment became more dependent on performance criteria; and follow-up studies evaluated the durability of change after formal treatment was terminated. These were among the most significant clinical contributions of the behavioral period.

Important changes also occurred in the concepts of treatment for preschool children who show early signs of stuttering. Even though it was not intended by Johnson, the effect of his theory had been to make clinicians afraid to intervene with preschoolers for fear of creating a problem from what was just a form of normal behavior. Findings from the behavioral period suggested that calling attention to disfluencies would not necessarily cause them to become more severe and, if done appropriately, could be an effective form of treatment.

> In an ingenious clinical experiment with RCTO, Martin and his colleagues provided a treatment condition in which two preschool children who stuttered spoke with a puppet. The puppet was mounted inside an illuminated stage box. Whenever the children stuttered, the stage lights went out, and the puppet became silent for 10 seconds. During these sessions, which were done with each child individually, the children's stuttering reduced "essentially to zero." Just as important, the reduction generalized to everyday speaking situations. *(Martin, Kuhl, & Haroldson, 1972)*

Current Status

Why did experimental research concerning the effects of stimulus consequences on stuttering begin to fade in the early 1980s? Among many possible reasons is the following: Early work had focused on the operant model, proposing that stuttering is controlled by its immediate environmental consequences. When this model became discredited, not only the model, but the findings themselves were rejected. **As a consequence, some of the most important results of this period have not received the attention they deserve.** Among them are: (1) the quite consistent experimental and clinical effects of RCTO, particularly when it is self administered (Martin & Haroldson, 1982); (2) the value of self-evaluation to maintaining treatment effects (Ingham, 1982); and (3) the positive clinical effects of modeling, watching others respond positively to treatment procedures (Martin & Haroldson, 1977).

These findings do more than *demonstrate* the effectiveness of certain clinical procedures. They suggest *the reason:* that the treatment conditions may be most effective when they alter how people think about their behavior and come to realize what they can do to change (Bandura, 1986). **This puts stuttering squarely within the grasp of contemporary social cognitive learning theory. It holds that people learn complex behavior principally from observation. They control their behavior from within because of what they understand, their motivation, and their expectations. Now, Johnson's ideas from long ago about the importance of meaning and beliefs in stuttering can be joined with experimental outcomes of the behavioral period to form a cornerstone for future studies of nature and treatment.**

Timing and Coordination of Speech Movements

Basic Concepts

Beginning with papers published in the late 1960s and extending through two books, Wingate brought fresh new concepts to bear on evidence about stuttering that had been accumulating since the 1930s (Wingate, 1969a, 1969b, 1970, 1976, 1988). With penetrating logic and a systematic unfolding of ideas, Wingate analyzed his own and earlier work concerning the location and variability of stutter events. In doing so, he determined a direction for research and theory that predominates to this day.

Initially, Wingate concluded that stuttering occurred, not on a sound, but when the speaker *tries to move to the succeeding sound* (Wingate, 1969a). Stuttering was, he said, a "phonetic transition" disorder, a breakdown in the flow of speech from one sound to the next. At about the same time, he analyzed conditions that induced fluency in persons who stutter: for example, metronome-timed speech, choral speaking, masking noise, and delayed auditory feedback (Wingate, 1969b, 1970). Wingate concluded that these conditions (and others that increased fluency in stutterers) could be accounted for by a single factor: "changes in vocalization" (Wingate, 1970, p. 870). By this he meant that speakers altered their manner of producing voice in these conditions, usually by prolonging vocalization or producing a rhythmic pattern of emphasized, or stressed, syllables.

Later, Wingate (1976, 1988) asserted that stuttering resulted from defective speech "prosody," the pattern of stressed syllables that we create while speaking by varying the pitch, duration, and intensity of voice. The stressing of syllables, he said, enables fluent speech by providing a rhythmic structure that helps to *organize* and *time* speech movements, somewhat like a bass drum serves to time the instruments and the steps of a marching band. He pointed out that defective prosody could account for stuttering's tendency to occur on stressed syllables, on word and syllable onsets that begin with consonants, on prominent words, and on initial words of sentences, all of which place special demands on prosody for their appropriate expression. Although these observations about the location of stutter events had been made 50 years earlier during the Johnson era, they were believed at that time to reveal the stutterer's need to avoid stuttering on important words. Now, Wingate, and others as well, saw the location of stutter events in new light: in relationship to the processes required for normal speech production. This interpretation was buttressed by the knowledge that so-called normal speech errors or "slips of the tongue" (e.g., "heft lemisphere" for "left hemisphere") also tend to occur in these same locations.

It remained, however, for Wingate to explain the source of the problem. Although the speech prosody defect is revealed in a breakdown of movement, he sought a *source* for the defect in earlier stages of *speech programming* (Wingate, 1988). Wingate believes that people who stutter have difficulty with the encoding processes by which words and their representative sounds are retrieved from memory and assembled into a program that controls the sequence of speech movements. Movements break down and stutter events occur particularly between the initial consonant and vowel of syllables, because, at that point, precise timing is necessary in order for the separately assembled sounds to be joined by fluent "coarticulated" movements. Stressed syllables are especially vulnerable to fracture because their fluent production requires the most exact timing of speech movements.

Other theories similar to Wingate's were developed during this period. Some theorists, like Wingate, believe the source lies in early stages of *programming* speech movements. Others prefer to think that the source lies at the point of *executing* those movements. However, **what all of these contemporary ideas have in common is their search for failures in normal speech production processes to account for the source of fluency interruptions.**

Research

Using Wingate's ideas as a springboard, research in the 1970s began to turn to the question of vocal control and timing in persons who stutter. For example, were their voice or speech initiation times different from normally fluent speakers? Were the movements of their vocal folds abnormal in some way when they stuttered? Even when they were "fluent," were their voice offset and onset times different from people who did not stutter? (See Adams, Freeman, & Conture, 1984; Starkweather, 1982.)

From studies of vocal control, interest expanded to the study of other speech movements involving e.g., the lips, jaw, and tongue. This work was concerned particularly with the speed, duration, relative timing, and coordination of movements. Techniques of measurement and performance tasks became more sophisticated. Studies began to measure multiple neuromuscular systems simultaneously (e.g., lips, jaw, and voice together) or to evaluate movement patterns in nonspeech systems (e.g., the eyes and fingers). (See Peters & Hulstijn, 1987; Peters, Hulstijn, & Starkweather, 1991.)

As the work progressed, a pattern began to emerge: **People who stutter, adults and quite often children as well, are usually slower and more variable than normally fluent speakers in many speech and nonspeech sequential movement tasks. Even more intriguing, when programming demands increase, persons who stutter require even more time and tend to make more errors as well.**

Treatment

The era concerned with speech timing and coordination has not had the revolutionary impact on treatment that characterized the two periods dominated by learning theory. Nonetheless, there have been important developments that affect particularly the work with preschool children who show early signs of stuttering.

Renewed emphasis is being placed on procedures to help reduce time pressure and complexity in parent-child conversations. Examples include modeling of slower speaking rates, less complex and shorter utterances, and longer pause intervals between utterances. Similar procedures have been used before, but now they are guided by a better foundation of theory and research concerning the requirements for producing fluent speech. Within this framework, they recognize that **in young disfluent children speech motor control processes may be insufficiently established to meet consistently the extraordinary demands of fluent speech.**

Current Status

Today, interest in speech motor control continues to drive much of the theory and research about stuttering. As the work continues to search for source factors of fluency interruption, the focus has shifted somewhat from timing failures that originate at the point of *executing* speech movements to those that originate at the time of *programming* those movements. More than ever before, models that explain how speech is programmed normally are being used as the basis for asking research questions and designing studies to answer them (Peters, Hulstijn, & Starkweather, 1991).

Perspective on Speech Motor Control and Learning

You will recall we spoke of the stuttering episode as having two principal components: (1) an interruption of fluency and (2) the speaker's reaction thereto. Although an individual episode of stuttering may be described as an *event* of movement, that does not necessarily mean that stuttering can be fully characterized as a *disorder* of movement. To characterize the disorder, we must account for a broader set of known conditions, for example, the episodic nature of stuttering at its onset, its persistence in only a small fraction of those who show early signs, the changes in its overt features over time, its enormous variability in different speaking circumstances, and post-treatment relapse which sometimes occurs years after apparently successful treatment has been completed. Here, our concern is not only with isolated events of *fluency failure,* but with what determines how the speaker reacts to these events and why these reactions do, or do not, persist.

Speech motor control is focused primarily on sources of fluency interruption that may underlie stutter events, particularly in young children when stuttering usually begins. Learning, on the other hand, is concerned principally with explaining the speaker's reactions to these interruptions: what form the reactions take, how they change over time and circumstances, what role they have in causing the problem to become chronic, and why they are often so resistant to change in older children and adults. From this point of view, we can see how explanations that focus on speech motor control and on learning are both needed to help understand the nature of this complicated disorder.

✦ SUMMARY AND CONCLUSIONS

You may be saying to yourself, "Stuttering is just too confusing. I'm becoming exhausted from thinking about it. There is too much research, and the results are too contradictory. There are too many explanations, each somewhat plausible, but none sufficient to fully explain the problem. Even the individual who stutters is inconsistent and, in certain circumstances, doesn't stutter at all!" If you are feeling this way, a review of some principal *observations* and *inferences* from this chapter should help alleviate your distress.

Observations

- ◆ The earliest speech characteristics of stuttering are not completely distinctive. Children who speak normally often produce the same disfluencies that children with beginning signs of stuttering do.

- ◆ Children's early disfluencies are often whole- and part-word repetitions that occur on the first words of sentences or clauses.

- ◆ Stuttering usually begins during the preschool years at a time when language and speech development are at a point of greatest acceleration, a period when the demands on encoding processes that enable fluent speech are very high.

- ◆ At their onset, the signs of stuttering are often episodic — they come and go, sometimes with no apparent explanation. Most children who go through this episodic phase do not develop a chronic stuttering problem.

- ◆ The speech characteristics of stuttering take many years to develop. They usually do not emerge full blown.

- ◆ Stutter events tend to occur on principal parts of speech, on the first three words of sentences, on syllables that receive vocal stress, at word or syllable onsets, on words that begin with consonants versus vowels, and at the point where syllable-initial consonant and vowel are joined. What we call "slips of the tongue" also occur in the same places.

- ◆ Virtually all persons who stutter speak fluently during so-called fluency-inducing conditions such as choral speaking or metronome-timed speech.

- ◆ The frequency of stuttering is highly variable in different speaking situations. Most people who stutter can speak much more fluently, for example, when talking to themselves, animals, or young children.

◆ Stuttering is reported to exist throughout the world, but it is considerably more prevalent in societies that are competitive and place a high premium on verbal expression.

◆ Stuttering runs in families. You are much more apt to stutter if you have a first-degree relative who stutters.

◆ Both members of a twin set are more likely to stutter when they are identical, but this does not always happen.

◆ The occurrence of stuttering in males versus females is about 3:1.

◆ No common personality disorder or profile has been found among persons who stutter.

◆ Time-out is the contingent stimulus that has most consistently reduced the frequency of stuttering. Its effects are more enduring when the stimulus is self-administered by the speaker.

◆ In speech motor control tasks, people who stutter often do not show the degree of left hemispheric dominance expected of normally fluent speakers.

◆ People who stutter are usually slower, more variable, and commit more errors in various speech and non-speech sequential movement tasks.

Inferences

◆ At their onset, early signs of "stuttering" reveal a condition of fluency breakdown which, to some extent, is apparently experienced by most preschool children.

◆ During the preschool years, children's speech disfluencies seem to reflect a lack of efficiency in the normal processes by which speech motor control is achieved and fluent speech is sustained.

◆ The frequent failure of early signs of stuttering to develop into a chronic disorder suggests that it may be as important to determine why stuttering persists in a few youngsters as to explain why it occurs at all.

◆ Changes in the observable characteristics of stuttering over time suggest the importance of learning and environmental influences to help account for the development and persistence of the disorder.

✦ Both genetic and environmental influences have a role to play in the occurrence of stuttering. Although the genetic link is clearly important, it appears to be neither a necessary nor sufficient condition to account for the disorder.

✦ Stuttering is not a manifestation of underlying personality disturbance. However, personality theory may some day have something to tell us about why the disorder persists in certain cases and why some people who stutter become so handicapped by their disability while others do not.

✦ When contingent stimuli reduce the frequency of stuttering, they may do so because they call the speaker's attention to what he is doing that he has the ability to change.

✦ Interruptions of fluency that lead to stutter events seem best understood as a breakdown in the encoding and/ or execution of speech movements.

✦ Speaker reactions to fluency interruptions appear to produce most of the observable features of stutter events. Although motor in character, the types and persistence of these reactions seem heavily dependent on individual learning and environmental circumstances.

✦ Although we can describe the severity of stuttering in terms of what we observe about the frequency and duration of stutter *events,* this does not necessarily account for the severity of the *disorder.* To do this we must consider the *handicap,* how stuttered speech affects the feelings, attitudes, and adjustment of the speaker.

In recent years, theories of speech motor control have been dominant as models for understanding the nature of stuttering in relation to fluent speech. In the meantime, less attention has been given to theories of learning, personality, and the environment. But it is certain that to comprehend stuttering as a *disorder of human communication* we ultimately will have to understand how all of these factors interact.

And so, we come to the end of our story. Fluent speech is arguably our most complex and amazing natural achievement as human beings. When it goes awry and leads to the disorder of stuttering, we should not expect simple explanations. This sentiment was captured long ago in the memoirs of a lifelong stutterer: Whoever can solve the problem of stuttering, can solve all the important troubles of the human race (Van Riper, 1971).

◆ REFERENCES

Adams, M. R., Freeman, F. J., & Conture, E. G. (1984). Laryngeal dynamics of stutterers. In R. F. Curlee & W. H. Perkins (Eds.), *Nature and treatment of stuttering: New directions* (pp. 89– 131). San Diego: College-Hill Press.

Andrews, G., Craig, A., Feyer, A.-M., Hoddinott, S., Howie, P., & Neilson, M. (1983). Stuttering: A review of research findings circa 1982. *Journal of Speech and Hearing Disorders, 48,* 226–246.

Bandura, A. (1986). *Social foundations of thought and action.* Englewood Cliffs, NJ: Prentice-Hall.

Bloodstein, O. (1987). *A handbook on stuttering.* Chicago: National Easter Seal Society.

Flanagan, B., Goldiamond, I., & Azrin, N. H. (1958). Operant stuttering: The control of stuttering behavior through response-contingent consequences. *Journal of Experimental Analysis of Behavior, 1,* 173–178.

Flanagan, B., Goldiamond, I., & Azrin, N. H. (1959). Instatement of stuttering in normally fluent individuals through operant procedures. *Science, 130,* 979–981.

Frick, J. (1951). *An exploratory study of the effect of punishment (electric shock) upon stuttering behavior.* Unpublished doctoral dissertation, University of Iowa, Iowa City.

Ingham, R. J. (1982). The effects of self-evaluation training on maintenance and generalization during stuttering treatment. *Journal of Speech and Hearing Disorders, 47,* 271–280.

Ingham, R. J. (1984). *Stuttering and behavior therapy.* San Diego: College-Hill Press.

James, J. E., Ricciardelli, L. A., Rogers, P., & Hunter, C. E. (1989). A preliminary analysis of the ameliorative effects of time-out from speaking on stuttering. *Journal of Speech and Hearing Research, 32,* 604–610.

Johnson, W. (1930). *Because I stutter.* New York: Appleton-Century-Crofts.

Johnson, W. (1933). An interpretation of stuttering. *Quarterly Journal of Speech, 19,* 70–77.

Johnson, W. (1938). The role of evaluation in stuttering behavior. *Journal of Speech Disorders, 3,* 85–89.

Johnson, W. (1946). *People in quandaries.* New York: Harper & Brothers.

Johnson, W., Brown, S., Curtis, J., Edney, C., & Keaster, J. (1956). *Speech handicapped school children.* New York: Harper & Row.

Johnson W. (1955a). The descriptive principle and the principle of static analysis. In W. Johnson & R. R. Leutenegger (Eds.), *Stuttering in children and adults* (pp. 432–447). Minneapolis: University of Minnesota Press.

Johnson, W. (1955b). The time, the place, and the problem. In W. Johnson & R. R. Leutenegger (Eds.), *Stuttering in children and adults* (pp. 3–25). Minneapolis: University of Minnesota Press.

Johnson, W. (1959). *The onset of stuttering.* Minneapolis: University of Minnesota Press.

Martin, R. R., & Haroldson, S. K. (1977). Effect of vicarious punishment on stuttering frequency. *Journal of Speech and Hearing Research, 20,* 21–26.

Martin, R. R., & Haroldson, S. K. (1982). Contingent self-stimulation for stuttering. *Journal of Speech and Hearing Disorders, 47,* 407–413.

Martin, R. R., Kuhl, P., & Haroldson, S. K. (1972). An experimental treatment with two preschool stuttering children. *Journal of Speech and Hearing Research, 15,* 743–752.

Martin, R. R., & Siegel, G. M. (1966). The effects of response-contingent shock on stuttering. *Journal of Speech and Hearing Research, 9,* 340–352.

Martin, R. R., St. Louis, K., Haroldson, S. K. & Hasbrouck, J. (1975). Punishment and negative reinforcement of stuttering using electric shock. *Journal of Speech and Hearing Research, 18,* 478–490.

Moore, W. H. (1990). Pathophysiology of stuttering: Cerebral activation differences in stutterers vs. nonstutterers. In J. A. Cooper (Ed.), *Research needs in stuttering: Roadblocks and future directions* (ASHA Reports, 18). Rockville, MD: American Speech-Language-Hearing Association.

Orton, S. T. (1927). Studies in stuttering. *Archives of Neurology and Psychiatry, 18,* 671–672.

Peters, H. F. M., & Hulstijn, W. (Eds.). (1987). *Speech motor dynamics in stuttering.* New York: Springer-Verlag.

Peters, H. F. M., Hulstijn, W., & Starkweather, C. W. (Eds.). (1991). *Speech motor control and stuttering.* New York: Elsevier.

Prins, D. (1991). Theories of stuttering as event and disorder: Implications for speech production processes. In H. F. M. Peters, W. Hulstijn, & C. W. Starkweather (Eds.), *Speech motor control and stuttering* (pp. 571–580). New York: Elsevier.

Prins, D., & Hubbard, C. P. (1988). Response contingent stimuli and stuttering: Issues and implications. *Journal of Speech and Hearing Research, 31,* 696–709.

Rosenfield, D., & Nudelman, H. (1987). Neuropsychological models of speech disfluency. In L. Rustin, H. Purser, & D. Rowley (Eds.), *Progress in the treatment of fluency disorders* (pp. 3–19). New York: Taylor & Francis.

Sheehan, J. G. (1953). Theory and treatment of stuttering as an approach-avoidance conflict. *Journal of Psychology, 36,* 27–49.

Sheehan, J. G. (1970). *Stuttering: Research and theory.* New York: Harper & Row.

Starkweather, C. W. (1982). *Stuttering and laryngeal behavior: A review* (ASHA Monographs, No. 18). Rockville, MD: American Speech-Language-Hearing Association.

Travis, L. E. (1931). *Speech pathology.* New York: D. Appleton & Company.

Travis, L. E. (1978). Neurophysiological dominance. *Journal of Speech and Hearing Disorders, 43,* 275–278. (Reprinted from *Speech pathology* by L. E. Travis, 1931, D. Appleton & Company, New York.)

Van Riper, C. (1937). The effect of penalty upon frequency of stuttering spasms. *Journal of Genetic Psychology, 50,* 193–195.

Van Riper, C. (1957). Symptomatic therapy for stuttering. In L. E. Travis (Ed.), *Handbook of speech pathology* (pp. 878–897). New York: Appleton-Century-Crofts.

Van Riper, C. (1958). Experiments in stuttering therapy. In J. Eisenson (Ed.), *Stuttering: A symposium* (pp. 273–393). New York: Harper & Brothers.

Van Riper, C. (1971). *The nature of stuttering.* Englewood Cliffs, NJ: Prentice-Hall.

Van Riper, C. (1973). *The treatment of stuttering.* Englewood Cliffs, NJ: Prentice-Hall.

Van Riper, C. (1982). *The nature of stuttering* (2nd ed.). Englewood Cliffs, NJ: Prentice-Hall.

Wingate, M. E. (1964). A standard definition of stuttering. *Journal of Speech and Hearing Disorders, 29,* 484–489.

Wingate, M. E. (1969a). Sound and pattern in artificial fluency. *Journal of Speech and Hearing Research, 12,* 677–687.

Wingate, M. E. (1969b). Stuttering as a phonetic transition defect. *Journal of Speech and Hearing Disorders, 34,* 107–108.

Wingate, M. E. (1970). Effect on stuttering of changes in audition. *Journal of Speech and Hearing Research, 13,* 861–873.

Wingate, M. E. (1976). *Stuttering theory and treatment.* New York: Irvington.

Wingate, M. E. (1988). *The structure of stuttering: A psycholinguistic analysis.* New York: Springer-Verlag.

Wischner, G. J. (1950). Stuttering behavior and learning: A preliminary theoretical formulation. *Journal of Speech and Hearing Disorders, 15,* 324–335.

Wischner, G. J. (1952). An experimental approach to expectancy and anxiety in stuttering behavior. *Journal of Speech and Hearing Disorders, 17,* 139–154.

◆ GLOSSARY

Accessory features of stuttering: distinctive audible and visible characteristics of stutter events that result from excessive effort and tensing.

Adaptation, spontaneous recovery, and consistency of stuttering: the tendency for stutter events to: (a) decline in frequency about 50% from the first to the fifth consecutive oral reading of a passage; (b) return to their original frequency within several hours following adaptation; and (c) occur on the same words when a passage is re-read aloud.

Associated features of stuttering: effects of stuttered speech on the adjustment of the individual.

Cerebral dominance: the control of one side of the brain, or the other, over certain functions. For speech, the left cerebral hemisphere is normally dominant.

Core features of stuttering: part-word or sound repetitions and prolongations that mark the occurrence of stutter events; may exist without accessory features.

Episodic stuttering: the tendency for earliest signs of stuttering to be intermittent during the preschool years.

Fluency inducing conditions: conditions that almost uniformly eliminate the occurrence of stuttering; for example, choral speaking and speaking to the beat of a metronome.

Fluent speech: characterized by the continuity or blending of words within phrases and a rapid rate which, in adults, is about 15 sounds per second.

Operant theory: an explanation of learning that attributes behavior change to the occurrence of environmental consequences.

Overlap phenomenon: the occurrence of the same speech disfluencies in normally speaking preschool children and children believed to show signs of early stuttering.

Psycholinguistic encoding processes (speech programming): mental actions by which words are retrieved from memory and assembled into a code that can direct the movements of speech structures.

Social-cognitive theory: an explanation of learning that attributes behavior change to the meaning of environmental consequences.

Stutter event: an occurrence during speech which is interpreted to consist of (a) a fluency interruption perceived by the speaker and (b) the speaker's coping reactions.

Stuttering disorder: characterized by the chronic occurrence of stutter events and their potentially handicapping effects on the speaker.

Sound Information: Scientific Substrates of Hearing*

CHARLES I. BERLIN, Ph.D.

This chapter is organized around three segments:

✦ Real case histories and the historic and scientific underpinning of the diagnosis and management.

✦ A collection of some questions about hearing in people and other animals which interest some of the general public. I compiled this list by asking high school and college students, people from the public at large (via a Computer Bulletin Board), friends and their families, what questions about hearing excited them enough to want to know more.

✦ WIMWIGs, which stands for **What I Meant . . . What I Got**.

---

*I had planned a different title for this chapter based on the first WIMWIG experience I had with a normal hearing secretary who had a jaundiced view of life; she produced transcription very different from what I had intended. Thus the acronym "What I Meant . . . What I Got." Based on one of her prize confusions I was going to call this chapter: Hearing Science, or: This work is Ridiculously Dumb . . . and the Calibrations are in a Mess.

I had just finished a scientific review of a very well done article and I dictated into my not-so-high-fidelity machine: "This work is meticulously done." She typed "this work is ridiculously dumb." Then, later in the critique, I commented that "the calibrations were in RMS" (an acronym for Root-Mean-Square). She typed "the calibrations are in a mess."

I wonder what would have happened if I hadn't proofread the critique before it went out? At any rate, this incident started me keeping a journal of bizarre auditory misperceptions that evolved from combinations of poor fidelity systems, poor perception, and different vocabulary stores that people brought to the work place. I named them WIMWIGs for this chapter, and they will appear from time to time as a reminder that this hearing business has lots of good fun and humor in it, as well as great personal satisfaction.

This chapter was written to tell you about hearing science and audiology as fields of study. It starts with a birth announcement which really represents the "death" of an expected child and the rebirth of a different one. It takes you from the extreme views of deafness as a tragedy to deafness as simply a cultural difference. Case histories will introduce you to a variety of patient problems one might encounter in the course of audiologic practice. The chapter also takes you through a series of answers to questions about basic and applied hearing science in humans and other animals. The chapter closes with "what it takes" to be a hearing scientist, followed by my own very personal commentary about the germinal importance of interpersonal communication in helping us all to "listen better" to each other whether with the ear, the eye — or the heart.

Birth Announcement . . . before we knew.

Announcing the birth of Dorothy Jane Crosby.
Stanford class of 2009, track, academic all-American, BS in pre-astronautics, Cum Laude . . .

2008 Olympics (Decathlon), Miss Florida, Senate hopeful.

Joined us July 23, 1988 at 5:43 PM.

"Your child is deaf. I know she's only 2 years old but we have tests that tell us even at birth if a child's inner ears are damaged. There are . . . ." The practitioner droned on, but we didn't remember hearing much. When your dreams shatter, there is no sound, just the slow motion vision of icebergs sliding off a glacier, making huge soundless waves and looking so calm — unless you happen to be swimming under the iceberg.

That's what it was like the day we learned that our beautiful two-year old had a hearing problem. It was hard to wrap our minds around the word 'deaf' immediately, but in recent months we had become increasingly aware that Dorothy Jane didn't seem to hear.

> . . . This wasn't happening to us, these things always happen to other people, — this was *not* happening! God, are you really sure you've picked the right family? Can we talk?
>
> Somehow we drove home and began the process of grieving . . . how could this be true, searching for strength, blaming ourselves for not knowing sooner, imagining what the future would bring, crying over our shattered dreams, and mourning for our poor little girl who couldn't possibly have a happy or normal life now.
>
> I'm glad to say that time was to prove us wrong on many counts . . . with time we were able to move through the initial emotional firestorm toward acceptance and a pragmatic plan for the future.
>
> For the first few weeks, I would awake and have to remember: "Oh yes, Dorothy will be deaf again today." It's not something you eventually recover from, like chicken pox.
>
> Adapted from the book *Silent Dancing* written by Osmond Crosby as a chronicle of his family's experience with deafness.

In the section that follows you will learn why Dorothy can't hear much, how she uses her residual hearing along with a system called Cued Speech to communicate in English with normal hearing people.

◆ FIRST, SOME INFORMATION ABOUT THE EAR

Figure 14–1 shows a picture of the ear, divided into three basic parts: outer, middle, and inner ears. When you have damage or disease to the outer or middle ears you have a so-called **conductive hearing loss**, in which sound is poorly conducted to the inner ear. Its treatments are usually surgical and/or medical. To hear better you simply have to make things louder or completely remove the obstacles and mechanical obstructions.

If the hair cells and/or nerve fibers in the inner ear are damaged this results in what has been called either **nerve deafness** or **sensorineural hearing loss**. Both names are somewhat incomplete and potentially misleading in their descriptions; we will clarify them for you later on. But in either hair cell or nerve loss the clarity of the signal is distorted and simply "making it louder" often can't do the job. Fortunately, we have learned how to make only some signals louder without exceeding the thresholds of discomfort, and

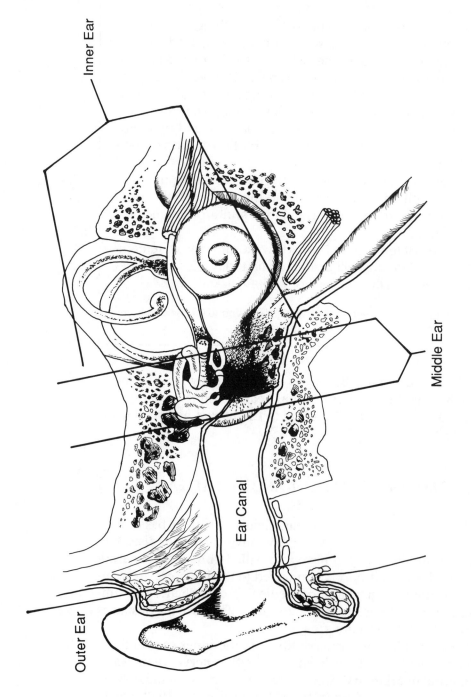

Inner Ear

Middle Ear

Ear Canal

Outer Ear

Figure 14–1. The three basic divisions of the ear: the outer, middle, and inner ear.

with new technology many people with hearing losses once thought to be unmanageable can be greatly helped.

The **outer ear** focuses sound down the ear canal to the ear drum membrane. This focus makes the sound a little stronger in critical speech-understanding ranges above 2000 Hz before it even reaches the ear drum membrane.

The ear drum membrane is like the skin on a kettle drum. It vibrates to the sounds which hit it and transmits those vibrations to the bones in the middle ear. If the ear drum membrane is torn you will neither go deaf nor have a serious hearing loss simply from the perforation. However, if left untreated, infection and scarring can cause far more hearing loss than the rupture of the ear drum membrane itself.

The **middle ear** has three bones in it which help bring sound efficiently to the inner ear where it is converted into a special electrical and neural code and sent to the brain. The existence of the middle ear was reported 450 years ago (see later).

The **inner ear**, or **cochlea**, has over 20,000 hair cells packed into what looks like a coiled snail shell about the size of your little fingernail. It is the organ system that is usually damaged when people mistakenly say "You have nerve deafness." Usually we have hair cell loss rather than nerve loss, and we'll tell you more about how we can tell one from the other later in this chapter.

All of these intricate structures of the inner ear are determined by the products of genes; thus an abnormal gene can lead to an ear that has difficulty transducing sound into neural energy and hence a sensorineural hearing loss.

◆ USEFUL FACTS ABOUT SOUND AND HEARING

There are three dimensions to sound: frequency, intensity, and time and you can remember them with the acronym F-I-T.

Frequency, reported in Hertz (Hz), represents the rate at which segments in the sound repeat themselves. Young humans are said to hear air-borne sound between about 20 Hz and 20,000 Hz. However, by bone conduction most humans (even many so-called "deaf" patients) can sense very powerful ultra-high frequency sounds past 30,000 Hz.

How well you hear in the range from 250 Hz to 3000 Hz predicts for the most part your ability to understand speech in quiet. Two-hundred fifty Hz is about one octave *below* middle C on the piano, while 3000 Hz is close to the eleventh white note from the top of the piano. A normal hearing person should be able to hear both of those notes when they are played softly even if the piano is over 60 feet away!

The higher the frequency the higher the Hz number; many people say the "pitch is higher" when the frequency increases. Keep in mind however that frequency and pitch are not the same thing, any more than heaviness and weight are the same. Weight is an objective number generated by a scale or other device, which generates a different sense of "heaviness" depending on who or what is trying to lift the object in question. In sound, certain frequencies have no "pitch" at all if they are outside the range of human hearing. Similarly, if the frequency of say a 17,000 Hz sound were to be doubled, its pitch won't change much at all provided it is intense enough to remain audible.

Intensity is the power per unit area exerted by a sound. It usually is expressed in decibels (dB), a number representing the logarithm of a ratio between two numbers. Thus:

$$dB = 10 \times \text{Log Output Power/Reference Power}$$

$$30 \text{ dB} = 10 \times \text{Log } 1000/1 \text{ (where the log of } 1000 = 3)$$

Thus 30 dB represents 1000 times more power than 0 dB and 40 dB represents *10,000 times* more power than 0 dB. Zero dB doesn't mean "quiet" or "nothing"; it really means "1," the starting point of the scale. If you want to know more about how that scale works, see the references at the end of the chapter.

"Time" in this context can mean either elapsed time (usually expressed in thousandths of a second) or phase of onset, that is, where in its own cycle of operation the sound starts and/or finishes. That's something like a Ferris wheel ride, in which you can measure the start from when your chair is at the bottom, at "9 o'clock," "3 o'clock," and so on. "Time" also can refer to rise and fall time, the notion of how fast a sound starts and/or finishes.

More of these facts will come up when the cases warrant.

✦ THE FIRST CASE

D.J.'s diagnosis was late in coming. She probably was hearing impaired from birth, but her parents, who are very well-educated and very sophisticated, were not sensitized to her problem. They probably also believed, like many others, that it is difficult if not impossible to test the hearing of a young baby. This is an unfortunate myth, as is evidenced by these related questions that people asked.

When do babies really start to hear?

Babies actually hear while they are in the womb. Their ears have developed by the second trimester, and, even though they live "under water," they hear through bone conduction. The next time you are in a swimming pool or bathtub, put your head under water and tap the side of the pool or tub with a hard object. You'll see what a crisp and sharp sound you hear (unless of course you have a hearing loss). Babies can hear sounds that are delivered directly to their mothers' abdomen for months before they are born. They also can hear most fairly loud sounds including music that normal hearing people can hear.

After they are born, babies can be seen to give a startle response (a blink or a "jump") in response to a sharp clap or loud noise in the nursery. Normal babies turn to the voice of a caretaker much more readily if they can see the face, and do so more regularly if the person is talking on the right side of the baby than on the left side. This behavior is probably related to the dominance of the left side of the brain for speech and language.

Babies' brain structures take about a year to develop more fully and prepare them to handle most of the sounds that reach their ears. However, the parts of the brain that deal with the combined understanding and expression of language are not fully developed until around puberty.

How can you tell if a newborn baby hears normally?

Two tests used by audiologists, one called **auditory brainstem response** (ABR) testing and the other called **otoacoustic emissions**, are now widely recommended as screening tests for hearing in newborns. During the ABR, a brief pulse is delivered to the ear and electric sensors pick up tiny electrical activity generated inside the lower brainstem in response to the clicks. An averaging computer adds up all the minute responses from the brain, extracts the response from sound-irrelevant background activity in the brain, and displays a set of waveforms whose locations in subsequent time are mathematically predictable for normal ears.

The click-evoked otoacoustic emissions test measures minuscule acoustic echoes given off by the hair cells of the inner ear. When a brief sound is introduced into the inner ear, the outer hair cells produce a small echo which can be recorded by ultrasensitive microphones placed in the ear canal. This too depends on averaging computers to extract the small signal from a wide array of irrelevant background noises.

When both tests show normal results, the child is clearly not a candidate for hearing aids or conventional amplification and can be considered likely to develop normal speech and hearing.

D.J., and later her sister Carina, were diagnosed as hearing impaired with the use of auditory brainstem response audiometry. D.J.'s hearing loss of between 90 and 100 dB (1,000,000,000 to 10,000,000,000 times poorer than normal) probably was caused by a defective gene leading to a loss of both outer and some inner hair cells; I concluded that because her sister Carina also has a hearing loss, and the likelihood of two siblings having hearing loss without a gene being involved is slim. However, I could be wrong. (See later on the sections re: genes.)

D.J.'s hearing loss is so great that for practical purposes she hears almost nothing. However, she is not *totally* deaf. To get an idea of what she hears, make a fist and put it over your mouth with the thumb and forefinger side next to your mouth. Open the mouth-side of your fist enough to put your lips into it, and then, with your fist keeping your mouth and lips from moving normally, try to talk. The muffled sound you generate is an approximation of what she hears with hearing aids, but as muffled as it sounds, this distorted speech can be used surprisingly well to learn to understand speech. Just keep in mind that people speak as they hear and a congenitally hearing impaired person will almost always speak with an "accent" unique to that person's hearing abilities.

Get a friend who has normal hearing to help you with this demonstration. Cover your mouth as I described in the previous paragraph and speak the words *railroad, cowboy, baseball*, and *hotdog*. Ask your friend to repeat your words. Some people will immediately be able to understand the words; others will need some practice. If needed, give your friend some practice by saying the four words clearly, and then muffle them with your fist. Then scramble the order, but make it clear that you will be using only those four words. What should happen is that your friend will be able to guess most, if not all, of the words. Now if you can suddenly and unexpectedly switch languages to a language your friend doesn't know or expect, his or her comprehension should drop markedly. This explains in part why hearing impaired children like D.J. need to learn the *language* they are to use as early as possible in their lives. If the language is to be English, the child needs as much help as possible to learn the structure of the language. One way to make English visible to the deaf is with a system called **Cued Speech**, invented by Dr. R. Orin Cornett. This is the system that the Crosby family elected to use with D.J. It helped her learn to read English at well above the second grade level by the time she was 5 years old, even though she could not at the time speak very clearly.

Like most hearing parents of deaf children, the Crosby family went through some agonizing decisions about how to raise and educate D.J. After weighing the arguments for and against using **American Sign Language**, they opted for hearing aid use and cued speech.

They were fortunate to have a school system that offered them many choices.

> After our two days visiting Fairfax County, we spent an evening with Sue Schwartz and Joan Miller in Maryland. Sue had edited the book Choices in Deafness, which was the pivotal book in our initial learning process. In Choices, the statement that we would read about deaf people who had grown up with *very* different educational methods, yet *all* had a success story to tell, was *exactly* what we needed to hear as "newly diagnosed" parents. (Crosby, in press, p. 23)

The family, in all their pain, needed to go through the grief of losing the child they had expected, and the joy of mobilizing their "new" child toward learning a language. Their pain was not lessened by the mismanagement they suffered at the beginning of their odyssey.

Crosby (in press) wrote in his journal:

> The test that indicated complete deafness for Dorothy Jane is called an "ABR," an Auditory Brainstem Response test. [Au: Misleading advice was given based on a test that was incorrectly interpreted by a physician trained in neurology instead of hearing.] . . . we were unfortunate to encounter a doctor who was either unaware of what he didn't know or was unwilling to admit it. . . . This neurologist never mentioned hearing aids and knew nothing of the options available to us. All he could do was mumble something about trying to find a sign language class. When the doctor told us he had never diagnosed a child as deaf as ours, it never occurred to me that this was because children with this sort of hearing loss are usually evaluated by audiologists and ENT specialists.
>
> When Dr. Berlin used the standard time interval of ten milliseconds he got the same results [Au: as the Neurologist]. However, when he lengthened the interval to both 15 and 25 milliseconds, he found a response of 85–90 dB in the high frequency range . . . and detected a response at 75–80 dB in the lower frequencies. This was still on the borderline of profoundly deaf (we learned that it's unlikely that she'll ever use a regular telephone), and he told us that even this little bit of hearing could deteriorate. But it was a starting point, a happy surprise after the bleak forecast that followed the earlier ABR test. Hearing aids often help people with this amount of hearing to perceive sounds,

words, language and their own voice. The possibility that spoken English could be our daughter's first language was now real and worth pursuing.

The bottom line was that Dr. Berlin fitted D.J. with ear molds and hearing aids . . . the challenge now became to convince her that sticking something into ears and leaving them there all day was a reasonable thing to do. (Crosby, in press, p. 9)

There is a bright scenario now for D.J.; her Dad, in his predictably loving and tender way, has written about it.

Birthday Girl
July 23, 1992

Four years ago You were born

Four years ago Your eyes were wise and knowing

Four years ago we were filled with hopes and dreams

Four years ago I told everyone that you would go to Stanford

Four years ago I told everyone that you would be an astronaut

Four years ago We didn't know.

Today I wished you Happy Birthday without speaking,
you said "new shoes" with your hands and face

Today you have a little sister . . .
she wears hearing aids too

Today We know more than then

Today we don't know where the journey leads

Today you can still be an astronaut or go to Stanford if you want

Today I'm filled with hopes and dreams

Some are different . . . many are the same.

Happy Birthday — dear, perfect child. (Crosby, in press, p. 19)

When can you be sure a baby is really talking?

Babies imitate what they hear in their environments. When what they say appears to be random we call it "babbling." However, careful analysis suggests that it is not nearly as random as we might think. Even deaf babies of signing parents "babble" with their hands and fingers. See Chapter 4 by Kuhl on perceptual development for additional information.

WIMWIG

"The patient is deaf" became "the patient is death" — maybe not so far from the truth for some people.

The kernel of D.J.'s story focuses on the human elements of deafness. The professionals who work with this family have to know lots about the biology and physics of deafness to advise the family technically. They also must be sensitive to the human issues of helping a family deal with their feelings. So a professional in this area would do well to first learn the science but keep the humanistic elements in balance.

◆ HOW IMPORTANT ARE GENES IN OUR ABILITY TO HEAR?

When someone has trouble hearing, a genetic problem is likely to play an important role in the cause. All of our characteristics are determined to a greater or lesser extent by the genes we inherit from our parents. They provide the code for thousands of the proteins that are responsible for our appearance, our health, and our behavior. The structure and shape of our ears and the functioning of our nerves and hair cells are controlled by the genes. If a gene that influences our ability to hear is abnormal, then hearing impairment may occur. Both D.J. and Carina have hearing problems. If more than one child in a family is affected, the most likely cause is a defective gene. For example, an abnormality in a gene that is important in prenatal development causes a dominant disease called Waardenburg syndrome. Children who have one copy of this abnormal gene have severe hearing impairment as well as other problems. Many people who have both hearing and visual impairment have a genetic disease called Usher syndrome. This disease is recessive, which means that individuals who are affected have *two* copies of the defective gene — they inherited one copy from their father and one copy from their mother. (Syndrome-based communication disorders are discussed in detail in Chapter 8.) Geneticists are performing research to isolate genes that cause hearing problems. When a gene is identified, the abnormal protein can be determined, and effective therapies based on the underlying defect can be developed. Often research on animals is helpful. You may be surprised to know that mice and humans have many genes in common. Thus, a gene on the 19th chromosome of the mouse that causes recessive deafness, identified recently by Dr. Bronya Keats in our laboratory, is homologous to the 9th chromosome of humans, and probably causes a similar type of recessive deafness. Many people affected by hearing loss may be helped through genetic research, which is on the cutting edge of health science in this decade. The human Genome project, designed to outline the entire library of human genetic material, has been called by some a project of the magnitude and ultimate importance of Columbus' voyage to the New World.

◆ MORE ABOUT WHAT WENT INTO THE EARLY DIAGNOSIS OF DEAFNESS

What is especially heartening is that today we can evaluate much of the auditory function of a young full-term baby within hours after its birth by using two tools developed by two people who made their initial discoveries from outside the mainstream of hearing science or audiology. The two tools are ABR and otoacoustic emissions; the two men are Donald Jewett and David Kemp, respectively.

The ABR

A (now) orthopedist named Donald Jewett along with colleagues Romano and Williston (1970), published a germinal paper on auditory brainstem response which has now become the gold-standard test for evaluating hearing in infants. The discovery of this response is rightfully shared with an Israeli group (Sohmer & Feinmesser, 1967) and two Japanese colleagues (Yoshie & Ohashi, 1970). All of these workers in turn built their observations and tests on the discovery of electrical activity in the cochlea, which was the 1930–1950 work of Drs. E. Glen Wever and his associates, Bray, Lawrence, Vernon, and others. The electrical recording from the inner ear (electrocochleography) was attempted in people in 1933 but was finally successfully performed in humans at the Johns Hopkins Hospital in the mid-1960s. I was a post-doctoral fellow at Hopkins at the time, supported by a National Institute of Health (NIH) fellowship, to study "Medical Audiology" with scientists, physicians, and engineers also supported by NIH. Our team of engineers and audiologists wheeled hundreds of pounds of recording gear into the operating room to record from the inner ears that the surgeons (Drs. Robert

Ruben, Al Lieberman, and John Bordley) had exposed for electrode access. These were exciting times when we could diagnose cochlear deafness in the operating room with great assurance. Now thousands of audiologists, neurologists, and otolaryngologists in the country have access to this computer-driven technology and can perform either **electrocochleography** or ABR in the office.

Otoacoustic Emissions

David Kemp was a petroleum engineer who was assigned in the mid-1970s to work at the Institute of Laryngology and Otology in London after his petro-geology work in the North Sea was terminated. Geologists who search for oil have a highly developed technology for creating minor underground explosions and searching for aberrant echoes from the earth's crust which might indicate oil deposits. Having no other assignment, Kemp applied his echo technology to the ear and discovered something no "right thinking" traditionally trained hearing scientist would have bothered to seek — an active process in the ear which actually generates sounds of its own either spontaneously or as an echo in response to incoming sounds. These echoes, now called otoacoustic emissions, can be used to screen for normal function of the inner ear in newborn infants. They also tell us much about how the hair cells work (Kemp, 1978).

WIMWIG

"The child had poor phrasing" became "The poor child was freezing!"

✦ HISTORICAL PERSPECTIVE

The ancients believed that when we saw anything it was because a light shone from the eye to illuminate the object, and when we heard something it was because a sound was made by the sympathetic vibration of a reservoir of air captured behind the ear drum membrane.

It wasn't until the Renaissance that men started to search for the truth by experimentation and observation rather than by word-of-mouth or written pronouncements. Vesalius, in 1543, described how he was cleaning out a skull to prepare a skeleton when a small bone happened to fall out of the ear; he quickly found a second ossicle still in place, but missed the third and smallest bone in the human body. He had uncovered the "hammer" (malleus) and "anvil" (incus) but had missed the "stirrup" (or stapes, pronounced stape-eez). Just a few years later the Italian scholar Ingrassia discovered the third bone and named it after its stirrup-like shape.

Eustachio, in around 1560, described a tube that connected the middle ear space to the nasal passages. This is the tube that gets blocked when you rapidly change altitude in an airplane or elevator. This was a very significant finding because it meant that no sealed pocket of air could exist in the middle ear. Undaunted, anatomists continued to look for the "magic pocket of resonating air" assuming it would be found somewhere else.

Many anatomists followed the lead of Gabriello Fallopio who opened the round window and peered through it. He found a coiled labyrinth of bone, cartilage, and membrane but believed that the pocket of air resided in the cochlea, even though he and many others saw fluid coming out of the cochlea. No one could believe that all these years of searching for the resonating pocket of air that made sounds emanate from the ear were useless! It is ironic that Kemp's (1978) report that the ear does make sounds of its own (see section on otoacoustic emissions), supported the belief but for reasons far removed from anything imagined centuries ago.

The concept of the resonating air pocket was finally demolished in the winter of 1777 when a scientist-physician named Phillipp Friedrich Meckel put a fresh temporal bone in the frozen ground overnight to see if he could test Cotugno's 1760 statement that "the ear was full of fluid and not air." The next morning he was elated to find that the inner ear was filled with frozen fluid. Cotugno was right! There was fluid in the cochlea and not air as the ancients had believed for 2200 years! (Wever, 1961).

The excitement of making a truly new discovery defies description; I wish you that joy in your life. It is then you also will see that we all stand on the shoulders of our predecessors, so that we have broader scope and vision because of both the insights and mistakes of our predecessors.

Until the 1500s it was generally believed the deaf were uneducable, and they often were put outside of the city walls, along with others deemed to be intellectually inferior, and left to die. It was not until the mid-1700s that a systematic attempt to educate the deaf with a hand language was introduced in France by the French abbe de l'Epee. At about the same time de l'Epee's German contemporary Heinicke stressed an oral approach to the deaf which employed speech and lip reading as essential tools. Both groups were only modestly successful in educating their so-called "deaf" patients well before anyone had developed ways of truly measuring the extent and nature of the auditory impairment.

In our times the invention of the telephone actually represented Alexander Graham Bell's *failure* to make an electronic hearing aid that would compensate for a family member's severe hearing loss! (Stevens & Warshofsky, 1965). Bell's father, Melville Bell, was a teacher of the deaf. To this day the telephone constitutes one of the biggest obstacles to easy accessibility for the deaf; to the culturally deaf it is one of the most despised products of hearing culture. Some deaf-culture-sensitive normal hearing roommates of signing deaf students at Gallaudet University have been known to use only a teletype or relay service rather than their own normal ears and speech to communicate with their normal-hearing family members.

Whistles used by Galton, Urbantschitsch, single stringed instruments, and various sirens and mechanical oscillators were used as mechanical hearing testing devices by people like C. C. Bunch before the widespread availability of electricity. (Stevens & Warshofsky, 1965)

The first systematic electronic hearing tests for medical purposes were performed in the late 1920s and early 1930s at the Johns Hopkins Medical Institutions by one of my teachers, Stacy Guild. Guild was an anatomist who used a (then) new invention, the Western Electric 1-A battery driven audiometer to test the hearing of dying patients at the bedside. He and his associates went into the hospital, tested the patients for their hearing sensitivity between 125 Hz and 16,384 Hz and then collected and processed their cochlear bones after the patients died. He developed an anatomical system for quantifying the damage (see as a modern example Schuknecht, 1974) which illustrates the difference between a normal inner ear and a pathological ear, lacking hair cells and nerve fibers.

What causes hearing loss or deafness?

First we should discriminate between hearing loss and deafness. *Hearing loss* implies something less than total absence of hearing sensation, while *deafness*, to many, implies literally and figuratively *absolutely* no ability to hear. Such truly "stone deaf" people are very rare, but in the past many patients were classified that way who either couldn't be tested accurately or chose to remain non-verbal and not use their ears for communication.

The two most common types of hearing loss, conductive and sensory, are caused by diseases in the outer/middle and inner ear, respectively. Conductive loss follows accumulation of fluid, debris, or infectious material in the middle ear, or occasionally by the simple impaction of wax (cerumen) in the external ear. About half of all early childhood inner ear hearing losses have a genetic origin. The other half come from combinations of acquired diseases like meningitis or German measles, or systemic conditions like prematurity or jaundice.

WIMWIG

"Brainstem Response" became "Brainstorm Response."

How can we fix it? Can you transplant or implant an artificial ear to help deaf people hear?

For people who heard in childhood, and developed normal speech and hearing before they became deaf, we first try hearing aids and/or **assistive listening devices**. Such a listening device is like an FM radio which both the patient and the target speaker use in tandem. The voice of the speaker, which at the mouth exceeds 105 dB sound pressure, is delivered by radio or a similar carrier directly to the ear of the hearing-impaired person. If this helps, and it often does, we can save the patient thousands of dollars in medical and surgical costs. To see what that might sound like, ask a friend to talk (quietly) into your ear; notice how clear and crisp every sound is and how your friend can whisper and still be understood even if there's lots of noise in the room. That's because you have improved something called the "**signal-to-noise ratio**." The higher that ratio is the easier it is for most people to understand you. However, if you talk directly into the ear of a person who is hearing-impaired, and they don't understand you, it is unlikely that a hearing aid or an assistive listening device alone will manage their problem completely.

If neither an aid nor assistive device works at all, we often recommend **cochlear implants**. These are digitally programmable devices which come in two parts. One part is implanted under the skin, into the snail-shell-like cochlea. The implanted part is made of electrodes and receivers that can accept instructions and information through the skin, change speech signals into electrical impulses, and deliver those impulses to the appropriate zone in the cochlea. The second part can be worn on the belt and contains the power supply and the microcomputer that analyzes incoming speech and changes it into electrical impulses to be used inside the cochlea.

Implanting people, especially children, who have *never* heard is increasingly coming under fire from the deaf community. And with some good reason, although there are excellent case examples of congenitally deaf children who are making good progress in speaking English with implants. **The deaf community feels these children should be raised with pride in their deafness and live primarily**

with their "own kind," a viewpoint which clearly raises controversy among hearing parents who want their children to live within their own family values and influence.

Are there deaf people who don't want to hear or speak? If so, why?

Yes. Years ago, when people were diagnosed as deaf, there were no hearing devices or technological support that worked as well as what we have today. In fact, many people who by today's standards could have used hearing aids and learned to communicate in the dominant culture using English found themselves as members of the signing deaf culture. And many seem quite comfortable with that choice. Many felt misunderstood and looked down upon by members of the speaking culture. Stung and angry at what they call the arrogance of the hearing world, an attitude which they felt degraded and discounted them as fully worthy and capable citizens, many now prefer the combined isolation and comfort of their own culture. They ask that hearing people who wish to feel comfortable in their society use *their* dominant language (American Sign Language) and learn to employ it at as early an age as possible to ensure fluency and a "native" accent. They vigorously oppose cochlear implantation of children recommended (usually) by hearing parents and professionals; they feel it takes away childrens' freedom of choice to join and communicate in a culture in which they would be welcomed as peers, instead of defective self-apologetic underperformers. Even more, they fear that research might identify the basic genetic defects that lead to the majority of cases of profound hearing loss. Such research might literally eliminate their culture. It is an argument often as heated and emotional as our current agony about abortion. However, none but the most militant want us to stop research that will help acquired deafness, or less severe forms of hearing loss. Yes, some people may choose deafness and ASL as their cultural right; but clear-thinking scientists must be supported to continue their research to allow all people to have a choice.

Which is more important to people, eyesight or hearing?

Helen Keller, who lost both her eyesight and hearing when she was around 2, commented on her condition by suggesting that her blindness isolated her in part from *things* around her. Her deafness was more serious to her because it isolated her from *people*. (See the brief discussion of Martin Buber's ideas of differentiating people from things near the end of this chapter.)

However, many members of the culturally deaf community who have never had hearing view their lack of audition as more of a cultural difference than a "handicap." They in fact resent the "colonialism" they feel is imposed on them by hearing people who want the deaf to be "just like them." Deafness, to a family that has always had deaf members, is simply not the tragedy you read about in the opening lines of this chapter. They argue, with considerable justification if we apply only past experiences, that a deaf child might always be considered an outsider, or a defective example of a hearing child, until the child joins the deaf community, embraces its culture and language (American Sign Language), and becomes a full, proud, well-connected citizen of a world in which he or she can participate fully as a respected peer instead of an underachieving outsider.

WIMWIG

"Visual Evoked Response" became "Official Revoked Response."

How does the inner ear change vibration into nerve impulses?

The **cochlea**, which comprises part of the inner ear, looks like a coiled snail shell (from which it gets its name) containing three compartments. When vibrations reach the inner ear they compress the fluids in two of the comparatively unyielding pair of compartments, the scala vestibuli and the scala tympani. **Scala** means "steps," "staircase," or "level" in Italian, as in La Scala, the multilevel opera house of Milan. **Scala vestibuli** means the level closest to the balance organ, while **scala tympani** means the level closest to the membrane called the round window. The organ of Corti contains two types of hair cells, outer hair cells and inner hair cells. The outer hair cells have contractile properties while the inner hair cells do not.

The middle compartment of the cochlea (aptly named **scala media**) contains the outer and inner hair cells and nerve fibers of the organ of Corti which change the mechanical oscillations of the tissues into electrochemical impulses carrying information to the brain. Most if not all of the sensory fibers of the inner ear are driven by the action of the inner hair cells; as of 1994 we believe the outer hair cells act like some form of preliminary sensor and then a preamplifier or assistive device to activate the inner hair cells and the nerve fibers attached to them.

The inner ear analyzes sound in part based on the mechanical properties of its hair cells and the basilar membrane on which the hair cells rest. There are at least two processes (see Figure 14–2), an active process below 60 dB and a passive process above 60 dB. In

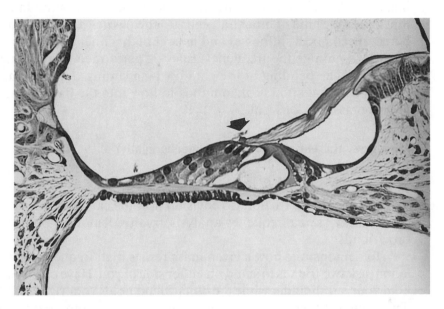

A

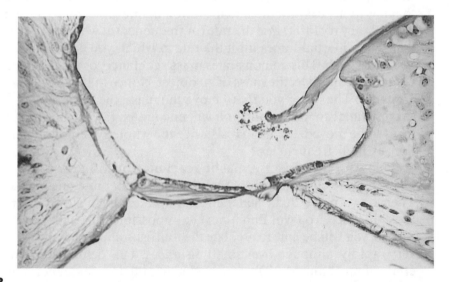

B

Figure 14–2. A. Cross-section of the developing mouse cochlea showing structures of the organ of Corti. **B.** Cross-section of mouse cochlea highlighting absence of organ of Corti. (Courtesy of Dr. D. B. Webster, Louisiana State University Kresge Laboratory)

the active process, the sharply tuned outer hair cells whose tips are embedded in the tectorial membrane move and contract, modifying, tuning, and possibly sharpening the nature of the stimulation that bends the cilia of inner hair cells. In the passive process, the inherent mechanical stiffnesses and masses of the inner ear structures seem to dominate the frequency analysis performed by the inner hair cells. The bending of the cilia opens a sliding trap-door-like mechanism that allows calcium ions to flow into the hair cell and force potassium ions out.

How does the ear analyze sound mechanically?

There are three factors to the mechanical analysis of vibration: mass, stiffness, and friction. To envision how the ear might use mass versus stiffness in a frequency analysis, try this demonstration with two friends:

To demonstrate how a given mass resists high frequency oscillation, ask two friends to stand on either side of you. Have one friend hold your left shoulder while the other friend holds your right shoulder. Then ask them to slowly push you back and forth alternately moving you towards one friend and away from the other. Notice that it is pretty easy for them to move you in one direction or the other until they try to *increase* the rate (or frequency) at which they push you. Then inertial forces limit the rate at which you can be moved back and forth. This demonstrates **mass reactance**, or the resistance to motion caused by the mass of an object. Notice that two rules will apply: (1) The faster you try to move the mass, the more reactance (or resistance to movement) you will encounter. (2) The heavier the mass to be moved, the more resistance the whole system has to motion at high frequencies.

Now for the converse, **elastic reactance** or stiffness. Ask your two friends to clasp all four of their hands together into one big ball. Then try to move their clenched fists up and down slowly over a large distance. You will find it next to impossible. But, with just two fingers, you will be able to oscillate the fourfist complex up and down very rapidly, although over small distances. This demonstrates the effect of mechanical stiffness on rejecting the low frequencies but passing the high frequencies.

These demonstrations sketch the mechanical rules of impedance: heavy masses reject high frequencies; light stiff systems reject low frequencies while easily accepting high frequency oscillations. This is the principle behind the massive strings on the piano producing bass sounds and the stiff short strings producing high pitches when they are struck with hammers. Similarly, bass speakers in high fidelity systems will be large, flexible, and massive, whereas so-called tweeters will be small and stiff.

Now then, the soft tissue portion of the **organ of Corti** in the human inner ear is 33–37 mm long and coiled around the inside of the bony cochlea we described earlier. It is graded in stiffness from the stiff end (the basal turn) to the comparatively massive apical end. The hair cells themselves also are graded in height and mass in a similar fashion, with the shortest, stiffest cells at the basal end gradually being replaced by taller heavier cells as one moves towards the apex of the cochlea.

The active processes of contraction and electrical activity generated by the outer hair cells seem to contribute to the fine tuning, sharp hearing in noise, and exceptionally keen sensitivity of the normal human ear.

One problem with this strictly mechanical description of how the inner ear might make a frequency analysis of incoming sound, is that the description doesn't account for many important facts we know about how sharply tuned both the hair cells and the nerve fibers themselves seem to be. We know that the outer and inner hair cells interact with one another, but we don't know exactly how and what the forces and mechanical shearing effects are exactly. Even more important, there are animals like lizards which have very different inner ear structures than mammals, but still have much of the same tuning properties in their hearing nerves. If we assume that a basilar membrane and a tectorial membrane are so important to the analysis of sound, then how do animals without these structures perform inner ear frequency analyses? This constitutes one of the exciting questions of hearing science in 1994.

In the years to come I hope someone reading this book will help us learn more about how the ear works. However, we have reviewed enough to understand that D.J. lost most of her hair cells, her sister Carina lost fewer hair cells but both lost more hearing in the high pitches (basal turn) than in the more apically analyzed low pitches.

By contrast, the next case was at first a "mystery"; she and other people like her have been misdiagnosed as "autistic" or "retarded" or "hysterical" in the absence of precise audiologic assessment. As you will see, she lost hair cells someplace other than the basal turn.

✦ A MYSTERY CLARIFIED
in *Time* Magazine, September 13, 1982

In an article entitled "Help for High Frequency Hearers" the unusual story of Karyl Ann Mirmelstein spurred a nationwide search for patients with "Ultra-audiometric Hearing."

After a bout with measles, three-year-old Karyl Ann Mirmelstein of Newport News, Va. seemed strangely unresponsive. Her mother consulted a number of doctors, who variously attributed the child's behavior to sibling rivalry with her baby sister, a learning disability, and even mental retardation. "I knew this couldn't be true," says Rona Mirmelstein. "I could see that Kam was very bright, perhaps more so than most children." (p. 63)

Kam in fact could hear sounds like the hissing of steam, and even the faint sounds of someone behind her whispering, but she seemed to be unable to understand everyday speech without lip-reading.

To get an idea of what Kam could hear, simply repeat only the consonants in the sentence: "She stopped going to beach parties last year" without using your voice. It should sound like *Sh stp ko ta peatch bpahteez lst hea*.

Clearly, she could hear, but not understand. Because most clinicians were familiar with hearing loss that was worse in the high frequencies, they had difficulty understanding the impact and clinical symptoms of someone who heard normally in the extremely high pitches but almost not at all in the low pitches.

People who listened to Kam talk knew something was "different," but many ascribed her manner of speaking to a foreign accent; some even went so far as to ask her if she came from Ireland or Scotland.

Physiologically, the hair cells at the basal end of her cochlea (the high frequency sensitive region) functioned normally, while the low frequency sensitive cells located more apically were affected.

More from the *Time* Magazine Article

Using special equipment (Berlin and his staff were) able for the first time to provide a precise diagnosis of Kam's problem: "ultraaudiometric hearing," that is, the capacity to hear, but only at extremely high frequencies.

With the help of . . . (Mead Killion at Knowles Electronics, J. K. Cullen Jr PhD and Henry Halperin MD who designed and built the first prototype we) produced . . . (a device) with two channels. . . . One channel amplifies high-pitched sounds; the other shifts lower pitches upward into the range heard by ultraaudiometrics.

For Kam the device opened up a bustling world, both rauc-ous and musical. Recounting her first experience in her diary she wrote: "All voices sounded like jabberwocky because they were so different." As she adjusted, however, she found that, "I was able to understand my cousin despite the fact that he has a low voice and a mustache. Later she rediscovered music: "I put Exodus on the stereo. SO stirring was the music that I suddenly began to cry in an almost hysterical way. The beauty of the sound was almost torture — I simply couldn't get enough of it." (*Time*, September 13, 1982, p. 63)

Also published in the scientific literature: Berlin et al. 1978, *Otolaryngology, Head and Neck Surgery* and in *Volta Review*, 1982, *84* (7), 352–363.

The "mystery" in this case was multi-faceted. In the early 1960s when Kam was a child, objective measures of hearing were not commonly available. Guesses and opinions substituted for data about her hearing; it was almost like the age of belief about the magic air reservoir. Her hearing loss had an island of normal high-frequency hearing with almost no usable low-frequency hearing; this violated the prevailing cochlear theory of the day, von Bekesy's **traveling wave theory**. The theory, which had earned von Bekesy the Nobel prize, said that sounds were translated into pitches through a base-to-apex traveling wave which always displaced the high-frequency end of the cochlea before it activated the low-frequency end. Thus it predicted high-frequency hearing loss easily from basal turn cochlear damage. However, the theory also predicted that an isolated island of normal hearing in the high frequencies, with virtually no usable hearing in the low frequencies, was impossible. The basal turn high-frequency cells also were supposed to respond to fairly intense low tones and give the patient some usable hearing before things got intense enough to stimulate the damaged or absent apical cells.

Like the many ancients before us who didn't recognize that the fluid coming out of the cochlea violated the air-reservoir theory, we barely sensed the significance of this case. An *active* process, where the normal basal turn hair cells were hypersensitized to respond to faint sounds, explained the data very well; however, at the time I wrote the first papers on this hearing loss (1978), studies on the active process of hearing and otoacoustic emissions (a hallmark of that active process) had just begun. Hearing science was undergoing a fascinating and exhilarating upheaval, and this case put our clinical research group on a productive new course.

Of course, as you might expect, there were many reports in the literature which made it clear that we had only a sketchy understanding of the workings of the inner ear. Separate groups had reported that dogs, cats, and people's ears could emit sound *spontaneously*. Recall that Kemp's great discovery was that ears generated an echo when stimulated by sound; others had already reported that ears could generate sound all by themselves. Scientist were asking: "Where does the energy come from to support an 'active' process of hair cell micromechanics?"

The secrets are now being revealed. The walls of each outer hair cell are composed of interlaced molecular structures that have contractile and motile properties. The hair cell seems to have micromotors all along the cell wall which change its length in response to electrochemical events. The stereocilia themselves have a trap-door-like opening for ions to pass through, and little tip links which seem to control what looks like a sliding trap door opening into the cilia. The mechanics of this delicate system are often disabled during acute noise exposure. Scientists, supported by the newly created National Institute of Deafness and Other Communication Disorders, have demonstrated the micromechanics of this system in a remarkable series of papers and films. Leaders in this area are building a map of the molecular properties of the hair cell that will lead to many rational and effective treatments for types of hearing loss we haven't even yet categorized. Most of these scientists have come to the study of the ear from disciplines as far removed from one another as engineering, medicine, psychology, zoology, physics, optics, physiology, biochemistry, pharmacy, and pharmacology, and some from audiology. All have brought an unending curiosity and perseverance to the questions of exactly how the cochlear system works.

Still other scientists had discovered that the hair cells in the inner ears of birds and other nonmammalian species regenerate after noise-induced trauma and some labs are reporting that mammalian ears can undergo some regeneration; they also are finding that certain drugs including retinoic acid can facilitate hair cell growth at least in test tube conditions. The future of medical remediation of some hearing loss may well lie in this research area; but there will be no future without young scientists to continue tugging at the strings which will unravel these mysteries.

Why do my ears ring and my ears feel full after a rock concert? What does it mean? Will it get better?

There are three warning signs that you are in a dangerous noise: (1) You have to shout to be heard; (2) You're left with a dullness and fullness in your ears; (3) You're left with tinnitus or a ringing in the ear.

The ringing in your ear is called *tinnitus*, pronounced /tin-night'-us/ or sometimes /tin'-knit-us/. There are many causes of tinnitus, but all seem to point to the general problem faced by most people who have hearing loss. Most have suffered hair cell loss and this appears to be liberating too much transmitter substance from some of the inner ear structures. The ear-fullness and the tinnitus usually run together and warn you that your ear has been overstimulated; fortunately it usually goes away after 36 to 72 hours of rest. But it should be a warning not to overexpose your ears. If you find yourself in a dangerously noisy area, either leave, or use ear protectors. We now have ear protection devices which do more than just block out harmful noises; some newer forms of protectors are "high fidelity" devices which allow all the sounds to come in as uniformly as before, but simply weakened slightly to protect the ear. Still another type uses phase-cancellation of engine noise or similar repetitive noise inside an electronically active ear phone. There are even ear protection devices for hunters which are said to allow the sound of the environment through unimpeded, but "shut off" when a sharp impulse like a gunshot reaches the device. Whatever your choice, protect your ears and the hair cells in them — they are likely to be your only set unless you are a bird or lizard.

While many of us approach the question of how the ear works from the view of the patient first, most approach the question from the general laboratory ethic of simple curiosity.

WIMWIG

"Self-instructional materials" became "Self-destructional materials".

✦ CONDUCTIVE HEARING LOSS

Heather had chronic ear infections ever since she was an infant. She often complained of pain in her ears, and at times had fevers as high as 104° Fahrenheit. She was treated with antibiotics on a regular basis and finally, at age 38 months, had pressure equalization (PE) tubes put in her ear drum membranes. Her language was slightly delayed and her parents felt that she wasn't progressing in speech and language at a rate comparable to her two older siblings. She was in fact just as intelligent, alert, malleable, and agreeable as her siblings, but her language and speech were just not quite as highly advanced as the rest of her development.

To get an idea of what Heather heard, simply put your fingers in your ears and listen to the radio or TV. Then take your fingers out of your ears and count up to 10 out loud. At the number 5 put your fingers back in your ears. Notice how loud your own voice seemed to you when you blocked your ears? The expected response is to then speak more softly. Thus, a number of related things affected Heather's communication. She spoke very softly and often could not be heard, yet she turned the TV up very loud and disturbed the other members of her family. She was speaking softly to others because of how loud her voice sounded to her. She turned up the TV because she had to overcome the blockage in her ears. Now add to that blocked-up feeling, a sense of weakness, helplessness, pain, fatigue, and frustration, and you have some idea of what young children with chronic middle ear disease experience. They also miss a lot more school than most children because of their chronically weakened and fatigued state. Children with problems like these are best treated by pediatric otolaryngologists (surgeons who treat childrens' diseases of the ear, nose, throat, head, and neck).

Middle ear disease is probably the single most common ailment of childhood and its proper management has stirred up considerable controversy. Primary care physicians (in this case pediatricians) are in my experience more likely to recommend antibiotics to treat middle ear disease and are less inclined to suggest surgery with PE tubes than are otolaryngologists. The scientific evidence that antibiotics, such as Amoxicillin, are effective in curing infectious middle ear effusion is highly controversial; on the other hand, the idea that chronic severe middle ear effusion can ultimately cause hearing loss and delay of language and speech is clear. The uncertainties with respect to the effects of conductive hearing loss involve:

1. Are there central nervous system problems caused by auditory deprivation?

2. Is there a critical age at which auditory deprivation is most destructive?

3. Can middle ear toxins ultimately cause inner ear deafness?

4. How much hearing loss, and for how long, will interfere with language acquisition?

Animal research has some answers.

1. Mice reared in silence, or with one of their ears given an artificial conductive loss, show a characteristic underdevelopment of portions of the lower brainstem. This underdevelopment can be overcome when and if the animals receive suitable sound stimu-

lation for a long enough time (Webster & Webster, 1977; Webster, 1988).

2. This phenomenon seems to be different with different species. Animals like mice, who do not hear until 21 days after birth, are much more likely to show the effects of auditory deprivation than are guinea pigs who hear normally at birth. Animals like the guinea pig that hear at birth are called "precocial," whereas those that develop hearing after birth, like the gerbil and the mouse, are called "altricial."

3. There also is no doubt that toxins from bacteria in the middle ear can enter the inner ear and cause severe and permanent hearing loss. We don't really know exactly how much hearing loss, or for how long, will interfere with language acquisition. However, whatever ultimate answers are revealed by research, the loss of productivity and concurrent misery caused by middle ear disease is a significant national concern and requires the utmost respect and scientific effort. Animals, and how they hear, however, are essential pieces of the puzzle about hearing loss. So let us leave human hearing studies for a while and address some common questions about animal hearing.

✦ HEARING IN OTHER ANIMAL SPECIES

What animals have "the best" hearing? (See Webster et al. [1992] for much more information on hearing in other animal species.)

The earliest mammals seem to have had very good hearing for frequencies between 10,000 and 40,000 Hz, a hearing range that overlaps very little with the human range of 20 Hz to about 16,000 Hz. Some, like the cat, can respond to sound pressures below −10 dB!

If we mean the most sensitive to faint sounds, we also have to ask, "In what frequency ranges and in what medium (e.g., air vs. water)?" Some bats hunt insects by echolocation, using sets of high frequency 60,000 to 120,000 Hz frequency-varying signals; insects that want to survive have to know when the bat sounds have hit them so that evasive maneuvers can start. Some moths, crickets, and mantises can hear the bat sounds and have startle or escape responses which help them survive. So bats and insects have the widest range of high-frequency hearing out past 100,000 Hz.

What about hearing in dolphins and whales?

Dolphins and some whales also use ultrasonic clicks and whistles to navigate and echolocate under water. Their hearing systems are extremely elaborate; but, remarkably, some are said to shift their frequency ranges to communicate with humans in our own frequency range. Their echolocation signals are broad frequency clicks containing energy ranging as high in frequency as 200,000 Hz. They also communicate (to one another?) in the frequency ranges from 4000 to 12,000 Hz. (Scientists, incidentally, don't really feel the common terms "dolphin," "whale," and "porpoise" represent real distinctions. They prefer the general term *cetaceans* to represent all three, and the term *odontocete* for toothed whales and *mysticete* for baleen whales which sift plankton through their teeth.)

WIMWIG

I meant to give an address as "New South Wales" in Australia. I got back "New South Whales."

Some undersea mammals can hear frequencies as low as 1/2 to 1/10 Hz which travel long distances under water and in fact can travel from one end of the Pacific Rim to the other. They may use these sound areas for communication or just plain "singing." Some porpoises hear from frequencies as low as 150 Hz to frequencies as high as 150,000 Hz. Do they win the prize for undersea hearing over the widest frequency ranges? Probably. But check the kangaroo rat next.

Kangaroo rats who live in the desert can actually hear the tiny low-frequency sounds made by a rattlesnake as it rears its head back for a strike. As the faint low pitched "whoosh" reaches its ears, the kangaroo rat leaps backwards in a reflexive avoidance maneuver. If you plug its ears, the rodent can't avoid the snake in the dark of the desert night.

Are snakes really deaf?

No. Like many other animals including birds, snakes just don't have easily visible ears. But they do hear, mostly in the low frequencies like their relatives the lizards. (They are called *Lepidosauria*; *lepido* means scale, so the scientific name means scaly lizards.)

What about other reptiles like lizards, turtles, and so on?

They also hear primarily in the low frequencies; but turtles belong to the order *Chelonia* from its Greek name *Chelone* with an ancestral connection that differs from snakes, crocodiles, and birds. In general, mammals are high frequency animals, while reptiles and birds hear better in the low frequencies.

How do fish hear?

Only animals with backbones (vertebrates) and insects have evolved specialized receptors for hearing. Fish hear with an organ containing hair cells which detect motion in the water around them. The organs are sensitive to displacements near the fish (so-called "near field" receptors which biologically are obviously more important in predator avoidance) and to sound waves traveling long distances through the water (so-called "far field" receptors). Some fish use a swimbladder which has gas (usually air) in it as a form of sound focusing drum; others have what are called Weberian ossicles, or small bones related to the ones we have in our own ears, to help bring sound to the nervous system for analysis. The problem is that the velocity of sound in water is about 4.5 times faster than in air. That, coupled with the fact that water is roughly 800 times denser than air, means that pressure-related hearing is impossible for fish without a swimbladder and they must use something called particle displacement for near-field "hearing." This problem occurs because the wavelengths of sounds in water are many times longer and larger than the fish themselves, and therefore pass right over or through the fish without causing a pressure differential on one side of the fish relative to the other. In contrast, animals that hear in air can use a pressure differential across the ear drum membrane to bring sound to the inner ear.

Virtually all fish studied have best hearing in the low frequencies below 1000 Hz, some as low as 100 Hz, and some can respond to sounds as faint as 19 to 24 dB SPL, extrapolated to the same scale as humans.

Some fish also make sounds, usually with their swimbladders, or with other structures strengthened by the swimbladder. These sounds are generally of low frequency content between 25 and 250 Hz. Because the underwater environment is a noisy one, some fish have evolved a communication system that depends on the temporal pattern rather than the frequency content of the "vocalization."

WIMWIG

". . . hearing loss" . . . became . . . "Herring walls."

What do birds hear like?

In contrast to fish, birds are highly vocal animals, but their hearing organs are very similar to those of crocodiles and all have a single middle ear bone. It is the mass and flexibility characteristics of this single lever system that give the bird hearing that is basically best in the low frequencies below 4000 Hz. Some birds can hear infra-sonic sounds of much less than 1 Hz and may use them for navigation. The barn owl, which localizes sound exceedingly well in the dark and can capture mice by sound, has an exceptionally well-organized basal (stiff) cochlear area and probably has the best high-frequency hearing of any bird. Its upper limit is still lower than that of most mammals.

Humans and most other mammals have two types of hair cells in the cochlea, outer hair cells and inner hair cells. Birds have two types of hair cells as well, called Tall Hair Cells and Short Hair Cells. Whether the two different types of hair cells have the same purpose and function in birds and mammals is still not clear. The suggestion has been made that the different hair cells in the bird may have other (nonauditory) functions.

For example, there is some evidence that pigeons, especially, and other migrating birds can hear infrasound which helps them navigate over long distances in the air. Scientists have suggested that the navigating sense is aided by infra-sonic cues from crashing surf and similar sounds which the birds can hear over long distances and use as a localization guide. They might also use the hair cells as pressure sensing devices to tell them about altitude or even wind direction or force.

Can we regrow any parts of the ear that die or don't develop?

Birds, and some lizards, have the capacity to regrow inner ear hair cells. Until recently we didn't think this could be accomplished in mammals. But now scientists have shown that with the use of Retin-A and calf serum some mammalian inner ear cells can be grown in a test tube. Other workers have shown that in some deaf mice hair cells regrow spontaneously only in the low-frequency zone, but we still don't know how or why and how to stimulate such regrowth. The sciences of tissue culture and genetics are being focused on this fascinating problem.

How about hearing in mice, dogs, cats, and other land-based mammals?

Like most land-based mammals, mice, dogs, and cats have sensitive high-frequency hearing, ranging from about 15 Hz up to 65,000 Hz for dogs and cats. Mice, on the other hand, have poor low-frequency hearing, being insensitive to any but the most powerful sounds below 1000 Hz. They are, however, sensitive to low-frequency air displacements which they sense with their vibrissae (whiskers) and can move quickly to avoid predators large enough to displace lots of air, no matter how silently.

One of the upper limits determining which sounds reach the inner ear is set by the mass of the middle ear ossicles. The heavier they are, the harder it is for an animal to hear high-pitched sounds. Therefore you might correctly reason that mice, dogs and cats, whose middle ears are much lighter than humans, can transmit high frequencies to the inner ear for analysis much more readily. Don't conclude from that, however, that human babies hear better in high frequencies than adults. The human middle and inner ears do not change in mass or overall size after birth or with aging. The changes in hearing with age have to do with inner ear damage to hair cells, mechanical or disease-related damage to the ear drum membrane or ossicles, or genetic susceptibility, not to changes in the size of the structures with maturity.

Why do crickets make all that noise at night?

They are producing mating and territorial sounds. The American tree crickets of the genus *Oecanthus* emit sounds as a function of the air temperature; you can deduce the temperature of the air in Fahrenheit by counting the number of chirps in 15 seconds and adding 39. If you have a thermometer and no watch, you can use the cricket as a timer by multiplying the temperature by 4 and subtracting 160 to find the chirps per minute.

When animals sing or make calls, do they learn their song or is it inherited? Or both?

Birds are the most vocal of animals, and some actually have inherited calls. We know that because if they are deafened their calls don't change. Other birds that are deafened never develop normal vocalizations. Some birds reared away from their natural habitats copy the calls of other birds. Some birds are such good mimics that they have been known to mimic the sound of passing trucks or other highway noises and mislead human listeners into thinking there is a highway nearby. Of course, birds that mimic human speech do so without using tongue, lips, and teeth as we do. They imitate a "close-enough" temporal and frequency pattern so that the ear of the listener perceives that true speech has been generated.

Almost all birds and other vocalizing animals have some form of "regional accent." For example the crows and green tree frogs of Pennsylvania have different enough calls from the crows and frogs of Europe that they have difficulty communicating with one another. Contrastively, if a barking tree frog and a green tree frog produce offspring, the calls they produce are a combination containing elements of the vocalization of both types of frogs.

How do scientists learn all this material about animal hearing?

Some of it is deduced mathematically from the mechanical characteristics of the ear and auditory system. Other material is deduced from the animals' behavior and especially their vocal output. This is based on the somewhat reasonable but not universally valid assumption that animals will not emit sounds they cannot hear. Humans make many sounds that they cannot hear, and even have parts of their vocal output which are inaudible to them. It is certainly possible for an animal to emit a click (which contains many frequencies because of its very brief rise and fall time) which has frequency content that the animal does not use. But, for the most part, organisms do not make much purposeful sound that doesn't have some adaptive value.

Another way to learn is to observe and manipulate animal behavior; some animals have been conditioned to perform tasks which, when carefully structured with systems of reward and punishment, can reveal to the scientists something about what the animal uses auditorily.

Scientists also study the bioelectric activity of animals with microelectrodes, stimulating the ear with sound and watching the response patterns of neural elements in the ear and nervous system, or "spearing" the cells with highly charged microelectrodes to study their electromechanical properties. Some scientists study the biochemical environment of the inner ear and nerve fibers; others study the genetics of hearing. The study of molecular pharmacology and molecular genetics promises to offer many new insights into the management and understanding of the causes of deafness.

Other scientists use behavioral training methods and/or so-called evoked potentials to see what sounds generate responses from the animal or gross electrical responses from the animals' nervous systems. Some scientists are actively studying a relatively new phenomenon in the ear called otoacoustic emissions which we talked about earlier in this chapter. This a true acoustic echo produced by the normal ear when it is struck by a sound to which the hair cells respond. The scientists then use this echo to study important mechanical characteristics of the inner ear.

As noted earlier, some of the same techniques are applied to study the hearing of humans and especially newborn babies, which is one of the many practical reasons why scientists use animals in their work.

WIMWIG

"Barcelona Spain" became "Barcelona's Pain."

"Vertebral artery" became "verbal artery."

"Person-to-person for Lydia" became a transatlantic call "Person to person for Libya."

Back to the Human Side

What skills do I need to become a scientist who studies hearing?

Scientists nowadays who make original contributions to their fields usually have doctoral degrees (Ph.D.s). Some scientists have M.D. degrees (clinical physician's degrees which also prepare them to treat patients either medically or surgically) in addition to or instead of their Ph.D. degrees. The Ph.D. degree is the highest degree a university offers and means essentially a "Doctor of Science." The M.D. degree means literally a Doctor of Medicine and is offered by medical schools exclusively to those who wish to practice medicine. The holders of the Ph.D. are usually scientists in their particular fields. All are entitled to be called "Doctor," despite the common American usage that "doctors" are physicians. It is interesting to note that in England surgeons specifically ask to be called "Mister" in recognition of their professional descendence from barbers. In America, lawyers who hold the J.D. degree (Juris Doctor) are also entitled to be called "Doctor" but generally avoid the practice.

Curiosity and perseverance are two very useful personality traits for any scientist. Orderly and systematic habits of solving problems and an ability to focus intently on important questions also are quite useful. If you have acquired computer expertise, knowledge in biology, zoology, experimental psychology, chemistry, physics, mathematics, engineering, electronics or related technical areas, you will have a special advantage. Today, an ability to work well with groups of other scientifically minded people, and to lead and coordinate group efforts, are also important personality traits, as is the ability to communicate clearly and concisely. But above all seeking knowledge for its own sake will carry the deepest and most gratifying rewards.

What skills do I need to become an audiologist?

Most audiologists today hold the master's degree (M.A., M.S., or M.C.D.) and clinical certification from the American Speech-Language-Hearing Association. This degree and its concomitant clinical certification would prepare you for patient care; many very successful and respected private practitioners hold masters' degrees and are fine clinicians.

If you want to be a private practitioner in the future, an Au.D. degree (a specific doctorate in audiology) would ultimately be the best degree to work for. However, as of the fall of 1993 there was only one authorized program for this degree in the United States. It is offered at Baylor Medical Center in Houston under the direction of Dr. James Jerger, the first President and Founder of the American Academy of Audiology. Neither the Au.D. nor the master's degree are meant to prepare you to be a scientist, any more than an M.D. prepares one for scientific inquiry. But no group has a monopoly on clear thinking and methodical data collection and analysis.

The clinical degree should prepare you to understand the workings of the ear and prepare you to understand and use new findings and principles as they reach the literature. Although clinical degrees are not meant to prepare you to make original experimentally based discoveries in the laboratory, as often happens, many important and useful observations and discoveries will undoubtedly be made during the course of clinical practice.

How long does the training take and how well does it pay?

Master's degree programs in speech-language pathology or audiology which prepare you either to work for others or start your own practice, now require about 2 to 3 years of post-graduate study, depending whether you come from a discipline within or outside communication disorders. Beginning salaries for graduates in 1993 ranged from $26,000 to $30,000. Note that private practitioners with good business acumen are known to make $150,000 to $250,000 per year by hiring others, and developing service contracts with nursing homes, school systems, insurance companies, and HMOs to give fee-for-service benefits. Some audiologists perform intra-operative monitoring including auditory, somatosensory, and electroneuronography procedures, billing insurance companies and patients based on the need of the surgeons to monitor specific surgical procedures. Some practitioners make even more money by dispensing hearing aids as part of their practices.

Doctoral programs in hearing sciences, like all true Ph.D. degrees, require a dissertation that makes an original contribution to the scientific knowledge base of the discipline. Completing that arduous training can take anywhere from 3 to 7 years or more. Many scientists pursue post-doctoral training for 1 to 3 years after they have completed their doctorates to better prepare them to compete in the grant-acquisition arena. Built on a background of anatomy, physiology, experimental design, and statistics, as well as instrumentation and acoustics, such rigorous training prepares a student for a research-based academic career, with salaries appropriate to the levels of professorship and institution served. Most of the successful scientists in the area have come from backgrounds of engineering, mathematics, physics, biology, zoology, anatomy, physiology, and psychology rather than the clinical service orientation. While beginning instructors or assistant professors might start at $40,000 to $45,000, some full professors with either clinical supplementary pay or consulting practices report that they make as much as $130,000 to $185,000 per year. Today, the success of a scientist is often measured by the nature and quality of his or her peer-reviewed grant funding and publications.

WIMWIG

"Deafness and heart disease" became "Deafness and hard diseases."

✦ AND MOST IMPORTANT OF ALL

Why don't my parents (or spouse or children) *listen* to me?

There are none so deaf as those who will not hear. This is the essence of the difference between the physiology of the ear ("hearing" in its most elementary form) and the ability of the intellect to sense and the willingness of the spirit to respond to cues, feelings and attitudes carried by what we say and how we say it. Most of us can be marvelous "listeners" if and when we truly care about the feelings being expressed, and the person doing the expressing. Probably the best example I have ever read on how to respect the spirit of others, instead of treating them like "things to manipulate," comes from the work of Martin Buber (e.g., *I and Thou* and *Between Man and Man*). Because it was translated from the German, many people find it difficult reading, but to me his works carry a truly powerful message, well worth the hours I spent on extracting his key ideas.

Even more powerful messages which reach the primitive need for emotional connection and communication of true feelings are carried in the book *Holding Time* by Martha Welch, M.D. Welch outlines a set of principles on how to establish trusting warm connection between children and parents. These principles also can work as well for adult couples, who use body closeness and tight holding, along with verbal expressions of deep unvarnished fears coupled with joys in a context of mutual security. Many of her very powerful and influential ideas were developed from the study of comparative biology of communication between mammalian mothers and their offspring, and they have been used successfully to treat autism as well as language delays in otherwise healthy children.

Finally, if you find communication difficult with a spouse or significant other of the opposite sex, you might enjoy reading a linguist's view of some of the bases for miscommunication between the sexes. Dr. Deborah Tannen suggests that the genders literally speak "different languages."

All three of these authors are cited in our Suggested Readings Section.

✦ SUMMARY

This chapter was written to interest you in hearing science and audiology as fields of study. It starts with the "death" of an expected child and the rebirth of a different one. It takes you from the extreme views of deafness as a tragedy to deafness as simply a cultural difference. The case histories introduce you to a variety of patient problems one might encounter in the course of practice. The chapter also takes you through a series of answers to questions about basic and applied hearing science in humans and other animals which many lay people in my experience and surveys have wanted to know. Peppered throughout the work are examples of what I called WIMWIGs, funny misperceptions of dictated materials. I called them WIMWIGs as an acronym for: **What I Meant versus What I Got**. It closes with "what it takes" to contribute to audiology and hearing science, followed by my own very personal commentary about the germinal importance of interpersonal communication in helping us all to "listen better" to each other whether with the ear, the eye — or the heart.

✦ ACKNOWLEDGMENTS

Thanks to my many colleagues who helped review and shape this chapter, and to my survey-respondents, friends and their children, and my own family whose questions I tried to answer. Support also came from NIDCD Grants DC-P01-000379; DC-T32-00007 and BMDR 1549, Kam's Fund for Hearing Research, and the Lions of Louisiana.

◆ REFERENCES

Berlin, C. I., Wexler, K. F., Jerger, J. F., Halperin, H. R., & Smith, S. (1978). Superior ultra-audiometric hearing: A new type of hearing loss which correlates highly with unusually good speech in the "profoundly deaf." *Otolaryngology, 86*(1), 111–116.

Berlin, C. I. (1986) Electrocochleography: An historical overview. In Ferraro, J., *Seminars in Hearing, 7*(3) 241–246.

Jewett, D., Romano, M., & Williston, J. (1970). Human auditory evoked potentials: Possible brainstem components detected on the scalp. *Science, 167*, 1517–1518.

Kemp, D. T. (1978) Stimulated acoustic emissions from within the human auditory system. *Journal of the Acoustical Society of America, 64*, 1386–1391.

Schuknecht, H. L. (1974). *Pathology of the ear.* Cambridge, MA: Harvard University Press.

Sohmer, H., & Feinmesser, M. (1967). Cochlear action potentials recorded from the external ear in man. *Annals of Otology, Rhinology, and Laryngology, 76*, 427–435.

Stevens, S. S. & Warshofsky, F. (1965). Sound and hearing. *Life Science Library*, Time, Inc.

Webster, D. B. (1962). A function of the enlarged middle ear cavities of the kangaroo rat, Dipodomys. *Physiological Zoology, 35*, 248–255.

Webster, D. B. (1988). Sound amplification negates central effects of a neonatal conductive hearing loss. *Hearing Research, 32*, 193–195.

Webster, D. B., & Webster, M. (19XX). Neonatal sound deprivation affects brainstem auditory nuclei. *Archives of Otolaryngology, 103*, 392–396.

Wever, E. G. (1961). *Theory of hearing.* New York: John Wiley & Sons.

◆ SUGGESTED READINGS

On Hearing Science

Altschuler, R., Bobbin, R. P., & Hoffman, D. (Eds.). (1986). *The neurobiology of hearing: The cochlea.* New York: Raven Press.

Durrant. J., & Lovrinic, J. (1984). *The bases of hearing science.* Baltimore: Williams & Wilkins.

National Institute of Deafness and other Communication Disorders (NIDCD). *Strategic Plan for Hearing Research.* Published every three years beginning in 1991. (Available from the NIDCD at the National Institutes of Health, Bethesda, MD.)

Webster, D. B., Fay, R. R., & Popper, A. N. (Eds.). (1992). *The evolutionary biology of hearing.* New York: Springer-Verlag.

On Deafness

Crosby, O. (in press). *Silent Dancing.*

Schwartz, S. (1989). *Choices in deafness: A parent's guide.* Rockville, MD: Woodbine House.

On Interpersonal Communication

Buber, M. (1970). *I and thou.* Walter Kaufmann, Trans. New York: Charles Scribner's Sons. (Original work published in German in 1923).

Buber, M. (1965). *Between man and man.* Ronald Gregor Smith, Trans. New York: Macmillan. (Original work published 1936 with "The Question to the Single One."

Tannen, Deborah. (1990). *You just don't understand.* New York: Ballantine Books.

Welch, M. (1988). *Holding time.* New York: Simon & Schuster.

◆ GLOSSARY

ABR: Auditory Brainstem Response, also called BAER (brainstem auditory evoked response); a record of the synchronous discharge of auditory nerve fibers in response to a click or brief tone burst. It is the most commonly available procedure for assisting in the diagnosis of hearing impairment in young infants and children. It can also be used to uncover hidden damage to the auditory nervous system.

ALD: Assistive Listening Device. A system that makes communication with the hearing-impaired more effective by improving the signal-to-noise ratio. The referees at NFL games switch on their FM systems when they want to be heard over the din of the crowd. Similarly, when a hearing-impaired person needs to get the clearest possible signal from the person talking, the best thing to do is to place the microphone for the ALD next to the mouth of the speaker, and deliver the signal with as little distortion as possible to the ear of the listener. Some ALDs are FM radio systems, in the form of miniature sending and receiving stations. Others use infra-red modulation technology, still others are simply hand-held amplifiers attached to a set of earphones. These latter are marketed under various names including Whisper 2000, Listen-Aider, Pocket-talker, Chaparral. The Chaparral system makes use of FM and related technology for music, TV, as well as everyday speech enhancement.

ASL: American Sign Language. The major language system used by the culturally Deaf in this country. It is a noble and respectable language of its own, with a unique spatial grammar, and syntax; however, it is *not* English articulated with the hands.

Cochlea: the coiled snail shell-like organ which contains the organ of Corti and the other auditory structures which change sound to neural energy in the inner ear. It is structured so that high-frequency sounds coming into the cochlea are analyzed at the stiff, basal turn of the cochlea, while low frequency tones are analyzed mostly at the apex at low intensities; the analysis of all signals seems to spread toward the stiff basal end as the intensity of the signals increases.

Cochlear implant: a device placed inside the cochlea to stimulate the organ of Corti and/or the residual nerve fibers in the cochlea. As of 1994 the 3 most commonly used types of implants are: a 23-channel Australian-made device, a 6–8 channel American-made device, and a single channel American device.

Conductive hearing loss: a hearing loss caused by obstruction to the normal sound-conducting mechanism of the outer and/or middle ears. Usually treatable by medicine or surgery. Relatively easy to manage with hearing aids, since direct amplification usually does the job.

Cued Speech: a system for making all the sounds of speech visible. In English it utilizes eight handshapes, placed in four different locations around the face, to remove any ambiguity about what is seen and heard by the person with a hearing impairment. Invented by physicist R. Orin Cornett, Ph.D., of Gallaudet College, it requires only 12 cues to ensure one-time communication. Two of its special strengths are that it allows virtually everything to be discussed as it happens around the hearing-impaired child and thus allows the child to learn much more language than is formally taught. Secondly, it supports a high likelihood that the child who uses it will be a fluent reader. It has been adapted for use in 53 languages and major dialects.

Elastic reactance: the rejection of low frequency vibrations as a result of the stiffness of the vibrating object. Elastic reactance goes up drastically as the frequency of the attempted motion *decreases*.

Electrocochleography: the recording of the synchronous electrical discharge of the compound VIIIth nerve Action Potential to a click or brief tone burst. Used initially as a clinical test for deafness, now used primarily to differentiate between various types of inner ear diseases.

Frequency: the speed with which a given motion repeats itself. Usually expressed in Hertz (Hz) or cycles per second. Thus a 512 Hz tone is one whose primary components repeat themselves 512 times per second; 512 Hz is roughly middle C on the piano. Four hundred and forty (440) Hz is the tone to which European symphony orchestras adjust the tuning of all their instruments. Thus a tone of 2000 Hz sounds much higher in pitch than a tone of 500 Hz, although keep in mind that pitch and frequency are *not* the same phenomena.

Inner ear: the structures of the ear which include the cochlea, the semicircular canals, the cochlear and vestibular labyrinths, the organ of Corti, the auditory nerve, and so on.

Intensity: the physical strength of a sound, expressed in decibels relative to a reference power of 10^{-16} watts/cm^2.

Mass reactance: the loss of energy which occurs when a mass is moved back and forth at a high frequency. The greater the mass, the more difficulty one encounters trying to move it back and forth at rapid rates. Moving a mass back and forth at low frequencies is considerably easier.

Middle ear: the segment of the ear that contains the ossicles, the opening to the Eustachian tube, parts of the facial nerve and related structures, the stapedius and tensor tympani tendons, and so forth. The entire middle ear is correctly called the ear drum, whereas the tympanic membrane which separates the middle ear from the outer ear is correctly called the ear drum *membrane*. Common usage mistakenly applied the term "ear drum" to the tympanic membrane only.

Nerve deafness: a term properly reserved for a type of hearing loss in which the hearing nerve itself is damaged. Unfortunately it has been misused as a generic term for *any kind* of inner ear hearing loss; the net effect of this semantic error is to mislead many patients with hair cell-based hearing losses to conclude erroneously that "they have dead hearing nerves and nothing can be done for them."

OAE: Otoacoustic emissions. Sounds (usually echoes) from the hair cells of the inner ear which are only seen when the hearing organ is intact. There are four types of emissions: transient-evoked, distortion-product, spontaneous, and stimulus-following. Only the first two are commonly used for clinical purposes.

Organ of Corti: the structure in the middle scala of the cochlea that contains the hair cells, supporting cells, nerve fibers, and membranes that turn mechanical displacement into neural codes that code sound for the brain to interpret.

Outer ear: the pinna and ear canal leading to the ear drum membrane.

Scala media: the middle compartment in the cochlea which contains the organ of Corti. It is bordered at the top by Reissner's membrane and at the bottom by the basilar membrane. The major space in the scala media is filled with a fluid called endolymph, but the cells in the organ of Corti are protected from that fluid by a tight network called the reticular lamina. The cells of the organ of Corti are probably surrounded by perilymphatic fluid from the scala tympani.

Scala tympani: the lower compartment of the cochlea which begins at the round window and contains fluid called perilymph.

Scala vestibuli: the upper compartment of the cochlea which is closest to the vestibular organs. It begins just past the oval window and vestibule of the bony cochlea.

Sensorineural hearing loss: the generic term for inner ear hearing loss when the diagnostician cannot be sure whether there is hair cell damage or nerve damage or both.

Signal-to-noise ratio: the ratio in decibels between the signal one wishes to hear (usually speech) and any interfering noises.

Time: usually elapsed time expressed in milliseconds (thousandths of a second); sometimes used to mean rise and fall time, that is, the number of milliseconds before a signal reaches, or drops from, its full plateau value.

Traveling Wave Theory: Georg von Bekesy's Nobel Prize-winning work led to this theory of frequency analysis in the cochlea which ascribes the ability of the ear to analyze sounds strictly to the mechanical gradient of stiffness along the organ of Corti.

Hearing Disorders

JAMES JERGER, PH.D.
BRAD STACH, PH.D.

After completing this chapter, you should understand:

◆ How we hear.

◆ How we test hearing.

◆ The nature of hearing disorders.

◆ Hearing rehabilitation.

This overview of hearing disorders begins with a brief discussion of the hearing mechanism, including relevant structures of the middle ear, the cochlea, the auditory nerve, and the central auditory pathways. The next section describes the various methods for measuring auditory status and function, including pure-tone, speech, immittance, otoacoustic emission, and auditory evoked potential audiometric techniques. The third section defines and describes the three major kinds of hearing disorder, conductive hearing loss, sensorineural hearing loss, and central auditory processing disorder. Finally, the fourth section summarizes intervention strategies for auditory rehabilitation, including conventional hearing aids, assistive listening devices, cochlear implants, speech reading, and auditory training.

Have you ever been able to identify people by hearing their footsteps? What an amazingly intricate system the hearing mechanism must be to allow such a feat! When the shoe strikes the floor, sound is generated by the outward movement of air pressure waves. These waves reach the eardrum, which vibrates at a rate and magnitude proportional to the nature of the wave. The eardrum transforms this vibration into mechanical energy in the middle ear, which in turn converts it to hydraulic energy in the inner ear. The hydraulic energy stimulates the sensory cells of the inner ear, which in turn stimulate the auditory nerve fibers. From these fibers electrical impulses travel to the brainstem and auditory cortex. But the passive reception of auditory information is only the beginning. The listener brings to bear on these electrical events attention to the sound, differentiation of the sound from background noise, and experience with similar sounds. The listener then puts all of these aspects of hearing into the context of the moment, and the footstep is identified as belonging to a certain individual.

That a sound as simple as a footstep can be identified is testimony to the exquisite sensitivity of the auditory system. Now imagine the intricacy of identifying the many sounds that have been molded together to create speech. The sounds of speech are made up of pressure waves that by themselves carry no meaning. When these sounds are put together in a certain order and processed by a normally functioning auditory system, they take on the characteristics of speech, which is then processed further to reveal the meaning of what has been said.

When you think about the auditory system, it is easy to become amazed that it serves both as an obligatory sense and as a very specialized means of communication. That is, the auditory system simultaneously monitors the environment for events that might alert the listener to danger, opportunity, or change, while focusing on the processing of acoustic events as complicated as speech. The important continual environmental monitoring, the intricacy of turning pressure waves into meaningful constructs, and the complexity of doing all this at once speaks to the extraordinary capability of the auditory system.

Cast in this light, it becomes possible to imagine what can happen when something goes wrong with the auditory system. Our experience in dealing with disordered auditory systems has taught us a great deal about their nature. One lesson that we have learned is that the system is fragile. Genetic flaws, noise exposure, certain drugs, and even the natural aging process can all result in permanent changes in the auditory system. A second lesson is that the auditory system is so rich in complexity that even substantial damage to it can be overcome with proper care and treatment. A third lesson is that, left untreated, the hearing impairment that results from auditory system damage can have a substantial impact on communication ability. In children, this can result in serious problems in the ability to develop verbal language. In adults, it can result in career restrictions. In the elderly, it can result in limitations to quality of life.

In this chapter, we will summarize what we know about how we hear, what causes impairment in hearing, how we measure hearing and hearing impairment, and how these impairments can be effectively treated.

✦ HOW WE HEAR

The auditory sense is obligatory. We simply cannot turn it off. In lower life forms, the main function of the auditory system is protection. Because it is obligatory, it is constantly assessing the surroundings for danger, as prey, and opportunity, as predator. In higher life forms, it takes on an increasingly important communication function, whether used for mating calls or talking on the telephone.

The auditory system is highly complex. It is a very sensitive system that can detect the smallest of pressure waves. In addition, it is a very precise system that can effectively differentiate very small changes in the nature of sound. It is also a system with a very large dynamic range. For example, the difference in the sound energy that can just barely be detected by the human ear and the sound energy that causes pain is on the order of 100 million to one.

The Nature of Sound and Hearing

Philosophers used to debate whether a tree that fell in a forest made a sound if no one was there to hear it. The question is of interest because it serves to illustrate the difference between the physical properties that we know as *sound* and the psychological properties that we know as *hearing*.

Sound is a common type of energy that occurs as a result of pressure waves that emanate when some force is applied to a sound source. For example, a hammer being applied to a nail results in pressure waves that propagate through the air, the hammer, the nail, and the wood. Sound results from the compression of molecules in the medium through which it is traveling. In this example, the sound that moves through the air results from a disturbance of air molecules. Groups of molecules are compressed, which, in turn, compress adjacent groups of molecules. This results in waves of pressure that emanate from the source.

Sound is characterized in two majors ways, **intensity** and **frequency**. An air molecule that is displaced will be moved a certain distance, return past its original location to an equal displacement in the opposite direction, and then return to its starting point. The total displacement can be thought of as one cycle in the movement of the molecule. The magnitude of the cycle, or the distance that the molecule moves, is called its intensity. The higher the force or magnitude of the compression wave, the higher the intensity of the signal. Intensity is expressed in units called decibels (dB). One of the most common referents for decibels is known as **hearing level** (HL), which represents intensity in relation to average normal hearing. Thus, 0 dB HL would refer to the intensity of a signal that could just barely be heard by the human ear. Human hearing ranges from 0 dB HL to the threshold of pain, around 140 dB HL. Normal conversational speech occurs at around 40 to 50 dB HL, and the point of discomfort is approximately 90 dB HL.

The second major method used to characterize sound is by its frequency. *Frequency* is the speed of vibration, or the number of cycles that a particle executes in a specified period of time. Frequency is expressed in cycles-per-second or Hertz (Hz). Human hearing in young adults ranges from 20 Hz to 20,000 Hz. The "A" key on the piano has a frequency of 440 Hz. The most important frequencies for the understanding of speech range from 250 to 8000 Hz.

In its most basic form, a tone of a single frequency, acoustic energy can be described by its intensity at that frequency. For more complex sounds, the interaction of intensity and frequency is referred to as the **spectrum of speech**. The spectral content of a speech signal is the distribution of energy across the various frequencies at any given moment in time. (See chapter by Stevens.)

The psychological correlates of these physical measures of sound are **loudness**, **pitch**, and **quality**. Loudness is the psychological correlate of intensity. Low intensity sounds are perceived as "soft" or "faint" sounds, while high intensity sounds are perceived as "loud." Pitch is the psychological correlate of frequency. Low frequency sounds are perceived as "low" in pitch, and high frequency sounds as "high" in pitch. Quality and type of sound are the psychological correlates of the spectral content of the signal.

The Outer and Middle Ear

Figure 15–1 shows a schematic diagram of the peripheral auditory system. The outer ear serves to collect sound waves and funnel them

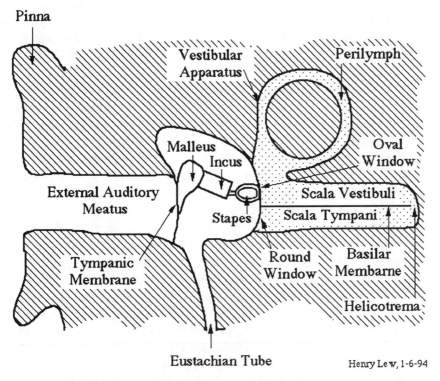

Henry Lew, 1-6-94

Figure 15–1. Schematic drawing of the peripheral auditory system, including the outer ear, the middle ear, and the inner ear or cochlea. Sound energy enters the external auditory canal and sets the tympanic membrane into vibration. This vibratory energy is transmitted through the three middle ear bones (ossicles), the malleus, incus, and stapes. The vibration of the footplate of the stapes sends waves through the fluid system of the inner ear or cochlea.

to the middle ear. The outer ear has two main components, the pinna and the ear canal. The pinna is the visible portion of the ear, consisting of skin-covered cartilage. In lower animals, the pinnae are very important and move as a way of aiding in the localization and collection of sound. In humans, the pinnae serve a more minor role in sound collection. The pinnae are important for sound localization in the vertical plane, for front-back localization, and for protection of the outer or external ear canal.

The external ear canal directs sound to the eardrum or **tympanic membrane**. It also serves to protect the tympanic membrane by the narrowness of its opening. Glands in the ear canal secrete a wax-like substance, called **cerumen**, which lubricates the ear canal and also protects the ear from intrusion by foreign objects, creatures, and so forth.

The tympanic membrane lies at the end of the external auditory canal. It is a membrane made of several layers of skin embedded into the bony portion of the canal. The membrane is fairly taut, much like the head of a drum. Sound waves strike the tympanic membrane, and it vibrates with a magnitude proportional to the intensity of the sound wave and at speeds proportional to its frequency content.

Beyond the tympanic membrane lies the middle ear cavity. The cavity is air-filled. Air in the cavity is kept at atmospheric pressure via the **Eustachian tube**, which leads from the cavity to the back of the throat. If air pressure changes suddenly, as it does when ascending or descending in an airplane, the cavity will have relatively more or less pressure than in the ear canal, and a feeling of fullness will result. Swallowing ordinarily opens the Eustachian tube, allowing the pressure to equalize.

Attached to the tympanic membrane is the **ossicular chain**, a series of three small bones, the **malleus**, **incus**, and **stapes**, which transfer the vibration of the tympanic membrane to the inner ear or **cochlea**. The malleus is attached to the tympanic membrane. The ossicular chain is suspended in the middle ear cavity by tendons. The stapes is attached to the **oval window**, which is an opening into the cochlea. When the tympanic membrane vibrates, it pushes and pulls the malleus, which vibrates the incus and, in turn, the stapes. The footplate of the stapes covers the oval window and is loosely attached to the bony wall of the fluid-filled cochlea. The middle ear serves as a means of matching the energy transfer from air to fluid. That is, air pressure waves vibrate the tympanic membrane, which vibrates the ossicles and sets the fluid of the cochlea into motion. If the middle ear did not exist, the air pressure waves would have to set the fluid of the cochlea into motion directly, and a substantial amount of energy would be lost in the process. Perhaps the best way to understand this is to understand why fish do not need a middle ear. Because the sounds that fish hear are propagated through water, the energy waves travel as fluid motion and set the inner ear fluids into motion directly. Very little loss of energy results. But, in humans, the energy waves are air-borne and need to be transformed into mechanical energy before being converted to hydraulic energy. The mechanical action of the middle ear serves as an efficient energy converter from air to fluid.

The Cochlea

Figure 15–2 shows an anatomical diagram of the important structures within the inner ear or cochlea. The **cochlea** is the sensory end-organ of hearing. Here, the sound waves, transformed into mechanical energy by the middle ear, set the fluid of the cochlea into motion in a manner consistent with their intensity and frequency. The cochlea is a fluid-filled space within the temporal bone, which resembles the shape of a snail shell. Suspended within this fluid-filled space is another fluid-filled space, known as the **cochlear partition**. The cochlear partition is cordoned off by two membranes. **Reissner's membrane** serves as the cover of the partition, and the

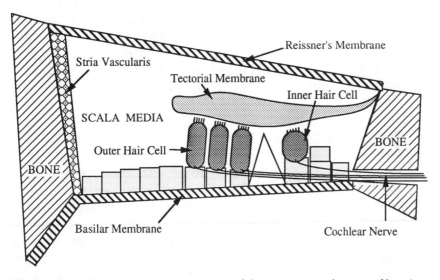

Figure 15–2. Schematic representation of the sensory end organ of hearing in the inner ear. The cochlear wave motion causes a shearing action between the small hairs (cilia), projecting from the upper surfaces of the hair cells, and the tectorial membrane. The cilia of the outer hair cells are actually embedded in the tectorial membrane. Bending of these cilia stimulates a chemical reaction which triggers the auditory nerve fibers.

basilar membrane serves as the base. Riding on the basilar membrane is **organ of Corti**, which contains the sensory cells of hearing. The sensory cells are of two types, outer hair cells and inner hair cells. **Outer hair cells** are elongated in shape and have small hair, or cilia, attached to their top. These cilia are embedded into the **tectorial membrane** which covers the organ of Corti. There are three rows of outer hair cells throughout most of the length of the cochlea. The outer hair cells are innervated by both afferent and efferent fibers of the nervous system. **Inner hair cells** are also elongated and have an array of cilia on top. Inner hair cells stand in a single row, and their cilia are in proximity to, but not in direct contact with, the tectorial membrane. The inner hair cells are innervated primarily by afferent, or sensory, fibers of the auditory nerve.

As the stapes vibrates in and out of the oval window, the fluid in the cochlea is set into a traveling wave-like motion. This traveling wave proceeds down the course of the cochlear partition, growing in magnitude, until it reaches a certain point of maximum displacement (see Figure 14–2 in the chapter by Berlin). For higher frequencies, this occurs closer to the oval window, nearer the basal end of the cochlea. For lower frequencies, it occurs farther from the oval window, at the apical end of the cochlea. When the traveling wave reaches its point of maximum height, the basilar membrane is displaced. At the point of basilar membrane displacement the inner hair cells are stimulated, sending neural impulses to the auditory nerve. Sensitivity of the inner hair cells appears to be controlled to some extent by the outer hair cells. For low intensity sound, the outer hair cells appear to move the tectorial membrane and change the distance between the membrane and the cilia of the inner hair cells, enhancing their sensitivity.

The Eighth Cranial Nerve

The auditory portion of the **eighth cranial nerve** exits the cochlea through the external auditory canal. Nerve fibers from the basal end of the cochlea are on the outside of the nerve bundle, and fibers from the apical end are in the center. Just after the nerve fibers exit the cochlea, a branch of nerve fibers from the vestibular system joins with the cochlear branch to form the eighth cranial nerve. The cochlear branch of the nerve consists of some 30,000 nerve fibers, which carry information to the brain stem.

As the inner hair cells of the cochlea are stimulated, they create chemical changes that trigger electrical impulses in the nerve fibers. These impulses travel up the eighth nerve until they reach their first synapse, which occurs at the cochlear nucleus.

The Central Auditory System

Figure 15–3 shows a schematic diagram of the central auditory nervous system. The central system is best described by its various nuclei. Each nucleus serves as a relay station for neural information from the cochlea and eighth nerve to other nuclei in the auditory nervous system and to nuclei of other sensory and motor systems (see Chapter 8, by Kent, for more information). All eighth nerve fi-

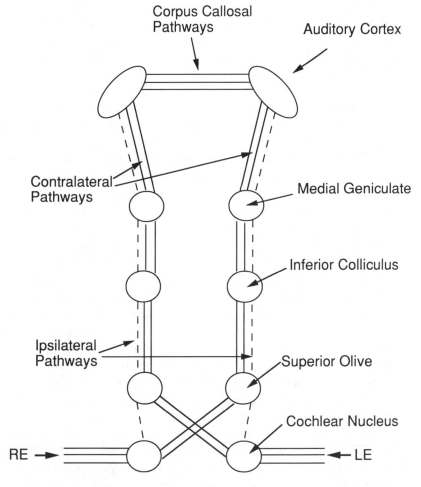

Figure 15-3. Schematic representation of the afferent auditory pathways in the central nervous system. Each auditory nerve terminates in the cochlear nuclei. From here, neural signals ascend on the same side of the brain (ipsilateral path) or on the opposite side (contralateral path). Thus both ears are represented at each auditory cortex. The contralateral pathway from each ear, however, is dominant. The right and left auditory areas at the cortical level are connected through pathways in the corpus callosum.

bers synapse at the **cochlear nucleus** on the same (ipsilateral) side of the brain. From the cochlear nucleus, approximately 75% of the nerve fibers cross over to the contralateral side of the brain. Some fibers terminate on the **medial nucleus of the trapezoid body** and some on the **medial superior olive**. Others proceed to nuclei beyond the superior olivary complex. Of the 25% that travel on the ipsilateral side of the brain, some terminate at the medial superior olive, some at the lateral superior olive and others at higher level nuclei. From the superior olivary complex, neurons proceed to the lateral lemniscus, the inferior colliculus, and the medial geniculate body. Nerve fibers may synapse on any of these nuclei or proceed beyond. Also, at each of these nuclei, some fibers cross over from the contralateral side of the brain. From the medial geniculate, nerve fibers proceed in a tract called auditory radiations to the auditory cortex in the temporal lobe.

This simplified explanation of the central auditory nervous system belies its rich complexity. For example, sound that is processed through the right cochlea has multiple, redundant pathways to both the right and left cerebral hemispheres. What begins as a pressure wave striking the tympanic membrane sets into motion a complex series of neural responses spread throughout the auditory system.

Much of the rudimentary processing of sound begins in the lower brainstem. For example, initial processing for sound localization occurs at the superior olivary complex where small differences between sounds reaching the two ears are detected. As another example, a simple reflex arc that triggers a contraction of the stapedius muscle occurs at the level of the cochlear nucleus. This reflex occurs when sound reaches a certain loudness and causes the stapedius muscle to contract, resulting in a stiffening of the ossicular chain.

Processing of speech information occurs throughout the central auditory system. The primary location for processing of speech information, however, occurs in the left cerebral hemisphere of most humans. Speech that is detected by the right ear proceeds through the dominant contralateral auditory channels directly to the left hemisphere. Speech that is detected by the left ear, however, must proceed through the dominant contralateral channel to the right hemisphere and then, via the corpus callosum, to the left hemisphere. Thus, in most humans, the right ear is dominant for the processing of speech information.

Hearing

Our ability to hear relies on this very sophisticated series of structures that process sound. The pressure waves of sound are collected by the pinna and funneled to the tympanic membrane by the external auditory canal. The tympanic membrane vibrates in response to the sound which sets the ossicular chain into motion. The mechanical movement of the ossicular chain then sets the fluids of the cochlea in motion, causing the hair cells on the basilar membrane to be stimulated. These hair cells trigger neural impulses through the auditory nerve to the auditory brainstem. From the brainstem, networks of neurons act on the neural stimulation, sending signals to the auditory cortex.

Although the complexity of these structures is remarkable, so too is the complexity of their function. All of this processing is obligatory and occurs constantly. The system is sensitive in its ability to detect very soft sounds, to detect very small changes in sound characteristics, and has a very large dynamic range. And when we call on our auditory system to do the complicated task of listening to speech, it does so even under extremely adverse conditions.

✦ HOW WE TEST HEARING

The general term for all of the techniques involved in the measurement of hearing is "audiometry." Audiometric methods fall into five major categories:

1. Pure-tone audiometry

2. Immittance audiometry

3. Otoacoustic emission audiometry

4. Speech audiometry

5. Evoked-potential audiometry

In the following sections we discuss each of these five methods of hearing measurement, then relate the results to site of disorder and type of hearing loss.

Pure-tone Audiometry

The purpose of pure-tone testing is to establish threshold sensitivity across the frequency range important for human communication. **Threshold sensitivity** is usually measured for a series of discrete sinusoids or **pure tones** (i.e., sounds in which all the energy is concentrated at a single frequency). The object of pure-tone audiometry is to determine the lowest intensity of such a sinusoid that the listener can "just barely hear," that is, his threshold of hearing for that sound. When such thresholds have been measured at a number of different sinusoidal frequencies, the results can be illustrated graphically, in a frequency versus intensity plot, to show how threshold sensitivity changes across the frequency range. Such a graph is called an "**audiogram**." In clinical pure-tone audiometry we usually measure thresholds at sinusoidal frequencies over the range from 250 Hz, at the low end, to 8000 Hz, at the high end. Within this range threshold is tested at octave intervals in the range below 1000 Hz and at half octave intervals in the range above 1000 Hz. Thus the "audiometric" frequencies for conventional pure-tone audiometry are 250, 500, 1000, 1500, 2000, 3000, 4000, 6000, and 8000 Hz.

The concept of threshold, as the "just-audible" sound intensity, is somewhat more complicated than it seems at first glance. The problem is that, when a sound is very faint, the listener may not hear it every time it is presented. When sounds are fairly loud we can present them over and over and the listener will almost always respond to them. Similarly, when sounds are very faint we can present them over and over and the listener will almost never respond to them. But when the sound intensity is in the vicinity of the listener's threshold he or she may not respond consistently. The same sound intensity might produce a response after some presentations but not after others. Knowing that this will almost always be the case, what we look for is the sound intensity that produces a response from the listener about 50% of the time. This is the classical notion of a sensory threshold. Within the range of sound intensities over which the listener's response falls from 100% to 0%, we seek the intensity level where response accuracy is about 50%.

In clinical audiometry sound intensity is expressed, on a decibel (dB) scale, relative to "average normal hearing." The zero point on this scale of sound intensities is the sound intensity corresponding to the mode of the distribution of threshold intensities measured on a large sample of persons with normal hearing. Such a decibel scale of sound intensities is called the "**hearing threshold level**" or simple "hearing level" scale, and is abbreviated as the HL scale. An audiogram, then, is a plot of the listener's threshold levels at the various test frequencies, where frequency is expressed in Hertz or Hz units and the threshold intensity is expressed on the HL decibel or dB scale. Figure 15–4 shows an example of such a plot. The zero line, running horizontally across the top of the graph, is the sound intensity corresponding to average normal hearing at each of the test frequencies. Figure 15–4 shows that, for this listener, the threshold at 1000 Hz is 30 dB HL.This means that when 1000 Hz sinusoidal signals were presented to the listener, and the intensity was systematically altered, the threshold, or intensity at which the

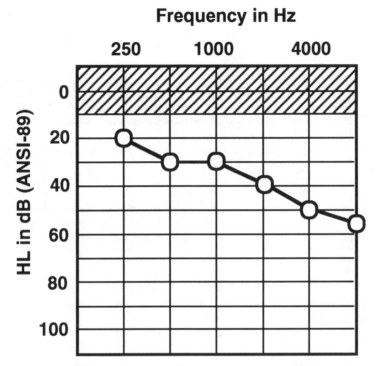

Figure 15-4. How hearing thresholds for pure tones are graphically represented. Each circular symbol represents the lowest intensity level (threshold) at that test frequency that the person being tested could just hear.

sound was heard about 50% of the time was at an intensity level 45 dB more intense than would be required for a person with average normal hearing.

There are two modes by which pure-tone test signals can be presented to the auditory system: through the air route via earphones or directly to the bones of the skull via a small vibrator. When the test signals are presented via earphones, via the air route, we are testing by "**air conduction**." Through the use of earphones or simular devices sinusoidal, or pure-tone, test signals can be presented either to the right ear or left ear. Thus an audiogram can be generated separately for each ear. On the other hand, when the test signals are presented by vibrator, via the bone route, we are testing by "**bone conduction**." The complete pure-tone audiogram, then, consists of four different plots: the air conduction and bone conduction curves for the right ear and the air and bone curves for the left ear. Figure 15-5 illustrates how such air-conduction and bone-conduction thresholds are plotted on an audiogram form.

Because the two ears are not completely isolated from one another, special precautions must be taken when testing one ear to be

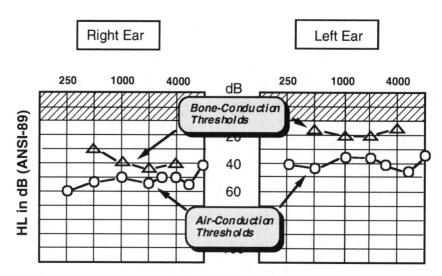

Figure 15–5. One of several possible methods for recording audiometric results. Circles are used to represent air-conduction thresholds, triangles to represent bone-conduction thresholds. Results for each ear are plotted on separate graphs for clarity and ease of analysis.

certain that the other ear is not participating in the response. This is particularly the case with unilateral losses where one ear is much more impaired than the other. In such a case the better ear may hear loud sounds presented to the poorer ear. The most common method of prevention is to "mask" the nontest ear with an interfering sound so that it cannot "hear" the test signal being presented to the test ear. In the case of air-conduction testing this can usually be accomplished with little difficulty. In the case of bone-conduction testing, however, masking can often be a major problem because of the minimal isolation between ears via bone conduction.

The pure-tone audiogram tells us a number of important things about a person's hearing loss:

Degree of loss. The HL scale extends from 0 to 110 dB. Where does sensitivity lie within this range? Is the loss mild (20–40 dB), moderate (40–70 dB), severe (70–95 dB), or profound (>95 dB)?

Shape of loss. Is the loss about the same at all test frequencies (flat audiometric contour), does the degree of loss increase as the curve moves from the low-frequency region to the high-frequency region (downward sloping contour), or does the degree of loss decrease as the curve moves from the low- to the high-frequency end (upward sloping contour).

Interaural symmetry. Is the loss about the same in both ears or is one ear substantially better than the other?

Is the loss conductive, sensorineural, or mixed? These are the three major categories of peripheral hearing loss. Conductive losses result from problems in the external ear canal or, more typically, from disorders of the middle-ear vibratory system (see Chapter 14 by Berlin). Sensorineural losses result from disorders in the inner ear or the auditory nerve. The audiometric signature of a conductive hearing loss is reduced sensitivity via the air-conduction route, but relatively normal sensitivity via the bone-conduction route. This is because the air-conduction loss reflects disorder along the entire chain of events from middle ear to inner ear to auditory nerve (i.e., both the conductive and the sensorineural systems). The bone-conduction loss, however, reflects only disorder in the inner ear and auditory nerve, because the bone-conducted signal goes directly to the cochlea, in effect bypassing the external and middle ear portions of the auditory system. (Strictly speaking, this is not quite true. Changes in middle-ear dynamics do affect bone-conduction sensitivity in predictable ways. But as a first approximation this is a useful way of thinking about the difference between conductive and sensorineural audiograms.) Comparison of the air- and bone-conduction threshold curves, then, tells us the broad category of loss. In a pure conductive loss there is reduced sensitivity by air conduction but relatively normal sensitivity by bone conduction. In a pure sensorineural loss, however, both air- and bone-conduction sensitivity are reduced equally. Finally, if there is loss by both air and bone conduction, but more loss by air than by bone, then the loss is categorized as "mixed" (i.e., there is both a conductive and a sensorineural component).

Later in this chapter we will present the audiograms typically associated with some common types of conductive, sensorineural, and mixed hearing losses.

Immittance Audiometry

Immittance is a physical characteristic of all mechanical vibratory systems. Very roughly, it is a measure of how readily the system can be set into vibration by a driving force. The ease with which energy will flow through the vibrating system is called its "**admittance.**"

The reciprocal concept, the extent to which the system resists the flow of energy through it, is called its "**impedance**." Immittance is a term meant to encompass both of these concepts. If the vibrating system can be forced to oscillate under little applied force, we say that the admittance (i.e., energy flow through the system) is high and the impedance is low. On the other hand, if the system resists being set into oscillation until the driving force is relatively high, then we say that the admittance of the system is low and the impedance is high.

Because conductive hearing loss is caused by changes in the transmission characteristics of the middle ear vibratory system, it is not surprising that the measurement of immittance plays an important role in clinical audiologic evaluation. There are three components in the clinical immittance battery: the tympanogram, the static immittance, and the acoustic reflex.

Tympanogram

The **tympanogram** is a graphic representation of how the immittance of the middle-ear vibratory system changes as air pressure is varied in the external ear canal. When the air pressure is the same on both sides of the tympanic membrane (i.e., when the air pressure in the external ear canal is the same as the air pressure in the middle-ear cavity), then the immittance of the normal middle-ear vibratory system is at its optimal peak and energy flow through the system is maximal. But if the air pressure in the external ear canal is either more than (positive pressure) or less than (negative pressure) the air pressure in the middle ear space, then the immittance of the system changes and energy flow is diminished. In the normal system the effect is quite precipitous. As soon as the air pressure changes even slightly below or above the air pressure producing maximum immittance, the energy flow drops quickly and steeply to a minimum value. Figure 15–6 plots immittance against air pressure in the external canal of a person with normal middle ear function. Air pressure is expressed as negative or positive relative to atmospheric pressure. The unit of measure of air pressure is the **decaPascal**, or daPa. The unit of measure of immittance is the **millimhO**, or mmhO. Such a plot of immittance against air pressure is called a tympanogram. In the case of the normal system, shown in Figure 15–6, the tympanogram has a characteristic shape. There is a sharp peak in immittance in the vicinity of 0 daPa of air pressure, and a rapid decline in immittance as air pressure moves away from 0, either in the negative or positive direction. This characteristically normal shape is designated **type A**.

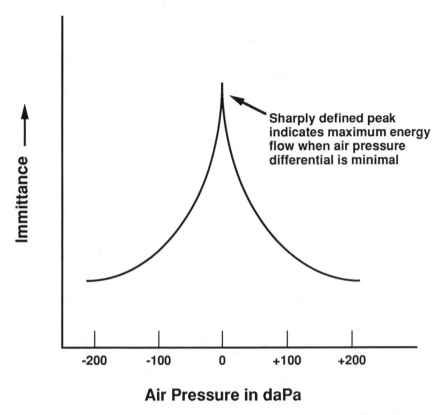

Figure 15–6. The tympanogram, a graphic representation of how the immittance of the middle-ear system changes as air pressure is varied in both the positive and negative directions in the external ear canal.

The clinical value of tympanograms derives from the fact that middle-ear disorder modifies the shape of the tympanogram in predictable ways. If, for example, the middle-ear space is filled with fluid (as in otitis media), then the tympanogram will lose its sharp peak and become relatively flat or only slightly rounded. This is due to the mass loading of the ossicular chain by the fluid present in the middle ear. This tympanogram shape is designated **type B**.

Another common cause of middle-ear disorder is faulty Eustachian tube function. The Eustachian tube connects the middle-ear space to the nasopharynx. It is ordinarily collapsed, but when you swallow, the tube briefly opens up, allowing fresh air to reach the middle ear. If for some reason the tube doesn't open when you swallow, or it is blocked at the nasopharyngeal orifice, then the air in the middle-ear space will not be replenished as it is used up. The result will be a loss of air pressure in the middle-ear space relative to the pressure in the external ear canal. This pressure differential will retract the tympanic membrane, sometimes causing severe pain. The effect on the tympanic membrane is to move the sharp peak away from 0 air pressure and well into the negative air pressure region. This occurs simply because it is necessary to add enough negative pressure in the external canal to match the negative pressure in the middle-ear space. When this balance has been achieved, energy flow through the middle-ear system will be at its maximum and the tympanogram will be at its peak. This tympanogram shape, normal in shape but with the peak at substantial negative air pressure, is designated **type C**.

Anything that causes the ossicular chain to become stiffer, thereby causing a reduction in energy flow through the middle ear, will simply attenuate the peak of the tympanogram. The shape will remain normal or **type A** but the entire tympanogram will become shallower. Such a tympanogram is designated **type A_s**, to indicate that the shape of the tympanogram is normal, with the peak at or near 0 daPa of air pressure, but with significant reduction in the height at the peak. The subscript "s" denotes "stiffness" or "shallowness." Such tympanograms are characteristic of otosclerosis, a disease of the bone surrounding the footplate of the stapes.

Finally, if there is a break or discontinuity in the chain of three bones connecting the tympanic membrane to the cochlea, the tympanogram will retain its normal shape but the peak will be much greater than normal. With the heavy load of the cochlear fluid system removed, the tympanic membrane will be much more free to respond to forced vibration. Hence energy flow at this point in the system will be greatly enhanced, resulting in a very deep tympanogram. Such a shape is designated **type A_d** to indicate that the shape of the tympanogram is normal and the peak is at or near 0 daPa of air pressure, but the height is significantly increased. The subscript "d" denotes "deep" or "discontinuity."

Figure 15–7 shows examples of each of these five tympanogram types. Their diagnostic value lies in the information they convey about changes in the physical status of the middle ear. When such information is viewed in relation to the results of acoustic reflex threshold testing, the combination can be extremely useful in evaluating disorder at all levels of the auditory system.

Static Immittance

In contrast to the dynamic measure of middle-ear function represented by the tympanogram, the term **static immittance** refers to the immittance of the middle-ear system when it is at rest. It can be viewed as simply the absolute height of the tympanogram at its peak.

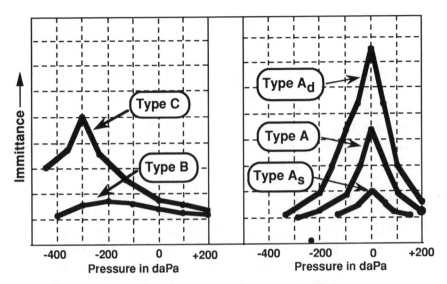

Figure 15–7. Clinical types of tympanograms. Type A tympanograms are characterized by a sharply defined peak at or near 0 decaPascals (daPa) of air pressure. In the type C tympanogram, the peak is still sharply defined but it has shifted well into the region of negative air pressure. In the type B tympanogram, the peak is either rounded or lost, resulting in a relatively flat or dome-shaped configuration.

The static immittance is measured by comparing the immittance when the air pressure is at 0, or at the air pressure corresponding to the peak, with the immittance when the air pressure is raised to positive 200 daPa. It is convenient to express these immittance measures as equivalent volumes of air in cubic centimeters (cc). When the air pressure is at +200 daPa, this measure is equivalent to the volume of air in the external ear canal. The contribution from the middle-ear system is negligible. This volume varies from about 0.5 cc to 1.5 cc in children and adults. When the air pressure is at 0 daPa, however, the measured volume is larger because it now includes the equivalent volume of the middle-ear system, that is the immittance of the middle-ear vibratory system expressed as an equivalent volume of air that would produce the same change in sound pressure level in the external canal. The static immittance, then, is the difference between the volume measurements at the two different air pressures. In adults without middle-ear disorder the difference ranges between 0.3 and 1.6 cc. There are two diagnostic applications of static immittance measurement. First, values below 1.3 cc or above 1.6 cc are strong evidence of middle-ear disorder. but this range is so large that many of the milder forms of conductive loss will fall within the normal range. If the static immittance falls outside the normal range, one can safely predict middle-ear disorder. But values within the normal range by no means exclude the possibility of middle-ear disorder.

The second, and perhaps more useful clinical application of the static immittance measure lies in its ability to detect small perforations of the tympanic membrane. Recall that the first volume measurement taken, with the air pressure in the external canal at +200 daPa, is actually measuring the volume of air in the external ear canal. If there is any aperture in the tympanic membrane through which air can travel, then the procedure will measure not only the volume of air in the external canal but, in addition, the much larger volume of air in the middle-ear space. Thus if the first volume measurement in the static immittance procedure is considerably larger than 1.5 cc (e.g., 4.5 or 5.0 cc), it must mean that there is a perforation in the tympanic membrane through which air can pass. This method for detecting perforations is actually more sensitive to small perforations than visual inspection of the tympanic membrane, even under magnification.

Acoustic Reflex

The "**acoustic reflex**" is the name we give to the reflexive contraction of the **stapedius muscle** in response to acoustic stimulation. The stapedius muscle connects the head of the stapes to the posterior wall of the middle ear. When it contracts it exerts an inward pull on the head of the stapes, thereby stiffening the ossicular chain so that energy flow through the middle ear system is slightly reduced. This slight change in immittance can be detected by the circuitry of the immittance audiometer. Thus if we present a sound to the ear and note a synchronized change in immittance, we know that the stapedius muscle has contracted. By varying the sound intensity, we can find the lowest sound level that produces a change in immittance. This is the "threshold" of the acoustic reflex. In persons with normal hearing and normal middle-ear systems this threshold will be reached for pure tones at an HL ranging from 70 to 100 dB. The average HL is about 85 dB. These ranges are constant across the frequency range from 500 to 4000 Hz. The diagnostic value of the acoustic reflex threshold lies in the way these thresholds are modified by auditory disorder.

When we present a single sound to the auditory system, there are actually four different acoustic reflex thresholds to be measured. This is because we can present the sound to either the right or the left ear and, whichever ear we stimulate, both stapedius muscles will contract. Thus for each ear of stimulation there are two reflexes, crossed and uncrossed, to consider. The term "**crossed acoustic reflex**" (CAR) denotes the situation in which sound is presented to one ear and the reflex is detected in the opposite or contralateral ear. The term "**uncrossed acoustic reflex**" (UCAR) denotes the situation in which sound is presented to one ear and the reflex is detected in the same or ipsilateral ear. Thus, for any frequency of stimulation there are four reflexes to consider, the right-to-left CAR, the left-to-right CAR, the right UCAR, and the left UCAR. There is considerable diagnostic information in the relationships among these four threshold levels. In general, however, the principles underlying the interpretation of subtle reflex abnormalities are beyond the scope of this chapter.

Otoacoustic Emission Audiometry

In recent years it has been discovered that the sensory hair cells of the inner ear actually expand and contract under stimulation. As they respond to incoming sounds they create outgoing sounds which travel from the cochlea, back through the middle ear, and out into the external ear canal. These sounds, created by the movements of the hair cells and emitted from the sensory apparatus, are called "**otoacoustic emissions**." Of the various types of emissions, the most useful for audiologic evaluation is the class called **evoked otoacoustic emissions** or EOAEs. Such emissions can be evoked by two kinds of eliciting signals, clicks and tone bursts. When a click is used the emission evoked is itself a click which can be recorded shortly after the onset of the eliciting click. The second kind of evoked emission is the distortion product created by the introduction of two different pure tones simultaneously into the ear canal. Because the cochlear mechanism is not linear, the presentation of two pure tones, f_1 and f_2, creates energy, or distortion products, at other frequencies which are combinations of, or differences between, the two eliciting tones. The most robust distortion product is the frequency $2f_1 - f_2$. It is called the **distortion-product evoked otoacoustic emission**, or DPEOAE. To measure DPEOAEs across the range of frequencies of interest in audiometry, a pair of tones at a constant frequency ratio, usually 1:2, is swept upward over the frequency region from 500 to 8000 Hz. The recording apparatus filters out the energy of the stimulating-frequency pair and records only the energy at the $2f_1 - f_2$ distortion-product frequency. The amplitude of this DPEOAE is typically displayed as a function of the f_2 frequency along with the noise floor of the recording system. If the EOAE is evoked by a click, the emission can be spectrally analyzed to show the frequency distribution of the emitted energy.

The basis for the clinical application of EOAEs is the fact that these emissions have been shown to be extremely sensitive to the status of the outer hair cells. When damage in the outer hair cells is sufficient to cause a sensorineural hearing loss of as little as 20–30 dB, the amplitude of the EOAE will be greatly attenuated or even abolished. The EOAE is, therefore, a very sensitive indicator of even very mild sensory loss due to outer hair cell damage. Perhaps the most important clinical application of EOAEs lies in screening the hearing of newborn babies and young children. The technique is rapid, objective, and inexpensive, and the EOAE is typically quite robust in babies. If it is absent, there is the strong presumption of hearing loss. There are, however, two problems with this application. First, to record emissions it is necessary to have a relatively quiet test situation. This requirement may be difficult to achieve in the noisy environments typical of newborn nurseries and neonatal intensive care units. Second, the EOAE is sensitive to the status of the middle-ear mechanism. Even mild conductive loss may abolish the emission. These two problems are the bases for a high false-positive rate, which complicates the economics of widespread screening programs.

The second clinical application lies in the differentiation between cochlear and retrocochlear sites of disorder. Because the EOAE is determined by outer hair cell status, it will not be affected by auditory disorders central to the cochlea. Thus the combination of a sensorineural hearing loss and relatively normal EOAEs allows the clinician to rule out a cochlear site in favor of a retrocochlear site.

Speech Audiometry

Speech audiometry is a key component of audiologic assessment for several reasons. First, it is concerned with the kinds of auditory signals used in everyday communication. Thus it can tell us, in a more realistic manner than signals like pure tones and clicks, how the auditory disorder affects the communicative problems of daily living. Second, the influence of speech processing can be detected at virtually every level of the auditory system. Thus, diagnostic tests based on speech materials can be constructed to examine processing throughout the auditory system, including the middle ear, the cochlea, the auditory nerve, the brain-stem pathways, and the auditory centers in the cerebral hemispheres. Third, there is a predictable relationship between a person's hearing for pure tones and his or her hearing for speech. Speech audiometric testing, therefore, can serve as a crosscheck on the validity of the pure-tone audiogram.

The materials of speech audiometry include nonsense syllables (e.g., "pa, ta, ka, ga"), single-syllable, or monosyllabic, words (e.g., "cat, tie, lick"), two-syllable, or spondee, words (e.g., "northwest, cowboy, firefly"), sentences containing key words (e.g., "*Open* your *window before* you *go* to *bed*"), sentences with the key word at the end (e.g., "The old train was powered by *steam*"), and synthetic syntax sentences (e.g., "Go change your car color is red").

Materials like these have been used to explore three dimensions of speech understanding: (a) threshold sensitivity, (b) suprathreshold speech understanding, and (c) central auditory processing.

Threshold Sensitivity

The preferred materials for the measurement of speech threshold are the **spondee words**. In theory, almost any materials could be used but the spondee words have the advantage that, with only small individual adjustments, they can be made "homogeneous with respect to audibility," that is, all just heard at about the same speech intensity level. This greatly helps in establishing a threshold for speech. By presenting a series of spondee words and systematically varying the intensity, one can determine the level at which the individual just hears about 50% of the test items. The clinical value of this **spondee threshold** (ST) is that it should agree closely with the pure-tone thresholds averaged across 500, 1000, and 2000 Hz. If both the pure-tone intensity levels and the speech intensity levels are expressed on a hearing threshold level (HL) decibel scale, the degree of hearing loss for speech (threshold HL) should agree with the degree of hearing loss for pure tones in the 500–2000 Hz region. The latter average HL is called the **pure-tone average**, or PTA. In clinical practice the ST and the PTA should be in fairly close agreement, differing by perhaps no more than ±6 dB. If, for example, the PTA is 42 dB, the ST should be somewhere between 36 and 48 dB. If there is a larger discrepancy between the two numbers, then one or the other is probably an invalid measure. In the case of malingering (nonorganic hearing loss), for example, the ST may be substantially less than the PTA. In some kinds of central auditory problems, moreover, the ST may be substantially more than the PTA.

Suprathreshold Speech Understanding

In the past, the most popular sets of materials for the measurement of suprathreshold speech understanding have been the monosyllabic, phonemically balanced word lists. These 50-word lists were compiled during World War II as test materials for comparing the speech transmission characteristics of aircraft radio receivers and transmitters. The words were selected from newspaper articles and arranged into 50-word lists. Each list was characterized by the fact that all of the sounds of English, the "phonemes," were represented in their relative frequency of occurrence in the language. Hence the lists were considered to be phonemically balanced and became known as **PB lists**. Raymond Carhart, one of the early pioneers of audiologic evaluation, adapted the PB lists to audiologic testing. He reasoned that if you first established the threshold for speech, the ST, then presented a PB list at a level 25 dB above the ST, the percent correct word repetition for a PB list would tell you something about how well the individual could understand speech in that ear. This measure, the PB score at a constant suprathreshold level, came to be called the "**discrimination score**," on the assumption that it was proportional to the individual's ability to "discriminate" among the individual sounds of speech. Carhart later adapted the measure to the evaluation of hearing aid performance by presenting the PB lists at suprathreshold levels via loudspeaker in the sound-treated room. This basic speech audiometric paradigm, a PB score at a defined sensation level about the ST, formed the framework for audiologic and aural rehabilitation procedures which are still in use today. Subsequent modifications of the original PB lists include the W-22 lists, developed at the Central Institute for the Deaf (CID), and the NU-6 lists, developed at Northwestern University. More recently, however, newer and more sophisticated speech audiometric techniques have been introduced. A novel procedure employing sentences with variable context is the **speech-perception-in-noise (SPIN) test**. In SPIN the test item, a single word, is the last word of a sentence. There are two types of sentences, those in which word identification is aided by context (e.g., "Let's decide by tossing a *coin*") and those in which context is not as helpful (e.g., "I'm glad you heard about the *bend*"). Sentences are presented to the listener against the background of competing multi-talker babble. Another sentence-based procedure is the **synthetic sentence identification (SSI) test**. Artificially created, seven-word sentences (e.g., "Agree with him only to find out") are presented to the listener against a background of the competing continuous discourse of a single talker. Both SPIN and SSI may be used, either alone or in combination with PB lists, to evaluate suprathreshold speech understanding.

Another recent modification of Carhart's original paradigm has been the exploration of speech understanding across the patient's entire dynamic range of hearing rather than at just a single supra-threshold level. Lists of words or sentences are presented at three to five different intensity levels, extending from just above the speech threshold to the upper level of comfortable listening. In this way a "performance versus intensity" or **PI function** is generated for each ear. The shape of this function often has important diagnostic significance. In most cases the PI function rises slowly, as speech intensity is increased, to an asymptotic level representing the best speech understanding that can be achieved in the test ear. In some cases, however, there is a paradoxical "rollover" effect, in which the function declines substantially as speech intensity increases beyond the level producing the maximum performance score. In other words as speech intensity increases, performance rises to a maximal value, then declines or "rolls over" sharply as intensity continues to increase. This **rollover effect** is commonly observed when the site of the hearing loss is central to the sensory structures of the cochlea (i.e., in the auditory nerve or the auditory pathways in the brain stem). Some examples of performance versus intensity functions for speech materials are shown in the next section.

Central Auditory Processing

Some problems in speech understanding appear to be based not on the distortions introduced by peripheral hearing loss but on deficits resulting from disorders in the auditory pathways in the central nervous system. Perhaps the most effective speech materials for the study of such central auditory processing disorders are the various **dichotic tests**. In the dichotic paradigm two different speech targets are presented simultaneously to the two ears (e.g., the word "boy" to one ear and the word "duck" to the other ear). The patient's task is determined by the instructions. In the "free report" mode the patient repeats back both words in any order. In the "directed report" mode the patient reports only the word heard in the precued ear. Over a list of such word pairs the right ear is precued on half of the trials, the left ear on the other half. In each mode there are two scores, one for targets correctly identified from the right ear, the other for targets correctly identified from the left ear. The patterns of results among these four scores can reveal both cognitive and specifically auditory processing deficits.

Dichotic tests have been constructed using nonsense syllables, monosyllabic words, staggered spondee words, and synthetic-syntax sentences. Examples of dichotic test results in central processing disorders are shown in the next section.

Auditory Evoked Potential Audiometry

By means of computer averaging it is possible to extract the tiny electrical voltages, or potentials, evoked in the brain by acoustic stimulation. These electrical events are quite complex and can be observed over a fairly broad time interval after the onset of stimulation. For audiological purposes it is convenient to group the **auditory evoked potentials** (AEPs) into three categories, based loosely on the latency ranges over which the potentials are observed. The three categories are often labeled as "early," "middle," and "late." The early potentials occur in the first 10–15 milliseconds (msec) following signal onset. They consist of a series of five positive peaks or waves collectively called the "**auditory brainstem response**" or ABR (see Figure 15-8). The five waves, occurring over the latency range from about 2 to 6 msec, are generated by the auditory nerve and by structures in the caudal brain stem ranging from the cochlear nucleus to the region of the inferior colliculus. The most robust peak, the fifth wave, has the important property that it can be observed at intensity levels close to auditory threshold. Thus, it can be used very effectively to estimate hearing sensitivity in babies, young children, and other difficult-to-test persons. A second important property of the ABR is that the time intervals between peaks are prolonged by auditory disorders central to the cochlea. This property makes the ABR extremely useful for differentiating cochlear from retrocochlear sites of disorder.

The **middle-latency response** (MLR) is characterized by two successive positive peaks, the first (P_a) at about 25–35 msec, the second (P_b) at about 40–60 msec. There is good evidence that the MLR is generated by structures at the level of primary auditory cortex. Although the MLR is the most difficult AEP to record in clinical patients, it shows promise as an aid to the identification of central auditory processing disorders.

The "**late**" or "**vertex**" **potential** (LVR) is characterized by a negative peak (N_1) at a latency of about 80–100 msec followed by a positive peak (P_2) at about 170–200 msec. This potential is greatly affected by subject "state." It is best recorded when the patient is awake and carefully attending to the sounds being presented. There is an important developmental effect on the LVR during the first 8–10 years. In older children and adults, however, it is robust and relatively easy to record. In children or adults with relatively normal auditory sensitivity, abnormality or absence of the LVR is associated with central auditory processing disorder.

Figure 15-8 shows examples of the ABR, MLR, and LVR waveforms as they would appear in a person with normal auditory function. Taken as a whole, this family of evoked responses is quite ver-

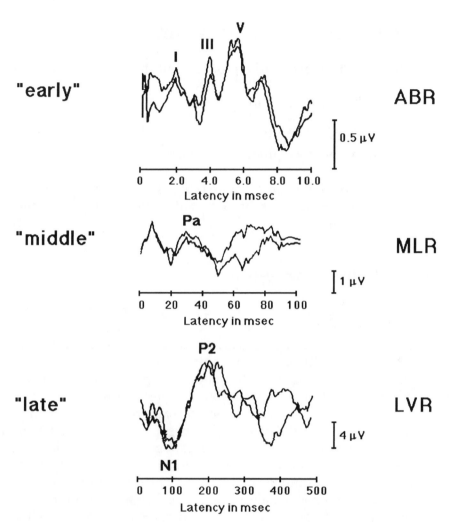

Figure 15-8. The family of auditory evoked potentials, categorized according to the latency periods in which they appear. The "early" or ABR waveform is characterized by three major peaks corresponding to evoked electrical activity at the level of the auditory nerve (wave I), the superior olivary complex (wave III), and the region of the inferior colliculus (wave V). ABR activity occurs in the first 10–15 msec after signal onset. The most prominent feature of the "middle" or MLR waveform is a positive peak (P_a) at 30–35 msec after signal onset. The "late" or LVR waveform shows a negative peak (N_1) at 80–100 msec, followed by a positive peak at 180–200 msec (P_2).

satile. Both ABR and LVR can be used to estimate auditory sensitivity independently of behavioral response. In addition, ABR can be used to differentiate cochlear from retrocochlear site of disorder. Finally, the array of all three responses is an effective tool for exploring central auditory processing disorders.

✦ NATURE OF AUDITORY DISORDERS

Auditory disorders can be grouped into three large categories:

1. Conductive hearing loss

2. Sensorineural hearing loss

3. Central auditory processing disorder

In the following sections we first discuss the types of disorder in each category, then present case studies illustrating typical audiometric findings.

Conductive Hearing Loss

Anything that interferes with the normal vibratory movements of the ossicular chain can produce conductive hearing loss. In children the most common cause is a build-up of fluid in the middle-ear space, usually because of faulty Eustachian tube function. The Eustachian tube connects the middle-ear space to the nasopharynx. Normally each time you swallow, the Eustachian tube opens and permits fresh air to reach the middle-ear space. If for any reason there is blockage of the tube at the nasopharyngeal end, the air in the middle-ear space cannot be exchanged. In short order the tissues lining the walls of the middle ear will begin to exude fluid. As this fluid rises within the middle ear it will eventually reach the level of the tympanic membrane and interfere with its normal vibration, causing a mild conductive hearing loss. Eventually the rising fluid will reach the ossicular chain and interfere with ossicular vibration. This will cause further increase in the degree of conductive hearing loss. Finally, if the fluid is not drained off promptly via ventilating tubes, and is allowed to remain in the middle ear for an extended period, it will develop a glue-like consistency and form permanent adhesions between the ossicles and the walls of the middle ear. At this point it may be necessary to intervene surgically to reverse the hearing loss.

Another common cause of mild conductive hearing loss in children is perforation of the tympanic membrane, caused either by a rupture due to excessive outward fluid pressure or by the insertion of ventilating tubes. Fortunately, such hearing losses are mild and almost always reversible.

In adults the most common cause of conductive hearing loss is otosclerosis, a disease of the bone surrounding the footplate of the stapes. As the abnormal bone growth proliferates around the mar-gin of the oval window, it causes a progressive conductive hearing loss due to interference with the normal vibratory mode of the stapes footplate. The disease is more common in women than in men and is often exacerbated by pregnancy. Fortunately the conductive hearing loss can be virtually eliminated by a surgical procedure called a "stapedectomy" in which the immobilized stapes bone is removed and replaced by a prosthesis.

Other causes of conductive hearing loss in adults include tumors growing in the middle-ear space, barotrauma when the barometric pressure on each side of the tympanic membrane is not properly equalized during ascent or descent in the air (e.g., an airplane during takeoff and landing) or underwater, discontinuity of the ossicular chain, either from trauma or erosion, and perforation of the tympanic membrane. Another common cause of conductive hearing loss, in both children and adults, is the excessive build-up of cerumen (earwax) in the external auditory canal. In some individuals cerumen can rapidly increase to the point where it blocks the canal or loads down the tympanic membrane. Such losses can, of course, be completely reversed by cleaning the cerumen out of the external canal.

The following case studies illustrate audiometric findings in a child with otitis media and in an adult with otosclerosis.

Case Study 1: Conductive Hearing Loss due to Otitis Media

The first example of conductive hearing loss is a 5-year-old boy who has had recurring bouts of otitis media since the age of 18 months. His hearing has fluctuated dramatically over this period, as the fluid level in the middle ear space rose and fell in response to antibiotic therapy. At the time of the audiogram, his parents felt that his hearing was poorer than it had ever been in the past. Figure 15–9A shows the results of pure-tone audiometry and speech audiometry. The air-conduction audiogram shows a moderate loss in both ears, but greater in the right ear. The PTA is 55 dB in the right ear and 40 dB in the left ear. Bone-conduction sensitivity, however, is well within the normal range on both ears. For speech audiometry pediatric versions of both word and sentence testing against a background of speech competition were used. Note that, once the conductive loss has been overcome by raising the speech intensity to relatively high levels, his speech understanding is normal. The PI functions rise rapidly to a maximum of 100% correct recognition and do not roll over with further increase in speech intensity.

Figure 15–9B shows the results of immittance audiometry. On the right ear the tympanogram is relatively flat and would be classi-

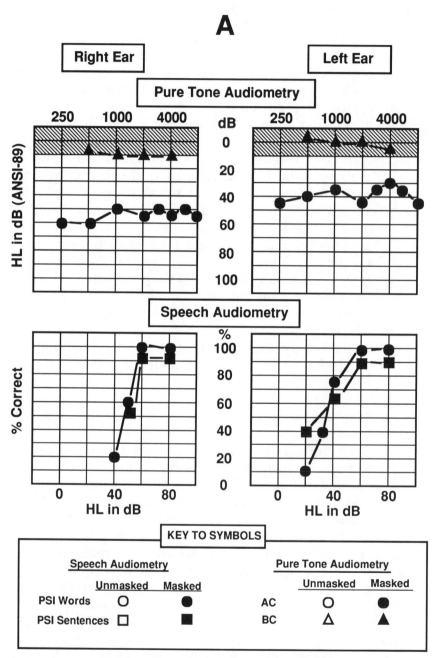

Figure 15–9. Audiometric findings in a 5-year-old boy with chronic otitis media. **A.** Pure-tone and speech audiometric results. **B.** Immittance results. Because of the possibility of cross-hearing from the nontest ear, all testing must be carried out with a masking noise in the contralateral ear. The filled symbols indicate that such contralateral masking was present. NR indicates no acoustic reflex response at a signal presentation level of 110 dB HL.

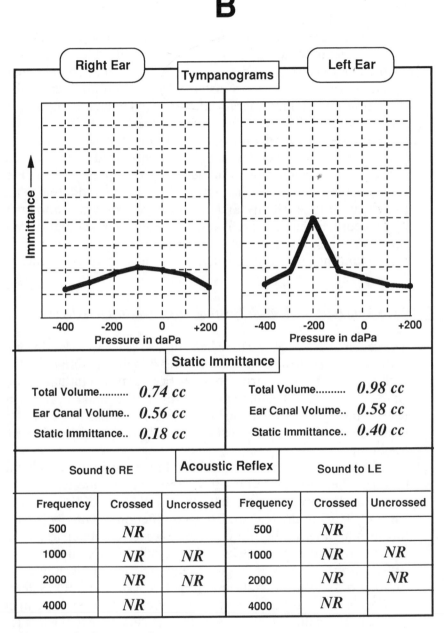

B

Figure 15–9 *(continued)*

fied as type B. On the left ear the tympanogram retains its sharp peak, but the peak is displaced substantially in the negative direction. This tympanogram would be classified as type C. The static immittance is well below the normal range on the right ear, 0.18 cc, but within the normal range on the left ear, 0.40 cc. No acoustic reflexes were recorded from either ear in either the crossed (CAR) or uncrossed (UCAR) modes.

All of these audiometric findings are entirely predictable from the middle-ear pathology. In the right ear the fluid level has caused such a mass loading of the ossicular chain and reduction in energy transmission that there is a substantial loss in auditory sensitivity, a flattening of the tympanogram, and inability to record any acoustic reflexes. In the left ear the effect is not as great. There is perhaps less fluid and the tympanogram shows that the ossicular chain can vibrate appropriately when air pressure is equalized on the two sides of the tympanic membrane. But because of the pressure imbalance there is a loss in energy transmission through the middle ear, a mild loss in auditory sensitivity, an abnormal tympanogram, and inability to record any acoustic reflexes. Because this is a straightforward problem in middle-ear mechanics, there is no difficulty with speech understanding once the sensitivity loss has been overcome.

Case Study 2: Conductive Hearing Loss due to Otosclerosis

The second case of conductive hearing loss is a 36-year-old woman with otosclerosis. She first noticed a hearing problem in her left ear at the age of 21. The hearing loss has been getting gradually worse. At the age of 25 she began to notice a loss in the right ear. It, too, has been getting gradually worse. She has been pregnant twice and has noticed a slight increase in the loss in both ears following each pregnancy.

Figure 15–10A shows the results of pure-tone and speech audiometry. The air-conduction audiogram shows a moderate loss in both ears, but greater in the left ear. The PTA is 35 dB in the right ear and 50 dB in the left ear. Bone-conduction sensitivity is within the normal range for both ears. Note, however, the notch in the bone conduction curves at 2000 Hz. This does not mean that there is a 15 dB sensorineural loss at this test frequency. It is a mechanical by-product of the stapes fixation and its effect on the fluid system in the cochlea. This is the characteristic bone-conduction curve in otosclerosis. It is called "Carhart's Notch" in deference to the late Raymond Carhart who first described the phenomenon. Figure 15–10A also shows PI functions for both PB words and SSI sentences. Once the sensitivity loss has been overcome by raising the speech intensity level, the PI functions climb rapidly to 100% on both ears, indicating that there is no problem with suprathreshold speech understanding.

Figure 15–10B shows the results of immittance audiometry. On both ears the tympanogram is a relatively shallow type A with a well-

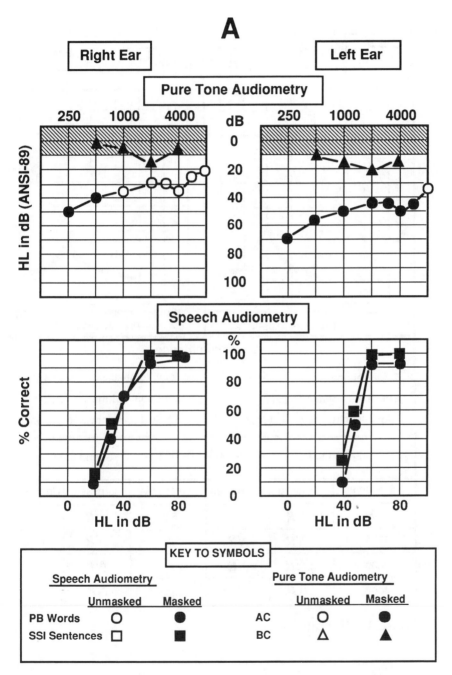

Figure 15–10. Audiometric findings in a 36-year-old woman with otosclerosis. **A.** Pure-tone and speech audiometric results. **B.** Immittance results. Note presence of Carhart's "notch" in both bone-conduction curves.

B

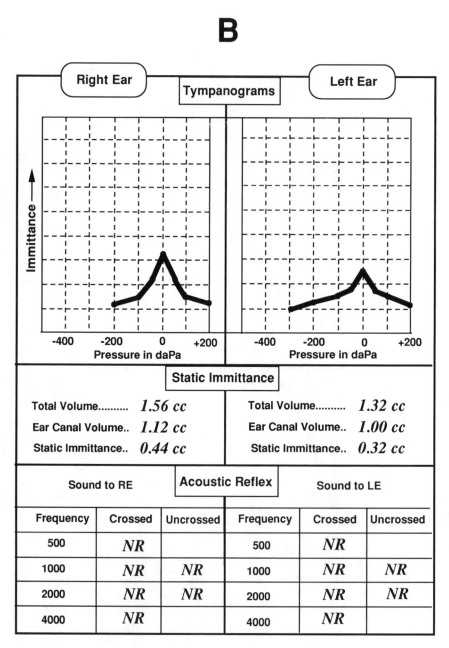

Figure 15–10 *(continued)*

defined peak but considerably reduced amplitude. On both ears the static immittance is at the low end of the normal range, 0.32 cc on the left ear and 0.44 cc on the right ear. No acoustic reflexes can be recorded from either ear in either the crossed (CAR) or uncrossed (UCAR) modes.

Sensorineural Hearing Loss

The relatively broad sensorineural category encompasses any hearing loss resulting from damage to the sensory structures of the inner ear or to the neural structure, the auditory nerve, connecting the inner ear to the central auditory pathways in the brain. In babies and young children the principal cause of sensorineural loss is hereditary deafness. Other causative factors include anoxia at birth, neonatal jaundice, meningitis, high fever illnesses, and ototoxic drugs.

In adults the most common source of sensorineural loss is the aging process. Throughout life there is a gradual but progressive loss of sensitivity to high frequency sounds due to degeneration of hair cells in the most basal portion of the cochlea. The process actually begins in the third decade (20–29 years) but initially involves only very high frequencies. As aging continues, however, the sensitivity loss moves downward on the frequency scale. By the seventh decade (60–69 years) the loss will have begun to involve the frequency region important for understanding speech and some hearing difficulty, called "**presbyacusis**," will begin to be experienced. By the ninth decade (80–89 years) many elderly persons will experience significant presbyacusis hearing problems requiring intervention and rehabilitation. There is, however, considerable variation in this aging effect among elderly persons. At any given age one can identify persons with relatively normal hearing and persons with varying degrees of loss ranging from mild to severe. We cannot predict how aging will affect a single individual, but we can predict, with confidence, that as age increases the proportion of persons with hearing in the normal range will decline progressively and the proportion with significant hearing problems will increase.

A second common cause of sensorineural loss in adults is exposure to excessive noise. The exposure may be occupational or recreational. Occupational risks include noisy work environments, military weaponry, accidental explosions, and aircraft noise. Recreational risks include the gunfire associated with hunting and target practice, loud music, auto racing, and, in the more northern climates, the use of snowmobiles. Prolonged exposure to high levels of noise causes the hair cells, the sensory structures in the inner ear, to degenerate and disappear. The damage begins in the basal turn of the cochlea, initially affecting sensitivity in the 4000–6000 Hz region. As the exposure continues, however, the damage spreads both upward and downward on the frequency scale. When the frequency range from 1000 to 3000 Hz becomes involved, socially handicapping hearing loss begins. Other common causes of sensorineural hearing loss in adults include ototoxic drugs, Meniere's disease, and tumors of the auditory nerve.

The vast majority of sensorineural losses are due to sensory rather than neural damage. The outer and inner hair cells, mounted within the organ of Corti, are responsible for as much as 95% of all sensorineural loss. Such losses are, furthermore, benign and usually medically or surgically untreatable. Neural damage, on the other hand, although comparatively rare, may be life-threatening. As it grows ever larger a tumor of the auditory nerve may invade the cerebellopontine angle and ultimately the brain stem itself where it may threaten structures vital to survival unless it is promptly removed by the neurotologic surgeon. It is important, therefore, to differentiate sensory from neural losses.

The following cases illustrate audiometric findings in patients with two kinds of sensorineural hearing loss; noise-induced and auditory-nerve tumor. They illustrate how the acoustic reflex, the evoked otoacoustic emissions, and the ABR can assist in the differentiation of sensory from neural disorder.

Case Study 3: Sensorineural Hearing Loss from Occupational Noise Exposure

The first case of sensorineural hearing loss is a 36-year-old seaman who has worked for the past 8 years on a high-speed supply boat ferrying goods and services from shore to personnel on platform oil rigs in the Gulf of Mexico. The boat is powered by twin 230-horsepower diesel engines. At full speed the noise level at any place on the boat varies between 110 and 115 dBA. Our patient spends 24 hours a day on the boat for 4 consecutive days. He is on a 4-day-on, 4-day-off cycle. Shortly after beginning work on the supply boat, he began to notice a ringing sound in the left ear at the end of each cycle of duty. More recently, he notices the ringing sound in the right ear as well. After 6 months his wife complained that she had to repeat things a lot before he heard them. His hearing has been getting gradually worse over the last 3 years. He has been issued ear protection devices but he doesn't like to use them.

The results of pure-tone and speech audiometry are summarized in Figure 15–11A. There is a high-frequency sensitivity loss in both ears, but greater in the left ear. The loss is greatest at 4000 Hz, somewhat less at the neighboring frequencies of 3000 and 6000 Hz. Moreover the loss is equal by air conduction and bone conduction. There is no gap between the air- and bone-conduction curves as we saw in the conductive losses. Interweaving air- and bone-conduction curves are the signature of sensorineural hearing loss. On speech audiometry, PI functions for both PB words and SSI sentences rise to a maximum which falls short of the 100% level. Maximum scores

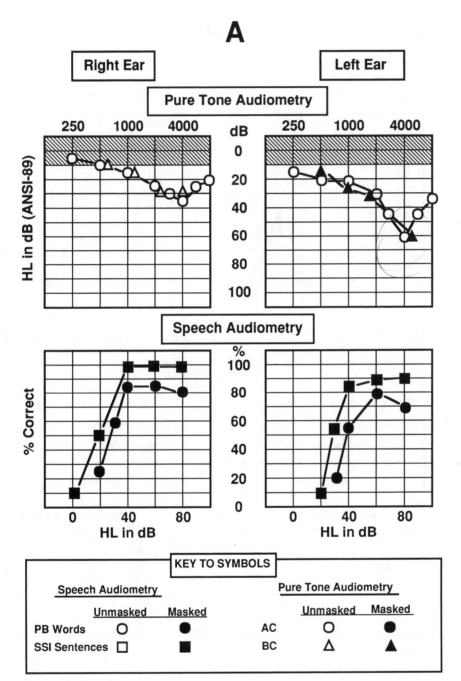

Figure 15–11. Audiometric findings in a 36-year-old man with noise-induced hearing loss. **A.** Pure-tone and speech audiometric results. **B.** Immittance results. **C.** Distortion-product otoacoustic emissions. **D.** Auditory brain stem responses. Note mild loss in word recognition scores due to loss of high-frequency sensitivity. Because this is a cochlear disorder, immittance findings and ABR results are all within normal limits while otoacoustic emissions are attenuated or absent.

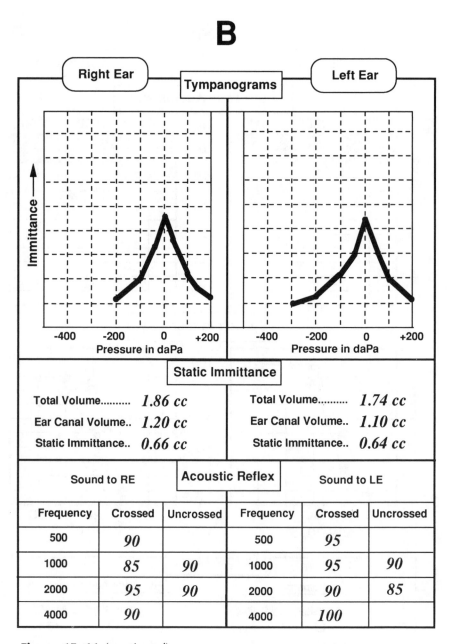

B

Sound to RE			Acoustic Reflex	Sound to LE		
Frequency	Crossed	Uncrossed		Frequency	Crossed	Uncrossed
500	90			500	95	
1000	85	90		1000	95	90
2000	95	90		2000	90	85
4000	90			4000	100	

Figure 15–11 *(continued)*

are slightly poorer in the left ear where the loss is greater. Finally, the maximum score for words is slightly below the maximum score for sentences, reflecting the greater dependence of word understanding on high-frequency sensitivity. In general, however, speech understanding is not yet drastically affected by the loss. We may anticipate, however, that if exposure continues, the sensitivity loss will

C

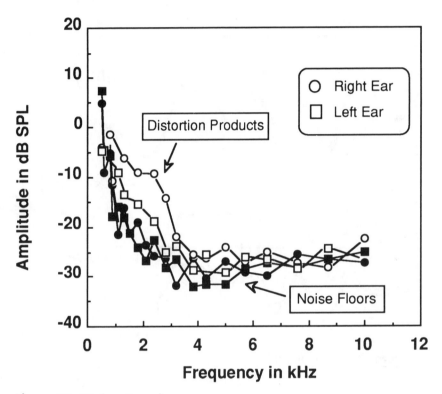

Figure 15-11 *(continued)*

involve lower frequencies and there will be a further decline in speech recognition scores.

The results of immittance audiometry are summarized in Figure 15–11B. The tympanograms are normal, type A, in both ears. The peak is sharply defined and located in the region of 0 daPa of air pressure. Both crossed and uncrossed reflexes are elicited at appropriate intensity levels. Finally, the static immittance is within the normal range, 0.66 cc for the right ear and 0.64 cc for the left ear. Because this is a sensorineural rather than a conductive loss it is not surprising that all immittance findings are normal.

Figure 15–11C summarizes results of distortion-product otoacoustic emission (DPOAE) testing. There are no measurable emissions above 3000 Hz from either ear, a result consistent with the extensive damage to outer hair cells caused by the excessive noise exposure.

D

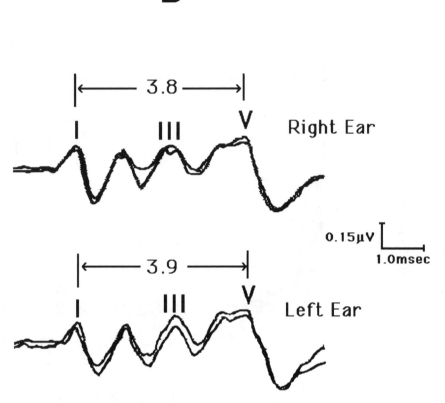

Figure 15–11(continued)

Figure 15–11D shows ABR waveforms from both ears in response to clicks presented at an intensity level of 80 dB HL. Waves I, III, and V are present at latencies either within the normal range or consistent with the high-frequency sensitivity loss.

In summary, noise-induced hearing loss is characterized by bilateral sensorineural loss with interweaving air- and bone-conduction audiometric curves, normal immittance findings, deficits in speech understanding that are predictable from the pattern of sensitivity loss, DPOAEs that are either greatly reduced in amplitude or absent, and relatively well-formed ABR waveforms with peaks at normal or expected latencies.

Case 4: Sensorineural Hearing Loss from Acoustic Tumor

The second case of sensorineural hearing loss is a 54-year-old man who complains of a hearing loss in the left ear. He reports that it came on gradually about 6 months ago and has been getting slowly but steadily worse. There is also a constant buzzing sound in his left ear. Radiologic imaging studies have revealed a small, space-occupying tumor in the left internal auditory canal. After surgical removal the tumor is identified as a vestibular schwannoma, arising from the vestibular portion of the eighth cranial nerve and exerting pressure on the auditory portion of the nerve.

Figure 15–12A summarizes pure-tone and speech audiometric findings. There is a unilateral loss in auditory sensitivity on the left side. The loss is greater for high frequencies than for low, but affects the entire audiometric frequency range. The air- and bone-conduction curves interweave. Speech audiometric results show that, on the unaffected right ear, the PI functions for both PB words and SSI sentences rise rapidly to the 100% level and remain there up to the highest intensity level tested. On the left ear, however, both PI functions are grossly abnormal. The PB word function reaches a maximum of only 65%, then rolls over dramatically and returns to 35% at the highest intensity. The SSI sentence function shows a similar pattern but with an even lower maximum score. These very poor speech understanding scores on an ear with only a relatively mild sensorineural loss are consistent with neural rather than sensory disorder. When the auditory nerve is damaged, the ability of the auditory system to transform the complex sounds of speech into the neural code of the central nervous system may be severely compromised. Thus the combination of a mild sensorineural loss and very poor speech understanding is a neural rather than a sensory sign.

Figure 15–12B summarizes immittance findings. Both tympanograms are normal, type A, and static immittance values of 0.64 cc and 0.72 cc are within the normal range. When signals are presented to the unaffected right ear both the crossed right-to-left and the right uncrossed acoustic reflex thresholds are observed at expected intensity levels. But when signals are introduced to the affected ear, neither crossed nor uncrossed reflexes can be elicited at equipment limits (110 dB HL). This result is in marked contrast to the reflex thresholds measured in the previous case of noise-induced loss. The difference is consistent with the differing sites of disorder. In the case of noise-induced loss, the damage was in the sensory cells in the cochlea and reflexes were elicited at normal levels. In the case of the acoustic tumor, however, the damage is in the neural portion of the peripheral auditory system. Even mild losses at this site frequently abolish the acoustic reflex. Thus absence of the reflex in a patient with only mild or moderate sensorineural loss is a retrocochlear sign.

Figure 15–12C summarizes distortion-product otoacoustic emission (DPOAE) amplitudes across the audiometric frequency range.

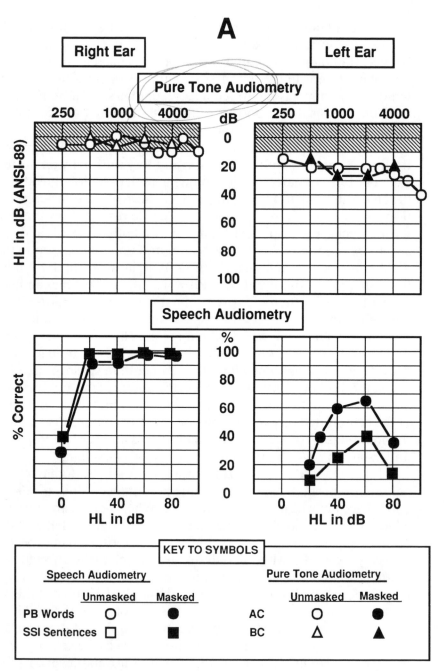

Figure 15–12. Audiometric findings in a 54-year-old man with a left acoustic tumor. **A.** Pure-tone and speech audiometric results. **B.** Immittance results. **C.** Distortion-product otoacoustic emissions. **D.** Auditory brain stem responses. Note very poor performance on tests of speech understanding on the left ear in spite of relatively mild sensitivity loss. Because this is an auditory nerve disorder, immittance and otoacoustic emission results are relatively normal, but the ABR shows a significantly prolonged interval between waves I and V.

B

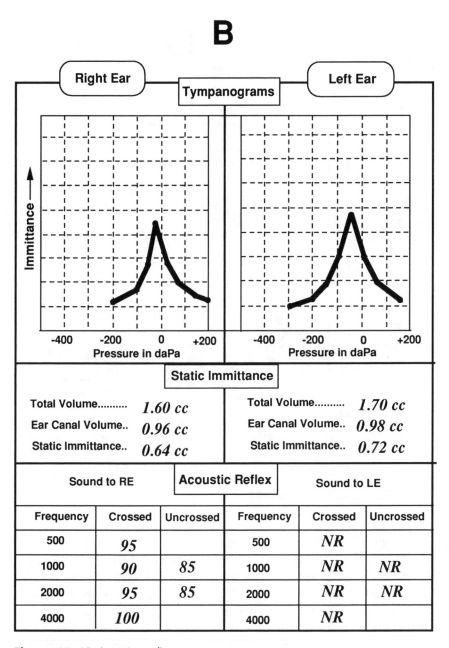

Figure 15–12 *(continued)*

On the unaffected right ear, emissions are robust and well above the noise floor. On the affected left ear, the amplitude is somewhat reduced but still larger than would be expected if the sensitivity loss were entirely cochlear. Note, for example, that the degree of loss on the left ear of the present case and on the right ear on the previous case of noise-induced loss is about equivalent. In the ear with noise-

C

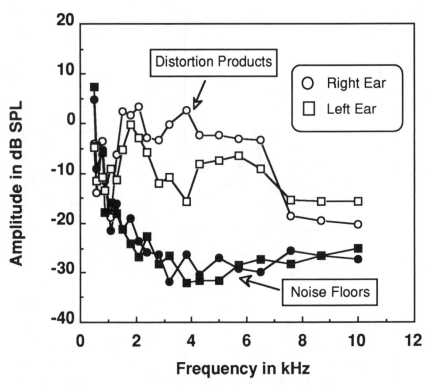

Figure 15–12 *(continued)*

induced loss this degree of loss was sufficient to abolish all DPOAEs, but in the ear with the acoustic tumor distortion-product amplitudes are well above the noise floor. In the face of moderate sensorineural loss, absence of DPOAEs is a cochlear sign, whereas presence of DPOAEs is a neural or retrocochlear sign.

Figure 15–12D shows ABR waveforms for both ears of the tumor patient. On the unaffected right ear the response is well formed. All five waves are present at expected normal latencies. In addition the interpeak latency intervals are normal. The latency interval between waves I and V, for example, is 4.1 msec. The expected normal range for this interval is between 3.6 and 4.4 msec. On the affected left ear, however, there is a marked prolongation of the interval between waves I and V. The observed value of 5.2 msec is well outside the normal range. Such prolongation of interpeak intervals indicates that neural conduction time between the generators respon-

D

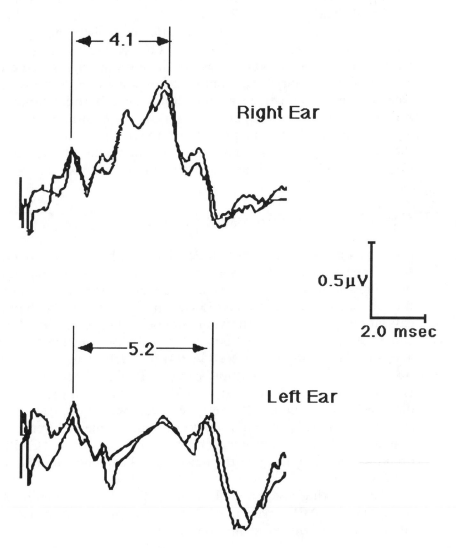

Figure 15–12 *(continued)*

sible for waves I and V is abnormally slowed, a sign of neural rather than sensory disorder. In the case of the patient with noise-induced loss there is no slowing of neural conduction time because the neural structures are not involved.

In summary, the vast majority of sensorineural hearing loss is due to sensory damage within cochlear structures. Air- and bone-conduction curves interweave, speech understanding is predictable from the degree and pattern of sensitivity loss, immittance results are usually within normal limits, otoacoustic emissions are usually abolished, and the ABR is normal. It is the case, however, that a small percentage of sensorineural loss is neural, due to involvement of the auditory nerve. Because such losses may be due to life-threatening causes, it is important to differentiate between sensory and neural loss. In the latter, the air and bone curves will also be interweaving, but on all other measures there will be significant differences from sensory loss. Immittance audiometry may show elevated or absent acoustic reflex thresholds, speech understanding scores may be extremely poor with rollover of PI functions, otoacoustic emissions may be present in spite of sensitivity loss, and the ABR may reflect delayed neural conduction time between auditory nerve and caudal brain stem structures.

Central Auditory Processing Disorder

Some persons with auditory disorders have neither conductive nor sensorineural loss. Auditory sensitivity, the ability to hear very faint pure tones, is not affected. Thus the pure-tone audiograms are quite normal. But, because of damage to the central structures which process auditory input, these individuals appear to have hearing difficulties. In young adults the most common causes of such **central auditory processing disorders** (CAPD) are cerebrovascular insult, trauma to the skull, and multiple sclerosis. In elderly persons there is accumulating evidence that some degree of central processing disorder may accompany the peripheral component of presbyacusis. Finally, there is accumulating evidence that some children with academic achievement problems may suffer from a form of CAPD even though there may be little neurological evidence of obvious brain disease.

The following case studies illustrate audiometric findings in two patients with CAPD, a young adult with multiple sclerosis and an adolescent boy with academic problems.

Case Study 5: CAPD from Multiple Sclerosis

The patient is a 28-year-old woman who was diagnosed with multiple sclerosis at the age of 24. She has visual problems and transient muscle weakness. For the past 2 years she has complained of difficulty in hearing from the right ear. Sounds are described as "muffled" and "far away." There is no obvious problem with the left ear.

Figure 15–13A shows the results of pure-tone and speech audiometry. Hearing sensitivity is well within normal limits and symmetric. There is no obvious hearing sensitivity loss in either ear. The results of speech audiometry show that, on the left ear, PI functions for both words and sentences rise quickly to the 90–100% level and show no significant rollover. On the right ear, however, both PI functions are grossly abnormal. The word function rises to a maximum of only 65%, then rolls over to 35% at the highest speech intensity tested. The sentence function never exceeds 40%. This combination of poor speech understanding and normal auditory sensitivity is one of the characteristic signatures of CAPD. Whenever a person with a normal audiogram complains of difficulty in speech understanding, the possibility of CAPD must be pursued.

Figure 15–13B shows the results of immittance audiometry. Both tympanograms are normal, type A, and static immittance values are within the normal range. On acoustic reflex testing, however, an interesting pattern emerges. Uncrossed reflexes are intact from either ear, but no crossed reflexes can be elicited. This pattern of results is consistent with a lesion in the brain stem in the area of the trapezoid body where the contralateral reflex pathways cross the brain stem. A lesion at this site typically spares the uncrossed reflexes but abolishes the crossed reflexes.

Figure 15–13C shows the results of otoacoustic emission testing. Not unexpectedly, emissions are robust from both ears because this is not a problem at the level of the sensory structures in the inner ear.

Finally, Figure 15–13D shows ABR waveforms. Morphology is somewhat degraded in both ears, but worse in the right ear. On the left ear one can identify waves I, III, and V, but the interpeak interval between waves I and III is abnormally prolonged. The normal expected range for this interpeak interval ranges from 1.6 to 2.4 msec, but in this patient the interval is 3.2 msec. On the right ear, the ear the patient complains about, we can identify wave I, wave II, and perhaps wave III but all later waves have disappeared. This selective loss of late wave is a characteristic ABR finding in disorders involving the auditory pathways in the brain stem.

In summary, this patient with multiple sclerosis shows classic signs of CAPD. The pure-tone audiogram is normal, but there is very poor speech understanding, absence of crossed reflexes, and grossly abnormal ABR.

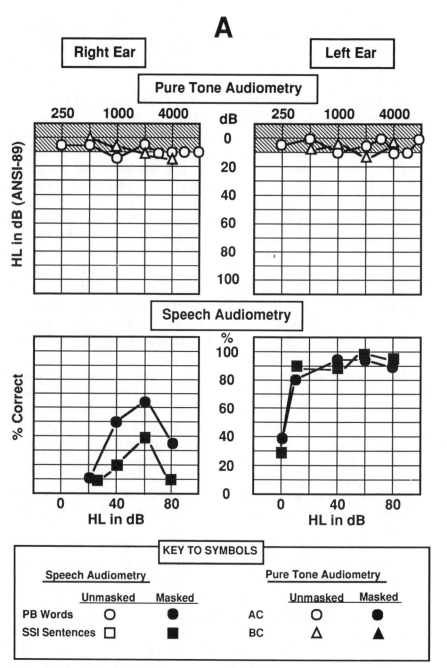

Figure 15–13. Audiometric findings in a 28-year-old woman with multiple sclerosis. **A.** Pure-tone and speech audiometric results. **B.** Immittance results. **C.** Distortion-product otoacoustic emissions. **D.** Auditory brain stem responses. Note deficit in speech understanding in right ear in spite of normal sensitivity for pure tones, a characteristic sign of central processing disorder. Normal otoacoustic emission results, combined with abnormal right ABR (absence of waves IV and V) and absence of crossed acoustic reflexes, indicate that problem is in the lower brain-stem auditory pathways.

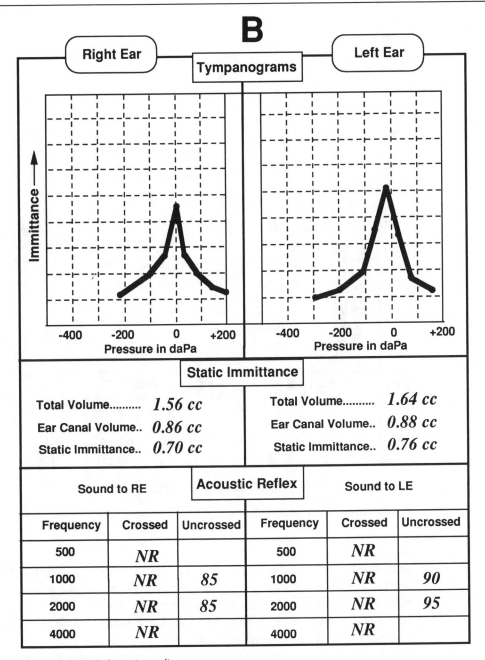

B

| Right Ear | Tympanograms | Left Ear |

Static Immittance

Right Ear	Left Ear
Total Volume.......... *1.56 cc*	Total Volume.......... *1.64 cc*
Ear Canal Volume.. *0.86 cc*	Ear Canal Volume.. *0.88 cc*
Static Immittance.. *0.70 cc*	Static Immittance.. *0.76 cc*

Acoustic Reflex

Sound to RE			Sound to LE		
Frequency	Crossed	Uncrossed	Frequency	Crossed	Uncrossed
500	*NR*		500	*NR*	
1000	*NR*	*85*	1000	*NR*	*90*
2000	*NR*	*85*	2000	*NR*	*95*
4000	*NR*		4000	*NR*	

Figure 15–13 *(continued)*

Case Study 6: CAPD in a Child

The patient is an 11-year-old boy whose parents are concerned about his poor academic achievement. He is repeating the 5th grade and not doing too well. His teacher feels that, at times, he doesn't seem to be hearing everything she says. He misses critical instructions

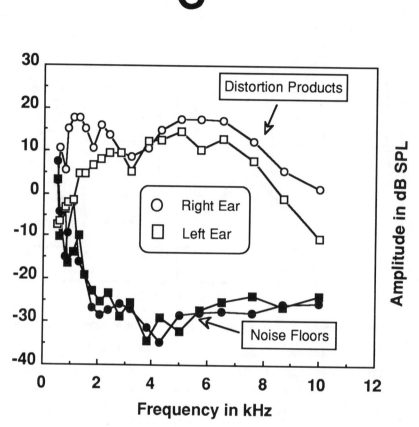

Figure 15-13 *(continued)*

and doesn't seem to be achieving at a level consistent with his potential. His mother wants to be sure that he doesn't have a hearing loss. The boy doesn't think he has a hearing loss but admits that, when the classroom is noisy, he does have trouble following the teacher's instructions and assignments.

Figure 15-14A shows the results of pure-tone and speech audiometry. Air- and bone-conduction thresholds are all within normal limits, but performance on tests of speech understanding is poor. On the right ear, the maximum PB score is a reasonable 86%, but there is considerable rollover of the PI function (30%). The maximum SSI score is only 30%. On the left ear the maximum PB score is 90%, but rollover is 50%. The maximum SSI score is only 45%. This combination of normal pure-tone thresholds and poor performance on tests of speech understanding is strongly suggestive of a central auditory processing deficit.

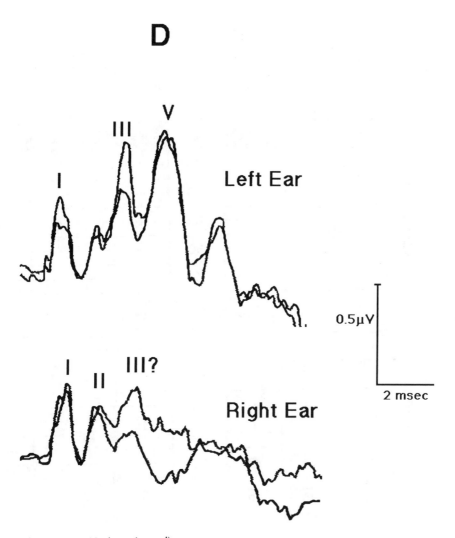

Figure 15-13 *(continued)*

Figure 15–14B summarizes the results of immittance audiometry. All results are within normal limits. Figure 15–14C summarizes DPOAE testing. Again, emissions are robust and well within normal limits. This combination of normal tympanograms, normal acoustic reflexes, and normal otoacoustic emissions rules out middle ear, inner ear, auditory nerve, and lower brain stem disorder. The auditory problem suggested by the poor speech understanding scores must lie at a higher level in the auditory system.

Figure 15–14D shows the results of auditory evoked potential testing. Waveforms are displayed for all three AEPs: the ABR, MLR, and LVR. ABR waveforms are normal. Waves III and V are clearly evident and all interpeak intervals are within normal limits. This re-

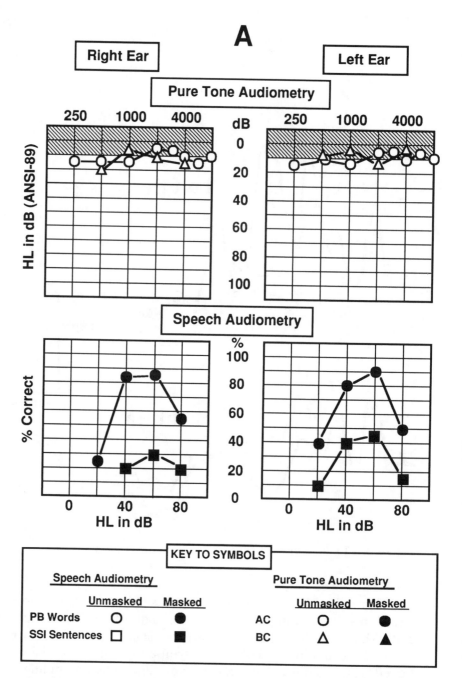

Figure 15-14. Audiometric findings in an 11-year-old boy with central auditory processing disorder of unknown etiology. **A.** Pure-tone and speech audiometric results. **B.** Immittance results. **C.** Distortion-product otoacoustic emissions. **D.** Auditory evoked potentials, including ABR, MLR, and LVR. The combination of normal immittance, normal otoacoustic emissions, and normal ABR, along with abnormal MLR and LVR waveforms, suggests an auditory processing problem at a relatively high brain-stem or cortical level.

B

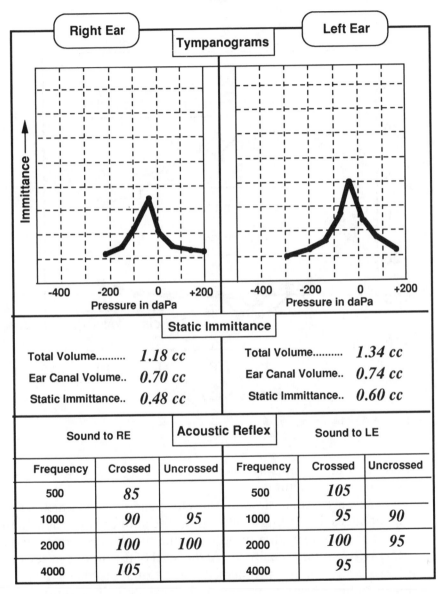

Figure 15–14 *(continued)*

sult is consistent with the acoustic reflex results in ruling out a lower brain-stem site. But both MLR and LVR waveforms are abnormal. Neither the positive peak, P_a of the MLR nor the N_1 and P_2 peaks of the LVR can be identified. These AEP abnormalities are consistent with an auditory disorder at a relatively high level in the

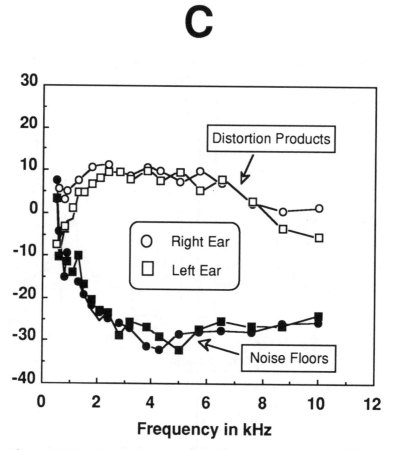

Figure 15-14 *(continued)*

central auditory pathways, perhaps involving auditory cortex and more central structures.

These six case studies show how the pattern of audiometric findings changes depending on the site of the auditory disorder. At the most peripheral site, the middle ear, the problem is largely one of decreased auditory sensitivity. At the level of the inner ear, sensitivity loss is still a major problem, but additional problems in speech understanding begin to appear. At the next level, the auditory nerve, sensitivity loss is no longer the major symptom. Now we find disproportionately poor speech understanding, elevated or absent acoustic reflexes, and prolonged neural conduction time. Finally, at the level of the central auditory pathways, there is no problem at all with auditory sensitivity, but speech understanding is disproportionately even poorer, acoustic reflex abnormalities are unique, and neural conduction time is greatly compromised. There are, in this sense, unique audiometric correlates of the various sites of auditory disorder.

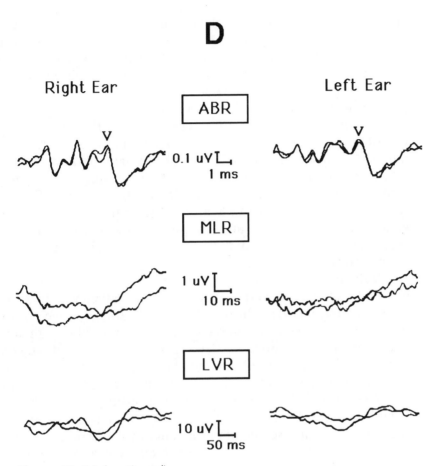

D

Figure 15-14 *(continued)*

◆ AUDITORY REHABILITATION

The most prevalent type of auditory disorder is a loss of hearing sensitivity. If the disorder causing the sensitivity loss cannot be managed by surgery, the most appropriate treatment consists of amplification, followed by some form of aural rehabilitation. The most common form of amplification is the conventional hearing aid. In some cases, other assistive listening devices may be used to supplement or substitute for hearing aid use. In individuals with a profound loss of hearing, a cochlear implant may be appropriate.

Hearing Instruments

The first step in the rehabilitation process is the use of a hearing aid. When hearing aids were first developed, they were relatively large in size and relatively inflexible in terms of their amplifying characteristics. Hearing aid use was restricted almost exclusively to individuals with substantial conductive hearing loss. Today's hearing aids are much smaller in size, and their output characteristics can be programmed at will. Hearing aids are now widely used by persons with sensorineural hearing loss.

Candidacy for amplification is fairly straightforward. If the degree of the patient's hearing impairment is sufficient to cause a communication disorder, the patient is a candidate for amplification. Thus, even if the hearing loss is mild, if it is causing difficulty with communication, the patient is likely to benefit from amplification. If a patient has a conductive hearing loss, it can usually be treated medically or surgically. If all attempts at medical or surgical treatment have been exhausted, the same rule of candidacy as for sensorineural hearing loss applies.

If the patient's hearing loss is about the same in both ears (i.e., bilaterally symmetric), it is desirable to fit the patient with two (binaural) hearing aids. Benefits from binaural hearing aids include improvement in sound localization and hearing speech better in noisy environments. In addition, evidence exists that the use of only one hearing aid in patients with bilateral hearing loss may have a long-term detrimental effect on the ear that is not fitted with an aid.

The process of obtaining hearing aids begins with a thorough audiological assessment. Following this, prudent health care would suggest a medical assessment to rule out any active pathology that might contraindicate hearing aid use. After medical clearance, impressions of the ear and ear canal are made for customizing the hearing aid device. When the device is received from the manufacturer, the hearing aid is adjusted and fitted to the patient, and an evaluation is made of the patient's performance with the aid. After successful fitting and dispensing, several follow-up appointments are usually scheduled to make minor adjustments or discuss any problems related to hearing aid use.

Conventional Hearing Aids

A hearing aid is an electronic amplifier that has three main components: a microphone, an amplifier, and a loudspeaker. The microphone has a diaphragm which moves in response to the pressure waves of sound. As it moves, it converts the acoustic signal into an electric signal. The electric signal is boosted by the amplifier and then delivered to the loudspeaker. The loudspeaker then converts the electric signal back into an acoustic signal to be delivered to the ear. A battery is used to provide power to the amplifier. Most hearing aids have external controls as well, including an intensity control and certain controls for shaping the amplifier's frequency response. Hearing aids may also contain a telephone or t-coil. A **t-coil** allows the hearing aid to pick of electromagnetic signals directly, bypassing the hearing aid microphone. This allows direct input from devices such as telephone receivers.

The three main components of the hearing aid are packaged in several ways. The most common types of conventional hearing aids are known as **behind-the-ear** (BTE), **in-the-ear** (ITE), and **in-the-canal** (canal) **hearing aids**. Examples of these three types are shown in Figure 15–15. In the BTE hearing aid (A) the microphone, amplifier, and loudspeaker are housed in a case that is worn behind the ear. The aid is held in place by a plastic hook that fits over the top of the ear. Amplified sound is delivered to the ear canal through a tube that leads to a custom-fitted earmold. An ITE hearing aid (B) has all of the components contained in a custom-fitted case that fits into the outer ear. A canal hearing aid (C) is a smaller version of the ITE, which fits mostly into the ear canal.

Although the decision on which type of hearing aid to wear may be based on cosmetic considerations, at least three other factors must be considered. First, there is the matter of acoustic feedback. If the amplified sound emanating from a loudspeaker is directed back into the microphone of the same amplifying system, the result is acoustic feedback or whistling of the hearing aid. Most people are familiar with this concept from experiences listening to public address systems. If the amplified sound of a public address system gets routed back into the microphone, a rather loud and annoying "squeal" occurs. One way to control feedback on hearing aids is to separate the microphone and loudspeaker by as much distance as possible. This solution favors the BTE hearing aid, wherein the output of the loudspeaker is in the ear canal and the microphone is behind the ear. Another solution is to attempt to seal off the ear canal so that the amplified sound cannot escape and be re-amplified. The tradeoff here is usually between size of the hearing aid and amount of output intensity that is desired. The higher the intensity of output, the more likely it is that feedback will occur. Thus, if a person has a more severe hearing loss, greater output intensity is required, and greater separation of the microphone and loudspeaker will be necessary. Thus, canal hearing aids are generally used for milder hearing losses and BTE hearing aids for more severe hearing losses. There are two other factors, however. Because the BTE is larger in size, the number and size of electronic components that can be included are greater. Therefore, a BTE hearing aid can provide more sophisticated sound processing than smaller ITE instruments. The final consideration is related to durability of the instruments.

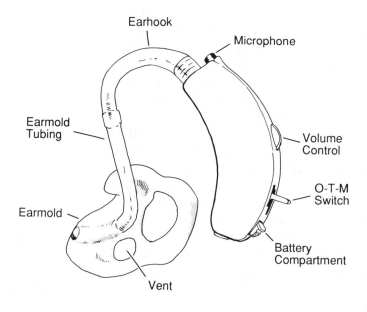

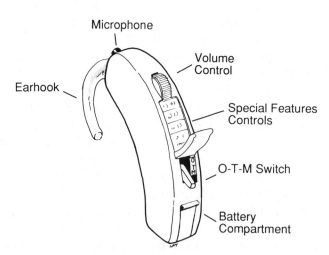

Figure 15–15. The three main types of hearing aids. **A.** Behind-the-ear (BTE), **B.** In-the-ear (ITE), and **C.** In-the-canal (ITC). (From Shimon, D. *Coping with hearing loss and hearing aids.* [1992]. San Diego: Singular Publishing Group, pp. 104, 106, 108. Reprinted with permission.)

In a canal instrument, all of the electronic components are placed in the ear canal and subject to the detrimental effects of perspiration and cerumen. BTE hearing aids, therefore, tend to be more durable.

The acoustic output characteristics of hearing aids are described in terms of amplification gain, frequency response, and output limiting. **Gain** of the hearing aid is the amount of sound that is added

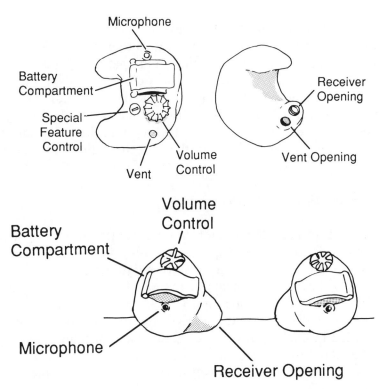

Figure 15-15 *(continued)*

to the input signal. If a speech signal enters the hearing aid at 50 dB and is amplified to 90 dB, the amount of gain is 40 dB. The **frequency response** of a hearing aid is the amount of gain as a function of frequency. Because most hearing losses are greater at some frequencies than at others, the ability to manipulate gain selectivity in different frequency regions is important. **Output limiting** refers to the maximum intensity of the amplified signal. If a signal of 100 dB were delivered to a hearing aid that had 40 dB gain, the output would be 140 dB without output limiting. Such a signal could be very damaging to the cochlea. It is necessary, therefore, to limit the maximum intensity level that the aid can generate.

A hearing aid is selected and fitted based on the individual's degree of hearing loss, the audiometric configuration of the loss, and estimates of the intensity levels at which sound is perceived to be uncomfortably loud. The first step in the selection process is to shape the hearing aid's frequency response to approximate some predetermined target. The target is based on any of a number of rules. In general, these rules state that the amount of gain at a certain frequency should be about one half to one third the number of decibels of the hearing loss at that frequency. Thus, a loss of 60 dB at 2000 Hz would require gain of from 20 to 30 dB at that frequency. The frequency response of the hearing aid is then adjusted to the target. Output limiting is set in relation to the patient's loudness discomfort level. Final verification of the aid's response characteristic is often made by speech audiometry. The patient is tested while wearing the hearing aid and listening to speech signals through loudspeakers. The hearing aid then is adjusted for listening comfort and for optimal performance on the speech audiometric measures.

Assistive Listening Devices

Amplification systems other than conventional hearing aids have been designed for more specific listening situations. These devices are collectively known as **assistive listening devices** or ALDs. Among the devices considered to be ALDs are personal amplifiers, FM systems, telephone amplifiers, and television listeners. In general, these devices are designed to enhance an acoustic signal imbedded in background noise by the use of a remote microphone. Instead of building the microphone into the receiver, it is physically separated from the receiver so that it can be moved closer to the signal source.

At least three categories of patients can benefit from the use of ALDs. One category includes patients who simply do not receive sufficient benefit from conventional hearing aids. As a general rule, individuals who have more severe hearing losses often find that supplementing hearing aid use with ALDs is necessary under certain circumstances. Other individuals, because of communication demands in their work place or social life, welcome the additional use of ALDs. A second category includes individuals who have amplification needs so specific that the general use of a hearing aid is not indicated. For example, some individuals feel that communication problems occur only when viewing television or attending church. For those individuals, an ALD tailored to that particular need is often an appropriate alternative to a conventional hearing aid. A final category is patients who have hearing disorders due to changes in central nervous system function. The resulting central auditory processing disorder is not necessarily accompanied by a loss in hearing sensitivity, but rather is characterized by difficulty in understanding speech in background noise. For these patients, use of a remote microphone for enhancement of signal-to-noise ratio is more appropriate than amplification from a conventional hearing aid.

A **personal amplifier** consists of a microphone that is connected to an amplifier box by a cord. The microphone is usually held by the person who is talking. The signal is then routed to a small box, which is usually about the size of a deck of cards. The box contains the battery, amplifier electronics, and volume control. The loud-speaker is typically a set of lightweight headphones or an ear-bud transducer. By separating the microphone from the amplifier, it can be moved close to the signal of interest. In doing so, the signal-to-noise ratio is enhanced, which can be of great benefit to those with hearing impairment.

Another type of ALD is a **personal FM system**. Such systems carry the concept of the remote microphone a step further. In this case, the microphone is connected to an FM transmitter. Signals are then sent to a receiver via FM radio waves. The person who is talking wears the microphone and transmitter. The listener wears the receiver. The receiver is coupled to the listener's ear via earphones or to hearing aid t-coils via a neck loop that transmits the signal. The advantage of an FM system over a personal amplifier is that the microphone can be moved a significant distance from the listener. This type of system works well in a restaurant, at church, in a class-room, and in similar places.

Other types of ALDs include those used specifically for talking on the telephone or for television viewing. Telephone amplifiers are available in several forms. Some handsets have built-in amplifiers with a volume control. There are also portable telephone amplifiers that can be attached to any telephone. The telephone receiver can also be adapted to transmit over FM waves to a personal FM system. Television listeners are similar in concept to the FM system. In this case, however, the transmitter is connected directly to the television. Audio signals from the television are transmitted, either by FM or by infrared light waves, to a dedicated receiver that is worn by the patient.

Cochlear Implants

Individuals who have severe or profound deafness and who cannot benefit from conventional amplification are candidates for a **cochlear implant**. Profound deafness results from a loss of hair cell function in the cochlea. As a result, neural impulses are not generated, and electrical activity in the auditory nerve is not initiated. A cochlear implant is designed to stimulate the auditory nerve directly. An electrode is surgically implanted into the cochlea. The electrode is attached to an electronic circuit which is implanted in the temporal bone. Acoustic signals are received via a microphone attached to a sophisticated amplifier. The amplifier then sends signals to the electrode via the implanted circuitry. When the electrode receives a signal, it applies an electrical current to the cochlea, thereby stimulating the auditory nerve.

Cochlear implants have been shown to be valuable in two groups of patients. Adults, who have lost their hearing adventitiously, can derive substantial benefit from a cochlear implant, especially as an aid to lipreading. Young children whose hearing loss is too severe to permit significant benefit from conventional hearing aid use can also benefit substantially from a cochlear implant.

Other Devices

Other assistive devices available for individuals with hearing impairment have been designed to replace what is typically an acoustic signal with a different type of signal that can be perceived by one of the other senses. One of the most commonly used assistive device is a text telephone. Communication over the telephone lines is achieved by typing messages. Another type of assistive device is closed captioning of television shows. Closed captioning presents the dialogue of a television show as text along the lower edge of the television screen. Other assistive devices include alerting devices, such as alarm clocks, fire alarms, and doorbells, which are designed to flash a light or vibrate a bed when activated.

Aural Rehabilitation

Adults

Following the completion of hearing aid fitting, a **hearing aid orientation** program is usually implemented. Such a program consists of informational counseling of both the patient and the patient's family. Topic areas include the nature of hearing and hearing impairment, the components and function of the hearing aid, and care and maintenance of the hearing aid. One of the most critical aspects of the hearing aid orientation is a discussion of reasonable expectations of hearing aid use and strategies for adapting to different listening environments. The hearing aid orientation program also provides an opportunity to discuss and demonstrate other assistive devices that might be of benefit to the patient.

In some programs, groups of patients with hearing impairment are brought together for orientation. Such groups serve at least two important functions. First, they provide a forum for expanded dissemination of information to patients and their families. Second, they provide a support group that can be very important for sharing experiences and solutions to problems.

Auditory training and **speechreading** are treatment methods that are sometimes used following the dispensing of hearing aids. Auditory training programs are designed to bring awareness to the hearing task and to improve listening skills. Speechreading, or lip-reading, programs are designed to enhance the skills of patients in supplementing auditory input with information that can be gained from lip movements and facial expressions.

Children

The goal of any treatment program for children is to ensure optimal acquisition of speech and language. In children with mild hearing sensitivity losses, such a goal can be accomplished by the careful fitting of hearing aids, good orientation of parents to hearing loss and hearing aids, and very careful attention to speech and language stimulation during the formative years. For more severe hearing losses, the task is more difficult and the decisions more challenging.

For many years there has been controversy about the best methods of communication development training for children with severe and profound hearing losses. One school of thought champions the **oral approach**, in which the child is fitted with hearing aids, or a cochlear implant, and undergoes very intensive training in oral/aural communication. The goal is to help the child to develop oral skills that will allow for a mainstreamed education and life style. Another school of thought champions the **manual approach**. In the manual approach the child learns sign language as the method of communication. The goal is to help the child develop language through a sensory system that is not impaired. Yet another school of thought champions the idea of combining oral and manual communication in a "**total communication approach**," emphasizing language development without regard to the sensory system. This approach seeks to maximize both language learning and oral communication. Although the topic of education of deaf children has always been controversial, the acrimony among proponents of these differing approaches has grown in recent years with the advent of cochlear implantation. Implants are proving to be a successful alternative to conventional hearing aid use, particularly in terms of ease of learning language. Many individuals who subscribe to the manual philosophy consider such an approach to be near heresy, however, because of their contention that deafness is an attribute not a disorder.

Irrespective of strategy, the most important components of a rehabilitation program are early identification and early intervention. The sooner a child is identified, the sooner the channels of communication required for language development can be opened.

◆ SUMMARY

After a hearing disorder has been identified a number of intervention strategies are available. The most common is the use of a conventional hearing aid or aids. The three main types of conventional aids in current use are BTE (mounted behind the pinna), the ITE (mounted within the auricle), and the canal (fitted entirely within the ear canal). For certain listening situations it is useful to supplement, or even to replace, the conventional aid with an assistive listening device, an amplification system characterized by the fact that the microphone is remote from the receiver for improved signal-to-background-noise ratio. For individuals whose hearing losses are so severe that they do not benefit from conventional amplification systems, the cochlear implant is proving a viable alternative. Other intervention strategies include traditional courses in speechreading and auditory training. Finally, there are special, and frequently controversial, issues associated with intervention strategies for hearing-impaired children.

◆ SUGGESTED READINGS

Hannley, M. (1986). *Basic principles of auditory assessment.* San Diego: College-Hill Press.

Jerger, S., & Jerger, J. (1981). *Auditory disorders.* Boston: Little, Brown.

Martin, F. (Ed.). (1981). *Medical audiology.* Englewood Cliffs, NJ: Prentice-Hall.

Martin, F. (1991). *A study guide: Introduction to audiology* (2nd ed.). Englewood Cliffs, NJ: Prentice-Hall.

Northern, J., & Downs, M. (1991). *Hearing in children* (4th ed.). Baltimore: Williams & Wilkins.

Speaks, C. (1992). *Introduction to sound: Acoustics for the hearing and speech sciences.* San Diego: Singular Publishing Group.

◆ GLOSSARY

Admittance: a technical term quantifying ease of energy flow through a vibratory system. Unit of measure is the acoustic mhO.

Air conduction: a general name for the test paradigm in which sound is presented to the listener via an earphone coupled to the ear.

Assistive Listening Device (ALD): amplification system in which the pick-up microphone is remote from the receiver/amplifier.

Audiogram: a graphic representation of an individual's hearing threshold levels via air- and bone-conduction at various test frequencies. The two ears may be represented on separate graphs or on the same graph.

Auditory Brainstem Response (ABR): a series of 5–7 positive potentials occurring in the first 10 msec after signal onset. Each peak is identified with a specific region of the afferent auditory system, extending from the auditory nerve itself to the medial geniculate body.

Auditory evoked potentials: small electrical potentials superimposed on the steady-state electrical activity of the brain in response to auditory input. Usually detectable only by signal averaging.

Auditory nerve: *See* **Eighth cranial nerve**.

Auditory training: systematic training to improve listening skills.

Basilar membrane: membrane which forms one wall of cochlear partition. Supports organ of Corti.

Bone conduction: a general name for the test paradigm in which sound is presented to the listener via a vibrator coupled to the skull.

BTE: conventional hearing aid mounted "behind-the-ear," between the upper and posterior surfaces of the pinna and the skull.

Central auditory processing: processing of raw sensations into meaningful percepts. Creation of auditory space.

Central Auditory Processing Disorder (CAPD): a disorder in the central processing of auditory input. Manifested by difficulty in understanding speech, especially in difficult listening situations, and difficulty in separating foreground speech targets from background speech competition, usually in spite of normal auditory sensitivity.

Cerumen: a wax-like substance present in the external ear canal.

Cochlea: fluid-filled, membranous structure within the bony labyrinth of the temporal bone. Comprised of three parallel canals: the scala vestibuli, scala media (cochlear partition), and scala tympani. Named for its overall similarity to a snail shell (cochlea in Latin).

Cochlear implant: a personal amplification system in which auditory input is converted to electrical signals which are applied to one or more electrodes implanted within the cochlea.

Cochlear nucleus: nucleus in the lower brain stem where all auditory nerve fibers synapse with second-order neurons of the ascending auditory pathways.

Cochlear partition: one of three canals, or scalae, within the cochlea. Bounded by Reissner's membrane, basilar membrane, and spiral ligament.

Dichotic: two different (uncorrelated) acoustic signals are delivered to the two ears simultaneously.

Dichotic test: a test in which the listener must identify one or both of two dichotically presented signals.

Discrimination score: percent of monosyllabic words correctly repeated when presented at an intensity well above the spondee threshold.

Distortion-Product Evoked Otoacoustic Emissions: acoustic energy created by stimulating the cochlea with two pure tones (f_1 and f_2). As a result of cochlear non-linear processes, energy is created at several frequencies that are combinations of the two stimulating frequencies. The most easily recorded is the $2f_1 - f_2$ distortion product (technically, the cubic distortion product).

Eighth cranial nerve: the cranial nerve subserving hearing and balance. Consists of two branches. The vestibular branch connects the sensory structures in the vestibular labyrinth to the vestibular pathways in the brain. The cochlear branch (auditory nerve) connects the sensory structures in the organ of Corti with the auditory pathways in the brain.

Eustachian tube: tubular structure connecting the nasopharynx with the middle ear.

Evoked Otoacoustic Emissions: faint sounds generated by nonlinear cochlear processes in response to acoustic stimulation. They can be detected by placing sensitive recording equipment within the ear canal.

Frequency: a physical dimension of sound relating to rate of oscillation, measured in cycles per second (Hertz).

Frequency response: relation between amplitude and frequency. In hearing aids, the relation between gain and frequency.

Gain: degree of amplification of a hearing aid. Difference between input intensity and output intensity. Specific to frequency.

Hair cells: hair cells provide the link between mechanical movement of the basilar membrane and excitation of auditory nerve fibers. Small hair-like structures (cilia) protrude from the upper surfaces of the cells. Nerve fibers terminate on the cell bodies. There are three rows of outer hair cells. They are innervated, in complex fashion, by only a small percentage of the totality of available nerve fibers. There is one row of inner hair cells. They are innervated, in relatively point-to-point fashion, by the vast majority (about 95%) of auditory nerve fibers.

Hearing Threshold Level (HTL) or Hearing Level (HL): a decibel scale of sound intensity in which the reference, or zero point, is the intensity corresponding to average normal hearing for the particular acoustic signal under consideration. Usually defined by the mode of the distribution of hearing threshold levels in a sample of the general population of young adults.

Immittance: a general term referring collectively to concepts of admittance and impedance.

Impedance: a technical term quantifying opposition to energy flow through a vibratory system. Unit of measure is the acoustic Ohm.

Incus: second of the three small bones constituting the ossicular chain. Named incus (Latin for anvil) because of its anvil-like shape.

Inner hair cells: *See* **Hair cells**.

Intensity: a physical dimension of sound relating to magnitude, measured either in terms of pressure exerted (Pascals) or energy expended (Watts).

In-the-Canal: conventional hearing aid mounted entirely within the external ear canal.

ITE: conventional hearing aid mounted entirely "in-the-ear," within the auricle.

Late or Vertex Response (LVR): an auditory evoked potential characterized by a negative peak (N_1) at a latency of about 80–100 msec, followed by a positive peak (P_2) at about 170–200 msec.

Loudness: the psychological correlate of intensity.

Malleus: first, or outermost, of the three small bones constituting the ossicular chain. Named malleus (Latin for hammer) because of its hammer-like shape.

Manual approach: educational philosophy for deaf children that emphasizes the use of sign language and finger spelling for the early development of language skills.

Medial nucleus of the trapezoid body: nucleus in the lower brain stem where some second-order neurons synapse with third-order neurons of the ascending auditory pathways. Important region for mediating crossed acoustic reflex.

Medial superior olivary body: nucleus in the lower brain stem where some second-order neurons synapse with third-order neurons of the ascending auditory pathways. Important region for comparing inputs from the two ears.

Middle-Latency Response (MLR): an auditory evoked potential characterized by a positive peak in the latency range from 30–35 msec. Identified with primary auditory cortex.

Oral approach: educational philosophy for deaf children that emphasizes the use of amplification, speech reading, and auditory training to develop oral/aural skills which will encourage a mainstream lifestyle.

Organ of Corti: spiral shaped structure mounted on basilar membrane within the cochlear partition. Contains the inner and outer rows of hair cells.

Ossicular chain: the chain of three ossicles (malleus, incus, and stapes) connecting the tympanic membrane with the cochlea.

Outer hair cells: *See* **Hair cells**.

Output limiting: setting an upper limit to the output of a hearing aid, usually by peak clipping or amplitude compression.

Performance vs. Intensity (PI) function: curve relating percent correct score to speech intensity. Useful for all types of speech test materials. Ordinarily, performance increases monotonically with increasing intensity.

Personal amplifier: assistive listening device in which the remote microphone is hard-wired to the receiver/amplifier.

Personal FM system: assistive listening device in which the remote microphone transmits to the receiver/amplifier via an FM radio wave.

Pitch: the psychological correlate of frequency.

Presbyacusis: the progressive loss in auditory function associated with the aging process. Often misspelled as "presbycusis."

Pure-Tone Average (PTA): average of the hearing threshold levels at 500, 1000, and 2000 Hz. Should agree with the spondee threshold.

Quality: the psychological correlate of spectrum.

Reissner's membrane: membrane which forms one wall of cochlear partition. Separates cochlear partition from scala vestibuli.

Rollover effect: paradoxic decrease in PI function at high speech levels. A characteristic of retrocochlear disorder.

Spectrum: the distribution of intensity across the frequency range.

Speech-Perception-in-Noise (SPIN) Test: a sentence test of suprathreshold speech understanding. Key word is the last word of the sentence. Consists of 50 sentences; 25 in which context helps to identify last word (high context), and 25 in which sentence context is not particularly helpful (low context).

Speech reading: supplementing auditory input with information from lip movements and facial expression.

Spondee threshold: intensity level at which listener correctly repeats 50% of spondee words.

Spondee word: a two-syllable word with equal stress on each syllable. Widely favored for measurement of speech threshold.

Stapes: third, or innermost, of the three small bones constituting the ossicular chain. Named stapes (Latin for stirrup) because of its stirrup-like shape.

Synthetic Sentence Identification (SSI) test: a sentence test of suprathreshold speech understanding. Test sentences were constructed synthetically according to probabilities governing word sequence. A closed set of 10 sentences is presented against a background of continuous speech competition.

T-coil: special hearing aid input channel permitting the aid to pick up electromagnetic signals directly by induction rather than via the microphone. Useful for direct input devices such as telephone receivers.

Tectorial membrane: gel-like layer within the cochlear partition. Cilia of outer hair cells are embedded in the "membrane." Thus, displacement of hair cells results in shearing movement between upper surface of hair cell and tectorial membrane.

Threshold sensitivity: the faintest sound that the patient can just detect. The intensity level below which the patient almost never hears the sound, but above which he or she usually does hear the sound. Defined statistically as the level yielding a correct response on 50% of repeated trials.

Total communication approach: educational philosophy for deaf children that emphasizes language development without regard to sensory system.

Tympanic membrane: a tense, oval-shaped membrane terminating the external ear canal. The chain of ossicles links the tympanic membrane to the fluid system of the inner ear.

Tympanogram: graphic representation of how the immittance of the middle-ear system changes as air pressure is varied in the external ear canal. A dynamic measure of middle-ear function.

Pascal: unit of measure of pressure. Named after the French mathematician, Blaise Pascal.

decaPascal: 10 Pascals.

Ohm: unit of measure of impedance. Named for German scientist George Simon Ohm.

mhO: unit of measure of admittance. The reciprocal of impedance. Therefore Ohm spelled backwards.

millimhO: 1/1000 of a mhO.

Type A: denotes normal tympanogram. Sharply defined peak at or near zero air pressure.

Type B: denotes relatively flattened tympanogram without sharp peak. Usually associated with fluid in the middle-ear space.

Type C: denotes tympanogram in which peak has been shifted significantly in the direction of negative air pressure in the external ear canal. Usually associated with retraction of tympanic membrane due to faulty Eustachian tube function.

Type A$_s$: denotes tympanogram with normal shape but attenuated peak amplitude. Usually associated with increased stiffness of ossicular chain, as in otosclerosis.

Type A$_d$: denotes tympanogram with normal shape but amplified peak amplitude. Usually associated with discontinuity of ossicular chain.

Acoustic reflex: reflexive contraction of stapedius muscles in response to relatively loud sound input.

Stapedius muscle: muscle connecting neck of stapes bone with medial wall of middle ear. Contraction pulls stapes inward, slightly stiffening ossicular chain.

Crossed acoustic reflex: stapedius muscle contraction recorded with sound stimulus to one ear, and immittance recording probe in the other ear.

Uncrossed acoustic reflex: stapedius muscle contraction recorded with sound stimulus and immittance recording probe in the same ear.

A Vision for the Future

FRED D. MINIFIE, PH.D.
RICHARD M. FLOWER, PH.D.

After reading this chapter, you should:

◆ Understand the distinction between clinical and research careers in Communication Sciences and Disorders.

◆ Be aware of career opportunities for speech-language pathologists, audiologists, and communication scientists.

◆ Be able to describe some of the specific research needs in the field of Communication Sciences and Disorders.

◆ Be able to make an informed decision as to whether a career in Communication Sciences and Disorders would be of interest to you.

This chapter discusses the personal attributes necessary for successful clinical careers in speech-language pathology and audiology, or in scientific careers in the discipline of Communication Sciences and Disorders. Readers are informed of outstanding career opportunities available to caring individuals who wish to enter one of the "helping professions" of speech-language pathology or audiology. Similar opportunities are described in the sciences undergirding clinical practice, where innovative problem solvers are needed to advance basic and applied knowledge in the field. Finally, readers are presented with a review of many of the research questions yet to be answered in Communication Sciences and Disorders.

If this book has done its job, it has provided you with an introductory look at the discipline of Communication Sciences and Disorders and the professions of Speech-Language Pathology and Audiology. It now should be clear to you that this field is relatively young as academic disciplines go, having begun in 1926. By comparison to the fields of mathematics, medicine, astronomy, and others that date from prehistory, Communication Sciences and Disorders is a young discipline. It has experienced rapid growth in its youthful existence but still has many areas in which knowledge and growth are yet incomplete. Even though sufficient knowledge has been gained for the establishment of effective programs for the diagnosis and remediation of many speech, language, and hearing disorders, much research must be done and much knowledge must yet be obtained before this field reaches its maturity. Thus, one of the goals of this book is to provoke bright young minds to consider the possibility of embarking on useful careers in Communication Sciences and Disorders.

If you are a "caring person" who honestly wants to be of assistance to other human beings who are in need, perhaps you might want to consider a career as a speech-language pathologist or audiologist. These careers would allow you to provide direct assistance to individuals with communicative impairments. As you have learned from this book communication is the primary avenue through which we, as human beings, are able to find fulfillment in the various aspects of our lives. Communication is the channel through which we reveal ourselves to those around us. For this reason, it is not an overstatement to conclude that human communication is intrinsically tied to our success in the personal, social, business, and spiritual aspects of our lives. In a very real sense, we are what we are able to communicate. For those of us who understand this relationship, it is particularly tragic when we observe someone who experiences a communication disorder, because we understand the profound effects it may have on so many aspects of that person's life. It is reassuring to know that the efforts of speech-language pathologists and audiologists allow many communicatively impaired patients to experience significant changes in their communication abilities — changes that allow them to achieve greater fulfillment in their lives. In this field nothing can be more rewarding, and personally satisfying, than knowing that you have been instrumental in helping someone overcome a communication disorder.

For a clinician to be truly effective in diagnosis and treatment of communication disorders, he or she must have two important characteristics. First, the clinician must "have his or her heart in the right place." That is, the clinician must have a genuine concern for the patient and honestly care whether the patient will improve. Most of us have an intuitive understanding of the positive effects brought about by human caring, but when used in a clinical setting, human caring can take on a powerful role in the success of treatment. In some cases honest human caring plays a primary role in a patient's improvement. Perhaps no force is greater than human caring in a clinical setting because it creates a proper atmosphere for acceptance and change.

The second characteristic of effective clinicians is that they must have a firm knowledge of communication disorders and their treatment. Effective clinicians must understand: (1) the nature of normal human communication, (2) the nature of communication disorders, and (3) the effects of specific treatments on the communication abilities of patients with specific communicative disorders. Because communication disorders are extraordinarily complicated, the clinician's need for new information is never ending.

You learned in Chapter 1 that in 1994 the entry level credential for clinical practice as a speech-language pathologist or audiologist is awarded following a Clinical Fellowship Year after completion of a master's degree in speech-language pathology or audiology. It is fair to say that in these fields a master's level of academic preparation provides only the foundation for lifelong learning. Indeed, most clinical practitioners continue to participate in programs of lifelong learning to ensure that their knowledge is current and appropriate. What does it take to be successful as a clinician? Considering the wide range of intellectual challenges in Communication Sciences and Disorders, it is not surprising that a wide range of individuals have been successful in this field. But the persons who are most successful in clinical careers in speech-pathology or audiology usually are compassionate human beings, who are self-starters, and are intellectually and emotionally capable of applying knowledge creatively in clinical settings.

On the other hand, if you have an interest in one or more of the topic areas discussed in this book, but harbor thoughts about contributing new information to the "knowledge of our times," perhaps you might want to consider a career in research in some aspect of Communication Sciences and Disorders. Those interests can often be combined with interests that lead to a career in academic teaching at the college or university level. The development of the scholarly credentials necessary to embark on a research career usually involves completion of a doctoral degree (Ph.D.) and may require special postdoctoral research experience. Of course, it is possible to combine clinical and research interests in a career. Scientists with applied research interests are in high demand in this field. Students contemplating the pursuit of a doctoral education in Communication Sciences and Disorders should recognize that, as in other scholarly research careers, only the best students are admitted, but the rewards and personal fulfillment are great for those who complete Ph.D. programs in this field.

◆ PREPARING FOR THE FUTURE

For any scientific or clinical field to survive, it is imperative that its members engage in activities designed to provide new understandings of the theories embraced by the discipline, develop new theories, and apply the new information to previously unresolved problems in the field. These are the characteristics of growing and vital disciplines that are actively preparing for the future. It would be a tragic mistake for specialists in Communication Sciences and Disorders to fail to recognize that there are rapid advances in basic knowledge occurring in many related fields. Knowledge will not stand still. So the reality is that scientific disciplines and professional fields, if they are to survive, must actively contribute to the "knowledge of the times" and not merely be "users of current knowledge." The sad but historically proven fact is that fields that choose simply to use the knowledge of their day, soon become slaves to yesterday's knowledge and yesterday's technologies. Thus, in our rapidly changing world of science, it is imperative that the field of Communication Sciences and Disorders take control of its future by developing the knowledge base necessary for the delivery of clinical services in the future. What we choose to do in the immediate time ahead will determine the long-range viability of our discipline.

How can (should) the field of Communication Sciences and Disorders prepare for the future? If we are to develop our clinical science, most certainly we must develop a cadre of clinical scientists. What kind of scientists do we need? How many will be needed?

These are among the genuine imponderables that currently face this field. We cannot say with surety what type of scientists we need, because we don't know what type of science will be needed during the next decades. But if we were to list the wide range of scientists that could be used by this field, it would include: neuroscientists, linguists, physiologists, acousticians, psychoacousticians, otolaryngologists, audiologists, speech-language pathologists, developmental psychologists, learning specialists, geneticists, voice specialists, gerontologists, specialists in early childhood, electrical engineers, computer scientists, and others. No two scientists are alike.

From a distance science can be organized into a coherent framework, but in practice, research is as varied as the approaches of individual researchers.

The National Academy of Sciences, *On Being a Scientist*, 1989 (p. 2)

Scientists are people of very dissimilar temperaments doing different things in different ways. Among scientists are collectors, classifiers, and compulsive tidiers-up; many are detectives by temperament and many are explorers; some are artists and others are artisans. There are poet-scientists and philosopher-scientists and even a few mystics.

Sir Peter Medawar, *The Art of the Soluble*, 1967 (p. 132)

I cannot guess at the things we will need to know from science to get through the time ahead, but I am willing to make a prediction about the method: we will not be able to call the shots in advance. We cannot say that we need this sort or that sort of technology, therefore we should be doing this sort or that sort of science. It does not work that way. We will have to rely, as we have in the past, on science in general, and on basic undifferentiated science at that, for the new insights that will open up new opportunities for technological development. Science is useful, indispensable sometimes, but whenever it moves forward, it does so by producing a surprise; you cannot specify the surprise you

(continued)

> *would like. Technology should be watched closely, monitored, criticized, even voted in or out by the electorate, but science itself must be given its head if we want it to work.*
>
> Lewis Thomas, M.D., *Late Night Thoughts on Listening to Mahler's Ninth Symphony*, 1984 (p. 28)

As diverse and idiosyncratic as are the sciences underlying human communication and its disorders, there are some issues on which we can agree. First, we can agree that scientific knowledge emerges from a process that is intensely human, with all of the foibles, virtues, and limitations imposed by humanity. Indeed, it might be surprising to some readers to learn that progress in Communication Sciences and Disorders, as in other scientific disciplines, is sometimes not so much the product of scientific investigation as it is the product of value-laden judgments, personal desires, and even a researcher's personality and style. This is true of progress in the basic areas of science as well as in the clinical sciences. They are all human processes.

When scientific knowledge moves ahead most rapidly, it is characterized by research that is theory-driven. Scientists seem to be most productive when they engage in systematic, thematic, and programmatic research missions. In this way, the scientist can delve in depth with issues in a narrow range of endeavor. When this proven formula for success as a scientist is followed, the scientist knowingly runs the risk of becoming so narrow in focus that she or he may lose sight of the general applicability of the knowledge gained in her or his research. The trick is to keep a balanced perspective. Is it possible to realize the more rapid gains achieved through a focused program of research, while keeping the broad needs of the field in perspective?

Elizabeth Kennan argues that university training programs are exemplified by a

> *retreat into smaller truths, the truths of various disciplines — content to ignore, whenever possible, those of our neighbors. Our professional fragmentation has suited the professional ambitions of our students. They have been left largely to pursue their specific interests without larger requirements, which is to say that they have studied the skills and techniques by which they hope to earn a living.*
>
> Elizabeth Kennan, "Liberal Education in a Post Modern World," 1989 (p. 33)

Roger Sale, in his 1989 essay "A Mind Lively and at Ease," presents the premise that

> Many academic disciplines have become so overwhelmed by the narrowness of their ideas that many of the professors are apt to say "There is just too much to know. I can only know a tiny bit of it." Thus, it is that in a university it is often knowledge that enslaves; when one is paralyzed by "all there is to know" one is thinking of knowing only as a matter of knowing expertly. Such a paralysis may drive one to more expert knowledge, but it will not lead to freedom. (p. 11)

In preparing for the future of Communication Sciences and Disorders, what is best course to follow? Should the field attempt to develop expert knowledge? Breadth of knowledge? How will future practitioners and researchers appreciate the contributions of their colleagues if they are trained so narrowly that they know only one small area?

We want you, as a reader, to consider the question of how to best prepare for the future of Communication Sciences and Disorders by thinking about two examples used by futurist Joel Barker in his video tape entitled "Discovering the Future: The Business of Paradigms." Those of you who have seen the popular video tape will already know that Joel Barker was heavily influenced by Thomas Kuhn's (1970) book *The Structure of Scientific Revolutions*. Indeed, Barker's use of the concept of paradigms directly stems from that influence. Two of his examples may help us understand a basic crisis that must be faced by all businesses, organizations, academic institutions, scientific disciplines, and clinical professions.

The first example is from the world of watchmaking. If asked what country in the world produced the most watches in 1965, you would likely respond, Switzerland. Indeed, in 1965 the watchmakers in Switzerland had a dominating 68% share of the world market. If you were to ask which country in the world produces the most watches in the 1990s, the answer would be Japan. In 1992, Switzerland held only a small (8%) share of the world market. What caused the change? Joel Barker provides a review of the chain of events in his video tape. We will paraphrase his commentary. Barker indicated that in 1968, there was a young scientist working in a research laboratory in a watch manufacturing company. The young man came up with a new idea about how to measure time. In his design, he used a quartz crystal and an electronic circuit that provided a much more precise measurement of time than did the elegant mechanical watches of the day which were designed to work with springs and gears. The young scientist took his idea to the owner of the watch manufacturing company where he was employed. He showed the owner his new idea and explained its operation. We do not know what the owner of the company said to the employee, except that he indicated that electronic watches were not the future of the watchmaking industry. He turned away his employee to think about other ideas. In fact, the watch manufacturer thought so little of the idea that he did not even seek to protect it with a patent. Because it was a novel idea, the owner permitted his company to display it at the next annual world exhibition of new watches. Interested observers from Seiko and Texas Instruments visited the exhibit area, and the rest is history. The employee had invented the concept of the liquid crystal that revolutionized the watchmaking industry. It is interesting to note that the employee worked for a Swiss watch manufacturer, so the idea could have propelled the Swiss into a new era of watchmaking that could have allowed them to become even more dominant in market share. However, because the owner of the company was so married to the paradigm of watch making that had served the Swiss so well in the past, he had blinders on when it came to seeing the value of a new idea.

The second example is a comparison of products manufactured in Japan in the 1950s with those manufactured in Japan in the 1990s. Typical American descriptors of Japanese products in the 1950s and early 1960s included such terms as "cheap, imitation, poor quality, low cost, junk," and so forth. In the 1990s typical descriptors included terms like "high cost, high quality, top-of-the-line," and "innovative"; and Japanese businesses were described with terms like "good management" and "dominant market share." In many cases the 1990's descriptors are complete opposites of the earlier ones. What happened? Something changed? Japanese businessmen implemented good management practices, and turned their businesses around; as a result their economy thrived, and Japan became a dominant economic world power. The impressive observation is that the Japanese realized that they needed to change and systematically went about overhauling their system of operation. They took control of their future by actively changing their assumptions and their practices.

Now, you may ask, what have these two examples to do with preparing for the future of the discipline of Communication Sciences and Disorders. The first example speaks to the issue of complacency and commitment to the status quo. The crisis that revolutionized the world of watchmaking is not too much different from the situation facing Communication Sciences and Disorders. As we indicated earlier in this chapter, this is a young field with many questions yet to be answered. Even though we have made great progress in this field since its inception, we must ask ourselves, "What changes need to be made today to ensure the continuance of this field and strengthen its future effectiveness in delivery of clinical services?" The second example speaks to how thoughtful changes can be instituted that can reshape and strengthen the business in which we are engaged. The example of Japanese business informs us that if we make thoughtful changes now, we can augur the future of the discipline.

At the conclusion of this book, we want to leave you with the question that Joel Barker leaves with his audiences. "What is it that is not now known, that if known would forever change the nature of your field?" Answering that question might lead you as a student into a productive new career. It could lead you into innovative and ground breaking patterns of clinical practice. It could lead you into a research career that would allow you to really make a difference by providing new knowledge. You might make the next important breakthrough in this field. The important point is, you should attempt to answer the question. Ask yourself, "Is there an important role for me in the field of Communication Sciences and Disorders?"

◆ RESEARCH: LOOKING TO THE FUTURE

We know that there are many answers to the question just asked. We won't pretend that we can answer the question for you. But we do want to provide you with a list of sample topics that need additional research as we prepare for the future. Think about these topics and add to the list as you continue your studies in this field. Hopefully, many of these issues will disappear from the list as they are addressed and answered by research.

Every provider of services to children and adults with speech, language, and hearing disorders is constantly plagued with unanswered questions — questions about the essential nature of communication processes, the identification and accurate description of communication disorders, and the most effective means of treating communication disorders. Those questions are at once a source of constant frustration and unceasing and intriguing challenges. In reality, therefore, every student of the discipline of Communication Sciences and Disorders is a constant seeker of answers to unanswered questions. Some speech-language pathologists and audiologists deal with questions as best they can in the day-to-day provision of clinical services. Others spend significant portions of their careers conducting formal research studies.

Research relating to the discipline of Communication Sciences and Disorders involves the efforts of scientists representing many different disciplines. Anatomists study structural characteristics of the organs that serve communication. Physiologists and neuroscientists study the processes involved in speech, language, and hearing. Linguists study the nature of languages and examine questions related to language acquisition and use. Psychologists study various issues related to communication behaviors. Often speech-language pathologists, audiologists, and speech and hearing scientists collaborate with these researchers, lending their special expertise to the research. But many speech-language pathologists, audiologists, and speech and hearing scientists conduct independent research seeking new information about human communication and communication disorders.

Few fields confront as many difficulties in conducting meaningful research. Of the many challenges to researchers in Communication Sciences and Disorders, two are particularly notable. First is the extreme complexity of human communication and its sensitivity — at any given moment — to a vast array of influences. Thus it becomes very difficult to isolate discrete elements for controlled studies. For example, in studying children's language, a researcher must account for all of the social and developmental factors that influence language acquisition and for all of the factors that may affect children's language comprehension and use in the particular situation in which data are gathered. Thus, designing research in this field is an extremely difficult task, and one must also use great caution in interpreting the implications of whatever findings emerge.

Second, important insights into many human functions and behaviors come from the study of animal models. However, except for some helpful information about hearing and some limited insights into certain anatomic and physiologic aspects of other communication processes, research involving animal models has limited applicability in the discipline of human communication and communication disorders. Despite these formidable obstacles, each year sees the emergence of some answers that may have immediate, or eventual application to the treatment of children and adults with speech, language, and hearing disorders.

Basic Research

For our purposes, basic research in this field can be defined as research that seeks to understand the myriad physiologic and behavioral factors that serve human communication. Such research may examine specific aspects of the anatomic structures involved in speech, language, and hearing and the essential physiology that serves those processes. For example, basic research studies may examine the structure and function of the auditory system, the component parts of the speech mechanism, or the structure and function of the areas of the brain responsible for directing communication processes. The 1990s have been termed the "Decade of the Brain" to focus attention on research on the sensory, motor, and cognitive functions of the brain. Perhaps no other area of research in communication sciences and disorders is potentially as important as research on the relationship between the structure and function of the brain and communication.

In recent years, substantial advances have been made in the technologies available for basic anatomic and physiologic research, in particular, technologies that are not invasive and permit detailed observation without disturbing normal function. Among these technologies are a variety of imaging techniques that permit studies of brain function and studies of movement of the structures — the larynx, the tongue, the soft palate — involved in speech production. Electrophysiologic technologies permit assessment of neural functions involved in hearing and the execution of speech movements through measuring the electrical activity generated by the central nervous system. New computer technologies have refined our ability to analyze the acoustic characteristics of speech and enabled us to conduct studies through devising models of speech and language comprehension and production.

Other basic research in human communication is essentially behavioral. It examines issues related to normal speech and language acquisition in children and the behaviors that comprise adult communication. This research examines such areas as the precursors of language during the first year of life, characteristics of children's speech and language at various stages of development, and relationships between the development of speech and language and social and cognitive development. As discussed in Chapters 3 and 5 by Kuhl and Bloom, there are many basic questions yet to be answered about the nature of development in speech perception and cognition.

On the other end of the age spectrum, we confront many unanswered questions about the relationship between structural and functional changes in aging individuals and their abilities to communicate. These issues are of considerable importance in understanding the nature of communication disorders among the elderly. The future undoubtedly will see rapid growth in concern for gerontologic communication disorders. The demographic data about the "graying of America" as the population becomes progressively older due to improved health care, fewer births, and so on, are undeniable. This leads to the logical conclusion that more communication disorders among older citizens will be seen in our patient caseloads than in the past. Thus, in the future this field is likely to be more concerned with mature communicators than it has in the past —

examining differences among speakers of different languages, characteristics of ordinary exchanges of information, factors that influence listener perceptions, and so on.

Members of the lay public often question the relevance of basic research because it sometimes has no immediate application to practical problems. For example, federal granting agencies are often challenged for their support of research that seems to deal exclusively with abstract, and even esoteric, questions. Yet the practical questions that trouble us often cannot be answered until we have a clearer understanding of normal human physiology and behavior. Better understanding of the diagnosis and treatment of communication disorders must often await better overall understanding of human communication.

Research on the Nature of Communication Disorders

Although we have accumulated considerable information about many types of communication disorders, a host of unanswered questions remain. Hearing loss is probably better understood than most communication disorders. Reasonably accurate methods are available to locate the site of the impairment responsible for the hearing loss in the auditory system. The severity of the loss can usually be measured in objective terms. The degree to which the underlying pathology can be treated medically is also reasonably well understood. Nevertheless many important questions remain unanswered.

Hearing losses that arise within the ear itself or in the peripheral nervous system are fairly well understood. But much less is known about the auditory problems that presumably result elsewhere in the auditory system. For example, relatively little is known about the implications of impairment to the auditory centers of the brain. Newly available technologies may facilitate important research in this area.

Despite the understanding we have acquired about the essential characteristics of hearing loss, there also are many unanswered questions about its social and developmental implications. These questions often are more important to clinical audiologists than are questions regarding essential pathology. Physiologically similar hearing impairments may have vastly different implications for different individuals. For example, hearing losses of the same kind and degree may influence development and learning in quite disparate ways in different children. Similarly, the social impact of hearing losses of the same magnitude will vary considerably from one adult to another. Answering some of these questions can have far-reaching implications for treatment planning.

A host of unanswered questions remain with respect to language disorders in both children and adults. Some children seem to encounter formidable problems in language acquisition, but for the most part the causes of those problems are unknown. We have only rudimentary understanding of the relationship between problems in early language development and overall cognitive development. Much more needs to be known, for example, about the relationship between problems in the acquisition of spoken language during the preschool years and later problems in the acquisition of written language skills.

We know that head injuries and strokes produce language impairments in adults, but we have limited understanding of the neurophysiologic bases of those impairments. Substantial differences occur between individuals in the recovery of language following insults to the central nervous system. Once again, our understanding of these differences is fragmentary at best.

Considerable research has been devoted to the problems some children encounter in acquiring the sound system of spoken language (i.e., in the acquisition of phonology). Presumably there are characteristic differences that can be classified and, hence, offer helpful guides for treatment; but much more research must be conducted to refine these classifications.

Stuttering has been more intensively researched than many speech disorders, yet, in many respects, it is one of the least understood. Does it represent a single diagnostic entity or is it merely the most apparent symptom of very different essential pathologies? Is stuttering a manifestation of fundamental organic differences in the central nervous system, or is it a learned behavior? These are among the many questions that undoubtedly will occupy researchers for some time to come.

New technologies are facilitating new research directions in the field of voice disorders. It is now possible to observe components of voice production much more precisely and hence identify more discretely the factors that account for aberrant voices. How stable are these acoustic measures of vocal function? Can they be applied usefully to the analysis of voice disorders? Are there special conditions that must be met before the data gathered can be of clinical value?

Not only do unanswered questions abound with respect to the communication disorders that are familiar to most speech-language pathologists and audiologists, but each year sees the addition of new challenges. Advances in medicine have resulted in the survival of once fatal conditions in high-risk newborns and in adults with massive strokes and head injuries, accounting for new populations of children and adults with communication disorders. The proliferation of substance abuse among pregnant women has produced a new group of children with developmental problems. A high proportion of patients with Human Immunodeficiency Virus (HIV) disease experience some kind of communication disorder during the course of that disease. If, as seems likely, HIV infection becomes a chronic, but manageable, condition, speech-language pathologists and audiologists may see a substantial new, but little-understood patient population. Therefore, even though answers may be found to the questions that have plagued us for many years, new questions are constantly emerging.

Research in Diagnosis

The findings of research about the nature of communication disorders obviously have implications for development of approaches to diagnosis. There are, nevertheless, important areas for research that relate specifically to diagnosis.

The major goal of research related to diagnosis is to evolve methods for the accurate description of communication disorders and to achieve information that will be helpful in planning treatment and formulating prognoses. There are also important secondary considerations. To be useful, diagnostic methods must be applicable within the practical limitations of clinical programs. Economic considerations are particularly important. Methods must not be so demanding of time or require such costly technologies that they cannot be applied in most settings. Furthermore, we must constantly ask whether the information yielded justifies the investment required.

During the past six decades excellent research has produced invaluable approaches to the description of hearing impairment. Nevertheless, unmet needs remain (e.g., for new and refined techniques for the assessment of hearing in infancy; more accurate description of impairments at higher levels in the auditory neural system, and more precise description of social handicaps incurred by hearing loss in an individual patient).

We have already noted that new technologies for acoustic analysis and for visualizing voice and speech production have made major contributions to the understanding of communication disorders. The application of these technologies in clinical diagnostic protocols is also an important and potentially productive area for research.

Test construction, particularly for the assessment of language disorders, is also a crucial endeavor. Among the important considerations are devising testing methods that accurately characterize a subject's real-life communication and methods that permit the assessment of actual language abilities without the undue influence of social and ethnic factors.

Thus far, too little research has been devoted to the validation of prognoses formulated on the basis of various diagnostic protocols. The economic realities of all health and human services fields are resulting in increasing limitations on which patients can be served. It is essential, therefore, that we refine our ability to predict the outcomes of whatever services are available.

Treatment Research

Treatment Research is concerned with such issues as the determination of whether providing treatment influences the acquisition or recovery of communication skills and the comparison of one approach to treatment with another. This is one of the most difficult types of research any investigator can pursue. Treatment programs are affected by all manner of influences. Therefore, it is extremely difficult to design research to ensure that whatever changes occur are indeed the result of whatever treatment is provided. Despite complexities, this area of research is crucial.

New technologies also have opened new opportunities for treatment research. For example, currently available equipment for the visual display of speech and voice characteristics may assist in improving the speech production of children and adults with profound hearing impairments and in the treatment of individuals with voice disorders. Computer programs can be devised to provide the intensive and expanded practice that most patients require for the acquisition or recovery of certain speech and language competencies. Studies of the application of these technologies have important implications for drawing conclusions about the effectiveness of various approaches to treatment. But they also have important economic implications: Do they enable speech-language pathologists and audiologists to use their time more efficiently in conducting treatment programs?

Other important areas of treatment research involve the collaboration with members of other professions. Frequently the total treatment program for children and adults with speech, language, and hearing disorders requires the collaboration of different specialists. For example,

◆ Many otolaryngologists and pediatricians believe that conservative approaches are preferable in the medical treatment of middle ear infections in children. Yet the use of these approaches may mean that a hearing loss is present for many weeks, or even months. Audiologists and speech-language pathologists are often concerned about the effects of such hearing losses on children's development and learning. This is an important area for collaborative research.

◆ The treatment of speech problems of children with cleft palate involves the close cooperation of many specialists, particularly surgeons, dentists, and speech-language pathologists. Many questions surround the comparative effectiveness of various approaches to treatment, the circumstances in which those approaches should be applied, and the sequence in which different steps in treatment should occur.

◆ There is preliminary — and fragmentary — evidence that certain drugs may facilitate language recovery in adults who have suffered strokes. Studies in this area require the collaborative efforts of neurologists, pharmacologists, and speech-language pathologists.

Research on Prostheses

Most people think of prostheses as mechanical devices to replace missing arms or legs. Actually, the term more broadly applies to all devices designed to compensate for impaired functions. Hearing aids probably represent the most familiar prosthetic devices in the field of communication disorders. Continuing research must be directed toward improving hearing aid performance and increasing precision in the selection of appropriate amplification for individual hearing aid users. Recently, "programmable" hearing aids have been developed which permit the user to modify the response of an aid to adapt to the situation in which it is being used.

In the past decade intensive research has resulted in the development of electronic devices that may be implanted surgically to provide direct stimulation to the auditory nerve in individuals with profound hearing impairments. Although there is a fairly substantial body of research regarding the use of these devices by adults with acquired hearing disorders, thus far there has been only limited study of their use by deaf children.

Prosthetic appliances may also be used by children and adults with speech disorders. When cleft palate or craniofacial defects cannot be corrected surgically, prosthetic appliances may be used to compensate for those defects. Appliances may also be used by patients who have suffered the loss of essential tissues and structures through cancer surgery. For example, cancer of the larynx may require surgical removal of the voice-producing mechanism, necessitating the use of a prosthetic appliance for voice production.

Some of the most intriguing research in recent years has focused on the development of so-called alternative and augmentative communication devices. Many of these devices are based on computer technologies. Children and adults who are unable to produce intelligible speech — usually because of severe neuromuscular problems — may use these devices to communicate successfully. Here is another example where advances in technology offer new and exciting opportunities for research in communication sciences and disorders and, ultimately, for improved treatment of children and adults with speech, language, and hearing disorders.

Students interested in exploring careers in science might be intrigued by the recent book *Complexity: The Emerging Science at the Edge of Order and Chaos* by M. Mitchell Waldrop (1992). You may discover, as have the authors of this chapter, that knowledge in fields such as this is self-organizing. The development of new information is not random and offers extraordinary challenges to scientists interested in describing its complex patterns of organization.

✦ CONCLUSION

Having just surveyed the many areas in which new information would prove helpful in advancing the quality of clinical practices in speech-language pathology and audiology, we have only scratched the surface. It is time to acknowledge that much more needs to be learned in this field. On the one hand, that may indicate that the field is not yet mature; on the other hand, it indicates that there are many opportunities for persons who are just entering the field. Is there a role for you in this field? That depends! How much do you wish to take control of your future? As the old General Electric TV commercial used to say: "The future is for those who prepare for it."

✦ REFERENCES

Barker, J. (1989). *Discovering the future: The business of paradigms.* [Videotape] Minneapolis/St. Paul: Charthouse International Learning Corporation.

Kennan, E. (1989). Liberal education in a post-modern world. In H. Costner (Ed.), *New perspectives on liberal education* (pp. 25–39). Seattle: University of Washington Press.

Kuhn, T. S. (1970). *The structure of scientific revolutions* (2nd ed.). Chicago: University of Chicago Press.

Medawar, P. B. (1967). *The art of the soluble.* London: Methuen.

National Academy of Sciences. (1989). *On being a scientist.* Washington DC: National Academy Press.

Sale, R. (1989). A mind lively and at ease. In H. Costner (Ed.), *New perspectives on liberal education* (pp. 3–23). Seattle: University of Washington Press.

Thomas, L. (1984). *Late night thoughts on listening to Mahler's Ninth Symphony.* New York: Bantam Books.

Waldrop, M. M. (1992). *Complexity: The emerging science at the edge of order and chaos.* New York: Simon & Schuster.

INDEX

INTRODUCTION TO

Communication Sciences and Disorders

EDITED BY
Fred D. Minifie, Ph.D.

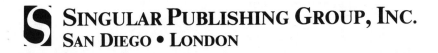

SINGULAR PUBLISHING GROUP, INC.
SAN DIEGO • LONDON

Singular Publishing Group, Inc.
401 West "A" Street, Suite 325
San Diego, California 92101-7904

19 Compton Terrace
London, N1 2UN, U.K.

e-mail: singpub@mail.cerfnet.com
Website: http://www.singpub.com

Typeset in 11/13 Times by CFW Graphics
Printed in the United States of America by McNaughton & Gunn

Library of Congress Cataloging-in-Publication Data

Introduction to communication sciences and disorders / edited by Fred
    D. Minifie.
       p.   cm.
    Includes bibliographical references and index.
    ISBN 1–56593–202–1
    1. Communicative disorders.   I. Minifie, Fred D.
    [DNLM: 1. Communicative Disorders. 2. Communication. WL 340
  I617 1994]
    RC423.I556   1994
    616.85'5—dc20
    DNLM/DLC
    for Library of Congress   94–3135
                                                         CIP

INTRODUCTION TO

Communication Sciences and Disorders

Microsoft®
Exchange Server 2003
UNLEASHED

Rand H. Morimoto, MCSE
Kenton Gardinier, MCSE, CISSP, MCSA
Michael Noel, MCSE+I, MCSA
Joe R. Coca Jr., MCSE

SAMS   800 East 96th Street, Indianapolis, Indiana 46240

Microsoft Exchange Server 2003 Unleashed

Copyright © 2004 by Sams Publishing

International Standard Book Number: 0-672-32581-0

Library of Congress Catalog Card Number: 2003111834

Printed in the United States of America

First Printing: December 2003

06   05   04   03   4   3   2   1

Trademarks

All terms mentioned in this book that are known to be trademarks or service marks have been appropriately capitalized. Sams Publishing cannot attest to the accuracy of this information. Use of a term in this book should not be regarded as affecting the validity of any trademark or service mark.

Warning and Disclaimer

Every effort has been made to make this book as complete and as accurate as possible, but no warranty or fitness is implied. The information provided is on an "as is" basis. The authors and the publisher shall have neither liability nor responsibility to any person or entity with respect to any loss or damages arising from the information contained in this book.

Bulk Sales

Sams Publishing offers excellent discounts on this book when ordered in quantity for bulk purchases or special sales. For more information, please contact

U.S. Corporate and Government Sales
1-800-382-3419
corpsales@pearsontechgroup.com

For sales outside of the U.S., please contact

International Sales
1-317-428-3341
international@pearsontechgroup.com

Associate Publisher
Michael Stephens

Acquisitions Editor
Neil Rowe

Development Editor
Mark Renfrow

Managing Editor
Charlotte Clapp

Project Editor
Sheila Schroeder

Copy Editor
Nancy Albright

Indexer
Larry Sweazy

Proofreader
Juli Cook

Technical Editor
James V. Walker, MCSE

Publishing Coordinator
Cindy Teeters

Interior Designer
Gary Adair

Cover Designer
Gary Adair

Page Layout
Susan Geiselman
Kelly Maish

Contributing Writers
Amanda Acheson, MCSE
Brian Peladeau, MCSE, CCNA
Chista Ashti, MCP, MCSE, CCNA
Chris Amaris, MCSE, CISSP, CCNA
Colin Spence
Ed Roberts, Windows Server
2003 MVP
Ilya Eybelman, MCSD, MCSE
Jeff Guillet, MCSE, MCP+I
Kathi Honegger
László Somi, CISSP, MCSE, MCNE
Peter Handley, CDE, MCSE

Contents at a Glance

Table of Contents

Foreword

About the Authors

Rand H. Morimoto, MCSE   Rand Morimoto has been in the computer industry for over 25 years and has authored, co-authored, or been a contributing writer for over a dozen books on Windows 2003, Security, Exchange 2000, BizTalk Server, and Remote and Mobile Computing. Rand is the president of Convergent Computing, an IT-consulting firm in the San Francisco Bay area that has been one of the key early adopter program partners with Microsoft, implementing beta versions of Microsoft Exchange Server 2003, SharePoint 2003, and Windows Server 2003 in production environments over 2 years before the product releases. Besides speaking at over 50 conferences and conventions around the world in the past year on tips, tricks, and best practices on planning, migrating, and implementing Exchange 2003, Rand is also a special advisor to the White House on cyber-security and cyber-terrorism.

Kenton Gardinier, MCSE, CISSP, MCSA   Kenton Gardinier is a senior consultant with Convergent Computing. He has designed and implemented technical and business-driven solutions for organizations of all sizes around the world for over 10 years. He has also led early adopter engagements, implementing products such as Windows Server 2003, Exchange Server 2003, and SharePoint Portal Server 2003 prior to the products' release for numerous organizations. Kenton is an internationally recognized author and public speaker. His speaking engagements include various industry-renowned conferences and Web casts. He has authored, co-authored, and contributed to several books on Windows, Exchange, security, performance tuning, administration, and systems management. Kenton has also written several magazine columns specializing in various technologies. He holds many certifications, including MCSE, CISSP, and MCSA.

Michael Noel, MCSE+I, MCSA   Michael Noel has been in the computer industry for over 10 years and has been working with the latest in Windows and Exchange technologies since the early versions of the software. Michael is the co-author of *Windows Server 2003 Unleashed* by Sams Publishing and has also been a contributing writer of books on Windows 2000, Exchange 2000, and Microsoft Operations Manager. Currently a senior consultant at Convergent Computing in the San Francisco Bay area, Michael has designed and implemented numerous large-scale technical projects with worldwide Active Directory and Exchange migrations, SharePoint Document Management and Portal Solutions, and high-availability solutions. Michael's experience in the area of real-world design and deployment and his level of involvement in Windows and Exchange server technologies from the beta stages supports his credentials in the field.

Joe R. Coca Jr., MCSE Joe Coca has been in the computer industry for over eight years and has been a contributing writer of several books, such as *Windows Server 2003 Unleashed* and *Windows 2000 Design and Migration*. In addition to writing, Joe has also been a guest speaker with the Enterprise Networking Association Conference and the president of a large user group in Silicon Valley and the San Francisco Bay area. As a consultant with Convergent Computing, Joe has designed and implemented various large Windows Server 2003 Active Directory and Exchange 2000 and 2003 environments, including several worldwide migrations from previous platforms to Microsoft Windows and Exchange Server.

Dedication

I dedicate this book to our new friend, Mrs. Cecilia Blackfield. You are an inspiration to all of us by sharing your decades of wisdom, leadership, friendship, and support. You have been such a great role model to show our children how hard work, dedication, and determination can lead to a wonderful life!

—Rand H. Morimoto, MCSE

This book is dedicated to my parents and parents-in-law for their love and for instilling in me the values that I will always cherish and carry with me.

—Kenton Gardinier, MCSE, CISSP, MCSA

This book is dedicated to my daughter Julia. Your smile fills my life with joy and happiness.

—Michael Noel, MCSE+I, MCSA

I dedicate this book to my three nephews: Vincent, Raymon, and Michael. Good luck in college and godspeed in your life journeys.

—Joe R. Coca Jr., MCSE

Acknowledgments

Rand H. Morimoto, MCSE   After finishing the Windows Server 2003 Unleashed book earlier this year, it was a lot of work to put together this Exchange Server 2003 Unleashed book. However, with many late nights and long weekends, along with the great assistance from many great supporters, we're glad to have this book out to share with others!

We want to thank Candy Hall for giving us the opportunity to write this book and a big thanks to Neil Rowe for your never-ending support of our work. To all those on the Sams Publishing team, including Mark Renfrow, Shiela Schroeder and Nancy Albright, thank you for your edits and changes to put all the words in the right order. Thank you to our technical editor, James Walker, for validating every page of content of the book for technical accuracy. We also want to thank all the consultants, consulting engineers, technical specialists, project managers, technical editors, and systems engineers at Convergent Computing who were valuable resources we called upon for thoughts, suggestions, best practices, tips, and tricks that made up the content of this book.

A big thank you to Microsoft for continuing to include us in your early adopter programs so we were able to get years of experience with Exchange Server 2003 before the product even shipped. Thank you to Susan Bradley, Jan Shanahan, and Patricia Anderson for including us in your program to support authors with internal Microsoft resources. What a great opportunity for us to have several different angles of support and assistance in the book writing process!

And thank you to our dozens of early adopter clients who, in many cases, were our guinea pigs as we worked together years before the product release, helping build case experience and knowledge of the technology.

Last but not least, to my wife Kim, thank you for taking care of the kids non-stop as I wrote evenings, nights, mornings, and on weekends. To Kelly and Andrew, thank you for being good while daddy wrote non-stop. Thank you to my parents, Ed and Vickie, for teaching me good work ethics. To my grandmother Mary, who continues to show me how courage and common sense lead to longevity. And to my brother Bruce and sister Lisa, thank you for all your support over the years! I never realized the support I got from my siblings until I started watching my own kids and how—between hits, fights, and screaming—there's really a love and support shared between brother and sister.

Kenton Gardinier, MCSE, CISSP, MCSA   There are truly so many people to extend my appreciation to, but first and foremost I would like to thank my wife Amy for always being there for me, having an incredible amount of patience, and making me an overall better person. Of course, I could not have asked for a better team to work with, both from Convergent Computing and from Sams. It is great to be a part of such a talented team!

I would also like to thank the many dedicated people at Microsoft for providing their resources and expertise, as well as our clients who helped us gain practical, real-world experience with Exchange Server 2003. It has truly been wonderful working closely with each and every one of you. You have greatly enhanced the content of this book.

Michael Noel, MCSE+I, MCSA   Thanks to everyone who assisted with the creation of this book. Special thanks go to the people of Convergent Computing, particularly Rand Morimoto, László Somi, and Pete Handley, who provided their technical insight and their valuable free time to assist. I would also like to thank the team at Microsoft who helped provide key pieces of information to really make this book shine. Most importantly, my deepest gratitude to the members of my family who suffered while I locked myself away to write this. Most notably in this group is my wonderful wife Marina, my beautiful daughter Julia, my parents Mary and George Noel, and my "other" parents Val and Liza Ulanovsky. I couldn't have made it through this without your love, support, and inspiration!

Joe R. Coca Jr., MCSE   I would like to thank the many friends and family members who have supported me over the past 10 years. A special thanks to Roger Ivy—your guidance and fatherly influence helped lead me to where I am today. Most of all, to my two sisters, Michelle and Carmen, your loving support and examples of hard work and dedication are truly my inspiration. Thanks also to Rand Morimoto for creating the opportunity to write this book.

We Want to Hear from You!

As the reader of this book, *you* are our most important critic and commentator. We value your opinion and want to know what we're doing right, what we could do better, what areas you'd like to see us publish in, and any other words of wisdom you're willing to pass our way.

As an associate publisher for Sams Publishing, I welcome your comments. You can email or write me directly to let me know what you did or didn't like about this book—as well as what we can do to make our books better.

Please note that I cannot help you with technical problems related to the topic of this book. We do have a User Services group, however, where I will forward specific technical questions related to the book.

When you write, please be sure to include this book's title and author as well as your name, email address, and phone number. I will carefully review your comments and share them with the author and editors who worked on the book.

Email: feedback@samspublishing.com

Mail: Michael Stephens
           Associate Publisher
           Sams Publishing
           800 East 96th Street
           Indianapolis, IN 46240 USA

For more information about this book or another Sams Publishing title, visit our Web site at www.samspublishing.com. Type the ISBN (excluding hyphens) or the title of a book in the Search field to find the page you're looking for.

Introduction

When my co-authors and I set out to write this book, we wanted to provide a fresh perspective on planning, designing, implementing, and migrating to an Exchange Server 2003 environment. The four of us (Rand, Mike, Kenton, and Joe) started working with Exchange Titanium more than 18 months prior to the product release to the public. We had several clients who were large beta implementers of Exchange Server 2003, and some of our clients have dozens of servers in production using the Exchange 2003 beta. With our clients having hundreds of thousands of mail users migrated to Exchange 2003 for months prior to product release, we have been fortunate to gain a breadth and depth of a broad Exchange 2003 install base. This provided us with the knowledge and experience behind the creation of this book.

Unlike some books that are merely a cut-and-paste of a previous Exchange 2000 edition of the book, the structure, organization, and content in this book was written from scratch. We felt it was important to outline and write information specific to the Exchange Server 2003 so that your review and use of this information is focused on the features and benefits of the Exchange 2003 environment. We also felt this approach would incorporate our true recommendations for best practices, tips, and tricks to get the most out of an Exchange Server 2003 messaging environment.

This book is organized into 10 parts, each part focusing on core Exchange Server 2003 areas, with several chapters making up each part:

- **Part I: Microsoft Exchange Server 2003 Overview**   This part provides an introduction to Exchange Server 2003, not only from the perspective of a general technology overview, but also to note what is truly new in Exchange Server 2003 that made it compelling enough for organizations to implement the technology in beta in a production environment. We also cover basic planning, prototype testing, and migration techniques, and provide a full chapter on the installation of Exchange Server 2003.

- **Part II: Microsoft Exchange Server 2003 Messaging**   This part covers the design of an Exchange Server 2003 messaging environment for small, medium, and large organizations. It also covers the integration of Exchange 2003 in a non-Windows environment. We understand that the implementation of Exchange is different for organizations of different sizes. Small organizations typically do not have the need for extensive routing groups and administrative groups, so the design illustrations focus on limited server environments. Exchange for large organizations frequently involves extensive front-end, back-end, and distributed user environments, so specific design recommendations are made for these types of organizations.

- **Part III: Microsoft Networking Services' Impact on Exchange**   This part covers DNS, Global Catalog and domain controller placement, Microsoft routing and remote access configuration, and Outlook Web Access configuration from the perspective of planning, integrating, migrating, and coexistence. Notes, tips, and best practices provide valuable information on features that are new in Exchange Server 2003. You explore what's new and different that you can leverage after a migration to Exchange Server 2003.

- **Part IV: Securing a Microsoft Exchange Server 2003 Environment**   Security is on everyone's mind these days, and Microsoft knew it and included several major security enhancements to Exchange Server 2003. We dedicate three chapters of the book to security, breaking the information into client-level security, such as remote client access, message encryption, and attachment encryption; server-level security, such as encrypted front-end and back-end server configuration, certificates, and privacy and antispam protection; and transport-level security, such as IPSec, http proxy, and system-to-system encrypted communications.

- **Part V: Migrating to Microsoft Exchange Server 2003**   This part is dedicated to migrations. We provide a chapter specifically on migrating from Windows NT4 to Windows Server 2003 as it applies to planning and preparing Active Directory with Exchange Server 2003 in mind. Other chapters in this part of the book address migrating Exchange 5.5 to Exchange Server 2003, Exchange 2000 to Exchange Server 2003, and compatibility testing of Exchange add-ins and components in a Windows 2003 and Exchange Server 2003 environment. These chapters are loaded with tips, tricks, and cautions on migration steps and best practices.

- **Part VI: Microsoft Exchange Server 2003 Administration and Management**   In this part, four chapters focus on the administration of an Exchange Server 2003 environment. This is where the importance of a newly written book (as opposed to a modified Exchange 2000 book) is of value to you, the reader. The administration and management of mailboxes, distribution lists, and sites have been greatly enhanced in Exchange Server 2003. Although you can continue to perform tasks the way you did in Exchange 2000, because of significant changes in replication, background transaction processing, secured communications, integrated mobile communications, and changes in Windows 2003 Active Directory, there are better ways to work with Exchange Server 2003. These chapters drill down into specialty areas helpful to administrators of varying levels of responsibility.

- **Part VII: New Mobility Functionality in Microsoft Exchange Server 2003**   Mobility is a key improvement in Exchange Server 2003, so this part focuses on enhancements made in the mobile phone and PDA replication tools to Exchange. Instead of just providing a remote node connection, Exchange Server 2003 provides true end-to-end secured anytime/anywhere access functionality. The wireless mobility functions provide access to Exchange, using mobile phone, wireless device, and PDA support. The chapters in this part highlight best practices on implementing and leveraging these technologies.

- **Part VIII: Client Access to Microsoft Exchange Server 2003**   This part of the book focuses on the enhancements to the Outlook Web Access client, various Outlook client capabilities, and Outlook for non-Windows systems. Outlook Web Access is no longer just a simple browser client, but one that can effectively be a full primary user client to Exchange. Different versions of the full Outlook client have varying levels of support in Exchange 2003 relative to security, XML-based forms support, data recovery, and information manageability. The chapters in this part of the book focus on providing details on leveraging the client capabilities.

- **Part IX: Client Administration and Management**   As many organizations choose to upgrade the client software on their desktop and mobile users, new capabilities in Windows Group Policies and various deployment techniques simplify the process. The two chapters in this part of the book cover best practices, tips, and techniques to automate the client administration and management process.

- **Part X: Fault Tolerance and Optimization Technologies**   The last part of the book addresses fault tolerance, data recovery, and system optimization in Exchange Server 2003. Exchange Server 2003 must be reliable, and Microsoft included several new enhancements in fault-tolerant technologies and data recovery to Exchange 2003. The four chapters in this part address system-level fault tolerance in leveraging clustering and network load balancing technologies, best practices in backup and restore procedures, tested procedures at recovering from a disaster, and capacity analysis and performance optimization of an Exchange 2003 environment. When these new technologies are implemented in an Exchange messaging environment, an organization can truly achieve better enterprise-level reliability and recoverability.

The real-world experience we have had in working with Exchange Server 2003 and our commitment to writing this book from scratch enables us to relay to you information that will be valuable in your successful planning, implementation, and migration to an Exchange Server 2003 environment.

PART I

Microsoft Exchange Server 2003 Overview

IN THIS PART

Exchange Server 2003 Technology Primer

Exchange Server 2003 is the latest release of the electronic messaging–focused application server products from Microsoft. Some are calling it a major service pack for Exchange Server 2000, and others are touting it as the strategic evolution of the Exchange messaging product's extension beyond just email and calendaring.

Because a migration from Exchange 5.5 or Exchange 2000 typically does not require a change in the Outlook client used by email users, many users might never know they were upgraded to Exchange 2003. However, when you look under the hood, Exchange Server 2003 is a major improvement of the Exchange messaging system, with significant changes that improve mobile user access, server reliability, message and server fault tolerance, and system scalability.

This chapter introduces the significant enhancements and diverse capabilities of the Exchange 2003 messaging system and references the chapters through the balance of this book that detail these improvements. The differences that Exchange Server 2003 adds to a messaging environment require a re-education so that design and implementation decisions take full advantage of the enhanced communications capabilities.

Using Exchange 2003 As an Email and Calendaring Solution

Exchange Server 2003 is a versatile messaging system, one that meets the needs of a variety of different business functions. Like earlier versions of Exchange, Exchange Server 2003 can provide all the basic email and calendaring functionality, but now it offers a lot more. An example of the Outlook 2003 client in Exchange 2003 is shown in Figure 1.1.

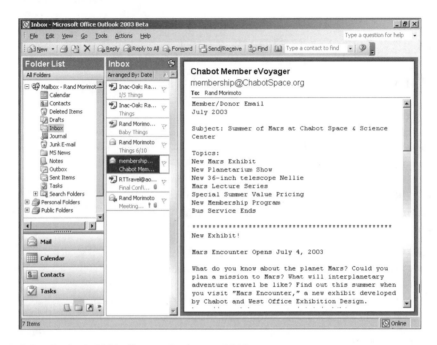

FIGURE 1.1   Outlook 2003 client to Exchange 2003.

Because Exchange Server 2003 provides a variety of different functions, an organization should choose how to best implement Exchange Server 2003 and the various messaging features to meet the needs of the organization. In small network environments with less than 50 users, an organization may choose to implement all the Exchange Server 2003 features on a single server. However in larger environments, multiple servers may be implemented to improve system performance and provide fault tolerance and redundancy.

Taking Advantage of Active Directory in Exchange

One of the major additions to the messaging system role introduced with the release of the Windows 2000 and Windows 2003 is Active Directory. Active Directory is more than a simple list of users and passwords for authentication into a network. It also is a directory that extends to other business applications. When fully leveraged, an organization can have its human resources (HR) department add an employee to the organization's HR software; then the HR software automatically creates a user in the Active Directory that generates a network logon, an email account, a voicemail account, and remote access capabilities—and links pager and mobile phone information to the employee. Likewise, if an employee is terminated, a single change in the HR software can issue automated commands to disable the individual's network, email, remote logon, and other network functions.

Exchange Server 2003 extends the capabilities of the Active Directory by integrating the email, mobile phone, and remote access functionality into a centralized administration tool. Organizations that purchase add-ins to Exchange—such as voicemail, pager, or faxing tools—expand the list of commonly managed resources.

Through the integration of better management tools, Exchange 2003 provides a more robust implementation of Active Directory and enables better scalability and redundancy to improve communication capabilities. Exchange Server 2003 effectively adds more reliability, faster performance, and better management tools to an enterprise, which can be leveraged as a robust text, data, and mobile communications system.

When planning the implementation of Exchange Server 2003, a network architect needs to consider which communication services are needed, and how they will be combined on servers or how they will be made redundant across multiple servers for business continuity failover. For a small organization, the choice to combine several server functions to a single system or to just a few systems is one of economics. The reason to distribute server services to multiple servers, however, also could be a decision for improving performance (see Chapter 33, "Capacity Analysis and Performance Optimization"), Exchange administration (see Chapter 18, "Exchange Server 2003 Mailbox, Distribution List, and Site Administration), creating redundancy (see Chapter 30, "System-Level Fault Tolerance"), and enabling security (covered in three chapters in Part IV, "Securing a Microsoft Exchange Server 2003 Environment").

Leveraging the Exchange 2003 As a Web Access Solution

A significant improvement in the Exchange 2003 Outlook Web Access (OWA) interface, shown in Figure 1.2, now provides organizations the ability to use OWA as their primary mail client for users. With previous versions of Exchange, organizations used the full Outlook client as the primary messaging client for their users. Outlook Web Access was limited in features and functions, leaving OWA as a secondary client for use when the primary client was unavailable or harder to access.

OWA 2003 adds spell-checking, forms, rules, pull-down menus, preview mode, and the ability to view other calendars and folders. These additions in OWA 2003 provide organizations the ability to make OWA 2003 the primary message client for their users, eliminating the need for a full desktop configuration, lowering the cost and effort of deploying desktop application software, and improving an organization's ability to provide access to mail from user's homes, from Internet kiosks, or from other remote locations.

The OWA 2003 client is covered in Chapter 26, "Everything You Need to Know about the OWA Client"; back-end server configuration of OWA is explored in Chapter 10, "Outlook Web Access 2003."

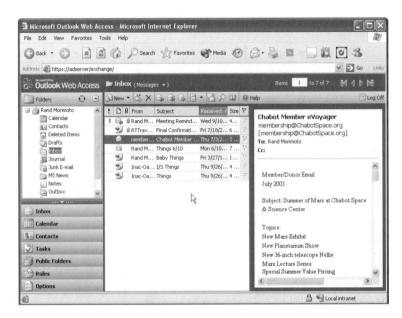

FIGURE 1.2   Outlook Web Access 2003.

Expanding into the New Wireless and Mobility Technologies

In addition to the Outlook Web Access client, Exchange 2003 also added new wireless and mobility technologies for the use of wireless phones and Pocket PC devices for access to mail and messaging, as shown in Figure 1.3. The new mobility technologies built in to Exchange 2003 minimize the need for users to have a separate mobile phone, PDA, and wireless email device lining their beltline. With multifunction mobile phones enabled with Pocket PC technologies, a user can have a single device that provides real-time email, calendar, contacts, and Internet access. Exchange 2003 provides real-time synchronization of information with mobile devices.

Although mobile device synchronization has existed for a few years, the utilities were typically add-ons to messaging systems that required additional costs and had complicated integration requirements. With mobility technologies built directly in to Exchange 2003, the licensing is part of the user cost, so a single-user license covers the cost of a full Outlook client, Web access client, and mobile phone or mobile device access client license. Because the mobility software is built directly in to Exchange 2003, there are no special installation or integration requirements. A user's mailbox is mobility-enabled, simplifying the process of providing mobile access to mail, calendars, contacts, and other Exchange system information.

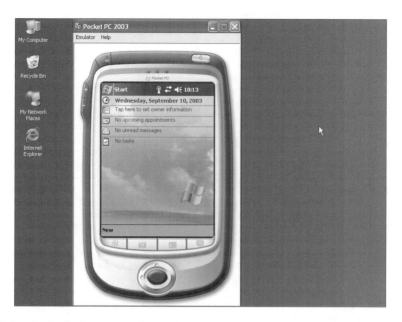

FIGURE 1.3   Outlook client on Pocket PC.

Mobility is covered in Part VII, "New Mobility Functionality in Microsoft Exchange Server 2003" in three chapters of the book: Chapter 22, "Designing Mobility in Exchange Server 2003," Chapter 23, "Implementing Mobile Synchronization in Exchange Server 2003," and Chapter 24, "Configuring Client Systems for Mobility."

Choosing the Right Time to Migrate to Exchange 2003

With the release of Exchange Server 2003, many organizations wonder when is the right time to migrate to the new messaging system. As with any technology, the decision typically starts with identifying the value of migrating versus the cost and effort to migrate.

This chapter introduces the many features and functions in Exchange Server 2003 that have helped other organizations plan a migration. Improvements in security, performance, and manageability provide benefits to organizations looking to minimize administration costs while providing more functionality to users.

The cost and effort to migrate to Exchange Server 2003 varies based on the current state of an organization's messaging environment and the features and functions of Exchange Server 2003 to be implemented. Some of the common states and needed functions are adding Exchange Server 2003 into an existing Exchange 5.5 or Exchange 2000 organization, doing a migration from Exchange 2000 to Exchange Server 2003, and migrating from Exchange 5.5 to Exchange Server 2003.

Adding an Exchange 2003 Server to an Existing Exchange Organization

Many organizations want to add a specific Exchange Server 2003 function, such as Outlook Web Access 2003, Outlook over HTTP, or mobile phone access. Functions such as these can be added on an Exchange Server 2003 server in an existing Exchange 5.5 or Exchange 2000 organization. This enables an organization to get Exchange Server 2003 application functionality fairly quickly and easily without having to do a full migration to Exchange Server 2003. In many cases, an Exchange Server 2003 server simply can be added to an existing network without impact. This provides extremely low messaging system impact, but provides an organization the ability to prototype and test the new technology, pilot it for a handful of users, and slowly roll out the technology to its client base as part of a regular system replacement or upgrade process.

Migrating from Exchange 2000 to Exchange 2003

For organizations that have already migrated to an Exchange 2000 and Active Directory environment, migrating to Exchange Server 2003 can provide access to several additional capabilities built on top of Windows 2003, such as mailbox recovery.

Fortunately, organizations that have already implemented Exchange 2000 or have already migrated from Windows NT4 to Windows 2000, have completed the hard part of their migration process. Effectively, Exchange Server 2003 uses the same Active Directory organizational structure that was created with Windows 2000, so forests, domain trees, domains, organizational users, sites, groups, and users all transfer directly into an Exchange Server 2003 organizational structure. If the organizational structure in Windows 2000 and Exchange 2000 meets the needs of the organization, the migration to Exchange Server 2003 is predominantly the moving of mailboxes from the old Exchange server to a new Exchange server.

Migrating from Exchange 2000 to Exchange 2003 requires a handful of preparatory steps. More details on the migration process from Exchange 2000 is covered in Chapter 16, "Migrating from Exchange 2000 to Exchange Server 2003."

Migrating from Exchange 5.5 to Exchange Server 2003

Organizations that still have Exchange 5.5 as their messaging environment, need to decide whether to migrate from Exchange 5.5 to Exchange 2000, or to migrate directly from Exchange 5.5 to Exchange Server 2003. Deciding factors include what features and functions in Exchange Server 2003 the organization wants and the cost and effort to migrate. Organizations do not have to migrate completely to Exchange Server 2003 to get Exchange Server 2003 functionality. An organization can choose to migrate just a couple of servers from Exchange 5.5 to Exchange Server 2003 without having to migrate the whole organization. This can be a first step for an organization to get Exchange Server 2003 functionality into its network.

If an organization has already begun its migration to Exchange 2000, it may choose to complete its Exchange 2000 migration and then implement Exchange Server 2003 in an in-place migration process later. As noted in the last section, "Migrating from Exchange 2000 to Exchange Server 2003," even if an organization has Exchange 2000 in its environment, it can migrate some of the Exchange 2000 servers to Exchange Server 2003 as an interim process. Of course, an organization can choose to migrate completely from Exchange 5.5 to Exchange Server 2003, and since the forest, domain, site, and other structural functions of Exchange 2000 and Exchange 2003 are identical, typically any planning done for a migration to Exchange 2000 can be applied to an organization's decision to migrate directly from Exchange 5.5 to Exchange Server 2003.

The planning, design, prototype, and migration steps to assist an organization in its migration from Exchange 5.5 to an Exchange Server 2003 environment is covered in Chapter 15, "Migrating from Exchange v5.5 to Exchange Server 2003."

Understanding the Two Versions of Exchange 2003

Exchange Server 2003 comes in two versions (as does Exchange 2000): Exchange 2003 Standard Edition and Exchange 2003 Enterprise Edition. This is similar to the naming designations used for Exchange 5.5 and Exchange 2000. Typically, the Standard Edition is used for either a small organization or as a utility server in a large environment. The Enterprise Edition has more expandability for larger organizations or those organizations that need to take advantage of some of the advanced capabilities of Exchange.

Getting to Know the Exchange 2003 Standard Edition

The Exchange Server 2003 Standard Edition is the basic message server version of the software. The Standard Edition supports one mailbox database up to 16GB. The Standard Edition has full support for Web access, mobile access, and server recovery functionality.

The Standard Edition is a good version of Exchange to support a messaging system for a small organization, as a front-end server for a larger environment, or as a bridgehead server for an Exchange organization. Many small and medium-sized organizations find the capabilities of the Standard Edition sufficient for most messaging server services, and even large organizations use the Standard Edition for message routing servers or as the primary server in a remote office. The Standard Edition meets the needs of effectively any environment wherein a server with a 16GB database is sufficient.

NOTE

Unlike Exchange 2000, which required an Enterprise Edition version of the messaging system for a server to be a front-end server, Exchange 2003 can run on a Standard Edition version of the messaging system. By enabling an organization to acquire a Standard Edition license of Exchange, the licensing cost can be significantly lowered for organizations that split their back-end mailbox server from their front-end client access server.

Expanding into the Exchange Server 2003 Enterprise Edition

The Exchange Server 2003 Enterprise Edition is focused at server systems that require more than a single 16GB Exchange messaging database. With support for up to 20 databases per server, the Enterprise Edition is the appropriate version of messaging system for organizations that have a lot of mailboxes or a lot of mail storage.

> **NOTE**
>
> Typically, organizations implementing Exchange Server 2003 Standard Edition install the messaging system on top of Windows Server (2000 or 2003) Standard Edition. Choosing to install the Standard Edition of Exchange 2003 on top of a Standard Edition of Windows limits the organization's ability to migrate the server to the Enterprise Edition of Exchange. Although an organization may choose to upgrade Exchange to the Enterprise Edition, the organization would also want to upgrade Windows to the Enterprise Edition, making it a challenging task to upgrade the version of the Exchange license.

Table 1.1 summarizes the differences between the Standard and Enterprise Editions.

TABLE 1.1   Exchange 2003 Standard Versus Enterprise Editions

Exchange 2003 Function	Standard Edition	Enterprise Edition
# of storage groups supported	1	4
# of databases per storage group supported	2 (1 private, 1 public)	5
Maximum database size	16GB	Unlimited (16TB maximum)
Clustering support	None	Up to 8-node
X.400 connector support	None	Included
OS support	Windows 2000 SP3+ or Windows Server 2003 Standard or Enterprise	Windows 2000 SP3+ or Windows Server 2003 Standard or Enterprise

Understanding How Improvements in Windows 2003 Enhance Exchange 2003

With the introduction of Windows Server 2003, Microsoft added several new features and functions to the operating system. Some of the features are general system enhancements, and other features directly add benefits and improvements for organizations using Exchange 2003. Enhancements in Windows 2003 improve user administration, security, data replication, and system performance.

Drag-and-Drop Capabilities in Administrative Tools

Many of the new administrative tools with Windows Server 2003, including the Exchange Server 2003 System Manager, provide drag-and-drop capabilities that enable administrators to select objects with a mouse and drag and drop the object to a new location. In

Windows 2000, an administrator would have to select the objects, right-click the mouse, select Move, and choose the destination from a menu or graphical tree. Although this might seem trivial, for any administrator reorganizing users between organizational units in the Active Directory Users and Computers utility, the ability to drag and drop objects can greatly simplify the time and effort it takes to organize and manage objects in the Active Directory.

Built-in Setup, Configuration, and Management Wizards

Other major additions to Windows 2003 that simplify tasks are a series of configuration and management wizards that come built in to the Windows 2003 and Exchange 2003 systems. Instead of having to walk through menus of commands to manually create or modify networking roles, the 2003 versions provide wizards that enable an administrator to add, modify, or remove system configurations. No doubt these wizards are a significant benefit to novices of the messaging system, because the questions in the wizards are typically simple to answer. However, even Windows experts find the wizards simplify the configuration process over manual installation tasks, because it is easier and faster to start with the base settings created by the wizard and then manually adjust changes.

Improvements in Security

Significantly more than just cosmetic updates are the security enhancements added to Windows Server 2003. During the middle of the development of the Windows Server 2003 product, Microsoft launched its Secured Computing Initiative (SCI), which stipulated that all products and solutions from Microsoft meet very stringent requirements for security. Although Exchange Server 2003 was already slated to have several new security enhancements, SCI created an environment where the Exchange Server 2003 product added and enhanced security significantly in the system environment.

Chapters 11, "Client-Level Security," 12, "Server-Level Security," and 13, "Transport-Level Security," of this book are focused on security in different core areas. Chapter 12 addresses some of the new defaults wherein most services are disabled on installation and must be enabled for access. Although this also might seem like a trivial change in a messaging system environment, it provides a relatively secured server immediately from initial installation. Previous versions of Exchange could easily take an hour going through all the unneeded features and manually locking down a server system. The server defaults and the functional or operational differences are noted in Chapter 12.

IPSec and Wireless Security Improvements

Transport-level security in the form of IPSec was included in Windows 2000; however, organizations have been slow to adopt IPSec security, typically because they don't understand how it works. Chapter 13 of this book addresses how IPSec is enabled in organizations, providing a high level of server-to-server, site-to-site, and remote user–to–LAN secured communications. Also covered in Chapter 13 is the new secured wireless LAN

(802.1X) technology that is built in to Windows Server 2003. Windows Server 2003 includes dynamic key determination for improvements in wireless security over the more common Wired Equivalency Protocol (WEP) that is used with standard 802.11 wireless communications. By improving the encryption on wireless communications, an organization can increase its confidence that Exchange Server 2003 can provide a truly secured messaging environment.

Performance and Functionality Improvements

A network end-user would likely never notice many new features added to Exchange Server 2003, and in many cases a network administrator would not even be aware that the technologies were updated and improved. These are technologies that help the network operate more efficiently and effectively so that a user might experience faster message transmission. (Although even if the network were able to respond twice as fast, many times a process that used to take three seconds to complete and now takes less than two seconds to complete is not something a user would particularly notice.) The key benefit typically comes in the area of overall network bandwidth demand improvements. For very large organizations, the performance improvements prevent the organizations from having to add additional servers, processors, or site connections; they gain system efficiencies from improvements in the core operating system and Exchange application.

Global Catalog Caching on a Domain Controller

One of the significant back-end improvements to Windows Server 2003 is the server's capability of caching Global Catalog (GC) information on domain controllers. In a Windows 2000 environment, for users to access the Global Catalog to view mail accounts and distribution lists, an organization typically put out a Global Catalog server to every site in the organization. This distributed Global Catalog server function minimized the ongoing traffic of users querying the catalog over a WAN connection every time they wanted to send an email to someone else in the organization. Directory replication occurred to Global Catalog, however, to keep the directory synchronized. With Windows Server 2003, an organization has the ability to place a domain controller in a remote location, and the Global Catalog information is cached to the remote system. This provides the best of both worlds: The directory information is readily available to remote users, but because it is just a cache of the information and not a fully replicated copy, synchronization and distribution of catalog information is done only when initially requested, and not each time a change is made to the directory.

Remote Installation Service for Servers

New to Windows Server 2003 is a server tool called Remote Installation Service for Servers, or RIS for Servers. RIS for Servers enables an organization to create images of server configurations, which can then be pushed up to a RIS server that can later be used to re-image a new system. RIS was standard with Windows 2000; however, it only supported the re-imaging of desktop systems.

RIS for Servers can be used several ways. One way organizations have leveraged RIS for Servers has been to create a new, clean server image with all of a company's core utilities installed. Every time the organization needs to install a new server, rather than starting from scratch with an installation CD, it can use the template RIS server installation. The image could include service packs, patches, updates, or other standard setup utilities.

RIS for Servers can also be used as a functional disaster recovery tool. After a server has been configured as an Exchange 2003 server with the appropriate program files and parameters configured, the organization can then run the RIPrep to backup the Exchange server image to a RIS server. In the event of a system failure, the organization can recover the server image from the state of the system before system failure.

> **NOTE**
>
> Creating RIS images for production servers requires planning and testing before relying on the system function for successful disaster recovery. Certain applications require services to be stopped before RIPrep is run. Chapter 32, "Recovering from a Disaster," addresses steps to conduct system server recovery.

RIS for Servers is a versatile tool that helps organizations quickly build new servers or recover from application server failures. Besides being covered in Chapter 32, RIS for Servers is also covered in detail in Chapter 3, "Installing Exchange Server 2003."

Scaling Reliability with 8-Node Clustering

Another Windows 2003 enhancement that is supported in Exchange 2003 is the support for 8-node clustering. Previous versions of Exchange supported up to 2-node clustering, which enabled an organization to have two systems available to support a series of mailboxes. Windows 2003 supports 8-node clustering, so an organization can now have up to eight servers clustered for a combination of performance load balancing and real-time system failover.

With active clustering, the load of the users accessing mailboxes hosted on the cluster can be distributed across the active servers, thus providing improved performance to users accessing mail. With 2-node clustering, the load was distributed to just two systems, thus limiting realistic access to thousands of simultaneous mail access connections. By expanding to up to 8-nodes, an organization can now have several thousand users simultaneously connecting to the mail store, distributing the load to up to eight systems for much better scalability.

In addition to providing load balancing, clustering provides failover and fault-tolerance capabilities, enabling an organization to have several thousand mailboxes protected by real-time fault failover and recovery. Through the implementation of active and passive clustering, an IT organization can choose the level of system recovery.

Details on how to plan, test, and implement a clustered Exchange 2003 environment is covered in Chapter 30. That chapter also covers other tools, technologies, and techniques on methods of improving Exchange system reliability and mailbox recovery in the event of a system failure.

Improving Mailbox Recovery Through Volume Shadow Copy Services

A significant addition to Windows Server 2003 is the Volume Shadow Copy Service (VSS) technology. Volume Shadow Copy takes a snapshot of a network volume and places the copy onto a different volume on the network. After a mirrored snapshot has been taken, at any time, files from the read-only shadow can be accessed without complications typical of network volumes in use. Exchange 2003 is one of the first application server products that takes advantage of the Volume Shadow Copy Service. VSS is used to improve online backups of Exchange databases, and it provides the basis from which mailbox recovery capabilities are provided in an Exchange 2003 environment. There are two primary ways VSS provides better system management support in Exchange 2003:

- **Online Backup of Files**   VSS provides the ability to back up open files, such as Exchange EDB data. Backing up open files has always been a challenge for organizations. Old tape backup software skipped files in use because there was no easy way to back up the files being used by applications such as Exchange. Improvements in tape backup software now provide the ability for an organization to add an Exchange backup agent so that Exchange databases can be backed up. However, the process of backing up Exchange data during production usage time significantly slows down the normal access to messages in the Exchange database.

  Windows Server 2003 Volume Shadow Copy provides the ability to create a snapshot to another volume. With the read-only shadow volume available, tape backup software can now launch a backup on the shadowed version of the database without having to contend with database access on the primary disk volume of the network. Furthermore, because the database on the shadowed volume is not in use, the backup system does not have to stop, unlock a file, back up the file, and then relock the file for user access.

- **Simple Mailbox Recovery**   Volume Shadow Copy Service technology is also used in Exchange 2003 to provide administrators the ability to recover lost or damaged mailboxes. Rather than having to go back to the last tape backup on a system, a mail administrator can go to the Exchange System Manager and choose to recover a mailbox. More details on mailbox recovery is covered later in the section "Simplifying Mailbox Recovery Using Integrated Tools."

Reliability Enhancements in Exchange Server 2003

In addition to the enhancements in Windows Server 2003 that improve the functionality of Exchange 2003, there are several new enhancements added to Exchange 2003 specifically to improve messaging reliability. These enhancements include long-awaited tools for mailbox and database recoverability. The tools provide simple mail message and mailbox folder recovery to complete recovery of deleted or damaged mailboxes.

Simplifying Mailbox Recovery Using Integrated Tools

One of the major enhancements added to Exchange 2003 is the Mailbox Recovery Center, shown in Figure 1.4. This tool provides mail administrators the ability to recover a mailbox of individual users that might have been accidentally deleted or corrupted. The mailbox recovery tool is integrated directly in the Exchange System Manager administration tool, making it easy for administrators to provide mailbox recovery assistance to users in the organization.

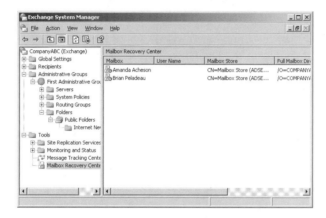

FIGURE 1.4   Mailbox Recovery Center in Exchange 2003.

The mailbox recovery tool and other disaster recovery tips and techniques are covered in Chapter 32.

Leveraging Recovery Storage Group Functionality

Any disaster recovery and system reliability plan includes techniques to plan, prepare, and implement system and data recovery. Exchange 2003 introduces the concept of a recovery storage group that is used as a spare data location where information can be recovered. The recovery storage group prepares the Exchange system for the capability of restoring and recovering mailboxes. Chapter 32 presents more details on the implementation of a recovery storage group.

Expanding on Manageability and Administration Benefits of Exchange 2003

Exchange 2003 introduced a series of functions that help Exchange administrators better manage and administer the Exchange environment. Some of those tools include improvements in the ExMerge utility for mailbox moves, the ability to create dynamic distribution lists, a simplified method of replication address lists between forests, step-by-step migration tools to upgrade from previous versions of Exchange, and better integration with Microsoft Operations Manager.

Improving the Speed of Mailbox Moves

For most Exchange administrators, the ExMerge utility is a familiar tool. When ExMerge first became available years ago, it was an Exchange Resource Kit of tools that enabled an administrator to export and import mailboxes. Over the years, Exchange administrators have found many occasions to export and import mailboxes—whether to back up a mailbox for future recovery, transfer the mailbox from one server or Exchange organization to another, or clean up a corrupt mailbox by exporting good messages and leaving bad messages behind.

Exchange 2003 introduces a completely revised version of the ExMerge utility. The new ExMerge utility now comes on the Exchange 2003 CD as part of the core utilities for Exchange, and the utility is now multithreaded. As a multithreaded tool, the utility can migrate multiple mailboxes at the same time, as shown in Figure 1.5, using more bandwidth and the capabilities of a server.

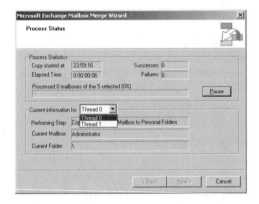

FIGURE 1.5   Multithreaded mailbox moves with the new ExMerge.

ExMerge is covered in more detail in Chapter 5.

Establishing Dynamic Distribution Lists

New to Exchange 2003 is the ability to dynamically create a mail distribution list. Prior to this feature, distribution lists were static groups in which members were added or deleted from a list. With dynamic group creation, a distribution list can be created by specifying LDAP query information. A group can be created that looks for all members who live in particular city, or a query created that looks for all individuals who live in California (CA), as shown in Figure 1.6, or a dynamic query created that looks for all individuals with manager, director, or VP in their title.

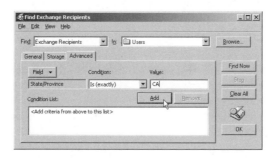

FIGURE 1.6   Setting a query-based distribution rule.

The dynamic lookup function requires that data fields serving as queries have consistent information or that the query takes into account matching for similarities—for example, matching for the words manager, mgr, or mngr if there is a lack of consistency in naming. However, the query-based group lookup is done through LDAP queries and can look in default or custom attribute fields to build a distribution list for users.

Query-based distribution lists are covered in Chapter 18.

Replicating Directories Between Forests

Although not new to Windows, Exchange 2003 formally introduces the Identity and Integration Feature Pack that synchronizes address book information between Exchange organizations. Before Exchange 2003, organizations were able to acquire a copy of Microsoft Metadirectory Service (MMS) under special license arrangements with Microsoft and with limited support. Because of the success of MMS in synchronizing directories between Active Directory forests, Identity and Integration Feature Pack (formerly known as MMS 3.0) is now freely downloadable from Microsoft.

With the inclusion of a synchronization wizard, Identity and Integration Feature Pack has the capability of synchronizing the address books between multiple Exchange forests, thus enabling an organization with multiple Active Directory forests to share directories. For more robust directory synchronization needs, Microsoft provides the Microsoft Identity and Integration Server (MIIS) that supports synchronization with non–Active Directory directories, such as LDAP, Novell NDS/e-Directory, and Exchange 5.5 Directory.

Chapter 18 explores more on the Identity and Integration Pack as well as directory replication.

Simplifying Migrations Using Structured Migration Tools

To help simplify the process of migrating from Exchange 5.5 and Exchange 2000 to Exchange 2003, Microsoft is providing an interactive step-by-step migration guide and migration tools. The interactive guide, shown in Figure 1.7, not only walks an administrator through the steps, but it also links each step to tools with applicable wizards and parameters needed for each migration step.

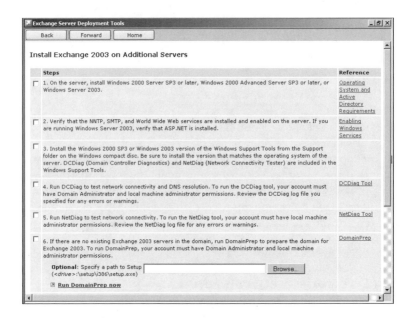

FIGURE 1.7   Step-by-step migration guide in Exchange 2003.

The tools can be launched manually to follow custom configuration steps; however, for organizations needing common tested procedures, the migration guide provides a simplified process.

The migration process from Exchange 5.5 is covered in Chapter 15; the migration process from Exchange 2000 is covered in Chapter 16.

Taking Advantage of Microsoft Operations Manager

Another management and administration tool that has been available from Microsoft to help Exchange administrators is the Microsoft Operations Manager, or MOM. Because manageability is so important to Exchange administrators to validate message routing, connect to the Internet, and monitor email traffic and spam, Microsoft includes the Exchange components for MOM with Exchange 2003. The Exchange 2003 agent for MOM, shown in Figure 1.8, includes over 1700 out of the box rules and a copy of the Microsoft knowledgebase.

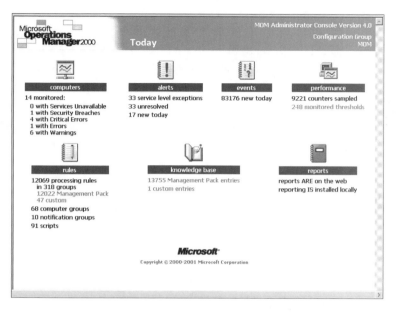

FIGURE 1.8   Microsoft Operations Manager for Exchange 2003.

The 1700 rules monitor and produce reports on everything from message traffic, server uptime, and replication statistics. The knowledgebase provides integrated access to debugging information for event errors or problem reports.

All this information helps an Exchange administrator gain better control for managing and administering the Exchange environment in an organization. Exchange Server 2003 management and maintenance practices are covered in Chapter 19, "Exchange Server 2003 Management and Maintenance Practices."

Improvements in Exchange 2003 Security

Security has been on the minds of most organizations, and very much so for the employees at Microsoft, which went through several secured computing initiative steps to improve security of all of its products. After designing Exchange 2003, Microsoft tested it repeatedly for security in the application code; Microsoft also integrated several security technologies either already present in Windows 2000 or new to Windows 2003 and Exchange 2003.

Establishing Security Between Front-end and Back-end Servers

All future products from Microsoft will include IP Security (IPSec) as an intra-domain/intra-forest secured communication standard. Rather than leaving the security between Exchange front-end and back-end servers to simple server-to-server communications, Microsoft now provides IPSec encryption between front-end and back-end servers.

By integrating IPSec's 168-bit encryption between servers, the security and integrity of information between servers in an Exchange forest is ensured. Security used to look at just external breaches, such as a hacker taking control of servers connected to the Internet. However with privacy of information—and legislation requiring security of personal information, healthcare patient information, or financial services data—organizations are leveraging the industry standard IPSec for server-to-server security even inside the firewall.

Chapter 13 covers IPSec security, along with securing internal and external Exchange servers.

Creating Cross-Forest Kerberos Authentication

Besides replicating directory information between forests, Windows 2003 provides the capability of creating cross-forest trusts and establishing cross-forest Kerberos authentication. Cross-forest Kerberos authentication provides the ability for an organization to share messages and attachments with trust-level security, which enhances secured communications.

You'll find more information on cross-forest Kerberos authentication in Chapter 5, "Designing an Enterprise Exchange Server 2003 Environment."

Restricting Distribution Lists to Authenticated Users

A minor function—but something that is a major enhancement for improved secured messaging interaction—is the ability to restrict distribution lists to authenticated users. With previous versions of Exchange, anyone could send an email to a distribution list if he knew the SMTP address name for the list. Although there were ways of blocking the ability for external access to distribution list message distribution, it was an all-or-nothing action.

With Exchange 2003, the Exchange administrator now has the ability to restrict distribution lists to authenticated users. An authenticated user in Exchange 2003 is someone who successfully logs on to an authorized domain or forest. With the implementation of authenticated user access to distribution lists, security is improved. Chapter 18 explores distribution lists.

Using Safe and Blocked Lists

Unwanted emails, or spam, account for over 30% of all emails transmitted over the Internet, and for some organizations, spam has extended beyond being a nuisance for users to delete. With inappropriate or undesired spam messages flashing pictures and displaying obscenities on screens of employees, spam has become a human resource issue. Exchange 2003 includes the ability to create lists for safe and blocked addresses, as shown in Figure 1.9, enabling Exchange administrators to control message flow. Although using safe and blocked lists is just a small step toward creating a spam-free environment, it is an effective method of implementing a more secure messaging environment.

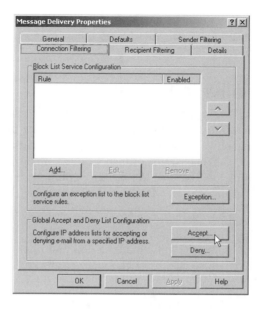

FIGURE 1.9   Safe and blocked lists in Exchange 2003.

Chapter 12 presents details on safe and blocked list functionality.

Filtering of Inbound Recipients Functionality

Filtering inbound recipients is a new feature built in to Exchange 2003. By being able to filter for inbound recipients, an organization can extend the restriction of desired or undesired message communications. The inbound recipient filter is covered in Chapter 12.

Blocking Attachments in Outlook Web Access (OWA)

Attachments in Outlook Web Access pose a threat for the distribution of viruses and message beaconing, which is a method spammers use to identify qualified email addresses. Outlook Web Access in Exchange 2003 provides the ability for the Exchange administrator to block attachments, thus minimizing the risk of the spread of viruses and awareness by spammers of valid email addresses. Chapter 12 covers attachment blocking in detail.

Supporting S/MIME for OWA Attachments

Included as part of the security functions built in to Exchange 2003 is the ability for organizations to send and receive attachments using S/MIME encryption. With previous versions of Exchange, in order to support certificates that enabled attachment encryption, the organization had to use the full Outlook client. With Exchange 2003, however, the

Outlook Web Access client now supports S/MIME attachments, thus providing the capability of securely communicating between email users. Chapter 13 explores S/MIME attachments in OWA.

Leveraging Mobility in Exchange 2003

As noted in an earlier section, "Expanding into the New Wireless and Mobility Technologies," Microsoft has included mobile communication capabilities for wireless phones and PDAs into Exchange 2003. This provides an organization the ability to enable users to access their email, calendars, and contacts from a wireless phone or Pocket PC device. Because the technology is built in to Exchange 2003, there is no need to add special software, servers, or integration with Exchange to provide this functionality. Mobility is now an integrated part of Exchange, providing access to users anytime and anywhere.

Additionally, mobility in Exchange 2003 includes a new and improved version of the Outlook Web Access Web client so that users can view, create, and manage their email, calendar, contacts, and public folder information from a Web browser.

Remote access to messaging information has been greatly enhanced with the added improvements of wireless and Web access communications.

Improving Outlook Web Access's Functionality

The first improvement in Exchange 2003 for remote and mobile access is a significant improvement to the Outlook Web Access client. Instead of organizations having to use the full Outlook client and full Windows desktop for users to check their email, the OWA in Exchange 2003 provides pull-down menus, spell-check, rules, filters, global address list access, and other functions that users want in their mail client.

With a more robust Web client for Exchange, organizations can choose to have OWA as the primary client for users, thus minimizing the need for setting up virtual private networks (VPNs), having laptops for all mobile users, or creating Citrix or Terminal Services farms for remote users. Outlook Web Access 2003 is covered in detail in Chapter 26.

Using Outlook 2003 over HTTPS

For organizations that still need the full Outlook client—possibly for integration with a client relationship management software—or power users with sophisticated access needs, Outlook 2003 combined with Exchange 2003 provides the ability to have a client-to-server connection over secured HTTP, as shown in Figure 1.10. This feature enables organizations to securely connect a full Outlook client to Exchange without having to set up a VPN, and without having to open up special ports for client/server access.

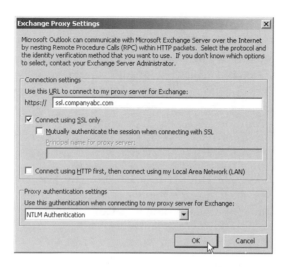

FIGURE 1.10   Outlook 2003 client configuration for secured HTTP access.

Setting up a remote full Outlook client can now take only a minute or two on a system running Outlook 2003, thus improving remote and mobile access while simplifying the security configuration process. Outlook 2003 over HTTPS improves an organization's ability to extend client access in a secured manner without the normal complexity of creating sophisticated client connections.

Chapter 11 explains secured client communication.

Leveraging ActiveSync for Exchange Replication

ActiveSync in Exchange 2003 is a utility that provides the synchronization of Exchange information to Pocket PC devices. Instead of having a cradle on each computer with a Pocket PC computer—or setting up ActiveSync for Pocket PC users to update their calendars, contacts, and other information—Exchange 2003 now includes ActiveSync as part of the core messaging system.

Pocket PC users with Ethernet, 802.11b wireless, or wireless phone connectivity can now synchronize security from their Pocket PC to Exchange 2003. Because ActiveSync is built in to Exchange 2003, there are no special server integration tools, dedicated sync gateway servers, or other devices necessary. All an organization needs is physical connectivity from either a wired or wireless Pocket PC device, and then the mobile devices can communicate with the Exchange environment.

Chapter 23 describes Pocket PC–ActiveSync integration.

Connecting Users Through Wireless Technologies

Besides synchronizing Pocket PC devices to Exchange 2003, the Exchange 2003 product also provides mobile phone connectivity to Exchange for devices supporting General Packet Radio Service (GPRS) or Single Carrier Radio Transmission Technology (1×RTT). In addition to GPRS and 1×RTT support, Exchange 2003 can also communicate with standard cellular phone or packet radio devices. Wireless phone connectivity in Exchange 2003 means that users with simple character-based phones can send and receive email messages and query calendars and contact lists from their mobile phones. Exchange 2003 also supports xHTML (WAP 2.x), cHTML, and HTML standards for mobile phone connectivity.

With Outlook Web Access 2003, Outlook over HTTPS, ActiveSync for Pocket PC devices, and mobile phone access, Exchange 2003 provides access to virtually any client device for access to information from anywhere. Chapter 23 explores mobile connectivity built in to Exchange 2003.

Performance Improvements in Exchange 2003

There are several additions to Exchange 2003 that help organizations better improve the performance of their Exchange servers. Exchange 2003 includes improvements such as better memory allocation and management through technologies that cache distribution lists and Global Catalog information as well as message notification suppression.

Performance improvements not only decrease the overhead of a server, enabling an organization to grow its organization, but performance improvements also enable an organization to minimize the number of servers needed in its environment. If an organization with five Exchange servers can decrease performance demands by 20%, the organization can eliminate an entire server from its network environment with no performance degradation seen by users.

Allocating Memory to Improve Performance

One of the improvements in Exchange 2003 is the ability to optimize the memory for servers greater than 1GB. This is actually a function of Windows 2003 memory management, which enables memory to be tuned between kernel and application memory. Rather than allocating memory equally between kernel and application memory, an organization can specifically allocate memory about 1GB to optimize kernel memory.

Chapter 33 covers tuning an optimization of memory and other recommendations based on best practices for optimizing a server configuration.

Using Caching on Distribution Lists

Exchange 2003 takes advantage of caching of information in several ways to improve system and message environment performance. One way caching improves Exchange is in its capability of caching Global Catalog information on domain controllers. Rather than requiring a Global Catalog server to query the directory for each lookup to the Global Catalog, Exchange 2003 takes advantage of Windows 2003 Global Catalog caching. When an Exchange client queries the Global Catalog, the response can now come from a cache off a domain controller, thus minimizing the need to query across a WAN connection to a remote Global Catalog server or to put a domain controller in each location.

Additionally, Exchange 2003 provides caching of distribution lists for email message distribution. By using the cache for distribution list information, fewer queries need to be made directly to the Global Catalog database, resulting in faster message transmission.

Chapter 33 explains caching distribution lists and Global Catalog information.

Controlling Message Notification

Exchange 2003 adds a new feature that enables the Exchange administrator to specify which message notifications get sent from an Exchange server. Normally when a message comes in to an Exchange server, if the Exchange server cannot find the recipient, a non-delivery receipt (NDR) is sent to the sender. However, with spam messages accounting for 30–50% of incoming messages for many organizations, the number of NDRs could be significant.

By controlling message notification, as shown in Figure 1.11, an Exchange administrator can designate what to do with message notification and can control the amount of responses generated from messages that might otherwise be undesired.

Controller message notification is a tuning and optimization function and is covered in Chapter 33.

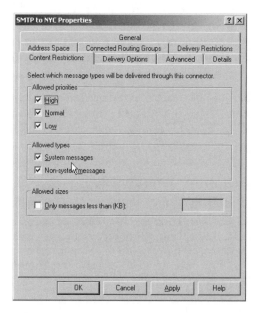

FIGURE 1.11   Controlling message notification in Exchange 2003.

Solidifying Core Technologies for Exchange 2003

Although this chapter has covered a variety of new features, functions, and capabilities built in to Exchange 2003, there are also a number of core technologies that Microsoft improved as well. Some of these core technology improvements come in the area of DNS improvements, reliable Global Catalog lookup improvements, tools, and strategies for successfully planning and migrating from Exchange 5.5 and Exchange 2000, and core technologies at leveraging Windows 2000 and Windows 2003 capabilities.

Solidifying DNS for Proper Message Routing

Domain Name System, or DNS, has been the core name resolution technology for Active Directory from which Exchange 2000 and Exchange 2003 extend the directory lookup scheme. Having a solid DNS infrastructure is critical to the success of proper email message routing. Organizations that do not clearly understand how to implement DNS, or integrate Active Directory DNS with existing Unix-based enterprise DNS systems, can impact efficient and effective message routing.

Chapter 7, "Domain Name System Impact on Exchange Server 2003," covers the basics as well as best practices and lessons learned at implementing DNS, which improves name resolution for an organization. Chapter 7 also addresses a core infrastructure need for reliable message routing and communications.

Deploying Global Catalogs for Reliable Directory Lookup

Global Catalogs are the directories used within an Active Directory or Exchange messaging environment for looking up other internal email users and distribution lists. Microsoft made changes in Windows 2003 on how Global Catalogs can be positioned in the Active Directory. The improvements in Global Catalog caching, replication of site information, and distribution list information have changed the way many organizations operate.

Chapter 8, "Global Catalog and Domain Controller Placement," covers new tips, tricks, and techniques on GC and DC placement, and provides a method in which the number of servers can be reduced, or at least optimize systems for better directory lookup and replication.

Completing a Migration to Windows 2003

Some organizations might still be running Windows NT4 or Exchange 5.5 and will take this opportunity to make a major upgrade to Windows 2003 and Exchange 2003. There are many reasons highlighted in this introduction chapter on why to upgrade to the latest Windows and Exchange systems, but Chapter 14, "Migrating from NT4 to Windows Server 2003," and Chapter 15 focus on specific areas for planning, prototype testing, and successfully completing the migration process.

Upgrading is not just getting the latest operating system and messaging system from Microsoft; the upgrade also provides the Exchange administrator with a more reliable messaging system with tools that help keep the system more secure, run more efficiently, and provide access from virtually anywhere and from any device in use in an organization.

Summary

This chapter highlighted the new features, functions, migration tools, and management utilities in Exchange Server 2003 that will help administrators take advantage of the capabilities of the new messaging system. An upgrade to Exchange Server 2003 is more than just a simple upgrade from one messaging system to another, because email hasn't changed much from version to version. This upgrade is an opportunity to benefit from the messaging system enhancements and the capabilities of the Windows Server 2003 and Exchange Server 2003. With these new tools, an organization can change the way users access the system remotely, improve security both in the background and at the client, and have the tools available to maintain, manage, and recover from a disaster.

The steps to proper planning and successful implementation are highlighted throughout this book, with tips, tricks, and best practices noted throughout the chapters.

Best Practices

This chapter highlighted the new features, functions, and core technologies built in to Exchange 2003. The following are best practices from this chapter:

- Use the step-by-step migration tools highlighted in Chapter 15 (for migrations from Exchange 5.5) and Chapter 16 (for migrations from Exchange 2000) to work through the upgrade process.

- Consider using the new Outlook Web Access 2003—not only as a Web browser client, but possibly as the primary mail client for many users, thus eliminating the need to support full desktop OSs and client software for users.

- Leverage the Outlook-over-HTTPS functionality covered in Chapter 11 to enable remote full client Outlook users connectivity to Exchange 2003 without the need to implement VPNs or other secured connection systems.

- Review Chapter 8 to determine whether you can decrease the number of domain controllers or Global Catalog servers on your network with an upgrade to Windows Server 2003, where GC and DC caching simplifies the requirement for domain controller placement.

- Test the mailbox recovery process highlighted in Chapter 32 to ensure that if you need to recover from mailbox deletion or corruption, you have successfully tested the functionality.

- Review your use of IPSec and whether you want to begin implementing server-to-server encryption to create a more secure networking environment. See Chapter 13 for more details on server-level security.

- Evaluate the use of RIS for Servers as a possible disaster recovery process to recover a failed Exchange server, or for adding additional Exchange servers to a network.

- Consider changing distribution lists to query-based distribution lists so that lookups can be dynamic instead of requiring manual addition and changes of users.

- If your organization needs to replicate directories with other Exchange organizations or with other directories, review Chapter 18 on Identify and Integration Feature Pack.

- For better Exchange server management, administration, and reporting, review Chapter 19 on tips and techniques on leveraging the Microsoft Operations Manager add-in that comes with Exchange 2003.

- To minimize spam and unwanted messaging, leverage the capabilities of safe and blocked lists, inbound recipient filtering, and attachment blocking, which is covered in more detail in Chapter 11 of this book.

- Consider using Exchange 2003's built-in remote and mobile capabilities for wireless phone and PDA device communications for messaging, calendaring, and contact communications.

- Review exiting enterprise configurations for network settings that may be modified or reconfigured with an upgrade to Windows 2003 and Exchange 2003.

CHAPTER 2

Planning, Prototyping, Migrating, and Deploying Exchange Server 2003

Messaging has evolved from an alternative to "snail mail" to an intricate communications and information storage environment. Exchange and Outlook users rely on it for formal and informal communications, keeping track of appointments, storing addresses and phone numbers, and (it's been said) receiving stock quotes, health tips, and urban myths. These tools are also available remotely in most environments, making them even more important at keeping the mobile professional productive and connected to his or her world.

It has become such a critical tool that the upgrade process should not be taken lightly. Although an upgrade from Exchange 5.5 or Exchange 2000 might at first appear to be a simple process, its success relies on your understanding of current issues with the messaging environment, defining both the objectives of the upgrade, and its potential effects on the user community. Adding more features and complexity to the messaging "ecosystem" might not result in ecstatic users, but reducing spam and the resulting impact on in-boxes might more than justify the cost of the upgrade. Reducing the number of milliseconds it takes to send an email probably won't get noticed, but being able to guarantee access to email anywhere and anytime should. An enthusiastic user community tends to generate support and momentum for projects, which extend the functionality of the messaging system.

Important decisions include whether the entire network operating system (NOS) needs to be upgraded (if Active Directory is not yet in place) or only a subset of it, and what other infrastructure components need to be changed or replaced.

The examples used in this chapter assume that the environments being migrated are primarily based on Exchange v5.5 or Exchange 2000, and except where noted that Active Directory is already in place. The same process can be applied to other messaging migration projects, such as GroupWise or Notes. The migration process is covered in detail in Chapters 14, "Migrating from NT4 to Windows Server 2003"; 15, "Migrating from Exchange v5.5 to Exchange Server 2003"; and 16, "Migrating from Exchange 2000 to Exchange Server 2003."

Initiation, Planning, Testing, and Implementation: The Four Phases to the Upgrade

This chapter presents a structured process for upgrading to Exchange Server 2003 and highlights some best practice recommendations to enhance the success of the project. The standard project management phases of *initiation*, *planning*, *testing*, and *implementation* can be used for organizations of any size. Between each phase is a "go/no go" step, in which the results of the phase are reviewed, and the decision-makers determine whether the project should move forward. Any problems that were encountered are assessed to determine whether they require attention before moving forward. This ensures that issues identified are addressed, rather than being overlooked, to inevitably crop up at the worst possible moment.

Documentation Required During the Phases

A number of documents are produced during each phase to ensure that it is well defined and ultimately successful. In the initiation phase the goals of the project can be identified and documented in a *Statement of Work* document. In the planning phase, more time and energy can be applied to detailing the end-state of the migration in a *Design* document. Although this document paints the picture of what the end-state looks like, the roadmap of how to get there is detailed in the *Project Schedule and Migration* documents. These documents are only drafts during this phase, because they need to be validated in the testing phase before they can be labeled "final."

The testing phase validates that the new technologies will effectively meet the organization's needs, and determines whether modifications to the project are needed. Any additional documents that would help with the implementation process, such as *Server Build* documents, *Business Continuity* or *Disaster Recovery* documents, and checklists for workstation configurations are also created during the testing phase. Finally, the appropriate *Maintenance* documents are created during the implementation phase. These phases and the documents to be created are discussed in more detail later in this chapter.

The following list summarizes the standard phases of an Exchange Server 2003 upgrade and the standard documents created in each phase:

- **Initiation Phase**   Statement of Work document

- **Planning Phase**   Design Document Draft, Migration Document Draft, and Migration Schedule Draft (Gantt Chart)

- **Testing Phase**   Design Document Final, Migration Document Final, Migration Schedule Final (Gantt Chart), Server Build Documents, Migration Checklists, and Training Documents for End-Users

- **Implementation Phase**   Maintenance Documents

For smaller projects, not all of these items are required, but it's important to have each document created *before* it is needed, to avoid show-stoppers during the migration process. For example, having a Statement of Work document that is well constructed and agreed upon in the initiation phase will smooth the way for the creation of the Design document and Migration document. A detailed Migration Schedule Gantt chart facilitates scheduling of resources for the actual work and clarifies the roles and responsibilities.

Initiation Phase: Defining the Scope and Goals

Upgrading to Exchange Server 2003 can be a simple process for basic messaging environments, or as challenging as a complete network operating system upgrade for more complex organizations. In most environments Exchange is implemented on multiple servers, and an upgrade will affect a number of other software applications. In fact, changes to the Exchange environment may affect the daily lives of the employees to a much greater extent than moving from NT to Windows Server 2003 (or even more than an upgrade from a non-Microsoft environment), because they will most likely receive a new Outlook client and change the way they access email remotely. With an operating system upgrade, the end-users often don't even know that anything has changed.

The upgrade process is also a great opportunity to help the business achieve its business objectives by leveraging the messaging components of the technology infrastructure and to help justify the never-ending IT expenses. Messaging, in essence, enables the sharing of information and access to data and other resources within the company to help the company deliver its products or services. With this critical purpose in mind, it makes sense to engage in a structured and organized process to determine the goals of the project, control the variables and risks involved, and make sure that a clear definition of the end-state has been crafted. The Statement of Work is the key deliverable from this phase that paints the overall picture of the upgrade project and gains support from the key decision-makers (and allocates an initial budget).

The Scope of the Project

Before the entire Statement of Work can be written, time should be allocated to define the scope of the project. The scope of the project simply defines what is included in the project and what is not. For a simpler environment this may be very easy to define—for example, an environment in which there is only one Exchange server used for email and scheduling, with a dedicated backup device and virus protection software. If this organization has not migrated to Active Directory yet, the scope might expand to include the upgrade of additional servers or simply upgrade the single server. A desktop upgrade might be included in the scope of the project if the features and benefits of Outlook 2003 are desired. In any case, it's important to clarify this level of detail at the beginning of the planning process. "Scope creep" is a lot more manageable if it can be predicted in advance!

> **NOTE**
>
> An example of a scope of work for a small organization is
>
> - Upgrade the Exchange 5.5 NT 4 Server to Exchange Server 2003 with Windows Server 2003.
> - Upgrade the Tape Back-up and Virus Protection software to Exchange Server 2003–compatible versions.
> - Upgrade the Outlook client to Outlook 2003 on all workstations.
> - Provide OWA access to all remote users.

In a larger company, "what's in" and "what's out" can be correspondingly more complicated. A company with multiple servers dedicated to Exchange functions—such as front-end and back-end servers, bridgehead servers, or servers dedicated to faxing or conferencing—requires the scope definition to get that much more detailed. Multiple sites and even different messaging systems complicate the scope, especially if the company has grown via mergers over the last few years.

> **NOTE**
>
> An example of a scope of work for a larger organization is
>
> - Upgrade the four Exchange 5.5 NT 4 Servers to two Exchange Server 2003 cluster pairs on Windows Server 2003, and upgrade the six NT file and print servers to two Windows Server 2003 cluster pairs.
> - Upgrade the Enterprise Tape Back-up and Virus Protection software on all servers to the latest versions that are Windows Server 2003–compatible and Exchange Server 2003–compatible.
> - Upgrade the Outlook client to Outlook 2003. Provide OWA access to all remote users.

The scope of work might change as the initiation phase continues and in the more detailed planning phase as the Design and Migration documents are created and reviewed. This is especially true for more complex migration projects after the detailed planning phase is completed and the all-important budget is created. At this point, the scope might need to be reduced, so that the budget requested can be reduced.

Identifying the Goals

As a next step in the initiation phase, it helps to spend time clearly identifying the goals of the project before getting too caught up in the technical details. All too often everyone runs up the whiteboard and starts scribbling and debating technology before agreeing on the goals. Although this conversation is healthy and necessary, it should be part of the planning phase, after the high-level goals for the project and initial scope have been defined. Even if there is a very short timeline for the project, the goals—from high-level business objectives, to departmental goals, to the specific technology goals—should be specified.

High-Level Business Goals

The vision statement of an organization is an excellent place to start because it tells the world where the company excels and what differentiates that company from its competitors. There will typically be several key objectives behind this vision, which are not so publicly stated, that can be related to the Exchange Server 2003 upgrade. These should be uncovered and clarified, or it will be difficult, if not impossible, to judge whether the project succeeds or fails from a business standpoint.

> **NOTE**
>
> High-level business goals that pertain to an Exchange Server 2003 upgrade can include better leveraging company knowledge and resources through efficient communications and collaboration, controlling IT costs to lower overhead and enable products to be more competitively priced, or improving security to meet governmental requirements.

Although this process sounds basic, it might be more difficult if the company hasn't documented or updated its business objectives in some time (or *ever*). Different divisions of larger companies might even have conflicting business goals, which can make matters more complicated. High-level business goals of a company can also change rapidly, whether in response to changing economic conditions or as affected by a new key stakeholder or leader in the company. So even if a company has a standard vision statement in place, it is worth taking time to review and ensure that it still accurately reflects the opinions of the key stakeholders.

This process helps clarify how the messaging upgrade fits into the overall company strategy and should help ensure that support will be there to approve the project and keep its momentum going. In this time of economic uncertainty, a project must be strategic and directly influence the delivery of the company's services and products; otherwise, the danger exists of a key stakeholder "pulling the plug" at the first sign of trouble or shifting attention to a more urgent project.

For example, a consulting organization might have a stated vision of providing the latest and greatest processes and information to its clients, and the internal goal could be to make its internal assets (data) available to all employees at all times to best leverage the knowledge gained in other engagements. The Exchange environment plays a key role in meeting this goal, because employees have become so dependent on Outlook for communicating and organizing information and many of the employees rely on portable devices and Pocket PCs.

A different company, one which specializes in providing low-cost products to the marketplace, might have an internal goal of cost control, which can be met by Exchange Server 2003 through reduction in the total server count and more cost-effective management to help reduce downtime. For this company, user productivity is measured carefully, and the enhancements in the Outlook 2003 client would contribute positively.

High-Level Messaging Goals

At this point the business goals that will guide and justify the Exchange upgrade should be clearly defined, and the manner in which Exchange Server 2003's enhanced features will be valuable to the company are starting to become clear. The discussion can now turn to learning from key stakeholders what goals they have that are specific to the messaging environment that will be put in place.

The high-level goals tend to come up immediately, and be fairly vague in nature; but they can be clarified to determine the specific requirements. A CEO of the company might simply state "I need access to my email and calendar from anywhere." The CTO of the same company might demand "zero downtime of the Exchange servers and easy administration." The CFO may want to "reduce the costs of the email system." If the managers in different departments are involved in the conversation, a second level of goals might well be expressed. The IT manager might want 4-node clustering, the ability to restore a single user's mailbox, and reduced user complaints about spam and performance. The marketing manager might want better tools to organize the ever-increasing amount of "stuff" in his employees' in-boxes and mail folders.

Time spent gathering this information helps ensure that the project is successful and the technology goals match up with the business goals. It also matters who is spearheading the process and asking the questions, because the answers might be very different if asked by the president of the company rather than an outside consultant who has no direct influence over the career of the interviewee.

NOTE

An example of some high-level messaging goals include a desire to have no downtime of the Exchange Servers, access to email and calendars from anywhere, better functionality of the OWA client, and increased virus and spam protection.

A specific trend or theme to look for in the expression of these goals is whether they are focused on fixing and stabilizing or on adding new functionality. When a company is fixated on simply "making things work properly," it might make sense to hold off on implementing a variety of new functionality (such as video conferencing or providing Windows-powered mobile devices such as Pocket PCs) at the same time.

Business Unit or Departmental Messaging Goals

After these higher-level goals have been identified, the conversations can be expanded to include departmental managers and team leads. The results will start to reveal the complexity of the project and the details needed to complete the statement of work for the migration project. For an Exchange upgrade project to be completely successful, these individuals, as well as the end-users, need to benefit in measurable ways.

Based on the business and technology goals identified thus far, the relative importance of different departments will start to become clear. Some organizations are IT-driven, especially if they are dependent on the network infrastructure to deliver the company's products and services, Others can survive quite well if technology isn't available for a day or even longer.

> **NOTE**
>
> An example of some departmental goals include a desire to ensure encrypted transmission of human resource and personnel emails, an OWA client that has the same functionality as the Outlook client, and support for SmartPhone and Pocket PC devices. The IT department might also like better mailbox recovery tools and Exchange-specific management tools that can be used from MOM.

All departments use email, but the sales department might also receive voicemails through the Outlook client and updates on product pricing, and thus need the best possible reliability and performance. This includes ensuring that viruses don't make it into employee in-boxes and that spam be reduced as much as possible.

Certain key executives are rarely in the office and aren't happy with the existing Outlook Web Access client. They also carry BlackBerry wireless devices and need to make sure that they remain fully functional during and after the upgrade.

The marketing department uses the email system for sharing graphics files via public folders, which have grown to an almost unmanageable size, but this enables them to share the data with strategic partners outside of the company. This practice won't change, and the amount of data to be managed will continue to grow over time.

The finance and human resources departments are very concerned about security and want to make sure that all email information and attached files are as safe as possible when traveling within the organization, or being sent to clients over the Internet.

The IT department has a very aggressive service level agreement (SLA) to meet and is interested in clustering, reducing the number of servers that need to be managed, and improving the management tools in place. In addition, Exchange Server 2003's integration with Active Directory will facilitate the management of users and groups and additions and changes to existing user information.

In the process of clarifying these goals, the features of the Exchange messaging system that are most important to the different departments and executives should become apparent.

A user focus group might also be helpful, which can be comprised of employee volunteers and select managers, to engage in detailed discussions and brainstorming sessions. In this way the end-users can participate in the initial planning process and help influence the decisions that will affect their day-to-day work experience. New features offered by the Outlook 2003 client include the Exchange Cached Mode, optimized network traffic with data compression, and an improved Outlook 2003 client and OWA capabilities.

Other outcomes of these discussions should include an understanding of which stakeholders will be involved in the project and the goals that are primary for each person and each department. A sense of excitement should start to build over the possibilities presented by the new technologies that will be introduced to make managers' lives easier and workers' days more productive.

Initiation Phase: Creating the Statement of Work

Executives generally require a documented Statement of Work that reflects strategic thinking, an understanding of the goals and objectives of the organization, and a sense of confidence that the project will be successful and beneficial to the company. The document needs to be clear and specific and keep its audience in mind, which generally means not going into too much technical detail. This document also needs to give an estimate of the duration of the project, the costs involved, and the resources required.

The initial scope of work might have changed and evolved as discussions with the executives, managers, and stakeholders reveal problems that weren't obvious and requirements that hadn't been foreseen. Although the scope started out as a "simple Exchange upgrade" it might have expanded to include an upgrade to Active Directory, the addition of new features for remote access to the messaging environment, or management and business continuity features.

The following is a standard outline for the Statement of Work document:

1. Scope of Work
2. Goals
3. Timeline and Milestones
4. Resources
5. Risks and Assumptions
6. Initial Budget

The following sections cover the different components of the Statement of Work. This document is arguably the most important in the entire process because it can convince the executives who hold the purse strings to move forward with the project—or, of course, stop the project in its tracks.

Summarizing the Scope of Work

At this point in the initiation phase, a number of conversations have occurred that have clarified the basic scope of the project, the high-level business goals as they pertain to the messaging upgrade, and the more specific goals for each department and of key stakeholders. Armed with this wealth of information, the lead consultant on the project should now organize the data to include in the Statement of Work and get sign-off to complete the phase and move to the more detailed planning phase.

The Scope section of the Statement of Work document should answer these essential questions:

- How many Exchange and Windows servers need to be upgraded?

- Where do these servers reside?

- What additional applications need to be upgraded (especially backup, virus protection, disaster recovery [DR], and remote access) as part of the project?

- What additional hardware needs to be upgraded or modified to support the new servers and applications (especially tape backup devices, storage area networks, routers)?

- Will the desktop configurations be changed?

The answers to these questions may still be unclear at this point, and require additional attention during the planning phase.

Summarizing the Goals

As discussed earlier, a number of conversations have been held previously on the topic of goals, so there may be a fairly long list of objectives at this point. A structure to organize these goals is suggested in the following list:

- Business continuity/disaster recovery (Clustering, Storage, Backup and Restore)

- Performance (Memory Allocation Improvements, Public Folders, Email)

- Security (Server, Email)

- Mobility (Outlook Web Access, Pocket PC and SmartPhone Support)

- Collaboration (Real-time Collaboration—replacement for Exchange Instant Messaging—SharePoint Portal)

- Serviceability (Administration, Management, Deployment)

- Development (Collaboration Data Objects, Managed API)

By using a framework such as this, any "holes" in the goals and objectives of the project will be more obvious. Some of the less glamorous objectives, such as a stable network, data recovery abilities, or protection from the hostile outside world, might not have been identified in the discussions. This is the time to bring up topics that might have been missed, before moving into the more detailed planning phase.

It might also be valuable to indicate what will be corrected by the upgrade ("pain points") and what new capabilities will be added.

Summarizing the Timeline and Milestones

A bulleted list of tasks is typically all that is needed to help define the time frame for the upgrade (more complex projects might benefit from a high-level Gantt chart of no more than 10–20 lines). The time frame should be broken down by phase to clarify how much time is to be allocated for the planning phase and testing phases. The actual implementation of the upgrade also should be estimated.

Depending on the complexity of the project, a time frame of 1–2 months could be considered a "short" time frame, with 2–4 months offering a more comfortable window for projects involving more servers, users, and messaging-related applications. Additional time should be included if an outside consulting firm will assist with part or all of the project.

Because every project is different, it's impossible to provide rules for how much time to allocate to which phase. Experience has shown that allocating additional time for the planning and testing phase helps the upgrade go more smoothly, resulting in a happier user base. If little or no planning is done, the testing phase will most likely miss key requirements for the success of the project. Remember also to allocate time during the process for training of the administrative staff and end users.

The key to successfully meeting a short timeline is to understand the added risks involved and define the scope of the project so that the risks are controlled. This might include putting off some of the functionality that is not essential, or contracting outside assistance to speed up the process and leverage the experience of a firm that has performed similar upgrades many times. Hardware and software procurement can also pose delays, so for shorter time frames, they should be procured as soon as possible after the ideal configuration has been defined.

Some upgrades can actually take place over a single weekend; then on Monday morning users show up for training and are up and running on the new messaging platform.

Summarizing the Resources Required

Typical roles that need to be filled for an Exchange Server 2003 upgrade project include

- Project Sponsor
- Exchange Server 2003 Design Consultant
- Exchange Server 2003 Technical Lead
- Exchange Server 2003 Consulting Engineer

- Project Manager

- Systems Engineer(s)

- Technical Writer

- Administrative Trainer

- End-user Trainer

The organization should objectively consider the experience and skills as well as available time of internal resources before deciding whether outside help is needed. For the most part, few companies completely outsource the whole project, choosing instead to leverage internal resources for the tasks that make sense and hiring external experts for the planning phase and testing phases. Often internal resources simply can't devote 100% of their energy to planning and testing the messaging technologies, because their daily duties will get in the way. Contracted resources, on the other hand, are able to focus just on the messaging project.

The resulting messaging environment needs to be supported after the dust settles, so it makes sense for the administrative staff to receive training in the early phases of the upgrade (such as planning and testing) rather than after the implementation. Many consultants provide hands-on training during the testing and implementation phases.

For larger projects, a team may be created for the planning phase, a separate team allocated for the testing phase, and a third team for the implementation. Ideally the individuals who perform the testing participate in the implementation for reasons of continuity. Implementation teams can benefit from less-experienced resources for basic server builds and workstation upgrades.

Summarizing the Risks and Assumptions

More time is spent discussing the details of the risks that could affect the successful outcome of the project during the planning phase; but if there are immediately obvious risks they should be included in the statement of work.

Basic risks could include

- Existing Exchange problems, such as corrupt database, lack of maintenance

- Lack of in-house expertise and bandwidth for the project

- Using existing hardware that might not have enough RAM, storage capacity, or processor speed

- WAN or LAN connectivity issues, making downtime a possibility

- A production environment that cannot experience any downtime or financial losses will occur

- Customized applications that interface with Exchange Server and that need to be tested and possibly rewritten for Exchange Server 2003

- Short timeline that will require cutting corners in the testing process

Summarizing the Initial Budget

The decision-makers will want to start getting a sense for the cost of the project, at least for the planning phase of the project. Some information might already be quite clear, such as how many servers need to be purchased. If the existing servers are more than a few years old, chances are they need to be replaced, and price quotes can easily be gathered for new machines. Software upgrades and licenses can also easily be gathered, and costs for peripheral devices such as tape drives or SANs should be included.

If external help is needed for the planning, testing, and implementation, some educated guesses should be made about the order of magnitude of these costs. Some organizations set aside a percentage of the overall budget for the planning phase, assuming outside assistance, and then determine whether they can do the testing and implementation on their own.

As mentioned previously, training should also not be forgotten—for both the administrative staff and the end-users.

Getting Approval on the Statement of Work

After the initial information has been presented in the Statement of Work format, formally present and discuss it with the stakeholders. If the process has gone smoothly this far, the Statement of Work should be approved, or, if not, items that are still unclear can be clarified. After this document has been agreed on, a great foundation is in place to move forward with the planning phase.

Planning Phase: Discovery

The planning phase enables the Exchange Server 2003 design consultant time to paint the detailed picture of what the end-state of the upgrade will look like, and also to detail exactly how the network will evolve to this new state. The goals of the project are clear, what's in and what's out are documented, the resources required are defined, the timeline for the planning phase and an initial sketch of the risks are anticipated, and the budget is estimated.

Understanding the Existing Environment

If the organization has multiple Exchange servers in place, third-party add-on applications, multiple sites, complex remote access, or security requirements, a network audit makes sense. If an outside company is spearheading the planning phase, this is its first real look at the configuration of the existing hardware and network, and it is essential to help create an appropriate end-state and migration process. Standard questionnaires are helpful to collect data on the different servers that will be affected by the upgrade.

The discovery process typically starts with onsite interviews with the IT resources responsible for the different areas of the network and proceeds with a hands-on review of the network configuration. Focus groups or whiteboarding sessions can also help dredge up concerns or issues that might not have been shared previously. External consultants often generate better results because they have extensive experience with network reviews and analysis and with predicting the problems that can emerge midway through a project.

Network performance can be assessed at the same time to predict the level of performance the end-users will see and whether they are accessing email, public folders, or calendars from within the company, from home, or from an Internet kiosk in an airport.

Existing network security policies might be affected by the upgrade, and should be reviewed. If AD is being implemented, group policies—which define user and computer configurations and provide the ability to centralize logon scripts and printer access—can be leveraged.

Anyone using Exchange is familiar with the challenges of effectively managing the data that builds up, and in grooming and maintaining these databases. The existing database structure should be reviewed at least briefly so the Exchange Server 2003 design consultant understands where the databases reside, how many there are and their respective sizes, and whether regular maintenance has been performed. Serious issues with the database(s) crashing in the past should be covered. Methods of backing up this data should also be reviewed.

Desktop configurations should be reviewed if the upgrade involves an upgrade to the Outlook client. If there are a variety of different desktop configurations, operating systems, and models, the testing phase might need to expand to include these.

Disaster recovery plans or service level agreements (SLAs) can be vital to the IT department's ability to meet the needs of the user community, and should be available for review at this time.

What remote and mobile connections to the messaging system are currently in use? OWA is used by most organizations, as well as Terminal Services, or VPNs. The features in Exchange Server 2003 may enable the organization to simplify this process; VPNs might no longer be needed because Outlook can be accessed via HTTP.

Although the amount of time required for this discovery process varies greatly, the goals are to fully understand the messaging infrastructure in place as the foundation on which the upgrade will be built. New information might come to light in this process that will require modifications to the Statement of Work document.

Understanding the Geographic Distribution of Resources

If network diagrams exist, they should be reviewed to make sure they are up to date and contain enough information (such as server names, roles, applications managed, switches, routers, firewalls, IP address info, gateways, and so forth) to fully define the location and function of each device that plays a role in the upgrade. These diagrams can then be modified to show the end-state of the project.

Existing utility servers—such as bridgehead servers, front-end servers, DNS naming servers, and DHCP or WINS servers—should be taken into account.

Has connectivity failure been planned for a partial or fully meshed environment? Connections to the outside world and other organizations need to be reviewed and fully understood at the same level, especially with an eye toward the existing security features.

Companies with multiple sites bring added challenges to the table. As much as possible, the same level of information should be gathered on all the sites that will be involved in and affected by the messaging upgrade. Also, a *centralized* IT environment has different requirements from a *distributed* management model.

If time permits, the number of support personnel in each location should be taken into account, as well as their ability to support the new environment. Some smaller sites might not have dedicated support staff and network monitoring, and management tools, such as MOM or SMS, might be required.

How is directory information replicated between sites, and what domain design is in place? If the company already has Active Directory in place, is a single domain with a simple organizational unit (OU) structure in place, or are there multiple domains with a complex OU structure? Global Catalog placement should also be clarified.

The answers to these questions directly shape the design of the solution, the testing phase, and the implementation process.

Planning Phase: Creating the Design Document

When the initial discovery work is complete, attention can be turned to the Design document itself, which paints a detailed picture of the end-state of the network upgrade. In essence, this document expands on the Statement of Work document and summarizes the process that was followed and the decisions that were made along the way.

The second key deliverable in the planning phase is the Migration document, which tells the story of how the end-state will be reached. Typically, these documents are separate, because the Design document gives the "what" and "why" information, and the Migration document gives the "how" and "when" information.

Collaboration Sessions: Making the Design Decisions

The planning phase kicked off with discovery efforts and review of the networking environment, and additional meetings with the stakeholders and the Project Team should be scheduled for collaborative discussions. This process covers the new features that Exchange

Server 2003 offers and how these could be beneficial to the organization as a whole and to specific departments or key users. Typically, several half-day sessions are required to discuss the new features and whether implementing them makes sense.

Ideally, quite a bit of thought has already gone into what the end-state will look like, as reflected in the Statement of Work document, so everyone attending these sessions will be on the same page in terms of goals and expectations for the project. If they aren't, this is the time to resolve differing opinions, because the Design document is the blueprint for the results of the messaging upgrade.

The collaborative sessions should be led by a consultant with hands-on experience in designing and implementing Exchange Server 2003 solutions. Agendas should be provided in advance to keep the sessions on track (see Figure 2.1 for a sample agenda) and enable attendees to prepare specific questions. A technical writer should be invited to take notes and start to become familiar with the project as a whole, because that individual will most likely be active in creating the Design document and additional documents required.

Agenda – Exchange 2003 Design

1. Goals and Objectives
    a. Overall Project Goals
    b. Department Goals
    c. Requirement for Scalability
    d. Need for Fault Tolerance / Redundancy

2. AD Topolgy
    a. Forests/Domains/Sites/GCs
    b. OUs/Groups/Users
    c. DNS/DDNS

3. Exchange 2003 Architecture
    a. Mailbox Server Placement
    b. Public Folder Servers
    c. Connector Servers
    d. OWA
    e. Global Catalog Placement
    f. Administrative Groups
    g. Routing Groups
    h. Mixed Mode vs. Native Mode
    i. Server Loading
    j. Server Sizing
    k. Client Performance over WAN
    l. High Availability

4. Exchange 2003 Database
    a. Storage Group Design
    b. Databases
    c. Log Files
    d. Database Sizing
    e. Users per server
    f. Mailbox Sizing
    g. Mailbox Cleanup
    h. Backup – Storage Group

    i. Restore – Database
    j. Service Level Agreements

5. Connectors
    a. Recipient Synch
    b. Bulletins/Public Folders Synch
    c. Configuration Synch
    d. One-way or Two-way

6. Security Model
    a. Groups
    b. Administrators
    c. Enterprise Administrators
    d. OWA/FE Servers

7. Administrative Model
    a. Server Administration
    b. View-Only Administrator
    c. Administrator
    d. Full Administrator
    e. User Administration
    f. Delegation
    g. System Policy
    h. Recipient Policy

8. Application Integration
    a. BlackBerry

9. Exchange Clients
    a. Outlook 2003/Outlook 2000 / XP
    b. OWA/HTTP-DAV/HTTPS
    c. POP3/SMTP
    d. IMAP4

FIGURE 2.1   Sample Exchange Server 2003 design agenda.

The specifics of the upgrade should be discussed in depth, especially the role that each server will play in the upgrade. A diagram is typically created during this process (or an existing Visio diagram updated) that defines the locations and roles of all Exchange 2003 Servers and any legacy Exchange Servers that need to be kept in place.

The migration process should be discussed as well, although often organizations prefer to discuss the minutiae of the migration *after* the Design document has been completed. Why spend hours discussing how to get to end-state A when the budget ends up being too high, and a design B needs to be crafted?

Disaster Recovery Options

A full disaster recovery assessment is most likely out of the scope of the messaging upgrade project, but the topic should be covered at this phase in the project.

Most people would agree that the average organization would be severely affected if the messaging environment were to go offline for an extended period of time. Communications between employees would have to be in person or over the phone, document sharing would be more complex, communication with clients would be affected, and productivity of the remote work force would suffer. Employees in the field rarely carry pagers any more, and some have even discarded their cell phones, so many employees would be hard to reach. This dependence on messaging makes it critical to adequately cover the topic of disaster recovery as it pertains to the Exchange messaging environment.

Existing service level agreements (SLAs) should be reviewed and input gathered on the "real" level of disaster recovery planning and testing that has been completed. Few companies have spent the necessary time and energy to create plans of action for the different failures that could take place, such as power failures in one or more locations, Exchange database corruptions, or server failures. A complete disaster recovery plan should include offsite data and application access as well.

Design Document Structure

The Design document expands on the content created for the Statement of Work document defined previously, but goes into greater detail and provides historical information on the decisions that were made. This is helpful if questions come up later in the testing or implementation process, such as "Whose idea was that?" or "Why did we make that decision?"

The following is a sample table of contents for the Exchange Server 2003 Design document:

1. Executive Summary

2. Goals and Objectives

   - Business Objectives

   - Departmental Goals

3. Background

- Overview of Process

- Summary of Discovery Process

4. Exchange Design

- Exchange 2000 Design Diagram

- Exchange Mailbox Server Placement (where do they go)

- Organization (definition of and number of Exchange Organizations)

- Administrative Groups (definition of and number of)

- Routing Groups (definition of and number of)

- Storage Groups (definition of and number of)

- Mixed Mode Versus Native Mode (choice and decision)

- Global Catalog Placement (definition and placement)

- Recipient Policies (definition and usage)

- Front-end and Bridgehead Servers (definition and usage, includes remote access)

- Server Specifications (recommendations and decisions, role for each server defined, redundancy, disaster recovery options discussed)

- Virus Protection (selected product with configuration)

- Administrative Model (options defined, and decisions made for level of administration permitted by administrative group)

- System Policies (definition and decisions on which policies will be used)

- Exchange Monitoring (product selection and features described)

- Exchange Backup/Recovery (product selection and features described)

5. Budget Estimate

- Hardware and Software Estimate

Executive Summary

The Executive Summary should summarize the high-level solution for the reader in under one page by expanding upon the scope created previously. The importance of the testing phase can be explained and the budget summarized.

Design Goals and Objectives

Goals and objectives have been discussed earlier in this chapter and should be distilled down to the most important and universal goals. They can be broken down by department if needed. The goals and objectives listed can be used as a checklist of sign-off criteria for the project. The project is complete and successful when the goals are all met.

Background

In the background section, the material gathered in the discovery portion of the planning phase should be included in summary form (details can always be attached as appendixes); also helpful is a brief narrative of the process the project team followed to assemble this document and make the decisions summarized in the design portion of the document.

Design

The design section defines how the Exchange Server 2003 environment will be configured. Exchange Server 2003 was designed to be extremely flexible in how it can be added to the network. In Figure 2.2, the possibilities are listed for Exchange 5.5, Exchange 2000, Exchange Server 2003, Windows NT, Windows 2000, and Windows Server 2003. This flexibility can be very important if there are third-party applications used to extend the functionality of the current version of Exchange that are not available for Exchange Server 2003 or that have been written specifically for a previous version of Exchange or to control the costs of the overall upgrade. For instance, a unified messaging solution currently in place on Exchange 2000 could simply be left as is while the rest of the messaging environment is upgraded to Exchange Server 2003.

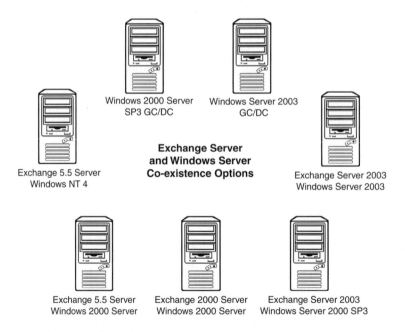

FIGURE 2.2   Exchange and Windows server coexistence.

NOTE

Note also that Exchange 5.5 and 2000 cannot run directly on servers running Windows 2003 Server; they can, however, operate in a Windows Server 2003 Active Directory environment.

Additional information on the options for coexistence of different Windows Server Operating Systems and Exchange Server versions is covered in Part II, "Microsoft Exchange Server 2003 Messaging."

Technical Advantages of Exchange Server 2003 Running on WS2003

Exchange Server 2003 can run on Windows 2000 and Windows Server 2003, but the latter provides a number of technical advantages. Note that Exchange Server 2003 cannot be run on Windows Server 2003 Web Edition.

Using Exchange Server 2003 with Windows Server 2003 provides memory tuning, database snapshot through Volume Shadow Copy Services (VSS), secured HTTP support for Outlook 2003, OWA compression support, IPSec support between front-end and back-end clusters, object quotas, and SID filtering. If Windows Server 2003 Enterprise is the platform, there is support for up to 8-way PIII or P4 processors, and up to 8-node clustering.

If the Enterprise version of Exchange Server 2003 is used, the 16GB database limit is removed; instead of 1 mailbox store, there can be up to 20 databases per server.

Future chapters cover these topics in greater detail, especially in Parts III, "Microsoft Networking Services' Impact on Exchange"; IV, "Securing a Microsoft Exchange Server 2003 Environment"; VI, "Microsoft Exchange Server 2003 Administration and Management"; VII, "New Mobility Functionality in Microsoft Exchange Server 2003"; and X, "Fault Tolerance and Optimization Technologies."

Agreeing on the Design

When the document is complete, it should be presented to the project stakeholders and reviewed to make sure that it fully meets their requirements, and to see whether any additional concerns come up. If there were significant changes since the initiation phase's Statement of Work document, they should be highlighted and reviewed at this point. Again, it is valuable in terms of time and effort to identify any issues at this stage in the project, especially when the Migration document still needs to be created.

Some organizations choose to use the Design document to get competitive proposals from service providers, and having this information levels the playing field and results in proposals that promise the same end results.

Creating the Migration Document

With the Design document completed and agreed to by the decision-makers, the Migration document can now be created. There are always different ways to reach the desired Exchange Server 2003 configuration, and the Migration document presents the method best suited to the needs of the organization—in terms of timeline, division of labor, and cost—based on the goals and objectives defined in the initiation and planning processes. The Migration document makes the project real; it presents specific information on "who does what" in the actual testing and migration process, assigns costs to the resources as applicable, and creates a specific timeline with milestones and due dates.

The Migration document should present enough detail about the testing and upgrade process that the resources performing the work have guidance and understand the purpose and goals of each step. The Migration document is not a step-by-step handbook of how to configure the servers, implement the security features, and move mailboxes. The Migration document is still fairly high level, and the resources performing the work need real-world experience and troubleshooting skills.

Additional collaborative meetings might be needed at this point to brainstorm and decide both on the exact steps that will be followed and when the testing and upgrade will be (see Figure 2.3).

Part V, "Migrating to Microsoft Exchange Server 2003," provides additional information about the various strategies and processes for moving from previous versions of Exchange to Exchange Server 2003.

The Project Schedule

A *project schedule* or *Gantt Chart* is a standard component of the Migration document, and it presents tasks organized by the order in which they need to be completed, in essence creating a detailed roadmap of how the organization will get from the current state, test the solution, and then implement it.

Other important information is included in the project schedule: resources assigned to each task, start dates and durations, key checkpoints, and milestones. Milestones by definition have no duration and represent events such as the arrival of hardware items, sign-off approval on a series of tasks, and similar events. Some additional time should be allocated (contingency time) if possible during the testing phase or between phases, in case stumbling blocks are encountered.

A good rule of thumb is to have each task line represent at least four hours of activities; otherwise, the schedule can become too long and cumbersome. Another good rule is that a task should not be less than 1% of the total project, thus limiting the project to 100 lines. The project schedule is not intended to provide detailed information to the individuals performing the tasks, but to help schedule, budget, and manage the project.

Agenda – Exchange 2003 Migration Planning

1. Goals and Objectives

2. Project Management
    a. Benefits of Phased Approach
    b. Phase 1 - Design/Planning
    c. Phase 2 - Prototype
    d. Phase 3 - Pilot
    e. Phase 4 - Implement
    f. Phase 5 - Support
    g. Timeline, Milestones
    h. Resource Requirements
    i. Risk Management
    j. Checkpoints

3. Migration Planning
    a. ForestPrep/DomainPrep
    b. Site Replication Service (SRS)
    c. Existing Mail PO Infrastructure/Routing
    d. PO Consolidation
    e. PO Pre-migration Maintenance
    f. Client Personal Folders Renaming
    g. One-to-one Mailbox Mapping
    h. Exchange Security Groups
    i. Universal Groups, DL, and Native Mode
    j. Move Mailboxes
    k. Migrating Mobile Users
    l. Direct/Gradual/Rolling Upgrade
    m. NTDSNoMatch Option
    n. Switching to Native Mode

4. Deployment Tools
    a. Scripting
    b. Built-in Exchange Migration Wizard
    c. Third-party

5. Building
    a. Normalize Environment

    b. Datacenter First
    c. Branch Offices Second
    d. Deployment Strategies
    e. Staged vs. Scripted vs. Manual

6. Documentation
    a. Design/Plan
    b. As-builts
    c. Build Guides
    d. Migration Guides
    e. Administration Guides
    f. Maintenance Guides
    g. Disaster Recovery Guides
    h. User Guides/Informational Updates

7. Training
    a. Users
    b. Administrators
    c. Migration Team
    d. Technical Experts

8. Communications
    a. Migration Team
    b. Executives and Management
    c. Administrators
    d. Users
    e. Methods
    f. Frequency
    g. Detail Level

9. Administration and Maintenance
    a. Administration
    b. Maintenance
    c. Disaster Recovery
    d. Guides
    e. Periodic Schedules
    f. Daily / Weekly / Monthly
    g. Planned Downtime
    h. Checklists
    i. Testing

FIGURE 2.3   Migration session agenda.

To create a project schedule, a product such as Microsoft Project is recommended, which facilitates the process of starting with the high-level steps and then filling in the individual tasks. The high-level tasks, such as those shown in Figure 2.4, should be established first and can include testing the server configurations and desktop designs, performing one or more pilot implementations, the upgrade or migration process, and the support phase.

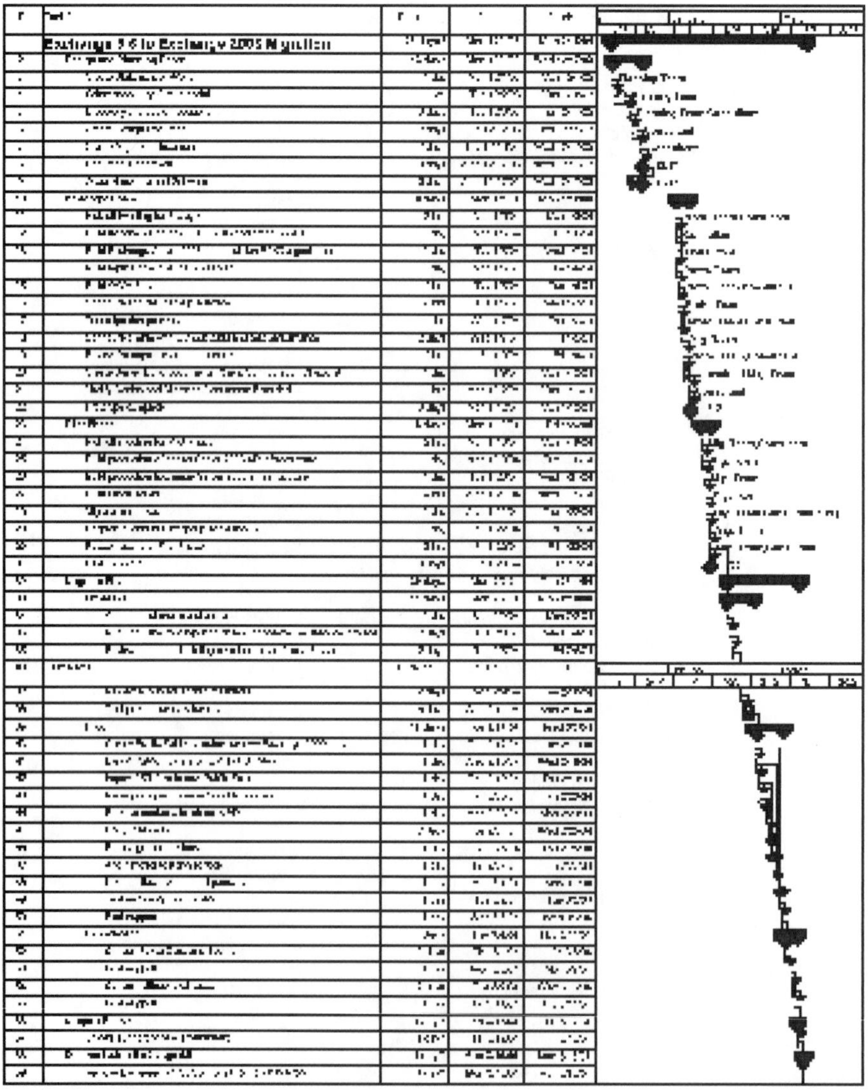

FIGURE 2.4   Sample project schedule.

Dependencies can also be created between tasks to clarify that Task 40 needs to be completed before Task 50 can start. A variety of additional tools and reports are built in to see whether resources are overburdened (for example, being expected to work 20 hours in one day), which can be used for *resource leveling*. A *baseline* can also be set, which represents the initial schedule, and then the *actuals* can be tracked and compared to the baseline to see whether the project is ahead or behind schedule.

Microsoft Project is also extremely useful in creating budgetary information and creating what-if scenarios to see how best to allocate the organization's budget for outside assistance, support, or training.

If the timeline is very short, the Gantt chart can be used to see if multiple tasks take place simultaneously or if this will cause conflicts.

Create the Migration Document

With the project schedule completed, the Migration document will come together quite easily, because it essentially fills out the "story" told by the Gantt chart. Typically the Migration document is similar to the structure of the Design document (another reason why many organizations want to combine the two), but the Design document relates the design decisions made and details the end-state of the upgrade, and the Migration document details the process and steps to be taken.

The following is a sample table of contents for the Migration document:

1. Executive Summary

2. Goals and Objectives of the Migration Process

3. Background

4. Summary of Migration-Specific Decisions

5. Risks and Assumptions

6. Roles and Responsibilities

7. Timeline and Milestones

8. Training Plan

9. Migration Process

   - Hardware and Software Procurement Process

   - Prototype Proof of Concept Process

   - Server Configuration and Testing

   - Desktop Configuration and Testing

   - Documentation Required from Prototype

   - Pilot Phase(s) Detailed

   - Migration/Upgrade Detailed

   - Support Phase Detailed

   - Support Documentation Detailed

10. Budget Estimate

- Labor Costs for Prototype Phase

- Labor Costs for Pilot Phase

- Labor Costs for Migration/Upgrade Phase

- Labor Costs for Support Phase

- Costs for Training

11. Project Schedule (Gantt Chart)

The following sections delve into the information that should be covered in each section. Part V of this book provides in-depth information on the steps involved in migrating to Exchange Server 2003 from Exchange 5.5 or Exchange 2000, and Part IX, "Client Administration and Management," provides details on the client configuration options and processes.

Executive Summary

As with the Design document, the executive summary section summarizes what the Migration document covers, the scope of the project, and the budget requested.

Goals and Objectives of the Migration Process

The goals and objectives of the migration overlap with those of the overall project, but should focus also on what the goals are for use and development of internal resources, and the experience of the user community. A goal of the overall project could be "no interruption of messaging services," and this would certainly be a goal to include in the Migration document.

Subphases of the Migration document have their own specific goals that might not have been included in the Design document. For example, a primary goal of the prototype phase, which takes place in a lab environment so it won't interfere with the production network, is to validate the design and to test compatibility with messaging-related applications. Other goals of the prototype phase can include hands-on training for the migration team, creating documents for configuration of the production servers, and creating and validating the functionality of the desktop configurations.

Background

A summary of the migration-specific decisions should be provided to answer questions such as "Why are we doing it that way?" Because there is always a variety of ways to implement new messaging technologies—such as in-place upgrades instead of buying new hardware—and a number of conversations will have taken place during the planning phase, it is worth summarizing them early in the document.

Risks and Assumptions

Risks pertaining to the phases of the migration should be detailed, and typically are more specific than in the Design document. For example, a risk of the prototype phase might be that the hardware available won't perform adequately and needs to be upgraded. Faxing, virus protection, or backup software might not meet the requirements of the Design document and thus need upgrading. Custom-designed messaging applications, or Exchange add-ons might turn out not to be Exchange Server 2003–compatible.

Roles and Responsibilities

The Design document focuses on the high-level "who does what"; the Migration document should be much more specific, because the budget for labor services is part of this deliverable. Rather than just defining the roles (such as project sponsor, Exchange Server 2003 design consultant, Exchange Server 2003 technical lead, and project manager) the Migration document specifically indicates the level of involvement of each resource throughout the prototype, pilot, and migration phases. The project sponsor should stay involved throughout the process, and regular project status meetings keep the team on the same page.

The project manager is expected to keep the project on time, on budget, and within scope, but generally needs support from the project sponsor and key stakeholders involved in the project. Depending on how the project manager role is defined, this individual may be either a full-time resource, overseeing the activities on a daily basis, or a part-time resource, measuring the progress, ensuring effective communications, and raising flags when needed. A cautionary note: Expecting the project manager to be a technical resource—such as the Exchange Server 2003 technical lead—can lead to a conflict of interest and generally does not yield the best results. Projects tend to be more successful if even 10% of an experienced Project Manager's time can be allocated to assist.

Timeline and Milestones

Specific target dates can be listed, and should be available directly from the project schedule already created. This summary can be very helpful to executives and managers, whereas the Gantt Chart contains too much information. Constraints that were identified in the discovery process need to be kept in mind here, because there might be important dates (such as the end of the fiscal year), seasonal demands on the company that black out certain date ranges, and key company events or holidays.

Training Plan

Will training happen during the prototype testing process in a hands-on fashion for the project team, or will classroom-style training be required? Will the end-users be trained while their desktops are being upgraded, or be left with a training document, or be directed to a training video on the network? If management tools are being added to the environment, who will train the appropriate resources on how to effectively use them and not be overwhelmed by false alarms?

Migration Process

The project schedule Gantt chart line items should be included and expanded upon so that it is clear to the resources doing the work what is expected of them. The information does not need to be on the level of step-by-step instructions, but it should clarify the process and results expected from each task. For example, the Gantt chart might indicate that an Exchange Server needs to be configured, and in the Migration document, information would be added about which Service Pack is to be used for the NOS and for Exchange, how the hard drives are to be configured, and which additional applications (virus protection, tape backup, faxing, network management) need to be installed.

If the Gantt chart lists a task of, for example, "Configure and test Outlook 2003 on sales workstation," the Migration document gives a similar level of detail: Which image should be used to configure the base workstation configuration, which additional applications and version of Office should be loaded, how is the workstation to be locked down, and what testing process should be followed (is it scripted or will an end-user from the department do the testing)?

Documentation also should be described in more detail. The Gantt chart might simply list "Create as-Built documents," with *as-built* defined as "a document containing key server configuration information and screen shots so that a knowledgeable resource can rebuild the system from scratch."

Sign-off conditions for the prototype phase are important and should be included. Who needs to sign off on the results of the prototype phase to indicate that the goals were all met and that the design agreed upon is ready to be created in the production environment?

Similar levels of information are included for the pilot phase and the all-important migration itself. Typically during the pilot phase, all the upgraded functionality needs to be tested, including remote access to email, voicemail access, BlackBerry and personal information managers, and public folders.

After the Exchange Server 2003 infrastructure is fully in place, what level of support will be provided? If an outside firm has assisted, will it leave staff onsite for a period of time to hold users' hands and troubleshoot any issues that crop up?

If documentation is specified as part of the support phase, such as Exchange maintenance documents, disaster recovery plans, or procedural guides, expectations for these documents should be included to help the technical writers make sure the documents are satisfactory.

Budget Estimate

At this point in the process the budgetary numbers should be within 10–20% of the final costs, bearing in mind any risks already identified that could affect the budget. Breaking the budget into prototype, pilot, migration, support, and training sections helps the decision-makers understand how the budget will be allocated and make adjustments if needed. No matter how much thought has gone into estimating the resources required and risks that could affect the budget, the later phases of the project may change based on the outcome of the prototype phase or the pilot phase.

The Prototype Phase

Exchange Server 2003 offers a wealth of new features when compared to Exchange Server 2000 or Exchange 5.5, including database backup through Volume Shadow Copy Service (VSS), public folder store replication improvements, Outlook 2003 Cached Exchange Mode, cross-forest Kerberos authentication, front-end and back-end Kerberos authentication, secured HTTP access from Outlook 2003, public folder search capabilities, and Exchange-specific events for use with MOM. Other features are upgrades from Exchange Server 2000 capabilities—such as Outlook Mobile Access (OMA), which is a rewrite of Mobile Information Server—and some of the previous functionality—such as Exchange Conferencing Server—are not supported on the Windows Server 2003 platform.

Depending on the design that was decided on by the organization, the prototype phase varies greatly in complexity and duration. It is still critical to perform a prototype, even for the simplest environments, to validate the design, test the mailbox migration process, and ensure that there won't be any surprises during the actual upgrade. The prototype lab should be isolated from the production network via a VLAN or physical separation to avoid interfering with the live users.

The prototype phase also gives the project team a chance to get acquainted with the new features of Exchange Server 2003 and any new add-on applications that will be used, and to configure the hardware in a pressure-free environment. If an external company is assisting in this phase, informal or formal knowledge transfer should take place. Ideally, the prototype lab exactly mirrors the final messaging configuration so that training in this environment will be fully applicable to the administration and support skills needed after the upgrade.

What Is Needed for the Lab?

At a bare minimum, the lab should include a new Exchange Server 2003 Server, one each of the standard desktop and laptop configurations, the tape drive that will be used to back up the public and private information stores, and application software as defined in the Design document. Connectivity to the Internet should be available for testing OWA and mobile access.

Additional information on testing applications and devices for compatibility with Exchange Server 2003 is provided in Chapter 17, "Compatibility Testing for Exchange Server 2003."

Existing data stores should be checked for integrity and then imported to Exchange Server 2003 to ensure that the process goes smoothly. Exchange Server 2003 comes with improved mailbox migration tools, which are more resistant to failure when corrupt mailboxes are encountered and are multithreaded for better performance.

> **NOTE**
>
> The recommended route for customers with Exchange 5.5 Servers to get to Exchange 2003 is to install an Exchange 2003 Server into the site and move mailboxes. If Exchange 2000 is already in place, an in-place upgrade process can be used (SP3 needed for both the Exchange and the NOS), but Exchange should actually be upgraded to Exchange Server 2003, and then Windows 2000 should be upgraded to Windows Server 2003. Note that in this case, Mobile Information Server, Instant Messenger, and/or Chat should be uninstalled.

If site consolidation or server consolidation are goals of the project, the prototype lab can be used for these purposes. Multi-forest connectivity can now be tested, but this requires an IIFP server in one or more of the forests to enable directory synchronization.

Exchange Server 2003 also comes with a number of new tools to aid in the testing and migration process, which are covered in detail in Chapter 17. These include a prescriptive guide that walks through the deployment process, preparation tools that scan the topology and provide recommendations, and validation tools.

For more complex environments and larger companies, the lab should be kept in place even after the upgrade is completed. Although this requires the purchase of at least one additional Exchange Server and related software, it provides a handy environment for testing patches and upgrades to the production environment, performing offline database maintenance, and in worst case scenarios, a server to scavenge from in times of dire need.

After the lab is configured to match the end-state documented in the Design document, representative users from different departments with different levels of experience and feature requirements should be brought in and given a chance to play with the desktop configurations and test new features and remote access. Input should be solicited to see whether any changes need to be made to the client configurations or features offered, and to help get a sense for the training and support requirements.

Disaster Recovery Testing

Another important testing process that can be performed prior to implementation of the new solution on the live network is business continuity or disaster recovery testing. Ideally this was covered in the design process and DR requirements were included in the design itself.

Documentation from the Prototype

During the prototype phase, a number of useful documents can be created that will be useful to the deployment team during the pilot and production upgrade phases, and to the administrators when the upgrade is complete.

As-built documents capture the key configuration information on the Exchange Server 2003 systems so that they can easily be replicated during the upgrade or rebuilt from scratch in case of catastrophic failure. Generally the as-built documents include actual screenshots of key configuration screens to facilitate data entry.

Assuming that DR requirements for the project were defined as suggested previously, this is a perfect time to summarize the testing that was performed in the lab and record the steps a knowledgeable administrator should take in the failure scenarios tested.

Final Validation of the Migration Document

When the testing is complete, the migration plan should be reviewed a final time to make sure that the testing process didn't reveal any show-stoppers that will require a change in the way the upgrade will take place or in the components of the final messaging solution.

The end-users who have had a chance to get their feet wet and play with the new Outlook 2003 client and learn about the new capabilities and enhanced performance of Exchange Server 2003 should be spreading the word by now, and the whole company should be excited for the upgrade!

The Testing Phase: Validating the Plan to a Limited Number of Users

With the testing completed, the Exchange Server 2003 upgrade team has all the tools needed for a successful upgrade, if the steps outlined so far in this chapter have been followed. The Design document is updated based on the prototype testing results so that the end-state that the executives and decision-makers are expecting has been conceptually proven. Unpleasant surprises or frantic midnight emails requesting more budget are nonexistent. The roadmap of how to get to the end-state is created in detail, with the project schedule outlining the sequential steps to be taken and the Migration document providing the details of each step. Documentation on the exact server configurations and desktop configuration are created to assist the systems engineers who will be building and configuring the production hardware.

The project team has gained valuable experience in the safe lab environment, so it is brimming with confidence and excited to forge ahead. End-users representing the different departments, who tested and approved the proposed desktop configurations, are excited about the new features that will soon be available.

To be on the safe side, a rollback strategy should be clarified, in case unforeseen difficulties are encountered when the new servers are introduced to the network. Disaster recovery testing can also be done as part of the first pilot, so that the processes are tested with a small amount of data and a limited number of users.

The First Server in the Pilot

The testing phase officially starts when the first Exchange 2003 Server is implemented in the production environment. The same testing and sign-off criteria that were used in the lab environment can be used to verify that the server is functioning properly and coexisting with the present Exchange servers. Surprises might be waiting that will require some troubleshooting, because the production environment will add variables that weren't present in the lab, such as large quantities of data consuming bandwidth, non-Windows servers, network management applications, and applications that have nothing to do with messaging but may interfere with Exchange Server 2003.

The migration of the first group of mailboxes is the next test of the thoroughness of the preparation process. Depending on the complexity of the complete design, it might make sense to limit the functionality offered by the first pilot phase to basic Exchange Server 2003 functionality, and make sure that the foundation is stable before adding on the higher-end features, such as voicemail integration, mobile messaging, and faxing. The first server should have virus protection software and tape backup software installed. Remote access via OWA is an important item to test as soon as possible, because there can be complexities involved with DMZ configurations and firewalls.

Choosing the Pilot Group

The first group of users—preferably more than 10—represents a sampling of different types of users. If all members the first pilot group are in the same department, the feedback won't be as thorough and revealing as if different users from different departments with varied needs and expectations are chosen. It's also generally a good idea to avoid managers and executives in the first round, no matter how eager they are, because they will be more likely to be the most demanding, be the least tolerant of interruptions to network functionality, and have the most complex needs.

Although a great deal of testing has taken place already, these guinea pigs should understand that there will most likely be some fine tuning that needs to take place after their workstations are upgraded; they should allocate time from their workdays to test the upgrades carefully with the systems engineer performing the upgrade.

After the initial pilot group is successfully upgraded and functional, the number of users can be increased, because the upgrade team will be more efficient and the processes fine-tuned to where they are 99% error free.

For a multisite messaging environment, the pilot process should be carefully constructed to include the additional offices. It might make sense to fully implement Exchange Server 2003 and the related messaging applications in the headquarters before any of the other locations, but issues related to WAN connectivity might crop up later, and then the impact is greater than if a small pilot group is rolled out at HQ and several of the other offices. It is important to plan where the project team and helpdesk resources will be, and they ideally should travel to the other offices during those pilots, especially if no one from the other office participated in the lab testing phase.

The helpdesk should be ready to support standard user issues, and the impact can be judged for the first few subphases of the pilot. Issues encountered can be collected and tracked in a knowledgebase, and the most common issues or questions can be posted on the company intranet or in public folders, or used to create general training for the user community.

Gauging the Success of the Test Phase

When the test phase is complete, a sampling of the participants should be asked for input on the process and the results. Few companies do this on a formal basis, but the results can be very surprising and educational. Most employees should be informed of when the upgrade will take place, that no data will be lost, and that someone will be there to answer questions immediately after the upgrade. Little changes to the workstation environment—such as the loss of favorites or shortcuts, or a change in the network resources they have access to—can be very distressing and result in disgruntled pilot testers.

A project team meeting should be organized to share learning points and review the final outcome of the project. The company executives must now make the go/no go decision for the full migration, so they must be updated on the results of the pilot process.

The Implementation

When the test phase is officially completed and any lingering problems have been resolved with the upgrade process, there will typically be 10–20% of the total user community upgraded. The project team will have all the tools it needs to complete the remainder of the upgrade without serious issues. Small problems with individual workstations or laptops will probably still occur but the helpdesk is probably familiar with how to handle these issues at this point.

A key event at this point is the migration of large amounts of Exchange data. The public and private information stores should be analyzed with `eseutil` and `isinteg`, and complete backup copies should be made in case of serious problems. The project team should make sure that the entire user community is prepared for the migration and that training has been completed by the time a user's workstation is upgraded.

It is helpful to have a checklist for the tasks that need to be completed on the different types of workstations and laptops so that the same steps are taken for each unit, and any issues encountered can be recorded for follow-up if they aren't critical. Laptops will most likely be the most problematic because of the variation in models, features, and user requirements, and because the mobile employees often have unique needs when compared to workers who remain in the office. If home computers need to be upgraded with the Outlook 2003 client and if, for instance, the company VPN is being retired, these visits need to be coordinated.

As with the pilot phase, the satisfaction of the user community should be verified. New public folders or SharePoint discussions can be started, and supplemental training can be offered for users who might need some extra or repeat training.

Decommissioning the Old Exchange Environment

As mentioned previously, some upgrades require legacy Exchange servers to be kept online, if they are running applications that aren't ready or can't be upgraded right away to Exchange Server 2003. Even in environments where the Exchange 5.5 or 2000 Servers should be completely removed, this should not necessarily be done right away.

Supporting the New Exchange Server 2003 Environment

After the dust has settled and any lingering issues with users or functionality have been resolved, the project team can be officially disbanded, and possibly receive some extra monetary reward for the extra hours and a job well done. If they haven't been created already, Exchange Server Maintenance documents should be created to detail the daily, weekly, monthly, and quarterly steps to ensure that the environment is performing normally and the databases are healthy.

If the prototype lab is still in place, this is an ideal testing ground for these processes and for testing patches and new applications.

Summary

Exchange used to mean email and scheduling to the average user, but it has grown to become a critical business communications and collaboration tool. Email must be available at any hour of the day, and must be protected from viruses and spam. Calendars must be accessible to co-workers for scheduling meetings, or for company resources—such as conference rooms—to be allocated. Public folders enable company information to be shared on an as-needed basis and are replacing intranets in many organizations. The new productivity tools in Outlook 2003 make it an even more valuable tool for the average user.

The Outlook client has become an invaluable filing cabinet for the average user and a way of listening to voicemails, reading faxes, and keeping up on industry news. More "road warriors" can be fully functional because of their ability to access the network remotely, but email and scheduling access are major requirements. Any change to the Exchange messaging environment has an impact on every user on the network, and many organizations worry more about an Exchange upgrade than an NOS.

With these added features comes complexity in how the Exchange environment is configured and how it integrates with the network as a whole. An organization can have multiple Exchange Mail servers, front-end servers to provide OWA access, bridgehead servers to connect sites, and conferencing and mobile information servers.

Exchange Server 2003 was designed to be very flexible in how it can be integrated with the existing messaging environment. Exchange 5.5, 2000, and 2003 can coexist, and Exchange Server 2003 can be installed on Windows 2000 Server (with some limitations) or Windows Server 2003. This flexibility requires a phased implementation that starts with creating a scope for the project (what's in, what's out), understanding the goals from a business standpoint and a technology standpoint, and creating a more detailed Statement of work document. As the process moves forward, time should be spent on discovery of the existing environment and collaborative design sessions to agree on what the end result of the migration will be. After the design is documented and agreed on by the company executives and project stakeholders, a roadmap needs to be created to detail how to get from point A to point Z. A project schedule in the form of a Gantt chart paints the high-level picture, and a Migration document tells the details of the resources required, the specifics of the tasks to be performed, and the risks involved.

After all this documentation, lab testing is essential to prove the conceptual design and train the project team on the new technologies and prepare any documents needed for the migration. Assuming no show-stoppers are encountered in the testing process, Exchange Server 2003 can be introduced to the production network on a pilot basis, with a handful of users with different needs. When this process is complete and any snags are resolved, the full migration can be performed, with a high level of confidence that no major problems will be encountered. Upon completion of the migration, maintenance procedures should be created to ensure that the new messaging ecosystem is optimized and tuned.

The process can be summarized by saying that a thorough understanding of the needs of the organization, an assessment of the current environment, and a structure design and testing process yield more successful results.

Best Practices

This chapter focuses on the planning, prototype testing, migration, and deployment overview for a Microsoft Exchange 2003 implementation. The following are best practices from this chapter:

- An upgrade to Exchange 2003 should follow a process that keeps the project on schedule. Set up such a process with a four-phase approach, including initiation, planning, testing, and implementation.

- Documentation is important to keep track of plans, procedures, and schedules. Create some of the documentation that could be expected for an upgrade project, including a statement of work document, a design document, a project schedule, and a migration document.

- Key to the initiation phase is the definition of the scope of work. Create such a definition, identifying the key goals of the project.

- Make sure that the goals of the project are not just IT goals, but also include goals and objectives of the organization and business units of the organization. This ensures that business needs are tied to the migration initiative, which can later be quantified to determine cost savings or tangible business process improvements.

- Set milestones in a project that can ensure that key steps are being achieved and the project is progressing at an acceptable rate. Review any drastic variation in attaining milestone tasks and timelines to determine whether the project should be modified or changed, or the plans reviewed.

- Allocate skilled or qualified resources that can help the organization to better achieve technical success and keep it on schedule. Failure to include qualified personnel can have a drastic impact on the overall success of the project.

- Identify risks and assumptions in a project to provide the project manager the ability to assess situations and proactive work and avoid actions that might cause project failures.

- Plan the design around what is best for the organization, and then create the migration process to take into account the existing configuration of the systems within the organization. Although understanding the existing environment is important to the success of the project, an implementation or migration project should not predetermine the actions of the organization based on the existing enterprise configuration.

- Ensure that key stakeholders are involved in the ultimate design of the Exchange 2003 implementation. Without stakeholder agreement on the design, the project might not be completed and approved.

- Document decisions made in the collaborative design sessions as well as in the migration planning process to ensure that key decisions are agreed upon and accepted by the participants of the process. Anyone with questions on the decisions can ask for clarification before the project begins rather than stopping the project midstream.

- Test assumptions and validate procedures in the prototype phase. Rather than learning for the first time in a production environment that a migration will fail because an Exchange database is corrupt or has inconsistencies, the entire process can be tested in a lab environment without impacting users.

- Test the process in a live production environment with a limited number of users in the prototype phase. Although key executives (such as the CIO, or IT Director) want to be part of the initial pilot phase, it is usually not recommended to take such high-visibility users in the first phase. The pilot phase should be with users that will accept an incident of lost email or inability to send or receive messages for a couple days while problems are worked out. In many cases, a pre-pilot phase could include the more tolerant users, with a formal pilot phase including insistent executives of the organization.

- Migrate, implement, or upgrade after all testing has been validated. The production process should be exactly that, a process that methodically follows procedures to implement or migrate mailboxes into the Exchange 2003 environment.

CHAPTER 3

Installing Exchange Server 2003

This chapter explains the basic installation of a new Exchange 2003 server. In this latest version of Exchange, Microsoft has taken a big step in improving the installation process to make it a lot more intuitive than previous versions of Exchange. The tools included on the installation CD walk you through the preinstallation tasks to verify the environment prior to installing the server.

When you execute `setup.exe`, you are not launched immediately into the installation program. You are taken through a step-by-step checklist of tasks prior to launching the setup executable.

This chapter does not present upgrading or migrating from previous versions of Exchange and other messaging platforms. You read about migrations in Chapters 14, "Migrating from NT4 to Windows Server 2003"; 15, "Migrating from Exchange 5.5 to Exchange Server 2003"; and 16, "Migrating from Exchange 2000 to Exchange Server 2003."

Preparing for Implementation of Exchange 2003

Several tasks should be done prior to installing Exchange 2003. The choice of running Exchange 2003 on Windows 2000 or Windows 2003 affects the preinstallation steps that need to take place and the functionality of Exchange. Some tasks are optional, such as forest prep and domain prep (automatically done when setup is run), but most tasks are requirements that would stop the install process, such as having a Global Catalog available on the network or not having the NNTP service installed on the server where you are installing Exchange.

Implementing Active Directory

Before you install Exchange Server 2003 on your network you need to make sure that Active Directory is properly deployed. The Active Directory infrastructure and DNS need to be healthy and without replication errors prior to installing your first Exchange 2003 server. It is so important to perform health checks and verification steps in your environment prior to installation that the Exchange development team has designed the installation program to include these steps. Exdeploy walks you through all the preinstallation health checks before running the setup program for Exchange 2003.

Realizing the Impact of Windows on Exchange

Because Windows is the base infrastructure for Exchange 2003, take into account key factors prior to implementing Exchange:

- Global Catalog placement

- Windows Mixed versus Native Mode

- Group type used

- Extension of the forest schema

- Preparation of the Active Directory domain

Global Catalog Placement

One item to review is the placement of Global Catalogs within the Active Directory site configuration. The importance of the Global Catalog server cannot be overstated. The Global Catalog is used for the address list that users see when they are addressing a message. If the Global Catalog server is not available, the recipient's address will not resolve when users address a message, and the message will immediately be returned to the sender.

One well-equipped Global Catalog server can support several Exchange 2003 servers on the same LAN segment. There should be at least one Global Catalog server in every Active Directory site that contains an Exchange 2003 server. For large sites, two Global Catalogs are much better and provide redundancy in the event the first Global Catalog server is unavailable.

For optimization, plan on having a Global Catalog server close to the clients to provide efficient address list access. Making all domain controller servers Global Catalog servers is recommended for single Active Directory domain models, and it's also not a bad idea for Active Directory designs that use a placeholder domain as the forest root with one or two first-level domains. A good Active Directory site design helps make efficient use of bandwidth in this design. This design helps reduce some of the overhead with multiple Global Catalogs in every Active Directory site.

> **NOTE**
>
> When implementing Exchange 2003 in a Windows 2003 environment, because of a significant infrastructure improvement in Windows 2003 Active Directory, the domain controllers (DCs) now support the caching of Global Catalog information. So although the recommendation in this chapter is to place a Global Catalog server in every site, an organization can choose to install just a domain controller in remote sites when Windows 2003 Active Directory has been implemented.

The Active Directory Replication Monitor (ReplMon) can be used to help determine the number of Global Catalogs in the Active Directory forest. To start the Active Directory Replication Monitor, click Start, All Programs, Windows Support Tools, Command Prompt, and then run `replmon.exe`. Use the Edit menu to add a monitored server. When the server is displayed, right-click the server and select Show Global Catalog Servers in Enterprise.

> **TIP**
>
> To access the Windows 2003 support tools, install them from the Windows 2003 CD. Go to the original CD, select Support, Tools, and run the `Suptools.msi` installer, which installs the Windows 2003 support utilities into the \Program Files\Support Tools\ directory.

Choosing Between Active Directory Mixed and Native Mode in Exchange 2003

If the domain that will host Exchange 2003 is or was in mixed mode, a message may be displayed during domain prep saying that the domain might possibly be insecure because of the Pre-Windows 2000 Compatible Access group. This is just a warning, and the installation of Exchange can proceed with just the understanding that Exchange may be insecure due to the current configuration of the domain.

Members of the Pre-Windows 2000 Compatible Access group will be able to see the members of groups that have their membership marked as hidden. In order to secure group membership, users and groups must be removed from this group before installing Exchange 2003. It is not necessary to resolve this security issue prior to installing Exchange 2003, because the removal of objects from this group can be done soon after Exchange 2003 has completed installation.

> **NOTE**
>
> Frequently, confusion occurs when Exchange implementers hear that Windows Active Directory must be in Native Mode for the organization to be able to implement Exchange 2000 or Exchange 2003. That's not true. As covered in Chapter 15, during a migration, if the destination domain is not in Native Mode, certain public folder group attributes are not migrated properly. Workarounds are covered in Chapter 15, so Exchange 2003 *can* be implemented in a Mixed Mode domain structure if that fits the needs of the organization.

Selecting a Windows 2000/Windows 2003 Group Model

Groups can be a big issue in Exchange 2003, especially in multidomain Windows 2000 or Windows 2003 Active Directory environments. Exchange 2003 uses Windows 2000 groups in place of the distribution lists that were used in Exchange 5.5. Distribution lists in Exchange 5.5 have been replaced by distribution groups in Active Directory. A Windows 2000 or Windows 2003 distribution group is the same as an Exchange 5.5 distribution list except it cannot be assigned permissions on an access control list. This means the strategy to secure calendars, public folders, and resources in Exchange 5.5 has to be redesigned for Exchange 2003. There are two major issues with groups that architects and administrators need to be concerned about:

- Visibility

- Permissions

Viewing Group Membership with Visibility

Visibility enables users to view the membership of the group. This is obviously an important requirement when sending an email to a group of users, because the users would like to see the list of recipients to whom they are sending the message.

Here is the way the group types affect visibility:

- **Domain Local** Domain membership is not in the Global Catalog. Users in a domain can see the membership of domain local groups only from their own domain. They can see the group entry for domain local groups from other domains in the Global Address List (GAL), but they cannot see the members.

- **Global** Domain membership is not in the Global Catalog. Users in a domain can see the membership of global groups only from their own domain. They can see the group entry for global groups from other domains in the Global Address List but they cannot see the members.

- **Universal** Domain membership is in the Global Catalog. Users can see the membership of the group no matter where the group resides.

In a single domain model or a domain model that uses a placeholder for the forest root and just one first-level domain, this issue is fairly simple to solve. Any group model will work in this design as long as all mailbox-enabled users reside in the same domain. If the plan is to add more domains later, universal groups should be used because of their flexibility. Another option would be to use domain local groups and then convert them to universal groups after the additional domains are installed.

Permissions

Security groups are required for assigning permissions to calendars, public folders, and resources. A security group type of domain local, global, or universal must be selected to control permissions on objects. Because controlling access to collaboration objects is essential, it's best to avoid distribution groups to reduce confusion for end-users and administrators. If the organization is supporting multiple mail platforms, it might be forced to support the distribution group as a representation of the foreign mail system's mailing list, but try to avoid using them for collections of Exchange 2003 users.

For full functionality, the best solution is to use universal security groups. This provides the ability to see group membership across all domains and to assign permissions to calendars, file shares, public folders, and other resources—all with the same group. In larger environments, there are some obvious challenges with using universal groups that are mostly political because of the segmentation of which group controls email, directory, and file resources.

The second challenge with universal security groups is that the Active Directory domain must be in native mode to support universal security groups. This means all DCs in the domain must be running Windows 2000 or Windows 2003 Active Directory and not Windows NT 4.0.

The last challenge with using universal security groups is that they incur a replication penalty. If the group membership changes for one user, the entire group is replicated to all DCs in the local domain and to all Global Catalogs in the forest. This usually does not make or break a design decision to use universal security groups, but architects need to keep it in mind if they have remote Global Catalogs across bandwidth-choked links. The way Active Directory handles group membership changes might change in future revisions of the product.

> **NOTE**
>
> The way Active Directory handles group membership changes could be a problem for organizations that use in-house applications or third-party applications that automatically rebuild Universal Security Group membership daily, depending on list size, rebuild frequency, and the number of lists.
>
> Although Active Directory in Windows 2000 had a practical limit of 5,000 users for a single group membership, Active Directory in Windows 2003 has extended that far beyond 5,000 users. If very large lists are required, you can choose to use nested lists and keep each individual list to a functionally limited basis.

Extending the Active Directory Schema

The first step to the actual implementation of Exchange 2003 is to extend the Active Directory schema. The **schema** comprises the rules that apply to the directory and controls what type of information can be stored in the directory. It also describes how that information is stored in the directory—such as string, string length, integer, and so on. Exchange 2003 almost doubles the amount of attributes in the Active Directory schema.

Extending the schema is the easiest part of the installation, but it is also the place where many organizations make mistakes. To extend the Active Directory schema, use the /forestprep switch on setup.exe for Exchange 2003 or follow the steps outlined in the deployment tool. A few tips to note before extending the Active Directory schema:

- The schema must be extended on the server that holds the Schema Master FSMO role. By default, the first server installed in the forest contains the Schema Master; however, this role could have been moved to another server. To locate which server contains the Schema Master FSMO role, use the Active Directory Schema MMC snap-in, right-click the Active Directory Schema icon under the console root, and select Operations Master.

TIP

To use the Active Directory Schema MMC snap-in, the adminpak.msi file must be installed on the server. Use the run command and execute adminpak.msi to install the adminpak. After the adminpak is installed, open the MMC from the run prompt by executing MMC; then use the Add/Remove snap-in option from the Console menu to add the Active Directory Schema MMC snap-in.

- The account used to extend the schema must be a member of the schema admins group and domain admins or enterprise admins groups. The schema admins and enterprise admins groups are available only in the first domain in the forest. If the messaging group does not control the forest root domain, this process must be delegated to the group that does.

- A schema change forces a full replication of domain databases and Global catalog information in Active Directory. Many administrators are scared of full replications and have heard stories of bandwidth-saturated WAN links due to schema extensions. However, when a full replication occurs, the directory information is compressed before it is sent across the network. The actual amount of data sent across the wire will be approximately 15–20% of the actual Active Directory database size.

NOTE

For Windows NT 4.0 organizations still in the Active Directory planning stages, to get an approximate size of the Active Directory database size multiply the Windows NT 4.0 SAM database by a factor of 3. This is a good ballpark estimate to use for the database size that will be seen immediately after migration. To calculate the size after implementing Exchange 2003 and other new directory information, use the AdSizer tool from Microsoft, available at http://www.microsoft.com/downloads/.

Preparing the Windows 2000 or Windows 2003 Domain

The second step in preparing to install Exchange 2003 is to prepare the Windows 2000 or Windows 2003 domain that will host the Exchange servers or mailbox-enabled users. To prepare the Windows 2000 or Windows 2003 domains, use the /domainprep switch on setup.exe for Exchange 2003 or follow the steps outlined in the deployment tool.

The account used to prepare the Windows 2000 or Windows 2003 domains must be a member of the domain admins group in the domain where the /domainprep command is being run. Running domainprep performs the following operations on the domain:

- Creates the global security group Exchange Domain Servers

- Creates the domain local security group Enterprise Exchange Servers

- Adds the Exchange Domain Servers group to Enterprise Exchange Servers group

- Grants appropriate rights to the domain controller used for the Recipient Update Service

For domains that will host mailbox-enabled users and not host Exchange servers, administrators have the choice of running domainprep or manually creating a Recipient Update Service for the domain in Exchange System Manager. If the domain will never host Exchange servers, the Recipient Update Service should be manually created. If the domain will eventually host Exchange servers, domainprep should be used.

Preparing to Install Exchange 2003

After a solid Windows 2000/Windows 2003 infrastructure has been put in place, Exchange 2003 can be planned for implementation. The installation preparation process follows standard project methodology, which includes planning, prototype testing, implementing, and ongoing support.

Planning Your Exchange 2003 Installation

Chapter 1, "Exchange Server 2003 Technology Primer," covers the differences between the Exchange 2003 Standard Edition and the Enterprise Edition, and why an organization would choose one version over the other for a server. Chapters 4, "Exchange Server 2003 Design Concepts," and 5, "Designing an Enterprise Exchange Server 2003 Environment," of this book address the planning and design of an Exchange 2003 implementation for a small/medium versus a medium/large organization, respectively.

Choosing to Install Exchange in Either a Test or Production Environment

When installing Exchange 2003 for the first time, the organization should make the decision whether the implementation will be exclusively a test environment implementation, or whether the test will be simply a preinstallation of a future production environment. It is typically suggested to have the first implementation of Exchange 2003 be one of building a completely isolated test environment.

Having a test environment isolates test functional errors so that if there are any problems in the testing phase, they will not be injected into the existing networking environment. Any decision to move forward or hold back the implementation of Exchange will not change the impact the decisions have for the organization.

Many times when an organization begins to install Exchange as if it is a test environment, it loads an evaluation copy of the Windows or Exchange license on a low-end hardware system. Then because it has so much success from the initial tests, the organization puts the system into a production environment. This creates a problem because the system is built on expiring licenses and substandard hardware. When committed to being solely a test environment, the results should be to rebuild from scratch, and not put the test environment into position as a full production configuration.

Prototyping Your Exchange 2003 Installation

When the decision is made to build in a test or production environment, build Exchange 2003 in the expected environment. If the system will be solely a test configuration, the implementation of Exchange 2003 should be in an isolated lab. If the system will be used in production, the implementation of Exchange 2003 should be focused on building the appropriate best-practice server configuration, which will give the organization a better likelihood of a full production implementation success.

Some of the steps an organization should go through when considering to build a test Exchange environment include

- Building Exchange 2003 in a lab
- Testing email features and functions
- Verifying design configuration
- Testing failover and recovery

Much of the validation and testing should occur during the test process. It's a lot easier testing a disaster recovery rebuild of Exchange in an exclusively test environment than to test the recovery of an Exchange server for the first time during a very tense server rebuild and recovery process after a system crash. Additionally, this is a good time to test application compatibility, as covered in Chapter 17, "Compatibility Testing for Exchange Server 2003," before migrating to a full messaging environment and then testing to see whether a third-party fax, voicemail, or paging software will work with Exchange 2003.

Another item to test during the prototype testing phase is directory replication in a large multisite environment to ensure that the Global Catalog is being updated fast enough between sites. And of course, security is of concern for many organizations these days, and the appropriate level of security for the organization should be tested and validated. Many times the plan for securing mailbox or public folder access sounds great on paper, but when implemented, is too limiting for the average user to get functionality from the service. Slight adjustments in security levels help minimize user impact while strengthening existing security in the organization.

Conducting Preinstallation Checks on Exchange 2003

When it comes to the actual installation of Exchange 2003, you can run setup manually or you can create an unattend file so that the install can be automated for a branch office with no technical staff at the site. There are also different configurations of Exchange, such as Mailbox Server, Public Folder Server, Front-end Server, Back-end Server, and Bridgehead Server. This section covers the preinstallation tasks prior to installing the first Exchange server in the environment.

There are some changes in the Exchange 2003 setup program when compared to Exchange 2000. These changes include identical schema files in the Active Directory connector and Exchange 2003 setup, meaning that the schema gets updated only once when using the ADC. Exchange 2003 also does not require full permissions at the organizational level when installing your second Exchange server. After the first Exchange server is installed, all subsequent servers can be installed with administrative group–level permissions instead of organizationwide permissions. The setup program will no longer contact the Schema FSMO Role holder, as it did with Exchange 2000 setup.

Verifying Core Services Installation

When installing Exchange 2003 on a Windows 2000 SP3 server, you must make sure that IIS, NNTP, and SMTP are installed and running. This can be done by checking the services applet within administrative tools from the Start menu. The setup program looks for IIS, NNTP, and SMTP services before it begins the install and fails if they are not present. If you are installing on a Windows 2000 SP3 server, the Exchange 2003 setup program will automatically install and enable ASP.NET and .NET framework for you.

If you are installing Exchange Server 2003 on a Windows Server 2003 server, none of these services are enabled by default. You have to enable these services manually prior to running the Exchange 2003 setup program.

TIP

In a new server installation, only the required services are enabled by default. If you are upgrading a server to Exchange 2003, it will retain the services status of the server. We recommend checking services postinstallation and disabling those that you are not using (for example, POP3, IMAP, NNTP).

Preparing the Forest

The forest prep process extends the Active Directory schema to include the Exchange 2003 classes and attributes required for the application to run. In order to run the forest prep process, you must have the following permissions by belonging to these groups: enterprise admins, schema adminis, domain admins, and local administrator on the Exchange server. During the forest prep process, you assign an account that has full Exchange administrator rights to the organization object in Exchange 2003.

> **NOTE**
>
> Notice that you no longer have to enter an organization name for Exchange during the forest prep process. This is now entered only at the point of installation.

Preparing the Domain

The domain prep process creates groups and permission within the Active Directory forest so that Exchange 2003 can modify user attributes. To run the `domainprep` setup parameter you must be a member of the domain admins and local administrator groups.

The groups that are created during this process are Exchange domain servers and Exchange enterprise servers. The Exchange domain servers group is a domain global security group and the Exchange enterprise servers group is a domain local security group.

Reviewing All Log Files

Each of the utilities that you execute has some output in its respective log files. Review the log file after running each utility to ensure no errors are encountered.

Performing an Interactive Installation of Exchange Server 2003

When installing Exchange Server 2003 for the first time in an environment, the easiest way to conduct the installation is to insert the Exchange 2003 CD and follow the step-by-step installation instructions. This section of the chapter focuses on the step-by-step installation of a basic Exchange Server 2003 server.

> **NOTE**
>
> For those who have installed previous versions of Exchange, the setup program now has a new switch that can be used during installation. Running setup with a `/ChooseDC {dcname}`, followed by the name of a domain controller, tells the setup program to look for a specific DC to write schema changes to or check for permissions and groups.

To install the first Exchange server in an organization using the interactive installation process of Exchange Server 2003, use the following steps:

1. Insert the Exchange 2003 CD (Standard or Enterprise).

2. Autorun should launch a splash screen with options for Resources and Deployment Tools. (If autorun does not work, select Start, Run. Then type **CDDrive:\setup.exe** and click OK.)

3. Click on Exchange Deployment Tools.

4. At the Deployment Tools welcome screen, click on Deploy the first Exchange 2003 Server.

5. Click on New Exchange 2003 installation.

6. Verify that your server has met all the operating system and Active Directory requirements. (Click on the reference link in the right column.)

7. Check that your server is running NNTP, SMTP, and World Wide Web Services. If you're running Windows 2003, you also need ASP.NET. (Check the reference link to the right of the window for details.)

8. Install the Windows 2003 Support Tools to use the preinstallation utilities (located on the Windows 2003 CD under \support\tools\).

9. Run DCDiag and view the log file output. Click on the reference link to the right for details. The syntax is

   ```
   DCDiag /f: log file /s:domain controller
   ```

10. Run NetDiag and view the log file output in netdiag.log.

11. Click Run Forestprep Now.

12. Click Next.

13. Read the license agreement, and then click I agree if you agree with the licensing. Click Next.

14. Click Next to accept the default administrator account.

15. Click Finish when the forest prep is done.

The next step is to run the domain prep on the domain that will hold the Exchange servers and user accounts. To prepare the domain, use the following steps:

1. Click Run Domainprep Now.

2. Click Next.

3. After reading the license agreement, click I agree, and then click Next.

4. Click Next again.

5. Click Finish.

After the domain has been prepared, it's time to install the Exchange messaging system:

1. Run Setup Now.

2. Click Next.

3. Select I agree after agreeing with the licensing requirements, and then click Next.

   In the Component Selection window, the default will be Typical for Microsoft Exchange, Install for Microsoft Exchange Messaging and Collaboration Services, and Install for Microsoft Exchange System Management Tools. The configuration screen should look something like Figure 3.1.

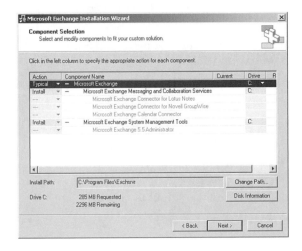

FIGURE 3.1   Component Selection screen for installation.

4. Click Next.

5. Select Create New Exchange Organization and click Next.

6. Type the Exchange organization name and click Next.

7. Select I agree that I have read and will be bound by the license agreements for this product.

8. Click Next.

9. If you already created the admin group and routing group structure, you will be prompted to select where to install this server. Choose an administrative group and click Next. Then choose a routing group and click Next.

10. Review the Installation Summary and click Next.

11. If you are installing in a Mixed Mode domain, you will get a security warning. Click OK to the security group warning.

12. Click on Finish.

13. Click on OK if prompted to reboot.

Performing a Scripted Installation of Exchange Server 2003

If you want to install Exchange with automation instead of manually choosing options, you can create an unattend file to run along with the setup program. This method is frequently used to script a standard series of configuration steps so that a script can be sent to branch offices, allowing local system administrators the option of installing the server onsite with minimal intervention.

Creating the unattend Install File

To create an unattend installation file, use the following steps:

1. Insert the Exchange CD.

2. Close the autorun splash screen.

3. Click on Start and choose Run.

4. Type

   ```
   cddrive:\setup.exe /createunattend drive:\filename.ini
   ```

   supplying your drive and filename—for example:

   ```
   F:\setup.exe /createunattend d:\e2kunattend.ini
   ```

5. Click Next.

6. Select I agree and click Next.

7. Select the Exchange components you want to install, change or keep the installation path, and click Next to continue.

8. Keep the default installation, type **create a new Exchange organization**, and click Next.

9. Type an organization name and click Next.

10. Choose I agree on the license agreement page and click Next.

11. Review the installation summary and click Next to accept and continue.

12. You should get a window that says the unattend file was successfully created. Click Finish.

13. Review the unattend file that you created; it is an .ini file and is around 14KB bytes.

Running `setup` in Unattended Mode

After the script file has been created, execute the script file:

1. Insert the Exchange CD.

2. Close the autorun splash screen.

3. Click on Start and choose Run.

4. Type

   `cddrive:\setup.exe /unattendfile filename.ini`

   The setup program will run automatically with no input required. You will see the progress window as it runs through the installation process. When the install is complete, the installation wizard will close.

5. Verify that the installation was successful by looking in the Start menu programs and checking for Exchange services.

Completing the Installation of Exchange 2003

After the first Exchange 2003 server has been installed, the Exchange environment will likely need to be customized to meet the needs and requirements of the organization. The custom options include

- Creating administrative groups

- Creating routing groups

- Creating storage groups

- Creating additional mailbox databases

- Creating a public folder store

Creating Administrative Group and Routing Group Structure

By default, the Exchange installation program will create an administrative group and routing group called first administrative group and first routing group. If your company wants to create an administrative group structure prior to installing Exchange, it can do so by installing the Exchange System Manager and creating the group structure.

Setting Administrative Views

To begin managing and administering the administrative groups and routing groups in Exchange 2003, Administrative Views needs to be configured. To enable Administrative Views, follow these steps:

1. Start the Exchange System Manager.

2. Right-click and select Properties on the Exchange organization.

3. On the properties page, select Display routing groups and Display administrative groups, as shown in Figure 3.2.

4. Click OK.

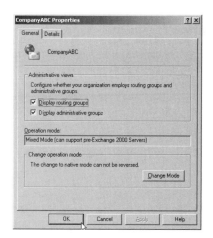

FIGURE 3.2   Enabling administrative views.

Creating Administrative Groups

For a clean installation of Exchange, the organization is set up in a single administrative group. The Exchange administrator can create additional administrative groups to delegate the administration of the organization to other administrators. To create an additional administrative group, follow these steps:

1. Start Exchange System Manager.

2. Right-click Administrative Groups and select New Administrative Group, as shown in Figure 3.3.

3. Type the name of the group and click OK.

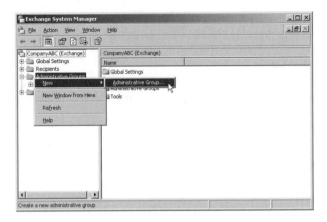

FIGURE 3.3   Adding an administrative group.

For many organizations that have multiple sites or multiple administrators, the common practice is to share administrative duties; all administrators in the organization can add, delete, or modify users in all sites. This is frequently used as a backup administration function when one administrator is not available—any other administrator in the organization can provide assistance. When administration tasks are shared, the organization may choose to have a single administrative group.

Creating Routing Groups

The default installation of administrative groups is to create a single administrative boundary; routing groups also create a single boundary for mail delivery. Routing groups are created to control message flow. A routing group connector then connects routing groups. A new routing group is usually created when there is a transition in bandwidth, such as from a LAN to a WAN. Servers separated by a WAN link or highly saturated or unstable LAN link are usually contained in separate routing groups.

In every routing group one server is identified as the routing group master (RGM). This server is responsible for propagating link state information to other servers in the routing group. The RGM is responsible for tracking which servers are up or down in their own routing group and propagating that information to the RGM servers in other routing groups on the network. Only two states are tracked for the message link, which are up or down.

Routing groups also affect a client's connection to a public folder. When a client attempts to access a public folder, the client uses the copy of the folder on its home server if it exists. If the folder cannot be located on the home server, the client uses a copy in its home server's routing group. If a copy is not available in the local routing group, clients attempt to locate the folder in a remote routing group. The arbitrary cost assigned to the routing group connector by the administrator determines which routing group is selected first.

If the organization has only a single location, a complicated routing structure is unnecessary. However, routing groups can enable the Exchange administrator(s) to throttle the routing of messages between servers and sites. This may be done if an organization has a very low bandwidth between sites and wants to prevent large attachments from saturating the limited bandwidth between locations. Standard messages could be sent throughout the day; however, messages with large attachments can be delayed until the evening when bandwidth is more readily available.

To create an additional routing group, follow these steps:

1. Start Exchange System Manager.

2. Expand the administrative groups/administrative group name.

3. Right-click on Routing Groups, and then select New Routing Group, as shown in Figure 3.4.

4. Type the routing group name and click OK.

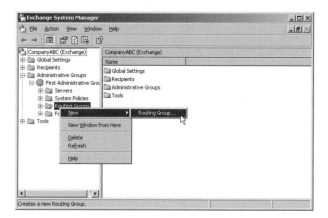

FIGURE 3.4   Adding a routing group.

You can also rename any new administrative group you create and any of the routing group names after the first server is installed in your organization. To do so, right-click, select Properties, and choose Rename.

Creating Storage Groups

Storage groups are collections of Exchange databases that the Exchange server manages with a separate process. Each storage group shares a set of transaction logs. Log files are not purged until the entire storage group has been backed up. All databases in the storage group are also subject to the Circular Logging setting on the storage group. Exchange 2003 Standard Edition supports a single storage group on a server, and a total of four storage groups are supported on each Exchange 2003 Enterprise Edition server.

NOTE

Circular logging is a process that can be enabled to save disk space by overwriting transaction logs. Enabling circular logging is dangerous because, in the event the database fails and has to be restored from tape, a replay of the information in the logs might not contain all the messages since the last backup. For data integrity and recovery reasons, Exchange administrators should never enable circular logging on the storage group. Instead, they should allocate sufficient disk space for the transaction logs and verify that a successful backup of the storage group is being performed each night. Running a *full* backup and then flagging the tape backup software to purge the log files is the best practice of ensuring that the database has been properly backed up and logs have been cleared.

As an administrator, you should create additional storage groups when

- **You can use separate physical transaction log drives to increase performance**   Putting an additional storage group on the same physical transaction log drive might actually reduce performance because of transaction log management and should be considered only if the first storage group is full.

- **You need to back up multiple databases simultaneously**   Databases are backed up at the storage group level. Using multiple storage groups allows simultaneous backups of each storage group.

- **The first storage group already has the maximum number of databases supported**   When another database is required on a server where the first storage group has the maximum number of supported databases, an additional storage group has to be created.

To create a new storage group, right-click the Exchange server in Exchange System Manager and select New, Storage Group. A set of options, as shown in Figure 3.5, is shown:

- **Name**   The name of the storage group appears in Exchange System Manager and Active Directory Users and Computers when managing users.

- **Transaction log location**   Put transaction logs on a different drive than the databases that will be part of this storage group; if the hard drive that the database is on crashes and you have to restore the database from tape, the logs are not affected by the database drive hardware failure. This method can improve data integrity and recoverability.

- **System path location**   The system path is the location of temporary files, such as the checkpoint file and reserve logs.

- **Log file prefix**   The log file prefix is assigned to each log file and is automatically assigned by the server.

- **Zero out deleted database pages**   This option clears deleted data from the drive, and although that process creates additional overhead, it also increases security.

- **Enable circular logging**   Never enable this setting. Make sure the backup jobs are completing successfully to prevent filling the transaction log drive.

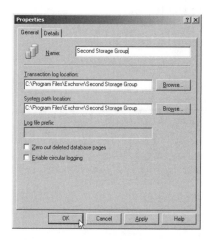

FIGURE 3.5   Options for creating a new storage group.

Managing Databases

Exchange 2003 Enterprise allows five databases per storage group. The number of databases can be any combination of public and private stores. Exchange 2003 stores data in two types of databases:

- **EDB**   Stores rich text messages and Internet Message headers.

- **STM**   Stores all MIME content. Stores audio, voice, and video as a stream of MIME data without conversion. This reduces the amount of space for storage and reduces the overhead on the server by not converting the data. Message bodies from the Internet messages are also stored in the STM database; the message header is converted to rich text format and stored in the EDB database.

A feature in Exchange 2003 mailbox and public store databases is full-text indexing. In earlier versions of Exchange, every folder and message was searched when users initiated a search. In Exchange 2003, the administrator can configure an index that is updated and rebuilt periodically. This enables fast searches for Outlook 2003, Outlook XP, and Outlook 2000 users. The following attachment types are also included in the index: doc, xls, ppt, html, htm, asp, txt, and eml (embedded MIME messages). Binary attachments are not included in the index. To initiate a full-text index, right-click the Mail or Public store and select Create Full Text Index.

Creating Additional Mailbox Stores

New mailbox stores should be created when the size of the existing mailbox store is growing too large to manage. To create a new mailbox store, right-click the storage group and select New, Mailbox Store. When creating a new mailbox store, the options to configure appear as tabs, as shown in Figure 3.6:

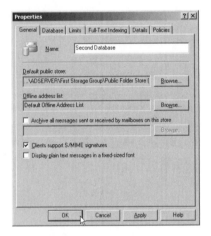

FIGURE 3.6   Options for creating a new database.

- **General**   Defines the database name, the offline address book to use, message archiving, whether digitally signed messages are allowed, and plain text display.

- **Database**   Sets the location for the EDB and STM databases. These should be stored on a hardware RAID 5 or 0+1 drive. Also controls the online database maintenance schedule.

- **Limits**   Configures the message storage limit at which users are warned that sending and receiving are prohibited. Also sets the deleted items and mailbox policy.

- **Full-Text Indexing**   Configures how often the full-text index is updated and rebuilt.

- **Details**   Notes any information about the configuration that is manually keyed in to this page by an administrator or Exchange server manager.

- **Policies**   Defines the system mailbox store policies that apply to the mailbox store.

Three entries are listed below the mailbox store that can provide the administrator information regarding the status of the store:

- **Logons**   Last logon time, last access time, client type used to log on, and the Windows 2000 or Windows 2003 account that was used.

- **Mailboxes**   Number of items in the mailbox, mailbox size, and last log on and log off time.

- **Full-Text Indexing**   Index information, such as location, size, state, number of documents, and the last build time.

Creating a Public Folder Store

Unlike the mailbox store, new public stores should be created only when there is a need for a new public folder tree, because each public folder store needs to be associated with a public folder tree. Public folder trees can be created under the folders container in each storage group. Only one public store from each Exchange server can be associated with a public folder tree. To create a new public store, right-click the storage group and select New, Public Store. The majority of the tabs are identical to those of the mailbox store. The following are tabs that contain unique public folder store settings:

- **Replication**   Sets the replication schedule, interval, and size limit for public folder replication messages.

- **Limits**   Includes an age limit setting for the number of days for folder content to be valid.

The entries listed below the public folder store provide the administrator information regarding the status of the store:

- **Logons**   Last logon time, last access time, client type used to log on, and the Windows 2000 or Windows 2003 account that was used.

- **Public Folder Instances**   Information about folders that are being replicated to other servers.

- **Public Folders**   Folder size, number of items, creation date, and last access time.

- **Replication Status**   Replication status of each folder in the public folder store—for example, In Sync indicates that the folder is up to date.

- **Full-Text Indexing**   Index information, such as location, size, state, number of documents, and the last build time.

Performing Postinstallation Configurations

After Exchange 2003 has been installed and customized, there are a few cleanup and implementation steps you should take:

- Disable unnecessary services.

- Remove information stores that won't be used.

- Set up routing group connections.

- Enable logging and message tracking.

- Delete mailbox and public folder stores.

Disabling Services

Although Exchange 2003 does a much better job by not automatically installing dozens of different utilities and services the way previous versions of Exchange did, it still installs some default services that might not be used by the organization. For security and administration purposes, if a service is not used, it should be disabled. To disable services that are commonly unused—such as IMAP, POP3, NNTP, or SMTP—do the following:

1. Select Start, All Programs, Administrative Tools, Services.

2. Scroll down to the IMAP4 Service.

3. Double-click on the service.

4. Under the Startup Type section, choose Disabled.

5. Under the Service Status section, click Stop.

6. Repeat steps 1–5 for POP3, NNTP, and SMTP, as applicable.

> **NOTE**
>
> If IMAP, POP3, and NNTP are used on a server, such as a front-end system hosting remote mail users, those services should not be disabled. It's common on back-end servers where IMAP or POP3 is not used that the service could be disabled; it's also common for organizations that use Exchange just for email and do not need NNTP on any of their servers. For servers or systems that are not routing mail, such as those set up solely as Exchange System Manager administration servers, the SMTP service should be disabled.

Removing Information Stores

By default, an information store that holds Exchange databases is created on each Exchange server installed in the organization. However, dedicated front-end servers that are just the Web front-end systems do not require information stores or databases. In those cases, the information stores should be deleted. To delete the information stores that are unneeded on front-end servers, follow these steps:

1. Select Start, All Programs, Microsoft Exchange, System Manager.

2. Navigate to Administrative Groups, Administrative Group Name, Servers, Server Name, Storage Groups.

3. Right-click on the mailbox store and choose Delete.

4. Click Yes.

5. Click OK and delete the database files manually.

> **CAUTION**
>
> Before deleting any database or information store, unless you are positive the database or infor-mation store is completely empty and unused, you might want to do a full backup of the data-base, store, and system—in case a user's mailbox was inadvertently hosted on the system. Sometimes during an early implementation of Exchange, an organization might start with just one or two servers in a pilot test environment. If a mailbox was stored on one of the test servers, it might eventually become the front-end server for the organization. Backing up a system is safer than making assumptions and regretting the decision later. Using the NTBackup utility covered in Chapter 31, "Backing Up the Exchange Server 2003 Environment," is a quick way to back up a system.

Setting Up Routing Group Connectors

Routing group connectors should be used in situations where there is greater than 64KB of available bandwidth between the routing groups. If there is not sufficient bandwidth, SMTP or X.400 connectors should be used to connect the routing groups. Routing group and routing group connector designs should follow the organization's physical connectiv-ity links. Four basic routing group connector strategies can be implemented based on the organization's physical network links:

- **Full Mesh** In a full mesh all routing groups connect to all other routing groups. Unless there are only a few routing groups the administrative overhead for imple-mentation becomes unbearable. This design can also be a waste of administrative resources if there isn't the WAN link redundancy to support the design.

- **Partial Mesh** A partial mesh tries to create the benefits of a full mesh without the added administrative overhead. If the WAN design is a partial mesh, build the routing groups to follow the partial mesh.

- **Hub and Spoke** In a hub and spoke design one routing group becomes the center of the universe and all other routing groups connect to it. In larger networks there can be multiple hubs in the enterprise, and the hubs are joined together in a full or partial mesh. This design is simple to implement and maintain but creates a single point of failure at the hub. This design is an option for locations that do not have any WAN link redundancy.

- **Linear**   In a linear design routing groups connect to only one other routing group in a straight line. Linear designs are not recommended.

To create a new routing group, follow these steps:

1. Navigate to Administrative Groups, Admin Group I, Routing Groups, HO, as shown in Figure 3.7.

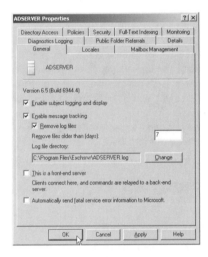

FIGURE 3.7   Traversing the Exchange System Manager for routing groups.

2. Right-click Connectors and choose New Routing Group Connector.

3. Type a name for the connector, as shown in Figure 3.8.

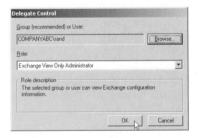

FIGURE 3.8   Routing group configuration screen.

4. Click These servers can send mail over the connector, and click Add to choose a server or check Any local server can send mail over the connector.

The General tab of the routing group connector defines a few significant items that administrators should understand when configuring the connector:

- **Connect this routing group with** Specifies the destination routing group for the RGC.

- **Cost** Arbitrary cost assigned by the administrator, which can be used to control which connector is used first if multiple connectors exist.

- **Server** Allows any server, or specifies specific servers allowed, to transfer mail to the destination routing group. By specifying specific servers, a bridgehead server is nominated. By specifying multiple servers, backup bridgehead servers are identified. The order of the servers in the list specifies which server is used first.

- **Do not allow public folder referrals** Disables the user's ability to access public folder content that is homed in the routing group connected to that server.

5. Click on the Remote Bridgehead tab and click Add to choose a server. After entering the bridgehead server selection, you will see a screen similar to Figure 3.9.

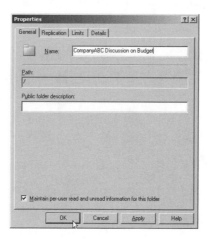

FIGURE 3.9 Bridgehead server configuration.

6. Click OK.

7. Select Yes to create a routing group connector in the remote routing group.

Enabling Logging and Message Tracking

Logging and message tracking are common functions enabled by Exchange administrators early on in an Exchange implementation to help the administrator validate that messages are flowing through the environment. By enabling the logging and message tracking function, the administrator can then run a report to find out which route a message took to get from one server to another, and how long it took for the message to be transmitted.

Many administrators never use the logging and message tracking function and simply assume that messages are getting from point A to point B successfully. In many environments, although messages reach their destination, they are routed from one site to another and once around the globe before being received by a mail user in the same site facility. Misconfigured routing group connectors, DNS errors, or other networking problems are often the cause. So it's usually helpful to monitor messages to ensure that they are being routed and processed as expected.

To enable logging and message tracking, follow these steps:

1. Open Exchange System Manager.

2. Navigate to Administrative Groups, Admin Group I, Servers, Server Name.

3. Right-click on the server object and choose Properties.

4. Select Enable subject logging and display and enable message tracking.

5. Type a number indicating days to keep the message tracking log files, as shown in Figure 3.10.

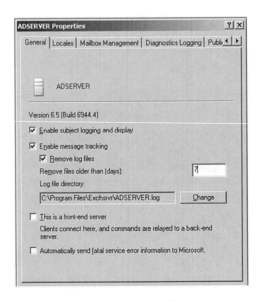

FIGURE 3.10   Configuring logging for message tracking.

Dismounting and Deleting Public Folder Stores

Unused public folder stores should be removed for security and administration purposes. Frequently, organizations that separate mailbox servers from front-end servers from public folder servers do not need public folder databases on the front-end or mailbox servers.

To dismount and delete public folder stores, follow these steps:

1. Expand the servers and storage group.

2. Right-click the public folder store and choose Dismount.

3. Click Yes to dismount the store.

4. Right-click the public folder store and choose Delete.

5. Click Yes twice.

6. Click Yes to delete the store.

7. Select OK to the message that says you have to select another public folder store for the system folders and that public folder store will have to be dismounted and remounted for the changes to take effect.

8. Choose a new public folder store for this server's system folders.

9. Click OK. You have to manually delete the database files for the store by going to the mdbdata directory and deleting pub1.edb and pub1.stm.

10. Right-click the mailbox store and choose Dismount.

11. Click Yes to dismount the store.

12. Right-click the mailbox store and choose Delete.

13. Click Yes.

14. Click OK. You have to manually delete the database files again as previously stated.

> **CAUTION**
>
> Unless you are positive that the database or information store is empty, you should do a full backup of the database, store, and system, in case the public folder store hosted the authoritative copy of the public folder information.

Using System Policies to Manage Mailbox and Public Stores

Many of the settings that can be manually set on each mail and public store can be set through a system policy to simplify the settings configuration. Standardizing Exchange server settings in a large deployment was always tough for Exchange Server 5.5 because each setting had to be manually set on every server. With a system policy, the mail and public store settings for limits, deleted item retention, and so on can be set through the policy, and the policy can be applied to the stores. Each administrative group has its own set of policies for the stores. When a policy is applied, the setting that the policy overrides displays as grayed out on the mailbox or public store. Administrators have the choice of choosing for which property pages for the mail or public store they want to configure policies.

To configure and apply a policy, follow these steps:

1. In the Exchange System Manager, in the Administrative Groups container, right-click on the administrative group you want to manage and select New, System Policies Container.

2. Right-click on the System Policies container and select New. Then select either Mailbox policy, Public store policy, or Server policy.

3. When a properties pages appears, enter a name you want to identify with this policy.

> **NOTE**
>
> Because the icon for the Mailbox or Public policies are the same, name the policy something descriptive to indicate it's a Mailbox or Public store policy.

4. Right-click the new policy and select Add Mailbox Store, Add Public Store, or Add Server, and then select the appropriate store or server. Click on OK to complete this task.

5. To force the policy to be applied immediately to all stores, right-click the policy and select Apply Now.

After the policy is created, it can be modified by right-clicking the policy and selecting Properties.

Best Practices for Configuring Storage Groups and Databases

After configuring hundreds—if not thousands—of storage groups and databases in beta and production environments, the following best practices have been determined:

- Keep databases small to keep restore and maintenance intervals short. The database size is organization-specific and depends on the speed that maintenance and restores run on the server hardware and the organization's Service Level Agreements for messaging services.

- Choose to create additional databases before creating additional storage groups to avoid overhead on the server for log file management.

- Use no more than four databases per storage group. This will leave one database position open in each storage group for offline database maintenance.

- Do not use circular logging.

- Verify that a successful backup is performed every day and the logs have been purged.

- Use full backups every day if possible.

- Periodically verify the backup using an isolated lab.

- Leave online system maintenance on and stagger the database maintenance times so that all databases and storage groups aren't trying to run maintenance at the same time.

- Do not use the prohibit-send option when configuring storage limits as a courtesy to end-users.

- Keep deleted items for at least seven days and deleted mailboxes for 30 days. Use the option to not remove the items permanently until the store is backed up.

Delegating Administration in Exchange 2003

The delegation of permissions can occur at the organizational or administrative levels. There are three levels of permissions that exist in Exchange 2003:

- **Exchange Full Administrator**   This level enables the administrator to add, delete, modify, and rename objects, with the ability to change security permissions. These rights are granted to global messaging administrators and at the administrative group where boundary of control changes.

- **Exchange Administrator**   This administrator level offers the add, delete, modify, and rename objects permissions. However, this level cannot change security permissions. This level is usually the standard level granted to individuals who need to manage or administer Exchange on a regular basis.

- **Exchange View Only Administrator**   With this level, you can view the configuration settings in Exchange System Manager. This level is usually granted to administrators who provide operational support (reviewing logs, creating reports, validating connectivity, and message routing) and do not necessarily need to change settings or configurations directly.

It's easier to delegate administration to a group than to a user. To delegate administration, right-click the administrative group or organization and select Delegate Control to launch the Delegation Wizard. Select the group or user from the Active Directory object picker dialog box and set the Exchange administration role, as shown in Figure 3.11. Then click Next and Finish to apply the permissions throughout the Exchange organization.

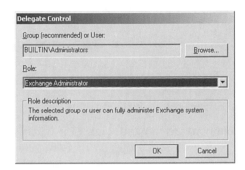

FIGURE 3.11   Delegating administration to an AD group.

> **NOTE**
>
> Being an Exchange Full Administrator or Exchange Administrator also requires that the group or user be a member of the server local administrator group. View-only administrators only need to be able to log on locally to the Exchange server. The Exchange Administration Delegation Wizard will not set permissions on the server itself, so permissions on the server must be set manually through Computer Management.

Configuring Additional Server Services

In addition to basic Exchange servers that host mailboxes for user email accounts, there are other Exchange Server 2003 services that can be configured:

- Bridgehead servers
- Front-end servers
- Public folder servers
- SMTP mail routing servers

Installing a Bridgehead Server

A **bridgehead server** is a routing server that accepts mail from another server and then distributes the mail to the next server in the route. Similar to the hub-and-spoke system used by airlines to prevent having to fly nonstop flights to and from every single city around the world, the bridgehead server minimizes the site-to-site direct-traffic flow by focusing mail between bridgehead servers.

Many times administrators with high-speed WAN bandwidth question why they wouldn't just have all Exchange servers route mail directly to all other Exchange servers. An example gives the best explanation: If a manager in the United States sends a message with a 20MB attachment to managers in 10 different European offices, 200MB of mail is routed between continents. However, if the organization had a bridgehead server in the U.K., only one 20MB message, with attachment, would go between the U.S. and the U.K. Then the message would be distributed from the U.K. to the rest of the European sites. Even between local sites with a T1 line, the belief is that there is plenty of bandwidth between the sites and users can send any size email because it's a local office. So unless attachment restrictions are placed on servers, a user could send a 40MB attachment to dozens of offices, taking up hundreds of megabytes of bandwidth. A bridgehead server can consolidate bandwidth between an East Coast and West Coast connection, minimizing traffic across the country.

To configure a bridgehead server, from the Remote Bridgehead tab on the routing group connector Properties page, a target server can be specified that will receive messages in the destination routing group. Multiple servers can be specified, and connections to the server are attempted in the order of the servers listed in the remote bridgehead list.

The Delivery Restrictions, Content Restrictions, and Delivery Options tabs are used to control which users can send messages and of what type across the connection. The Delivery Options tab includes the option of scheduling large messages across a specific message route during a specific period of time. For example, large attachments from one site to another site that has a slow connection can schedule all attachments of a certain size to be transported later in the day or evening. Using this option for messages greater than a few megabytes on busy or slow links can keep mail flowing without clogging the link.

When the connector is configured, the administrator is then prompted to create a corresponding connector in the remote routing group. The administrator should keep this in mind when naming the connector, because automatically configured connectors in the remote routing group will use the same name as the connector configured in the local routing group.

Routing group connectors are not the only option for administrators to link routing groups. The SMTP and X.400 connectors also can be used for linking. Both connectors have a Connected Routing Groups tab that can be used to connect routing groups when bandwidth is limited or other services, such as encryption, are required.

Enabling SSL for Services on Front-end Servers

You can enable most of the protocols on the front-end server from within the Exchange System Manager. To enable SSL for POP3, IMAP4, SMTP, and NNTP, use the following steps:

1. Open Exchange System Manager.

2. Navigate to Administrative Groups, Servers, Protocols.

3. Select a protocol and expand it.

4. Right-click on the protocol and choose Properties.

5. Click on the Access tab.

6. Under Secure Communications, click on Certificate.

7. Select Next.

8. Select Create a new certificate and click Next.

9. If you have an internal Certificate Authority (CA), you can choose Send the request immediately to a CA; otherwise, choose Prepare now and send later, and then click Next.

10. Type a name for the certificate, choose the bit length, and click Next.

11. Type the organization name and unit and then click Next.

12. Type a common name for the Website or fully qualified DNS name.

13. Type the country, state, and city, and then click Next. (Do not use abbreviations.)

14. Type a path and filename for the CSR file and click Next.

15. Review the summary and click Next.

16. Click Finish.

If your organization uses a third-party certificate authority such as Verisign, Tharte, or others, send the CSR file created in the previous steps to the third-party certificate authority to have a valid certificate file created. After a certified file is issued by the third-party CA, do the following:

1. Open Exchange System Manager.

2. Navigate to Administrative Groups, Servers, Protocols.

3. Select a protocol and expand it.

4. Right-click on the protocol and choose Properties.

5. Click on the Access tab.

6. Under Secure Communications, click on Certificate, and then click Next.

7. Choose Process the pending request and install the certificate, and then click Next.

8. Click and browse to select the certificate file you received from the third-party CA, and click Next.

9. Review the summary of the certificate to verify that it is correct and click Next.

10. Click Next on the confirmation screen.

Managing Public Folders

Public folders are collaboration objects in Microsoft Exchange that can be used to share information with a group of individuals in the organization, and are the basis of workflow applications.

Public folders can be created either through the Outlook 2003, Outlook XP, or Outlook 2000 client or through Exchange System Manager. To create folders through the Exchange System Manager, locate the folders container in the administrative group. Right-click the default public folder tree and select New, Public Folder. The tabs, shown in Figure 3.12, are for the following:

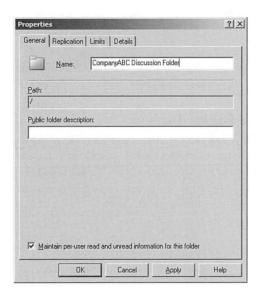

FIGURE 3.12   Tab options when creating a public folder.

- **General**   Contains the option of configuring an address list display name to be different from the folder name and whether folder content read and unread information is tracked for each user.

- **Replication**   Controls which public folder stores receive a copy of the folder and at what frequency the information is replicated.

- **Limits**   Configures the storage, deletion, and age limit settings. These settings can be inherited from the public store database settings or from a public store system policy.

- **Details**   Allows for the entry of administrative notes.

To mail-enable the folder, right-click the folder in Exchange System Manager and select Mail Enable. After the folder is mail-enabled, right-click the folder and select Properties to view the following tabs:

- **Exchange General**   Displays the folder's alias and the public folder tree that contains the folder. Options also exist for Delivery Restrictions and Delivery Options, which are inherited from the Exchange organization.

- **Email Addresses**   Lists email addresses for the object, which are defined in the Recipient Policies from Exchange System Manager. This includes the SMTP, X.400 address, and addresses for other mail platforms.

- **Exchange Advanced**   Includes settings that control address list visibility and the custom attributes.

Folders can also be created in Outlook 2003, Outlook XP, or Outlook 2000 by accessing the Public Folders, All Public Folders container.

Creating New Public Folder Trees

MAPI clients can use only the default public folder tree, so this process does not apply to organizations that use only the Outlook 2003, Outlook XP, or Outlook 2000 client. Only Web-based clients can use other public folder trees. Organizations might want to consider creating a new public folder tree to support customized Web-based applications that use the Web store capabilities of the public store. Creating new public folder trees is a four-step process:

1. Create the tree.

2. Create a public store associated with the tree.

3. Link the tree with the public store by using the Associated Public Store dialog box when creating the store.

4. Mount the public store.

To create new public folder trees, use Exchange System Manager to locate the folders container in the administrative group. Right-click the folders container and select New, Public Folder Tree; enter the name of the folder tree. The second step is to create a public folder store by right-clicking a storage group and selecting New, Public Store. The third step is to use the Browse button to select the new public folder tree as the associated public folder tree when creating the public store. The final step is to mount the store. To mount the store, choose Yes when prompted to mount the store.

> **NOTE**
>
> To mount stores created on remote servers, Active Directory must complete replication of the store configuration information.

Using Dedicated Public Folder Servers

Many Exchange 5.5 organizations used dedicated public folder servers to support their folder installations and keep the load of collaboration applications and repositories off their mail servers. This is still an acceptable practice; however, do not remove the private store from the dedicated public folder server if the organization plans to administer the public folder tree on the server from Exchange System Manager. To configure dedicated public folder servers, leave the mailbox store unpopulated or permanently dismount the mailbox store by marking the store with the Do not mount this store at start-up option on the Database tab of the mailbox store.

Designing Public Folder Trees

The first level of the public folder tree is called top-level public folders. In most organizations, the top few levels of the public folder structure are designed with some hierarchy in mind. This is done to organize the information and also to control the replication of information across the network. It might not be efficient to replicate the entire public folder tree to every server in the organization if the information is needed in only certain areas of the company. Generally, the first few levels are designed with a department or geographic organization. Most Exchange administrators usually lock down the top-level folders to prevent the hierarchy from being corrupted by users. To lock down the top-level folders, set the following permissions:

1. Right-click the Public Folder tree under the folders container in the administrative group and select properties.

2. Click the Security tab.

3. Select the Everyone group.

4. Select the Deny option for the Create top level public folder permissions.

Understanding Public Folder Replication

Public folder replication enables information that's created in one folder to be replicated to all other public stores configured on its Replication tab. Public folders operate in a multimaster replication hierarchy where every public store has a read and write copy of the folder. By default, a public folder inherits the replication schedule from the public store Replication tab or the public store system policy that is applied to the server.

Plan on spending some time developing the replication scheme for the public folder hierarchy. Not all information in the tree needs to replicate immediately. Exchange administrators should make sure that top-level folder administrators understand which folders replicate more quickly than others and should be used for time-sensitive information.

System Folders

The Exchange system folders control many of the underlying components of the Exchange organization, such as storing the Offline Address Book and the public free and busy time information that users see when they create meeting requests. The Exchange system folders include EForms Registry, Events Root, Nntp Control Folder, Offline Address Book, Schedule+ Free Busy, StoreEvents, and System Configuration. Administrators might need to view information about the system folders when troubleshooting problems on the server. By default, the system folders are not displayed in Exchange System Manager. To view system folders, follow these steps:

1. Open Exchange System Manager.

2. In Exchange System Manager, expand the Folders container.

> **TIP**
>
> For Native Mode Exchange environments, use the Folders container under Administrative Group.

3. Right-click Public Folders.

4. Select View System Folders.

SMTP Connectors and Virtual Servers

SMTP is the primary message routing protocol used in Exchange 2003 and is the backbone of many other services, such as OWA, POP3, and IMAP. Exchange 2003 uses the base SMTP service configuration provided by IIS and extends its functionality to link state routing, advanced queuing engine, and enhanced message categorization. Many of the features that are added to the base SMTP service are Exchange-specific commands.

Two basic components need to be configured for SMTP on the Exchange 2003 server: the SMTP Virtual Server and the SMTP Connector. The SMTP Virtual Server is used to define settings—such as the domain and authentication—for connections. Multiple SMTP virtual servers can be used on a physical server to support the needs of different groups in the organization. The purpose of the SMTP connector is to use SMTP to route external mail. The SMTP Connector is the replacement for the Internet Mail Service in Exchange 5.5. The connector defines how that mail is delivered and any restrictions on messages or connectivity that apply to the delivery.

Creating SMTP Connectors

The following process assumes the connector is being installed to send messages to the Internet.

To install the SMTP connector, right-click the routing group's connectors container and select New, SMTP Connector. To configure the connector, use the following steps:

1. On the General tab enter a descriptive name for the connector, such as **SMTP(Internet)**.

2. Select the method to deliver the SMTP messages, either DNS or smart host. If you're using a smart host, it's better to use a hostname rather than an IP address; an IP address change in the organization will not cause mail routing to fail as long as DNS properly resolves the name to another IP address. If you're using IP addresses, they must be enclosed in brackets ([ ]). Multiple smart hosts can be entered but must be separated by semicolons (;) or commas (,).

3. Add a server in the local routing group as the local bridgehead. This will be the server responsible for delivering SMTP messages in this routing group.

4. Add an address space entry. If this connector will route all mail to the Internet, create an SMTP address entry and leave the default setting to send all addresses. If there are multiple connectors with the same address space entry, the cost can be modified to set one of the connectors to a higher or lower priority. The higher the cost, the lower the priority.

5. Set Connector Scope for Entire Organization or the routing group. If using Entire Organization, all servers in the organization can send messages through this connector.

6. Set the advanced settings for security if necessary. For sending mail to servers on the Internet, set the option for HELO instead of EHLO for ensured interoperability.

The General tab of the SMTP connector is configured to deliver SMTP mail to the Internet. The other tabs on the SMTP connector can be configured as needed, but most organizations leave the settings as the default when configuring connectors to send SMTP mail to the Internet.

Creating SMTP Virtual Servers

In most Exchange organizations, it's not necessary to create additional SMTP virtual servers. Unless the organization is supporting multiple domain names that require different settings or POP3 and IMAP users that require secured SMTP relays, creating additional SMTP virtual servers is not necessary.

To create a new SMTP Virtual Server, right-click the SMTP protocol container and select New, SMTP Virtual Server. The wizard then prompts for the name of the virtual server and the IP address. It's best to use a descriptive name for the virtual server, such as the domain name (in this example, smtp.companyabc.com). Only IP addresses that have been configured on the server's LAN adapters appear in the IP address selection box.

The following tabs are available for the SMTP Virtual Server:

- **General**   The General tab can be used to limit the number of connections and the connection timeout and contains the IP address and port number combinations configured for the virtual server. When you're adding additional IP addresses, the Enable Filter option can be used to apply message filters that have been configured in the Message Delivery options under the Global container for the organization. Logging for the SMTP connection can also be enabled here.

- **Access**   The Access tab controls the Authentication mechanism in place and can be used to enable secure communication under the Certificate and Communication buttons. Connections and SMTP message relaying can also be controlled.

- **Messages**   The Messages tab controls the number of messages that can be transferred and the handling of nondelivery reports. A setting that's really helpful during mail migrations is the Forward all mail with unresolved recipients to host option, which enables mail for the same domain name to be delivered to another mail platform that may have been previously responsible for the SMTP domain name for the Exchange organization.

- **Delivery**   The Delivery tab configures outbound message retry intervals, authentication, DNS, and smart host configuration information.

Securing SMTP Mail Relays

The Relay button on the Access tab of the SMTP Virtual Server is responsible for controlling the capability for remote hosts of relaying SMTP messages off the Exchange SMTP server. Open SMTP mail relays are a target for spammers, who use the open relay to send unsolicited email messages anonymously.

By default, SMTP message relaying is not enabled. Only the hosts specifically entered in the relay configuration can relay SMTP messages. By selecting the option All Except the List Below, you open the relay to any server on the Internet. The check box Allow All Computers which Successfully Authenticate to Relay is an override for the lists of hosts listed above the check box that are either allowed or not allowed to relay. This check box is selected by default and will allow POP3 and IMAP clients to relay SMTP messages off the server as long as they can authenticate.

To configure Outlook Express for authentication, use the Servers tab of the mail account and mark the check box under the Outgoing Mail Server for My Server Requires Authentication. The Settings button enables the user to enter a different account or use the same account as the Incoming Mail Server.

If the organization needs to support POP3 and IMAP users, the next step in configuring the SMTP relay is to select the authentication method under the Authentication button on the Access tab. If this SMTP virtual server will be used for all SMTP connections, the

Anonymous Access selection should remain on. If only POP3 and IMAP users will use this virtual server, Anonymous Access should be disabled.

The most secure method to access the SMTP server over the Internet is to remove the Integrated Windows Authentication method and enable the check box for Requires TLS Encryption. In order to select Requires TLS Encryption, you must install a certificate on the server, which can be obtained through the Certificate button on the Access tab for the SMTP virtual server. After the certificate is installed, encryption can be required under the Communication button on the Access tab of the SMTP virtual server.

Select the Require Secure Channel check box under the Communication button if this server will be used to relay messages exclusively for POP3 and IMAP clients. If this server is receiving SMTP mail for the organization, connections will be rejected if they cannot support SSL.

In order to use TLS security for sending messages, the POP3 and IMAP clients need to support TLS or SSL. To configure Outlook Express for SSL, use the Advanced tab of the POP3 or IMAP mail account and select This Server Requires a Secure Connection (SSL).

Testing the Exchange 2003 Installation

After Exchange 2003 has been installed and appears to be working, or at least nothing has reported an error that would indicate a problem with the installation, there are a few things that can be tested to validate the installation. Some of these steps involve actually setting up a test user, testing the sending and receiving of email from a test user, checking the flow of mail between servers, and checking to make sure the Outlook Web Access function is working properly.

Creating a Mailbox

The easiest way to confirm whether Exchange is working properly is to create a mailbox and test sending and receiving email. To create a mailbox, use the following steps:

1. Click on Start, All Programs, Microsoft Exchange, Active Directory Users and Computers.

2. Right-click on the user account you want to create a mailbox for, select All Tasks, and then select Exchange Tasks.

3. At the Welcome to Exchange Tasks screen, click Next to bypass the welcome page. You can disable the welcome page by clicking on the box next to Do not show this welcome page again.

4. Verify that Create mailbox is highlighted and click Next.

5. Accept the default or type an alias name for the user, server name, and mailbox store name.

6. Click Next to continue.

7. Click Finish. (You can click on the box next to View detailed report when this wizard closes if you want to see the full report of the mailbox creation.)

Testing Mail Flow Using OWA

Another test can involve whether the user can log on to Outlook Web Access. Successful OWA access validates that the Web services are working properly, that the front-end and back-end servers are communicating properly, and that the organization's firewall supports the passing of OWA traffic. To test mail flow using Outlook Web Access, follow these steps:

1. Open Internet Explorer and go to http://{*servername*}/exchange.

2. Log in as an Exchange user and send messages to another Exchange user.

3. Open a second Internet Explorer window and log in as the other Exchange user.

4. Verify that mail has been received by the second user.

5. Send a reply to the first user and confirm that the messages were successfully sent and received.

> **NOTE**
>
> More specific details on using Outlook Web Access is covered in Chapter 26, "Everything You Need to Know About Outlook Web Access Client."

Installing the Exchange System Manager

If you have an administrative machine and you want to install the Exchange System Manager on it to perform administrative tasks for Exchange, you can install the Exchange System Manager program locally.

> **NOTE**
>
> When installing the Exchange System Manager only, you still are required to have the IIS SMTP and NNTP service installed on your PC. However, for a standalone administration system, the IIS, SMTP, and NNTP services are not required after installation and should be disabled after the installation is complete.

To install the Exchange System Manager program, follow these steps:

1. Insert Exchange 2003 CD (Standard or Enterprise).

2. Autorun should launch a splash screen with options for Resources and Deployment Tools. (If autorun does not work, select Start, Run. Then type **CDDrive:\setup.exe** and click OK.)

3. Click on Exchange Deployment Tools.

4. At the Deployment Tools welcome screen, click on Install Exchange System Management Tools only.

5. Review the prerequisite options, and when you comply with the initial configuration, click on Run Setup now.

6. Click Next.

7. Review the license agreement, and when in agreement, select I Agree, and then click Next.

8. In the component selection window, confirm that the Microsoft Exchange System Management tools option has been selected.

9. Click Next to begin the installation of the tools.

10. Click Finish when done.

Summary

Microsoft has simplified the process for installing the Exchange Server product, and Exchange Server 2003 is the easiest-to-install Exchange version to date. As with any simplified installation process, however, it's important to understand the steps leading to a successful installation so that any appropriate planning or preparation is done prior to the live installation. Additionally, because Exchange Server 2003 includes many new functions that extend beyond basic email messaging and calendaring, getting the first Exchange 2003 server installed properly sets the foundation for a successful enterprise rollout of the Exchange messaging system.

Best Practices

The following are best practices from this chapter:

- Review Chapter 1 to understand the common reasons organizations plan and deploy the Exchange 2003 messaging system.

- Leverage the planning and design details in Chapters 4 and 5 of this book to prepare the business for an appropriate messaging system design and configuration.

- The easiest way to install the first Exchange 2003 server in a new environment is to follow the interactive installation process initiated by an autorun automatic load from the Exchange Server 2003 CD.

- For an organization that will be installing many Exchange servers and wants to ensure an identical build between servers, creating an unattended installation script can ensure that a common installation process is followed.

- After installing Exchange 2003, consider locking down services that may not be needed—such as POP3, IMAP, and the like—which can improve security on the Exchange server.

- Create additional Exchange databases when the database file size begins to reach 15–20GB, to keep data backup, maintenance, and recovery to a more manageable level.

- Use system policies to minimize the effort it takes to manage servers individually when a single change in a group policy can automatically make changes on all servers simultaneously.

- Use a bridgehead server to minimize the traffic between site boundaries that can be better served by managed message transmission and routing.

- SMTP relaying should be enabled only when absolutely necessary, and when enabled should be properly locked down. This prevents spammers from gaining unauthorized access to relay spam messages.

PART II

Microsoft Exchange Server 2003 Messaging

IN THIS PART

Exchange Server 2003 Design Concepts

Formulating a Successful Design Strategy

The fundamental capabilities of Exchange Server 2003 are impressive. Improvements to security, reliability, and scalability enhance an already road-tested and stable Exchange platform. Along with these impressive credentials comes an equally impressive design task. Proper design of an Exchange Server 2003 platform will do more than practically anything to reduce headaches and support calls in the future. Many complexities of Exchange may seem daunting, but with a proper understanding of the fundamental components and improvements, the task of designing the Exchange Server 2003 environment becomes manageable.

This chapter focuses specifically on the Exchange Server 2003 components required for design. Key decision-making factors influencing design are presented and tied into overall strategy. All critical pieces of information required to design Exchange Server 2003 implementations are outlined and explained. This chapter does not focus on migration from existing platforms to Exchange Server 2003, which is instead covered in Chapters 15, "Migrating from Exchange v5.5 to Exchange Server 2003," and 16, "Migrating from Exchange 2000 to Exchange Server 2003."

Getting the Most Out of Exchange Server 2003 Functionality

Designing Exchange Server used to be a fairly simple task. When an organization needed email and the decision was made to go with Exchange Server, the only real decision to make was how many Exchange servers were needed. Primarily, organizations really needed only email and eschewed any "bells and whistles."

Exchange Server 2003, on the other hand, takes messaging to a whole new level. No longer do organizations require only an email system, but other messaging functionality as well. After the productivity capabilities of an enterprise email platform have been demonstrated, the need for more productivity improvements arises. Consequently, it is wise to understand the integral design components of Exchange before beginning a design project.

Significant Changes in Exchange Server 2003

There have been two major areas of improvement in Exchange Server 2003. The first is in the realm of user access and connectivity. The needs of many organizations have changed and they are no longer content with slow remote access to email and limited functionality when on the road. Consequently, many of the improvements in Exchange focus on various approaches to email access and connectivity. The improvements in this group focus on the following areas:

- **Outlook Web Access (OWA)**   The Outlook Web Access (OWA) client is now almost completely indistinguishable from the one that debuted in Exchange 5.5. Improvements over the Exchange 2000 OWA client are also impressive, with support for nearly all functionality that exists in the standard Outlook client. In fact, from first glance, there are no distinguishable differences between the two clients.

- **Outlook Mobile Access (OMA)**   Outlook Mobile Access (OMA) was developed to fill the vast, growing niche of mobile phone, pager, and PDA Internet access to email. Because the screen sizes on these clients are much smaller and the connection requirements so different, a mail client more suited for these conditions was created. OMA simplifies and streamlines Exchange mail access from these clients and adds an additional access option to Exchange.

- **Outlook 2003 Offline Improvements**   One major improvement in client access for Exchange 2000 comes in the form of improvements to the "heavy" Outlook client. In addition to improved MAPI compression, Outlook 2003 dramatically improves offline and slow-link connections to make it more feasible to access Exchange from remote locations. In addition, the concept of "RPC over HTTP" enables Outlook 2003 access to Exchange data across the HTTP or HTTPS ports, reducing the need for cumbersome VPN connections.

The second major area of improvement in Exchange Server 2003 has been in the area of back-end improvements. End-users are not aware of these improvements, but they make the Exchange Administrator's job much easier. These improvements include the following:

- **New Deployment Tools**   One of the major problems that Microsoft had with Exchange 2000 was the steep learning curve associated with its deployment. In general, Microsoft products had always been easy to set up, with wizards showing the way. With Exchange 2000, however, the complexity of deployment required command-line `forestprep` and `domainprep` commands; manual Active Directory Connector ADC setup; and confusing concepts, such as Config_CAs, the Site Replication Service, and schema extensions. With Exchange Server 2003, all of these requirements are still present, but the means with which they are accomplished have been streamlined. A step-by-step process known as the Exchange Deployment Wizard leads an administrator through the installation process, reducing the potential for error or major directory issues.

- **Administrative Tool Improvements**   The development team for Exchange Server 2003 listened to Exchange administrator feedback and drastically improved the functionality and capabilities of the Exchange System Manager administrative toolset. Enhanced queue viewing capabilities, move mailbox tool enhancements, dynamic distribution list functionality, and (drum-roll please) the ability to run Exchange System Manager on Windows XP have greatly simplified the job of the Exchange Administrator.

- **Database Backup and Restore Capabilities**   The overall backup and restore functionality of Exchange has been improved in Exchange Server 2003. New Enhancements, such as the Volume Shadow Copy Service, the Mailbox Recovery Center, and the Recovery Storage Group concept help position Exchange Server 2003 for simplified and enhanced backup and restore capabilities.

It is important to incorporate the concepts of these improvements into any Exchange design project, because their principles often drive the design process.

Exchange and Operating System Requirements

Exchange Server 2003 has some specific requirements, both hardware and software, that must be taken into account when designing. These requirements fall into several categories:

- Hardware requirements
- Operating system
- Active Directory
- Exchange version

Each requirement must be addressed before Exchange Server 2003 can be deployed.

Hardware Requirements

Design your Exchange hardware to scale out to the user load, which is expected for up to three years from the date of implementation. This helps retain the value of the investment put into Exchange. Specific hardware configuration advice is offered in later sections of this chapter.

Operating System

Exchange Server 2003 is optimized for installation on Windows Server 2003. The increases in security and the fundamental changes to Internet Information Services (IIS) in Windows Server 2003 provide the basis for many of the improvements in Exchange Server 2003. However, Exchange Server 2003 also can be installed on Windows 2000. The specific compatibility matrix, which indicates compatibility between Exchange versions and operating systems, is illustrated in Table 4.1.

TABLE 4.1   Exchange Version Compatibility

Version	Windows NT 4.0	Windows 2000	Windows 2003
Exchange 5.5	Yes	Yes	No
Exchange 2000	No	Yes	No
Exchange 2003	No	Yes	Yes

Active Directory

Exchange originally maintained its own directory. With the advent of Exchange 2000, however, the directory for Exchange was moved to the Microsoft Active Directory, the enterprise directory system for Windows. This gave greater flexibility and consolidated directories, but at the same time increased the complexity and dependencies for Exchange. Exchange Server 2003 uses the same model, with either Windows 2000 or Windows Server 2003 Active Directory as its directory component.

> **NOTE**
>
> Active Directory is loosely modeled on the original Exchange 5.5 Directory. Administrators familiar with the Exchange 5.5 Directory will notice similarities between the environments, particularly in the replication engines.

Exchange Version

As with previous versions of Exchange, there are separate Enterprise and Standard versions of the Exchange Server 2003 product. The Standard version supports all Exchange Server 2003 functionality with the exception of the following key components:

- **Greater than 16GB Mailbox Store**   The standard version of Exchange Server 2003 can support only a single database of up to 16GB in size. Organizations with small numbers of users or strict storage limits can use this version of Exchange without problems, but larger organizations require the Enterprise version because databases may increase to larger than 16GB.

There is no direct upgrade path from the Exchange Standard version to the Enterprise version. Only a mailbox migration procedure that can transfer mailboxes from a Standard version server to an Enterprise version server will be able to accomplish an upgrade. Consequently, it is important to make an accurate determination of whether the Enterprise version of the software is needed.

- **Multiple Mailbox Database Stores**   One of the key features of Exchange Server 2003 is the capability of the server to support multiple databases and storage groups with the Enterprise version of the software. This capability is not supported with the Standard version of the product.

- **Clustering Support**   Exchange Server 2003 clustering is available only when using the Enterprise version of the software. Support for up to an 8-way active-active or active-passive cluster on Windows Server 2003 is available.

- **X.400 Connectors**   Although becoming increasingly less common, the ability to install and configure X.400 Connectors for remote site connectivity is available only in the Enterprise version of the software.

Scaling Exchange Server 2003

The days of the Exchange server "rabbit farm" are gone. No longer is it necessary to set up multiple Exchange server implementations across an organization. Exchange 2000 originally provided the basis for servers that could easily scale out to thousands of users in a single site, if necessary. Exchange Server 2003 enables even more users to be placed on fewer servers through the concept of site consolidation.

Site consolidation enables organizations that might have previously deployed Exchange servers in remote locations to have those clients access their mailboxes across WAN links or dial-up connections by using the enhanced Outlook 2003 or Outlook Web Access clients. This solves the problem that previously existed of having to deploy Exchange servers and Global Catalog (GC) servers in remote locations, with only a handful of users, and greatly reduces the infrastructure costs of setting up Exchange.

Having Exchange Server 2003 Coexist with an Existing Network Infrastructure

Exchange is built upon a standards-based model, which incorporates many industry-wide compatible protocols and services. Internet standards—such as DNS, IMAP, SMTP, LDAP, and POP3—are built in to the product to provide coexistence with existing network infrastructure.

In a design scenario, it is necessary to identify any systems that require access to email data or services. For example, it might be necessary to enable a third-party monitoring application to relay mail-off of the SMTP engine of Exchange so that alerts can be sent. Identifying these needs during the design portion of a project is subsequently important.

Identifying Third-Party Product Functionality

Microsoft built specific hooks into Exchange Server 2003 to enable third-party applications to improve upon the built-in functionality provided by the system. For example, built-in support for antivirus scanning, backups, and spam filtering exist right out of the box, although functionality is limited without the addition of third-party software. The most common additions to Exchange implementation are

- Antivirus

- Backup

- Spam filtering

- Fax software

Active Directory Design Concepts for Exchange Server 2003

After all objectives, dependencies, and requirements have been mapped out, the process of designing the Exchange Server 2003 environment can begin. There are several key areas where decisions should be made:

- Active Directory design

- Exchange Server placement

- Global Catalog placement

- Client access methods

Understanding the Active Directory Forest

Because Exchange Server 2003 relies on the Windows Server 2003 Active Directory for its directory, it is subsequently important to include Active Directory in the design plans. In many situations, an Active Directory implementation, whether based on Windows 2000 or Windows Server 2003, already exists in the organization. In these cases, it is necessary only to plan for the inclusion of Exchange Server into the forest.

If an Active Directory structure is not already in place, a new AD forest must be established. Designing the Active Directory forest infrastructure can be complex, and can require nearly as much thought into design as the actual Exchange Server configuration itself. Subsequently, it is important to understand fully the concepts behind Active Directory before beginning an Exchange 2003 design.

In short, a single "instance" of Active Directory consists of a single Active Directory forest. A forest is composed of Active Directory trees, which are contiguous domain namespaces in the forest. Each tree is composed of one or more domains, as illustrated in Figure 4.1.

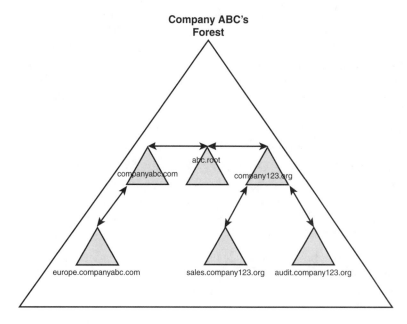

FIGURE 4.1   Multi-tree forest design.

Certain cases exist for using more than one Active Directory forest in an organization:

- **Political Limitations**   Some organizations have specific political reasons that force the creation of multiple Active Directory forests. For example, if a merged corporate entity required separate divisions to maintain completely separate IT infrastructures, more than one forest would be necessary.

- **Security Concerns**   Although the Active Directory domain serves as a de facto security boundary, the "ultimate" security boundary is effectively the forest. In other words, it is possible for user accounts in a domain in a forest to hack into domains within the same forest. Although these types of vulnerabilities are not common and are difficult to do, highly security-conscious organizations should implement separate AD forests.

- **Application Functionality**   A single Active Directory forest shares a common directory schema, which is the underlying structure of the directory and must be unique across the entire forest. In some cases, separate branches of an organization require that certain applications, which need extensions to the schema, be installed. This might not be possible or might conflict with the schema requirements of other branches. These cases might require the creation of a separate forest.

- **Exchange-Specific Functionality**   In certain circumstances, it might be necessary to install Exchange Server 2003 into a separate forest, to enable Exchange to reside in a separate schema and forest instance. An example of this type of setup would be an organization with two existing Active Directory forests that creates a third forest specifically for Exchange and uses cross-forest trusts to assign mailbox permissions.

The simplest designs often work the best. The same principle applies to Active Directory design. The designer should start with the assumption that a simple forest and domain structure will work for the environment. However, when factors such as those previously described create constraints, multiple forests can be established to satisfy the requirements of the constraints.

Understanding the Active Directory Domain Structure

After the Active Directory forest structure has been laid out, the domain structure can be contemplated. As with the forest structure, it is often wise to consider a single domain model for the Exchange 2003 directory. In fact, if deploying Exchange is the only consideration, this is often the best choice.

There is one major exception to the single domain model: the placeholder domain model. The placeholder domain model has an isolated domain serving as the root domain in the forest. The user domain, which contains all production user accounts, would be located in a separate domain in the forest, as illustrated in Figure 4.2.

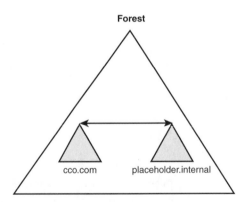

FIGURE 4.2   The placeholder domain model.

The placeholder domain structure increases security in the forest by segregating high-level schema-access accounts into a completely separate domain from the regular user domain. Access to the placeholder domain can be audited and restricted to maintain tighter control on the critical schema. The downside to this model, however, is the fact that the additional domain requires a separate set of domain controllers, which increases the infrastructure costs of the environment. In general, this makes this domain model less desirable for smaller organizations, because the tradeoff between increased cost and less security is too great. Larger organizations can consider the increased security provided by this model, however.

Reviewing Active Directory Infrastructure Components

There are several key components of Active Directory that must be installed within an organization to ensure proper Exchange Server 2003 and Active Directory functionality. In smaller environments, many of these components can be installed on a single machine, but all need to be located within an environment to ensure server functionality.

The Domain Name Service (DNS) Impact on Exchange Server 2003 Design

In addition to being tightly integrated with Active Directory, Exchange Server 2003 is intrinsically linked with the Domain Name Server (DNS). DNS serves as the lookup agent for Exchange Server 2003, Active Directory, and most new Microsoft applications and services. DNS translates common names into computer-recognizable IP addresses. For example, the name www.cco.com translates into the IP address of 12.155.166.151. Active Directory and Exchange Server 2003 require that at least one DNS server be made available so that name resolution properly occurs.

Given the dependency that both Exchange Server 2003 and Active Directory have on DNS, it is an extremely important design element. For an in-depth look at DNS and its role in Exchange Server 2003, see Chapter 7, "Domain Name System Impact on Exchange Server 2003."

DNS Namespace

Given Exchange Server 2003's dependency on DNS, a common DNS namespace must be chosen for the Active Directory structure to reside in. In multiple tree domain models, this could be composed of several DNS trees, but in small organization setups, this normally means choosing a single DNS namespace for the AD domain.

There is a great deal of confusion between the DNS namespace in which Active Directory resides, and the email DNS namespace in which mail is delivered. Although they are often the same, in many cases there are differences between the two namespaces. For example, CompanyABC's Active Directory structure is composed of a single domain named abc.internal, and the email domain to which mail is delivered is companyabc.com. The separate namespace, in this case, was created to reduce the security vulnerability of maintaining the same DNS namespace both internally and externally (published to the Internet).

For simplicity, CompanyABC could have chosen companyabc.com as its Active Directory namespace. This choice increases the simplicity of the environment by making the Active Directory login User Principal Name (UPN) and the email address the same. For example, the user Pete Handley is pete@companyabc.com for login, and pete@companyabc.com for email. This option is the choice for many organizations, because the need for user simplicity often trumps the higher security.

Global Catalog Caching and GC/DC Placement

Because all Exchange directory lookups use Active Directory, it is vital that the essential Active Directory Global Catalog information is made available to each Exchange server in the organization. For many small offices with a single site, this simply means that it is important to have a full Global Catalog server available in the main site.

Recall that the Global Catalog is an index of the Active Directory database that contains a partial copy of its contents. All objects within the AD tree are referenced within the Global Catalog, which enables users to search for objects located in other domains. Every attribute of each object is not replicated to the Global Catalogs, only those attributes that are commonly used in search operations, such as first name and last name. Exchange Server 2003 uses the Global Catalog for the email-based lookups of names, email addresses, and other mail-related attributes.

Windows Server 2003 domain controllers and sites enable the concept of Universal Group Membership Caching, which enables a standard (non Global Catalog) domain controller to cache the membership of commonly referenced universal groups in the organization. Because this is one of the most common types of objects that are looked up using the Global Catalog, the addition of this functionality enables the placement of domain controllers in remote sites without a local Global Catalog, as illustrated in Figure 4.3.

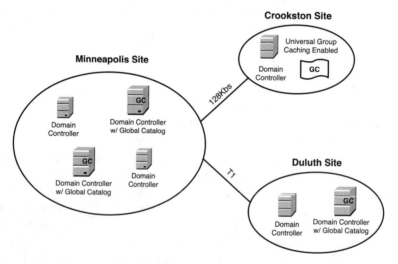

FIGURE 4.3   Global Catalog and domain controller placement.

Because full Global Catalog replication can consume more bandwidth than standard domain controller replication, it is important to design a site structure to reflect the available WAN link capacity. If a sufficient amount of capacity is available, a full Global

Catalog server can be deployed. If, however, capacity is limited, universal group membership caching can be enabled to reduce the bandwidth load. The important factor to keep in mind is that any local Exchange server must have an available copy of Global Catalog information nearby so that performance can be optimized.

Multiple Forests Design Concepts Using Microsoft Identify Integration Server 2003 (MIIS2003)

Microsoft Identify Integration Server 2003 (MIIS2003) enables out-of-the-box replication of objects between two separate Active Directory forests. This concept becomes important for organizations with multiple Exchange implementations that want a common Global Address List for the company. Previous iterations of MIIS required an in-depth knowledge of scripting to be able to synchronize objects between two forests. MIIS 2003, on the other hand, includes built-in scripts that can establish replication between two Exchange Server 2003 AD forests, making integration between forests easier. For more information on using MIIS with Exchange Server 2003, see Chapter 6, "Integrating Exchange Server 2003 in a Non-Windows Environment."

Determining Exchange Server 2003 Placement

Previous versions of Exchange essentially forced many organizations into deploying servers in sites with greater than a dozen or so users. With the concept of site consolidation in Exchange Server 2003, however, smaller numbers of Exchange servers can service clients in multiple locations, even if they are separated by slow WAN links. For small and medium-sized organizations, this essentially means that one or two servers should suffice for the needs of the organization, with few exceptions. Larger organizations require a larger number of Exchange servers, depending on the number of sites and users. Designing Exchange Server 2003 placement must take into account both administrative group and routing group structure.

Designing Administrative Groups

An Exchange Server 2003 administrative group is a logical assortment of Exchange Servers that are administered by the same IT team. A single administrative group can encompass multiple physical locations, depending on the administrative requirements of the organization. For example, in Figure 4.4, CompanyABC has two administrative groups, one for the IT team in North America, and one for the team in Europe.

Administrative groups enable the simple delegation of granular administrative rights to specific groups. In CompanyABC's case, this means that specific rights can be granted to the IT team in Europe to administer only European servers, and not North American servers—and vice versa.

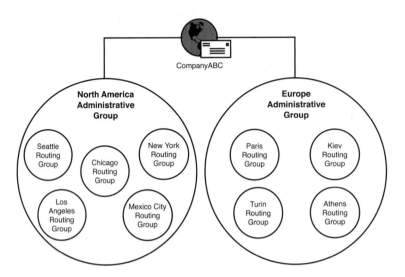

FIGURE 4.4   Multiple administrative groups in Exchange 2003.

Planning Routing Group Topology

The concept of the routing group in Exchange enables a distinction to be made between administration of servers and the actual physical sites in which servers are located.

> **NOTE**
>
> Administrative groups and routing groups in Exchange 5.5 were not separate concepts, but both existed in the form of the Exchange 5.5 site. Consequently, administrative groups and routing groups in Exchange Server 2003 cannot be separated from each other unless the Exchange organization is running in Exchange 2003 native mode.

Figure 4.4 shows that CompanyABC used multiple routing groups within the two administrative groups that have been created. Subsequently, designing administrative group and routing group structure for an organization simply requires outlining the administrative needs and the physical routing restrictions in place in the organization. In many cases, a single administrative group is all that is required, because single IT teams often manage organizations of this size. On the same thread of reasoning, it is often the case that a single routing group can encompass all the servers in a small organization, especially when taking into account the site consolidation strategies mentioned in the previous sections of this chapter.

Examining Public Folder Design Concepts

The public folder structure in Exchange Server 2003 is, for better or worse, the main storehouse of publicly accessed information in the messaging infrastructure. For example, departmental calendars or contact lists can be stored in Exchange public folders.

The Exchange Server 2003 public folder store is a separate database, which is used to store public folder information. In a small or medium-sized organization, a single public folder store can be created and used. In larger organizations, multiple servers can contain multiple public folder stores, each configured to contain a read/write replica of public folder information for redundancy purposes.

Environment Sizing Considerations

In some cases with small organizations, the number of users is small enough to warrant the installation of all Active Directory and Exchange Server 2003 components on a single server. This scenario is possible, as long as all necessary components—DNS, a Global Catalog domain controller, and Exchange Server 2003—are installed on the same hardware.

Identifying Client Access Points

At its core, Exchange Server 2003 essentially acts as a storehouse for mailbox data. Access to the mail within the mailboxes can take place through multiple means, some of which may be required by specific services or applications in the environment. A good understanding of what these services are and if and how your design should support them is warranted.

MAPI Client Access with Outlook 2003

The "heavy" client of Outlook, Outlook 2003, has gone through a significant number of changes, both to the look and feel of the application, and to the back-end mail functionality. The look and feel has been streamlined based on Microsoft research and customer feedback. Although it might take some getting used to, the layout and configuration is much more efficient, making checking email, scheduling, and other messaging features easier to accomplish.

On the back end, Outlook 2003 improves the MAPI compression that takes place between an Exchange Server 2003 system and the Outlook 2003 client. The increased compression helps reduce network traffic and improve the overall speed of communications between client and server.

In addition to MAPI compression, Outlook 2003 introduces the ability to run in a slow-link mode, which automatically detects slow connections between client and server and adjusts Outlook functionality to match the speed of the link. When a slow link is detected, Outlook downloads only email header information. When emails are opened, the entire email is downloaded, including attachments if necessary. This drastically reduces the amount of bits across the wire that are sent, because only those emails that are required are sent across the connection.

The Outlook 2003 client is the most effective and full-functioning client for users who are physically located close to an Exchange Server. With the enhancements in slow-link functionality, however, Outlook 2003 can also be effectively used in remote locations. The decision about which client to deploy as part of a design should keep these concepts in mind.

Outlook Web Access (OWA)

The Outlook Web Access (OWA) client in Exchange Server 2003 has been revamped and optimized for performance and useability. There is now very little difference between the full function client and OWA. With this in mind, OWA is now an even more efficient client for remote access to the Exchange Server. The one major piece of functionality that OWA does not have, but the full Outlook 2003 client does, is offline mail access support. If this is required, the full client should be deployed. Aside from this, however, the improvements in OWA make this a difficult choice.

Outlook Mobile Access (OMA)

Microsoft anticipates that the wireless messaging market will expand by leaps and bounds in the coming years. The company subsequently has invested heavily in gearing its technologies toward wireless access methods. Exchange Server 2003 is one of those technologies, and the introduction of Outlook Mobile Access (OMA) gives an indication of Microsoft's push into this arena.

OMA enables wireless devices, such as handheld organizers, wireless phones, and other small-screen appliances to have an access method to Exchange mailbox data that is customized to the uniquely small reading areas of these devices. The OMA client enables an optimized mail experience, and is ideal for those types of clients that use wireless devices.

The POP3 Protocol

Exchange Server 2003 enables access to email via the older, but industry-standard POP3 Protocol. POP3 is often used with clients such as Outlook Express and Eudora, and is limited in its functionality beyond basic mail retrieval. If a specific need exists to maintain POP3 functionality, this protocol can be designed into the environment. If there is no distinct need to use it, it should be disabled to minimize potential security risks.

The IMAP Protocol

Similar to POP3, the IMAP protocol is an older industry standard that relates to mail sending and retrieval. Many Unix mail clients, such as PINE, use IMAP for mail. As with the POP3 protocol, unless a specific need exists to support IMAP clients, the IMAP protocol should be disabled.

Simple Mail Transport Protocol (SMTP)

The Simple Mail Transfer Protocol (SMTP) is an industry-standard protocol that is widely used across the Internet for mail delivery. The SMTP protocol is built in to Exchange servers and is used by Exchange systems for relaying mail messages from one system to another, which is similar to the way that mail is relayed across SMTP servers on the Internet. Exchange is dependent on SMTP for mail delivery and uses it for internal and external mail access.

> **NOTE**
>
> Previously, Exchange 5.5 (and earlier) used the X.400 protocol to relay messages internally from one Exchange Server to another. This feature changed in Exchange 2000 and later in Exchange Server 2003, where X.400 is used only for backward compatibility with Exchange 5.5 systems.

By default, Exchange Server 2003 uses DNS to route messages destined for the Internet out of the Exchange topology. If, however, a user wants to forward messages to a smarthost before they are transmitted to the Internet, an SMTP connector can be manually set up to enable mail relay out of the Exchange system. SMTP connectors also reduce the risk and load on an Exchange Server by offloading the DNS lookup tasks to the SMTP smarthost. SMTP connectors can be specifically designed in an environment for this type of functionality.

RPC over HTTP Protocol

The new access protocol added to Exchange Server 2003 is the RPC over HTTP protocol, which enables standard Outlook 2003 access across firewalls. The Outlook 2003 client encapsulates RPC packets into HTTP or HTTPS packets and sends them across standard Web ports (80 and 443), where they are then extracted by the Exchange Server 2003 system. This technology enables Outlook to communicate using its standard RPC protocol, but across firewalls and routers that normally do not allow RPC traffic. The potential uses of this protocol are significant, because many situations do not require the use of cumbersome VPN clients.

Configuring Exchange Server 2003 for Maximum Performance and Reliability

After decisions have been made about Active Directory design, Exchange Server placement, and client access, optimization of the Exchange Server itself helps ensure efficiency, reliability, and security for the messaging platform.

Designing an Optimal Operating System Configuration for Exchange

As previously mentioned, Exchange Server 2003 operates best when run on Windows Server 2003. The enhancements to the operating system, especially in regard to security, make Windows Server 2003 the optimal choice for Exchange. Unless clustering or network load balancing is required, which is rare for smaller organizations, the Standard version of Windows Server 2003 can be installed as the OS.

> **NOTE**
>
> Contrary to popular misconception, the Enterprise version of Exchange can be installed on the Standard version of the Operating System, and vice versa.
>
> Although there has been a lot of confusion on this concept, both versions of Exchange were designed to interoperate with either version of Windows.

Avoiding Virtual Memory Fragmentation Issues

Windows Server's previous iterations have suffered from a problem with virtual memory (VM) fragmentation. The problem would manifest itself on systems with greater than 1GB of RAM, which run memory-intensive applications such as SQL Server or Exchange. The Advanced Server Edition of Windows 2000 enabled a workaround for this problem, in the form of a memory allocation switch that allocated additional memory for the user kernel.

Windows Server 2003 includes the capability of using this memory optimization technique in both the Standard and the Enterprise versions of the software, so that the switch can now be used on any Windows Server 2003 system with more than 1GB of physical RAM. The switch is added to the end of the boot.ini file, as illustrated in Figure 4.5.

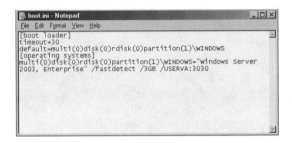

FIGURE 4.5   boot.ini parameter switch setting.

The /3GB switch tells Windows to allocate 3GB of memory for the user kernel, and the /USERVA:3030 switch optimizes the memory configuration, based on tests performed by Microsoft that determined the perfect number of megabytes to allocate for optimal performance and the least likely instance of VM fragmentation.

Configuring Disk Options for Performance

The single most important design element, which improves the efficiency and speed of Exchange, is the separation of the Exchange database and the Exchange logs onto a separate hard drive volume. Because of the inherent differences in the type of hard drive operations performed (logs perform primarily write operations, databases primarily read), separating these elements onto separate volumes dramatically increases server performance. Keep these components separate in even the smallest Exchange server implementations. Figure 4.6 illustrates some examples of how the database and log volumes can be configured.On Server1, the OS and logs are located on the same mirrored C:\ volume and the database is located on a separate RAID5 drive set. With Server2, the configuration is taken up a notch, with the OS only on C:\, the logs on D:\, and the database on the RAID5 E:\ volume. Finally, Server3 is configured in the optimal configuration, with separate volumes for each database and set of logs. The more advanced a configuration, the more detailed and complex the drive configuration can get. However, the most important factor that must be remembered is to separate the Exchange database from the logs wherever possible.

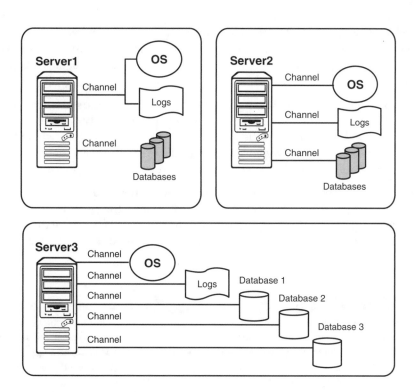

FIGURE 4.6 Database and log volume configuration.

Working with Multiple Exchange Databases and Storage Groups

The Enterprise version of Exchange Server 2003 not only enables databases of larger than 16GB, it also enables the creation of multiple separate databases on a single server. This concept gives great flexibility in design while enabling reduced downtime and increased performance.

A storage group is a logical grouping of databases that share a single set of logs. Each Exchange Server 2003 Enterprise system can handle a maximum of 4 storage groups per server, and each storage group can contain a maximum of 5 databases. This means that each server could theoretically hold up to 20 databases.

In practice, however, each instance of a storage group that is created uses a significant amount of resources, so it is wise to create additional storage groups only if absolutely necessary. Multiple databases, on the other hand, can solve several problems:

- **Reduce Database Restore Time**   Smaller databases take less time to restore from tape. This concept can be helpful if there is a group of users who require quicker recovery time (such as management). All mailboxes for this group could then be placed in a separate database to provide quicker recovery time in the event of a server or database failure.

- **Provide for Separate Mailbox Limit Policies**   Each database can be configured with different mailbox storage limits. For example, the standard user database
could have a 200MB limit on mailboxes, and the management database could have a
500MB limit.

- **Mitigate Risk by Distributing User Load**   By distributing user load across
multiple databases, the risk of losing all user mail connectivity is reduced. For
example, if a single database failed that contained all users, no one would be able to
mail. If those users were divided across three databases, however, only one-third of
those users would be unable to mail in the event of a database failure.

- **Provide for a Recovery Storage Group**   Exchange Server 2003 provides a
concept called a recovery storage group, which enables the creation of a special
storage group to which entire databases can be restored. This can be run on a
production mail server and can greatly simplify the task of restoring mailbox data to
production accounts.

> **NOTE**
>
> One disadvantage to multiple databases is that the concept of single-instance storage is lost
> across databases. Single-instance storage occurs when only one copy of an email message sent to
> multiple people is stored on the server, dramatically reducing the space needed to store mass
> mailings. Each separate database must keep a copy of mass mailings, however, which increases
> the aggregate total size of the databases.

Clustering for Exchange Server 2003

Exchange Server 2003 is configured to use Windows Server 2003 clustering for enhanced
redundancy and increased uptime. Clustering can be set up with up to 8 cluster nodes
with the Enterprise version of Windows Server 2003. Clustering is an expensive option,
but one that will increase reliability of the Exchange Server 2003 implementation.

> **NOTE**
>
> Microsoft no longer recommends a full active-active clustering configuration. Consequently, at
> least 1 cluster node should be configured as passive. With 8-way clustering, this means that 7
> nodes can be active, and 1 node passive.

Monitoring Design Concepts with Microsoft Operations Manager

The enhancements to Exchange Server 2003 do not stop with the improvements to the
product itself. New functionality has been added to the Exchange Management Pack for
Microsoft Operations Manager (MOM) that enables MOM to monitor Exchange servers for

critical events and performance data. The MOM Management Pack is preconfigured to monitor for Exchange-specific information, and enable administrators to proactively monitor Exchange servers.

Backup and Restore Design Concepts and the Volume Shadow Copy Service

The backup and restore functionality for Exchange Server 2003 has been enhanced via integration with the Volume Shadow Copy Service (VSS) of Windows Server 2003. VSS enables an Exchange database to be backed up via snapshots of the database, which create full data images that can be used for restores. This functionality can also be leveraged by software companies that create backup software for Exchange to further improve the capabilities for Exchange Server 2003 backup and restore.

Uncovering Enhanced Antivirus and SPAM Features

Exchange Server 2003 provides an improved Anti-Virus API (AVAPI), which enables preemptive identification of potential viruses in email attachments. The improved AVAPI can be integrated with antivirus software for Exchange written by third-party software companies and helps secure an Exchange environment.

Securing and Maintaining an Exchange Server 2003 Implementation

One of the greatest advantages of Exchange Server 2003 is its emphasis on security. Along with Windows Server 2003, Exchange Server 2003 was developed during and after Microsoft's Trustworthy Computing initiative, which effectively put a greater emphasis on security over new features in the products. In Exchange Server 2003, this means that the OS and the application were designed with services "Secure by Default."

With Secure by Default, all nonessential functionality in Exchange must be turned on if needed. This is a complete change from the previous Microsoft model, which had all services, add-ons, and options turned on and running at all times, presenting much larger security vulnerabilities than was necessary. Designing security effectively becomes much easier in Exchange Server 2003, because it now becomes necessary only to identify components to turn on, as opposed to identifying everything that needs to be turned off.

Patching the Operating System Using Software Update Services

Although Windows Server 2003 presents a much smaller target for hackers, viruses, and exploits by virtue of the Secure by Default concept, it is still important to keep the OS up to date against critical security patches and updates. Currently, two approaches can be used to automate the installation of server patches. The first method involves configuring the Windows Server 2003 Automatic Updates client to download patches from Microsoft and install them on a schedule. The second option is to set up an internal server to coordinate patch distribution and management. The solution that Microsoft supplies for this functionality is known as Software Update Services (SUS).

SUS enables a centralized server to hold copies of OS patches for distribution to clients on a preset schedule. SUS can be used to automate the distribution of patches to Exchange Server 2003 servers, so that the OS components will remain secure between service packs. Software Update Services may not be necessary in smaller environments, but can be considered in medium-sized to large organizations that want greater control over their patch management strategy.

Using Front-End Server Functionality

The OWA component of Exchange Server 2003 can be further secured and optimized through the use of a dedicated Exchange Server 2003 front-end server. A front-end server is an Exchange server that acts as a proxy for mail access. No working databases are kept on a front-end server; the front-end server relays requests from clients to the back-end Exchange mailbox server.

In Figure 4.7, the front-end server SFEX01 is set up in the DMZ of CompanyABC's firewall. Secure Sockets Layer (SSL) encryption is used by clients to access the front-end server. The front-end server then relays client requests from the Internet to the back-end SFEX02 server. This configuration helps secure the back-end server and also offloads the data decryption responsibilities from the back-end mailbox servers. For more information on front-end/back-end design, see Chapter 10, "Outlook Web Access 2003."

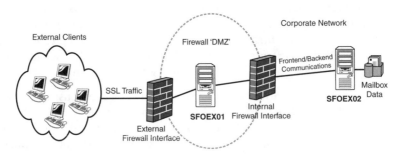

FIGURE 4.7   Front-end/back-end Exchange server configuration.

Implementing Maintenance Schedules

Exchange uses the Microsoft JET Database structure, which is effectively the same database engine that has been used with Exchange from the beginning. This type of database is useful for storing the type of unstructured data that email normally carries, and has proven to be a good fit for Exchange Server. Along with this type of database, however, comes the responsibility to run regular, scheduled maintenance on the Exchange databases on a regular basis.

Although online maintenance is performed every night, it is recommended that Exchange databases be brought offline on a quarterly or, at least, semiannual basis for offline maintenance. Exchange database maintenance utilities, `eseutil` and `isinteg`, should be used to compact and defragment the databases, which can then be mounted again in the environment.

Exchange databases that do not have this type of maintenance performed run the risk of becoming corrupt in the long term, and will also never be able to be reduced in size. Consequently, it is important to include database maintenance into a design plan to ensure data integrity.

Using Antivirus and Backup Solutions

It has become a must for organizations to employ antivirus and backup solutions for Enterprise email applications. As previously mentioned, one of the major advantages of Exchange is that the OS and the application itself support advanced backup and antivirus technologies that can be tied into by third-party software resellers. This third-party support is broad, and should be part of any Exchange design.

Summary

Exchange Server 2003 offers a broad range of functionality and improvements to messaging and is well suited for organizations of any size. With proper thought for the major design topics, a robust and reliable Exchange email solution can be put into place that will perfectly complement the needs of any organization.

When Exchange design concepts have been fully understood, the task of designing the Exchange Server 2003 infrastructure can take place.

Best Practices

The following are best practices from this chapter:

- Use the site consolidation strategies to reduce the number of Exchange servers to deploy.

- Separate the Exchange log and database files onto separate physical volumes whenever possible.

- Install Exchange Server 2003 on Windows Server 2003.

- Use the \3GB and \USERVA:3030 switches in the boot.ini file of any Exchange Server 2003 server with greater than 1GB of RAM.

- Integrate an antivirus and backup strategy into Exchange Server design.

- Keep a local copy of the Global Catalog close to any Exchange servers.

- Implement quarterly or semiannual maintenance procedures against Exchange databases by using the ISINTEG and ESEUTIL utilities.

- Keep the OS and Exchange up to date through service packs and software patches, either manually or via Software Update Services.

- Keep the Active Directory design simple, with a single forest and single domain, unless a specific need exists to create more complexity.

- Identify the client access methods that will be supported and match them with the appropriate Exchange Server 2003 technology.

- Implement DNS in the environment on the AD domain controllers.

- Use an external (published) Active Directory DNS namespace if simplicity is important, or use an internal (nonpublished) Active Directory DNS namespace if security is more important.

CHAPTER 5

Designing an Enterprise Exchange Server 2003 Environment

Exchange Server 2003 was designed to accommodate the needs of multiple organizations, from the small Mom-and-Pop businesses to large multinational corporations. In addition to the scalability features present in previous versions of Exchange, Exchange Server 2003 offers more opportunities to scale the back-end server environment to the specific needs of any group.

This chapter addresses specific design guidelines for organizations of various sizes. Throughout the chapter, specific examples of small, medium, and large organizations are presented and general recommendations are made. This chapter assumes a base knowledge of design components that can be obtained by reading Chapter 4, "Exchange Server 2003 Design Concepts."

In this chapter, sample companies have been chosen to illustrate how Exchange Server 2003's design principles can be applied to organizations of varying sizes. Each major section of the chapter details the best practice design decisions taken by each of these organizations, to more effectively illustrate the common approaches to Exchange Server 2003 design. The end of the chapter summarizes the design decisions taken by each organization.

Designing for Small Organizations— Company123

Small businesses account for a large portion of the install base for Exchange. Consequently, a great deal of work went into creating a more cost-effective Exchange model that works for smaller organizations. In addition to the advanced feature set of Exchange 2000, Exchange Server 2003 offers more opportunities to scale the implementation to fit the size of the organization deploying it.

The example of a small organization, for the purposes of this chapter, is Company123. Company123 is the manufacturer of a line of boutique microfiber towels and distributes its product through various resellers. Company123 has 13 employees in its San Francisco headquarters and another 3 in an office in London. As part of a messaging deployment for Company123, the decision was made to deploy Exchange Server 2003. The specific design decisions reached by Company123 are detailed in later sections.

Designing for Midsize Organizations—OrganizationY

The heart of the target market for Exchange is the realm of the midsize organization. Exchange has always been a good choice for organizations of this size, and recent improvements in design components make it an even better match.

The example of a midsize organization is OrganizationY. OrganizationY is a software company headquartered in Manchester, Missouri. OrganizationY is composed of approximately 1200 users, 500 in Manchester, 300 in Los Angeles, 100 in Saint Petersburg, Russia, and an additional 300 scattered in various smaller locations worldwide. OrganizationY determined that Exchange was best suited for its messaging needs and designed an Exchange Server 2003 infrastructure using the design criteria outlined in later sections.

Designing for Large Organizations—CompanyABC

One of the last, heavily fought realms for "frontiers" in the messaging world is that of the large, enterprise organizations. Microsoft has invested considerable resources into expanding the install base of Exchange Server into this arena, and has fixed many of the problems with Exchange that previously kept it geared toward small and midsize organizations.

The example of a large organization for the purposes of this chapter is CompanyABC. CompanyABC is a large, multinational medical services company headquartered in Minneapolis. A total of 9000 users worldwide work for CompanyABC, with major centers in San Francisco, Dallas, New York, Paris, Moscow, Tokyo, and Singapore. Multiple smaller offices are spread around the globe. CompanyABC recently acquired a competitor, effectively doubling its size, but requiring thought into integration of the new environment. The decision to deploy Exchange Server 2003 was based on the improvements made to Exchange in areas of site consolidation, clients, and total cost of ownership. Specific design decisions reached by CompanyABC are outlined in later sections.

Designing Active Directory for Exchange Server 2003

Active Directory is a necessary and fundamental component of any Exchange Server 2003 implementation. That said, organizations of any size do not necessarily need to panic about setting up Active Directory in addition to Exchange, as long as a few straightforward design steps are followed. The following areas of Active Directory must be addressed to properly design and deploy Exchange Server 2003:

- Forest and Domain Design

- AD Site and Replication Topology Layout

- Domain Controller and Global Catalog Placement

- DNS Configuration

Forest and Domain Design

Because Exchange Server 2003 uses Active Directory for its underlying directory structure, it is necessary to link Exchange with an Active Directory forest.

In many cases, an existing Active Directory forest and domain structure is already in place in organizations considering Exchange Server 2003 deployment. In these cases, Exchange can be installed on top of the existing AD environment, and no AD design decisions need to be made. Exchange Server 2003 can be installed on either a Windows 2000 or Windows Server 2003 Active Directory implementation.

In some cases, there may not be an existing AD infrastructure in place, and one needs to be deployed to support Exchange. In some specific cases, Exchange may be deployed as part of a separate forest by itself, as illustrated in Figure 5.1. This is often the case in an organization with multiple existing AD forests.

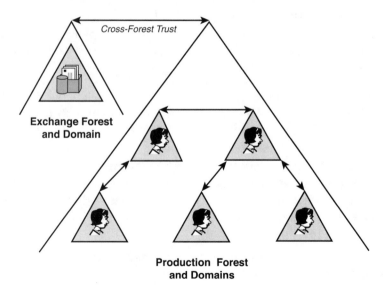

FIGURE 5.1   Multi-forest Exchange configuration.

In any case, AD should be designed with simplicity in mind. A single-forest, single-domain model, for example, will solve the needs of many organizations. If Exchange itself is all that is required of AD, this type of deployment is the best practice to consider.

In some cases, a separate domain called a **placeholder root domain** can be established to increase overall forest security by segregating rights to the AD schema into a separate domain from the normal domain accounts. This model increases security, but also requires the deployment of more domain controllers for the additional domain.

> **NOTE**
>
> The addition of Exchange Server 2003 into an Active Directory forest requires an extension of the AD forest's Active Directory schema.
>
> Considerations for this factor must be taken into account when deploying Exchange onto an existing AD forest.

Microsoft has gotten serious recently about support for Exchange Server across multiple forests. This was previously an onerous task to set up, but the ability to synchronize between separate Exchange organizations has been simplified through the use of Microsoft Identify Integration Server 2003. MMIS now comes with a series of preconfigured scripts to replicate between Exchange forests, enabling organizations which, for one reason or another, cannot use a common forest to unite the email structure through object replication.

AD Site and Replication Topology Layout

Active Directory sites should mirror existing network topology. Where there are pools of highly connected AD domain controllers, for example, Exchange sites should be created to optimize replication. Smaller organizations have the luxury of a simplified AD site design. In general, the number of sites is small—or, in most cases, composed of a single physical location. Small organizations should subsequently configure their Active Directory implementation with a single AD Site. Midsize and larger organizations may require the creation of multiple Active Directory sites to mirror the WAN connectivity of the organization.

Domain Controller and Global Catalog Placement

In small or midsize organizations, there are effectively two options regarding domain controller placement. The first option involves using the same physical server for domain controller and Exchange Server duties. This option is feasible for smaller organizations because its impact on the server is minimal.

The second option is to separate the Active Directory domain controller duties onto a separate physical server from Exchange Server 2003. This option is more expensive, but has the advantages associated with distributed computing. As the anticipated load on the server increases with the number of users using the system, this option becomes necessary.

Configuring DNS

Because AD and Exchange are completely dependent on DNS for lookups and overall functionality, configuring DNS is an important factor to consider. In the majority of cases, DNS is installed on the domain controller(s), which enables the creation of Active Directory–Integrated DNS Zones. AD-Integrated Zones enable DNS data to be stored in AD with multiple read/write copies of the zone available for redundancy purposes. Although using other non-Microsoft DNS for AD is supported, it is not recommended. See Chapter 7, "Domain Name System Impact on Exchange," for more information on third-party DNS scenarios.

The main decision regarding DNS layout is the decision about the namespace to be used within the organization. The DNS namespace is the same as the AD domain information, and it is difficult to change later. The two options in this case are to configure DNS to use either a published, external namespace that is easy to understand, such as cco.com, or an internal, secure namespace that is difficult to hack into, such as cconet.internal. In general, the more security-conscious an organization, the more often the internal namespace will be chosen.

Active Directory Design Decisions for Small Organizations

Company123 did not have an existing Active Directory infrastructure in place, so design decisions regarding AD were necessary. Because its needs were not complex, however, the AD design decisions were not complex. Small organizations rarely need to spend a great deal of time worrying about Active Directory forests, trees, and domains. In reality, the vast majority of these small organizations use a single-forest, single-domain model for their Active Directory.

In Company123's case, the size of the company dictated a simple Active Directory design. Because it had no specific need for a complex forest design, it settled for a single-forest, single-domain AD design, as illustrated in Figure 5.2.

In Company123's case, 12 of the 15 employees are physically located in the San Francisco headquarters. An additional 3 employees are located in a London office, but it was determined that the number of employees in this location was too small to warrant the creation of a second AD Site. A single San Francisco site was created for AD.

When the decision about domain controller placement arose, Company123 chose the simple structure of having a single domain controller for the entire forest. This meant that there were no decisions to be made regarding Global Catalog placement either, because the first domain controller is, by default, a Global Catalog server. In addition, most small organizations opt to have their domain controller on the same hardware as their Exchange Server, which is the configuration chosen by Company123.

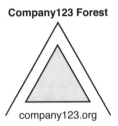

FIGURE 5.2   Single-forest, single-domain Active Directory design.

Company123 installed and configured DNS on the single server chosen as the domain controller and Exchange server for the organization. A single forward lookup zone for the AD domain was created (`company123.org`) and a reverse lookup zone was created for the subnet (`10.0.0.0/24`), as illustrated in Figure 5.3.

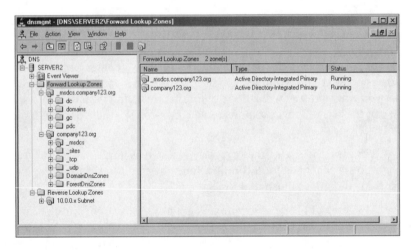

FIGURE 5.3   Forward lookup and reverse lookup zone configuration.

The DNS namespace chosen for the Active Directory domain was the same as the external DNS namespace registered to Company123 on the Internet: `company123.org`. This option was less secure, but because the security needs of Company123 were not great, the decision was made to assume the same namespace for convenience purposes and therefore not confuse the end-users.

Midsize Organization AD Design Decisions

OrganizationY already had an Active Directory domain infrastructure in place and wanted to integrate Exchange Server 2003 into the forest. The AD domain structure used a placeholder root structure, which isolated the schema master role and increased security for the organization, as illustrated in Figure 5.4.

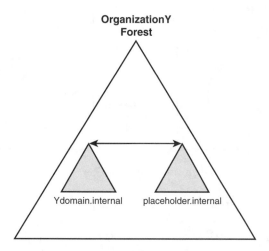

FIGURE 5.4   Placeholder root Active Directory design structure.

OrganizationY had three major locations, so separate Active Directory sites had been configured for each location to optimize replication traffic. In advance of the Exchange Server 2003 project, the two largest sites—Manchester and Los Angeles—were allocated full Global Catalog servers. The St. Petersburg site was allocated domain controllers, but with the Universal Group Caching options enabled for the site. This ensured that the Exchange servers would have fast access to Global Catalog information from each site.

The primary user domain used an internally published DNS namespace named Ydomain.internal. DNS Zones were configured for both the placeholder root domain (placeholder.internal) and the user resource domain (ydomain.internal). The local copy of the zone was configured as AD-Integrated, and the other domain zone was configured as a stub zone, as illustrated in Figure 5.5. This enabled the highest level of security along with the most efficient levels of replication.

Large Organization AD Design Decisions

CompanyABC was faced with a complex Active Directory problem. Separate AD forests had already been deployed in two locations within the company, and it was determined to be too complex an undertaking to consolidate the AD forests into a single forest for Exchange.

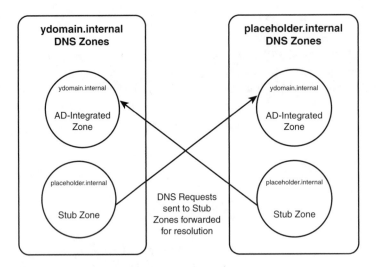

FIGURE 5.5   AD-integrated and stub zone configuration.

CompanyABC was left with the decision to either deploy Exchange Server 2003 in two locations and synchronize the address lists between them using Microsoft Identify Integration Services (MIIS) 2003, or deploy a dedicated forest for Exchange. The second option was chosen, and CompanyABC designed a completely separate AD forest for Exchange, but with cross-forest transitive trusts established between the forests, as illustrated in Figure 5.6.

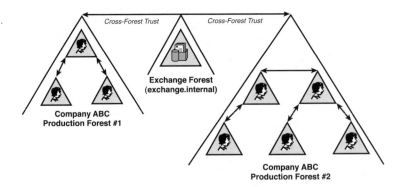

FIGURE 5.6   Multiple Active Directory forest with cross-forest trusts.

The AD Site structure was set up to follow existing WAN topology, with Active Directory sites for Minneapolis, San Francisco, Dallas, New York, Paris, Moscow, Tokyo, and Singapore. Each site contained Global Catalog domain controllers for fast Exchange access.

As evident in Figure 5.6, CompanyABC chose a single domain model with a DNS name-space of exchange.internal for the Exchange forest. All external forest accounts would be granted permissions to their mailboxes across the cross-forest trusts.

Determining Hardware and Software Components

Justifying hardware and software purchases is often a difficult task for organizations of any size. It is therefore important to balance the need for performance and redundancy with the available funds available in the budget, and thus deploy the optimal Exchange server hardware and software configuration.

Server Number and Placement

Exchange scales very well to a large number of mailboxes on a single machine, depending on the hardware chosen for the Exchange server. Exchange Server 2003 also does not require dedicated systems for connectors, as did some previous versions. Subsequently, Exchange Server 2003 is optimal for organizations that want to limit the amount of servers that are deployed and supported in an environment.

Exchange 2000 previously had one major exception to this concept, however. If multiple sites required high-speed access to an Exchange server, multiple servers were necessary for deployment. Exchange Server 2003, on the other hand, introduces the concept of site consolidation, which enables smaller sites to use the Exchange servers in the larger sites through the more efficient bandwidth usage present in Outlook 2003 and the OWA and OMA technologies.

Server Redundancy and Optimization

The ability of the Exchange server to recover from hardware failures is more than just a "nice-to-have" feature. Many server models come with an array of redundancy features, such as multiple fans and power supplies, and mirrored disk capabilities. These features incur additional costs, however, so it is wise for smaller organizations to perform a cost-benefit analysis to determine what redundancy features are required. Midsize and larger organizations should seriously consider robust redundancy options, however, because the increased reliability and uptime is often well worth the up-front costs.

One of the most critical but overlooked performance strategies for Exchange is the concept of separating the Exchange logs and database onto separate physical drive sets. Because Exchange logs are very write-intensive, and the database is read-intensive, having these components on the same disk set would degrade performance. Separating these compo-nents onto different disk sets, however, is the best way to get the most out of Exchange.

In addition to separating the Exchange database onto a striped RAID5 set, the SMTP component used by Exchange can be optimized by moving it to the same partition as the database. By default, the SMTP component is installed on the system (OS) partition, but can be easily moved after an Exchange server has been set up. You can easily move the SMTP folder by accessing the Messages tab under the default SMTP Virtual Server in Exchange System Manager, as illustrated in Figure 5.7.

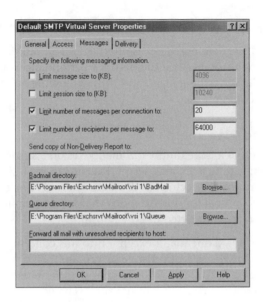

FIGURE 5.7   Moving the SMTP folder in ESM.

Server Memory and Processor Recommendations

Exchange Server is a resource-hungry application that, left to its own devices, will consume a good portion of any amount of processor or memory that is given to it. Although it operates best with multiple processors and more RAM, small organizations may not need the enhanced performance that this investment brings. The amount of processors and RAM required should reflect the budgetary needs of the organization. In general, 1GB of RAM and dual processors is a good rule of thumb for smaller organizations, but a single processor and as low as 500MB of RAM could also work.

Midsize and larger organizations should consider multiprocessor servers and greater amounts of RAM—2GB or 4GB. This will help increase the amount of mailboxes that can be homed to any particular server.

> **NOTE**
>
> Any Exchange Server 2003 system with greater than 1GB of physical RAM should include the /3GB /USERVA=3030 switches in the boot.ini file, which optimize the memory allocation for these systems.

Server Operating System Considerations

Exchange Server 2003 is optimized for use with Windows Server 2003, and it is therefore logical to place Exchange on a server with the new OS installed. Exchange Server 2003 takes advantage of the increased security and feature set of Windows Server 2003, and is therefore the recommended approach for small organizations deploying Exchange.

> **NOTE**
>
> Although it is preferable to install Exchange Server 2003 on Windows Server 2003, this does not mean that the entire network needs to be Windows Server 2003–only. All other servers, including Exchange 2000 and Windows 2000 Active Directory, can coexist in the environment at the same time.

The base OS for Exchange, Windows Server 2003, comes in two versions, Enterprise and Standard. Some midsize and larger organizations could deploy the Enterprise version of the Windows Server 2003 product, namely for clustering support. If this functionality is not required, the Standard version of the OS should be sufficient.

Small organizations, on the other hand, will almost exclusively require only the Standard version, rather than the Enterprise version, of the Windows Server 2003 product. The Enterprise version is required for concepts such as server clustering and support for more than four processors, which are seldom required for small server deployments.

Designing Clustering and Advanced Redundancy Options

In larger organizations, the need to ensure a very high level of reliability is paramount. These organizations often require a level of uptime for their email that equates to "5 nines" of uptime, or 99.999% uptime a year. For this level of redundancy, a higher level of Exchange redundancy is required than the standard models. For these organizations, support may be warranted.

> **NOTE**
>
> Clustering in Windows Server 2003 supports up to 8 nodes. It is now Microsoft's recommendation, however, that at least 1 node in a cluster be set up in passive mode for the most effective failover strategy. For more information on using clustering with Exchange Server 2003, see Chapter 30, "System-Level Fault Tolerance."

Small Organization Hardware and Software Design Decisions

Because 12 of the 15 employees were located in San Francisco, Company123 deployed a single Exchange Server 2003 system, running on the same hardware as the Active

Directory and DNS components. It was designed to enable the three London users to access Exchange using the slow-link and offline capabilities of Outlook 2003.

Company123 decided to deploy server hardware with RAID redundant disks and dual power supplies and fans. Because messaging was a critical aspect for the company, the additional cost was determined to be warranted for the small organization. In addition, the Exchange database, SMTP engine, and Exchange logs were separated onto different physical drive sets, as illustrated in Figure 5.8. This helped Company123 to get the most out of its hardware investment.

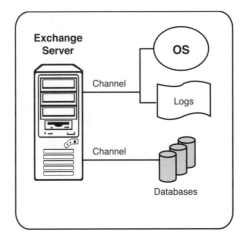

FIGURE 5.8   Separating Exchange components on separate drive sets.

Company123 purchased enterprise-level server hardware with dual processors and 1GB of RAM. Because it was deploying all Active Directory and Exchange components on a single machine, it decided to invest in hardware so that its Exchange implementation would be relevant for several years to come.

The decision was made to deploy its Exchange Server using Windows Server 2003 Standard Edition, because the company wanted the optimal OS configuration for Exchange and didn't have any need for server clustering support.

Midsize Organization Hardware and Software Design Decisions

OrganizationY determined that Exchange mailbox servers would run in two sites, Manchester and Los Angeles, and that the St. Petersburg location and all other smaller sites would connect to these Exchange servers using the improved slow-link functionality in Outlook 2003. This significantly reduced hardware and support expenditures because the number of servers that would have been required was reduced to two for the entire organization, as illustrated in Figure 5.9.

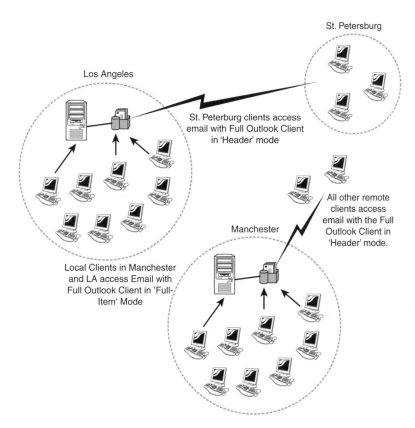

St. Petersburg

Los Angeles

St. Peterburg clients access
email with Full Outlook Client
in 'Header' mode

All other remote
clients access
email with the Full
Outlook Client in
'Header' mode.

Manchester

Local Clients in Manchester
and LA access Email with
Full Outlook Client in 'Full-
Item' Mode

FIGURE 5.9   Exchange organization with a reduction of servers.

Each server was optimized for the Exchange role with 4GB of RAM, quad processors, redundant fans and power supplies, and RAID controllers providing redundant disks. Each server had a separate RAID set for the OS, a separate one for the logs, and a RAID5 set for the database and SMTP folder, as illustrated in Figure 5.9.

The servers were installed with Windows Server 2003 Standard Edition. Because clustering was determined to be unnecessary, the Standard Edition of Windows sufficed.

Large Organization Hardware and Software Design Decisions

CompanyABC deployed Exchange mailbox servers in the largest sites: Minneapolis, San Francisco, Dallas, New York, Paris, Moscow, Tokyo, and Singapore. All other users within the organization were configured to use the mailbox servers in these locations for email access.

The largest site, Minneapolis, clustered its Exchange mailbox Servers into a 4-node cluster, with 3 active nodes and 1 passive node. The server hardware for these cluster nodes was composed of enterprise grade servers with redundant fans and power supplies, 4GB of

RAM, quad processor, and RAID redundant disks. The disk arrays were configured with separate RAID sets for the OS, Logs, and Databases/SMTP Folder, as illustrated in Figure 5.10.

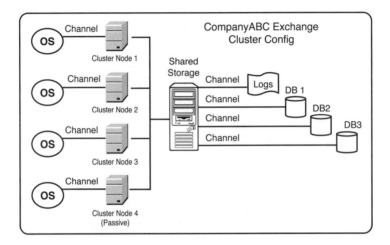

FIGURE 5.10   Separate drive sets for an Exchange 2003 configuration.

The servers in the other large sites were configured with the same hardware, but without clustering capabilities. Windows Server 2003 Standard Edition was installed on all servers with the exception of the clustered servers, which were installed with the Enterprise version of the software.

Designing Exchange Infrastructure

After Active Directory and the physical OS has been chosen and deployed, the Exchange infrastructure can be set up and optimized for the specific needs of the organization. With these needs in mind, there are several things that can be done to optimize an Exchange Server 2003 setup, as detailed in the following sections.

Exchange Version and Org Name

When installing Exchange, the choice of Exchange version needs to be made. As with Windows Server 2003, there are two versions of Exchange, Standard and Enterprise. The Standard version enables all Exchange Server 2003 functionality except the following:

- Multiple databases
- Databases larger than 16GB
- Clustering support
- X.400 Connectors

In smaller organizations, nearly all implementations of Exchange require only the Standard version; the advanced feature set of the Enterprise Edition is geared toward larger deployments. The critical factor that pushes the midsize-to-large organizations to the Enterprise version, however, is the 16GB database limit. Some organizations require large mailbox sizes and could potentially require multiple databases larger than 16GB. Because this functionality is available only with the Enterprise version of the software, it must be installed.

> **CAUTION**
>
> Because the standard version of Exchange does not support databases larger than 16GB, keep track of the size of the private database store, ensuring that it stays well below the 16GB limit. The database will shut down if it reaches this limit.

When installing the first Exchange Server 2003 system, the setup program prompts for the creation of the Exchange Organization. The information entered in the Exchange Organization is fairly trivial, because end-users do not access this information. However, the Exchange Organization is unique across the forest and should reflect the name of the organization that will use the Exchange Server 2003 implementation.

Administrative Group and Routing Group Structure

Exchange Server 2003 continues with the Exchange 2000 concept of separating the administration of servers with the physical location of those servers. In other words, Exchange servers could exist in multiple sites but be administered by the same group. The administration of Exchange servers is subsequently facilitated through the creation of administrative groups, and the physical server routing facility is facilitated through routing groups.

In a nutshell, administrative groups in Exchange Server 2003 should be established to designate administrative boundaries for Exchange components. In other words, if the entire organization is centrally administered, there should be only a single admin group for the entire organization. If there is a separate admin group—for servers in Europe, for example—multiple admin groups can be created to provide eased delegation of administration.

Routing groups, on the other hand, are used to optimize replication between "islands" of high connectivity, similar to the concept of Active Directory and Exchange 5.5 sites. Servers within the same routing group communicate with each other faster and more often, and Exchange systems in remote routing groups can be configured to replicate information on a scheduled basis.

Public Folder Structure and Replication

Public folders in Exchange have a somewhat mixed relationship with administrators and users. Many organizations widely use the group calendaring and posting features of public folders, but others maintain a public folder database with little or no data in it.

Public folder architecture for small organizations is usually quite simple; because there is normally only one Exchange server, only one public folder instance is possible. If there is more than one server and fast access to public folder information is required, it may be necessary to create a second public folder instance.

Midsize-to-large organizations, on the other hand, can take advantage of the ability to have multiple read/write copies of public folder trees by deploying public folder instances in various servers across the organization. This ensures fast public folder access for users.

Exchange Databases and Storage Groups

As previously mentioned, the Enterprise version of Exchange enables the concept of multiple databases, up to a maximum of 20. This enables a greater amount of design freedom and gives administrators more flexibility. A maximum of four production storage groups can be created, and each storage group can contain up to five databases.

> **NOTE**
>
> Exchange Server 2003 introduces a concept called a recovery storage group, which enables the restoration of mailbox data to a completely separate storage group from the regular mail data. An Exchange Recovery storage group can be installed as a fifth storage group on the Enterprise version of Exchange, but it also can be used on the Standard version.

Exchange Recovery Options

Deploying Exchange requires considerable thought about backup and recovery solutions. Because Exchange is a live, active database, special considerations need to be taken into account when designing the backup strategy for email.

Microsoft designed Exchange Server 2003 to use the new backup APIs from Windows Server 2003. These APIs support the Volume Shadow Copy service, which enables Exchange databases to be backed up through creation of a "shadow copy" of the entire disk at the beginning of the backup. The shadow copy is then used for the backup, so that the production disk is not affected.

> **NOTE**
>
> The Windows Server 2003 backup utility can be used to back up Exchange using the traditional online backup approach. Volume Shadow Copy requires a third-party solution that has been written to support the new Windows Server 2003 backup and restore APIs.

Exchange Server 2003 also includes support for the concept of a recovery storage group, which is an additional storage group (available with either Standard or Enterprise Exchange) and which can be used on a running server to restore databases and mailboxes "on the fly." This streamlines the mailbox recovery process, because restore servers are no longer a necessity. For more information on backup and recovery options, see Chapter 31, "Backing Up the Exchange Server 2003 Environment."

Exchange Antivirus and Antispam Design

Viruses are a major problem for all organizations today. Email is especially vulnerable, because it is typically unauthenticated and insecure. Consequently, design of an Exchange implementation should include consideration for antivirus options.

Exchange Server 2003 improves upon the Virus Scanning Application Programming Interface (VSAPI) that was introduced in Exchange 2000. The enhanced VSAPI 2.5 engine enables quarantine of email messages, as opposed to simply attachments, and enables virus scanning on gateway servers. Third-party virus products can be written to tie directly into the new VSAPI and use its functionality.

Spam, unsolicited email, has become another major headache for most organizations. In response to this, Exchange Server 2003 has some built-in antispam functionality that enables email messages to contain a spam rating. This helps determine which emails are legitimate, and can be used by third-party antispam products as well.

Exchange Monitoring Solution

Email services are required in many organizations. The expectations of uptime and reliability are increasing, and end-users are beginning to expect email to be as available as phone service. Subsequently, the ability to monitor Exchange events, alerts, and performance data is optimal.

Exchange Server 2003 is a complex organism with multiple components, each busy processing tasks, writing to event logs, and running optimization routines. There are several methods of monitoring Exchange, the most optimal being Microsoft Operations Manager (MOM). MOM is essentially a monitoring, alerting, and reporting product that gathers event information and performance data, and generates reports about Microsoft servers. An Exchange-specific management pack for MOM contains hundreds of pre-packaged counters and events for Exchange Server 2003. Use of the management pack is ideal in midsize and larger environments to proactively monitor Exchange.

Although close monitoring of multiple Exchange servers is best supported through the use of MOM, this may not be the most ideal approach for smaller organizations because MOM is geared toward medium and large organizations. Exchange monitoring for small organizations can be accomplished through old-fashioned approaches, such as manual reviews of event log information, performance counters using perfmon, and simple SNMP utilities to monitor uptime, which is the approach taken by Company123.

Small Organization Exchange Infrastructure Design Decisions

In small organizations such as CompanyABC, it is typical for a single group (or single individual) to administer the entire organization, so a single administrative group should suffice. In addition, there may be only one site (or a small number of sites) and Exchange Server 2003 can be configured with a single routing group for each site. Because of its size, Company123 used a single routing group and a single administration group, as illustrated in Figure 5.11.

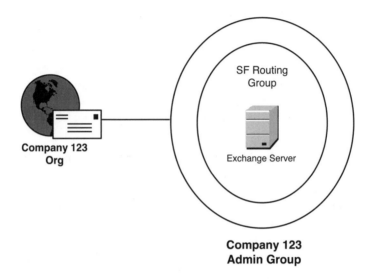

FIGURE 5.11   Routing group and admin group design for a small organization.

The Exchange infrastructure was deployed at Company123 with Exchange Standard Edition on its single server. The Exchange organization was named Company123 for simplicity.

Because Company123 was using the Standard version of Exchange Server 2003, it did not require additional thought into database or storage group design. Following this logic, it deployed a single private information store, a single public information store, and a single storage group.

Midsize Organization Exchange Infrastructure Design Decisions

Administration within OrganizationY is centralized, and required the creation of a single admin group for the Exchange Organization. The Exchange organization was named OrganizationY and the routing group structure was divided into separate routing groups for Manchester and Los Angeles, as illustrated in Figure 5.12.

Each Exchange Server in the organization used the Enterprise version of Exchange, because support for large and multiple databases was required. A third-party backup and antivirus solution were chosen to protect the mail data. The Exchange servers were each configured with three private store databases for mailboxes, and one public folder store, as illustrated in Figure 5.12. Users were distributed across the databases by practice group—with management in one database and marketing in another, for example. This helped OrganizationY shorten recovery time for certain groups while also enabling separate mailbox limits and database options.

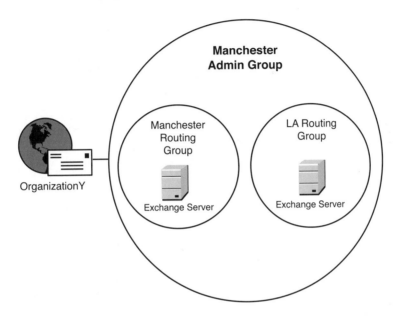

FIGURE 5.12 Routing group and admin group design for a mid-size organization.

Microsoft Operations Manager was deployed in the Manchester location to monitor all AD and Exchange servers and provide for proactive systems management.

Large Organization Exchange Infrastructure Design Decisions

CompanyABC was divided into two separate IT Teams. One IT team managed the parent company, which included the Minneapolis, San Francisco, Moscow, and Tokyo offices. The second IT team managed the company that had been acquired, which included the Dallas, New York, Paris, and Singapore offices. Consequently, two administrative groups were created and a total of eight routing groups were created, as illustrated in Figure 5.13. The Exchange organization was named CompanyABC.

All servers across the entire organization were installed with the Enterprise version of Exchange to enable large databases, as illustrated in Figure 5.13. The user base was distributed across the databases alphabetically to ease the administration of the mailboxes. Each site contained a local copy of the public folder tree to ensure quick response time. Finally, third-party antispam, antivirus, and backup solutions were put in place to protect Exchange.

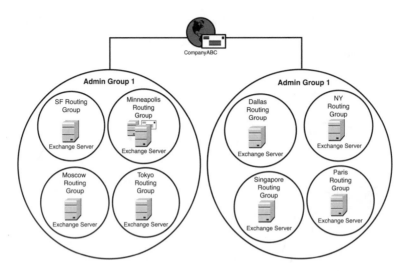

FIGURE 5.13   Routing group and admin group design for a large organization.

Microsoft Operations Manager was deployed with the Exchange Server 2003 Management Pack and configured to monitor all components of Active Directory and Exchange Server 2003.

Integrating Client Access into Exchange Server 2003 Design

Although the Exchange Server is a powerful systems component, it is only half the equation for an email platform. The client systems compose the other half, and are a necessary ingredient that should be carefully determined in advance.

Client Access Methods

Great effort has been put into optimizing and streamlining the client access approaches available in Exchange Server 2003. Not only have traditional approaches such as the Outlook client been enhanced, but support for nontraditional access with POP3 and IMAP clients is also available. The following options exist for client access with Exchange Server 2003:

- **Outlook 2003**   The full Outlook 2003 client has been streamlined and enhanced. MAPI communications with Exchange 2003 systems have been compressed, and the addition of slow-link detection enables speedy mail retrieval for remote users.

- **Outlook Web Access (OWA)**   The Outlook Web Access (OWA) client is now nearly indistinguishable from the full Outlook 2003 client. The one major component missing is offline capability, but nearly every other Outlook 2003 functionality is part of OWA.

- **Outlook Mobile Access (OMA)**   Outlook Mobile Access (OMA) is a version of Outlook Web Access, which has been optimized for use on handheld devices, such as cellular phones, PDAs, and other small-screen units.

TIP

OMA functionality can be tested from an Internet Explorer 6.0 client by accessing the following:

```
http://servername/oma
```

where *servername* is the name of the Exchange Server where OMA is running. This is a useful trick if a real OMA client is not available for testing purposes.

- **Post Office Protocol (POP3)**   The Post Office Protocol (POP3) is a legacy protocol that is supported in Exchange 2003. POP3 enables simple retrieval of mail data via applications that use the POP3 protocol. Mail messages, however, cannot be sent with POP3 and must use the SMTP engine in Exchange. By default, POP3 is not turned on and must be explicitly activated.

- **Interactive Mail Access Protocol (IMAP)**   Legacy Interactive Mail Access Protocol (IMAP) access to Exchange is also available, which can enable an Exchange Server to be accessed via IMAP applications, such as some Unix mail clients. As with the POP3 protocol, IMAP support must be explicitly turned on.

NOTE

Exchange Server 2003 supports the option of disallowing MAPI access or allowing only specific Outlook clients MAPI access. This can be configured if an organization desires only OWA access to an Exchange server. It can also, for security reasons, stipulate that only Outlook 2003 can access the Exchange server. The registry key required for this functionality is the following:

```
Location:HKLM\System\CurrentControlSet\Services\MSExchangeIS\ParametersSystem
Value Name: Disable MAPI Clients
Data Type: REG_SZ
String: Version # (i.e. v4, v5, etc)
```

See Microsoft Technet Article 288894 for more information:

```
(http://support.microsoft.com/default.aspx?scid=KB;EN-US;288894)
```

Each organization will have individual needs that determine which client or set of clients will be supported. In general, the full Outlook 2003 client offers the richest messaging experience with Exchange Server 2003, but many of the other access mechanisms, such as Outlook Web Access, are also valid. The important design consideration is identifying what will be supported, and then enabling support for that client or protocol. Any methods that will not be supported should be disabled or left turned off for security reasons.

Front-End Server Design

As noted, Exchange Server 2003 enables an Exchange Server to act as a proxy agent for mail, which is also known as a front-end server. Front-end servers relay client requests back to the back-end mailbox store, and they serve two main purposes. First, front-end Exchange systems serve to protect the mailbox store from direct attacks from the Internet. Second, front-end servers offload processor-intensive activities, such as decryption of SSL client traffic.

By default, all Exchange Server 2003 systems have front-end capabilities built in, which effectively means that organizations can use a single Exchange server without the need to deploy a dedicated front-end system, if not required. In most cases for small businesses, this would be the preferred option to spending more on a second Exchange server. Larger and midsize organizations may want to deploy front-end technology as part of a design to increase security and scalability.

> **NOTE**
>
> Once it has been enabled via Mobile Services in Exchange System Manager, OMA can be tested to verify its functionality. Microsoft removed the requirement that front-end servers use the Enterprise version of the Exchange license; however, current Exchange 2000 front-end servers do not have a direct mechanism to downgrade to the Standard version of Exchange 2003 and save the Enterprise license for another system. To accomplish this, the server has to be rebuilt from scratch.

Small Organization Client Access Design Decisions

Company123 deployed the full Outlook 2003 client for all of its users, to take advantage of the full-featured set offered by the application. The users in the London office use Outlook in the auto-detected slow-link header mode, which enables them to more efficiently use their slower access.

Since it was a small organization and did not require the security and scalability of a dedicated front-end server, Company123 opted to use a single Exchange server with front-end support.

Midsize Organization Client Access Design Decisions

OrganizationY used a mixed approach to client access. The majority of users in the main Manchester and Los Angeles sites were given full Outlook 2003 clients for access to the Exchange servers. Users in St. Petersburg, however, accessed mail through Outlook Web Access for most individuals, and the full Outlook 2003 client for traveling users who required offline access. Users in smaller sites across the organization used a combination of the two technologies, with some individuals using Outlook Mobile Access from cell phones and other handheld devices, as illustrated in Figure 5.14.

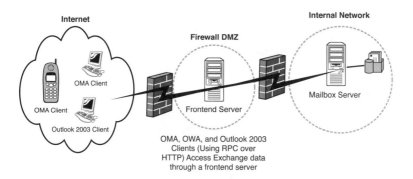

FIGURE 5.14 Outlook Mobile Access from handheld devices.

A dedicated front-end server was set up in the DMZ of the firewall in Manchester to enable Internet access to corporate email. This enabled remote users to access their corporate email from any location on the Internet by using RPC over HTTP capabilities in the Outlook 2003 client. The traffic was encrypted through SSL to protect the data. This design model gave great flexibility and accessibility to users across the organization.

Large Organization Client Access Design Decisions

CompanyABC was configured to enable access to email from several different client access mechanisms. The preferred client was established as Outlook 2003, but MAPI access from downlevel Outlook clients (XP/2000/98) was also provided. POP3 and IMAP access were also given to specific offices that had special needs. In addition, access to Outlook Web Access was provided for all mailboxes through a series of load-balanced front-end servers, as illustrated in Figure 5.15.

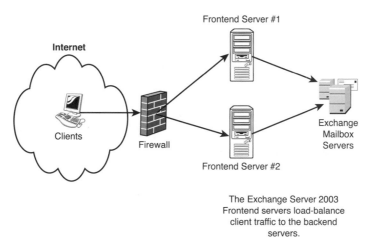

FIGURE 5.15 Load balancing Outlook Web Access.

The slow-link caching and improved OWA client greatly increased CompanyABC's capabilities to consolidate email services to its largest sites and subsequently helped decrease the total cost of ownership for the entire organization.

Summarizing Design Examples

Every organization is unique, but there are certain similarities that organizations of varying sizes possess. In general, the following company examples can be used as a starting point to match its needs to the needs of any similar organization. The following sections summarize the design decisions presented by the sample organizations in this chapter.

Summarizing the Sample Small Organization Design Model

As illustrated throughout this chapter, Company123 followed a best practice model from small organizations for its Exchange Server 2003 design strategy. Each organization is unique, and there might be other factors that would change some of these design decisions, but they are presented to give a better understanding of how the needs of a sample small organization fit into Exchange Server 2003 design.

In summary, the following key design elements were implemented as part of Company123's small organization Exchange Server 2003 design:

- **Forest and Domain Design**   Single forest/Single domain—company123.org

- **AD Site and Replication Topology Placement**   Single site

- **AD Domain Controller and Global Catalog Placement**   Single domain controller/Global Catalog server

- **DNS Layout**   AD-integrated company123.org zone

- **Server Number and Placement**   Single Exchange Server 2003 system, on same hardware as AD domain controller

- **Server Redundancy and Optimization**   RAID1 drive set for OS and Logs; RAID5 drive set for database and SMTP folder

- **Server Memory and Processor**   1GB RAM, single processor

- **Server Operating System**   Windows Server 2003 Standard Edition

- **Exchange Version and Org Name**   Exchange Server 2003 Standard Edition/org name: Company123

- **Administrative Group and Routing Group Structure**   Single admin group/single routing group

- **Public Folder Structure and Replication**   Single public folder store

- **Exchange Database and Storage Group Structure**   Single private folder store/single public folder store

- **Exchange Monitoring Solution**   Manual monitoring via event log parsing and using perfmon counters

- **Client Access Methods**   Outlook 2003 client for all users; Outlook 2003 in slow-link header mode for remote users

- **Front-end Server Design**   Single Exchange Server with front-end capabilities

Summarizing the Sample Midsize Organization Design Model

OrganizationY is fairly typical of the run-of-the-mill, midsize organization in today's environment. The following design decisions can be useful in designing Exchange Server 2003 for these types of organizations:

- **Forest and Domain Design**   Used existing placeholder root domain AD structure with placeholder domain (`placeholder.internal`) and user resource domain (`ydomain.internal`)

- **AD Site and Replication Topology Placement**   Separate AD sites for three main locations

- **AD Domain Controller and Global Catalog Placement**   Full Global Catalogs in two largest sites; universal group caching enabled in third site

- **DNS Layout**   AD-integrated zones for local DNS trees; stub zone for separate tree in the forest

- **Server Number and Placement**   Exchange Servers in Manchester and Los Angeles; all other sites to access Exchange using auto-detected slow-link capabilities of Outlook 2003 or OWA

- **Server Redundancy and Optimization**   Redundant fans and power supplies; RAID sets for OS, logs, and database

- **Server Memory and Processor**   4GB RAM, quad processors

- **Server Operating System**   Windows Server 2003 Standard Edition

- **Exchange Version and Org Name**   Exchange Server 2003 Enterprise Edition

- **Administrative Group and Routing Group Structure**   Single admin group; two routing groups (Manchester, Los Angeles)

- **Public Folder Structure and Replication**   Two public folder instances, one for each routing group

- **Exchange Database and Storage Group Structure**   Three private store databases for each Exchange Server, divided by practice group; single production storage group

- **Exchange Monitoring Solution**   MOM deployed

- **Client Access Methods**   Outlook 2003 client for most users, OWA for Internet users

- **Front-end Server Design**   Single front-end server deployed for RPC over HTTP access to Exchange from the Internet

Summarizing the Sample Large Organization Design Model

The complexities of larger organizations were not lost on the Exchange design team. Exchange Server 2003 was built upon the lessons learned by large organizations with Exchange 2000 and is consequently a better product. The sample large organization shown in this chapter is not unique, and some of the following design strategies can be used for similar designs:

- **Forest and Domain Design**   Separate, dedicated AD forest (`exchange.internal`) for Exchange with cross-forest transitive trusts to the two existing AD production forests

- **AD Site and Replication Topology Placement**   AD sites for each large location

- **AD Domain Controller and Global Catalog Placement**   Full Global Catalog servers in each AD site

- **DNS Layout**   Single AD-integrated DNS zone (`exchange.internal`)

- **Server Number and Placement**   Exchange Mailbox Servers in each major location; 4-node Exchange cluster with one passive node in Minneapolis

- **Server Redundancy and Optimization**   Redundant fans and power supplies; RAID drive sets; cluster in Minneapolis

- **Server Memory and Processor**   4GB RAM, quad processors

- **Server Operating System**   Windows Server 2003 Standard for non–cluster systems; Windows Server 2003 Enterprise for cluster nodes

- **Exchange Version and Org Name**   Exchange Server 2003 Enterprise Edition

- **Administrative Group and Routing Group Structure**   Two admin groups, 8 routing groups

- **Public Folder Structure and Replication**   Public folder instance in each routing group

- **Exchange Database and Storage Group Structure** Three private stores on each mailbox server, divided alphabetically; single storage group for each server

- **Exchange Monitoring Solution** Microsoft Operations Manager deployed for all AD and Exchange System monitoring needs

- **Client Access Methods** Preferred client Outlook 2003; support for older MAPI clients, OWA, OMA, IMAP, and POP3

- **Front-end Server Design** Dual load-balanced front-end servers to provide for remote RPC over HTTP Internet access to Exchange data

Summary

Exchange Server 2003 offers a broad range of functionality and improvements to messaging and is well-suited for organizations of any size. With proper thought into the major design topics, a robust and reliable Exchange email solution can be put into place that will perfectly complement the needs of organizations of any size.

In short, Exchange easily scales up to support thousands of users on multiple servers, and it also scales down very well. Single Exchange server implementations can easily support hundreds of users, even those that are scattered in various locations. This flexibility helps establish Exchange as the premier messaging solution for organizations of any size.

Best Practices

- Try to create an Active Directory design that is as simple as possible. Expand the directory tree with multiple subdomains and forests at a later date if needed.

- Even if the organization has high bandwidth between sites, create a site to better control replication and traffic between sites.

- When possible, DNS in an organization should be Microsoft DNS; however, Windows 2003 (and Windows 2000) also can be integrated with non-Microsoft DNS.

- Minimize the number of servers needed by consolidating services into as few systems as possible.

- Use the /3GB /USERVA=3030 switch in boot1.ini to optimize system memory in an Exchange Server with more than 1GB of RAM.

- If the organization does not have a third-party antispam software program, enable the Microsoft Exchange 2003 antispam functionality to minimize unwanted mail.

CHAPTER 6

Integrating Exchange Server 2003 in a Non-Windows Environment

$\mathbf{B}$y using Active Directory for its own directory system, Exchange Server 2003 reduces the amount of administration required in an Exchange environment by eliminating a redundant directory. But beyond the boundaries of Active Directory, organizations have needed the capabilities of further extending their directories, ideally reducing the maintenance required to a single administrative point. When a new employee starts, for example, a single entry would then ideally create a mailbox, enter the new employee into an HR database, create a Unix account, create a Novell Directory Services (NDS) account, and the like.

These types of capabilities and integration in non-Windows environments have become more streamlined and capable with the release of several new tools that possess these types of metadirectory capabilities. The use of these tools in an Exchange Server 2003 environment can greatly reduce the administrative overhead associated with having multiple directories, and subsequently make it less costly to operate.

This chapter focuses on the integration of Exchange Server 2003's directory system, Active Directory, with non-Windows environments, such as Unix, Novell, and Lightweight Directory Access Protocol (LDAP) directories. Various tools that can be used to accomplish this are presented, and the pros and cons of each are analyzed.

Synchronizing Directory Information with Microsoft Identity Integration Services (MIIS) 2003

In most enterprises today, each individual application or system has its own user database or directory to track who is permitted to use that resource. Identity and access control data reside in different directories as well as applications such as specialized network resource directories, mail servers, human resource, voice mail, payroll, and many other applications.

Each has its own definition of the user's "identity" (name, title, ID numbers, roles, membership in groups). Many have their own password and process for authenticating users. Each has its own tool for managing user accounts, and sometimes its own dedicated administrator responsible for this task. Further, most enterprises have multiple processes for requesting resources and for granting and changing access rights. Some of these are automated, but many are paper-based. Many differ from business unit to business unit, even when performing the same function.

Administration of these multiple repositories often leads to time-consuming and redundant efforts in administration and provisioning. It also causes frustration for users, requiring them to remember multiple IDs and passwords for different applications and systems. The larger the organization, the greater is the potential variety of these repositories and the effort required to keep them updated.

In the past, Microsoft has provided a number of tools and services to provide coexistence with other directories and to migrate users to Active Directory. For Novell NetWare and eDirectory environments, these tools include Services For NetWare (SFNW), Gateway Services For NetWare (GSNW), and the broader support provided by Microsoft Metadirectory Services 3.0. Microsoft's latest metadirectory solution to provide coexistence and migration support is Microsoft Identity Integration Server (MIIS) 2003.

Understanding MIIS 2003

MIIS is a system that manages and coordinates identity information from multiple data sources in an organization, enabling you to combine that information into a single logical view that represents all of the identity information for a given user or resource.

MIIS enables a company to synchronize identity information across a wide variety of heterogeneous directory and non-directory identity stores. This enables customers to automate the process of updating identity information across heterogeneous platforms while maintaining the integrity and ownership of that data across the enterprise.

Password management capabilities enable end-users or helpdesk staff to easily reset passwords across multiple systems from one easy-to-use Web interface. End-users and helpdesk staff no longer have to use multiple tools to change their passwords across multiple systems.

There are actually two versions of MIIS. The first version, known as the Identity Integration Feature Pack for Microsoft Windows Server is free to anyone licensed for Windows Server 2003 Enterprise Edition. It provides functionality to integrate identity information between multiple Active Directory forests or between Active Directory and Active Directory Application Mode (ADAM).

The second version requires a separate licensing scheme and also requires SQL Server 2000 Enterprise for the back-end database. This version is known as the Microsoft Identity Integration Server 2003—Enterprise Edition. It provides classic metadirectory functionality that enables administrators to synchronize and provision identity information across a wide variety of stores and systems.

Understanding MIIS 2003 Concepts

It is important to understand some key terms used with MIIS 2003 before comprehending how it can be used to integrate various directories. Keep in mind that the following terms are used to describe MIIS 2003 concepts but might also help give you a broader understanding of how metadirectories function in general:

- **Management Agent (MA)**   An MIIS 2003 management agent is a tool used to communicate with a specific type of directory. For example, an Active Directory management agent enables MIIS 2003 to import or export data and perform tasks within Active Directory.

- **Connected Directory (CD)**   A connected directory is a directory that MIIS 2003 communicates with using a configured MA. An example of a connected directory is a Microsoft Exchange 5.5 directory database.

- **Connector Namespace (CS)**   The connector namespace is the replicated information and container hierarchy extracted from or destined to the respective connected directory.

- **Metaverse Namespace (MV)**   The metaverse namespace is the authoritative directory data created from the information gathered from each of the respective connector namespaces.

- **Metadirectory**   Within MIIS 2003, the metadirectory is made up of all the connector namespaces plus the authoritative metaverse namespace.

- **Attributes**   Attributes are the fields of information that are exported from or imported to directory entries. Common directory entry attributes are name, alias, email address, phone number, employee ID, or other information.

MIIS 2003 can be used for many tasks but is most commonly used for managing directory entry identity information. The intention here is to manage user accounts by synchronizing attributes, such as login ID, first name, last name, telephone number, title, and department. For example, if a user named Jane Doe is promoted and her title is changed from manager to vice president, the title change could first be entered in the HR or Payroll databases; then through MIIS 2003 management agents, the change could be replicated to other directories within the organization. This ensures that when someone looks up the title attribute for Jane Doe, it is the same in all the directories synchronized with MIIS 2003. This is a common and basic use of MIIS 2003 referred to as **identity management**. Other common uses of MIIS 2003 include account provisioning and group management.

> **NOTE**
>
> MIIS 2003 is a versatile and powerful directory synchronization tool that can be used to simplify and automate some directory management tasks. Because of the nature of MIIS 2003, it can also be a very dangerous tool—management agents can have full access to the connected directories. Misconfiguration of MIIS 2003 management agents could result in data loss, so careful planning and extensive lab testing should be performed before MIIS 2003 is released to the production directories of any organization. In many cases, it might be prudent to contact Microsoft consulting services and certified Microsoft solution provider/partners to help an organization decide whether MIIS 2003 is right for its environment, or even to design and facilitate the implementation.

Exploring MIIS 2003 Account Provisioning

MIIS enables administrators to easily provision and de-provision users' accounts and identity information, such as distribution, email and security groups across systems, and platforms. Administrators will be able to quickly create new accounts for employees based on events or changes in authoritative stores such as the human resources system. Additionally, as employees leave a company they can be immediately de-provisioned from those same systems.

Account provisioning in MIIS 2003 enables advanced configurations of directory management agents, along with special provisioning agents, to be used to automate account creation and deletion in several directories. For example, if a new user account is created in Active Directory, the Active Directory MA could tag this account. Then, when the respective MAs are run for other connected directories, a new user account could be automatically generated.

One enhancement of MIIS 2003 over MMS is that password synchronization is now supported for specific directories that manage passwords within the directory. MIIS 2003 provides an application programming interface (API) accessed through the Windows Management Interface (WMI). For connected directories that manage passwords in the directory's store, password management is activated when you configure the management agent in Management Agent Designer. In addition to enabling password management for each management agent, Management Agent Designer returns a system name attribute using the WMI interface for each connector space object.

Outlining the Role of Management Agents (MAs) in MIIS 2003

A management agent links a specific connected data source to the metadirectory. The management agent is responsible for moving data from the connected data source and the metadirectory. When data in the metadirectory is modified, the management agent can also export the data to the connected data source to keep the connected data source synchronized with the metadirectory. Generally, there is at least one management agent for each connected directory. MIIS 2003, Enterprise Edition, includes management agents for the following identity repositories:

- Active Directory

- Active Directory Application Mode (ADAM)

- Attribute-value pair text files

- Comma-separated value files

- Delimited text files

- Directory Services Markup Language (DSML) 2.0

- Exchange 5.5

- Exchange 2000 and Exchange Server 2003 Global Address List (GAL) synchronization

- Fixed-width text files

- LDAP Directory Interchange Format (LDIF)

- Lotus Notes/Domino 4.6/5.0

- Novell NDS, eDirectory, DirXML

- Sun/iPlanet/Netscape directory 4.x/5.x (with "changelog" support)

- Microsoft SQL Server 2000, SQL Server 7.0

- Microsoft Windows NT4 Domains

- Oracle 8i/9i

- Informix, dBase, ODBC and OLE DB support via SQL Server Data Transformation Services

Management agents contain rules that govern how an object's attributes are mapped, how connected directory objects are found in the metaverse, and when connected directory objects should be created or deleted.

These agents are used to configure how MIIS 2003 will communicate and interact with the connected directories when the agent is run. When a management agent is first created, all the configuration of that agent can be performed during that instance. The elements that can be configured include which type of directory objects will be replicated to the connector namespace, which attributes will be replicated, directory entry join and projection rules, attribute flow rules between the connector namespace and the metaverse namespace, plus more. If a necessary configuration is unknown during the MA creation, it can be revisited and modified later.

> **NOTE**
>
> For directories that do not manage passwords in the directory's store, password synchronization can sometimes be handled by a third party password synchronization product, such as Psynch (www.psynch.com).

Defining MIIS 2003 and Group Management

Just as MIIS 2003 can perform identity management for user accounts, it also can perform management tasks for groups. When a group is projected into the metaverse namespace, the group membership attribute can be replicated to other connected directories through their management agents. This enables a group membership change to occur in one directory and be replicated to other directories automatically.

Installing MIIS 2003 with SQL 2000

Both versions of MIIS 2003 require a licensed version of SQL Server 2000 with SP3 or greater to run, and an install of the product will prompt for the location of a SQL 2000 Server, as illustrated in Figure 6.1.

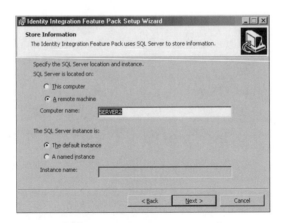

FIGURE 6.1   SQL install options with MIIS 2003.

Synchronizing Exchange Server 2003 with Novell eDirectory

Novell eDirectory and NDS environments are commonplace in business environments, and there is an increasing need to integrate them into deployed Exchange infrastructures. Several tools exist that can make this a reality, including the MIIS 2003 tools discussed. In addition, tools in the Microsoft-supplied Services for NetWare can be used to synchronize directory information between the two directory systems.

Understanding Novell eDirectory

Novell eDirectory is a distributed, hierarchical database of network information that is used to create a relationship between users and resources. It simplifies network management because network administrators can administer global networks from one location (or many) and manage all network resources as part of the eDirectory tree.

User administration is simplified because the users dynamically inherit access to network resources from their placement in the eDirectory tree. For example, eDirectory enables a user to dynamically inherit access to departmental resources, such as applications and printers, when that user is placed in the department's eDirectory container.

eDirectory information is typically stored on several servers, which are often at different locations. This enables information to be stored near the users who need it and provides efficient operation even if the users are geographically dispersed. Names are organized in a top-down hierarchy or tree structure. This helps users find resources in a structured manner. It also enables an administrator to administer a large network by delegating portions of the tree to local administrators.

The entries in an eDirectory database represent network resources available on the network and are referred to as objects. An object contains information that identifies, characterizes, and locates information pertaining to the resource it represents. eDirectory uses a single naming system that encompasses all servers, services, and users in an internetwork. In the past, names were administered separately on each server. Now, eDirectory enables information entered once to be accessible everywhere and lets a user log in once to access diverse, geographically separated resources.

An eDirectory database can be divided into logical partitions according to business needs, network use, geographical location, access time, and other factors. These partitions can be distributed to any server represented in the directory. When an eDirectory database is distributed to multiple servers, eDirectory maintains the equality of the distributed logical partitions by distributing object information changes to the appropriate servers.

Deploying MIIS 2003 for Identity Management with eDirectory

MIIS 2003 can be an effective tool for managing identities between Novell eDirectory environments and Active Directory. Identity information could include names, email and physical addresses, titles, department affiliations, and much more. Generally speaking, identity information is the type of data commonly found in corporate phone books or intranets. To use MIIS 2003 for identity management between Active Directory and Novell eDirectory, follow these high-level steps:

1. Install MIIS 2003.

2. Create a management agent for each of the directories, including an Active Directory management agent and a Novell eDirectory management agent.

3. Configure the management agents to import directory object types into their respective connector namespaces.

4. Configure one of the management agents—for example, the Active Directory MA—to project the connector space directory objects and directory hierarchy into the metaverse namespace.

5. Within each of the management agents, a function can be configured called attribute flow, which defines which directory object attributes from each directory will be projected into the respective metaverse directory objects. Configure the attribute flow rules for each management agent.

6. Configure the account-joining properties for directory objects. This is the most crucial step because it determines how the objects in each directory are related to one another within the metaverse namespace. To configure the account join, certain criteria can be used, such as employee ID or first name and last name combination. The key is to find the most unique combination to avoid problems when two objects with similar names are located—for example, if two users named Tom Jones exist in Active Directory.

7. After completely configuring the MAs and account joins, configure management agent run profiles to tell the management agent what to perform with the connected directory and connector namespace. For example, perform a full import or export of data. The first time the MA is run, the connected directory information is imported to create the initial connector namespace.

8. After running the MAs once, you can run them a second time to propagate the authoritative metaverse data to the respective connector namespaces and out to the connected directories.

These steps outline the most common use of MIIS 2003; these steps can be used to simplify account maintenance tasks when several directories need to be managed simultaneously. When more sophisticated functionality using MIIS 2003 is needed, such as the automatic creation and deletion of directory entries, extensive scripting and customization of MIIS 2003 can be done to create a more complete enterprise account provisioning system.

Using Microsoft Directory Synchronization Service to Integrate Directories

Microsoft Directory Synchronization Services (MSDSS), part of the Services for NetWare Toolkit, is a tool used for synchronization of directory information stored in the Active Directory and NDS. MSDSS synchronizes directory information stored in Active Directory with all versions of NetWare; MSDSS supports a two-way synchronization with NDS and a one-way synchronization with Novell 3.x bindery services.

Because Active Directory does not support a container comparable to an NDS root organization and because Active Directory security differs from Novell, MSDSS, in migration mode only, creates a corresponding domain local security group in Active Directory for each NDS organizational unit (OU) and organization. MSDSS then maps each Novell OU or organization to the corresponding Active Directory domain local security group.

MSDSS provides a single point of administration; with a one-way synchronization, changes made to Active Directory will be propagated over to NDS during synchronization. Synchronization from Active Directory to NDS allows changes to object attributes, such as a user's middle name or address, to be propagated. In two-way synchronization mode, changes from NDS to Active Directory require a full synchronization of the object (all attributes of the user object).

One of the key benefits to MSDSS is password synchronization. Passwords can be administered in Active Directory and the changes propagated over to NDS during synchronization. Password synchronization allows users access to Windows Server 2003 and Novell NDS resources with the same logon credentials.

The MSDSS architecture is made up of the following three components. These components manage, map, read, and write changes that occur in Active Directory, NDS, and NetWare bindery services:

- The configuration of the synchronization parameters is handled by the session manager.

- An object mapper relates the objects to each other (class and attributes), namespace, rights, and permissions between the source and target directories.

- Changes to each directory are handled by a DirSync (read/write) provider. LDAP is used for Active Directory calls and NetWare NCP calls for NDS and NetWare binderies.

In addition to the core components of MSDSS, the session configuration settings (session database) are securely stored in Active Directory. Specific scenarios for MSDSS include the following:

- A company is migrating directly from Novell to a Windows Server 2003 network. All network services—such as DNS, DHCP, and IIS services—are running on a single server. MSDSS can be used to migrate all users and files over to Windows Server 2003 after all services have been migrated.

- A company is gradually migrating from Novell to a Windows Server 2003 network. The network services—such as DNS, DHCP, and IIS—are installed on multiple servers and sites. MSDSS can be used to migrate and synchronize AD and NDS directories during the migration.

Installation of the Microsoft Directory Synchronization Service

Separate from the installation of the File and Print Services for NetWare (FPNW) is the installation of the MSDSS. This tool is not installed with the rest of the File and Print Services for NetWare tools; an organization may install FPNW on one server, whereas MSDSS will likely be installed only on a single server. Effectively, MSDSS does the synchronization between Active Directory and Novell NDS and eDirectory. MSDSS needs to be installed on a Windows domain controller to properly synchronize directory information between the two different network environments.

To install MSDSS on a Windows 2003 domain controller, follow these steps:

1. On the domain controller computer on which the MSDSS will be installed, insert the CD into the CD-ROM drive.

2. Go into the MSDSS directory on the CD-ROM (such as d:\msdss) and run the msdss.msi script package. This launches the installation wizard.

3. Choose to install the Microsoft Directory Synchronization Service.

NOTE

Installing MSDSS initiates an extension of the schema of the Active Directory forest. As with any schema update, the Active Directory should be backed up (see Chapter 31, "Backing Up the Exchange Server 2003 Environment," for details on doing a full backup of the Active Directory). Also with a schema update, because the update will replicate directory changes to all global catalogs throughout the organization, the replication should be done at a time when a Global Catalog synchronization can take place without impact on the normal production environment.

Synchronizing eDirectory/NDS with Active Directory Using Services for NetWare

For organizations that have both a Windows Active Directory and a Novell eDirectory (or NDS) environment, there are two primary methods of performing directory synchronization between the two directories. One method is using the Novell DirXML product, and the other method is using the MSDSS utility. With regard to synchronization of user accounts and passwords, both tools do the same job, and for the purpose of this book, the Microsoft solution will be the focus of this section. To set up directory synchronization with MSDSS, do the following:

1. Launch the MSDSS utility by selecting Start, Programs, Administrative Tools, Directory Synchronization.

2. Right-click on the MSDSS tool option and select New Session.

3. Click Next at the New Session Welcome screen.

4. At the synchronization and migration tasks screen, choose either NDS or Bindery for the type of service.

NOTE

Use the NDS option if Novell NetWare 4.x or higher running NDS or eDirectory is used. Use the Bindery option if Novell NetWare 3.2 or lower bindery mode is running on the Novell network.

---

5. Dependent on the synchronization option, choose either a one way (from Active Directory to NDS/Bindery), a two-way (AD to NDS/Bindery and back), or a migration from NDS/Bindery to Active Directory. Click Next.

6. For the Active Directory container and domain controller, choose the AD container to which objects will be synchronized, as well as the name of the domain controller that'll be used to extract and synchronize information, similar to the settings shown in Figure 6.2. Click Next.

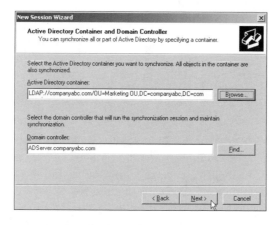

FIGURE 6.2   Setting server synchronization information settings.

7. For the NDS Container and Password, select the NDS container to and/or from which AD information will be synchronized. Enter a logon name and password for a supervisor account on Novell to access the Novell directory. Click Next.

8. On the initial reverse synchronization screen, select the password option to define passwords to be either blank, same as the username, set to a random value (that can be viewed in the log file), or set to an organizational default. Click OK after making the password option, and then click Next to continue.

9. Click Finish to begin the synchronization/migration process.

Implementing MSDSS

MSDSS runs on a Windows 2000 or Windows 2003 domain controller and replicates user account and password information between the Active Directory environment and a Novell eDirectory or NDS environment. MSDSS is a Windows service that synchronizes user account information between Active Directory and NetWare. The following are best practices determined in the implementation of MSDSS in an enterprise environment:

- Ensure that the Microsoft MSDSS server that is running on a Windows Active Directory domain controller and then Novell directory server are on the same network segment or have limited hops between each other.

- Because directory synchronization reads and writes information directly to the network directory, test the replication process between mirrored domain and directory services in a test lab environment before implementing MSDSS for the first time in a production environment.

- Monitor directory and password synchronization processing times to confirm the transactions are occurring fast enough for users to access network resources. If users get an authentication error, consider upgrading the MSDSS server to a faster system

- Password characteristic policies (requiring upper- and lowercase letters, numbers, or extended characters in the password, and password change times) should be similar on both the Microsoft and Novell environments to minimize inconsistencies in authorization and update processes.

Identifying Limitations on Directory Synchronization with MSDSS

Although directory synchronization can provide common logon names and passwords, MSDSS does not provide dual client support or any application-level linkage between multiple platform configurations. This means that if a Novell server is running IPX as a communication protocol and Windows is running TCP/IP, MSDSS does not do protocol conversion. Likewise, if an application is running on a Novell server requiring the Service Advertising Protocol (SAP), because Windows servers commonly use NetBIOS for device advertising, a dual client protocol stack must be enabled to provide common communications.

MSDSS merely links the logon names and passwords between multiple environments. The following are areas that need to be considered separate from the logon and password synchronization process:

- Protocols, such as TCP/IP and IPX/SPX, should be supported by servers and clients.

- Applications that require communication standards for logon authentication may require a client component to be installed on the workstations or servers in the mixed environment.

- Applications that were written for Novell servers (such as Network Loadable Modules [NLMs] or BTrieve databases) should be converted to support Windows.

- Login scripts, drive mappings, or other access systems compatible with one networking environment may not work across multiple environments, so those components should be tested for full compatibility.

- Backup utilities, antivirus applications, network management components, or system monitoring tools that work on one system should be purchased or relicensed to support another network operating configuration.

Backing Up and Restoring MSDSS Information

MSDSS configuration, tables, and system configurations are critical to the operations of the MSDSS synchronization tool. Microsoft provides a backup and restore utility that enables the storage and recovery of MSDSS information. To back up MSDSS, do the following:

1. Select Start, Programs, Administrative Tools, MSDSS Backup & Restore Utility. A screen similar to the one shown in Figure 6.3 should appear.

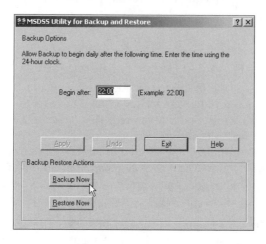

FIGURE 6.3   Backing up MSDSS information.

2. Either click on Backup Now to back up the MSDSS session directory, or change the default time when the MSDSS information should be backed up.

3. If it is required to back up the session directory information, the process will notify that the MSDSS service will need to be stopped. Choose Yes to continue.

4. Upon completion of the backup, there will be a prompt that the MSDSS service will need to be restarted. Choose Yes to restart the MSDSS service.

At any time, if the MSDSS session directory information gets corrupt or behaves erratically, the MSDSS information can be restored. To restore MSDSS, do the following:

1. Select Start, Programs, Administrative Tools, MSDSS Backup & Restore Utility.

2. Click on Restore Now to restore the MSDSS session directory.

3. When notified that the MSDSS service will need to be stopped, choose Yes to continue.

4. Upon completion of the restore, a final prompt will appear to signify that the MSDSS service will need to be restarted. Choose Yes to restart the MSDSS service.

Managing Identity Information Between LDAP Directories and Exchange Server 2003

LDAP Directories are commonplace today and can be found in many business environments. Unix applications in particular make wide use of the LDAP standard for directories. Along with this proliferation of LDAP directory structures comes a need to synchronize the information contained within them to an Exchange Server 2003 environment. The Enterprise version of MIIS 2003 contains MAs that support synchronization to LDAP directories. Consequently, a good understanding of LDAP concepts is required before synching between the environments.

Understanding LDAP from a Historical Perspective

To understand LDAP better, it is useful to consider the X.500 and Directory Access Protocol (DAP) from which it is derived. In X.500, the Directory System Agent (DSA) is the database in which directory information is stored. This database is hierarchical in form, designed to provide fast and efficient search and retrieval. The Directory User Agent (DUA) provides functionality that can be implemented in all sorts of user interfaces through dedicated DUA clients, Web server gateways, or email applications. The DAP is a protocol used in X.500 directory services for controlling communications between the DUA and DSA agents. The agents represent the user or program and the directory, respectively.

The X.500 directory services are application-layer processes. Directory services can be used to provide global, unified naming services for all elements in a network, translate between network names and addresses, provide descriptions of objects in a directory, and provide unique names for all objects in the Directory. These X.500 objects are hierarchical with different levels for each category of information, such as country, state, city, and organization. These objects may be files (as in a file system directory listing), network entities (as in a network naming service such as NDS), or other types of entities.

Lightweight protocols combine routing and transport services in a more streamlined fashion than do traditional network and transport-layer protocols. This makes it possible to transmit more efficiently over high-speed networks—such as ATM or FDDI—and media—such as fiber-optic cable.

Lightweight protocols also use various measures and refinements to streamline and speed up transmissions, such as using a fixed header and trailer size to save the overhead of transmitting a destination address with each packet.

LDAP is a subset of the X.500 protocol. LDAP clients are, therefore, smaller, faster, and easier to implement than X.500 clients. LDAP is vendor-independent and works with, but does not require, X.500. Contrary to X.500, LDAP supports TCP/IP, which is necessary for any type of Internet access. LDAP is an open protocol, and applications are independent of the server platform hosting the directory.

Active Directory is not a pure X.500 directory. Instead, it uses LDAP as the access protocol and supports the X.500 information model without requiring systems to host the entire X.500 overhead. The result is the high level of interoperability required for administering real-world, heterogeneous networks.

Active Directory supports access via the LDAP protocol from any LDAP-enabled client. LDAP names are less intuitive than Internet names, but the complexity of LDAP naming is usually hidden within an application. LDAP names use the X.500 naming convention called Attributed Naming.

An LDAP URL names the server holding Active Directory services and the Attributed Name of the object—for example:

```
LDAP:// Server1.fastportfolio.com/CN=LSomi, ,OU=Users,O=fastportfolio,C=US
```

By combining the best of the DNS and X.500 naming standards, LDAP, other key protocols, and a rich set of APIs, the Active Directory enables a single point of administration for all resources, including files, peripheral devices, host connections, databases, Web access, users, arbitrary other objects, services, and network resources.

Understanding How LDAP Works

LDAP directory service is based on a client-server model. One or more LDAP servers contain the data making up the LDAP directory tree. An LDAP client connects to an LDAP server and asks it a question. The server responds with the answer or with a pointer to where the client can get more information (typically, another LDAP server). No matter which LDAP server a client connects to, it sees the same view of the directory; a name presented to one LDAP server references the same entry it would at another LDAP server. This is an important feature of a global directory service such as LDAP.

Outlining the Differences Between LDAP2 and LDAP3 Implementations

LDAP 3 defines a number of improvements that enable a more efficient implementation of the Internet directory user agent access model. These changes include

- Use of UTF-8 for all text string attributes to support extended character sets

- Operational attributes that the directory maintains for its own use—for example, to log the date and time when another attribute has been modified

- Referrals enabling a server to direct a client to another server that might have the data that the client requested

- Schema publishing with the directory, enabling a client to discover the object classes and attributes that a server supports

- Extended searching operations to enable paging and sorting of results, and client-defined searching and sorting controls

- Stronger security through an SASL-based authentication mechanism

- Extended operations, providing additional features without changing the protocol version

LDAP 3 is compatible with LDAP 2. An LDAP 2 client can connect to an LDAP 3 server (this is a requirement of an LDAP 3 server). However, an LDAP 3 server can choose not to talk to an LDAP 2 client if LDAP 3 features are critical to its application.

> **NOTE**
>
> LDAP was built on Internet-defined standards and is composed of the following RFCs:
>
> - **RFC 2251** Lightweight Directory Access Protocol (v3)
> - **RFC 2255** The LDAP URL Format
> - **RFC 2256** A Summary of the X.500(96) User Schema for use with LDAPv3
> - **RFC 2253** Lightweight Directory Access Protocol (v3): UTF-8 String Representation of Distinguished Names
> - **RFC 2254** The String Representation of LDAP Search Filters

Using Services for Unix to Integrate Unix Environments with Exchange Server 2003

In addition to the MIIS 2003 directory synchronization tools available for synching to Unix-based directory systems, a series of tools is available from Microsoft to supply this functionality as well. The tools are known as Services for Unix (SFU), as illustrated in

Figure 6.4, and include advanced functionality that can be used to integrate Unix systems into an Exchange Server 2003 environment.

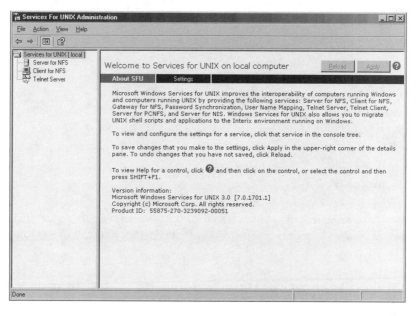

FIGURE 6.4   Services for Unix.

Services for Unix Defined

For many years, Unix and Windows systems were viewed as separate, incompatible environments that were physically, technically, and ideologically different. Over the years, however, organizations found that supporting two completely separate topologies within their environments was inefficient and expensive; much redundant work was also required to maintain multiple sets of user accounts, passwords, environments, and so on.

Slowly, the means to interoperate between these environments was developed. At first, most of the interoperability tools were written to join Unix with Windows, as evident with Samba, a method for Linux/Unix platforms to be able to access Windows NT file shares. Other interoperability tools were developed as well, but Microsoft was accused of pretending that Unix did not exist, and subsequently its Unix interoperability tools were not well developed.

The development of SFU for Windows Server 2003 signaled a change to this strategy. Microsoft developers spent a great deal of time developing tools for Unix that not only focused on migration, but also on interoperability. Long-awaited functionality—such as password synchronization, Unix scripts on Windows, joint security credentials, and the like—were presented as viable options and can be considered as part of a migration to, or interoperability scenario with, Windows Server 2003.

SFU is composed of several key components, each of which provides a specific integration task with different Unix environments. Any or all of these components can be used as part of SFU because the installation of the suite can be customized, depending on an organization's needs. The major components of SFU are as follows:

- Interix
- Gateway for NFS
- NFS Client
- NFS Server
- User Name Mapping
- Password Synchronization
- NIS Domains

Each component can be installed separately, or multiple components can be installed on a single server, as required. Each component is described in more detail in the following sections.

Understanding Services for Unix Prerequisites

SFU interoperates with various "flavors" of Unix but was tested and specifically written for use with the following Unix iterations:

- Sun Solaris 2.7
- Red Hat Linux 7.0
- Hewlett-Packard HP-UX 11
- IBM AIX 4.3.3

> **NOTE**
>
> SFU is not limited to Sun Solaris, Red Hat Linux, HP-UX, or IBM AIX. It actually performs quite well in various other similar Unix implementations, but has not been tested to the same degree as with the most common Unix versions.

SFU has some other important prerequisites and limitations that must be taken into account before considering it for use in an environment:

- The Server for NIS must be installed on an Active Directory domain controller.
- The NFS Client and Gateway for NFS components cannot be installed on the same server.

- Password synchronization requires installation on domain controllers in each environment.

- The Server for NIS Authentication component must be installed on all domain controllers in the domain in which security credentials will be used.

Outlining the Role of Interix As a Component of Services for Unix

There is one major change to the new version of SFU. Interix, a previously standalone product from SFU 2.0, has been integrated into the Services for Unix package. Interix is an extension to the Windows POSIX subsystem that enables the native execution of Unix scripts and applications in a Windows environment. Interix is not an emulation product, and all applications and scripts run natively in the built-in POSIX subsystem of Windows Server 2003.

Interix fills the gap between development on Unix platforms and development in Windows. It was written to enable programmers familiar with Unix to continue to use the most familiar programming tools and scripts, such as grep, tar, cut, awk, and many others. In addition, with limited reprogramming efforts, applications that run on Unix-based systems can be ported over to the Wintel platform, building on the low cost of ownership of Windows while retaining software investments from Unix.

Understanding Interix Scripting

The Korn and C Shells are both available in the Interix environment, and both behave exactly as they would in Unix. SFU also supports the single-rooted file system through these shells, which negates the need to convert scripts to support drive letters.

Outlining Interix Tools and Programming Languages

Interix supports all common Unix tools and utilities, with all the familiar commands such as grep, man, pr, nice, ps, kill, and many others. Each tool was built to respond exactly the way it is expected to behave, and Interix users can build or import their own customizable tools using the same procedures that they would in a Unix environment.

SFU streamlines the sharing of information between Unix and Windows Server 2003, allowing users from both environments to seamlessly access data from each separate environment, without the need for specialized client software. Using the Gateway for NFS, Server for NFS, and NFS Client enables this level of functionality and provides a more integrated environment.

Synchronizing Users with SFU

The goal of single sign-on, in which users on a network log in once and then have access to multiple resources and environments, is still a long way off. It is common for a regular user to maintain and use three or more separate usernames and associated sets of passwords. SFU goes a long way toward making Single Sign-on a reality, however, with the User Name Mapping and Password Synchronization capabilities.

Detailing User Name Mapping in SFU

User Name Mapping enables specific user accounts in Windows Server 2003 Active Directory to be associated with corresponding Unix user accounts. Because Exchange Server 2003 uses AD, it becomes easier to integrate Unix user accounts with their corresponding mailboxes in Exchange. In addition to mapping identically named user accounts, User Name Mapping enables the association of user accounts with different names in each organization. This factor is particularly useful considering the fact that Unix user accounts are case-sensitive, whereas Windows accounts are not. User Name Mapping, along with many components of Services for Unix, can be installed on a stand-alone server. In addition, User Name Mapping supports the ability to map multiple Windows user accounts to a single user account in Unix. This capability enables, for example, multiple administrators to map Windows Server 2003 Active Directory accounts with the Unix root administrator account.

Performing Password Synchronization with SFU

Going hand in hand with the User Name Mapping service, password synchronization enables those user accounts that have been mapped to automatically update their passwords between the two environments. This functionality allows users on either side to change their passwords and have the changes reflected on the mapped user accounts in the opposite platform.

As previously mentioned, password synchronization must be installed on all domain controllers on the Active Directory side because all the DCs must be able to understand the Unix password requests forwarded to them. In addition, password synchronization is supported "out of the box" in only the following Unix platforms:

- Solaris 7 and 8
- Red Hat Linux 6.2 and 7.0
- HP-UX 11

All other flavors of Unix require a recompile of the platform, which is made easier by the inclusion of make files and SFU source code.

Summary

Exchange Server 2003 running on Active Directory already goes far toward the goal of a single directory system for managing enterprise user accounts. The addition of advanced tools—such as MIIS 2003, Services for NetWare, and Services for Unix—further extends the capabilities of an organization to achieve this goal by providing for single metadirectory functionality. Proper use of these tools can significantly reduce the overhead associated with maintaining separate Exchange, Unix, NetWare, LDAP, and other directory implementations.

Best Practices

The following are best practices from this chapter:

- Use the Identity Integration Feature Pack version of MIIS 2003 for synchronizing information between various versions of Active Directory.

- Use the Enterprise version of MIIS 2003 for synchronization between non-AD directories, such as Novell eDirectory, LDAP, and Unix directories.

- Consider Services for NetWare when synching directories or integrating a Novell NetWare environment with Exchange Server 2003.

- Deploy Services for Unix to integrate Unix directories and functionality into an Exchange Server 2003 environment.

- Use Account Provisioning in MIIS 2003 to reduce the overhead associated with creating and deleting user accounts.

6

PART III

Networking Services' Impact on Microsoft Exchange

IN THIS PART

CHAPTER 7

Domain Name System Impact on Exchange Server 2003

Name resolution is a key component in any network operating system implementation. The capability of any one resource to locate other resources is the centerpiece of a functional network. Consequently, the name-resolution strategy chosen for a particular NOS must be robust and reliable and should conform to industry standards.

Name resolution plays a major part in any electronic mail environment. As mail travels from the sender to the recipient, servers that handle the mail need to be able to resolve the name of the destination. This concept is similar to the way that post offices handle mail that is routed from one destination to the next. Just as the post office relies on ZIP Codes to route the mail between regions, the electronic mail system uses DNS to resolve where the mail server responsible for handling mail for a particular destination is located.

This chapter gives an overview of the main components of the Domain Name System (DNS) and how it works. Particular focus is given to the interaction between DNS and Exchange Server 2003 environments. In addition, troubleshooting advice and best practices are outlined and defined.

Domain Name Service Defined

Network naming services were developed to overcome the obstacle of humans having to remember complex computerized addresses. The DNS is a distributed database indexed by domain names. Recall that each domain name exists as a path in a large inverted tree, the domain namespace. The structure of this tree is hierarchical.

All DNS implementations adhere to a specific set of criteria:

- Each node in the tree has a text label that can be up to 63 characters long.

- The root of the tree is labeled with a zero-length name.

- The full name of any node in the tree is the path from the node to the root, using the text labels separated by a dot. When the root node's label is printed, it appears as the name of the node, ending with a dot.

- An absolute domain name is also referred to as a **fully qualified domain name (FQDN)**.

- DNS specification requires that nodes under the same parent have different labels. This restriction guarantees that a single node is uniquely defined within the tree, regardless of its location in the structure.

How DNS Is Used

DNS is composed of two main components, clients and servers. The servers store information about specific components of the DNS structure and service requests, and the clients issue requests.

Each server contains a partial subset of the entire DNS namespace. These subsets are known as **zones**. DNS Servers can contain copies of either forward or reverse lookup zones. **Forward lookup zones** are used to resolve DNS names to IP addresses. For example, the forward lookup zone for microsoft.com resolves www.microsoft.com to its numerical IP address. **Reverse lookup zones** are responsible for resolving IP addresses to DNS names, or the reverse of the forward lookup zones.

The key to understanding how a DNS client resolves DNS queries is to understand the order in which name resolution occurs. The DNS client follows through these steps when resolving DNS names. If a match is found, the results are returned and no further steps are taken. If all steps have been exhausted, the client receives an error. Initially, the DNS client will attempt to resolve the request using local resources:

- The local cache, which is obtained from previous queries, is searched. The items in this cache remain until the Time-to-Live (TTL) period, which is set on each item, expires. Every time the DNS client is shut down, the cache is cleared.

- The local HOSTS file, which is stored in the %systemroot%\system32\drivers\etc directory is queried. The HOSTS file contains hostname-to-address mappings to enable manual hard-coding of DNS-to-IP addresses. These entries remain static and remain on the system even if it is rebooted.

When the client has exhausted all its locally available options, it sends a query to the DNS server for the record that it is seeking. The DNS server attempts to resolve the client's query the following way:

- If the query result is found in any of the zones for which the DNS server is authoritative, the server responds to the host with an authoritative answer.

- If the result is in the zone entries of the DNS server, the server checks its own local cache for the information.

If the local resources fail to provide an answer to the client's query it attempts to resolve the query by sending the request to other DNS servers in the form of a recursive query. This query is sent to either the server that is listed as a Forwarder, or to the set of servers set up in the DNS server's Root Hints file.

The DNS query is then sent around the Internet until it comes into contact with the DNS servers that are listed as being authoritative for the zone listed in the query. That DNS server then sends back the reply as either affirmative (with the IP address requested) or negative.

Who Needs DNS?

Not all situations require the use of the DNS. There are other name resolution mechanisms that exist beside DNS, some of which come standard with the operating system that companies deploy. Managing name servers in a domain sometimes is too much overhead. DNS makes life easier, but not all scenarios have the requirement of a complex name resolution structure.

In the past, an organization with a standalone, non-interconnected network could get away with using only host files or Microsoft's Windows Internet Naming Service (WINS) to provide NetBIOS-to-IP address name translation. Some very small environments could also use broadcast protocols such as NetBEUI to provide name resolution. In modern networks, however, DNS becomes a necessity, especially in mixed Windows/Unix environments.

In addition to local name translation, connecting to the Internet makes DNS connectivity a must. The World Wide Web, mail services, file transfer, and remote access services all use DNS services. Simply gaining access to the Internet does not, however, mean that every company or individual connecting to the Internet has to set up its own DNS server. Internet Service Providers (ISPs) can take care of managing DNS services on behalf of the user. A small organization might have a few hosts that access the Internet and might rely on its ISP to host those records. When a company wants to have more control over the domain and the name servers for that domain, it sets up its own DNS servers.

Types of DNS Servers

DNS is an integral and necessary part of any Windows Active Directory implementation. In addition, it has evolved to be the primary naming service for the Unix OS and the Internet. Because of Microsoft's decision to make Windows Server 2000 (and Windows Server 2003) Internet-compatible, DNS has replaced WINS as the default name resolution technology. Microsoft followed IETF standards and made its DNS server compatible with other DNS implementations.

Unix BIND DNS

Many organizations have significant investment in Unix DNS implementations. Microsoft Exchange heavily relies on Active Directory, and Active Directory heavily relies on DNS. Microsoft Active Directory can coexist and use third-party DNS implementations as long as they support active updates and SRV records. In some cases, organizations choose not to migrate away from the already implemented Unix DNS environment; instead, they coexist with Microsoft DNS. Companies using coexisting Unix and Microsoft DNS environments should consider the following:

- The Unix DNS installation should be at least 8.1.2.

- For incremental zone transfers, the Unix DNS implementation should be at least 8.2.1.

Third-Party (Checkpoint-Meta IP or Lucent Vital QIP) DNS

Third-party DNS implementations can provide significant enhancements in enterprise class IP management. They either provide integrated management of Unix, Linux, and Microsoft DNS and DHCP servers from a central location or can be used in place of the previously mentioned implementations. Latest versions fully support dynamic DNS updates, SRV records, and Incremental Zone Transfer, which should be considered a necessity if Active Directory uses the third-party DNS servers.

DNS Compatibility Between DNS platforms

DNS clients should, in theory, be able to query any DNS server regardless of who wrote that implementation. Active Directory, in particular, has some unique requirements from all DNS servers, however. Clients that authenticate to Active Directory look specifically for server resources, which means that the DNS server has to support SRV records. In Active Directory, DNS clients can dynamically update the DNS server with their IP address using Dynamic DNS. It is important to note that Dynamic DNS is not supported by all DNS implementations.

> **NOTE**
>
> In a mixed DNS environment, Microsoft specifically recommends using Microsoft DNS server as the primary DNS server and all others as secondary. Microsoft reasons that its implementation is the newest and more likely to be backward-compatible with older DNS implementations.

Examining DNS Components

As previously mentioned, name servers, or DNS servers, are systems that store information about the domain namespace. Name servers can have either the entire domain namespace or just a portion of the namespace. When a name server only has a part of the domain namespace, the portion of the namespace is called a zone.

DNS Zones

There is a subtle difference between zones and domains. All top-level domains, and many domains at the second and lower level, are broken into zones—smaller, more manageable units by delegation. A zone is the primary delegation mechanism in DNS over which a particular server can resolve requests. Any server that hosts a zone is said to be authoritative for that zone, with the exception of stub zones, defined later in the chapter.

A name server can have *authority* over more than one zone. Different portions of the DNS namespace can be divided into zones, each of which can be hosted on a DNS server or group of servers.

Forward Lookup Zones

A forward lookup zone is created to do forward lookups on the DNS database, resolving names to IP addresses and resource information. For example, if a user wants to reach the Exchange server named `mail.fastportfolio.com` and queries for its IP address through a forward lookup zone, DNS returns `66.70.211.11`, the IP address of the server.

Reverse Lookup Zones

A reverse lookup zone performs the opposite operation as the forward lookup zone. IP addresses are matched up with a common name in a reverse lookup zone. This is similar to knowing the phone number but not knowing the name associated with it. Reverse lookup zones must be manually created, and do not exist in every implementation. Reverse lookup zones are primarily populated with PTR records, which serve to point the reverse lookup query to the appropriate name.

TIP

It is good practice for the SMTP mail server to have a record in the reverse lookup zone. Spam control sites check for the existence of this record. It is possible to be placed on a spammer list if the site does not have a PTR record for the MX entry in the DNS reverse lookup zone.

Active Directory–Integrated Zones

A Windows 2003 DNS server can store zone information in two distinct formats: Active Directory–integrated, or standard text file. An Active Directory–integrated zone is an available option when the DNS server is installed on an Active Directory domain controller. When a DNS zone is installed as an Active Directory zone, the DNS information is automatically updated on other server AD domain controllers with DNS by using Active Directory's multimaster update techniques. Zone information stored in the Active Directory allows DNS zone transfers to be part of the Active Directory replication process secured by Kerberos authentication.

Primary Zones

In traditional (non–Active Directory–integrated) DNS, a single server serves as the master DNS server for a zone, and all changes made to that particular zone are done on that particular server. A single DNS server can host multiple zones, and can be primary for one and secondary for another. If a zone is primary, however, all requested changes for that particular zone must be done on the server that holds the master copy of the zone. As illustrated in Figure 7.1, `fastportfolio.com` is set up on `SERVER1` as the primary zone. On `SERVER2`, `development.fastportfolio.com` zone is located, and the server is the primary for that zone as well as for the `hq.fastportfolio.com` primary zone. `SERVER1` also holds a secondary zone copy of `development` and `hq` zone, for `fastportfolio.com`.

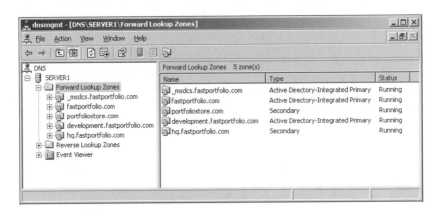

FIGURE 7.1   DNS primary and secondary zones.

Creating a new primary zone manually is a fairly straightforward process. The following procedure outlines the creation of a standard zone for the `fastportfolio.com` DNS namespace:

1. Open the DNS MMC snap-in (Start, Administrative Tools, DNS).

2. Navigate to DNS\<Servername>\Forward Lookup Zones.

3. Right-click Forward Lookup Zones and choose New Zone.

4. Click Next on the Welcome screen.

5. Select Primary Zone from the list of zone types available and click Next to continue.

6. Type the name of the primary zone to be created and click Next.

7. Because you're creating a new zone file, as opposed to importing an existing zone file, select Create a New File with This File Name and click Next.

8. Determine whether dynamic updates will be allowed in this zone. If not, select Do Not Allow Dynamic Updates and click Next to continue.

9. Click Finish on the Summary page to create the zone.

Secondary Zones

A secondary zone is established to provide redundancy and load balancing for the primary zone. Secondary zones are not necessary if the zone has been set up as the Active Directory, because the zone will be replicated to all domain controllers in the domain. With secondary zones, each copy of the DNS zone database is read-only, however, because all recordkeeping is done on the primary zone copy. A single DNS server can contain several zones that are primary and several that are secondary. The zone creation process is similar to the one outlined in the preceding section on primary zones, but with the difference being that the zone is transferred from an existing primary server.

Stub Zones (Delegated Zones)

The concept of stub zones is new in Microsoft DNS. A **stub zone** is a zone that contains no information about the members in a domain but simply serves to forward queries to a list of designated name servers for different domains. A stub zone subsequently contains only NS, SOA, and glue records. **Glue records** are A records that work in conjunction with a particular NS record to resolve the IP address of a particular name server. A server that hosts a stub zone for a namespace is not authoritative for that zone.

As illustrated in Figure 7.2, the stub zone effectively serves as a placeholder for a zone that is authoritative on another server. It allows a server to forward queries that are made to a specific zone to the list of name servers in that zone.

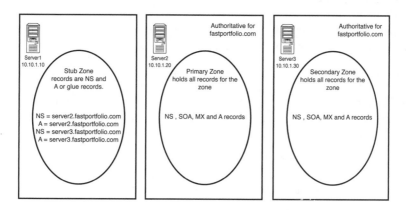

FIGURE 7.2   Stub zone.

DNS Queries

The primary function of DNS is to provide name resolution for requesting clients, so the query mechanism is one of the most important elements in the system. Two types of queries are commonly made to a DNS database: recursive and iterative.

Recursive Queries

Recursive queries are most often performed by resolvers, or clients that need to have a specific name resolved by a DNS server. Recursive queries are also accomplished by a DNS server if forwarders are configured to be used on a particular name server. A **recursive query** asks whether a particular record can be resolved by a particular name server. The response to a recursive query is either negative or positive.

Iterative Queries

Iterative queries ask a DNS server to either resolve the query or make best-guess referral to a DNS server that might contain more accurate information about where the query can be resolved. Another iterative query is then performed to the referred server and so on until a result, positive or negative, is obtained.

DNS Replication or Zone Transfer

Copying the DNS database from one server to another is accomplished through a process known as a **zone transfer**. Zone transfers are required for any zone that has more than one name server responsible for the contents of that zone. The mechanism for zone transfer varies, however, depending on the version of DNS and whether the zone is Active Directory–integrated.

Primary-Secondary (Master-Slave) (RW-RO)

The primary name server holds the authoritative copy of the zone. For redundancy and load sharing, a secondary or slave name server should be set up. The DNS name resolution does not care that it is dealing with a primary or secondary server.

The main difference between primary and secondary server is where the data comes from. Primary servers read it from a text file, and the secondary server loads it from another name server over the network via the zone transfer process. A slave name server is not limited to loading its data from a primary master name server; a slave server can load a zone from another slave server.

A big advantage of using a secondary name server is that only one set of DNS databases needs to be maintained, since all secondaries are read-only (RO) databases. All updates to the zone file have to be done at the server holding the primary zone file.

AD-Integrated Replication

One of the most significant changes from Windows 2000 Server to Windows Server 2003 is the location where the zone file is stored in Active Directory. Windows Server 2003 Active Directory–integrated zones are stored in the application partition, whereas in Windows 2000 Server the zones were part of the Global Catalog (GC). This change in the location of the zone file reduces cross-forest replication traffic, because the application partition is unique to each domain.

DNS Resource Records

In the DNS hierarchy, objects are identified through the use of **resource records (RR)**. These records are used for basic lookups of users and resources within the specified domain and are unique for the domain in which they are located. Because DNS is not a flat namespace, multiple identical RRs can exist at different levels in a DNS hierarchy.

Start of Authority Record

The **Start of Authority (SOA) record** indicates that this name server is the best source for information within the zone. An SOA record is required for each zone. The server referenced by the SOA record maintains and updates the zone file.

The SOA record also contains other useful information, such as the latest serial number for the zone file, the email address of the responsible person for the zone and Time to Live (TTL).

Host Records

A **host (A) record** is the most common form of DNS records; its data is an Internet address in a dotted decimal form (for example, `10.32.1.132`). There should be only one A record for each address of a host.

Name Server Records

Name Server (NS) records indicate which servers are available for name resolution for that zone. All DNS servers are listed as NS records within a particular zone. When slave servers are configured for the zone, they will have an NS record as well.

Mail Exchange Record

A **mail exchanger (MX) record** specifies a mail forwarder or delivery server for Simple Mail Transfer Protocol (SMTP) servers. MX records are the cornerstone of a successful Internet mail routing strategy.

One of the advantages of a DNS over HOSTS files is its support for advanced mail routing. LMHOST files allowed only attempts to deliver mail to the host's IP address. If that failed, they could either defer the delivery of the message and try again later or bounce the message back to the sender. DNS offers a solution to this problem, by allowing the setup of backup mail server records.

Backup mail server records are also MX records, but with a higher priority number as the primary MX record for the domain. In Figure 7.3, `whitehouse.gov` has two mail servers, one with priority `100` and one with priority `200`.

The preference values of MX determine the order in which a mailer uses a record. The preference value of an MX record is important only in relation to the other servers for the same domain. Mail servers will attempt to use the MX record with the lower number first; if that server is not available, they will try to contact the server with a higher number, and so on.

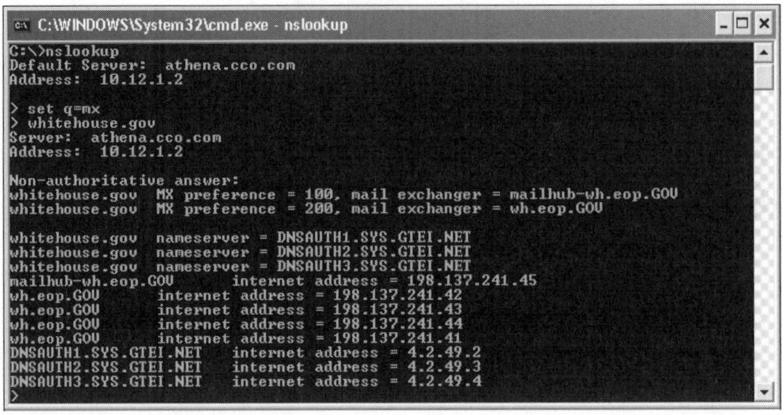

FIGURE 7.3   `whitehouse.gov` mail server entries.

MX record preference can also be used for load sharing. When several mail hosts have the same preference number associated with them, a sender can choose which mail server to contact first.

Mail routing based on preference numbers sounds simple enough, but there are major caveats that mail administrators have to understand. When troubleshooting mail routing problems, administrators use the following concepts to pinpoint the problem.

Mail routing algorithms based on preference numbers can create routing loops in some situations. The logic in mail servers helps circumvent this problem:

```
Companyabc.com  IN      MX      10      m1.companyabc.com
Companyabc.com  IN      MX      20      m2.companyabc.com
Companyabc.com  IN      MX      30      m3.companyabc.com
```

Using this example, if a message is sent from a client to LSomi@companyabc.com from an email address outside of companyabc.com, the mail server looks up the available mail server for companyabc.com based on the MX records set up for that domain. If the first mail server with the lowest priority is down (m1.companyabc.com), the mail server attempts to contact the second server (m2.companyabc.com). m2 will try to forward the message to m1.companyabc.com because that server is on the top of the list based on preferences. When m2 notices that m1 is down, it will try to contact the second server on the list, (itself), creating a routing loop. If m2 would try to send the message to m3, m3 would try to contact m1, then m2, and then itself, creating a routing loop. To prevent these loops from happening, mail servers discard certain addresses from the list before they decide where to send a message. A mailer sorts the available mail host based on preference number first, and then checks the canonical name of the domain name on which it's running. If the local host appears as a mail exchange, the mailer discards that MX record and all MX records with the same or higher preference value. In this example, m2 will not try to send mail to m1 and m3 for final delivery.

The second common mistake administrators have to look out for with an MX record is the alias name. Most mailers do not check for alias names; they check for canonical names. Unless an administrator uses canonical names for MX records, there is no guarantee that the mailer will find itself and create a mail loop.

Hosts listed as mail exchangers must have A records listed in the zone so that mailers can find address records for each MX record and attempt mail delivery.

Another common mistake when configuring mail hosts is the configuration of the hosted domain local to the server. ISPs and organizations commonly host mail for several domains on the same mail server. As mergers and acquisitions happen, this situation becomes more common. The following MX record illustrates that the mail server for companyabc.com is really the server mail.companyabc.com:

```
companyabc.com IN MX 10 mail.companyabc.com
```

Unless mail.companyisp.com is set up to recognize companyabc.com as a local domain, it will try to relay the message to itself, creating a routing loop and resulting in the following error message:

```
554 MX list for companyabc.com points back to mail.companyabc.com
```

In this situation, if mail.companyabc.com was configured not to relay messages to unknown domains, it would refuse delivery of the mail.

Service (SRV) Record

Service (SRV) records are RRs that indicate which resources perform a particular service. Domain controllers in Active Directory are referenced by SRV records that define specific services, such as the Global Catalog, LDAP, and Kerberos. SRV records are relatively new additions to DNS and did not exist in the original implementation of the standard. Each SRV record contains information about a particular functionality that a resource provides. For example, an LDAP server can add an SRV record indicating that it can handle LDAP requests for a particular zone. SRV records can be very useful for Active Directory because domain controllers can advertise that they can handle GC requests.

> **NOTE**
>
> Because SRV records are a relatively new addition to DNS, they are not supported by several downlevel DNS implementations, such as Unix BIND 4.1 and NT 4.0 DNS. It is therefore critical that the DNS environment that is used for Windows Server 2003's Active Directory has the capability of creating SRV records. For Unix BIND servers, version 8.1.2 or higher is recommended.

Canonical Name Record

A **canonical name (CNAME)** represents a server alias or allows any one of the member servers to be referred to by multiple names in DNS. The record redirects queries made to the A record for the particular host. CNAME records are useful when migrating servers, and for situations in which friendly names, such as `mail.companyabc.com`, are required to point to more complex, server-naming conventions, such as `sfoexch01.companyabc.com`.

CAUTION

Though DNS entries for MX records can be pointed to canonical (CNAME) host records, doing so is not advised, and is not a Microsoft recommended best practice. Increased administrative overhead and the possibility of misrouted messages can result. Microsoft recommends that mail/DNS administrators always link MX records to fully qualified principal names or domain literals. For further details, see Microsoft support article #153001.

Other Records

Other, less common forms of records that may exist in DNS have specific purposes, and there might be cause to create them. The following is a sample list, but it is by no means exhaustive:

- **AAAA**   Maps a standard IP address into a 128-bit IPv6 address. This type of record becomes more prevalent as IPv6 is adopted.

- **ISDN**   Maps a specific DNS name to an ISDN telephone number.

- **KEY**   Stores a public key used for encryption for a particular domain.

- **RP**   Specifies the Responsible Person for a domain.

- **WKS**   Designates a particular Well Known Service.

- **MB**   indicates which host contains a specific mailbox.

Multihomed DNS Servers

For multihomed DNS servers, an administrator can configure the DNS service to selectively enable and bind only to IP addresses that are specified using the DNS console. By default, however, the DNS service binds to all IP interfaces configured for the computer.

This can include

- Any additional IP addresses configured for a single network connection.

- Individual IP addresses configured for each separate connection where more than one network connection is installed on the server computer.

- For multihomed DNS servers, an administrator can restrict DNS service for selected IP addresses. When this feature is used, the DNS service listens for and answers only DNS requests that are sent to the IP addresses specified on the Interface tab in the Server properties.

By default, the DNS service listens on all IP addresses and accepts all client requests sent to its default service port (UDP 53 or TCP 53 for zone transfer requests). Some DNS resolvers require that the source address of a DNS response be the same as the destination address that was used in the query. If these addresses differ, clients could reject the response. To accommodate these resolvers, you can specify the list of allowed interfaces for the DNS server. When a list is set, the DNS service binds sockets only to allowed IP addresses used on the computer.

In addition to providing support for clients that require explicit bindings to be used, specifying interfaces can be useful for other reasons:

- If an administrator does not want to use some of the IP addresses or interfaces on a multihomed server computer

- If the server computer is configured to use a large number of IP addresses and the administrator does not want the added expense of binding to all of them

When configuring additional IP addresses and enabling them for use with the Windows 2003 DNS server, consider the following additional system resources that are consumed at the server computer:

- DNS server performance overhead increases slightly, which can affect DNS query reception for the server.

- Although Windows 2003 provides the means to configure multiple IP addresses for use with any of the installed network adapters, there is no performance benefit for doing so.

- Even if the DNS server is handling multiple zones registered for Internet use, it is not necessary or required by the Internet registration process to have different IP addresses registered for each zone.

- Each additional address might only slightly increase server performance. In instances when a large overall number of IP addresses are enabled for use, server performance can be degraded noticeably.

- In general, when adding network adapter hardware to the server computer, assign only a single primary IP address for each network connection.

- Whenever possible, remove nonessential IP addresses from existing server TCP/IP configurations.

Using DNS to Route SMTP Mail in Exchange Server 2003

Simple Mail Transfer Protocol (SMTP) has become the standard Internet protocol for electronic mail. Commonly used on Unix and Linux environments, and more recently in Windows, SMTP is used not only for mail delivery across the Internet, but also used within Active Directory as an alternative transport mechanism for site traffic.

Domains that want to participate in electronic mail exchange need to set up MX record(s) for their published zone. This advertises the system that will handle mail for the particular domain, so that SMTP mail will find the way to its destination.

Using DNS in Exchange 2003

Microsoft Exchange Server 2003 uses DNS exclusively for name resolution. In addition to talking to a DNS server for local name lookup, it also uses DNS to communicate over the Internet via SMTP mail services.

Each user has to authenticate to the Active Directory in order to access an Exchange mailbox. Exchange Server 2003 itself has information about authenticating other servers in the domain. This information can be found in Exchange System Manager under the Server Properties, Directory Access tab. The Exchange server obtains this information from the DNS server.

Understanding SMTP Mail Routing

Email is probably the most widely used TCP/IP and Internet application today, with the possible exception of the World Wide Web. SMTP defines a set of rules for addressing, sending and receiving mail between systems, based on the model of communication shown in Figure 7.4. As a result of a user mail request, the SMTP sender establishes a two-way connection with the SMTP receiver. The SMTP receiver can be either the ultimate destination or an intermediate (mail gateway). The SMTP sender generates commands that are replied to by the receiver. All this communication takes place over TCP port 25. When the connection is established, a series of commands and replies are exchanged between the client and server. This connection is similar to a phone conversation, and the commands and responses are equivalent to verbal communication.

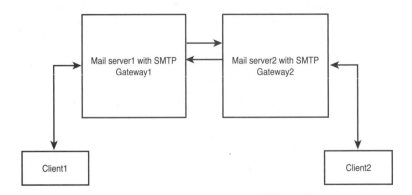

FIGURE 7.4   SMTP communications.

> **NOTE**
>
> In various implementations, there is a possibility of exchanging mail between the TCP/IP SMTP mailing system and the locally used mailing systems. These applications are called **mail gateways** or **mail bridges**. Sending mail through a mail gateway may alter the end-to-end delivery specification, because SMTP guarantees delivery only to the mail gateway host, not to the real destination host, which is located beyond the TCP/IP network. When a mail gateway is used, the SMTP end-to-end transmission is host-to-gateway, gateway-to-host, or gateway-to-gateway; the behavior beyond the gateway is not defined by SMTP.

Examining Client DNS Use for Exchange

Before users can access their mailboxes on an Exchange server, they must be authenticated. Authentication requires a DNS lookup in order to locate a domain controller on which the users' accounts can be authenticated.

Clients normally cannot deliver messages directly to destination mail hosts. They typically use a mail server to relay messages to destinations. Using SMTP, clients connect to a mail server, which first verifies that the client is allowed to relay through this server, and then accepts the message destined for other domains.

A client uses DNS to resolve the name of a mail server. For example, when configuring an Outlook mail client to connect to an Exchange server, only the short name and not the FQDN is used to connect to the server. The short name is resolved by DNS to the FQDN of the Exchange server to which the client is connected.

Understanding DNS Requirements for Exchange Server 2003

In Active Directory, all client logons and lookups are directed to local domain controllers and GC servers through references to the SRV records in DNS. Each configuration has its DNS and resource requirements. In a member server configuration, Exchange relies on other servers for client authentication and uses DNS to find those servers. In an Active Directory domain controller configuration, on the other hand, the Exchange server also participates in the authentication process for Active Directory.

Exchange 5.5 and E2k3 DNS/WINS Name Resolutions Requirements

Exchange 5.5 and NT4 use different name resolution orders when trying to resolve a name. NT4 relies on the local hostname, HOST, DNS NetBIOS name cache, WINS, B-Cast NetBIOS broadcasts, and the LMHOSTS file for name resolution. Windows 2000 and higher clients, on the other hand, use a significantly different approach for name resolution. Windows 2000 uses hostname resolution first, rather than NetBIOS name resolution techniques. In addition, a local cache is used to reduce network traffic.

Windows NT servers and Exchange 5.5 servers find Exchange 2003 servers via DNS, but name resolution might be slightly slower because of the order previously outlined. Windows 2003 and Exchange rely on DNS, so these servers must be part of a DNS name resolution schema. When older clients and servers are used that do not have DNS as the primary name resolution, it is best to add Windows 2003 servers and Exchange server to the WINS database statically—directly to the WINS database—or dynamically—adding the WINS server IP address under the TCP/IP configuration section.

> **TIP**
>
> When migrating from Windows NT4, one of the first tasks is to update the DNS server to a version that supports dynamic updates and, most importantly, SRV records.

DNS and SMTP RFC Standards

In 1984, Paul Mockapetris was responsible for designing the first DNS architecture. The result was released as RPC 882 and 883. These were superseded by RFC 1034 (Domain Names—concepts and facilities) and 1035 (Domain Names—implementation and specification) the current specifications of the DNS. RFCs 1034 and 1035 have been improved by many other RFCs, which describe fixes for potential DNS security problems, implementation problems, best practices, and performance improvements to the current standard.

RFC 2821 defines the SMTP, which replaced the earlier versions of RFC 821 and 822.

Virtual SMTP Servers

The SMTP protocol is an essential part of Exchange 2003 and Active Directory. Although Exchange 4.x and 5.x messaging is primarily based on X.400 mail transfer standards, Exchange 2000 and 2003 are native SMTP messaging systems. However, when an Exchange 2000/2003 server has to communicate to an Exchange 5.5 server, it still uses the MTA and x.400 for communication.

A single virtual SMTP server runs by default on all Exchange 2003 servers. In most cases, this is the SMTP server needed for external and internal communications. An administrator might want to install an additional SMTP virtual server for the following reasons:

- To maintain multiple domain namespaces on the same server
- To establish different authentication methods for different users or groups
- To configure different SMTP options to different users

Routing Groups

A **routing group** is a collection of servers that enjoy a persistent high-bandwidth connection and it's used to organize server communication based on bandwidth constraints. All servers within a routing group communicate with each other directly when transferring mail. This is also known as **mesh topology**. Reasons for setting up routing groups include the following:

- Low speed or unreliable connection between Exchange servers

- Administrators wanting more control over the message flow within the organization

- Fault tolerance or high availability between routing groups

Exchange messages can be routed from sender to recipient the following ways:

- With sender and recipient located on the same server

- With sender and recipient located in the same routing group

- Between routing groups

- To a server outside the Exchange organization

The preferred method for connecting routing groups in Exchange is via the routing group connector. Routing groups themselves do not use a particular protocol, but will use SMTP for all traffic to and from Exchange 2000/2003 servers and Remote Procedure Calls (RPCs) for Exchange 5.5 servers. Email routing between routing groups is funneled through the bridgehead server, which is fully configurable on a per–routing group basis.

Mixed Environment Mail Routing

Companies with multiple email systems usually use SMTP mail transport between these dissimilar systems. Microsoft Exchange 2003 can connect to any other RFC-compliant SMTP gateway. It also supports authenticated and secure transfer between SMTP gateways.

SMTP Mail Security, Virus Checking, and Proxies

Spamming and security issues are daily concerns for email administrators. As the Internet grows, so too does the amount of spam that mail servers have to confront. Unwanted messages not only can take up a lot of space on mail servers, but can also carry dangerous payloads or viruses. Administrators have to maintain a multilayered defense against spam and viruses.

There are several security areas that have to be addressed:

- Gateway security to control access to the mail server delivering messages to/from the Internet

- Mail database security where messages are stored

- Client mail security where messages are opened and processed

Gateway security is a primary concern for administrators because a misconfigured gateway can become a gateway used by spammers to relay messages. Unauthenticated message relay is the mechanism spammers rely on to deliver their messages. When a server is used for unauthenticated message relay, it not only puts a huge load on server resources, but also might get the server placed on a spam list. Companies relying on spam lists to control their incoming mail traffic refuse mail delivered from servers listed in the database; therefore, controlling who can relay messages through the mail relay gateway is a major concern.

Application-level firewalls allow mail proxying on behalf of the internal mail server. Essentially, mail hosts trying to connect to the local mail server have to talk to the proxy gateway, which is responsible for relaying those messages to the internal server. Going one step further, these proxy gateways can also perform additional functions to check the message they are relaying to the internal host or to control the payload passed along to the internal server.

This configuration is also helpful in stopping dangerous viruses from being spread through email. For example, dangerous scripts could potentially be attached to email, which could execute as soon as the user opens the mail. A safe configuration allows only permitted attachment types to pass through. Even those attachments have to pass virus checking before they are passed to an internal mail server. Figure 7.5 illustrates the schematics of how an application gateway works.

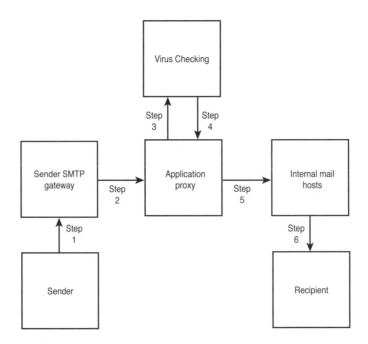

FIGURE 7.5   Application gateway.

The following process describes how one server contacts another server to send email messages that include virus checking:

1. The sender contacts its SMTP gateway for message delivery.

2. The SMTP gateway looks up the MX record for the recipient domain and establishes communication with it. The application proxy acting as the SMTP server for the recipient's domain receives the message. Before the recipient gateway establishes communication with the sender gateway, it can check whether the sender SMTP gateway is listed on any known spam lists. If the server is not located on any spam lists, communication can resume and the message can be accepted by the proxy server.

3. The application proxy forwards the message for virus checking.

4. After virus checking, the mail is routed back to the application proxy.

5. Mail is delivered to the internal SMTP gateway.

6. The recipient picks up the mail message.

> **NOTE**
>
> Application proxy and virus or spam checking might be done within the same host. In that case, steps 2–5 are done in one step without having to transfer a message to a separate host.

Third-party products can be used for virus checking not only at the gateway level, but also directly on an Exchange email database. Database level scans can be scheduled to run at night when the load is lower on the server; real-time scans can perform virus checking in real time before any message is written to the database.

The final checkpoint for any multilayered virus protection is on the workstation. The file system and the email system can be protected by the same antivirus product. Messages can be scanned before a user is able to open the message or before a message is sent.

Protecting email communications and message integrity puts a large load on administrators. Threats are best dealt with using a multilayered approach from the client to the server to the gateway. When each step along the way is protected against malicious attacks, the global result is a secure, well-balanced email system.

SMTP Server Scalability and Load Balancing

In a larger environment, administrators might set up more than one SMTP server for inbound and/or outbound mail processing. Windows Server 2003 and Exchange Server 2003 provide a very flexible platform to scale and balance the load of SMTP mail services. DNS and Network Load Balancing (NLB) are key components for these tasks.

Administrators should not forget about hardware failover and scalability. Multi-network interface cards are highly recommended. Two network cards can be teamed together for higher throughput, can be used in failover configuration, or can be load-balanced by using one network card for front-end communication and another for back-end services, such as backup.

Network design can also incorporate fault tolerance by creating redundant network routes and by using technologies that can group devices together for the purpose of load balancing and delivery failover. Load balancing is the process where requests can be spread across multiple devices to keep individual service load at an acceptable level.

Using NLB, Exchange Server SMTP processes can be handed off to a group of servers for processing, or incoming traffic can be handled by a group of servers before it gets routed to an Exchange server. The following example outlines a possible configuration for using NLB in conjunction with Exchange. Figure 7.6 illustrates the layout of the message flow.

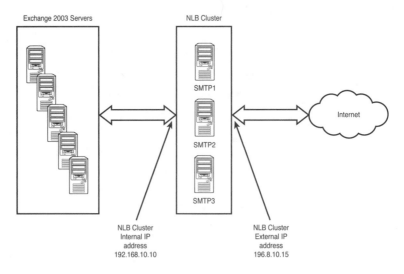

FIGURE 7.6   Message flow with NLB and Exchange Server 2003.

DNS, in this example, has been set up to point to the name of the NLB cluster IP address. Externally, the DNS MX record points to 196.8.10.15 as the mail relay gateway for companyabc.com. Exchange server uses smarthost configuration to send all SMTP messages to the NLB cluster. The NLB cluster is configured in balanced mode where the servers share equal load. Only port 25 traffic is allowed on the cluster servers. This configuration would offload SMTP mail processing from the Exchange servers because all they have to do is to pass the message along to the cluster for delivery. They do not need to contact any outside SMTP gateway to transfer the message. This configuration allows scalability because when the load increases, administrators can add more SMTP gateways to the cluster. This setup also addresses load balancing, because the NLB cluster is smart enough to notice whether one of the cluster nodes has failed or is down for maintenance. An additional ramification of this configuration is that message tracking will not work beyond the Exchange servers.

NOTE

Administrators should not forget about the ramifications of antivirus and spam checking software with NLB. These packages in gateway mode can also be used as the SMTP gateway for an organization. In an NLB clustered mode, an organization would need to purchase three sets of licenses to cover each NLB node.

A less used but possible configuration for SMTP mail load balancing uses DNS to distribute the load between multiple SMTP servers. This configuration, known as DNS round robin, does not provide as robust a message routing environment as the NLB solution.

Configuring DNS to Support Exchange Servers

Because DNS is already required and integrated with Active Directory before Exchange Server is installed, most companies already have a robust DNS environment in place. Exchange by itself accesses DNS servers to find resources on the local network, such as Global Catalog servers and domain controllers. It also uses DNS to search for MX records of other domains.

External DNS Servers for the Internet

The external DNS server for Exchange (or any other mail system) is responsible for giving out the correct MX and A records for the domain for which it is authoritative. Administrators should take security precautions regarding who can change these records—and how. Intentionally or accidentally changing these records can result in undelivered mail.

Most companies let their ISP host the external DNS entries for their domain. ISPs provide internal administrators with methods of managing DNS entries for their domain. In some cases it has to be done over the phone, but normally a secure Web interface is provided for management. Although this setup is convenient and ISPs usually take care of load balancing and redundancy, some companies opt to host their own zone records for the Internet. In this case companies have to host their own DNS server in-house with the ISP responsible only for forwarding all requests to their DNS server. When hosting an external DNS server, in-house administrators have to think about security issues and DNS configuration issues.

Internal DNS Servers for Outbound Mail Routing

Exchange SMTP gateways are responsible for delivering mail to external hosts. As with any name process involving resolving names to IP addresses, DNS plays a major part in successful mail delivery.

Exchange can route mail to outbound destinations two ways. One is by using smarthosts to offload all processing of messages destined to other domains. As seen in the previous section, an NLB cluster can be used to route Internet mail to its final destination.

The second way is the default, with Exchange Server 2003 taking care of delivering messages to other domains. In this scenario, Exchange queries DNS servers for other domains' MX records and A records for address resolution.

Internal DNS Servers for Internal Routing of Email Between Exchange Servers

Exchange 2003 depends entirely on SMTP for mail routing, both internally and externally. Internally, Exchange servers have to be able to resolve either the short name (for example, server1) or the FQDN (for example, server1.companyabc.com).

Troubleshooting DNS Problems

Troubleshooting is part of everyday life for administrators. DNS is no exception to this rule. Subsequently, understanding how to use the following tools to troubleshoot DNS will not only help avoid mistakes when configuring DNS-related services, but will also provide administrators with a useful toolbox to resolve issues.

Using Event Viewer to Troubleshoot

The first place to look for help when something is not working, or it appears that it is not working, is the system logs. With Windows Server 2003, the DNS logs can be conveniently accessed directly from the DNS MMC console. Parsing this set of logs can help the administrator troubleshooting DNS replication issues, query problems, and other issues.

For more advanced Event Log diagnosis, administrators can turn on Debug Logging on a per-server basis. Debugging should be turned on only for troubleshooting, because log files can fill up fast. To enable Debug Logging, follow these steps:

1. Open the DNS MMC snap-in (Start, Administrative Tools, DNS).

2. Right-click on the server name and choose Properties.

3. Select the Debug Logging tab.

4. Check the Log Packets for Debugging box.

5. Configure any additional settings as required and click OK.

6. Turn off these settings after the troubleshooting is complete.

Troubleshooting Using the `ipconfig` Utility

The `ipconfig` utility is used not only for basic TCP/IP troubleshooting, but can also be used to directly resolve DNS issues. These functions can be invoked from the command prompt with the correct flag, detailed as follows:

- `ipconfig /displaydns`   This command displays all locally cached DNS entries. This is also known as the DNS resolver cache.

- `ipconfig /flushdns`   This switch can be used to save administrators from a lot of headaches when troubleshooting DNS problems. This command flushes the local DNS cache. The default cache time for positive replies is 1 day; for negative replies, it is 15 minutes.

- `ipconfig /registerdns`   This flag informs the client to automatically re-register itself in DNS, if the particular zone supports dynamic zone updates.

NOTE

Client-side DNS caching is configurable in the registry via the following key:

`\\HKLM\System\CurrentControlSet\Services\DNSCach\Parameters`

`Set MaxCacheEnrtyTtlLimit = 1 (default = 86400)`

`Set NegativeCacheTim = 0 (default = 300)`

The first entry overwrites the TTL number in the cached address to 1 second, essentially disabling the local cache. The second entry changes the negative cache from 15 minutes to 0, essentially disabling the negative cache facility.

Monitoring Exchange Using Performance Monitor

Performance monitor is a built-in, often overlooked utility that enables a great deal of insight into issues in a network. Many critical DNS counters can be monitored relating to queries, zone transfers, memory use, and other important factors.

Using `nslookup` for DNS Exchange Lookup

In both Windows and Unix environments, `nslookup` is a command-line administrative tool for testing and troubleshooting DNS servers. Simple query structure can provide powerful results for troubleshooting. A simple query contacts the default DNS server for the system and looks up the inputted name.

To test a lookup for www.companyabc.com, type

`nslookup www.companyabc.com`

at the command prompt. nslookup can also be used to look up other DNS resource types—for example, an MX or SOA record for a company. To look up an MX record for a company type, use the following steps, as illustrated in Figure 7.7:

1. Open a command prompt instance.

2. Type **nslookup** and press Enter.

3. Type **set query=mx** (or simply **set q=mx**) and press Enter.

4. Type **microsoft.com** and press Enter.

FIGURE 7.7 nslookup MX query.

An MX record output not only shows all the MX records that are used for that domain, their preference number, and the IP address they are associated with; the name server for the domain is also displayed.

By default, nslookup queries the local DNS server the system is set up to query. Another powerful feature of nslookup is that it can switch between servers to query. This feature enables administrators to verify that all servers answer with the same record as expected. For example, if an organization is moving from one ISP to another, it might use this technique, because the IP addresses for its servers might change during the move. The DNS change takes an administrator only a few minutes to do, but replication of the changes through the Internet might take 24–72 hours. During this time, some servers might still use the old IP address for the mail server. To verify that the DNS records are replicated to other DNS servers, an administrator can query several DNS servers for the answer through the following technique:

1. Open a command prompt instance.

2. Type **nslookup** and press Enter.

3. Type **server <server IP address>** for the DNS server you want to query.

4. Type **set query=mx** (or simply **set q=mx**) and press Enter.

5. Type **microsoft.com** and press Enter.

Repeat from step 3 for other DNS servers.

nslookup can also help find out the version of BIND used on a remote Unix DNS server. An administrator may find it useful to determine which version of BIND each server is running for troubleshooting purposes. To determine this, the following steps must be performed:

1. From the command line, type **nslookup**, and then press Enter.

2. Type **server <server IP address>** for the IP address of the DNS server queried.

3. Type **set class=chaos** and then press Enter.

4. Type **set type=txt** and then press Enter.

5. Type **version.bind** and then press Enter.

If the administrator of the BIND DNS server has configured the server to accept this query, the BIND version that the server is running is returned. As previously mentioned, the BIND version must be 8.1.2 or later to support SRV records.

Troubleshooting with DNSLINT

DNSLINT is a Microsoft Windows utility that helps administrators diagnose common DNS name resolution issues. The utility is not installed by default on Windows Servers and has to be downloaded from Microsoft. Microsoft Knowledge Base Article—321046 contains the link to download this utility.

When this command-line utility runs, it generates an HTML file in the directory it runs from. It can help administrators with Active Directory troubleshooting and also with mail-related name resolution and verification. Running DNSLINT /d <domain_name> /c tests DNS information as known on authoritative DNS servers for the domain being tested; it also checks SMTP, POP3, and IMAP connectivity on the server. For the complete options for this utility, run DNSLINT /?.

Using dnscmd for Advanced DNS Troubleshooting

The dnscmd utility is essentially a command-line version of the MMC DNS console. Installed as part of the Windows Server 2003 Support tools, this utility enables administrators to create zones, modify zone records, and perform other vital administrative functions. To install the support tools, run the support tools setup from the Windows Server 2003 CD (located in the \support\tools directory). You can view the full functionality of this utility by typing **DNSCMD /?** at the command line, as illustrated in Figure 7.8.

FIGURE 7.8   dnscmd functionality.

Summary

DNS is the cornerstone of name resolution on the Internet and within Windows Server 2003 and Active Directory. Subsequently, it is also an integral part of any modern email solution, particularly with Exchange Server 2003. Without a solid understanding of DNS and the tie-ins DNS has with Exchange, both Active Directory and Exchange are destined to fail. A well-designed DNS implementation, on the other hand, helps keep both Exchange and Active Directory stable and reliable.

Best Practices

The following are best practices from this chapter:

- Use Windows 2000/2003 DNS or BIND 8.1.2 or higher to support SRV records.

- Administrators should set up redundant name resolution servers in the event that one server fails.

- Use caching-only DNS servers to help leverage load and minimize zone transfer traffic across WAN links.

- Make any DNS implementations compliant with the standard DNS character set so that zone transfers are supported to and from non–Unicode-compliant DNS implementations, such as Unix BIND servers. This includes a–z, A–Z, 0–9, and the hyphen (-) character.

- Set up multiple MX records for all mail servers for redundancy. ISPs usually function as a secondary mail relay gateway for the hosted domain.

- Always protect internal DNS servers and SMTP gateways by a firewall.

CHAPTER 8

Global Catalog and Domain Controller Placement

There is simply no way around it; Active Directory is a critical and necessary component of any Exchange Server 2003 deployment. When Exchange lost its directory component with the introduction of Exchange 2000, the result was a lot of grumbling about the learning curve associated with Active Directory. The advent of Windows Server 2003 and Exchange Server 2003, brought the optimization and simplification of the Active Directory environment. Lessons learned from Windows 2000 Active Directory have been integrated into the newest version of Active Directory, which is available with Windows Server 2003.

Notwithstanding the improvements, there is still a great deal of misunderstanding about Active Directory and its core components. The Global Catalog, for example, is a critical component of Exchange and requires a solid grasp of its concepts.

This chapter explains the relationship between Exchange Server 2003 and Active Directory and how the placement of domain controllers and global catalog servers affects it. Components of Exchange Server 2003 that access Active Directory are explained, and troubleshooting techniques for directory access problems are detailed. In addition, this chapter offers best practice recommendations for domain controller and Global Catalog placement and presents detailed fine-tuning information.

Active Directory Structure

Active Directory (AD) is a robust, standards-based Light Directory Access Protocol (LDAP) directory developed by Microsoft. In addition to serving as the central directory for Windows Server 2003, AD is also used to store the Exchange Server 2003 directory information. All Exchange attributes, such as email address, mailbox location, home server, and a whole range of other information used by Exchange is directly stored in Active Directory.

Exploring AD Domains

An Active Directory domain is the main logical boundary of Active Directory. In a standalone sense, an AD domain looks very much like a Windows NT domain. Users and computers are all stored and managed from within the boundaries of the domain. However, several major changes have been made to the structure of the domain and how it relates to other domains within the Active Directory structure.

Domains in Active Directory serve as a security boundary for objects and contain their own security policies. For example, different domains can contain different password policies for users. Keep in mind that domains are a logical organization of objects and can easily span multiple physical locations. Consequently, it is no longer necessary to set up multiple domains for different remote offices or sites, because replication concerns can be addressed with the proper use of Active Directory sites, which are described in greater detail later in this chapter.

Exploring AD Trees

An Active Directory tree is composed of multiple domains connected by two-way transitive trusts. Each domain in an Active Directory tree shares a common schema and Global Catalog. The transitive trust relationship between domains is automatic, which is a change from the domain structure of NT 4.0, wherein all trusts had to be manually set up. The transitive trust relationship means that because the asia domain trusts the root companyabc domain, and the europe domain trusts the companyabc domain, the asia domain also trusts the europe domain. The trusts flow through the domain structure.

Exploring AD Forests

Forests are a group of interconnected domain trees. Implicit trusts connect the roots of each tree into a common forest.

The overlying characteristics that tie together all domains and domain trees into a common forest are the existence of a common schema and a common Global Catalog. However, domains and domain trees in a forest do not need to share a common namespace. For example, the domains microsoft.com and msnbc.com could theoretically be part of the same forest, but maintain their own separate namespaces (for obvious reasons).

> **NOTE**
>
> Each separate instance of Exchange Server 2003 requires a completely separate AD Forest. In other words, AD cannot support more than one Exchange organization in a single forest. This is an important factor to bear in mind when examining AD integration concepts.

Understanding AD Replication with Exchange Server 2003

An understanding of the relationship between Exchange and Active Directory is not complete without an understanding of the replication engine within AD itself. This is especially true because any changes made to the structure of Exchange must be replicated across the AD infrastructure.

Active Directory replaced the concept of Primary Domain Controllers (PDCs) and Backup Domain Controllers (BDCs) with the concept of multiple domain controllers that each contain a master read/write copy of domain information. Changes that are made on any domain controller within the environment are replicated to all other domain controllers in what is known as **multimaster replication**.

Active Directory differs from most directory service implementations in that the replication of directory information is accomplished independently from the actual logical directory design. The concept of Active Directory sites is completely independent from the logical structure of Active Directory forests, trees, and domains. In fact, a single site in Active Directory can actually host domain controllers from different domains or different trees within the same forest. This enables the creation of a replication topology based on your WAN structure, and your directory topology can mirror your organizational structure.

From an Exchange point of view, the most important concept to keep in mind is the delay that replication causes between when a change is made in Exchange and when that change is replicated throughout the entire AD structure. The reason for these types of discrepancies lies in the fact that not all AD changes are replicated immediately. This concept is known as replication latency. Because the overhead required in immediately replicating change information to all domain controllers is large, the default schedule for replication is not as often as you might want. To immediately replicate changes made to Exchange or any AD changes, use the following procedure:

1. Open Active Directory Sites and Services.

2. Drill down to Sites, *sitename*, Servers, *servername*, NTDS Settings. The server name chosen should be the server you are connected to, and from which the desired change should be replicated.

3. Right-click each connection object and choose Replicate Now, as illustrated in Figure 8.1.

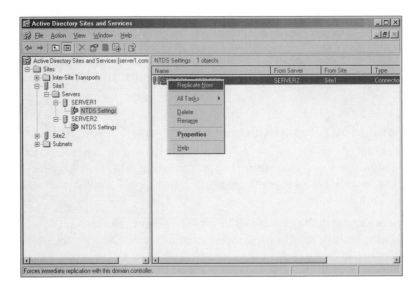

FIGURE 8.1   Forcing AD replication.

Examining the Role of Domain Controllers in AD

Exchange has always relied on domain controllers for authentication of user accounts. Mailboxes in Exchange 5.5 were controlled through the application of security from Windows NT 4.0 and, later, Active Directory domain accounts. It should come as no surprise, consequently, that Exchange Server 2003 also relies on Active Directory domain controllers for authentication purposes. Proper placement of DCs is also important.

Examining Domain Controller Authentication in Active Directory

To understand how Exchange manages security, an analysis of Active Directory authentication is required. This information aids in troubleshooting the environment, as well as in gaining a better understanding of Exchange Server 2003 as a whole.

Each object in Exchange, including all mailboxes, can have security directly applied for the purposes of limiting and controlling access to those resources. For example, a particular administrator may be granted access to control a certain set of Exchange Servers, and users can be granted access to mailboxes. What makes Exchange particularly useful is that security rights can be assigned not only at the object level but at the attribute level too. This enables granular administration, by allowing such tasks as a Telecom group being able to modify only the phone number field of a user, for example.

When a user logs in to a domain, the domain controller performs a lookup to ensure a match between the username and password. If a match is made, the client is then authenticated and given the rights to gain access to resources, including Exchange Server 2003 mailboxes.

Because the domain controllers provide users with the keys to access the resources, it is important to provide local access to domain controllers for all Exchange servers. If a local domain controller became unavailable, for example, users would be unable to authenticate to their mailboxes in Exchange, effectively locking them out.

Domain Controller Placement with Exchange Server 2003

As previously identified, Exchange relies heavily on the security authentication performed by Active Directory domain controllers. This concept is important for Exchange Server 2003 design, because placement of domain controllers becomes an important concept. In general, at least one Active Directory domain controller must be within close proximity to any Exchange Server to enable quick authentication for local users and mailboxes. In some smaller sites, this might mean placing the domain controller role on the physical Exchange server itself. It is important to note, however, that the separation of the domain controller function from Exchange is more ideal, gives the greatest performance boost, and should be considered in all but the smallest sites.

Other sites may deploy more than one Active Directory domain controller for user authentication. This enables the distribution of domain controller tasks, but also builds redundancy into the design. Because each DC is multimaster, if one goes down the other will be able to take over domain controller responsibilities.

> **NOTE**
>
> Although Active Directory domain controllers are multimaster, downlevel clients (Windows NT 4.0 and lower) still require access to a Windows NT Primary Domain Controller (PDC) equivalent. A single Windows 2000/2003 DC acts as the PDC Emulator for each domain, and is not multimaster for that role. If the AD DC with this role goes down, the downlevel clients are disrupted as if their NT PDC went down. Windows 2000/XP-and-higher clients do not have this problem, however, because they are able to take advantage of the multimaster DC approach.

Defining the Global Catalog

The Global Catalog is an index of the Active Directory database that contains a partial copy of its contents. All objects within the AD tree are referenced within the Global Catalog, which enables users to search for objects located in other domains. Every attribute of each object is not replicated to the Global Catalogs—only those attributes that are commonly used in search operations, such as first name, last name, and so on.

Global catalog servers, commonly referred to as GCs or GC/DCs, are Active Directory domain controllers that contain a copy of the Global Catalog. Locating a minimum of one Global Catalog server in each physical location is a wise move, because the Global Catalog must be referenced often by clients, and the traffic across slower WAN links would limit this traffic. In addition, technologies such as Exchange Server 2003 need fast access to Global Catalog servers for all user transactions, making it very important to have a Global Catalog server nearby.

Understanding the Relationship Between Exchange Server 2003 and the AD Global Catalog

In the past, an Exchange server could continue to operate by itself with few dependencies on other system components. Because all components of the mail system were locally confined to the same server, downtime was an all-or-nothing prospect. The segregation of the directory into Active Directory has changed the playing field somewhat. In many cases, downlevel clients no longer operate independently in the event of a Global Catalog server failure. Keep this in mind, especially when designing and deploying a domain controller and Global Catalog infrastructure.

> **NOTE**
>
> Because Outlook clients and Exchange can behave erratically if the Global Catalog they have been using goes down, it is important to scrutinize which systems receive a copy of the global catalog. In other words, it is not wise to set up a Global Catalog domain controller on a workstation or substandard hardware, simply to offload some work from the production domain controllers. If that server fails, the effect on the clients is the same as if their Exchange server failed.

Understanding Global Catalog Structure

The Global Catalog is an oft-misunderstood concept with Active Directory. In addition, design mistakes with Global Catalog placement can potentially cripple a network, so a full understanding of what the Global Catalog is and how it works is warranted.

As mentioned earlier, Active Directory was developed as a standards-based LDAP implementation, and the AD structure acts as an X.500 tree. Queries against the Active Directory must therefore have some method of traversing the directory tree to find objects. This means that queries that are sent to a domain controller in a subdomain need to be referred to other domain controllers in other domains in the forest. In large forests, this can significantly increase the time it takes to perform queries.

In Active Directory in Windows 2000/2003, the Global Catalog serves as a mechanism for improving queries. The Global Catalog contains a partial set of all objects (users, computers, and other AD objects) in the entire AD forest. The most commonly searched attributes are stored and replicated in the Global Catalog (that is, first name, username, email address). By storing a read-only copy of these objects locally, full tree searches across the entire forest are accomplished significantly faster. So, in a large forest, a server that holds a copy of the Global Catalog contains information replicated from all domains in the forest, as illustrated in Figure 8.2.

Creating Global Catalog Domain Controllers

With the exception of the first domain controller in a domain, all domain controllers in Active Directory are not Global Catalog servers by default; they must first be established as such through the following procedure:

1. Open Active Directory Sites and Services.

2. Navigate to Sites, *sitename*, Servers, *servername*.

3. Right-click NTDS Settings and then select Properties.

4. Check the box labeled Global Catalog, as indicated in Figure 8.3.

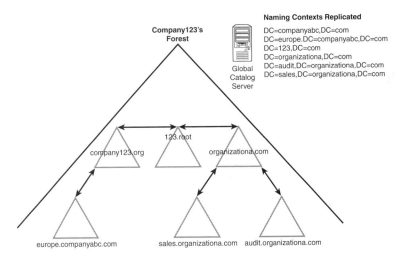

FIGURE 8.2   Global catalog replication.

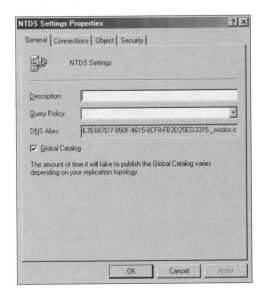

FIGURE 8.3   Creating a Global Catalog server.

After being made into Global Catalog servers, domain controllers then receive their read-only copy of the partial domain naming context from each domain in the forest. To remove a domain controller from Global Catalog duties, uncheck the box; the DC will no longer hold a copy of the GC information.

> **NOTE**
>
> In large forests, replicating a full set of Global Catalog information can be a time- and band-width-consuming activity. Schedule the creation of Global Catalog servers during periods of low network activity, such as over an evening or weekend.

Verifying Global Catalog Creation

When a domain controller receives the orders to become a Global Catalog server, there is a period of time when the GC information will replicate to that domain controller. Depending on the size of the Global Catalog, this could take a significant period of time. To determine when a domain controller has received the full subset of information, use the replmon (replication monitor) utility from the Windows Server 2003 support tools. The replmon utility indicates which portions of the AD database are replicated to different domain controllers in a forest, and how recently they have been updated.

replmon enables an administrator to determine the replication status of each domain naming context in the forest. Because a Global Catalog server should have a copy of each domain naming context in the forest, determine the replication status of the new GC with replmon. For example, the fully replicated Global Catalog server in Figure 8.4 contains the default naming contexts, such as Schema, Configuration, and DnsZones, in addition to domain naming contexts for all domains. In this example, both the companyabc.com domain and the europe.companyabc.com domain are replicated to the ELG-DC1 domain controller.

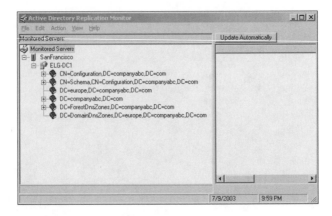

FIGURE 8.4   ReplMon GC creation verification.

Using Best Practices for Global Catalog Placement

The general rule of thumb with GC placement is to place at least one GC in close network proximity to any major service that requires use of the Global Catalog (3268) port. Exchange Server 2003 makes extensive use of this port, and it is therefore wise to include a local GC in any site that contains an Exchange Server.

These requirements do not mean that an unnecessary number of Global Catalog servers need to be deployed, however. In reality, the total number of GCs that need to be deployed can be reduced in many situations through the concept of site consolidation in Exchange Server 2003. This concept enables multiple physical sites to use a central Exchange Server or set of servers, as opposed to having Exchange Servers (and their corresponding GCs) deployed to each site. Site consolidation works by having remote clients use the improved client remote access capabilities of Outlook 2003, OWA, and OMA. For more information on site consolidation strategies, see Chapter 4, "Exchange Server 2003 Design Concepts."

Optimizing Global Catalog Promotion

As previously mentioned, domain controllers can easily be promoted or demoted into Global Catalog servers with a single check box. The ease of this operation should not be taken lightly, however, because there can be a significant impact on network operations during this procedure.

When promoting a domain controller to Global Catalog status, the server immediately writes SRV records into DNS indicating its status as a Global Catalog server. In the past, this would cause problems, because Exchange 2000 servers would immediately begin using the incomplete Global Catalog on a newly created GC server, which would yield improper results. Upon the release of Service Pack 2 for Exchange 2000 and subsequently Exchange Server 2003, a mechanism for detecting the readiness of a Global Catalog server was built into Exchange, specifically into the DSAccess service. This prevented Exchange from using those GCs until it received a full copy of the Global Catalog.

> **NOTE**
>
> After a domain controller has been promoted to Global Catalog status, the server will require a reboot at some point. Although an administrator who sets up a GC server will never be prompted to reboot, the Name Service Provider Interface (NSPI) service, which is used by Outlook for address book lookups, will not function properly until the newly promoted GC server has been rebooted. In general, Exchange should be able to proxy this service for the clients, but it is still a good idea to plan for a reboot of a GC shortly after its creation.

Exploring Global Catalog Demotion

Removing a Global Catalog server from production can also have a detrimental effect in certain cases. Outlook 2000-and-older clients, for example, experience lockup issues if the

Global Catalog server they have been using is shut down or removed from GC service. The loss of a GC server is the equivalent of the loss of an Exchange server, and should therefore not be taken lightly. Outlook 2002-and-greater clients, however, automatically detect the failure of their Global Catalog server and reroute themselves within 30 seconds. Scheduling Global Catalog or domain controller demotions for the off-hours, therefore, is important.

> **NOTE**
>
> If a production Global Catalog server goes down, downlevel (pre-2002) versions of Outlook can regain connectivity via a restart of the Outlook client. In some cases, this means forcing the closure of OUTLOOK.EXE and MAPISP32.EXE from the Task Manager or rebooting the system.

Deploying Domain Controllers Using the Install from Media Option

When deploying a remote site infrastructure to support Exchange Server 2003, take care to examine best practice deployment techniques for domain controllers in order to optimize the procedure. In the past, deploying domain controller and/or Global Catalog servers to remote sites was a rather strenuous affair. Because each new domain controller would need to replicate a local copy of the Active Directory for itself, careful consideration into replication bandwidth was taken into account. In many cases, this required one of these options:

- The domain controller was set up remotely at the start of a weekend or other period of low bandwidth.

- The domain controller hardware was physically set up in the home office of an organization and then shipped to the remote location.

This procedure was unwieldy and time-consuming with Windows 2000 Active Directory. Fortunately, Windows Server 2003 addressed this issue through use of the Install from Media option for Active Directory domain controllers.

The concept behind the media-based GC/DC replication is straightforward. A current, running domain controller backs up the directory through a normal backup process. The backup files are then copied to a backup media, such as a CD or tape, and shipped to the remote GC destination. Upon arrival, the dcpromo command can be run with the /adv switch (dcpromo /adv), which activates the option to install from media, as illustrated in Figure 8.5.

After the dcpromo command restores the directory information from the backup, an incremental update of the changes made since the media was created is performed. Because of this, you still need network connectivity throughout the DCPROMO process, although the amount of replication required is significantly less. Because some dcpromo operations have been known to take days and even weeks, this concept can dramatically help deploy remote domain controllers.

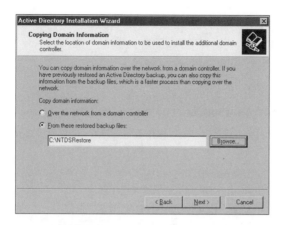

FIGURE 8.5   Install from media option.

Understanding Universal Group Caching for AD Sites

Windows Server 2003 Active Directory enables the creation of AD Sites that cache universal group membership. Any time a user uses a universal group, the membership of that group is cached on the local domain controller and is used when the next request comes for that group's membership. This also lessens the replication traffic that would occur if a Global Catalog was placed in remote sites.

One of the main sources of replication traffic is group membership queries. In Windows 2000 Active Directory, every time clients logged in, their universal group membership was queried, requiring a Global Catalog to be contacted. This significantly increased login and query time for clients who did not have local Global Catalog servers. Consequently, many organizations had stipulated that every site, no matter the size, have a local Global Catalog server to ensure quick authentication and directory lookups. The downside of this was that replication across the directory was increased, because every site would receive a copy of every item in the entire AD, even though only a small portion of those items would be referenced by an average site.

Universal Group Caching solved this problem because only those groups that are commonly referenced by a site are stored locally, and requests for group replication are limited to the items in the cache. This helps limit replication and keep domain logins speedy.

Universal Group Caching capability is established on a per site basis, through the following technique:

1. Open Active Directory Sites and Services.

2. Navigate to Sites, *sitename*.

3. Right-click NTDS Site Settings and choose Properties.

4. Check the Box labeled Enable Universal Group Membership Caching, as illustrated in Figure 8.6.

5. Click OK to save the changes.

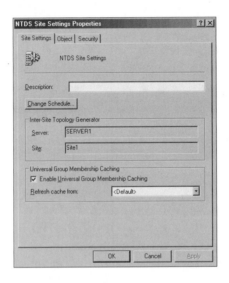

FIGURE 8.6   Universal group caching.

> **NOTE**
>
> Universal group (UG) caching is useful for minimizing remote-site replication traffic and optimizing user logins. Universal group caching does not replace the need for local Global Catalog servers in sites with Exchange 2000/2003 servers, however, because it does not replace the use of the GC Port (3268), which is required by Exchange. UG caching can still be used in remote sites without Exchange servers that use the site consolidation strategies of Exchange Server 2003 previously mentioned.

Exploring DSAccess, DSProxy, and the Categorizer

The relationship that Exchange Server 2003 has with Active Directory is complex and often misunderstood. Because the directory is no longer local, special services were written for Exchange to access and process information in AD. Understanding how these systems work is critical for understanding how Exchange interacts with AD.

Understanding DSAccess

DSAccess is one of the most critical services for Exchange Server 2003. DSAccess, via the dsacccess.dll file, is used to discover current Active Directory topology and direct Exchange to various AD components. DSAccess dynamically produces a list of published AD domain controllers and Global Catalog servers and directs Exchange resources to the appropriate AD resources.

In addition to simple referrals from Exchange to AD, DSAccess intelligently detects Global Catalog and domain controller failures, and directs Exchange to fail over systems dynamically, reducing the potential for downtime caused by a failed Global Catalog server. DSAccess also caches LDAP queries made from Exchange to AD, speeding up query response time in the process.

DSAccess polls the Active Directory every 15 minutes to identify changes to site structure, DC placement, or other structural changes to Active Directory. By making effective use of LDAP searches and Global Catalog port queries, domain controller and Global Catalog server suitability is determined. Through this mechanism, a single point of contact for the Active Directory is chosen, which is known as the Configuration Domain Controller.

Determining the DSAccess Roles

DSAccess identifies AD servers as belonging to one of four groups:

- **Domain Controllers**   Up to 10 domain controllers, which have been identified by DSAccess to be fully operational, are sorted into this group.

- **Global Catalog Servers**   Up to 10 identified Global Catalog domain controllers are placed in this group.

- **Configuration Domain Controller**   A single AD domain controller is chosen as the configuration domain controller to reduce the problems associated with replication latency among AD domain controllers. In other words, if multiple domain controllers were chosen to act as the configuration DC, changes Exchange makes to the directory could conflict with each other. The configuration domain controller role is transferred to other local DCs in a site every eight hours.

- **All Domain Controllers**   This group includes all identified domain controllers, Global Catalog servers, and the configuration domain controller. It often contains multiple listings for the same server if that server appears in more than one group.

The roles that have been identified by DSAccess can be viewed in the Directory Access tab of Exchange Server properties in Exchange System Manager, as illustrated in Figure 8.7. In addition, manual overrides can be performed in this dialog box as necessary.

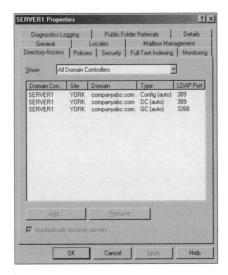

FIGURE 8.7   Directory access groups.

DSAccess went through a complete overhaul in Exchange 2000 Service Pack 2. In addition to integrating new GC promotion safeguards, DSAccess was also optimized to enable Exchange to more easily act as a front-end server in a DMZ environment. Specifically, the reliance on the RPC protocol was eliminated, making it easier to lock down this type of environment.

Understanding DSProxy

DSProxy is a component of Exchange that parses Active Directory and creates an address book for downlevel Outlook (pre–Outlook 2000 SR2) clients. These clients assume that Exchange uses its own directory, as opposed to directly using the Active Directory by itself, as Outlook 2000 SR2-and-greater clients do. The DSProxy service provides these higher-level clients with a referral to an Active Directory Global Catalog server, which they then use without accessing the Exchange servers directly. The newer Outlook clients do not refresh this information unless a server failure has occurred or the client is restarted.

DSProxy uses NSPI instead of LDAP for address list lookups, because NSPI is a more efficient interface for that type of lookup. Only Global Catalog servers support NSPI, so they are necessary for all client address list lookups.

Outlining the Role of the Categorizer

The SMTP Categorizer is a component of Exchange that is used to submit mail messages to their proper destination. When a mail message is sent, the Categorizer queries the DSAccess component to locate an Active Directory server list, which is then directly queried for information that can be used to deliver the message.

Although the Categorizer in Exchange gets a list of all Global Catalog servers from DSAccess, it normally opens only a single LDAP connection to a GC server to send mail, unless a large number of messages are queued for delivery.

> **TIP**
>
> Problems with the Categorizer are often the cause of DNS or AD lookup issues. When troubleshooting mail-flow problems, use message tracking in Exchange Server 2003 to follow the course of a message. If the message stops at the Categorizer, it is often wise to start troubleshooting the issue from a directory access perspective.

Understanding AD Functionality Modes and Their Relationship to Exchange Groups

Exchange Server 2003 and Active Directory functionality was designed to break through the constraints that limited Exchange 5.5 implementations. In order to accomplish this, however, levels of compatibility with downlevel NT domains and Exchange 5.5 organizations was required. These requirements stipulated the creation of several functional modes for AD and Exchange that limit the application of new functionality. Several of the limitations of the AD functional modes in particular impact Exchange Server 2003 itself, specifically Active Directory group functionality. Consequently, a firm grasp of these concepts is warranted.

Understanding Windows Group Types

Groups in Windows Server 2003 come in two flavors; security and distribution. In addition, groups can be organized into different scopes; machine local, domain local, global, and universal. It might seem complex, but the concept, once defined, is simple.

Defining Security Groups

The type of group that administrators are most familiar with is the security group. This type of group is used to apply permissions to resources en masse, so that large groups of users can be administered more easily. Security groups could be established for each department in an organization. For example, users in the marketing department could be given membership in a marketing security group. This group would then have permissions on specific directories in the environment. This concept should be familiar to anyone who has administered downlevel Windows networks, such as NT or Windows 2000.

Defining Distribution Groups in Exchange Server 2003

The concept of distribution groups in Windows Server 2003 was introduced in Windows 2000 with its implementation of Active Directory. Essentially, a distribution group is a group whose members are able to receive SMTP mail messages that are sent to the group. Any application that has the capability of using Active Directory for address book lookups can use this functionality in Windows Server 2003.

Distribution groups are often confused with mail-enabled groups, a concept in environments with Exchange 2000/2003. In addition, in most cases distribution groups are not used in environments without Exchange 2000/2003, because their functionality is limited to infrastructure that can support them.

> **NOTE**
>
> In environments with Exchange 2000/2003, distribution groups can be used to create email distribution lists that cannot be used to apply security. However, if separation of security and email functionality is not required, you can make security groups mail-enabled.

Mail-Enabled Groups in Exchange Server 2003

Exchange Server 2003 utilizes Active Directory mail-enabled groups to their full-extent. These groups are essentially security groups that are referenced by an email address, and can be used to send SMTP messages to the members of the group. This type of functionality becomes possible only with the inclusion of Exchange 2000 or greater. Exchange 2000 actually extends the forest schema to enable Exchange-related information, such as SMTP addresses, to be associated with each group.

Most organizations will find that the concept of mail-enabled security groups satisfies most of the needs, both security and email, in an organization. For example, a single group called Marketing, which contains all users in that department, could also be mail-enabled to allow users in Exchange to send emails to everyone in the department.

Explaining Group Scope

Groups in Active Directory work the way that previous group structures, particularly in Windows NT, have worked, but with a few modifications to their design. As mentioned earlier, group scope in Active Directory is divided into several groups:

- **Machine Local Groups**   Machine local groups, also known as local groups, previously existed in Windows NT 4.0 and can theoretically contain members from any trusted location. Users and groups in the local domain, as well as in other trusted domains and forests can be included in this type of group. However, local groups allow resources only on the machine they are located on to be accessed, which greatly reduces their useability. Machine local groups are not used by Exchange Server 2003 for security.

- **Domain Local Groups**   Domain local groups are essentially the same as local groups in Windows NT, and are used to administer resources located only on their own domain. They can contain users and groups from any other trusted domain and are typically used to grant access to resources for groups in different domains.

- **Global Groups**   Global groups are on the opposite side of domain local groups. They can contain only users in the domain in which they exist, but are used to grant access to resources in other trusted domains. These types of groups are best used to supply security membership to user accounts who share a similar function, such as the sales global group.

- **Universal Groups**   Universal groups can contain users and groups from any domain in the forest, and can grant access to any resource in the forest. With this added power come a few caveats: First, universal groups are available only in Windows 2000 or 2003 AD Native Mode domains. Second, all members of each universal group are stored in the Global Catalog, increasing the replication load. Universal group membership replication has been noticeably streamlined and optimized in Windows Server 2003, however, because the membership of each group is incrementally replicated.

Universal groups are particularly important for Exchange Server 2003. When migrating from Exchange 5.5 to Exchange 2003, for example, Exchange 5.5 distribution lists are converted into universal groups for the proper application of public folder and calendaring permissions. An AD domain that contains accounts that access Exchange 5.5 mailboxes must be in AD Native Mode before performing the migration. For more information on this concept, see Chapter 15, "Migrating from Exchange 5.5 to Exchange Server 2003."

Functional Levels in Windows Server 2003 Active Directory

Active Directory was designed to be backward-compatible. This helps to maintain backward compatibility with Windows NT domain controllers. Four separate functional levels exist at the domain level in Windows Server 2003, and three separate functional levels exist at the forest level:

- **Windows Server 2003 Mixed**   When Windows Server 2003 is installed in a Windows 2000 Active Directory forest that is running in Mixed Mode, Windows Server 2003 domain controllers will be able to communicate with Windows NT and Windows 2000 domain controllers throughout the forest. This is the most limiting of the functional levels, however, because certain functionality—such as universal groups, group nesting, and enhanced security—is absent from the domain. This is typically a temporary level to run in, because it is seen more as a path toward eventual upgrade.

- **Windows Server 2003 Native**   Installed into a Windows 2000 Active Directory that is running in Windows 2000 Native Mode, Windows Server 2003 runs itself at a

Windows 2000/2003 functional level. Only Windows 2000 and Windows Server 2003 domain controllers can exist in this environment.

- **Windows Server 2003 Interim**   Windows Server 2003 interim mode gives Active Directory the capability of interoperating with a domain composed of Windows NT 4.0 domain controllers only. Although a confusing concept at first, the Windows Server 2003 interim functional level does serve a purpose. In environments that seek to upgrade directly from NT 4.0 to Windows Server 2003 Active Directory, interim mode enables Windows Server 2003 to manage large groups more efficiently than if an existing Windows 2000 Active Directory exists. After all NT domain controllers have been removed or upgraded, the functional levels can be raised.

- **Windows Server 2003**   The most functional of all the various levels, Windows Server 2003 functionality is the eventual goal of all Windows Server 2003 Active Directory implementations. Functionality on this level opens the environment to features such as schema deactivation, domain rename, domain controller rename, and cross-forest trusts. To get to this level, first all domain controllers must be updated to Windows Server 2003. Only after this can the domains, and then the forest, be updated to Windows Server 2003 functionality.

As previously mentioned, it is preferable to convert AD domains into Windows Server 2003 Native Mode, or Windows Server 2003 Functional Mode before migrating Exchange 5.5 Servers that use those domains. The universal group capabilities that these modes provide for make this necessary.

To change domain or forest functional levels in Active Directory to the highest level for Windows Server 2003, follow these steps:

1. Open Active Directory Domains and Trusts from Administrative Tools.

2. In the left scope pane, right-click Active Directory Domains and Trusts and then click Raise Domain Functional Level.

3. In the box labeled Select an available domain functional level, select Windows Server 2003 and then choose Raise.

4. Click OK, and then OK again to complete the task.

5. Repeat the steps for all domains in the forest.

6. Perform the same steps on the forest root, except this time click Raise Forest Functional Level and follow the prompts.

After the domains and the forest have been upgraded, the Functional Mode will indicate Windows Server 2003, as shown in Figure 8.8.

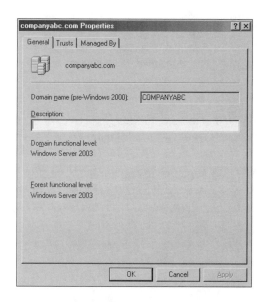

FIGURE 8.8   Windows Server 2003 functional forest.

NOTE

Domain rename functionality in a Windows Server 2003 functional forest was originally created to change only the name of forests with a default Windows Server 2003 schema. This precluded the ability to rename domains that had schema extensions for Exchange 2000/2003. Domain rename capability with Exchange Server 2003 forests, however, is slated to be included in Exchange Server 2003 Service Pack 1.

Exchange Server 2003 Functional Modes

Not to be confused with Windows Server 2003 functional modes, Exchange can be run under two operations modes:

- **Mixed Mode**   An Exchange Server 2003 Organization running in Mixed Mode can support Exchange 5.5 Servers as part of the organization. Exchange routing groups and administrative groups cannot be separated when running in this mode, however.

- **Native Mode**   Native Mode in Exchange Server 2003 supports both Exchange 2000 and Exchange 2003 servers. In addition, Native Mode Exchange organizations support multiple routing groups within the same administrative group.

> **NOTE**
>
> There is no difference in functionality between Exchange Server 2003 and Exchange 2000 from a functional mode perspective. There is no option to upgrade to an Exchange Server 2003-only mode.

To make the change from Exchange Mixed Mode to Native Mode, click the Change Mode button in the properties of the organization, as illustrated in Figure 8.9.

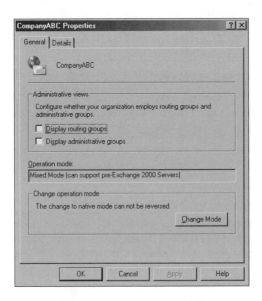

FIGURE 8.9 Switching to Exchange Server 2003 Native Mode.

Summary

Exchange Server 2003 is a powerful but complicated piece of technology. With the scalability and performance enhancements comes an increased degree of interdependence with other system components, most notably the Global Catalog. Access to the Global Catalog and AD domain controllers is critical and cannot be overlooked. A good Exchange deployment plan takes these factors into account.

Best Practices

The following are best practices from this chapter:

- Deploy at least one domain controller in each physical location with more than 10 users.

- Use the Install from Media option to deploy remote Global Catalog servers.

- Promote or demote Global Catalog servers and domain controllers during off-hours.

- Use Exchange Server 2003 site consolidation concepts to reduce the total number of deployed Exchange Servers and Global Catalog servers.

- Understand the role of DSAccess, DSProxy, and the Categorizer and how Global Catalog or domain controller failures can affect them.

- Place at least one GC in close network proximity to any major service (such as Exchange Server 2003) that requires use of the Global Catalog (3268) port.

- Ensure that at least one domain is in Windows 2003 Native mode or Windows Server 2003 functional modes before migrating to Exchange Server 2003.

- Do not use substandard or workstation hardware for Global Catalog servers, because failures can affect Outlook clients.

- Use Outlook 2002 or 2003 clients when possible to reduce the threat of client lockup in the event of GC failure.

- Use universal group caching for domain controllers in sites without local Exchange servers.

CHAPTER 9

Configuring Routing and Remote Access for Mobile Users

For organizations that want to extend Exchange 2003 to dial-up or VPN users, or to create secured tunnels between sites, the Windows 2003 Routing and Remote Access Service (RRAS) provides secured end-to-end connections. RRAS hasn't changed much between Windows 2000 and Windows 2003, but if administrators used Remote Access Server (RAS) in Windows NT4, they'll find drastic improvements in functions and options in the new RRAS technology.

Routing and Remote Access Service provides a secured remote access solution for mobile users. Although Exchange 2003 provides a greatly enhanced Outlook Web Access (covered in Chapter 26, "Everything You Need to Know About the OWA Client") and secured Outlook 2003 to Exchange 2003 RPC over HTTP (covered in Chapter 25, "Getting the Most out of the Microsoft Outlook Client"), which eliminate the need to create VPN tunnels between client and server, organizations still have client-to-server tunnel requirements.

Many users require some form of dial-up modem access for their email in locations where high-speed Internet is not available. Other users not only want to access Outlook information but also transfer files and access other applications over a VPN tunnel. RRAS provides these mobile user capabilities.

RRAS not only provides client-to-server tunneling, but also provides the ability for an organization to establish tunnels between networks for site-to-site tunneling. Rather than paying for expensive point-to-point lease-line connections or frame-relay lines, an organization can establish a tunnel between multiple sites over the Internet. With lower cost

DSL, CableModem, or remote satellite Internet connections, tunnels can secure internal messaging between sites using RRAS.

Windows Server 2003 Routing and Remote Access Features and Services

Windows Server 2003 builds on the Routing and Remote Access features that were provided by Windows NT 4.0 and Windows 2000. Routing and Remote Access in Windows Server 2003 includes all the features and services from all previous versions of the Windows server products combined.

The following features were provided by Windows NT 4.0:

- RIP version 2 routing protocol for IP

- Open Shortest Path First (OSPF) routing protocol for IP

- Demand-dial routing and routing over on-demand or persistent WAN links, such as analog phone, ISDN, or Point-to-Point Tunneling Protocol (PPTP)

- Internet Control Message Protocol (ICMP) router discovery

- Remote Authentication Dial-In User Service (RADIUS) client

- IP and IPX packet filtering

- PPTP support for router-to-router VPN connections

- Routing and RAS Admin administrative tool and the Routemon command-line utility

Windows 2000 expanded the remote access capabilities of the Windows line by adding support for the following features:

- Multiprotocol Routing and Remote Access Service that can route IP, IPX, and AppleTalk simultaneously

- Internet Group Management Protocol (IGMP) and support for multicast boundaries

- Network Address Translation (NAT), which simplifies small office or home office (SOHO) network connections to the Internet through addressing and name resolution components

- Layer 2 Tunneling Protocol (L2TP) over Internet Protocol Security (IPSec) support for router-to-router VPN connections and remote access

- Demand-dial routing that can route IP and IPX over on-demand or persistent WAN links, such as analog phone lines, ISDN, or over VPN connections that use either PPTP or L2TP over IPSec

- RRAS integration that provides the ability to integrate a firewall with RRAS and NAT functions

Windows Server 2003 continues the evolution of RRAS by adding some new features. The Routing and Remote Access Service for Windows 2000 and Windows Server 2003 features include the following:

- Point-to-Point Protocol over Ethernet (PPPoE) Dial-On-Demand

- Background Intelligent Transfer Service (BITS)

- NAT Transversal using Universal Plug and Play (UPnP)

- Improved administration and management tools that use a Microsoft Management Console (MMC) snap-in or the Netsh command-line tool

Using Point-to-Point Protocol over Ethernet Dial-on-Demand

The PPPoE dial-on-demand feature provides the option to use Point-to-Point Protocol over Ethernet (PPPoE) in a dial-on-demand network connection, which enables the use of PPPoE with the RRAS NAT feature to connect to the Internet. PPPoE enables an RRAS server to connect to the Internet through a common broadband medium, such as a single DSL line, wireless device, or cable modem. All the users over the Ethernet share a common connection.

Detailing the Background Intelligent Transfer Service 1.5

Background Intelligent Transfer Service (BITS) is a background file transfer mechanism and queue manager. File transfers through BITS are "throttled" to minimize the effect on system performance because of bandwidth consumed. File transfer requests are also persistent across network disconnects and workstation reboots until the file transfer is complete. When the transfer is complete, the application that requested the file transfer is notified of the completion. This feature enables low-priority download operations to complete in the background without affecting users' bandwidth.

Version 1.5 of BITS adds down-level client support through redistribution, file upload support, and optional advanced upload features. Background File Upload requires the BITS server application, which is included in Windows Server 2003 and is available for redistribution for Windows 2000-based servers.

Understanding NAT Transversal Using Universal Plug and Play

NAT Transversal technology was designed to enable network applications to detect the presence of a local NAT device. NAT Transversal provides a means for applications to create port mappings on local NAT devices, such as Internet Connection Sharing (ICS) and other Internet gateway devices that support UPnP. The applications can identify the external IP address and automatically configure port mappings to forward packets from the external port of the NAT to the internal port used by the network application. Independent Software Vendors (ISVs) can use this feature to develop applications that create port mappings on UPnP-enabled NAT devices.

Configuring Routing and Remote Access Service Architecture

Routing and Remote Access is built on a series of communications and management agents, transport protocols, forwarders, and APIs. These components have been built, expanded, and improved over the years to provide a secure, efficient, effective, and reliable communications system for client-to-server and server-to-server communications in a Windows networking environment.

Understanding the SNMP Agent

Windows Server 2003 RRAS supports the Simple Network Management Protocol (SNMP) Management Information Bases (MIBs). The SNMP agent provides monitoring and alerting information for SNMP management systems. The SNMP agent is a critical component to the reliability and manageability of RRAS as a cornerstone to remote and mobile communications.

Examining Management Applications

Management applications for RRAS include the Routing and Remote Access snap-in and the Netsh command-line utility. These applications help an organization better administer the remote and mobile communications environment.

Detailing Authentication, Authorization, and Accounting

AAA is a set of components that provides authentication, authorization, and accounting for RRAS when it is configured for the Windows authentication provider or the Windows accounting provider. The local AAA components are not used when RRAS is configured for the RADIUS authentication or accounting provider. The AAA components are also used by the Internet Authentication Service (IAS).

Understanding the Dynamic Interface Manager (Mprdim.dll)

The Dynamic Interface Manager component supports a Remote Procedure Call (RPC) interface for SNMP-based management functions used by management utilities such as the Routing and Remote Access snap-in. It communicates with the Connection Manager (CM) for demand-dial connections and configuration information to the router managers (such as the IP Router Manager and IPX Router Manager). The Dynamic Interface Manager also loads configuration information from the Windows Server 2003 Registry. In addition, it manages all routing interfaces, including local area network, persistent demand-dial, and IP-in-IP interfaces.

Working with the Connection Manager

The Connection Manager components manage WAN devices and establish connections by using the Telephony Application Programming Interface (Telephony API or TAPI). The

Connection Manager also negotiates PPP control protocols, including Extensible Authentication Protocol (EAP) and implements Multilink and Bandwidth Allocation Protocol (BAP).

Outlining the Role of the Telephony Application Programming Interface

The Telephony Application Programming Interface provides services to create, monitor, and terminate connections independently of hardware. The Connection Manager uses TAPI to create or receive demand-dial connections.

Conceptualizing the IP Router Manager (Iprtmgr.dll)

The IP Router Manager component obtains configuration information from the Dynamic Interface Manager. It loads and communicates configuration information to IP routing protocols, such as RIP for IP and OSPF supplied with Windows Server 2003. It also communicates IP packet filtering configuration information to the IP filtering driver and communicates IP routing configuration information to the IP forwarder in the TCP/IP protocol. The IP Router Manager also maintains an interface database of all IP routing interfaces. In addition, it initiates demand-dial connections for routing protocols by communicating with the Dynamic Interface Manager.

Configuring the IPX Router Manager (Ipxrtmgr.dll)

The IPX Router Manager obtains configuration information from the Dynamic Interface Manager and maintains an interface database of all IPX routing interfaces. It communicates IPX packet filtering configuration information to the IPX filtering driver and communicates IPX routing configuration information to the IPX forwarder driver. The IPX Router Manager loads and communicates configuration information to IPX routing protocols (RIP for IPX and SAP for IPX). In addition, it initiates demand-dial connections for routing protocols by communicating with the Dynamic Interface Manager.

Understanding Unicast Routing Protocols

RRAS provides the following four unicast routing protocols:

- **RIP for IP (iprip2.dll)**   The RIP for IP routing protocol communicates RIP for IP–learned routes by using the Route Table Manager. It also uses Winsock to send and receive RIP for IP traffic and exports management APIs to support MIBs and management applications through the IP Router Manager.

- **OSPF Routing Protocol (ospf.dll)**   The OSPF routing protocol communicates OSPF-learned routes by using the Route Table Manager. It uses Winsock to send and receive OSPF traffic and exports management APIs to support MIBs and management applications through the IP Router Manager.

- **RIP for IPX (ipxrip.dll)**   The RIP for IPX routing protocol communicates RIP for IPX–learned routes by using the Route Table Manager. It uses Winsock to send and receive RIP for IPX traffic. It also exports management APIs to support MIBs and management applications through the IPX Router Manager.

- **SAP for IPX (ipxsap.dll)**   The SAP for IPX routing protocol communicates SAP for IPX–learned routes by using the Route Table Manager. It uses Winsock to send and receive SAP for IPX traffic and also exports management APIs to support MIBs and management applications through the IPX Router Manager.

Describing IP Multicast Routing Protocols

The IP multicast routing protocol that RRAS uses is IGMP (versions 1, 2, and 3). IGMP communicates multicast group membership information to the Multicast Group Manager. It also uses Winsock to send and receive IGMP traffic and exports management APIs to support MIBs and management applications through the Multicast Group Manager.

Exploring the Role of the Route Table Manager (Rtm.dll)

The Route Table Manager maintains a user-mode route table for all routes from all possible route sources. It displays APIs for adding, deleting, and enumerating routes that are used by the routing protocols. The Route Table Manager also communicates only the best routes to the appropriate forwarder driver. The best routes are those that have the lowest preference level (for IP routes) and the lowest metrics. The best routes become the routes in the IP forwarding table and IPX forwarding table.

Using the Multicast Group Manager

The Multicast Group Manager maintains all multicast group memberships and communicates multicast forwarding entries (MFEs) in the IP Multicast Forwarder. It also reflects group membership between IP multicast routing protocols.

Conceptualizing the IP Filtering Driver (ipfltdrv.sys)

The IP filtering driver obtains configuration information from the IP Router Manager. It also applies IP filters after the IP forwarder has found a route.

Working with IP Unicast Forwarder

The IP Unicast Forwarder, a component of the TCP/IP protocol (Tcpip.sys), obtains configuration information from the IP Router Manager. It stores the IP forwarding table, a table of the best routes obtained from the Route Table Manager. It can also initiate a demand-dial connection and forward unicast IP traffic.

Using IP Multicast Forwarder

The IP Multicast Forwarder, which is a component of the TCP/IP protocol (Tcpip.sys), stores multicast forward entries obtained from IP multicast routing protocols through the Multicast Group Manager. It is based on multicast traffic received and communicates new source or group information to the Multicast Group Manager. It also forwards IP multicast packets.

Outlining the IPX Filtering Driver (Nwlnkflt.sys)

The IPX filtering driver obtains configuration information from the IPX Router Manager and applies IPX filters after the IPX forwarder driver has found a route.

Using the IPX Forwarder Driver (Nwlnkfwd.sys)

The IPX forwarder driver obtains configuration information from the IPX Router Manager and also stores the IPX forwarding table, a table of the best routes obtained from the Route Table Manager. The IPX forwarder driver can initiate a demand-dial connection and forward IPX traffic.

Examining Virtual Private Networks

A virtual private network (VPN) is the extension of a private network that encompasses links across shared or public networks, such as the Internet. A VPN enables data to be sent between two computers across the Internet in a manner that emulates a point-to-point private link. With a virtual private network, illustrated in Figure 9.1, a point-to-point link, or "tunnel," is created by encapsulating or wrapping the data with a header that provides routing information, enabling the data to travel through the Internet. A private link is created by encrypting the data for confidentiality; data packets that are intercepted while traveling through the Internet are unreadable without the proper encryption keys.

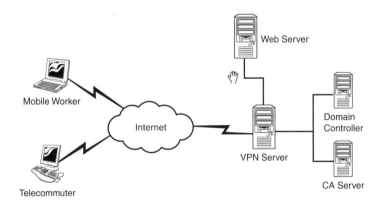

FIGURE 9.1   Virtual private networking across the Internet.

VPN technology provides corporations with a scalable and low-cost solution for remote access to corporate resources. VPN connections allow remote users to securely connect to their corporate networks across the Internet. Remote users would access resources as if they were physically connected to the corporate LAN.

Outlining Components Needed to Create a VPN Connection

A virtual private network connection requires a VPN client and a VPN server. A secured connection is created between the client and server through encryption that establishes a tunnel, as shown in Figure 9.2.

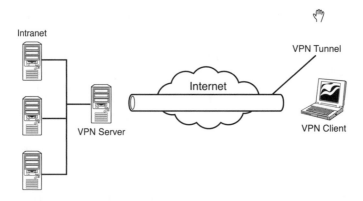

FIGURE 9.2   Establishing a VPN tunnel between a client and server.

Understanding the VPN Client

A **VPN client** is a computer that initiates a VPN connection to a VPN server. It can be a remote computer that establishes a VPN connection or a router that establishes a router-to-router VPN connection. Microsoft clients—including Windows NT 4.0, Windows 9x, Windows 2000, and Windows XP—can create a remote access VPN connection to a Windows Server 2003 system.

Windows NT Server 4.0, Windows 2000 Server, and Windows Server 2003–based computers running RRAS can create router-to-router VPN connections to a Windows Server 2003 VPN server. VPN clients can also be any non-Microsoft PPTP client or L2TP client using IPSec.

Working with the VPN Server

A VPN server is a computer that accepts VPN connections from VPN clients. It can provide a remote access VPN connection or a router-to-router VPN connection. The VPN server name or IP address must be resolvable as well as accessible through corporate firewalls.

Establishing Tunnel/VPN Connections

The tunnel is the portion of the connection in which data is encapsulated. The VPN connection is the portion of the connection where the data is encrypted. The data encapsulation, along with the encryption, provides a secure VPN connection.

> **NOTE**
>
> A tunnel that is created without the encryption is not a VPN connection, because the private data is sent across the Internet unencrypted and can be easily read.

Understanding Internet/Intranet Infrastructure

A shared or public internetwork is required to establish a VPN connection. For Windows Server 2003, the transit internetwork is always an IP-based network that includes the Internet as well as a corporation's private IP-based intranet.

Outlining Authentication Options to an RRAS System

Authentication in any networking environment is critical for validating whether the individual wanting access should be allowed access to network resources. Authentication is an important component in the Windows Server 2003 security initiative. Windows Server 2003 can authenticate a remote access user connection through a variety of PPP authentication protocols, including

- Password Authentication Protocol (PAP)

- Challenge Handshake Authentication Protocol (CHAP)

- Microsoft Challenge Handshake Authentication Protocol (MS-CHAP)

- MS-CHAP version 2 (MS-CHAP v2)

- Extensible Authentication Protocol-Message Digest 5 (EAP-MD5)

- Extensible Authentication Protocol-Transport Level Protocol (EAP-TLS)

Detailing Authentication Protocols for PPTP Connections

For PPTP connections, only three authentication protocols (MS-CHAP, MS-CHAP v2, and EAP-TLS) provide a mechanism to generate the same encryption key on both the VPN client and VPN server. Microsoft Point-to-Point Encryption (MPPE) uses this encryption key to encrypt all PPTP data sent on the VPN connection. MS-CHAP and MS-CHAP v2 are password-based authentication protocols.

Without a Certificate Authority (CA) server or smartcards, MS-CHAP v2 is highly recommended because it provides a stronger authentication protocol than MS-CHAP. MS-CHAP v2 also provides mutual authentication, which allows the VPN client to be authenticated by the VPN server and the VPN server to be authenticated by the VPN client.

If a password-based authentication protocol must be used, it is good practice to enforce the use of strong passwords (passwords greater than eight characters) that contain a random mixture of upper- and lowercase letters, numbers, and punctuation. Group Policies can be used in Active Directory to enforce strong user passwords.

Conceptualizing EAP-TLS Authentication Protocols

Extensible Authentication Protocol-Transport Level Protocol (EAP-TLS) is designed to be used along with a certificate infrastructure that uses user certificates or smartcards. With EAP-TLS, the VPN client sends its user certificate for authentication, and the VPN server sends a computer certificate for authentication. This is the strongest authentication method because it does not rely on passwords. Third-party CAs can be used as long as the certificate in the computer store of the IAS server contains the Server Authentication **certificate purpose** (also known as a **certificate usage** or **certificate issuance policy**). A certificate purpose is identified using an object identifier (OID). If the OID for Server Authentication is 1.2.3.7.6.5.7.8.1, the user certificate installed on the Windows 2000 remote access client must contain the Client Authentication certificate purpose (OID 1.2.3.7.6.5.7.8.2).

Working with Authentication Protocols for L2TP/IPSec Connections

For L2TP/IPSec connections, any authentication protocol can be used because the authentication occurs after the VPN client and VPN server have established a secure connection known as an IPSec security association (SA). Using either MS-CHAP v2 or EAP-TLS provides strong user authentication.

Choosing the Best Authentication Protocol

Very little time is spent by organizations to choose the most appropriate authentication protocol to use with their VPN connections. In many cases, the lack of knowledge about the differences between the various authentication protocols is the reason a selection is not made. In other cases, the desire for simplicity is the reason heightened security is not chosen as part of the organization's authentication protocol decisions. Whatever the case, the following suggestions will assist you in selecting the best authentication protocol for VPN connections:

- Using the EAP-TLS authentication protocol for both PPTP and L2TP connections is highly recommended if the following conditions exist in an organization. If a smartcard will be used, or if a certificate infrastructure that issues user certificates exists, EAP-TLS is the best and most secure option. Note that EAP-TLS is supported only by VPN clients running Windows XP and Windows 2000.

- Use MS-CHAP v2 and enforce strong passwords using group policy if you must use a password-based authentication protocol. Although not as strong a security protocol as EAP-TLS, MS-CHAP v2 is supported by computers running Windows XP, Windows 2000, Windows NT 4.0 with Service Pack 4 and higher, Windows ME, Windows 98, and Windows 95 with the Windows Dial-Up Networking 1.3 or higher Performance and Security Update.

Examining VPN Protocols

PPTP and L2TP are the communication standards used to manage tunnels and encapsulate private data. Data traveling through a tunnel must also be encrypted to be a VPN connection. Windows Server 2003 includes both PPTP and L2TP tunneling protocols.

To establish a tunnel, both the tunnel client and tunnel server must be using the same tunneling protocol. Tunneling technology can be based on either a Layer 2 or Layer 3 tunneling protocol that corresponds to the Open System Interconnection (OSI) Reference Model. Layer 2 protocols correspond to the Data-link layer and use frames as their unit of exchange. PPTP and L2TP are Layer 2 tunneling protocols that encapsulate the payload in a PPP frame before it is sent across the Internet. Layer 3 protocols correspond to the Network layer and use packets. IPSec tunnel mode is a Layer 3 tunneling protocol that encapsulates IP packets in an additional IP header before sending them across the Internet.

Tunneling Within a Windows Server 2003 Networking Environment

For Layer 2 tunneling technologies, such as PPTP and L2TP, a tunnel is similar to a session; both of the tunnel endpoints must agree to the tunnel and must negotiate configuration variables, such as address assignment or encryption or compression parameters. In most cases, data transferred across the tunnel is sent using a datagram-based protocol. A tunnel maintenance protocol is used as the mechanism to manage the tunnel.

Layer 3 tunneling technologies generally assume that all the configuration issues are preconfigured, often by manual processes. For these protocols, there may be no tunnel maintenance phase. For Layer 2 protocols (PPTP and L2TP), however, a tunnel must be created, maintained, and then terminated.

After the tunnel is established, tunneled data can be sent. The tunnel client or server uses a tunnel data transfer protocol to prepare the data for transfer. For example, as illustrated in Figure 9.3, when the tunnel client sends a payload to the tunnel server, the tunnel client first appends a tunnel data transfer protocol header to the payload. The client then sends the resulting encapsulated payload across the internetwork, which routes it to the tunnel server. The tunnel server accepts the packets, removes the tunnel data transfer protocol header, and forwards the payload to the target network. Information sent between the tunnel server and tunnel client behaves similarly.

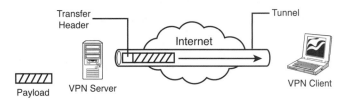

FIGURE 9.3 Tunneling the payload through a VPN connection.

Point-to-Point Tunneling Protocol

The Point-to-Point Tunneling Protocol (PPTP) is a Layer 2 protocol that encapsulates PPP frames in IP datagrams for transmission over the Internet. PPTP can be used for remote access and router-to-router VPN connections. It uses a TCP connection for tunnel maintenance and a modified version of Generic Routing Encapsulation (GRE) to encapsulate PPP frames for tunneled data.

Layer 2 Tunneling Protocol

Layer 2 Tunneling Protocol (L2TP) is a combination of the Point-to-Point Tunneling Protocol (PPTP) and Layer 2 Forwarding (L2F), a technology proposed by Cisco Systems, Inc. L2TP encapsulates PPP frames that are sent over IP, X.25, Frame Relay, and ATM networks. The payloads of encapsulated PPP frames can be encrypted and/or compressed. When sent over the Internet, L2TP frames are encapsulated as User Datagram Protocol (UDP) messages.

L2TP frames include L2TP connection maintenance messages and tunneled data. L2TP connection maintenance messages include only the L2TP header. L2TP tunneled data includes a PPP header and PPP payload. The PPP payload can be encrypted or compressed (or both) using standard PPP encryption and compression methods.

In Windows Server 2003, L2TP connections do not negotiate the use of PPP encryption through Microsoft Point-to-Point Encryption (MPPE). Instead, encryption is provided through the use of the IPSec Encapsulating Security Payload (ESP) header and trailer.

IP Security

IPSec was designed as an end-to-end mechanism for ensuring data security in IP-based communications. The IPSec architecture includes an authentication header to verify data integrity and an encapsulation security payload for both data integrity and data encryption. IPSec provides two important functions that ensure confidentiality: data encryption and data integrity. IPSec uses an authentication header (AH) to provide source authentication and integrity without encryption and the ESP to provide authentication and integrity along with encryption. With IPSec, only the sender and recipient know the security key. If the authentication data is valid, the recipient knows that the communication came from the sender and that it was not changed in transit.

Choosing Between PPTP and L2TP/IPSec

One of the choices to make when you're deploying Windows Server 2003–based VPNs is whether to use L2TP/IPSec or PPTP. Windows XP and Windows 2000 VPN client and server computers support both L2TP/IPSec and PPTP by default. Both PPTP and L2TP/IPSec use PPP to provide an initial envelope for the data and then append additional headers for transport through the Internet. PPTP and L2TP also provide a logical transport mechanism to send PPP payloads and provide tunneling or encapsulation so that PPP payloads based on any protocol can be sent across the Internet. PPTP and L2TP rely on the PPP connection process to perform user authentication and protocol configuration.

There are a few differences between the PPTP and L2TP protocols. First, when using PPTP, the data encryption begins after the PPP connection process is completed, which means PPP authentication is used. With L2TP/IPSec, data encryption begins before the PPP connection process by negotiating an IPSec security association. Second, PPTP connections use MPPE, a stream cipher that is based on the Rivest-Shamir-Aldeman (RSA) RC-4 encryption algorithm and uses 40-, 56-, or 128-bit encryption keys. Stream ciphers encrypt data as a bit stream. L2TP/IPSec connections use the Data Encryption Standard (DES), which is a block cipher that uses either a 56-bit key for DES or three 56-bit keys for 3-DES. Block ciphers encrypt data in discrete blocks (64-bit blocks, in the case of DES). Finally, PPTP connections require only user-level authentication through a PPP-based authentication protocol. L2TP/IPSec connections require the same user-level authentication as well as computer-level authentication using computer certificates.

Advantages of L2TP/IPSec over PPTP

Although PPTP users significantly outnumber L2TP/IPSec users, because of a higher level of security in L2TP/IPSec and several other benefits of L2TP/IPSec, organizations that seek to improve secured remote connectivity are beginning to implement L2TP/IPSec VPN as their remote and mobile access standard. The following are the advantages of using L2TP/IPSec over PPTP:

- IPSec provides per packet data authentication (proof that the data was sent by the authorized user), data integrity (proof that the data was not modified in transit), replay protection (prevention from re-sending a stream of captured packets), and data confidentiality (prevention from interpreting captured packets without the encryption key). PPTP provides only per packet data confidentiality.

- L2TP/IPSec connections provide stronger authentication by requiring both computer-level authentication through certificates and user-level authentication through a PPP authentication protocol.

- PPP packets exchanged during user-level authentication are never sent unencrypted, because the PPP connection process for L2TP/IPSec occurs after the IPSec security associations are established. If intercepted, the PPP authentication exchange for some types of PPP authentication protocols can be used to perform offline dictionary attacks and determine user passwords. If the PPP authentication exchange is encrypted, offline dictionary attacks are possible only after the encrypted packets have been successfully decrypted.

Advantages of PPTP over L2TP/IPSec

Although L2TP/IPSec is perceived to be more secure than a PPTP VPN session, there are significant reasons why organizations choose PPTP over L2TP/IPSec. The following are advantages of PPTP over L2TP/IPSec:

- PPTP does not require a certificate infrastructure. L2TP/IPSec requires a certificate infrastructure for issuing computer certificates to the VPN server computer (or other authenticating server) and all VPN client computers.

- PPTP can be used by all Windows desktop platforms (Windows XP, Windows 2000, Windows NT 4.0, Windows Millennium Edition [ME], Windows 98, and Windows 95 with the Windows Dial-Up Networking 1.3 Performance and Security Update). Windows XP and Windows 2000 VPN clients are the only clients that support L2TP/IPSec and the use of certificates.

IPSec functions at a layer below the TCP/IP stack. This layer is controlled by a security policy on each computer and a negotiated security association between the sender and receiver. The policy consists of a set of filters and associated security behaviors. If a packet's IP address, protocol, and port number match a filter, the packet is subject to the associated security behavior.

Installing and Configuring Routing and Remote Access

Unlike with most network services of Windows Server 2003, RRAS cannot be installed or uninstalled through the Add or Remove Programs applet in the Control Panel. After you install Windows Server 2003, Routing and Remote Access is automatically installed in a disabled state.

To enable and configure the Routing and Remote Access Service, log on using an account that has local administrator privileges. Then follow these steps:

1. Choose Start, Programs, Administrative Tools, Routing and Remote Access, as shown in Figure 9.4.

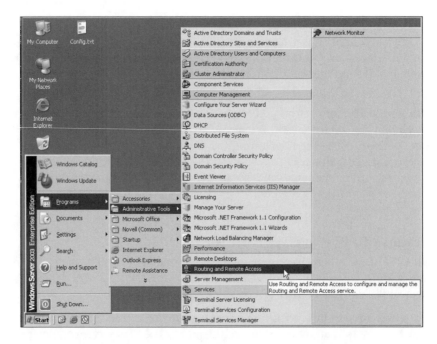

FIGURE 9.4   Launching the Routing and Remote Access administration tool.

2. For the local computer, right-click the server icon and select Configure and Enable Routing and Remote Access, as shown in Figure 9.5.

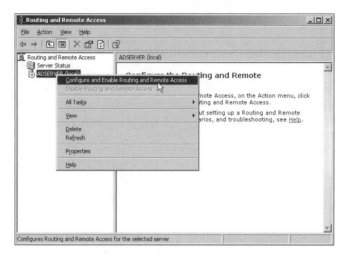

FIGURE 9.5   Configuring and enabling Routing and Remote Access.

3. For a remote computer, right-click the Server Status icon and click Add Server. In the Add Server property page, select the server you want to add. Then right-click the remote server icon and select Configure and Enable Routing and Remote Access.

4. Select the Custom Configuration option and then click Next.

5. Choose the options you want to configure in the Routing and Remote Access Server Setup Wizard, as shown in Figure 9.6.

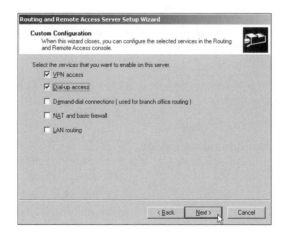

FIGURE 9.6   Choosing installation options in the Routing and Remote Access Server Setup Wizard.

6. After you complete the wizard steps, the remote access router is enabled and configured based on your selections in the wizard. To configure additional features, use the Routing and Remote Access snap-in.

Configuring Remote Access Clients

In a remote access networking environment, the server component is only half of the configuration, and the remote access clients need to be properly configured to complete the secured mobile access environment. There are many variations in remote access client systems that make choosing the right client configuration important.

A client system could vary based on the operating system—such as Windows 95/98, Windows NT4, Windows 2000, or Windows XP—or the client system could be a Macintosh, Unix system, or even a system at an Internet café or kiosk in an airport. The configuration of the client system also varies based on the type of information being transferred—such as email, files, or confidential database information.

This section covers the technologies available and the decisions that need to be made to choose the right configuration for remote access client systems.

Configuring the VPN Client

If you have a small number of VPN clients, you can configure the connections manually for each client. For an environment with 100 or more remote access VPN clients, it makes more sense to configure the remote access configuration automatically. Problems encountered when automatically configuring VPN connections for a large environment include the following:

- The organization has a variety of Windows desktop clients.

- End-users made configuration errors.

- A VPN connection might need a double-dial configuration, wherein a user must dial the Internet before creating a VPN connection with the organization's intranet.

The solution to these configuration issues is to use the Connection Manager, which contains the following features:

- Connection Manager Client Dialer

- Connection Manager Administration Kit

- Connection Point Services

Working with the Connection Manager Client Dialer

The Connection Manager client dialer is software that is installed on each remote access client. It includes advanced features that make it a superset of basic dial-up networking. CM simplifies the client configuration for the users by enabling them to do the following:

- Select from a list of phone numbers to use, based on physical location.

- Use customized graphics, icons, messages, and help.

- Automatically create a dial-up connection before the VPN connection is made.

- Run custom actions during various parts of the connection process, such as pre-connect and post-connect actions.

A customized CM client dialer package (CM profile) is a self-extracting executable file created by the Connection Manager Administration Kit. The CM profile can be distributed to VPN users via CD-ROM, email, Web site, or file share. The CM profile automatically configures the appropriate dial-up and VPN connections. The Connection Manager profile does not require a specific version of Windows and will run on the following platforms: Windows XP, Windows 2000, Windows NT 4.0, Windows Millennium Edition, and Windows 98.

Understanding the Connection Manager Administration Kit

The Connection Manager Administration Kit (CMAK) enables administrators to preconfigure the appearance and behavior of the CM. With CMAK, client dialer and connection software enables users to connect to the network using only the connection features that are defined for them. CMAK also enables administrators to build profiles customizing the Connection Manager Installation package sent to remote access users.

Connection Point Services

Connection Point Services (CPS) enables the automatic distribution and update of custom phone books. These phone books contain one or more Point of Presence (POP) entries, with each POP containing a telephone number that provides dial-up access information for an Internet access point. The phone books give users a complete POP list, which enables remote users to connect to different Internet access points when they travel. CPS also can automatically update the phone book when changes are made to the POP list.

CPS has two components:

- **Phone Book Administrator**   A tool used to create and maintain the phone book database and to publish new phone book information to the Phone Book Service.

- **Phone Book Service**   A Microsoft Internet Information Services (IIS) extension that runs on a Windows Server 2003 server configured with IIS. Phone Book Service automatically checks the current phone book and downloads a phone book update if required.

Single Sign-on Concepts

Single sign-on enables remote access users to create a remote access connection to an organization and log on to the organization's domain by using the same set of credentials. For a Windows Active Directory domain-based infrastructure, the username and password or a smartcard is used for both authenticating and authorizing a remote access connection and for authenticating and logging on to a Windows domain. You enable single sign-on by selecting the Logon by Using Dial-Up Networking option on the Windows XP and Windows 2000 logon property page and then selecting a dial-up or VPN connection to connect to the organization. For VPN connections, the user must first connect to the Internet before creating a VPN connection. After the Internet connection is made, the VPN connection and logon to the domain can be established.

Improving Remove Connectivity with NAT Transversal

Network Address Translation (NAT) Traversal is a set of capabilities that enables network-aware applications to discover they are behind an NAT device, learn the external IP address, and configure port mappings to forward packets from the external port of the NAT to the internal port used by the application. This process happens automatically, so the user does not have to manually configure port mappings. NAT Traversal relies on discovery and control protocols that are part of the Universal Plug and Play Forum–defined specifications. The UPnP Forum has a working committee focused on defining the control protocol for Internet gateway devices and defining the services for these devices. NAT and NAT Traversal will no longer be needed in an IPv6 world where every client has a globally routable IP address.

The significance of NAT Traversal is the ability of a privately addressed L2TP/IPSec client to access an RRAS system. In Windows 2000, although L2TP/IPSec was introduced, it was rarely used for remote users because individuals who connect to the Internet frequently connect through a private address public provider using NAT. As an example, when a user connects to the Internet from a hotel, airport, wireless Internet café connection, or the like, the host provider of Internet connectivity usually does not issue a public IP address. Rather the provider uses Network Address Translation, effectively providing the user a private 10.x.x.x address behind a proxy. With Windows 2000, the L2TP/IPSec client cannot traverse out of the private address space.

With Windows Server 2003, NAT Traversal enables the privately addressed L2TP/IPSec client to route outside the private address zone, thus enabling the client to gain VPN connectivity. In early implementations of Windows Server 2003, many organizations have migrated to this new OS specifically for the benefit of being able to set up an NAT Traversal RRAS system.

Using RRAS Tools and Utilities

Several tools and utilities are available for Windows Server 2003 Routing and Remote Access Service. The following utilities enable administrators to configure and obtain information for accounting, auditing, and troubleshooting RRAS:

- Routing and Remote Access MMC snap-in

- Netsh command-line tool

- Authentication and accounting logging

- Event logging

- Tracing

Routing and Remote Access MMC Snap-in

The Routing and Remote Access snap-in, shown in Figure 9.7, is located in the Administrative Tools folder. It is the primary management tool for configuring Windows Server 2003 RRAS.

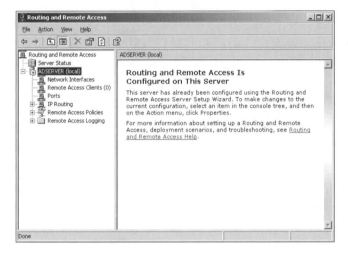

FIGURE 9.7   Administering RRAS through the Routing and Remote Access snap-in.

Within the RRAS snap-in is a series of floating windows that display table entries or statistics. After a floating window is displayed, you can move it anywhere on the screen, and it remains on top of the Routing and Remote Access snap-in. Table 9.1 lists the floating windows in the Routing and Remote Access snap-in and includes their location.

TABLE 9.1   Routing and Remote Access Floating Windows

Floating Window	Location	Description
TCP/IP information	IP Routing/General/Interface	Global TCP/IP statistics, such as the number of routes, incoming and outgoing bytes
Multicast boundaries	IP Routing/General/Interface	The contents of the TCP/IP multicast boundaries

TABLE 9.1   Continued

Floating Window	Location	Description
Multicast statistics	IP Routing/General	Statistics per group, such as the number of multi-cast packets received
Address translations	IP Routing/General/Interface	The contents of the Address Resolution Protocol (ARP) cache
IP addresses	IP Routing/General/Interface	The IP addresses assigned to routing interfaces
IP routing table	IP Routing/General/Static Routes	The contents of the IP routing table
RRAS clients	Remote Access Clients	The list of client connections, including local and remote addresses and TCP ports
UDP listener ports	Ports	The list of UDP ports on which the router is listening
Areas	IP Routing/OSPF	The list of configured OSPF areas
Link state database	IP Routing/OSPF	The contents of the OSPF link state database
Neighbors (OSPF)	IP Routing/OSPF	The list of neighboring OSPF routers and their state
Virtual interfaces	IP Routing/OSPF	The list of configured virtual interfaces and their state
Neighbors (RIP)	IP Routing/RIP	The list of neighboring RIP routers
DHCP Allocator information	IP Routing/NAT/Basic Firewall	Statistics on the number and types of DHCP messages sent and received
DNS Proxy information	IP Routing/Network Address Translation	Statistics on the number of types of DNS messages sent and received
Mappings	IP Routing/NAT/Basic Firewall/Interface	Contents of the Network Address Translation mapping table
Group table	IP Routing/IGMP	Global list of groups detected by using the IGMP routing protocol
Interface group table	IP Routing/IGMP/Interface	Interface list of groups detected by using the IGMP routing protocol
IPX parameters	IPX Routing/General	Global IPX statistics, such as the number of routes and services, packets received, and packets forwarded
IPX routing table	IPX Routing/Static Routes	The contents of the IPX routing table
IPX service table	IPX Routing/Static Services	The contents of the SAP service table
RIP parameters	IPX Routing/RIP for IPX	Global statistics on the RIP for IPX protocol
SAP parameters	IPX Routing/SAP for IPX	Global statistics on the SAP for IPX protocol

The Netsh Command-Line Tool

Netsh is a command-line and scripting tool used to configure Windows Server 2003 networking components on local or remote computers. Windows Server 2003 Netsh also enables you to save a configuration script in a text file for archiving or for configuring other servers. Netsh is installed with the Windows Server 2003 operating system.

Netsh is a shell that can support multiple Windows Server 2003 components through the addition of Netsh helper DLLs. A Netsh helper DLL extends Netsh functionality by providing additional commands to monitor or configure a specific Windows Server 2003 networking component. Each Netsh helper DLL provides a context or group of commands for a specific networking component. Subcontexts can exist within each context; for example, within the routing context, the subcontexts IP and IPX exist to group IP routing and IPX routing commands.

Netsh command-line options include the following:

- **-a** *<AliasFile>*   Specifies that an alias file be used. An alias file contains a list of Netsh commands and an aliased version so that the aliased command line can be used in place of the Netsh command. Alias files can be used to map commands to the appropriate Netsh command that might be more familiar in other platforms.

- **-c** *<Context>*   Specifies the context of the command corresponding to an installed helper DLL.

- *Command*   Specifies the Netsh command to carry out.

- **-f** *<ScriptFile>*   Specifies that all the Netsh commands in the file *ScriptFile* be run.

- **-r** *<Remote Computer Name or IP Address>*   Specifies that Netsh commands are run on the remote computer specified by its name or IP address.

You can abbreviate Netsh commands to the shortest unambiguous string. For example, typing the command **ro ip sh int** is equivalent to typing **routing ip show interface**. Netsh commands can be either global- or context-specific. You can issue global commands in any context and use them for general Netsh functions. Context-specific commands vary according to the context. Table 9.2 lists the global commands for Netsh.

TABLE 9.2 Netsh Commands

Command	Description
..	Moves up one context level
? or help	Displays command-line help
add helper	Adds a Netsh helper DLL
delete helper	Removes a Netsh helper DLL

TABLE 9.2   Continued

Command	Description
show helper	Displays the installed Netsh helper DLLs
online	Sets the current mode to Online
offline	Sets the current mode to Offline
set mode	Sets the current mode to Online or Offline
show mode	Displays the current mode
flush	Discards any changes in Offline mode
commit	Commits changes made in Offline mode
show machine	Displays the computer name on which the Netsh commands are carried out
exec	Executes a script file containing Netsh commands
quit or bye or exit	Exits Netsh
add alias	Adds an alias to an existing command
delete alias	Deletes an alias from an existing command
show alias	Displays all defined aliases
dump	Writes the configuration
popd	For a script, pops (fetches) a context from the stack
pushd	For a script, pushes (adds) the current context onto the stack

Netsh can function in two modes: Online and Offline. In Online mode, commands executed by Netsh are carried out immediately. In Offline mode, commands executed at the Netsh prompt are accumulated and carried out as a batch by using the commit global command. The flush global command discards the batch commands. Netsh commands can also run through a script. You can run the script by using the -f option or by executing the exec global command at the Netsh command prompt.

The dump command can be used to generate a script that captures the current RRAS configuration. This command generates the current running configuration in terms of Netsh commands. The generated script can be used to configure a new RRAS server or modify the current one.

For the Routing and Remote Access Service, Netsh has the following contexts:

- **ras**   Use commands in the ras context to configure remote access configuration.

- **aaa**   Use commands in the aaaa context to configure the AAA component used by both Routing and Remote Access Service and Internet Authentication Service.

- **routing**   Use commands in the routing context to configure IP and IPX routing.

- **interface**   Use commands in the interface context to configure demand-dial interfaces.

Authentication and Accounting Logging

The Routing and Remote Access Service can log authentication and accounting information for PPP-based connection attempts. This logging is separate from the events found in the system event log and can assist in tracking remote access use and authentication attempts. Authentication and accounting logging is useful for troubleshooting remote access policy issues; the result of each authentication attempt is recorded, as is the remote access policy that was applied. The authentication and accounting information is stored in a configurable log file or in files stored in the `%systemroot%\System32\LogFiles` folder. The log files are saved in Internet Authentication Service (IAS) or in a database-compatible format, which can enable database programs to read the log file directly for analysis. Logging can be configured for the type of activity you want to log (accounting or authentication activity). The log file settings can be configured from the properties of the Local File object in the Remote Access Logging folder in the Routing and Remote Access snap-in.

Event Logging

Windows Server 2003 RRAS also performs extensive error logging in the system event log. You can use information in the event logs to troubleshoot routing or remote access problems.

The following four levels of logging are available:

- Log errors only (the default).

- Log errors and warnings.

- Log the maximum amount of information.

- Disable event logging.

You can set the level of event logging on the General tab of the following property pages:

- IP Routing/General

- IP Routing/NAT/Basic Firewall

- IP Routing/OSPF

- IP Routing/IGMP

- IPX Routing/General

- Routing/RIP for IPX

- IPX Routing/SAP for IPX

NOTE

Logging uses system resources; therefore, you should use it sparingly to help identify network problems. After you identify the problem, reset the logging to its default setting (log errors only).

Tracing

RRAS for Windows Server 2003 provides extensive tracing capability that can be used to troubleshoot complex network problems. By enabling file tracing, you can record internal component variables, function calls, and interactions. File tracing can be enabled on various RRAS components to log tracing information to files. Enabling file tracing requires changing settings in the Windows Server 2003 Registry.

CAUTION

Do not edit the Registry unless you have no alternative. The Registry Editor bypasses standard safeguards, allowing settings that can damage your system or even require you to reinstall Windows.

Each installed routing protocol or component is capable of tracing, and each appears as a subkey, such as OSPF and RIPV2.

Similar to the authentication and accounting logging, tracing consumes system resources; therefore, you should use it sparingly to help identify network problems. After the trace is complete or the problem is identified, immediately disable tracing. Do not leave tracing enabled on multiprocessor computers.

The tracing information can be complex and detailed. Often, this information is useful only to Microsoft support engineers or network administrators who are experts in using the Windows Server 2003 Routing and Remote Access Service. To enable file tracing for each component, do the following:

1. Run `regedit.exe` and navigate to the following Registry key:

   `HKEY_LOCAL_MACHINE\SOFTWARE\Microsoft\Tracing\<Component>`

   (*Component* represents the component for which you want to enable file tracing.)

2. Select the component for which you want to enable file tracing.

3. Right-click the EnableFileTracing entry, click Modify, and then assign a value of **1** (the default value is **0**).

4. For the selected component, modify additional entries as needed:

   To set the location of the trace file, right-click the FileDirectory entry, click Modify, and then type the location of the log file as a path. The filename for the log file is the name of the component for which tracing is enabled. By default, log files are placed in the `%windir%\Tracing` directory.

   To set the level of file tracing, right-click the FileTracingMask entry, click Modify, and then type a value for the tracing level. The tracing level can be from **0** to **0xFFFF0000**. By default, the level of file tracing is set to **0xFFFF0000**, which is the maximum level of tracing.

To set the maximum size of a log file, right-click the MaxFileSize entry, click Modify, and then type a size for the log file. The default value is `0x00100000`, or 64KB.

Remote Access Scenarios

To help you better understand how Routing and Remote Access can be leveraged in an enterprise environment, we've created a couple of scenarios. The following two scenarios include mobile and home user access of RRAS and a site-to-site connected RRAS environment.

Remote Mobile and Home Users

Remote access users connecting from home or a hotel have several options. The connection options depend on the available hardware connection and the version of the Windows desktop operating system. The following are some options available to remote mobile and home users:

- **Dial-up Remote Access**   Remote and mobile users can access corporate network resources by dialing up to an RRAS server. The dial-up VPN client, shown in Figure 9.8, initiates a connection to an RRAS server to authenticate the user and then provides access to the corporate intranet.

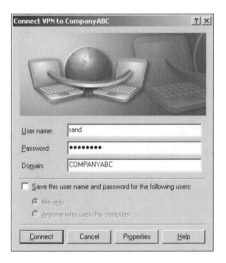

FIGURE 9.8   Using the dial-up window to connect to an RRAS server.

- **Windows Terminal Services (WTS)**   Windows Terminal Services provides remote and mobile users access to Windows-based programs running on a Windows Server 2003. With WTS, users can run programs, open and save files, and use corporate network resources as if they were installed on their local computers. Using

Windows Server 2003 WTS also enables users to access their local drives for file transfers, access serial devices, and print to their local printers. Remote home users can access the WTS server through direct dial-up, Internet Explorer (requires an ActiveX plug-in), and Windows Terminal Server Client. Terminal Services is covered in detail in Chapter 21, "Using Terminal Services to Manage Exchange Servers."

- **VPN Connection**   Remote and mobile users who have access to the Internet can create VPN connections to establish remote access connections to a corporate intranet. VPN remote access eliminates the need for long-distance calls to corporate RAS servers. Remote clients can use their connections to local ISPs to create VPN connections to their corporate office. The VPN software creates a virtual private network between the dial-up user and the corporate VPN server across the Internet. VPN clients have a choice of connecting by using PPTP or L2TP or having the connection automatically selected, as shown in Figure 9.9. As stated earlier in this chapter, PPTP is supported by a variety of Windows desktop platforms but does not have the level of security provided by L2TP/IPSec. L2TP/IPSec provides a higher level of data integrity and security but requires a certificate infrastructure.

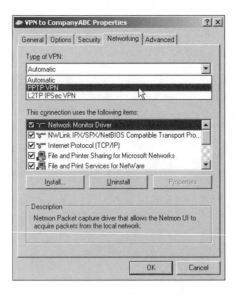

FIGURE 9.9   Choosing between the PPTP, L2TP, or automatic connection type.

Site-to-Site Connections

Organizations can also use VPN connections to establish routed and secure connections between geographically separate offices or other organizations over the Internet. A routed VPN connection across the Internet logically operates as a dedicated WAN link. The two methods for using VPNs to connect local area networks at remote sites are as follows:

- **Using Dedicated Lines to Connect Branch Offices**   Rather than using an expensive dedicated circuit between the branch offices, both the branch office RRAS servers can use a local dedicated circuit and local ISP to connect to the Internet. The VPN software uses the local ISP connections and the Internet to create a virtual private network between the branch office servers.

- **Using a Dial-Up Line to Connect Branch Offices**   Instead of having an RRAS server initiate a long-distance call to another RRAS server, the server at each branch office can call a local ISP to establish a connection to the Internet. The VPN software uses the Internet connection to create a VPN between the branch office servers across the Internet.

In both cases, the services that connect the branch offices to the Internet are local. The office routers that act as VPN servers must be connected to a local ISP with a dedicated line. This VPN server must be listening 24 hours a day for incoming VPN traffic.

Summary

For many users who want to access their Exchange email remotely without using the new Outlook Web Access or RPC over HTTP method of access, using a dial-up or VPN access through Routing and Remote Access Service provides a flexible and secure alternative. Additionally, for a solution of providing secure site-to-site communications, possibly over the Internet between multiple Exchange site locations, RRAS also provides the ability to tunnel between multiple locations.

With high-speed Internet connectivity in hotels, airports, cafés, homes, and office buildings, mobile users have relatively easy access to either Ethernet connections or wireless connections as they travel. By leveraging the technologies built in to Windows Server 2003, and extending the communications to Exchange 2003 messaging communications, users have several options to always keep in touch with their mail, calendar, contacts, and other corporate communications information.

Best Practices

The following are best practices from this chapter:

- Use the EAP-TLS authentication protocol for both PPTP and L2TP connections

- If a smartcard will be used, or if a certificate infrastructure that issues user certificates exists, use EAP-TLS.

- Use MS-CHAP v2 and enforce strong passwords using group policy if you must use a password-based authentication protocol.

- Use IPSec to provide per packet data authentication (proof that the data was sent by the authorized user), data integrity (proof that the data was not modified in transit), replay protection (prevention from resending a stream of captured packets), and data confidentiality (prevention from interpreting captured packets without the encryption key).

- L2TP/IPSec connections provide stronger authentication by requiring both computer-level authentication through certificates and user-level authentication through a PPP authentication protocol.

- PPTP does not require a certificate infrastructure. L2TP/IPSec requires a certificate infrastructure for issuing computer certificates to the VPN server computer (or other authenticating server) and all VPN client computers.

- Use PPTP for versions of Windows prior to Windows 2000 and Windows XP.

- For an environment with a hundred or more remote access VPN clients, configure the remote access solution automatically using the Connection Manager Administration Kit.

- Logging remote access activity uses system resources; therefore, use it sparingly to help identify network problems.

- Do not leave tracing enabled on multiprocessor computers.

CHAPTER 10

Outlook Web Access 2003

Beginning with Exchange 5.5, the Outlook Web Access (OWA) tool has offered users the ability to view email information from a Web browser. Early versions of the OWA client were cumbersome, lacked functionality, and didn't scale very well beyond a few hundred connections. With Exchange 2000, the OWA client was rewritten and improved, but still lacked many of the functional characteristics of the full Outlook client. The Outlook Web Access Client in Exchange Server 2003, however, is vastly improved and closer than ever to full Outlook client functionality.

As the OWA client has improved, the need for the Exchange Server infrastructure to support and streamline OWA has risen as well. In the past, many organizations removed or disabled OWA functionality for security or support reasons. With Exchange Server 2003, the arguments against using OWA are diminished, and it becomes more important to analyze how OWA can fit into a client access plan.

This chapter focuses on configuring an Exchange Server 2003 to support Outlook Web Access functionality. It focuses on best practices of front-end/back-end server configuration, including network load balancing (NLB) and front-end server upgrade considerations.

Understanding OWA and the Exchange Virtual Server

Unlike Exchange 5.5, every deployed Exchange 2000 and Exchange 2003 Server has OWA functionality built in via the HTTP virtual server component of IIS. The HTTP virtual server acts as a proxy to the Information Store, relaying requests made through OWA to the mailboxes. The IIS installation on each Exchange Server also handles POP3, IMAP4, NNTP, and SMTP access in a similar fashion, through virtual servers for each component, as illustrated in Figure 10.1.

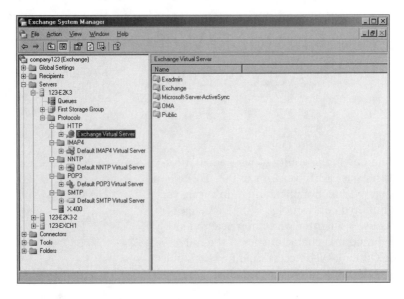

FIGURE 10.1   Virtual servers in Exchange Server 2003.

> **NOTE**
>
> For security reasons, the POP3, IMAP4, and NNTP Services are disabled in Exchange Server 2003. To enable these virtual servers, the services must first be started and set to run automatically. After this has been done, the virtual servers can be started to provide access via these protocols.

The virtual server concept is important because it provides the basis for more advanced and secure OWA designs.

Designing an OWA Infrastructure

All deployed Exchange Server 2003 systems will be running OWA, and there might be times you will not want to expose mailbox servers directly to HTTP access, especially from unsecured networks such as the Internet. In organizations with fewer security requirements, allowing Port 80 (or preferably encrypted SSL traffic over Port 443) through a firewall to the Exchange 2003 server will suffice. Larger or more security-conscious organizations might require an additional buffer of security, in the form of front-end/back-end server topology.

Designing an Exchange Front-end/Back-end OWA Architecture

The ability to configure front-end servers is a new concept introduced in Exchange 2000 and improved upon in Exchange Server 2003. Exchange 5.5 allowed an ASP-based front-end server for Outlook Web Access by enabling a dedicated IIS server to handle OWA client traffic, but Exchange 2000/2003 enables an increased degree of flexibility by offloading all protocols and enabling load balancing of those servers.

Front-end servers contain no mailboxes, and proxy HTTP, POP3, and IMAP traffic to a back-end server. They cannot, however, handle MAPI request in the same way, because MAPI clients must communicate directly with the server containing the client's mailbox. The term **back-end server** refers to any Exchange 2000/2003 server that contains the mailbox store and is configured to communicate with a front-end server for IMAP, HTTP, or POP3. Back-end servers could handle all the tasks that the front-end servers handle, but separating front-end/back-end responsibilities provides the following benefits:

- **Isolates the Servers Containing the Mailbox Store**   This enables the servers with mailboxes to remain in a secure network, and the front-end servers can be placed in the DMZ where an attack is more likely.

- **Offloads Processing Overhead for Encryption/Decryption Processes**   SSL-based encryption and decryption processes, which are used to secure HTTP, POP3, and IMAP, add 15% to 40% processor overhead to the Exchange Server and can be delegated to the front-end server.

- **Enables Multiple Servers to Have the Same Alias in DNS**   Using a DNS round-robin between Exchange servers with mailbox stores forces users to authenticate twice if the first server they are directed to does not contain their mailbox. This will not occur with front-end servers configured in a round-robin as long as all front-end servers can communicate directly with all mailbox store servers.

- **Enables Automatic Referrals to Public Folder Content for IMAP Clients** Many IMAP clients do not handle referrals to other servers. When an IMAP client needs folder content that might be available on another server, a front-end server will handle the referral and provide the public folder content for the IMAP client.

Front-end/Back-end Servers

When a client connects to a front-end server for HTTP access, the front-end server queries Active Directory to find the correct back-end server that contains the user's mailbox. The front-end server then sends the request to the back-end server, with the HTTP host header unmodified.

For the back-end server to respond to the front-end server's request, an HTTP virtual server must exist on the back-end server that is configured to communicate with the front-end server. Both the front-end server and back-end server must have identical HTTP virtual servers for this communication to take place. This is an important consideration because it effectively means that the back-end HTTP virtual server or servers must be enabled for front-end OWA to function properly. The back-end server treats the front-end server the same as it would a client who connected directly to the back-end server. When the back-end server responds to the client request, the communication travels through the front-end server unchanged.

> **NOTE**
>
> Each Exchange Server 2003 system can contain multiple HTTP virtual servers. This is useful in situations where an OWA server needs to respond to requests from OWA clients from multiple domains. For example, if a single OWA server will respond to `owa.companyabc.com`, `owa.company123.org`, and `owa.organizationy.com`, virtual servers need to be set up for each domain on both the front-end and back-end server, because the host header information does not change when proxying requests.

The following are a few facts to note regarding the communication between the front-end and back-end server:

- **Front-end and back-end servers communicate only over port 80.**   Trying to use any other port on the virtual server, such as 8080, will not work.

- **SSL cannot be used between front-end and back-end servers to secure communication.**   Use IPSec to secure traffic between front-end/back-end servers when it must traverse unsecured networks.

- **Front-end servers support only HTTP 1.1 basic authentication.**   If users will be connecting to the server over the Internet, SSL should be enabled on the front-end server to secure the session and the user's credentials.

- **When authenticating to the front-end server, users need to enter the domain name.**   User credentials need to be entered in the format domain/ username.

Planning for Front-end OWA Servers

The general recommendation from Microsoft is to plan for one front-end server for no more than four back-end servers. Front-end servers require fast processors to handle tasks such as encryption through SSL or IPSec, and they should also be configured with sufficient memory. Large disks are not required in the front-end servers because they have unpopulated mail store databases or no databases at all. The level of fault tolerance in the front-end server is really up to the organization. If features such as network load balancing are enabled, it might not be worth spending the extra dollars for RAID controllers, redundant fans, and network adapters. If NLB is not used, organizations should consider at least hardware RAID 1 disk configuration.

Securing Communications on Front-end Servers

If the front-end server will be used for Internet clients, the communication between the client and the server should be secured using SSL.

> **NOTE**
>
> For steps on configuring a front-end server for SSL see the section later in this chapter, "Using SSL to Secure Access to the Front-end Server."

If secure communication is needed between the front-end and back-end servers, IPSec can be implemented. The back-end server should be configured for Client (respond only) so that IPSec is not required for MAPI client access. On the front-end server, only HTTP traffic initiated by the front-end server on Port 80 should be configured for IPSec. IPSec firewalls will have to be opened for IP identifiers 50 and 51.

Understanding Authentication in Front-end/Back-end Servers

When connecting to the front-end server, the user can be authenticated in a number of places. Depending on the security policy for the organization, users can be authenticated at the back-end server or both the front-end and the back-end servers.

If the front-end server is enabled for authentication, the users can connect to the front-end server using an implicit logon or an explicit logon. This implicit logon is in the format of http://server/exchange and the explicit logon is in the form of http://server/exchange/username. When authentication is disabled on the front-end server, users must use the explicit logon and are authenticated by the back-end server only.

Users will always be authenticated on the back-end server regardless of the front-end configuration; however, if the front-end server is enabled for authentication, the authentication credentials are passed from the front-end server to the back-end server automatically, so users are prompted only once to authenticate. Behind the scenes, however, the servers process the authentication twice.

Not using authentication on the front-end server has a few disadvantages besides not being able to use implicit logons. When authentication is enabled, administrators can configure a simplified URL for OWA access, so users do not have to attach /exchange to the http://servername. To configure a simplified URL, open Internet Services Manager. Configure the Default Web Site Home Directory on the front-end server to A redirection to a URL and enter /**exchange** in the Redirect to box, as shown in Figure 10.2. Remember to mark the check box for A directory below URL entered; otherwise, the redirection will not work.

10

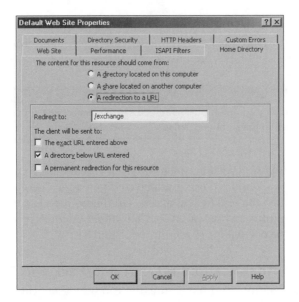

FIGURE 10.2   Configuring a simplified URL.

With authentication disabled on the front-end server, public folder requests cannot be load-balanced. When front-end servers authenticate the user, they know which public folder the user is configured for and make sure the user is connected to the correct public folder server. The front-end server can also query Active Directory and direct users to the appropriate public folder server for public folder applications. If a user requests content that is not available on the user's home public folder server, the front-end servers keep a cache of which public folder replicas exist on each public folder servers to get users to the content more quickly on subsequent requests.

To disable authentication on the front-end server, use Internet Services Manager and access the properties of each virtual directory in the HTTP virtual server on the front-end server. Use the Authentication button on the Access tab and uncheck Integrated Windows authentication and Basic authentication; then check Enable anonymous access, as shown in Figure 10.3. After this, enter the account to use for anonymous access.

> **NOTE**
>
> For security reasons, it is not generally recommended to disable authentication on the front-end server, because it leaves the back-end servers open to denial-of-service attacks, negating some of the protections that the front-end servers provide.

Configuring a Firewall for Front-end Servers

To use a front-end/back-end server configuration with firewalls, the front-end server must be able to initiate a connection to the back-end server. If the front-end server is behind a firewall, the organization's security policy must permit the front-end server to initiate the connection to the back-end server or the organization will not be able to use front-end/back-end servers.

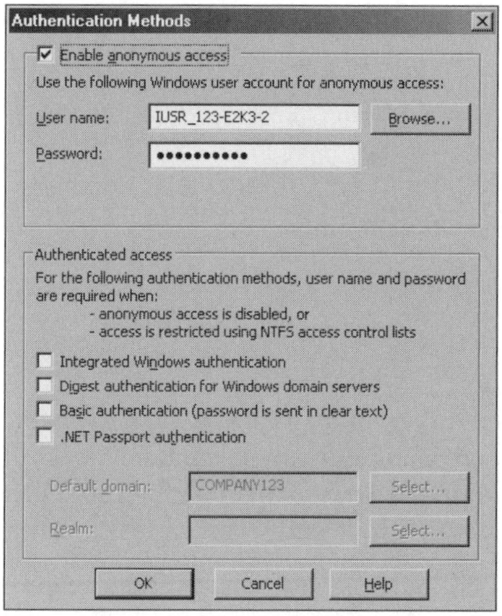

FIGURE 10.3   Disabling front-end server authentication.

For client access to the front-end server, the following ports must be open from the Internet to the front-end server or servers. If one or more of these protocols will not be supported, they can be disabled:

- **443/TCP HTTPS**   HTTP secured with SSL.

- **993/TCP IMAPS**   IMAP secured with SSL.

- **995/TCP POP3S**   POP3 secured with SSL.

- **25/TCP SMTP**   Required for relaying from POP3 and IMAP clients or receiving Internet mail from the outside. This is not required if SMTP mail is relayed from another location or not allowed.

> **NOTE**
>
> Although it is not normally recommended to allow non-encrypted traffic over the "normal" ports for HTTP, IMAP4, and POP3 (80, 143, and 110), it can be allowed, depending on the security requirements of the organization. In addition, if port 80 is open, clients need to be educated to access the server over an https:\\ connection. If this is not feasible, port 80 has to be opened, and a special Web page can be placed that automatically redirects clients to use the SSL port.

10

For the front-end server to communicate with the back-end server, the following ports must be open between the front-end server(s) and the internal network:

- 80/TCP HTTP

- 143/TCP IMAP

- 110/TCP POP3

- 25/TCP SMTP

- 389/TCP LDAP Access to Active Directory

- 3268/TCP Access to the Global Catalog

- 88/TCP Kerberos Authentication

- 88/UDP Kerberos Authentication

It's also recommended to open Port 53 for TCP and UDP to enable the front-end server to query DNS for the global catalog and domain controller records. If the DNS ports are not open, a host file can be used on the server. The host file should list all global catalog and domain controller servers that the front-end server needs to contact.

Exchange Server 2003 front-end servers have reduced their reliance on requiring RPC between the front-end servers and the AD domain controllers, but unfortunately have not completely divorced themselves from this role. Specifically, front-end servers require RPC for client authentication and to do queries to locate AD domain controllers and global catalog servers.

To support client authentication on the front-end server, the following additional ports should be opened:

- 135/TCP RPC Port Endpoint Mapper

- 1024+/TCP RPC Service Ports

- 445/TCP Netlogon

If it is not possible to open dynamic RPC ports between front-end servers and the AD domain controllers, it might be possible to force AD to communicate over specific ports through a Registry change on all domain controllers. Because this requires production domain controller changes that differ from general best practice, it is not normally recommended.

Disabling Unnecessary Services on the Front-end Server

Front-end servers require only a few services to operate. Listed are the services that are required by each protocol on the front-end server:

- **HTTP**   World Wide Web Publishing Service and Exchange System Attendant

- **POP3**   Exchange POP3, Exchange System Attendant, and Exchange Information Store

- **IMAP**   Exchange IMAP, Exchange System Attendant, and Exchange Information Store

> **NOTE**
>
> All Exchange services other than the HTTP, POP3, and IMAP services should be left disabled in the Services snap-in on the front-end servers. This ensures that the front-end server processes only the tasks necessary to be dedicated to service.

By default, in POP3 and IMAP configurations, the front-end server requires a storage group on the server even though it might not contain any databases. The storage group can be removed if the dependencies on the Exchange information store are removed in the Registry. To remove the POP3 and IMAP front-end servers' dependency on the Exchange Information Store, remove the MSExchangeIS entry from the DependOnService Registry entries in the following Registry keys:

HKEY_LOCAL_MACHINE\System\CurrentControlSet\Services\IMAP4SVC

HKEY_LOCAL_MACHINE\System\CurrentControlSet\Services\POP3SVC

When a firewall separates the front-end and back-end servers and the RPC ports are not open, the POP3 and IMAP dependency on the Exchange Information Store must be removed.

For HTTP, POP3, and IMAP configurations, all public folder store databases should be deleted from the server. Mail store databases can be left on the server as long as they do not contain any mailboxes. Leaving the mail store databases on the server enables the Internet Service Manager to be run against the server, so items such as the SSL configuration can be modified.

Front-end servers that receive mail from the Internet need to retain at least one private information store so non-delivery receipts (NDRs) can be sent to Internet users. If one store is not mounted, the message conversion cannot take place and the NDR messages become stuck in the local delivery queue. An information store database is also required if there are Exchange 5.5 servers in the same routing group to enable the MTA to transfer mail over RPC.

Reducing Server Configuration

As the number of front-end servers grows, the overhead of configuring each back-end server to communicate with the front-end servers grows too. Remember that each back-end server must have a corresponding HTTP virtual server for each front-end server. Using a single HTTP virtual server on the back-end server configured for all front-end servers is possible and can help reduce the HTTP virtual server configuration overhead with a large number of front-end servers. This technique can be used as long as the front-end server configurations are identical.

Two methods of configuring front-end/back-end servers exist. Organizations have the option of building new HTTP virtual servers on the front-end and back-end servers, or they can choose to use the default HTTP virtual servers that are created during the Exchange Server 2003 installation. The easiest method is to use the default virtual server configuration. Organizations should not consider creating new virtual servers and building a custom configuration unless they have been successful in the lab with front-end/back-end servers in the default virtual server configuration.

Configuring Network Load Balancing for Front-end Servers

A DNS-based round-robin can be used to load-balance between front-end servers by creating multiple A records for each front-end server with the same hostname—for instance, `mail.company.com`. This solution provides primitive load balancing and works well while all servers are online. The disadvantage to this solution is that the DNS will still return the IP address of a failed server in the round-robin.

A better solution for load balancing is to use the Network Load Balancing (NLB) feature of Windows Server 2003. NLB uses a virtual IP address for all connections to the front-end servers. NLB will not attempt to connect with an offline server. SSL can also be used on front-end servers in the NLB cluster to secure client communication. When using SSL and NLB, use the default Client Affinity setting of Single to preserve the client session state between a client and a specific node in the NLB cluster.

Configuring Front-end and Back-end Servers

Exchange 2000 previously required that all front-end servers run the Enterprise version of Exchange to be able to run as a front-end server. This is no longer the case in Exchange Server 2003, and the Standard version of the software will be able to run as a front-end server. To configure a front-end server, use Exchange System Manager to access the properties of the front-end server and click the check box This is a front-end server, as shown in Figure 10.4.

After the server has been made into a front-end server, the Exchange POP3, Exchange IMAP, and World Wide Web Publishing Service services must be restarted, as shown in the prompt in Figure 10.5.

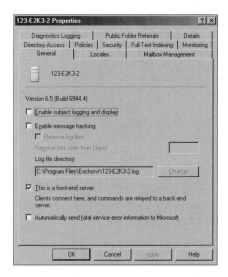

FIGURE 10.4 Creating a front-end server.

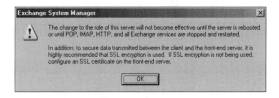

FIGURE 10.5 Finalizing front-end server creation.

Unless the front-end server will be accessed by an alias name, the configuration is complete. If the server will be accessed by one or more alias names, a custom virtual server and virtual directories need to be created on the front-end server, and a corresponding HTTP virtual server and virtual directories should be created on the back-end servers.

Using the Default HTTP Virtual Server for Internet Clients

Most organizations use front-end and back-end servers to support Internet clients, and this type of configuration is demonstrated in the following section. This section provides a best-practice solution to support Internet clients with the default HTTP Virtual server configuration. Much of the information in the industry regarding configuring front-end/back-end servers is conceptually crystal clear but extremely vague when it comes to the implementation. To complete the front back-end server configuration:

1. Verify that the This is a front-end server check box is marked in Exchange System Manager. Don't restart any services or reboot yet.

10

2. Create an alias name in the external DNS for the HTTP front-end server, such as `Web mail.companyabc.com`.

> **NOTE**
>
> This front-end server alias could also be used on the internal DNS, as if internal clients also will be using the front-end server.

3. Add the DNS alias as a Host Header to the Default Web site in Internet Service Manager on the front-end server.

4. Configure the simplified URL mentioned earlier in this section to automatically redirect clients to the `/exchange` Web site when they connect to the front-end server. Also mark this redirection as permanent.

5. In Internet Services Manager, disable Integrated Windows Authentication and verify that Basic Clear Text Authentication is selected on the Default Web site on the front-end server. Propagate these settings to the other Web sites on the front-end server when prompted after clicking Apply or OK.

6. Reboot the front-end server.

7. Do not make any changes to the back-end server's HTTP virtual server or virtual directory configuration.

8. Test the configuration internally.

9. Configure the Default Web Site for SSL authentication. See the section "Using SSL to Secure Access to the Front-end Server," later in this chapter.

10. Retest the configuration internally.

11. Optimize the front-end server by disabling unnecessary services and removing unnecessary databases.

12. Open port 443 for SSL access to the front-end server through the firewall and perform other firewall configurations if necessary.

13. Retest the front-end server access from the Internet.

Configuring the Back-end Server

If the organization chooses to use the default HTTP virtual server on the front-end server and internal and external HTTP clients will be serviced by the same front-end server, no configuration is necessary on the back-end server. However, if the front-end server is isolated from internal clients through a firewall, it might be necessary to have internal HTTP clients access the back-end server directly. If this is the case, it might be necessary to configure an alias name, such as webmail.companyabc.com in the internal DNS. Another option organizations may consider to support internal clients is to use the simplified URL mentioned earlier in this chapter and either SSL or Integrated Windows Authentication, the default authentication method for back-end servers.

As previously mentioned, it is possible to use one HTTP virtual server for all front-end servers with either the default or custom-configured HTTP virtual servers. With custom configurations, organizations also have the choice to configure one virtual server on the back-end server per front-end server. To configure additional HTTP virtual servers to support custom configurations, right-click on the HTTP protocol folder under the back-end server in Exchange System Manager and select New Virtual Server. Figure 10.6 shows a custom virtual server being configured for all front-end servers.

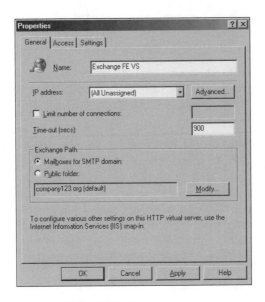

FIGURE 10.6   Configuring an HTTP virtual server.

The next step is to create the virtual directories. Create the virtual directories by right-clicking the HTTP virtual server and selecting New Virtual Directory. Two virtual directories should be created, one directory for mailboxes and the other for public folders. It's best to use the names Exchange and public if the virtual directories will allow access to all public folder trees and the entire domain for mailboxes. No other settings need to be changed when creating the virtual directories unless authentication needs to be disabled on the front-end server. The next step is to create the same HTTP virtual server and directories on every back-end server that contains mailboxes that will be accessed through the front-end server. Finally, verify that the HTTP virtual server and virtual directory configuration have been created on all front-end servers.

10

Using SSL to Secure Access to the Front-end Server

To use SSL to secure client access to the front-end server, the server requires a certificate. Certificates can be generated through Certificate Services or by a third-party CA. After the certificate is created, it should be installed on the Exchange virtual server that was created for the front-end server. If the default Exchange virtual server is being used for the front-end server, the certificate should be added to the default Web site.

> **NOTE**
>
> Ensure that the license logging service is running on the front-end server to allow more than 10 simultaneous SSL connections to the front-end server.

If you are using an HTTP virtual server other than the default on the front-end server, and if clients access the front-end server through a redirection on the default Web site, the certificate also should be installed on the default Web site.

To request and install a certificate, open Internet Services Manager and access the properties of the Web site. Select the Directory Security tab and click the Server Certificate button. This accesses the Web Server Certificate Wizard, which will step you through requesting or installing the certificate.

After the certificate is installed on the Web site, SSL must be enabled so that the server will accept requests only over SSL. To enable SSL, access the Web site properties through Internet Services Manager and select the Directory Security tab. Click the Edit button under Secure Communications and check the box for Require secure channel (SSL), as shown in Figure 10.7. Check the Require 128-bit encryption box only if the client's browsers support 128-bit encryption; otherwise, the client will be denied access.

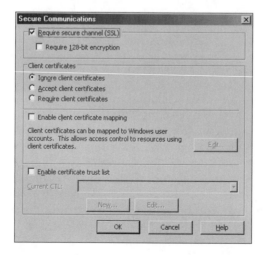

FIGURE 10.7   Enabling SSL for secure client access.

NOTE

Each virtual server instance that requires SSL needs to have a unique certificate associated with it, which is an important consideration when determining the number of virtual servers that will be required.

Upgrading Existing Exchange 2000 Front-end OWA Servers

There are several important factors to keep in mind when upgrading an Exchange 2000 front-end/back-end OWA configuration to Exchange Server 2003. First, before upgrading back-end mailbox servers, all front-end servers in an administrative group must be upgraded to Exchange Server 2003. The upgrade process on the Exchange back-end servers will actually stop if this situation is not corrected in advance. Consequently, it is important to upgrade or replace front-end servers as the first wave of an Exchange Server 2003 migration process.

The Exchange virtual server in Exchange 2000 runs on IIS 5, which cannot communicate with the IIS 6 Exchange virtual server in Exchange Server 2003. So, Exchange 2000 front-end servers would not be able to communicate with mailboxes on an Exchange Server 2003 system. Exchange Server 2003 front-end servers, on the other hand, are backward-compatible with IIS 5 and can subsequently communicate with back-end Exchange 2000 systems.

A second consideration to keep in mind when upgrading OWA front-end servers is that, during the setup process, Exchange Server 2003 will enable some of the Exchange services that might have been previously disabled. It is necessary to disable these services after the upgrade process to maintain the same level of security. The following services are affected by this:

- Exchange Information Store Service

- Exchange Message Tracking Agent (MTA) Service

- POP3 Service

- IMAP4 Service

NOTE

Because Exchange Server 2003 front-end servers do not require an Enterprise license of Exchange, it might be tempting to replace existing Exchange 2000 front-end servers, which required the Enterprise license, with Standard license versions to free the more expensive license. This concept can be achieved only if the front-end servers are rebuilt from scratch or replaced, however, because in-place upgrades of front-end servers cannot downgrade the license.

10

Summary

With the dramatic improvements to the OWA client functionality and look and feel, the need to deploy a robust and reliable Exchange Server 2003 OWA environment has become more acute. Building OWA support directly into each Exchange Server enables this functionality, but the security of the system can be questionable, as many exploits take advantage of Web services. With the concept of Exchange front-end/back-end technology, however, the security and flexibility of OWA can be achieved. By proxying OWA requests, front-end servers give a greater degree of design freedom and protect the valuable data stored in the mailboxes on the back-end servers. Consequently, when designing an Exchange Server 2003 environment, keep these factors in mind to take full advantage of the capabilities of OWA.

Best Practices

The following are best practices from this chapter:

- Use a front-end server in a DMZ firewall configuration for the most secure OWA client access from the Internet.

- Use SSL encryption wherever possible for client access from the Internet.

- Upgrade or replace all Exchange 2000 front-end servers before upgrading any back-end mailbox servers to Exchange Server 2003.

- Disable any unnecessary services or protocols on a front-end server.

- Use network load balancing to load-balance multiple front-end servers.

- Replace, rather than upgrade, existing Exchange 2000 front-end servers to recover expensive Exchange Enterprise licenses.

PART IV

Securing a Microsoft Exchange Server 2003 Environment

IN THIS PART

Client-Level Security

Security in general is often regarded as a significant and sometimes complex part of the network environment. Although some environments take security more seriously than others, it is a topic that must be properly addressed and implemented. Microsoft is continually tackling security head-on, ensuring that not only are known vulnerabilities not an issue but also that future threats can be avoided.

Microsoft's approach to security spans across its entire business product line, and Exchange Server 2003 is no exception. In fact, Microsoft has gone to great lengths to provide a rich array of security features at the client, server, and transport layers in Exchange Server 2003 to protect the messaging environment investment. This approach helps ensure that every link in the messaging chain is as secure as the other links.

Tips and Tricks for Hardening Windows

Exchange Server 2003 and its client counterparts are only as secure as the underlying operating system that supports them. The good news is that by default both Windows Server 2003 and Windows XP Professional are more secure than any other Windows operating system. Despite this fact, default installations are not going to magically secure any environment, so security customizations are almost always going to be recommended.

> **NOTE**
>
> Entire books have been dedicated to securing Windows operating systems, so it is unrealistic to assume that this chapter can thoroughly examine all—or even most—of the critical security policies, methodologies, and practices that should be considered for implementation in order to protect the network environment.

Securing Windows Server 2003 or Windows XP Professional can be broken down into smaller, more manageable components, including—but not limited to—authentication, access control, patch management, and communications. Organizations of all sizes should at least take these focal areas into consideration, especially when implementing new services or technologies.

Windows Server 2003 Security Improvements

Out of the box, Windows Server 2003 reduces its attack surface, making it more difficult from the start to gain unauthorized access. This reduction in the attack surface area stems from many improvements, including—but not limited to—the following:

- The number of services running by default is significantly reduced.

- Internet Information Services (IIS) has been completely overhauled and is no longer installed by default. In addition, group policies can be implemented that prevent rogue IIS installations.

- Access Control Lists (ACLs) have been redefined and are stronger by default.

- Security can be defined by server and user roles.

- Public Key Infrastructure (PKI) Certificate Services has been greatly improved and includes advanced support for automatic smart card enrollment, Certificate Revocation List (CRL) deltas, and more.

- Wireless security features, such as IEEE 802.1X, are supported.

Windows XP Professional Security Improvements

Windows XP Professional complements Windows Server 2003 from the client-computer perspective and supports the security features that are built in to Windows Server 2003. Among the notable security improvements built into Windows XP Professional are:

- Core system files and kernel data structures are protected against corruption and deletion.

- Software policies can be used to identify and restrict which applications can run.

- Wireless security features, such as IEEE 802.1X, are supported.

- Sensitive or confidential files can be encrypted using the Encrypting File System (EFS).

- Communications can be encrypted using IP Security (IPSec).

- Kerberos-based authentication is supported.

- Enhanced support for security devices, such as smart cards, are available.

Internet Connection Firewall Protection

Exchange Server 2003 for many environments is intended to provide access to messaging anytime and virtually anywhere. Many users must securely access their mail from not only corporate office locations but also from hotels, client sites, and other locations. As a result, users are often more susceptible to viruses and intrusions. To minimize security risks, client computers should have the Internet Connection Firewall (ICF) enabled (as shown in Figure 11.1), especially when they are directly connected to the Internet.

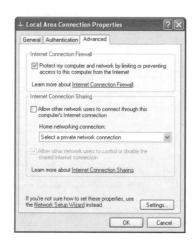

FIGURE 11.1   Enabling ICF to protect Windows XP.

As the name implies, ICF serves as a firewall for a single computer or a group of computers if the computer with ICF is also running Internet Connection Sharing. More specifically, ICF uses stateful packet inspection to monitor all communications to and from the computer and records which traffic originates from the computer or computers it is protecting (that is, outbound traffic). Consequently, ICF allows outbound traffic while stopping unsolicited inbound traffic.

Standardizing Security with Security Templates

Security templates are a practical and effective means to standardize an environment on security policies and configurations. These security templates can be customized to adhere to security requirements of the organization, and these security templates can be applied to client computers as well as to servers using the Security Configuration and Analysis Microsoft Management Console (MMC) snap-in.

> **TIP**
>
> Microsoft provides several security templates based on functional roles within the network environment that can easily be applied to client computers and the server. However, as a best practice, always customize the security template to ensure that application and operating system functionality is not broken or negatively affected.

This not only ensures that computers are identically configured with the same security configurations, but it also is an easy way to configure appropriate security measures for those computers that are not managed using Group Policy Objects (GPOs).

Using the Security Configuration and Analysis Tool

The Security Configuration and Analysis tool, shown in Figure 11.2, is a utility that can apply security templates to computers. It compares a computer's security configurations with a security template. When the computer's security configuration does not conform to the settings in the security template, it can be used to apply the modifications and standardize the computer's security configuration.

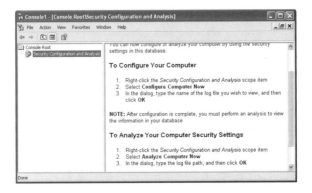

FIGURE 11.2   Using the Security Configuration and Analysis tool.

This utility has two modes of operation; analysis and configuration. It is always a good idea to analyze the computer prior to making any modifications, because it enables administrators to manually compare the differences and select which settings to change. To analyze a computer, do the following:

1. Start the MMC by typing **MMC** in the Start, Run menu.

2. From the File menu, select Add/Remove Snap-in and then click the Add button.

3. Choose the Security Configuration and Analysis snap-in and then click the Add button again.

4. Click the Close button to close and then the OK button to return to the MMC.

5. In the MMC, right-click the Security Configuration and Analysis snap-in and select Open Database.

6. Type a database name, select a location to store the database, and then click Open.

7. Choose a security template and then click Open.

8. Right-click the Security Configuration and Analysis snap-in and choose Analyze Computer Now. Click OK when done.

The tool displays which security settings are and are not in compliance with the security template settings. When the analysis is reviewed, you can choose to configure the system with the template setting by right-clicking the snap-in and choosing Configure Computer Now.

Customizing Security Templates

One of the primary purposes of customizing security templates is to ensure that the organization's specific security requirements are met. It is also a way to ensure that business requirements and goals that are supported through the use of applications and systems' functional roles are not compromised. Typically, the larger the organization, the more systems it has and thus there might be a need for more customized security templates. For instance, if there are different security and business requirements for the various Exchange Server 2003 functional roles, administrators can customize a security template for each of those roles.

> **TIP**
>
> Use security templates provided by Microsoft, the National Security Agency (NSA) or the National Institute of Standards and Technology (NIST) as baselines for customizing the organization's security templates.

Windows Server 2003 and Windows XP Professional are equipped with the Security Templates MMC snap-in that enables administrators to quickly and easily customize security templates to fit the requirements for specific systems. To begin using this tool, add the Security Templates MMC snap-in by following the steps outlined in the previous section "Using the Security Configuration and Analysis Tool."

When the Security Templates snap-in is expanded, it displays the default search path to where the built-in security templates are stored, which is the `%SystemRoot%\security\templates` directory. Other paths can be opened to display other security templates that may reside on the system. Either select New Template after right-clicking on the path, or as a best practice use the Save As selection after right-clicking an existing or baseline security template to create a new, customized template. After creating and naming the new security template, expand it to display all the security settings that can be modified, as shown in Figure 11.3. When the security template has been customized, save it to a network share and use the Security Configuration and Analysis tool to apply the template to the appropriate systems.

Keeping Up with Security Patches and Updates

Service packs (SPs) and hotfixes for both the operating system and applications are vital parts to maintaining availability, reliability, performance, and security. Microsoft packages these updates into SPs or as individual updates (hotfixes).

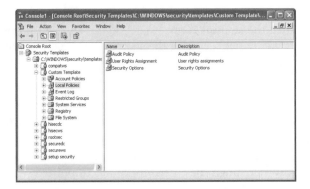

FIGURE 11.3   Using the Security Template MMC snap-in to customize a security template.

There are several ways an administrator can update a system with the latest SP: CD-ROM, manually entered commands, Windows Update, or Microsoft Software Update Services (SUS).

> **NOTE**
>
> Thoroughly test and evaluate SPs and hotfixes in a lab environment before installing them on production servers and client machines. Also, install the appropriate SPs and hotfixes on each production server and client machine to keep all systems consistent.

Windows Update

Windows Update is a Web site that scans a local system and determines whether there are updates to apply to that system. Windows Update is a great way to update individual systems, but this method is sufficient for only a small number of systems. If administrators choose this method to update an entire organization, there is an unnecessary amount of administration.

Software Update Services (SUS)

Realizing the increased administration and management efforts administrators must face when using Windows Update to keep up with security updates for anything other than small environments, Microsoft has created Software Update Services (SUS) to minimize administration, management, and maintenance of mid- to large-sized organizations. SUS communicates directly and securely with Microsoft to gather the latest security updates.

The security updates downloaded onto SUS can then be distributed to either a lab server for testing (recommended) or to a production server for distribution. After these updates are tested, SUS can automatically update systems inside the network.

> **NOTE**
>
> You can find more information on SUS and download the product from
> http://www.microsoft.com/windows2000/windowsupdate/sus/.

Client-Based Virus Protection

Viruses might be one of the most dangerous threats faced by computer systems. Many viruses are written to exploit specific vulnerabilities that might be present in clients and servers. Due to the large percentage of companies that use Microsoft products, many such viruses are specifically written to attack the Windows operating system. Consequently, it is extremely important to consider using an enterprise antivirus solution on all clients and servers. All the major antivirus manufacturers include robust scanners that detect, quarantine, or remove viruses.

An aggressive plan should be in place to keep antivirus signature files and engines up to date. Because virus outbreaks can wreak havoc worldwide in a matter of hours, rather than days, it is wise to have the antivirus solution check for updates daily.

Windows Lockdown Guidelines and Standards

Microsoft has gone to great lengths to provide secure and reliable products. Moreover, it has worked closely with companies, government agencies, security consultants, and others to address security issues in the computer industry. Through this concerted effort and teamwork, secure standards and guidelines have been developed for not just Microsoft products but also other leading vendors as well.

In addition to Microsoft security standards and guidelines, it is advisable that organizations use recommended best practices compiled by the National Institute of Standards and Technologies (NIST) and the National Security Agency (NSA). Both NIST and NSA provide security lockdown configuration standards and guidelines that can be downloaded from their Web site (http://www.nist.gov and http://www.nsa.gov respectively).

Exchange Server 2003 Client-Level Security Enhancements

As mentioned earlier, Exchange Server 2003 has many new and improved security features at the client level. At a glance, these features include—but are not limited to—the following:

- Support for MAPI (RPC) over HTTP or HTTPS and can be configured to use either Secure Sockets Layer (SSL) or NTLM-based authentication

- Support for authentication methods, such as Kerberos and NTLM

- Antispam features, such as safe and block lists, as well as advanced filtering mechanisms to control the amount of unwanted emails

- Protection against Web beaconing, which is used by advertisers and spammers to verify email addresses and determine whether emails have been read

- Attachment-blocking by Exchange Server 2003 before it reaches the intended recipient

- Rights management support, which prevents unauthorized users from intercepting emails

Securing Outlook 2003

Exchange Server 2003 and Microsoft Office 2003 are very well integrated, and the teaming provides a formidable security front. Both new and improved features help provide a safe and reliable messaging environment and are described in the following sections.

Securely Accessing Exchange over the Internet

In previous versions of Exchange (and Outlook), Outlook users that needed to connect to Exchange over the Internet needed to establish a VPN connection prior to using Outlook. The only alternative solution was to open all sorts of RPC ports to the Internet or make a few Registry modifications to statically map RPC ports. Either way presents more of a security risk for the Exchange messaging environments than most are willing to afford.

Now, with Exchange Server 2003 and Outlook 2003, Outlook 2003 users can connect securely over the Internet via an HTTPS proxy connection. This feature reduces the need for VPN solutions and keeps the messaging environment as secure as possible. VPN solutions are still viable and can be used to provide a host of other services for mobile users.

To enable this type of secure connectivity, do the following:

1. Within Outlook 2003, select E-mail Accounts from the Tools menu.

2. Select View or change existing email accounts and then click Next to continue.

3. Click Change and, on the next screen, click the More Settings button.

4. Under the Connection tab, check Connect to my Exchange mailbox using HTTP and then click the Exchange Proxy Settings button.

5. Type the URL. This can be the same URL as the OWA or Outlook Mobile Access (OMA) URL, as shown in Figure 11.4.

6. Verify that Connect using SSL only is checked. If SSL is not used, the connection will use HTTP and will not be secure.

7. Optionally, select whether this SSL connection requires mutual authentication. Mutual authentication ensures that both parties (the server and the client) are who they say they are.

8. Choose whether to use NTLM or Basic proxy authentication (NTLM is the strongest of the two and is used by default). The best practice is to use only NTLM to keep security at its highest.

9. Click OK when done.

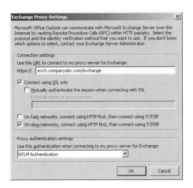

FIGURE 11.4   Configuring a secure Outlook 2003 connection to Exchange Server 2003 over the Internet.

NOTE

This feature requires several components before functioning. It requires that the client is running Windows XP Professional with Service Pack 1 or higher and that the server infrastructure is running Windows Server 2003 and Exchange Server 2003 (that is, mailbox, front-end, Global Catalog, and public folder servers).

TIP

Outlook 2003 users who will be using RPC over HTTPS as described in this section should be using Cached Exchange mode. Cached Exchange mode optimizes the communications between Exchange Server 2003 and Outlook 2003.

Encrypting Outlook 2003 and Exchange Server 2003 Communications

As a MAPI client, Outlook 2003 uses Remote Procedure Calls (RPCs) to communicate with Exchange Server 2003. RPCs are interprocess communications (IPC) mechanisms that, during the transfer of information, can either use or not use encryption. By default, Outlook 2003 does not use encrypted RPC communication. It is important to note that using this form of encryption is different from using RPC over HTTPS as described earlier in the section "Securely Accessing Exchange over the Internet Using Outlook." RPC over HTTPS is still required if the Outlook 2003 client needs to securely communicate over a public network such as the Internet.

In Figure 11.5, a user or administrator can enable encrypted RPC communication between Outlook 2003 and Exchange Server 2003 by simply checking the box within the Encryption section. To modify this setting, do the following:

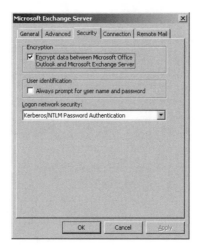

FIGURE 11.5   Enabling encrypted RPC communications in a LAN environment.

1. In Outlook 2003, click on E-mail Accounts from the Tools menu.

2. Select View or change existing email accounts and then click Next.

3. Click the Change button and, on the next window, click the More Settings button.

4. Select the Security tab and then check Encrypt data between Microsoft Office Outlook and Microsoft Exchange Server.

5. Click OK to close the window.

6. Click Next and then Finish when done.

Because encryption requires additional processing overhead, it is important to thoroughly test this feature prior to deploying it in a production environment.

Authenticating Users

By default, Outlook 2003 uses the credentials of the user who is logged onto the local computer to access the Outlook 2003 profile and mailbox. It first tries to use Kerberos for the authentication process and then NT LAN Manager (NTLM). Administrators can also set Outlook 2003 to use Kerberos Password Authentication or NTLM solely, as illustrated in Figure 11.6.

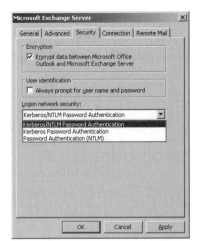

FIGURE 11.6 Configuring authentication options for Outlook 2003.

> **TIP**
>
> For stronger security, use Kerberos-only authentication. Use the Kerberos/NTLM or the NTLM options only for backward compatibility with older systems. Kerberos provides encryption of a user's credentials when communicating with Active Directory for authentication.

Although the default setting is a secure method of authenticating users, some users might still be prone to leave their computers unattended and therefore leave open the opportunity for someone to gain unauthorized access to the user's email. For instance, a user leaves to run an errand and forgets to lock the computer or log off. Someone in the office can then simply open Outlook 2003 and have full access to the user's mailbox.

Many organizations do not necessarily think that this is either a high security risk or the organization's responsibility but Outlook 2003 can be configured nonetheless to mitigate the chances of this occurring. Outlook 2003 can be configured to always prompt for the user's username and password before accessing the mailbox on Exchange Server 2003. To increase this level of security, do the following:

1. Within Outlook 2003, select E-mail Accounts from the Tools menu and then select View or change existing email accounts. Click Next to continue.

2. Click the Change button and, in the next window, click More Settings.

3. Go to the Security tab and then in the User identification section, check Always prompt for username and password.

Blocking Attachments

A common and often effective way for viruses and malicious scripts to spread is through email. When a user receives a message with an attachment, all the user needs to do is to try opening the virus for the virus to infect the computer.

As a result of this threat, Microsoft has incorporated attachment blocking in Outlook, and Outlook Web Access (OWA), to help prevent such infections. By default, Outlook does not block attachments with common Microsoft Office file formats—such as .doc, .xls, and .ppt—but it does block executables—such as .exe, .bat, and .vbs files. It is important to note that the common Microsoft Office file attachments that are not blocked by default can contain viruses. However, using an antivirus on the client computer can significantly reduce the chances of these types of attachments causing any harm.

Outlook does not provide any way for the end-user to unblock these attachments. If files with these file formats need to be shared, users must rename the file, zip the files in question, or place the files on a network share.

> **NOTE**
>
> If an Outlook 2003 user tries sending an attachment that is blocked by default, a warning message is displayed informing the user that the attachment may be unsafe and recipients using Outlook 2003 may not be able to open the attachment. It then asks the user if the attachment should be sent anyway.

Protecting Against Spam

If you have ever had an email account, odds are you have also been a victim of at least one spam message. If you have only had a few spam messages, you are one of the lucky ones. Unfortunately, having an email account somewhere is going to put you at risk of receiving unsolicited and often pornographic email messages.

> **NOTE**
>
> It has been estimated by many organizations that billions upon billions of spam messages will be sent in less than a year's time. In fact, some estimates predict that out of all of the Internet email messages, roughly 70% will be spam. Whatever the numbers turn out to be, it is definitely too high.

Spam does not just affect your patience and productivity. It affects companies, Internet service providers, and anyone else who is hosting messaging services. The battle against spam is just beginning, and legal battles are well underway against both known spammers and companies that host the messaging services. In some cases, employees are suing employers on grounds that the employer is not implementing strong enough measures to keep spam from entering someone's mailbox. In any scenario, spam and its effects cost the computer industry billions of dollars, which ultimately affects everyone relying on messaging.

Spam and Antispam Tools

Spam is not new to the Internet community. It has been around for many years and probably for many more to come. It has become more prevalent over the last several years because of the increasing number of people using the Internet—many of whom are using it for the first time. With more people and larger target audiences for spammers, spam has proven to be a corrupt but effective way of making profits.

> **NOTE**
>
> Spammers are becoming increasingly more creative and cunning. For instance, spammers frequently change email addresses, domain names, content, and more to get past a company's protective measures and into someone's mailbox. Some message content (for example, a word or phrase) that is not legitimate in one message may be legitimate in another.

Microsoft has provided at least some basic form of antispam technologies in Exchange since version 5.5 and Outlook 98. For example, junk mail filters were provided to help identify messages that had either offensive material or other keywords indicating the message was spam. This form of spam prevention placed most, if not all, of the responsibility on the end-user to block unwanted email messages.

Other methods of antispam technology relied on reverse DNS lookups and IP blocking features that helped verify who the sender was and determine whether the spam was coming from a legitimate source. These techniques are still employed with Exchange Server 2003, but they are also complemented by a host of other techniques to provide the most comprehensive coverage against spam as possible.

Protecting Against Web Beaconing

A common and very popular format for email messages is HTML. This is primarily because of the rich content that can be presented, including graphics, images, font formatting, and more. A less-known fact, however, is that HTML-based messages can also present security problems and annoyances because of the various code and hidden images that the message can contain.

Web beaconing is a term used to describe the method of retrieving valid email addresses and information on whether a recipient has opened a message. Advertisers, spammers, and the like thrive on Web beaconing to help them become more profitable and improve audience targeting. For instance, when an unsuspecting user opens an email message that contains a Web beacon, the user's email address and possibly other information is sent to the solicitor. The user is oblivious that personal information has been given.

Outlook 2003 can be used to block Web beacons and consequently prevent the user's email address from ending up in the wrong hands. By default, if Outlook 2003 suspects that the content of a message could be used as a Web beacon, it presents a pop-up window warning users that to help protect their privacy, links to images, multimedia, or other external content have been blocked. The text content of the email message is viewable by the user, and the user is then presented with an option to unblock the content. This enables the user to make a conscious decision of whether to display all the contents of the message.

Although the default setting is recommended because it is an excellent way to protect end-users from a barrage of unwanted emails and it helps minimize unsolicited emails, it is possible to disable this option. To change the default settings, do the following:

1. In Outlook 2003, select Options from the Tools menu.

2. Click on the Security tab and then click Change Automatic Download Settings.

3. In the Automatic Picture Download Settings window, choose whether to download pictures or other content automatically. Outlook 2003 can also be customized to automatically download content from safe lists or from Web sites listed in the trusted IE security zones, as illustrated in Figure 11.7.

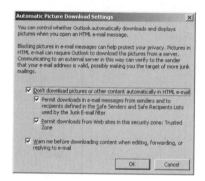

FIGURE 11.7   Configuring Automatic Picture Download Settings.

Filtering Junk Mail

As mentioned earlier, junk mail filtering has been available in earlier versions of Exchange and Outlook. This feature has been improved from earlier versions and minimizes the responsibility of end-users to configure junk mail filtering options. In fact, junk mail filtering is primarily controlled by Exchange Server 2003 administrators, but options can be set by the users. Most junk mail or spam is filtered before it reaches the user's mailbox.

> **TIP**
>
> Despite the fact that Exchange Server 2003 and Outlook 2003 have sound, practical spam fighting techniques and features built in, organizations should evaluate third-party antispam tools. Third-party tools provide advanced features and customizations that offer stronger protection against spam.

Outlook 2003 presents four levels of junk mail protection:

- **No Protection**   The only filtering that occurs is when email originates from the manually configured blocked senders list. This is fairly ineffective, considering that spammers change source email addresses constantly.

- **Low**   Safe and block lists are consulted with this level of protection, but Outlook 2003 also searches for key words and phrases in the message's subject and body.

- **High**   This uses the features of the low setting plus it is more aggressive with filtering. Users should not permanently delete suspected spam and should check the junk email folder more frequently to find possible false positives.

- **Safe Lists Only**   This setting is the most restrictive because it allows only messages from preapproved senders to be delivered to the inbox. Although this is a good option to have, it probably will not be one that is chosen very often. You might get a legitimate message from someone you do not know, or in many cases there might be a spam message from a trusted domain.

TIP

With any filtering level that you use, send mail to the Junk E-mail folder, at least initially, rather than deleting it. Use the high level to ensure that most, if not all, spam is filtered. Most of the false positives are likely to come from mailing lists and newsletters. If this is the case, it is easier to use this setting and unblock those mailing lists that are legitimate. Testing has shown that the high level setting cuts as much as 90% of spam out of a user's mailbox.

As illustrated in Figure 11.8, Outlook 2003 by default is set to Low to keep only the most obvious spam out. Any filtered messages are placed in the Junk E-mail folder unless the delete all junk email option is checked.

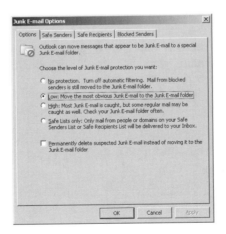

FIGURE 11.8   Outlook 2003 Junk E-mail filtering options.

Filtering with Safe and Block Lists

Outlook 2003 enables users to create and manage their own safe and block lists. A safe list is a list of email addresses or domains that are trustworthy; a block list contains those email addresses or domains that are always considered spam or junk mail.

There are actually two safe lists that Outlook 2003 users can create and manage: Safe Senders and Safe Recipients. The Safe Senders list is intended to store email addresses or domains of individual users, and the Safe Recipients list covers members of email lists or groups. An example of when the latter should be used is when you are a member of a discussion group where many members pass emails back and forth through the mailing list.

As the name implies, block lists can contain known spamming email addresses or domains. Depending on how your organization is taking a stance on spam, there might be only a few entries in this list.

Outlook 2003 also gives users the ability to import whitelists and blacklists, which are similar to safe lists and block lists, respectively. These lists may be quite large though and have been known to cause performance problems, because each message had to be checked and verified against the potentially large list that was imported.

> **NOTE**
>
> Outlook 2003 trusts the user's contacts by default. This keeps messages from those contacts away from the Junk E-mail folder.

Blocking Read Receipts

Most email applications, such as Outlook, enable users to request read receipts for the messages that they send. Read receipts tell the sender that the intended recipient has at least opened the email.

Outlook 2003 prompts a user by default on whether the user wants to send a read receipt if a message requests one. To ensure that users do not accidentally send read receipts, it is recommended to turn off sending read receipts and consequently turn off the prompting. To do so, use the following steps:

1. In Outlook 2003, select Options from the Tools menu.

2. Click the E-mail Options button to display the E-mail Options window.

3. Click the Tracking Options button to display the Tracking Options window and then select Never send a response.

4. Click OK three times to close all the options windows.

Information Rights Management in Office 2003

Information Rights Management (IRM) also known as Rights Management (RM) is an unprecedented new feature that enables users to create and control information. More specifically, it gives the creator of the specific information control over the following:

- What can be done with the information

- Who can perform actions or tasks with the information (for example, who can forward a specific message, print a document, or copy a file)

- The lifetime of the information (that is, the message expiration on a specific date)

IRM granularizes security for Microsoft Office 2003 Professional applications such as Word, Excel, PowerPoint, Outlook, and any other IRM-aware application. IRM is intended to complement other security technologies, such as S/MIME and PGP. It secures the contents of information (for example, documents and messages), but it does not provide authentication to the information. In addition, it is important to keep the appropriate access controls on the information as an added layer of security.

There is an IRM server component that resides on Windows Server 2003, and support is built into Office 2003 Professional. When implemented, Outlook 2003 users can use a toolbar icon to manage and secure their outgoing messages. For instance, user1 can send a message intended only for user2. Depending on the IRM settings for that message, user2 might be able to only read the message and not be able to forward it, copy it, or print it. This keeps the message's contents from falling into the wrong hands and is particularly useful for sensitive or confidential information.

Securing Outlook Web Access

OWA provides the interface for users to access their mail through Internet Explorer (IE). When compared to previous versions, OWA is far superior, not just in functionality but also in terms of security. At a quick glance, OWA provides the following security features and enhancements:

- Built-in S/MIME support

- Stripping of Web beacons, referrals, and other potentially harmful content from messages

- Attachment blocking

- OWA form-based (cookie) authentication

- Session inactivity timeout

- OWA infrastructure using IPSec and Kerberos

- Safe and block lists

Protecting Against Potentially Harmful Message Content

Outlook 2003 gives the option to read messages in HTML (default), rich text, and plain text formats. If these users are employing plain text format to read their messages, they are not at risk of Web beacons giving away their information. The messaging experience is not as rich, but security vulnerabilities are minimized. OWA users, on the other hand, are particularly susceptible to Web beacons because all messages are read using the HTML format.

This risk is easily thwarted, however, by keeping the default OWA setting of blocking external content in HTML messages. On the OWA Options page, there is a single check box under the Privacy and Junk E-mail Prevention section that helps prevent such a risk.

Blocking Attachments Through OWA

The concept and functionality of blocking attachments is similar to that of Outlook 2003. The implementation, however, is different; an administrator enables attachment blocking by modifying the Registry. To enable attachment blocking for OWA, do the following:

1. Start the Registry Editor by typing **regedit** in the Start, Run dialog box on the OWA server.

2. Locate the following Registry key:

   HKEY_LOCAL_MACHINE\SYSTEM\CurrentControlSet\Services\MSExchangeWeb\OWA

3. Create a new DWORD value by selecting New, DWORD Value from the Edit menu.

4. In the right window pane, type **DisableAttachments** for the name of the DWORD value.

5. Right-click DisableAttachments and select Modify.

6. Select Decimal and then type one of the following values for the configuration that is required:

   0 to allow all attachments
   1 to block all attachments
   2 to allow only attachments from the back-end servers

7. Click OK when done.

Using Safe and Block Lists

Like the Outlook 2003 features, many of the OWA counterparts match the functionality. This holds true when using safe and block lists. These lists are managed in the Options page within OWA. On the OWA Options page, locate the Privacy and Junk E-mail Prevention section and click on the Manage Junk E-mail Lists button to modify the Safe

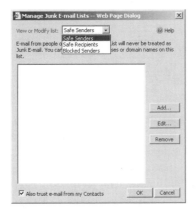

Senders, Safe Recipients, or Blocked Senders list, as illustrated in Figure 11.9.

FIGURE 11.9 Managing safe and block lists in OWA.

Using Digital Signatures and Encryption

Secure/Multipurpose Internet Mail Extensions (S/MIME) is used to digitally sign and encrypt messages. Digital signatures provide authentication, nonrepudiation, and data integrity; encryption keeps message contents confidential.

> **NOTE**
>
> S/MIME for Outlook 2003 and OWA can work with an organization's (for example, Windows Server 2003 Certificate Services) or outsourced Public Key Infrastructure (PKI) solution. The following sections on S/MIME assume that a PKI is in place. For information on implementing PKI for Exchange Server 2003, refer to Chapter 12, "Server-Level Security."

Simplified Fundamentals of Using Digital Signatures and Encryption

Digital signatures and encryption are fundamental components to S/MIME. S/MIME is in turn a small subset of PKI which has a large reach into many different security facets. For instance, PKI supports smart cards, SSL, user certificates, and much more. For the purposes of this chapter it is important to have an understanding of S/MIME and how it can be used to secure the messaging environment.

X.509 is a digital certificate standard that defines the format of the actual certificate used by S/MIME. The certificate identifies information about the certificate's owner and includes the owner's public key information. X.509 is the most widely used digital certificate and therefore has become the industry standard digital certificate. PKI products, such as Microsoft's Certificate Services included in Windows Server 2003, are products that generate X.509 digital certificates to be used with S/MIME capable clients.

The Signing Process

When a user chooses to sign a message, a random checksum is generated from and added to the message. The random checksum is the digital signature (also known as a digital ID). This signature is then encrypted using the user's private signing key. The user then sends the message to the recipient that includes three items: the message in plain text, the sender's X.509 digital certificate, and the digital certificate.

The recipient then checks its Certificate Revocation List (CRL) to see whether the sender's certificate is on the list. If the certificate is not on the list, the digital signature is decrypted with the sender's public signing key. If it is on the CRL, the recipient is warned that the sender's certificate has been revoked. Remember that the digital certificate included the sender's public signing key. The recipient's client then generates a checksum from the plain text message and compares it to the digital signature. If the checksums match, the recipient knows the sender is the one who sent the message. If they do not match, the recipient is warned that the message has been tampered with.

The Encryption Process

When a user chooses to encrypt a message, the client generates a random bulk encryption key that is used to encrypt the contents of the message. The sender then uses the recipient's public key to encrypt the bulk encryption key. This is referred to as a **lockbox**. If there are multiple recipients for the message, individual lockboxes are created for each recipient, using his or her own public encryption key. The contents of the lockbox (the bulk signing key) are the same, however. This saves the client the overhead of encrypting the message multiple times and still ensures that the message contents stay secure.

For this process to work, the sender must have a copy of the recipient's digital certificate. The certificate can be retrieved from either the Global Address List (GAL) or the sender's Contact list. The digital certificate contains the recipient's public encryption key, which is used to create the lockbox for the bulk encryption key.

When the recipient receives the message, he will use a private encryption key to decrypt the lockbox that contains the bulk encryption key used to encrypt the message contents. The bulk encryption key is then used to decrypt the message.

Configuring Outlook 2003 for Secure Messaging

To configure Outlook 2003 clients for secure messaging, do the following:

1. In Outlook 2003, click Tools, Options and select the Security tab.

2. Obtain a secure email certificate if one does not already exist by either choosing the Get a Digital ID option (to obtain the certificate from a third party) or by using the Certificate snap-in (`certmgr.msc`) to request one from the organization's PKI.

3. Select Options from the Tools menu and then click on the Security tab.

4. On the Security tab, click Settings to display the default security settings, as shown in Figure 11.10. Ensure that the Security Setting Preferences reflect the S/MIME settings.

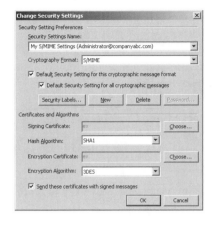

FIGURE 11.10   Verifying Outlook 2003 S/MIME settings.

5. Click OK.

6. Check Encrypt contents and attachments for outgoing messages and Add digital signature to outgoing messages.

7. Click OK when done.

Configuring OWA for Secure Messaging

Earlier versions of Outlook supported digital signatures and encryption, but OWA did not. The Exchange Server 2003 OWA version now supports these S/MIME features, using an S/MIME ActiveX control.

Users can download the S/MIME ActiveX control from Exchange Server 2003 by clicking on the Download button under the E-mail Security section on the OWA Options page. Two windows prompt the user to accept or decline the installation and execution of the S/MIME ActiveX control, as illustrated in Figure 11.11. Simply selecting Yes to both of these prompts allows the user to enable S/MIME.

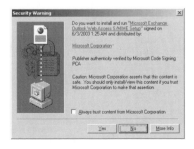

FIGURE 11.11   Accepting S/MIME certificates.

To configure default S/MIME settings for OWA, do the following:

1. Scroll down to the E-mail Security section on the OWA Options page.

2. Check Encrypt contents and attachments for outgoing messages and Add a digital signature to outgoing messages.

If these options are left unchecked, the OWA user can still use S/MIME on a per message basis.

Sending Secure Messages

To configure S/MIME on a per message basis in Outlook 2003, do the following:

1. Create a new message and then click the Options button within the message window.

2. Click the Security Settings button to display the Security Properties window.

3. Check either email security setting (Encrypt message contents and attachments or Add a digital signature to this message).

4. In the Security Settings section, select the appropriate S/MIME configuration and then click OK.

5. Click Close when done.

To configure S/MIME on a per message basis in OWA, do the following:

1. Create a new message and then click the Options button within the message window.

2. Check either email security setting (Encrypt message contents and attachments or Add a digital signature to this message), as shown in Figure 11.12.

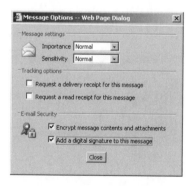

FIGURE 11.12   Using S/MIME for an individual message.

3. Click Close when done.

11

The easiest way to enable secure messaging with users outside of the Exchange 2000 organization is to send the user a digitally signed message. Outlook 2000 and later sends a copy of the sender's certificate with any signed message by default. The recipient of the signed message can then add the sender and certificate to the Contacts folder. When users receive an encrypted message they need to enter their security password to decrypt the message.

Summary

Keeping messaging clients secure is a critical facet to any Exchange environment and it involves careful planning, design, and testing in order to meet the requirements of the organization. Properly securing messaging clients and access to the messaging infrastructure requires security configurations of the operating system (both Windows Server 2003 and Windows XP Professional), Exchange Server 2003, and Microsoft Office 2003. This provides a robust, well-rounded, and secure solution.

Best Practices

The following are best practices from this chapter:

- Customize security templates to ensure that application and operating system functionality are not broken or negatively affected.

- Use security templates provided by Microsoft, the National Security Agency (NSA) or the National Institute of Standards and Technology (NIST) as baselines for customizing the organization's security templates.

- Keep servers and client computers up-to-date with the latest service pack and security updates.

- Consult Microsoft, NIST, and NSA security guidelines for securing the operating system.

- Use third-party antivirus software.

- Authenticate clients to the Exchange Server 2003 messaging infrastructure, using Kerberos whenever possible.

- Outlook 2003 users should use Cached Exchange mode if they will be using RPC over HTTPS connections over the Internet.

- Combine Exchange Server 2003, Outlook 2003, and third-party features to combat spam.

- Block all read receipts.

- Implement IRM.

- Use S/MIME to encrypt sensitive or confidential messages.

CHAPTER 12

Server-Level Security

Exchange Server 2003 server-level security involves a combination of policy, configuration, and practices. With any type of system, these aspects require thorough planning, designing, and testing. This includes, but is not limited to, the development of messaging-related security policies, standardization of Windows Server 2003 and Exchange Server 2003 security mechanisms, and implementing industry standard best practices.

Server-level security for the messaging environment is one of the most important considerations for a secure messaging environment because Exchange Server 2003 not only stores messaging data; it is a mission-critical form of communication. As a result, it is important to establish a server-level security plan and to gain a full understanding of the security capabilities of both the operating system that it is dependent on and Exchange.

Microsoft's Trustworthy Computing Initiative

Microsoft has undergone a vast transformation in regards to security. Microsoft seeks to provide server products, like Exchange Server 2003, that are "secure by design, secure by default, and secure by development." Every security aspect in virtually all of its server products is scrutinized. Specific features, vulnerabilities, and code have been analyzed to ensure that Exchange Server 2003 is as secure as possible.

Secure by Design

Microsoft's Trustworthy Computing Initiative is the cornerstone of Exchange Server 2003 development. The initiative began by providing security-focused training to the entire Exchange Server 2003 team and specially created cross-component, security-focused teams. These teams shared developer best practices to increase code quality and minimize the attack surface. Microsoft then performed code reviews to ensure that changes made to one feature set did not impose or create a security risk in others. This entire process is performed constantly.

In addition to constant code reviews, teams of security experts, called Red Teams, performed product testing and threat reviews. These teams essentially acted as hackers, attempting to compromise systems and exploit vulnerabilities based on function or feature.

Secure by Default

Another integral part of the security initiative was to minimize the attack surface areas possible with Exchange Server 2003. This translates to keeping default installations more secure. By minimizing the number of services and functions that are enabled by default, organizations are less likely to have features unknowingly enabled that may present a security risk. For instance, frequently used protocols are no longer enabled by default. These protocols include POP3, IMAP4, NNTP and Outlook Mobile Access (OMA). Other features, such as new user restrictions and messaging limitations, have also been enabled to reduce the likelihood that default installations are unsecure.

Secure by Deployment

Microsoft equips IT personnel with the necessary tools and documentation to securely and successfully deploy Exchange Server 2003. The deployment tools and documentation ensure that the network environment is healthy, properly configured, and ready to accept Exchange Server 2003.

Coupling these tools and documentation with the appropriate training helps prepare Exchange Server 2003 administrators. It gives them the necessary resources and knowledge to adequately secure the messaging environment based on the security requirements of the specific organization.

Building Communications and Community

Another focal point to the security initiative is building communications and community around all server products. This framework for encouraging the sharing of information is analogous to user groups where groups of IT professionals shared experiences, insights, and other pertinent knowledge. Communications and community can be fostered through a number of different mediums such as newsgroups, discussion lists, user groups, and security Web sites.

Assessing Your Risks

A key consideration for security is risk and the costs associated with securing information. This is not just about determining the monetary value of the information but equally important is assessing the different types of risks and the value of the information. Ask yourself how much would it cost the organization if the information was destroyed, altered, or stolen.

This is not an easy task; in fact, it is often a daunting one. While monetary values can easily be associated with some types of information, other information may be nearly impossible to assess. The important thing to remember is that it's essential to secure your resources and a balance must be struck between the cost of securing the information with the information's value.

Once the assessment process is initiated, it is important to begin analyzing possible security vulnerabilities for the service or functionality that the organization is offering. The following are some of the security risks to investigate and protect against for Exchange Server 2003:

- **Denial of Service**   A denial of service, or DoS, occurs when a user either maliciously or surreptitiously performs some action that causes a service interruption. The interruption may affect targeted users or the entire server. An example might be the "ping of death" or a specially crafted email header that consumes the entire Exchange server processing time.

- **Viruses or Trojan Horse Messages**   Viruses, email worms, and Trojan Horse messages are the bane of the messaging world. They can cause many hours of lost productivity, and keeping on top of this issue can be a full-time job. Thankfully, Exchange Server 2003 has numerous features that help administrators and antivirus vendors combat this problem.

- **Spam**   Unfortunately, unsolicited email (spam) is destined to be a part of the messaging community's life for a very long time—if not forever. It forces unwanted and frequently objectionable material into users' inboxes, costing Internet users billions of dollars annually. The reason is simple: Spam is a cheap way for mass-marketers to get their message out to a wide segment of people.

- **Intentional Attacks**   These attacks are usually targeted at a specific entity or messaging system. Attacks may occur to disrupt normal business operations or compromise a known vulnerability in the company's messaging system. The administrator should bear in mind that some intentional attacks are used to focus attention away from the "real" attack.

- **Message Spoofing**   Message spoofing is a tactic used by many email worms, such as KLEZ and BugBear, as well as some intentional attacks by malicious users. Message spoofing alters SMTP headers so that mail appears as though it came from a different address or messaging server. These messages are sometimes difficult and time-consuming to troubleshoot.

Designing a Secure Messaging Environment

The messaging environment is composed of much more than just the Exchange servers and client machines. Firewalls, network perimeters, accessibility options for users, security policies, and more are integral components that must be thoroughly designed as well.

Establishing a Corporate Email Policy

Corporate or organizational email policies are used to govern and enforce appropriate business use of the messaging environment. They are also used to provide grounds for investigations of inappropriate use of corporate email. It is recommended to establish these policies and get the business to approve them as soon as possible.

> **NOTE**
>
> Corporate email policies not only define how the system can and should be used; they also limit liability.

The following are possible considerations and guidelines to include in the corporate email policy:

- The policy should expressly state that the email system is not to be used for the creation or distribution of any offensive or disruptive messages, including messages containing offensive comments about race, gender, age, sexual orientation, pornography, religious or political beliefs, national origin, or disability. State that employees who receive any emails with this content should report the matter to their supervisor immediately.

- Employees should not use email to discuss competitors, potential acquisitions, or mergers, or to give their opinion about another firm. Unlawful messages, such as copyright infringing emails, should also be prohibited. Include examples and be clear about measures taken when these rules are breached.

- Include a list of "email risks" to make users aware of the potential harmful effects of their actions. Advise users that sending an email is like sending a postcard or letter; if they do not want it posted on the bulletin board, they should not send it.

- If the organization monitors the content of its employees' emails, it must mention this in the email policy. It is important to note that most states and countries are allowed to monitor employees' emails if the employees are cognizant that the messages are being monitored. Organizations should warn users that there is no expectation of privacy in anything they create, store, send, or receive on the company's computer system. In addition, organizations should warn employees that messages may be viewed without prior notice.

- Establish clear email retention policies.

- Include a point of contact for questions arising from the email policy.

The corporate email policy should be made available in a variety of different places on a variety of different mediums. For instance, include the corporate email policy on the intranet, in employee handbooks, and periodically in the company newsletter. The policy can also be included as users log into the messaging system using forms-based authentication.

Securing Exchange Server 2003 Through Administrative Policies

Similar to the corporate email policy for users, it is recommended to establish administrative policies that govern the operation and usage of the Exchange Server 2003 messaging system. Considerations for the organization's administrative policies include the following:

- Administrative and operator accounts should not have mailboxes.

- Grant permissions to groups rather than users.

- SMTP addresses should not match the User Principle Name (UPN).

- Require complex (strong) passwords for all users.

- Require users to close the browser when finishing an Outlook Web Access (OWA) session.

- Require Secure Sockets Layer (SSL) for HTTP, POP3, IMAP4, NNTP, and LDAP clients.

- Set policies globally and customize other user policies.

- Set storage limits and reply-to policies.

Using Email Disclaimers

Email disclaimers inform recipients of corporate legal information and policies. For all practical purposes, email disclaimers are used to reduce liability and caution recipients about misusing the information contained within the message. Email disclaimers can be tacked onto the bottom of all outgoing messages automatically when sent through a particular server.

The following is a sample email disclaimer:

> The information contained in this message is intended solely for the individual to whom it is specifically and originally addressed. This message and its contents may contain confidential or privileged information. If you are not the intended recipient, you are hereby notified that any disclosure or distribution, or taking any action in reliance on the contents of this information, is strictly prohibited.

TIP

The organization's legal department or representative should approve the contents of the email disclaimer. If there were ever a situation where the information could potentially be used in a court of law, the email disclaimer will hold more relevance under scrutiny.

Exchange Server 2003 SMTP event sinks are used to add email disclaimers to all outgoing mail or outgoing mail from a specific server. Third-party products are available as well but also come with a cost. To create an email disclaimer, follow these high-level steps:

1. Install the Exchange Software Development Kit (SDK).

2. Create an event sink using Visual Basic Script and save it as **EventSinkScript.vbs**.

3. Open the Command Prompt by typing **cmd** at the Start, Run menu dialog box and browse to the ...\Exchange SDK\SDK\Support\CDO\Scripts directory.

4. Register the event sink using the smtpreg.vbs script provided in the Exchange SDK. For example, at the command prompt, type

   ```
   cscript smtpreg.vbs /add 1 onarrival SMTPScriptingHost CDO.SS_
   SMTPOnArrivalSink "mail from=*@your-domain-here.com"
   ```

   Press Enter when done.

5. Type

   ```
   cscript smtpreg.vbs /setprop 1 onarrival SMTPScriptingHost Sink ScriptName
   ```

   ```
   "C:\EventSinkScript.vbs".
   ```

6. Test the SMTP event sink and email disclaimer.

For more information on creating an SMTP event sink for an email disclaimer, refer to Knowledge Base article 317680.

Exchange Server-side Security Improvements

Exchange Server 2003 has numerous product enhancements and new features including those that are security related. The following are some of the most notable server-level security features:

- **Distribution Lists Restricted to Authenticated Users**   You can allow only sending from authenticated users or specify which users can or cannot send mail to specified distribution lists.

- **Support of Real-Time Safe and Block Lists**   Reduce the amount of unsolicited mail delivered to your organization with connection filtering.

- **Inbound Recipient Filtering**   Reduce unsolicited email messages by filtering inbound messages based on the recipient. Messages that are addressed to users that are not found, or to whom the sender does not have the permissions to send, are rejected. This applies only to messages sent by anonymously authenticated users.

- **Kerberos Authentication Between a Front-end and Back-end Server**   To help ensure that credentials are securely passed from front-end to back-end servers, Exchange Server 2003 uses Kerberos delegation when sending user credentials.

- **Virus Scanning API 2.5**   Third-party antivirus products can run on servers running Exchange Server 2003 that do not have resident Exchange mailboxes. These products can be configured to send messages to the sender and to delete messages.

- **Antispam Integration with Outlook 2003 and Outlook Web Access**   You can upload the Safe and Block Senders List to Exchange Server 2003 for filtering.

- **Clustering Security**   Exchange Server 2003 clustering supports Kerberos authentication against an Exchange virtual server. Exchange Server 2003 also supports Internet Protocol Security (IPSec) between front-end servers and clustered back-end servers running Exchange.

- **Public Folder Permissions for Unknown Users**   Public folders, with distinguished names in ACLs that cannot be resolved to security identifiers, drop the unresolvable distinguished names.

- **Domain Users Denied Local Logon to Exchange Server 2003 Servers by Default**   When Exchange Server 2003 is installed on a member server, the domain users group is denied local logon rights in the local security configuration. This prevents non-administrators from logging on to the server even if they should gain physical or Remote Desktop access to the Exchange server.

- **Removal of Top-Level Public Folder Creation Permissions for Everyone and Anonymous Logon**   Exchange Server 2003 secures rampant public folder creation by removing the ability of these groups to create top-level public folders.

- **Maximum Message Size Limitations**   By default, Exchange Server 2003 limits public folder message sizes to 10MB. In addition, inbound and outbound messages have the same cap on message size.

- **Selected Services Disabled by Default**   With the exception of in-place upgrades, services such as POP3, IMAP4, and Outlook Mobile Access (OMA) are installed but disabled by default. Administrators must manually enable these services.

Security Roles in Exchange Server 2003

Exchange Server 2003 administration is determined through permissions and Exchange roles. Roles determine the level to which IT personnel can administrator Exchange objects within the Exchange Organization.

The Exchange Server 2003 roles work in conjunction with standard Windows Server 2003 groups and permissions structures. However, they are different and can be a bit confusing at first. For instance, the Exchange Full Admininstrator role is not found in Active Directory Users and Computers like a standard user or group would be. Rather, the

Exchange Server 2003 roles should be viewed as templates that can define how administrators manage and maintain Exchange.

In previous versions, permissions were set through applying rights to Active Directory users' and groups' Exchange objects property pages. Now, role-based administration is assigned using the Exchange Server 2003 Delegation Wizard.

> **NOTE**
>
> For more information on Exchange Server 2003 administration, refer to Chapter 18, "Exchange Server 2003 Mailbox, Distribution List, and Site Administration."

Depending on where and which roles are assigned, different levels of permissions can be applied to different Exchange server objects. Leveraging each of the three Exchange server administrative roles are

- **Exchange Full Administrator**   The Exchange Full Administrator role is the least restrictive of all three Exchange Server 2003 roles. Similar to Full Control, using this role allows administrators to manage Exchange objects (that is, add, delete, and change permissions and objects). Assign this role only to Exchange administrators who require complete access to the Exchange Server 2003 organization. The Exchange administrator with this role must also manually be added to the Exchange Server 2003 server's local administrators group.

- **Exchange Administrator**   This role is ideal for performing daily Exchange administration by allowing Exchange Server 2003 administrators the ability to add, change, or modify objects. This role cannot modify permissions of other Exchange administrative roles and it is recommended to place the administrator with this role into the server's local administrators group.

- **Exchange View Only Administrator**   The Exchange View Only Administrator role is the most restrictive of all exchange roles because it allows administrators to view Exchange objects only. Use this role to restrict administrative permissions between Exchange administrative groups.

Required Roles to Install Additional Exchange Server 2003 Servers

In previous versions of Exchange, the Exchange Full Administrator role was required to install additional Exchange servers in the organization. This is no longer required in Exchange Server 2003. Exchange Full Administrator rights at the administrative group level can now be delegated to allow other Exchange administrators to add new Exchange Server 2003 servers within their location. This reduces the amount of administrative overhead.

To delegate control to other Exchange administrators to install additional Exchange Server 2003 servers, do the following:

1. Open the Exchange System Manager (ESM) from the Start, All Programs, Microsoft Exchange menu by selecting System Manager.

2. Expand Administrative Groups and then right-click on the administrative group that requires delegated control and select Delegate Control.

3. In the Exchange Administration Delegation Wizard, click Next.

4. In the next window, shown in Figure 12.1, click Add to add the user or group who will add an Exchange Server 2003 server in the site.

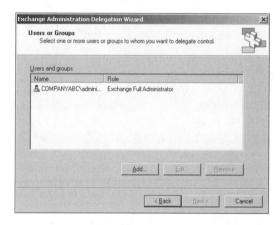

FIGURE 12.1   Using the Exchange Administration Delegation Wizard.

5. Select the role of Exchange Full Administrator and click OK.

6. Click Next and then Finish.

TIP

The user or group should also be a member of the local administrators group on the server. Run the Exchange Administration Delegation Wizard again on either the Organization or administrative group to view who has been delegated Exchange roles.

Tips, Tricks, and Best Practices for Hardening Windows Server 2003

Exchange Server 2003 is only as secure as Windows Server 2003. Therefore, it is imperative to secure Windows Server 2003 to ensure it conforms to the security standards for the organization.

Layered Approach to Server Security

Security works best when it is applied in layers. It is much more difficult to rob a house, for example, if a thief not only has to break through the front door, but also has to fend off an attack dog and disable a home security system. The same concept applies to server security: multiple layers of security should be applied so that the difficulty in hacking into a system becomes that much greater.

Windows Server 2003 seamlessly handles many of the security layers that are required, using Kerberos authentication, NTFS file security, and built-in security tools to provide for a great deal of security out of the box. Once Windows Server 2003 is secured according to the organization's requirements, Exchange Server 2003 security can be integrated to conform to the security requirements of the organization.

Physical Security Considerations

An Exchange Server 2003 server can be very restrictive in what resources are accessible but if the server is not physically secured, an unauthorized user or hacker can more easily gain unauthorized access. For example, simply unplugging the server can have serious repercussions even if the unauthorized user was not able to access messaging data.

Physical security should be a requirement for any organization because it is the most common cause of security breaches. Despite this fact, many organizations have loose levels, or no levels, of physical security for their mission-critical servers.

Servers should be physically secured behind locked doors, preferably in an environmentally controlled room. Other methods of physically securing servers includes hardware locking devices, video surveillance, and more.

Restricting Logon Access

All servers should be configured to allow only administrators to physically log in to the console. By default, Exchange Server 2003 does not allow any members of the domain users group local logon privileges. This prevents non-administrators from logging on to the server even if they can gain physical access to the server.

Auditing Security Events

Auditing is a way to gather and keep track of activity on the network, devices, and entire systems. By default, Windows Server 2003 enables some auditing, whereas many other auditing functions must be manually turned on. This allows for easy customization of the features the system should have monitored.

Auditing is typically used for identifying security breaches or suspicious activity. However, auditing is also important to gain insight into how the servers are accessed. Windows Server 2003's auditing policies must first be enabled before activity can be monitored.

Auditing Policies

Audit policies are the basis for auditing events on a Windows Server 2003 system. Depending on the policies set, auditing may require a substantial amount of server resources in addition to those resources supporting the server's functionality. Otherwise, it could potentially slow server performance. Also, collecting lots of information is only as good as the evaluation of the audit logs. In other words, if a lot of information is captured and a significant amount of effort is required to evaluate those audit logs, the whole purpose of auditing is not as effective. As a result, it's important to take the time to properly plan how the system will be audited. This enables the administrator to determine what needs to be audited and why without creating an abundance of overhead.

Audit policies can track successful or unsuccessful event activity in a Windows Server 2003 environment. These policies can audit the success and failure of events. The types of events that can be monitored include:

- **Account Logon Events**   Each time a user attempts to log on, the successful or unsuccessful event can be recorded. Failed logon attempts can include logon failures for unknown user accounts, time restriction violations, expired user accounts, insufficient rights for the user to log on locally, expired account passwords, and locked-out accounts.

- **Account Management**   When an account is changed, an event can be logged and later examined. Although this pertains more to Windows Server 2003 than Exchange Server 2003, it is still very relevant because the Exchange directory is stored in Active Directory.

- **Directory Service Access**   Any time a user attempts to access an Active Directory object that has its own System Access Control List (SACL), the event is logged.

- **Logon Events**   Logons over the network or by services are logged.

- **Object Access**   The object access policy logs an event when a user attempts to access a resource (for example, a printer or shared folder).

- **Policy Change**   Each time an attempt to change a policy (user rights, account audit policies, trust policies) is made, the event is recorded.

- **Privilege Use**   Privileged use is a security setting and can include a user employing a user right, changing the system time, and more. Successful or unsuccessful attempts can be logged.

- **Process Tracking**   An event can be logged for each program or process that a user launches while accessing a system. This information can be very detailed and take a significant amount of resources.

- **System Events**   The system events policy logs specific system events, such as a computer restart or shutdown.

The audit policies can be enabled or disabled through either the local system policy or Group Policy objects. Audit policies are located within the Computer Configuration\Windows Settings\Security Settings\Local Policies\Audit Policy folder, as shown in Figure 12.2.

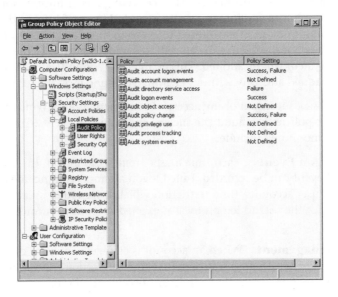

FIGURE 12.2   Windows Server 2003 audit policies.

Securing Groups

An important way to secure your messaging environment is by securing distribution and mail-enabled security groups. For instance, CompanyABC is a medium-sized company with 1,000 users. To facilitate company-wide notifications, the HR Department created a distribution group called "All Employees". All employees are members of the "All Employees" group. By default there are no message restrictions for new groups, meaning that anyone can send to this list. If CompanyABC has an Internet Mail SMTP Connector, this group will also have an SMTP address.

Consider what would happen if a new user sent an email to "All Employees" advertising a car for sale. Now imagine that the user sent it with a read receipt and delivery notification requested. This can have disastrous results if the server is unable to process this many requests at once.

In a similar scenario, intentions are not as innocent as the new user trying to sell a car. In fact, it can be an attempted denial of service (DOS) attack. An attacker sends an SMTP message to the "All Employees" group with a delivery notification receipt requested and spoofs the Return to address field as the same SMTP address as the distribution group. The effect is (1 + 1000 + 1000 * 1000) = 1,001,001 messages! Since a delivery notification receipt was requested, this single email results in over 1 million messages processed by the system.

Exchange Server 2003 now offers an easy solution for this problem by configuring message restrictions for the distribution group. To secure distribution groups so that only authenticated users can use it, do the following:

1. Open Active Directory Users and Computers from the Start, All Programs, Microsoft Exchange menu.

2. Right-click the distribution group and select Properties.

3. Select the Exchange General tab and under the Message restrictions section, check the check box to Accept messages: From authenticated users only.

4. Click OK when done.

An administrator could further restrict the usage of this group by allowing only a specific security group to use it. To restrict access to the distribution group to a specific user or group, do the following:

1. In the Active Directory Users and Computers snap-in, right-click the distribution group and select Properties.

2. Select the Exchange General tab and under the Message restrictions section, select the Only from radio button.

3. Click Add and enter the security group that has permissions to send to the distribution group.

4. Click OK when finished.

Keep Services to a Minimum

Depending on the role that an Exchange Server 2003 server will fulfill, not all services that are installed by default are necessary for the server to function. It is considered good practice to limit the number of entry points (services) into a server. Any services that are not required for the system to function should be disabled. Note that this can be performed using a customized security template.

Locking Down the File System

Files secured on Windows Server 2003 are only as secure as the permissions that are set on them. Subsequently, it is good to know that Windows Server 2003, for the first time in a Microsoft operating system, does not grant the Everyone group full control over share-level and NTFS-level permissions. In addition, critical operating system files and directories are secured, to disallow their unauthorized use.

Despite the overall improvements made, a complete understanding of file-level security is recommended to ensure that the file-level security of a server is not neglected.

> **NOTE**
>
> The Exchange Server 2003 installation process requires that partitions on the server are formatted as NTFS.

Using the Microsoft Baseline Security Analyzer

The Microsoft Baseline Security Analyzer (MBSA) is a tool that identifies common security misconfigurations and missing hotfixes via local or remote scans of Windows systems. MBSA provides users with the ability to scan a single Windows system and obtain a security assessment as well as a list of recommended corrective actions. Furthermore, administrators may use the MBSA tool to scan multiple functional roles of a Windows-based server on the network for vulnerabilities to help ensure systems are up-to-date with the latest security-related patches.

To run MBSA, do the following:

1. Download the latest security XML file to use with MBSA. (This is downloaded automatically if the server is connected to the Internet.) This file contains a list of current service packs and hotfixes that should be applied to a system.

2. Keep the default settings and scan the server(s).

Consulting Standards and Guidelines

As mentioned in Chapter 11, "Client-Level Security," Microsoft has gone to great lengths to provide secure and reliable products. Moreover, it has worked closely with companies, government agencies, security consultants, and others to address security issues in the computer industry.

In addition to Microsoft security standards and guidelines, it is advisable that organizations use recommended best practices compiled by the National Institute of Standards and Technologies (NIST) and the National Security Agency (NSA). Both NIST and NSA provide security lockdown configuration standards and guidelines that can be downloaded from their Web site (http://www.nist.gov and http://www.nsa.gov respectively).

Securing Servers with Security Templates

Security templates are a practical and effective means to apply security policies and configurations to Exchange Server 2003 servers. Although security templates are provided with Windows Server 2003, it is recommended to customize them prior to applying them using the Security Configuration and Analysis Microsoft Management Console (MMC) snap-in.

This not only ensures that computers are identically configured with the same security configurations but it also is an easy way to configure appropriate security measures for those computers that are not managed using GPOs.

> **NOTE**
>
> For more information on customizing and using security templates, refer to Chapter 11.

Keeping Up with Security Patches and Updates

Service packs (SPs) and hotfixes for both the operating system and applications, such as Exchange Server 2003, are vital parts to maintaining availability, reliability, performance, and security. There are several ways an administrator can update a system with the latest SP: CD-ROM, manually entered commands, Systems Management Server (SMS) Windows Update, or Microsoft Software Update Server (SUS).

> **NOTE**
>
> Thoroughly test and evaluate SPs and hotfixes in a lab environment before installing them on production servers. Also, install the appropriate SPs and hotfixes on each production server to keep all systems consistent.

Windows Update

Windows Update is a Web site that scans a local system and determines whether there are updates to apply to that system. Windows Update is a great way to update individual systems, but this method is sufficient for only a small number of systems. If administrators choose this method to update an entire organization, there would be an unnecessary amount of administration.

Software Update Services

Software Update Services (SUS) minimizes administration, management, and maintenance of mid- to large-sized organizations communicating directly and securely with Microsoft to gather the latest security updates and SPs (for Windows XP SP1 and Windows 2000 SP4 or higher).

The security updates downloaded onto SUS can then be distributed to either a lab server for testing (recommended) or to a production server for distribution. After these updates are tested, SUS can automatically update systems inside the network.

> **NOTE**
>
> You can find more information on SUS and download the product from
>
> `http://www.microsoft.com/windows2000/windowsupdate/sus/`

Hardening IIS

IIS is an integral part of Windows Server 2003 and it has come a long way from its predecessors especially in terms of security. Several key enhancements such as a reduced attack surface and enhanced application isolation deliver a robust and secure Web platform.

IIS installs only the features needed to fill its defined role or function. It works by turning off unnecessary features, much like the IISLockdown utility performed, thus reducing the attack surface available to attackers. For previous versions of Windows, the IISLockdown tool was available as a separate download. It is now, however, built into IIS. IIS maintains a UrlScan.ini file with a specific section for DenyUrlSequences and can limit the length of specific fields and requests. This functionality replaces some of the features of URLScan, a complementary component of using IISLockdown.

IIS Hardening Checklist

Although IIS does a good job at installing and enabling only what is needed, it is important to review IIS security configurations on the organization's Exchange Server 2003 servers. Table 12.1 summarizes key hardening aspects of IIS as well as presents other key recommendations for securing the Web components on the messaging server.

TABLE 12.1   IIS Hardening Checklist

Recommendation	Description
Enable logging using W3C. Use the extended properties sheet to add more info to the logs.	IIS logging can identify many different parameters and record them for later analysis. Add client IP address, username, method, URI Stem, HTTP status, Win32 status, User Agent, server IP address, and server port.
Set log file ACLs (admin— Full Control, system—Full Control, everyone—write, create).	This prevents someone from covering his tracks. Any log file that IIS generates will be stored in the %SystemRoot%\system32\LogFiles folder on the system partition. If the access control settings for these files are not secured, an attacker might cover up his actions on the server by deleting associated log entries.
Remove unused script mappings.	Unused script mappings—such as .htr, .ida, .htw, .idc, .printer, .shtm, .stm, and .shtml could be used to gain access to the system. If any script mappings within IIS are not being used, they should be removed.
Set appropriate directory permissions.	Set appropriate ACLs on virtual directories.

Other Hardening Techniques for Windows Server 2003

Although not all inclusive, Table 12.2 provides a quick checklist of recommended security precautions to take on an Exchange Server 2003 server.

TABLE 12.2   Windows Server 2003 Hardening Checklist

Recommendation	Description
Secure default Windows Repair Directory (`\%SystemRoot%\Repair`).	Set an appropriate level of access to this directory to prevent unauthorized access to system files.
Protect against data remnants.	The Recycle Bin saves a copy of a file when it is deleted through Windows Explorer. On critical servers this could pose a security risk. A sensitive file might be deleted; yet a copy of that file would remain in the Recycle Bin. To configure the Recycle Bin to prevent deleted files from being saved, use the following procedure: 1. Right-click the Recycle Bin icon on the desktop, and select Properties. 2. Check the box labeled Do not move files to the Recycle Bin. Remove files immediately on delete. 3. Click OK. 4. Empty the Recycle Bin of any preexisting files.

Automatically clear the pagefile before the system shuts down.	Virtual Memory support in Windows Server 2003 uses a system pagefile to swap pages from memory when they are not being actively used. On a running system, this pagefile is opened exclusively by the operating system and hence is well protected. However, to implement a secure Windows Server 2003 environment, the system pagefile should be wiped clean when the system shuts down. To do so, change the data value of the `ClearPageFileAtShutdown` value in the following Registry key to a value of **1**:
	`HKEY_LOCAL_MACHINE\SYSTEM\CurrentControlSet\Control\Session Manager\Memory Management`.
	If the value does not exist, add the following value:
	    Value Name: **ClearPageFileAtShutdown**
	    Value Type: **REG_DWORD**
	    Value: **1**

Rename the administrator account.	Renaming the administrator account helps prevent unauthorized access by using the default administrator account. In addition, consider establishing a decoy account named "Administrator" with no privileges. Scan the event log regularly to identify attempts to use this account.
Remove all unnecessary file shares.	Scrutinize all shares to determine whether they should be removed or shares should be locked down.

Securing by Functional Roles of the Server

Exchange Server 2003 servers can participate in various responsibilities in a given messaging environment. Some of these responsibilities may be intertwined due to budget constraints, business requirements, or technical justifications. No matter how the roles and responsibilities play out in the environment, it's important to secure them appropriately based on the roles of the server.

Some examples of the functional roles that Exchange Server 2003 servers can have within the messaging environment include, but are not limited to, the following:

- **Front-end Servers**   Front-end servers relay client requests to back-end servers and should not host information stores.

- **Connector and Relay Servers**   Connector or relay servers act as a bridge between different Exchange sites or organizations, as well as to foreign servers on different networks.

- **Back-end Servers**   Back-end servers refer to Exchange servers that are located on the internal network and do not directly face the Internet. These servers generally host information stores containing mailboxes or public folders.

Exchange Server 2003 Running on Domain Controllers

Some smaller messaging environments might consider implementing Exchange Server 2003 on a Global Catalog/domain controller (GC/DC) to save on costs and administration. On the contrary, this configuration can actually increase costs by increasing administration and maintenance, and potentially cause more downtime (both scheduled and unscheduled). An equally important reason for avoiding this configuration is to minimize security risks and other implications, such as the following:

- Clustering is not available.

- Performance is affected.

- DSAccess, DSProxy, and Global Catalog services will not be load-balanced or have failover capabilities.

- All services run under LocalSystem and might pose a greater chance of compromise.

- Exchange administrators require physical access to the DC.

- The server takes much longer to shut down.

Special Security Considerations for Exchange and Operating System Upgrades

If Exchange Server 2003 runs on top of Windows 2000 SP3, the admininstrator has the option of doing an in-place upgrade of the NOS to Windows 2003 Server. Because of the new security and functionality of Windows 2003, Exchange Server 2003 must make some adjustments to IIS 6.0 after the upgrade.

As the server starts up, it looks for a `/lm.ds2mb/61491` key in the IIS metabase. If the key does not exist, Exchange performs the following steps:

1. IIS switches from Compatibility Mode to Worker Process Isolation Mode.

2. Exchange ISAPI extensions are enabled and an Application Pool is created.

3. IIS creates the `/lm.ds2mb/61491` key in the metabase.

4. IIS automatically restarts the W3SVC service for the changes to take effect.

Each of these changes are logged in the Application Event Log.

Standardizing Exchange Server 2003 Servers

Organizations are challenged by varying IT infrastructure standards because all too often systems vary in the type of components used, how they are built, how they are configured, and more. The variations require significantly more administration and maintenance especially in mid to large size environments. The result of which increases the number of IT personnel needed to support such a solution and the associated IT expenditures.

Standardizing the messaging environment is in the organization's best interest not only to save on administration, maintenance, and troubleshooting but also to help promote a more secure environment. Standardization ensures that each server has been properly secured based on the role or function that it serves.

Standardizing Server Builds

When organizations build servers from scratch, typically the build parameters including security configurations are inconsistent. From an administration, maintenance, troubleshooting, and security point of view, this can be a nightmare. Each server must be treated individually and administrators must try to keep track of separate, incongruent configurations.

Protecting Exchange Server 2003 from Viruses

Exchange Server 2003 does not provide what is typically thought of as antivirus software (i.e. an application that gets installed and enabled to scan for viruses) but it does provide various tools and an Antivirus Application Program Interface (AVAPI) that help to protect the messaging infrastructure from viruses and worms. Third-party vendors, such as the ones listed in Table 12.3, can hook their antivirus applications into the AVAPI to gain access to messages as they are handled by Exchange.

TABLE 12.3   Third-Party Antivirus Products for Exchange Server 2003

Vendor/Product	Web Site
Sybari's Antigen for Exchange	http://www.sybari.com
Aladdin's eSafe Mail	http://ealaddin.com/esafe/mail
GFI MailSecurity for Exchange	http://www.gfi.com/mailsecurity
Panda Antivirus for Exchange Server	http://www.pandasecurity.com
Trend's ScanMail for Microsoft Exchange	http://www.trend.com
Symantec's AntiVirus/Filtering for Microsoft Exchange	http://enterprisesecurity.symantec.com
Softwin's BitDefender	http://www.bitdefender.com
Sophos MailMonitor for Exchange 2000	http://www.sophos.com

There are many mechanisms that can be used to protect the messaging environment from viruses and other malicious code. Most of third-party virus scanning products scan for known virus signatures as well as provide some form of heuristics to scan for unknown viruses. Other anti-virus products block suspicious or specific types of message attachments at the point of entry before a possible virus reaches the information store.

As alluded to, there are two fundamental ways for anti-virus products to keep viruses from affecting the information store:

- **Gateway Scanning**   Gateway scanning works by scanning all messages as they go through the SMTP gateway (typically to the Internet). If the message contains a virus or is suspected of carrying a virus, the antivirus product can clean, quarantine, or delete it before Exchange has to do any further processing. More specifically, a transport event sink takes the message and places it into a queue to be scanned.

- **Mailbox Scanning**   Mailbox scanning is useful to remove viruses that have entered the information store. For example, a new virus might make it into the Exchange information store before a signature file that can detect it is applied, so the virus is not detected by the gateway scanner. The information store can be rescanned after the new pattern file is installed, cleaning the viruses that made it in. If a user opens a virus-laden message, the mailbox scanner will clean it. A mailbox scanner will also scan messages created from the internal network so that if a user brings a floppy disk from home with an infected file that is then emailed to a colleague, the message will not go through the SMTP gateway but the mailbox scanner will detect and clean it upon submission to the mail store.

The New AVAPI 2.5 Specification

Exchange Server 2003 AVAPI is a new and improved version compared to earlier versions supported in Exchange's predecessors. Antivirus vendors use this specification to provide a robust solution against viruses, worms, and spam.

The more notable features of AVAPI version 2.5 in Exchange Server 2003 include the following:

- Gateway scanning occurs before mail even gets to the mailbox.

- The ability to clean, quarantine, or delete messages is available. (AVAPI version 2.0 supported removing the virus, but still delivered the message.)

- Additional message properties are now exposed.

- More detailed status codes are available to Outlook from vendor software.

- Guaranteed outbound scanning is offered.

Combating Spam

Spam is a global problem that affects everyone with an Internet-accessible email address. It is not just a frustration anymore; it affects many things including an organization's ability to be productive among other things. In Chapters 11 and Chapter 13, "Transport-Level Security," many methods and features such as blocking attachments, filtering, and preventing Web beaconing were examined to help prevent spam in the organization. To continue with that examination, the following sections describe common best practices to minimize or alleviate spam.

Use Blacklists

Many companies are unknowingly serving as open relays, which aid spammers by essentially permitting them to use the company's messaging system for unsolicited email. When a company or domain is reported as an open relay, the domain can be placed on a blacklist. This blacklist in turn can be used by other companies to prevent incoming mail from a known open relay source. Blacklists are useful because they can help prevent spam.

You can find some organizations that maintain blacklists at the following addresses:

- `http://www.dsbl.org`

- `http://www.mail-abuse.com`

- `http://www.spamcop.net`

- `http://ordb.org`

Report Spammers

Organizations and laws are getting tougher on spammers, but spam prevention requires users and organizations to report the abuse. Although this often is a difficult task because many times the source is undecipherable, it is nonetheless important to take a proactive stance and report abuses.

Users should contact the system administrator or help desk if they receive or continue to receive spam, virus hoaxes, and other such fraudulent offers. System administrators should report spammers and contact mail abuse organizations, such as the ones listed earlier in the section "Use Blacklists." System administrators must also use discretion based on the offense, the frequency, and the possible ramifications of various ways of dealing with the spam. For instance, if a few spam messages appear to originate from yahoo.com it might serve the company better to filter messages based on a message's language contents rather than blocking the entire domain.

Use a Third-Party Antispam Product

Microsoft has equipped users, system administrators, and third-party organizations with the tools necessary to combat spam. Using third-party products strengthens the company's defense and complements the tools that Microsoft provides in Exchange Server 2003. Third-party products also provide a multitude of features that help with reporting, customizations, and filtering mechanisms to keep only the unwanted mail away from the messaging environment and users.

Do Not Use Open SMTP Relays

By default, Exchange Server 2003 is not configured to allow open relays. If an SMTP relay is necessary in the messaging environment, take the necessary precautions to ensure that only authorized users or systems have access to these SMTP relays.

Use the Work Email Address for Work Only

Although this is self-expanatory, it is important to note that this policy and practice not only helps minimize spam in the workplace but it also helps prevent the messaging environment from being used for unauthorized purposes. It is recommended for everyone, including system administrators, to use a personal email address for subscribing to or signing up for non–business-related services.

Take Caution When Sharing Your Email Address

Whether you use your email address for business or non-business purposes, think twice before giving away your email address. Some people have gone so far as to not list their email address on business cards. Others use a secondary email address for those higher-risk situations. Take the time to determine the appropriateness of giving out your email address and be aware of the possible consequences.

Look for Privacy Statements and Mailing Options

When submitting information through an online form, look for a privacy statement and mailing options. Make sure the statement includes protection of all your information, including your email address, and make sure that you are not opting to be put on a mailing list.

Remove or "Unsubscribe" at Your Own Discretion

A general rule of thumb to follow is that if it looks like spam, it probably is. Removing your name or "unsubscribing" only validates your account and can result in more spam.

Summary

Securing Exchange Server 2003 from a server-level perspective is multifaceted. It involves proper planning and design, hardening Windows Server 2003, developing policies, implementing or enabling Exchange Server 2003 features, and much more. This chapter focused on the server-level aspects that promote a secure messaging environment.

Best Practices

The following are best practices from this chapter:

- Assess the messaging environment's risks.

- Establish a corporate email policy.

- Establish administrative policies.

- Use email disclaimers and have them approved by a legal representative.

- Plan and design Exchange Server 2003 security roles.

- Use a layered approach when hardening Windows Server 2003.

- Perform periodic security assessments.

- Keep updated with the latest service packs and hotfixes.

- Assess the functional role of the server and secure it accordingly.

- Do not install Exchange Server 2003 on a domain controller.

- Standardize Exchange Server 2003 security.

- Implement a mailbox and gateway antivirus scanner.

Transport-Level Security

Organizations of all sizes use Exchange Server 2003, not as simply an email system, but also for internal and external communications. This communication is vital to any organization and it must be efficient and secure. The level of security depends on the business, security policies, type and content of information being communicated, and which parties are communicating.

Securing external communication is vital—especially information that is transmitted over public networks such as the Internet. External communication is an important facet to address when considering transport-level security, but it is not the only important aspect to secure. Internal communication, whether it is internal employees sending messages or server-to-server interactions, are equally important. This chapter focuses on the mechanisms that exist to protect and encrypt information sent between computers on a network. New and improved transport security features in Windows Server 2003 and Exchange Server 2003 are examined.

The Onion Approach

Security is a relative term, because even the most secure infrastructures are subject to vulnerabilities, and an environment is only as secure as its weakest link. One of the best defenses, however, is deploying multiple layers of security on critical network data. Using multiple layers of security is often referred to as the onion approach, where different stages or layers of security are used to protect the information. Generally speaking, as the information becomes more sensitive or confidential, the number of onion layers increases to thwart unauthorized access.

The premise behind the onion approach is that if a single layer of security is compromised, the intruder will have to bypass the second, third, fourth, and so on layers of security to gain access to the information. For example, relying on a complex 128-bit "unbreakable" encryption scheme is worthless if an intruder uses simple social engineering to acquire the password or PIN from a validated user. Putting in a second or third layer of security makes it that much more difficult for intruders to break through all layers.

On the other hand, adding security layers also affects usability and sometimes even functionality. As the security layers are applied, the complexity increases for authorized users trying to gain access to the information. The key to providing multiple layers of security is that the information is worthwhile to protect and the mechanisms that are put into place are as transparent as possible to authorized users.

When working with Windows Server 2003 and Exchange Server 2003, there are many security facets to consider implementing. Transport-level security is just one of those facets, but it is an important one to consider for organizations of all sizes. Transport-level security also uses an onion approach, wherein multiple levels of authentication, encryption, and authorization can be implemented for an enhanced degree of security on a network.

Using Public Key Infrastructure with Exchange Server 2003

Public Key Infrastructure (PKI), in a nutshell, is an extensible infrastructure used to provide certificate-based services. It is a conglomeration of digital certificates, registration authorities, and Certificate Authorities that can be used to provide authentication, authorization, non-repudiation, confidentiality, and verification. A Certificate Authority (CA) is a digital signature of the certificate issuer.

PKI implementations are widespread and are becoming more of a critical component of modern networks. Windows Server 2003 fully supports the deployment of various PKI configurations. PKI deployments can range from simple to complex, as illustrated in Figures 13.1 and 13.2, with some PKI implementations using internal and external PKIs to supply a wide range of services and trust relationships with other entities. Although entire books are dedicated to PKI, this chapter focuses on how PKI can be used to secure Exchange Server 2003 implementations.

Certificate Services in Windows Server 2003

Windows Server 2003 includes a built-in Certificate Authority (CA) known as Certificate Services. Certificate Services can be used to create certificates and subsequently manage them; it is responsible for ensuring their validity. Certificate Services can also be used to trust outside PKIs, such as a third-party PKI, to expand services and secure communication with other organizations.

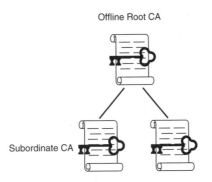

Offline Root CA

Subordinate CA

FIGURE 13.1   A simple PKI.

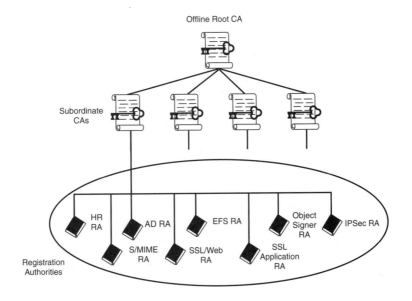

Offline Root CA

Subordinate CAs

HR RA
AD RA
S/MIME RA
EFS RA
SSL/Web RA
SSL Application RA
Object Signer RA
IPSec RA

Registration Authorities

FIGURE 13.2   A complex PKI.

The type of CA that you install and configure depends on the purpose or purposes of the Windows Server 2003 PKI. Certificate Services for Windows Server 2003 can be installed as one of the following CA types:

- **Enterprise Root Certification Authority**   The enterprise root CA is the most trusted CA in an organization and, if required in an organization, should be installed before any other CA. All other CAs are subordinate to an enterprise root CA. Enterprise root CAs store certificates in Active Directory (AD) by default.

- **Enterprise Subordinate Certification Authority**   An enterprise subordinate CA must get a CA certificate from an enterprise root CA but can then issue certificates to all users and computers in the enterprise. These types of CAs are often used for load balancing of an enterprise root CA; more importantly, using subordinates provides stronger security for the PKI.

- **Standalone Root Certification Authority**   A standalone root CA is the root of a hierarchy that is not related to the enterprise domain information, and therefore certificates are not stored in AD. Multiple standalone CAs can be established for particular purposes.

- **Standalone Subordinate Certification Authority**   A standalone subordinate CA receives its certificate from a standalone root CA and can then be used to distribute certificates to users and computers associated with that standalone CA.

Windows Server 2003 PKI can also be either online or offline. The key difference is the level of security that is required in the organization.

> **TIP**
>
> An enterprise root CA is the most versatile CA in Windows Server 2003 because it integrates tightly with AD and offers more certificate services. If you're unsure as to what CA to use, choose an enterprise root or subordinate CA for use with messaging. Most importantly, however, is that with any PKI there must be careful planning and design.

PKI Planning Considerations

Any PKI implementation requires thorough planning and design, as noted earlier. Possible planning and design considerations include the following:

- Multinational legal considerations, including creation and standardization of a formal Certificate Practice Statement (CPS)

- Policies and procedures for issuing, revoking, and suspending certificates

- PKI hardware identification and standardization, including employee badge integration

- Determination of CA hierarchy administration model

- Creation of a redundant CA infrastructure based on geographical location

- Policies and procedures for creation of CAs as subordinates and policy enforcers within a greater hierarchy including qualified subordination and cross-certification

- Policies and procedures for creation of Registration Authorities (RAs) and their placement within the CA hierarchy

- CA trust strategies

- Policies and procedures for maintaining the CA as a 7×24×365 operation

- Policies and procedures for key and certificate management, including—but not limited to—key length, cryptographic algorithms, certificate lifetime, certificate renewal, storage requirements, and more

- Policies and procedures for securing the PKI

- Published plans for providing high availability and recoverability

- Policies and procedures for integrating the CA with LDAP and/or Active Directory

- Policies and procedures for integrating with existing applications

- Policies and procedures for security-related incidents (for example, bulk revocation of certificates)

- Policies and procedures for delegation of administrative tasks

- Standards for PKI auditing and reporting

- Policies and procedures for change control

- Standards for key length and expiration of certificates

- Policies and procedures for handling lost certificates (that is, smartcard)

- Policies and procedures for safe distribution of the CA public key to end-users

- Policies and procedures for enrollment (for example, auto-enrollment, stations, and so forth)

- Policies and procedures for incorporating external users and companies

- Procedures for using certificate templates

As you can see from this list, implementing PKI is not to be taken lightly. Even if the organization is implementing PKI just for enhanced Exchange Server 2003 messaging functionality, the considerations should be planned and designed.

Installing Certificate Services

To install Certificate Services on Windows Server 2003, follow these steps:

1. Choose Start, Control Panel, Add or Remove Programs.

2. Click Add/Remove Windows Components.

3. Check the Certificate Services box.

4. A warning dialog box will be displayed indicating that the computer name or domain name cannot be changed after you install Certificate Services. Click Yes to proceed with the installation.

5. Click Next to continue.

6. The next screen enables you to create the type of CA required. Refer to the preceding list for more information about the different types of CAs that you can install. In this example, choose Enterprise Root CA and click Next to continue.

7. Enter a common name for the CA—for example, `TestCA`.

8. Enter the validity period for the Certificate Authority and click Next to continue. The cryptographic key will then be created.

9. Enter a location for the certificate database and then database logs. The location you choose should be secured to prevent unauthorized tampering with the CA. Click Next to continue. Setup will then install the CA components.

10. If IIS is not installed, a prompt will be displayed indicating that Web Enrollment will be disabled until you install IIS. If this box is displayed, click OK to continue.

11. Click Finish after installation to complete the process.

Fundamentals of Private and Public Keys

Encryption techniques can primarily be classified as either symmetrical or asymmetrical. **Symmetrical encryption** requires that each party in an encryption scheme hold a copy of a **private key**, which is used to encrypt and decrypt information sent between the two parties. The problem with private key encryption is that the private key must somehow be transmitted to the other party without it being intercepted and used to decrypt the information.

Asymmetrical encryption uses a combination of two keys, which are mathematically related to each other. The first key, the private key, is kept closely guarded and is used to encrypt the information. The second key, the **public key**, can be used to decrypt the information. The integrity of the public key is ensured through certificates. The asymmetric approach to encryption ensures that the private key does not fall into the wrong hands and only the intended recipient is able to decrypt the data.

Understanding Certificates

A **certificate** is essentially a digital document issued by a trusted central authority that is used by the authority to validate a user's identity. Central, trusted authorities such as VeriSign are widely used on the Internet to ensure that software from Microsoft, for example, is really from Microsoft, and not a virus in disguise.

Certificates are used for multiple functions, including, but not limited to, the following:

- Secure email
- Web-based authentication

- IP Security (IPSec)

- Secure Web-based communications

- Code signing

- Certification hierarchies

Certificates are signed using information from the subject's public key; identifier information such as name, email address, and so on; and the CA.

Certificate Templates

As mentioned earlier, there are multiple functions for certificates, and hence there are multiple types of certificates. In other words, one certificate may be used to sign code and another certificate used to provide support for secure email. This is a one-to-one relationship wherein a certificate is used for a single purpose. Certificates can also have a one-to-many relationship wherein one certificate is used for multiple purposes.

> **TIP**
>
> One of the best examples of a certificate that uses a one-to-many relationship is the user certificate. A User certificate by default provides support for user authentication, secure email, and the Encrypting File System (EFS), as shown in Figure 13.3.

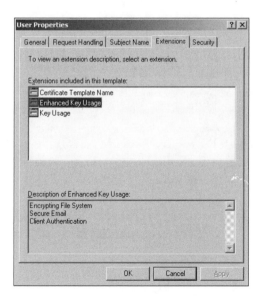

FIGURE 13.3   Default properties for the User certificate.

Windows Server 2003 contains a large number of certificates, and each has an assigned set of settings and purposes. In essence, certificates can be categorized into six different functional areas:

- **Server Authentication**   These certificates can be used to authenticate servers to clients as well as provide authentication between servers.

- **Client Authentication**   These certificates are used to provide client authentication to servers or server-side services.

- **Secure Email**   Users can digitally sign and encrypt email.

- **Encrypting File System**   These certificates are used to encrypt and decrypt files using EFS.

- **File Recovery**   These certificates are used for recovering encrypted EFS files.

- **Code Signing**   These certificates can sign content and applications. Code signing certificates help users and services trust code.

Customizing Certificate Templates

To customize a certificate template to be used in the network environment, use the Certificate Templates snap-in, as shown in Figure 13.4. To use this snap-in, do the following.

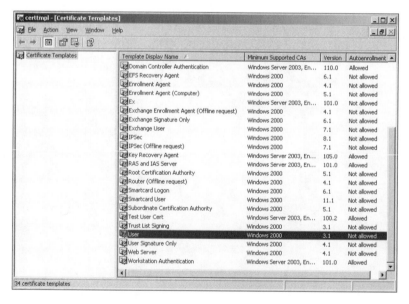

FIGURE 13.4   The Certificate Templates snap-in.

1. Open the Run dialog box from the Start menu and type **MMC**.

2. In the MMC console window, select Add/Remove Snap-in from the File menu.

3. Click the Add button and select the Certificate Templates snap-in.

4. Click Add and then click Close.

5. Click OK when done.

6. In the left pane, select Certificate Templates. This will display in the right pane all the available certificate templates.

7. Right-click the template to modify and select Duplicate Template. For this example, select the User certificate template.

8. Type the certificate template display name from within the General tab, as shown in Figure 13.5.

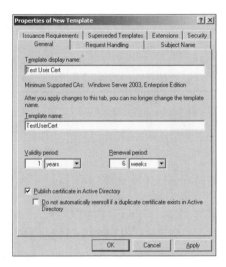

FIGURE 13.5   Customizing a certificate template.

9. Within the Request Handling tab, verify that the purpose of the certificate is to provide signature and encryption capabilities.

10. On the Issuance Requirements tab, select whether the certificate requires manager approval and the number of authorized signatures that are required. These options control how and when users can get the certificate.

11. On the Security tab, check which users will have enroll or auto-enroll rights. By default, the Domain Users group has enroll permissions.

12. Click OK when done.

Smartcards in a PKI Infrastructure

A robust solution for PKI can be found in the introduction of smartcard authentication for users. Smartcards are small devices that have a microchip embedded in them; this chip enables them to store unique information in each card. User login information, as well as certificates installed from a CA server, can be placed on a smartcard. When a user needs to log in to a system, the user places the smartcard in a smartcard reader or simply swipes it across the reader itself. The certificate is read, and the user is prompted only for a PIN, which is uniquely assigned to each user. After the PIN and the certificate are verified, the user can log in to the domain.

> **NOTE**
>
> Smartcards can also be used to complement the use of passwords. For instance, strong passwords can be used in addition to a PIN number if the organization's security policy dictates very strong authentication requirements.

Smartcards have obvious advantages over standard forms of authentication. It is no longer possible to simply steal or guess someone's username and password, because the username can be entered only via the unique smartcard. If stolen or lost, the smartcard can be immediately deactivated and the certificate revoked. Even if a functioning smartcard were to fall into the wrong hands, the PIN would still need to be used to properly access the system. Smartcards are fast becoming a more accepted way to integrate the security of certificates and PKI into organizations.

Certificate Enrollment

Users must first be issued certificates before they are able to sign or encrypt messages. How users obtain the certificates depends on the organization's security policy and procedures and the infrastructure that is in place to support certificate services. If the organization is using Windows Server 2003 Certificate Services, users can obtain certificates in the following manner:

- Auto-enrollment
- Using smartcards
- Using the Web enrollment form
- Using the MMC

> **NOTE**
>
> When using Windows Server 2003 Certificate Services (PKI), public keys are stored in the AD, which enables users in the AD to encrypt messages for others in the AD. Private keys, on the other hand, are typically stored on the user's computer or on a smartcard.

Use the following steps to request a certificate using the MMC:

1. Type **certmgr.msc** from the Start, Run command window.

2. In the Certificate Manager window, expand Certificates—Current User.

3. Right-click on Personal and select All Tasks, Request New Certificate.

4. Click Next in the Certificate Request Wizard and then select the User certificate. It is important to note that these certificates must be made available to the users. Refer to the section "Customizing Certificate Templates," earlier in this chapter, for more information on how to provide certificates to users.

5. Click Next and then type the friendly name for the certificate.

6. Click Next and then Finish when done.

In the Certificate Manager window, click on the Personal, Certificates folder to display the certificates that have been issued to the current user, as shown in Figure 13.6.

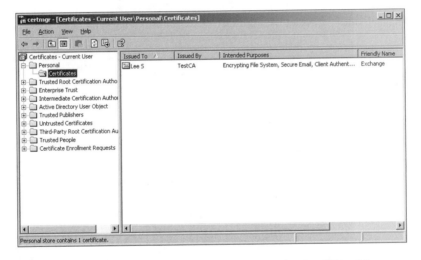

FIGURE 13.6   Displaying issued certificates of a user, using the Certificate Manager.

> **TIP**
>
> The Active Directory Users and Computers snap-in can be used to display which certificates have been issued to a user. Select Advanced Features from the View menu and then double-click the user. The certificates can be viewed on the Published Certificates tab, as illustrated in Figure 13.7.

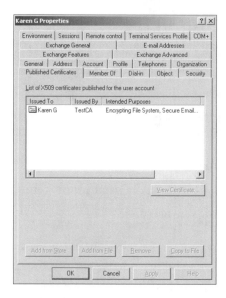

FIGURE 13.7   Displaying issued certificates of a user, using Active Directory Users and Computers.

Supporting S/MIME

Secure/Multipurpose Internet Mail Extensions (S/MIME) is used to digitally sign and encrypt messages. Digital signatures provide authentication, non-repudiation, and data integrity, and encryption keeps message contents confidential.

To support S/MIME, X.509 digital certificates are used. The certificate identifies information about the certificate's owner and includes the owner's public key information. X.509 is the industry standard for digital certificates. The Windows Server 2003 certificate templates that support S/MIME are Exchange User, Exchange Signature Only (for only digital signatures), Smartcard User, and User.

Supporting Digital Signatures

Signing a message generates a random checksum that is added to the message. The random checksum is the message's fingerprint or digital signature, which is then encrypted using the user's private signing key. The user then sends the message to the recipient that includes three items: the message in plain text, the sender's X.509 digital certificate, and the digital certificate.

The recipient checks the Certificate Revocation List (CRL) to see whether the sender's certificate is on the list. If the certificate is not on the list, the digital signature is decrypted with the sender's public signing key. If it is on the CRL, the recipient is warned that the sender's certificate has been revoked. The recipient's client then generates a checksum from the plain text message and compares it to the digital signature. If the checksums match, the recipient knows the sender is the one who sent the message. If they do not match, the recipient is warned that the message has been tampered with.

Message Encryption

The process of encrypting a message generates a random bulk encryption key that is used to encrypt the contents of the message. The sender uses the recipient's public key to encrypt the bulk encryption key. For this process to work, the sender must have a copy of the recipient's digital certificate. The certificate can be retrieved from either the Global Address List (GAL) or the sender's Contact list. The digital certificate contains the recipient's public encryption key, which is used to create the lockbox for the bulk encryption key.

When the recipient receives the message, he or she will use a private encryption key to decrypt and gain access to the bulk encryption key. The bulk encryption key is then used to decrypt the message. The Exchange User, Smartcard User, and User certificate templates have encryption and decryption capabilities.

Comparing PGP and S/MIME

Pretty Good Privacy (PGP) is similar to S/MIME because it can sign and encrypt messages. It is an alternative to using S/MIME.

Use PGP in the following situations:

- For single users or small workgroups

- If there are many different types of mail clients

Use S/MIME for the following situations:

- For larger environments

- For standardization

- If Outlook is the primary (or only) mail client

- If you want to make secure email transparent to the end-user

Protecting Communications with IP Security

IP Security (IPSec) is a mechanism or policy for establishing end-to-end encryption of all data packets sent between computers. IPSec operates at Layer 3 of the OSI model and subsequently uses packets for all traffic between computers participating in the IPSec policy.

IPSec is often considered to be one of the best ways to secure the traffic generated in an environment, and is useful for securing servers and workstations, both in high-risk Internet access scenarios and also in private network configurations as an enhanced layer of security.

Fundamentals of IPSec

As mentioned earlier, all traffic between participating computers (whether initiated by an application, the operating system, services, and so on) is encrypted. IPSec places its own header on each encrypted packet and sends the packets to the destination server to be decrypted. The primary advantage to this is that it helps prevent eavesdropping and discourages unauthorized access.

As you can imagine, IPSec requires additional processing overhead in order to efficiently encrypt and decrypt data as it moves among the participating computers. There are network interface cards (NICs) that have built-in support for IPSec and which offload much of the processing overhead. These NICs are highly recommended in a production environment.

Key IPSec Functionality

IPSec in Windows Server 2003 provides the following key functionality:

- **Data Privacy**   All information sent from one IPSec machine to another is thoroughly encrypted by such algorithms as 3DES, which effectively prevent the unauthorized viewing of sensitive data.

- **Data Integrity**   The integrity of IPSec packets is enforced through ESP headers, which verify that the information contained within an IPSec packet has not been tampered with.

- **Anti-Replay Capability**   IPSec prevents streams of captured packets from being re-sent, known as a "replay" attack.

- **Per Packet Authenticity**   IPSec uses certificates or Kerberos authentication to ensure that the sender of an IPSec packet is actually an authorized user.

- **NAT Transversal**   Windows Server 2003's implementation of IPSec now enables IPSec to be routed through current NAT implementations, a concept that will be defined more thoroughly in the following sections.

- **Diffie-Hellman 2048-Bit Key Support**   Virtually unbreakable Diffie-Hellman 2048-bit key lengths are supported in Windows Server 2003's IPSec implementation, assuring that the IPSec key cannot easily be broken.

IPSec NAT Transversal (NAT-T)

IPSec in Windows Server 2003 supports the concept of Network Address Translation Transversal (NAT-T). Understanding how NAT-T works requires a full understanding of the need for NAT itself.

Network Address Translation (NAT) was developed because not enough IP addresses were available for all the clients on the Internet. Because of this, private IP ranges were established (10.x.x.x, 192.168.x.x, and so on) to enable all clients in an organization to have a unique IP address in their own private space. These IP addresses were designed to not route through the public IP address space, and a mechanism was needed to translate them into a valid, unique public IP address.

NAT was developed to fill this role. It normally resides on firewall servers or routers to provide NAT capabilities between private and public networks. RRAS for Windows Server 2003 also provides NAT capabilities.

Because the construction of the IPSec packet does not enable NAT addresses, IPSec traffic has, in the past, been dropped at NAT servers, because there was no way to physically route the information to the proper destination. This posed major barriers to the widespread implementation of IPSec because many of the clients on the Internet today are addressed via NAT.

NAT Transversal, which is a new feature in Windows Server 2003's IPSec implementation, was jointly developed as an Internet standard by Microsoft and Cisco Systems. NAT-T works by sensing that a NAT network needs to be transversed and subsequently encapsulating the entire IPSec packet into a UDP packet with a normal UDP header. NAT handles UDP packets flawlessly, and they are subsequently routed to the proper address on the other side of the NAT.

NAT Transversal works well but requires that both ends of the IPSec transaction understand the protocol so as to properly pull the IPSec packet out of the UDP encapsulation. With the latest IPSec client and server, NAT-T becomes a reality and is positioned to make IPSec into a much bigger success than it is today.

Configuring IPSec

IPSec is built into Windows Server 2003 and is also available for clients. In fact, basic IPSec functionality can easily be set up in an environment that is running Windows Server 2003's Active Directory, because IPSec can use the Kerberos authentication functionality in lieu of certificates. Subsequently, it is a fairly straightforward process to install and configure IPSec between servers and clients, and should be considered as a way to further implement additional security in an environment.

Establishing an IPSec Policy

Although other policies can be customized to fit the organization's security requirements, three predefined IPSec policies are built into Windows Server 2003:

- **Server (Request Security)**   This policy option requests but does not require IPSec communications. Choosing this option enables the server to communicate with other non-IPSec clients, and is recommended for organizations with fewer security needs or those in the midst of, but not finished with, an implementation of IPSec.

- **Client (Respond Only)**   This option enables the configured client computer to respond to requests for IPSec communications.

- **Secure Server (Require Security)**   The most secure policy option is the Require Security option, which stipulates that all network traffic to and from the server must be encrypted with IPSec.

To establish a simple IPSec policy on a server, do the following:

1. Choose Local Security Policy from the Start, Administrative Tools menu.

2. Navigate to IP Security Policies on Local Computer.

3. In the right pane, right-click Server (Request Security) and select Assign.

To establish a simple IPSec policy on a Windows XP client, do the following:

1. Choose Local Security Policy from the Start, Administrative Tools menu. The Administrative Tools must be enabled in the Task Manager view settings.

2. Navigate to IP Security Policies on Local Computer.

3. In the right pane, right-click Client (Respond Only) and select Assign.

Transport Layer Security

Transport Layer Security (TLS) is another, lesser-known method of encrypting traffic. It is essentially a newer version of SSL and is used primarily to encrypt SMTP specific traffic, particularly SMTP connector–related traffic. TLS encryption can also be used with Basic or Integrated Windows Authentication to protect credentials as they are being transmitted.

Locking Down SMTP

SMTP is the de facto messaging standard—not only for Exchange Server 2003 but also for the industry. This service is not built into Exchange Server 2003 but rather is a service provided by Windows Server 2003. Nonetheless, SMTP security and other parameters can be easily configured through the Exchange System Manager (ESM).

General SMTP Security Best Practices

Some general security best practices for SMTP include, but are not limited to, the following:

- **Limit Message Size**   Limiting the size of incoming and outgoing emails not only helps save disk space on the Exchange Server 2003 server, it also minimizes Denial of Service (DoS) vulnerabilities.

- **Disable Auto-replies**   The classic out-of-office or on-vacation message that users may configure are essentially messages informing a hacker that "I'm not at home." Users are notorious for also giving information, such as contact information, in these auto-reply receipts that should not necessarily be shared with anyone that sends them an email.

- **Restrict User Access**   Allowing only authenticated users to send email prevents unauthorized users from using the system for spam or other nonapproved messaging.

- **Control SMTP Connections**   Controlling which IP addresses or domains that can send emails will greatly reduce spam, spam-relaying, and DoS attacks.

- **Hide the SMTP Greeting**   Hide the SMTP greeting so that hackers must work even harder to discover which messaging system they are trying to attack.

Configuring Message Delivery Limits

Message delivery limits prevent users from sending large messages through Exchange. Large messages tie up Exchange resources (processing time, queue availability, disk storage, and more) and if misused can be just as bad as experiencing a DoS attack. It also molds users into using better, alternative delivery methods, such as file shares, compression of attachments, and even document management portals. Exchange Server 2003 uses a 10,240KB (10MB) message size limit by default, and this can be easily set to smaller sizes.

Another important message delivery limit that can be used to secure Exchange Server 2003 involves the number of recipients that a message can be sent to at any one time. Limiting the maximum number of recipients limits internal users' ability to essentially spam the enterprise with large numbers of emails. Exchange Server 2003 limits the number of recipients per message to 5,000 recipients. Using public folders in addition to a limitation on the maximum number of recipients can also mold users into working more efficiently with Exchange Server 2003.

To configure Exchange Server 2003 message delivery limits, do the following:

1. Open the ESM by choosing System Manager from the Start, All Programs, Microsoft Exchange menu.

2. Expand Global Settings and then right-click Message Delivery and select Properties.

3. On the Defaults tab, adjust the limits for Sending message size or Receiving message size.

4. To control the number of recipients per message, adjust the Recipients limits setting.

TIP

Distribution Groups are expanded when evaluating the maximum recipients limit. It might be necessary to override some users (for example, the Human Resources (HR) department) with No Limit in Active Directory Users and Computers to allow them to use an All Employees distribution group.

Securing SMTP Virtual Servers

Security configuration parameters can be found within the SMTP virtual server's Property pages. To view the Property pages for a server's SMTP virtual server, do the following:

1. Open the ESM by choosing System Manager from the Start, All Programs, Microsoft Exchange menu.

2. Expand the Exchange Organization, the Administrative Group where the server resides, the Exchange Server 2003 server, the Protocols folder, and finally the SMTP folder.

3. Right-click the Default SMTP Virtual Server and select Properties.

Using Authentication Controls

All three of the supported authentication methods supported by the SMTP virtual server (that is, anonymous, Basic, and Integrated Windows Authentication) are enabled as illustrated in Figure 13.8. Although this configuration might appear to be completely insecure, it depends on the organization's security policy and whether the SMTP virtual server is accessible by a host on the Internet. Many SMTP hosts do not require usernames and passwords and instead rely on other methods to secure access. If the organization has only a small number of SMTP hosts accessing the SMTP virtual server, use either Basic with TLS or Integrated Windows Authentication.

CAUTION

Checking the option to resolve anonymous email might leave the messaging environment susceptible to spoofing. Spoofing is essentially the ability for an unauthorized user to masquerade as a valid or authorized user. It can give users and hackers the ability to forge messages as if they were being sent from a legitimate user.

These options are accessible by clicking the Authentication button on the Access tab within the SMTP virtual server's Property pages.

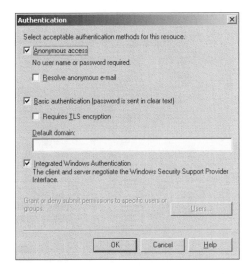

FIGURE 13.8   Authentication methods supported by SMTP virtual servers.

Securing Communications

Communications with the SMTP virtual server can be secured using digital certificates and encryption. More specifically, using encryption can be made a requirement through the use of TLS. To secure communications using TLS, do the following:

1. Within the SMTP virtual server's Property pages, select the Access tab.

2. Click on the Certificate button within the Secure communications section to start the Web Server Certificate Wizard. Click Next to bypass the welcome screen.

3. As illustrated in Figure 13.9, there are several options for obtaining a digital certificate, including creating a new one, assigning an existing certificate, importing, or copying a certificate from another site.

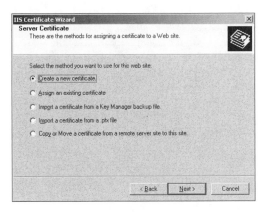

FIGURE 13.9   Requesting a digital certificate for the SMTP virtual server.

4. Click Next and then select the certificate to use. The options vary depending on the option chosen in the previous step.

5. Click Next and then review the certificate summary window.

6. Click Next and then Finish when done.

At this point, the certificate is installed but the secure communications is not enabled. To require encrypted communications, do the following:

1. Click on the now visible Communications button.

2. In the Security window check the check box to require encrypted communications.

3. Optionally, check the check box to require 128-bit encryption. This option is recommended when using TLS.

Restricting Access to the SMTP Virtual Server

Access to the SMTP virtual server can be restricted based on the IP address, subnet, or domain. These options are found by clicking the Connection button on the Access tab.

Controlling SMTP Relaying

SMTP relay servers deliver messages without regarding the recipient or sender. This functionality is very useful to many organizations, but if the relay is wide open, spammers can and will prey on it whenever possible so that thousands upon thousands of messages can be easily broadcast without ever disclosing their true point of origin. For instance, an organization might need to relay alerts and notifications from internal systems to users. A monitoring solution, such as Microsoft Operations Manager (MOM), can be configured to send email alerts to the administrator via a relay server if the Exchange server goes down. Another example would be to enable UNIX servers to relay backup reports and logs to administrators.

> **NOTE**
>
> Relaying can also be enabled on an SMTP connector if the Allow Messages to Be Relayed to These Domains option is checked on the Address Space tab of the SMTP connector's Property pages.

The good news is that Exchange Server 2003 must be manually configured to enable any SMTP relaying. However, more often than not many organizations still are unknowingly SMTP relays because of misconfigurations or carelessness.

As spam enters an organization, administrators can view the SMTP header to reveal the SMTP relay server from which the message originated. The spammed organization can then either complain to the organization that was used as a relay—or worse, add the SMTP relay server to a relay blacklist. These blacklists, which Exchange Server 2003 supports, help reduce spam but can wreak havoc for organizations that are unknowingly relaying because messages can be blocked so that spam is not further propagated using your SMTP relay.

If your organization must use relaying, there are security measures that can be taken to prevent SMTP relay abuse. Connection control methods, similar to what was described in the earlier section "Restricting Access to the SMTP Virtual Server," can restrict access to the SMTP relay based on IP addresses, subnets, and domains. Domain restrictions require reverse lookups, however, which can severely affect server performance. In addition to connection control, relaying can be controlled through the use of authentication methods.

Using Authentication to Secure a Relay Server

In Exchange 2003, the administrator can grant or deny relay permissions to specific users and groups. Relay permissions give the user the right to use the SMTP virtual server to send mail to a destination outside the organization. More specifically, relaying can be restricted using Discretionary Access Control Lists (DACLs), which enables more granularities with restrictions. Restricting relaying on SMTP virtual servers is useful to allow a group of users to relay mail to the Internet, but deny relay privileges for others

For outbound connections, authentication can be configured to control connections from the SMTP relay server to other messaging servers. These options can be located by doing the following:

1. Click the Delivery tab within the SMTP virtual server's Property pages.

2. Click Outbound Security to view the authentication options.

The authentication options for outbound security allow you to choose only one type of authentication to use, which is not the case for the inbound security settings. When either Basic or Integrated Windows Authentication is used, additional information must be supplied and the other servers must support authentication. If Basic is chosen, a username and password must be supplied by the SMTP relay server. On the other hand, if Integrated Windows Authentication is to be used, a valid account and password must be supplied. In either case, TLS can be used and is recommended.

Securing Routing Group Connectors

A collection of messaging servers connected via high-speed bandwidth (512KB or higher) in Exchange Server 2003 is defined as a **routing group**. By default, one routing group is created. Anytime a server is added to a routing group the connections between the servers are automatically configured.

Another purpose for the routing group is communicating with other routing groups through specialized connectors. When routing groups communicate with other routing groups, they do so through designated servers most commonly known as **bridgehead servers**. Exchange Server 2003 provides many such connectors that can connect to other Exchange servers as well as foreign messaging environments, such as Lotus Notes. The most common connector in Exchange Server 2003 is the SMTP connector. As the name implies, the SMTP connector uses the SMTP protocol, but other connectors use SMTP by default as well. Other commonly used routing groups include the X.400 and the routing group connectors.

> **NOTE**
>
> Routing group connector security is strong by default and there is minimal configuration. However, this connector does not support encryption unless the servers participate in an IPSec policy where all traffic is encrypted. If connector communications traffic flows through public networks, use the SMTP connector instead to support encrypted communications.

Using X.400

X.400 is a long-standing messaging standard that Exchange Server 2003 uses for compatibility with older or foreign messaging systems. It can be configured using either X.25 or TCP/IP.

From a security perspective, X.400 has been superceded by SMTP. One of the key reasons is because SMTP supports strong authentication whereas X.400's authentication is much weaker. For instance, X.400 supports the use of passwords, but the passwords are transmitted in plain text. Use the SMTP connector instead of the X.400 connector whenever possible.

Securing SMTP Connectors

Exchange Server 2003's SMTP connector can be used to connect to the Internet, to other Exchange servers, to other Exchange organizations, or to other messaging systems. With regard to security there are several key considerations to take in account, including content restrictions, authentication, encryption, and relaying.

Outbound Security Controls

Outbound security controls can be set on the SMTP connector and are very similar to those mentioned earlier in the section "Using Authentication Controls." These controls provide authentication (anonymous, Basic, and Integrated Windows Authentication) and encryption (using TLS) options. The basic difference between these options and those for the SMTP virtual server is that only one authentication method can be selected.

To configure outbound security controls for the SMTP connector, do the following:

1. In the ESM, expand the administrative and routing groups.

2. Under the defined routing group for the messaging environment, expand the Connectors folder to reveal the SMTP connector.

3. Right-click the SMTP connector and select Properties.

4. Click the Outbound Security button on the Advanced tab.

5. Select the authentication method and whether not the connector will use TLS. By default, the SMTP connector uses anonymous access.

Integrated Windows Authentication with TLS offers the strongest and securest form of authentication for outbound security and is therefore recommended.

Using the Internet Mail Wizard

The Internet Mail Wizard is designed to create a secure, reliable, nonrelaying Internet mail SMTP connector. This wizard is not only for inexperienced Exchange Server 2003 administrators, but it is also very useful for even the most experienced. It walks the administrator through the creation of an Internet mail SMTP connector.

To use the Internet Mail Wizard, do the following:

1. Open the ESM by choosing System Manager from the Start, All Programs, Microsoft Exchange menu.

2. Right-click the Exchange organization name and select Internet Mail Wizard.

3. Click Next twice to bypass the Welcome and Prerequisites for Internet Mail windows.

4. Select the Exchange Server 2003 server to create the SMTP connector. The wizard then checks whether the server meets the prerequisites. Click Next when it has completed and passed.

5. Choose whether this connector will send or receive Internet email, as shown in Figure 13.10 and then click Next.

6. Review the domains that will receive email for this Exchange organization and then click Next. Domains can be added or removed at this point if necessary.

7. Select the SMTP virtual server that will be the bridgehead for outbound Internet email and then click Next.

8. Specify whether to use DNS or a smarthost to send Internet email. If DNS will be used and the Exchange Server 2003 will not resolve DNS addresses, enter the external DNS servers. If a smarthost is used, enter the hostname or IP address enclosed in brackets (for example, [192.168.1.20]). Click Next to continue.

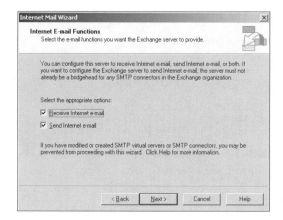

FIGURE 13.10   Using the Internet Mail Wizard.

9. Specify whether to allow delivery to all domains or to specific domains and then click Next.

10. Review the configuration and then click Next.

11. Click Finish when done. Optionally, check the check box to view a detailed configuration report.

Securing Other Exchange-Supported Protocols

Examining Exchange Server 2003 transport-level security would not be complete without discussing protocols other than SMTP. In addition to SMTP, Exchange Server 2003 supports the following:

- Network News Transfer Protocol (NNTP)

- Post Office Protocol version 3 (POP3)

- Internet Message Access Protocol (IMAP4)

Some notable security features Exchange Server 2003 provides regarding these protocols includes, but is not limited to, the following:

- These protocols are not enabled by default unless the system was upgraded from a previous version of Exchange that also had these services running.

- Each protocol runs as a service and the service is disabled by default.

- IMAP4 and POP3 support Basic authentication over SSL or TLS as well as NTLM-based authentication.

- NNTP supports anonymous (disabled by default), Basic authentication, Integrated Windows Authentication, and SSL client authentication.

- Each protocol supports secure, certificate-based communications.

- Each protocol can use connection controls (IP address or domain names) to grant or deny access.

Protecting Client–to–Front-end–Server Communications

When clients connect to an Outlook Web Access (OWA) server, the information must be protected to ensure that usernames, passwords, and messaging data are not susceptible to compromise. This protection can be accomplished through the use of SSL on the Internet Information Services (IIS) virtual server. SSL requires a digital certificate that can be supplied either by the organization's PKI or through a third-party, such as VeriSign.

Automatic SSL redirection

If SSL is used on the OWA server, clients connect to the OWA server by typing **https://<FQDN>** or **https://<FQDN>/exchange** to log on and use Exchange Server 2003 over the SSL connection. One of the biggest hassles for clients, however, is remembering to use https rather than just http. Using http means using the nonsecure URL.

Exchange Server 2003 provides a way to automatically redirect OWA clients to an SSL connection if they should use the non-secure URL. This prevents users from mistakingly trying to use the non-secure URL—not to mention keeps the number of helpdesk calls to a minimum if users are not able to gain access to email.

To configure automatic SSL redirection when form-based authentication is not in use, create a new HTM file called HTTPSRedirect.htm with the following contents:

```
<!DOCTYPE HTML PUBLIC "-//W3C//DTD HTML 4.01//EN"
"http://www.w3.org/TR/html4/strict.dtd">
<HTML><HEAD>
<meta http-equiv="refresh" content="0; url=https://webmail.companyabc.com">
</HEAD></HTML>
```

> **NOTE**
>
> In the examples provided, replace webmail.companyabc.com in the file contents with the Fully Qualified Domain Name (FQDN) of the organization's OWA server.

If you use form-based authentication, do the following:

1. Create a new HTM document called HTTPSRedirect.htm with the following content:

```
<!DOCTYPE HTML PUBLIC "-//W3C//DTD HTML 4.01//EN"
"http://www.w3.org/TR/html4/strict.dtd">
<HTML><HEAD>
<meta http-equiv="refresh" content="0;
url=https://webmail.companyabc.com/exchweb/bin/auth/owalogon.asp?url=
https://webmail.companyabc.com/exchange&reason=0">
</HEAD></HTML>
```

2. Save the file in `%SYSTEMROOT%\help\iisHelp\common\`.

3. From the Administrative Tools menu, open the Internet Information Services (IIS) Manager and expand the local computer.

4. Expand Web Sites and then right-click Default Web Site and choose Properties.

5. On the Custom Errors tab, select the HTTP Error 403;4 message entry and click the Edit button.

6. Ensure that the Message type is File and then click the Browse button and navigate to `%SYSTEMROOT%\Help\iisHelp\common\HTTPSRedirect.htm`.

7. Click Open and then click OK twice to close the Properties window.

8. Stop and restart the Default Web Site.

Locking Down Front-end and Back-end Server Communications

The very nature and capabilities of a front-end (FE) and back-end (BE) Exchange Server 2003 configuration lends itself to a more secure environment. An FE server hosts only the Internet Information Services (IIS) virtual server that provides the interface to users and communicates with the BE virtual server. It should not, by definition, host Exchange information stores containing messaging data. Only the back-end servers contain information stores so that messaging data is not easily accessible from outside the organization.

TCP and UDP Ports

Many organizations place FE servers in the perimeter network (also known as the DMZ) to segment the internal network from those servers requiring some degree of exposure to the Internet. As a result, ports must be opened on the firewall to enable for the FE and BE servers to communicate. Other ports might also be necessary depending on the services being offered and the configuration of the messaging environment.

Table 13.1 lists the common inbound ports to open to the OWA FE servers.

TABLE 13.1   Inbound Ports to the OWA FE

Protocol	TCP/UDP	Port Number
HTTP	TCP	80
HTTPS	TCP	443
SMTP	TCP	25
POP3	TCP	110
IMAP	TCP	143

Table 13.2 lists the commonly required ports between FE and BE Exchange Server 2003 servers. Some of these ports are optional, and the specific ports that the organization might require will vary depending on the messaging environment.

> **NOTE**
>
> SSL cannot be used between an FE and BE server. If the organization's security policy dictates that communication between the FE and BE servers is encrypted, implement IPSec.

TABLE 13.2   Commonly Used Ports Between FE and BE Exchange Servers

Protocol	TCP/UDP	Port Number
HTTP	TCP	80
DNS Lookup	TCP/UDP	53
Kerberos	TCP/UDP	88
Network Time Protocol(NTP)—optional	TCP	123
RPC End Point Mapper	TCP	135
LDAP	TCP/UDP	389
Server Message Block (SMB)	TCP	445
Link State Algorithm	TCP	691
Global Catalog	TCP	3268

The ports listed in Table 13.3 are optional.

TABLE 13.3   Optional Ports Between FE and BE Exchange Servers

Protocol	TCP/UDP/ID	Port/ID Number
POP3	TCP	110
IMAP	TCP	143
SMTP	TCP	25
RPC	TCP	1024+
IPSec	IP Protocol ID	50, 51
IPSec	UDP	500

> **TIP**
>
> To avoid having to leave a large number of RPC ports open, statically map them to a standard-ized port number. To statically map the port, create a registry key value called `TCP/IP Port` of type `REG_DWORD` in
>
> `HKEY_LOCAL_MACHINE\SYSTEM\CurrentControlSet\Services\NTDS\Parameters`.

Summary

Transport-level security is a major security consideration for any organization and can significantly impact server and client-level security methods. Securing the communica-tions between users and servers on a network is vital, and in some cases required by law. This chapter examined the various transport-level security methods supported by Windows Server 2003 and Exchange Server 2003 and provided best practices for securely configuring and effectively locking down an organization's transmission of data.

Best Practices

The following are best practices from this chapter:

- Thoroughly plan and design the organization's PKI.

- Use a User certificate when users require access to multiple certificate services.

- Customize certificate templates.

- Use smartcards.

- Use S/MIME to sign and encrypt messages.

- Use IPSec to encrypt communications between front-end and back-end servers.

- Limit SMTP message size.

- Use TLS to secure SMTP.

- Disable auto-replies.

- Control the distribution group maximum recipients limit.

- Use the strongest authentication methods possible.

- Avoid allowing anonymous access.

- Secure mail relay servers.

- Configure automatic SSL redirection.

- Open only ports that are absolutely necessary for communication.

PART V

Migrating to Microsoft Exchange Server 2003

IN THIS PART

Migrating from NT4 to Windows Server 2003

Before the many benefits of Exchange Server 2003 can be realized, the directory for Exchange, Microsoft's Active Directory, must be created and configured. In some cases where no existing infrastructure is in place, this involves designing and implementing an Active Directory infrastructure from scratch. Most environments, however, use an existing Windows 2000 or Windows NT domain infrastructure. Organizations wherein Windows 2000 Active Directory is deployed can upgrade to Windows Server 2003 Active Directory, or simply not upgrade before deploying Exchange. As Exchange Server 2003 can be installed on either directory platform, the decision is not critical.

With Windows NT 4.0 domains, however, you must upgrade to Active Directory to be able to support the directory requirements of Exchange Server 2003. This chapter details the options available for migrations from NT to Windows Server 2003 and explores the various pros and cons of each approach. In addition, step-by-step example best-practice migration strategies are presented and detailed.

Defining the Migration Process

Any migration procedure requires a defined procedure that details the reasons for migration, steps involved, fallback precautions, and other important factors that can influence the migration process. When these items have been finalized, the steps toward performing the migration implementation can be accomplished and the performance increases can be realized.

Defining Exchange Server 2003 Objectives

As part of any migration project, establishing project objectives are a critical but often overlooked aspect of a project. Without objectives, it becomes difficult to define whether a project has been successful. Although there are significant improvements between Windows NT 4.0 domains and Windows Server 2003 AD, the ultimate decision to upgrade might be to support Exchange Server 2003. As previously mentioned, Exchange Server 2003 requires a functional Windows 2000/2003 Active Directory implementation for its directory, and this might force an organization to upgrade.

> **NOTE**
>
> Although it is necessary for Exchange 2000/2003 to use an Active Directory forest for directory and authentication purposes, there is one scenario in which an existing NT 4.0 domain can be preserved, if desired or required. Exchange Server 2003 can be installed in a new, separate AD forest, with a manual trust established to the production NT domain. The NT domain accounts can then be granted full mailbox privileges to the Mailbox-enabled user accounts that can be created in the AD domain.

Establishing Migration Project Phases

After the decision has been made to upgrade, a detailed plan of the resources, timeline, scope, and objectives of the project should be outlined. Establishing a project plan, whether ad hoc or professionally drawn up, should be part of any migration plan, to assist in accomplishing the planned objectives in a timely manner with the correct application of resources.

A condensed form of the standard phases for a migration project is detailed as follows:

- **Discovery**   The first portion of a design project should be a discovery, or fact-finding portion. This section focuses on the analysis of the current environment and documentation of the results of the analysis. Current network diagrams, server locations, WAN throughputs, server application dependencies, and all other relevant sections should be detailed as part of the Discovery phase.

- **Design**   The Design portion of a project is a straightforward concept. All key components of the actual migration plan should be documented and key data from the Discovery phase should be used to draw up Design and Migration documents. The project plan itself would normally be drafted during this phase. This is especially true with Windows NT 4.0 because there are significant differences in structure between NT and Windows Server 2003.

- **Prototype**   The Prototype phase of a project involves the essential lab work to test the design assumptions that were made during the Design phase. The ideal prototype would involve a mock production environment that is migrated from Windows NT 4.0 to Windows Server 2003. Step-by-step procedures for migration can also be outlined and produced as deliverables for this phase.

- **Pilot**   The Pilot phase, or Proof-of-Concept phase, involves a production "test" of the migration steps, on a limited scale. For example, a single domain controller could be upgraded to Windows Server 2003 in advance of the migration of all other domain controllers.

- **Implementation**   The Implementation portion of the project is the full-blown migration of network functionality or upgrades to the operating system. This process can be done quickly or slowly over time, depending on the needs of an organization. Make the timeline decisions in the Design phase and incorporate them into the project plan.

- **Training and Support**   Learning the ins and outs of the new functionality that Windows Server 2003 can bring to an environment is essential towards the realization of the increased productivity and reduced administration that the OS can bring to an environment. Consequently, it is important to include a training portion in a migration project, so that the design objectives can be fully realized.

For more detailed information on the project plan phases of a migration, reference Chapter 2, "Planning, Prototyping, Migrating, and Deploying Exchange Server 2003."

In-Place Upgrade Versus New Hardware Migration

Because the underlying operating system kernel is similar between Windows NT 4.0 and Windows Server 2003, the possibility exists to simply upgrade an existing Windows NT Server in place. Depending on the type of hardware currently in use in a Windows NT 4.0 network, this type of migration strategy becomes an option. Often, however, it is more appealing to simply introduce newer systems into an existing environment and retire the current servers from production. This type of technique normally has less impact on current environments and can also support fallback more easily.

Which migration strategy to choose depends on one major factor: the condition of the current hardware environment. If Windows NT 4.0 is taxing the limitations of the hardware in use, it might be preferable to introduce new servers into an environment and retire the old Windows NT 4.0 servers. If, however, the hardware in use for Windows NT 4.0 is newer and more robust, and could conceivably last for another 2–3 years, it might be easier to perform in-place upgrades of the systems in an environment.

In most cases, a dual approach to migration is taken. Older hardware is replaced by new hardware running Windows Server 2003. Newer Windows NT 4.0 systems are upgraded in place to Windows Server 2003. Consequently, performing an audit of all systems to be migrated and determining which ones will be upgraded and which ones will be retired is an important step in the migration process.

Choosing a Migration Strategy

As with many technology implementations, there are two approaches that can be taken regarding deployment: a quick, "Big-Bang" approach, or a phased, slower approach. The

Big-Bang option involves quickly replacing the entire Windows NT 4.0 infrastructure (often over the course of a weekend) with the new Windows Server 2003 environment. The phased approach involves a slow, server-by-server replacement of Windows NT 4.0. Each approach has its advantages and disadvantages, and there are key factors of Windows Server 2003 to take into account before a decision is made.

Because there are fundamental structural changes between the NT domain structure and Active Directory, the argument of not maintaining two conflicting and redundant environments for long periods of time supports the Big-Bang approach. That said, there are situations in which the phased approach might be more appealing. Larger organizations with a heavy investment in Windows NT 4.0 might determine that a phased approach will help divide the upgrade into manageable components. Other risk-averse organizations might decide to minimize risk through the use of this strategy. Windows Server 2003 easily accommodates both migration options.

Exploring Migration Options

Migration to Windows Server 2003 can be precipitated by one of many factors. In the case of Exchange Server 2003, the necessity of an Active Directory infrastructure in place requires that the infrastructure be upgraded to support it. Other reasons also might justify the upgrade, such as improvements in reliability, scalability, and a lower Total Cost of Ownership (TCO). In any case, an upgrade from NT 4.0 to Windows Server 2003 can be done in several ways.

Upgrading a Single Member Server

The direct upgrade approach from Windows NT 4.0 to Windows Server 2003 is the most straightforward approach to migration.

The upgrade takes all settings on a single server and upgrades them to Windows Server 2003. If a Windows NT 4.0 Server handles WINS, DNS, and DHCP, the process upgrades all WINS, DNS, and DHCP components, as well as the base operating system. This type of migration is very tempting, and it can be extremely effective, as long as all prerequisites (mentioned later) are satisfied.

Often, upgrading a single server can be a project. The standalone member servers in an environment are often the workhorses of the network, loaded with a myriad of different applications and critical tools. Performing an upgrade on these servers would be simple if they were used only for file or print duties and if their hardware systems were all up-to-date. Because this is not always the case, it is important to detail the specifics of each server that is marked for migration.

Verifying Hardware Compatibility

Testing the hardware compatibility of any server that will be directly upgraded to Windows Server 2003 is critical. During the installation process is not the most ideal time to be notified of problems with compatibility between older system components and the drivers required for Windows Server 2003. Verify the hardware in a server for Windows Server 2003 on the manufacturer's Web site, or on Microsoft's Hardware Compatibility List (HCL).

Microsoft offers minimum hardware levels that Windows Server 2003 will run on, but it is *highly* recommended to install the OS on systems of a much higher caliber, as these recommendations do not take into account any application loads, domain controller duties, and so forth. The following is a list of Microsoft's recommended hardware levels for Windows Server 2003:

- 550MHz CPU

- 256MB RAM

- 1.5GB free disk space

It cannot be stressed enough that it is almost always recommended to exceed these levels to provide a robust computing environment.

> **NOTE**
>
> One of the most important features that mission-critical servers can have is redundancy. Putting the operating system on a mirrored array of disks, for example, is a simple yet effective way of increasing redundancy in an environment.

Verifying Application Readiness

Nothing ruins a migration process like a mission-critical application that will not work in the new environment. List all applications on a server that will be required in the new environment. Applications that will not be used or whose functionality is replaced in Windows Server 2003 can be retired and removed from consideration. Applications that have been verified for Windows Server 2003 can be designated as "safe" for upgrade. Delegate any other applications that might not be compatible but are necessary to another server, or force the upgrade to wait on that specific server.

In addition to the applications, the version of the operating system that will be upgraded is an important consideration in the process. A Windows NT 4.0 Server install can be upgraded to either Windows Server 2003 Standard Server or Windows Windows Server 2003 Enterprise. A Windows NT 4.0 Enterprise Edition install can be upgraded *only* to Windows Server 2003 Enterprise, however.

Backing Up and Creating a Recovery Process

It is critical that a migration does not cause more harm to an environment than good. A good backup system put in place is essential for quick recovery in the event of upgrade failure. Often, especially with the in-place upgrade scenario, a full system backup is the only way to recover, and you should detail fallback steps in the event of problems.

Standalone Server Upgrade Steps

After all considerations regarding applications and hardware compatibility have been thoroughly validated, the process of upgrading a standalone server can be accomplished. The following steps detail the process involved with this type of upgrade process:

1. Insert the Windows Server 2003 CD into the CD drive of the server to be upgraded.

2. The welcome page should appear automatically. If not, select Start, Run, and type **X:\Setup** (where **X:** is the CD drive).

3. Click on Install Windows Server 2003 Enterprise Server.

4. Select Upgrade from the drop-down box, as illustrated in Figure 14.1, and click Next to continue.

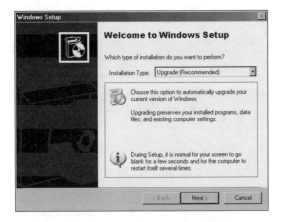

FIGURE 14.1   Upgrading to Windows Server 2003.

5. Click I accept this agreement at the License screen and click Next to continue.

6. The next dialog box prompts you to enter the 25-character product key. This number can be found on the CD case or in the license documentation from Microsoft. Enter it and click Next to continue.

7. The next prompt is crucial. It indicates which system components are not compatible with Windows Server 2003. It will indicate important factors such as the fact that IIS will be disabled as part of the install. IIS can be reenabled in the new OS, but is turned off for security reasons. Click Next after reviewing these factors.

8. The system then copies files and reboots, continuing the upgrade process. After all files have been copied, the system is then upgraded to a fully functional install of Windows Server 2003.

> **NOTE**
>
> Many previously enabled components, such as IIS, are turned off by default in Windows Server 2003. Ensure that one of the post-upgrade tasks performed is an audit of all services, so that those disabled can be reenabled.

Upgrading an NT 4.0 Domain Structure to Active Directory via the In-Place Upgrade Process

Upgrading an NT 4.0 domain environment to Windows Server 2003 Active Directory can be accomplished through two methods. As previously mentioned, the first method involves upgrading the domain structure in place. This method is more straightforward and easy to accomplish, but involves a greater degree of risk and does not immediately give the advantages of domain consolidation that can be achieved through the second option, which is migrating the domain accounts into a new AD structure.

This section details the steps required if the first option is chosen. The sample scenarios outlined assume a fairly simple environment, but the overall strategy can easily be ported into a more complex domain structure.

Upgrading the Windows NT4 Primary Domain Controller

Performing an in-place upgrade of a Windows NT 4.0 domain to Active Directory requires that the machine running the Primary Domain Controller (PDC) role be upgraded to Windows Server 2003. This can either be an existing domain controller, or a new one created solely for the purposes of the upgrade. To perform an in-place upgrade, insert the Windows Server 2003 installation CD-ROM into the CD-ROM drive of the PDC. Then following these steps:

1. If the server has autorun enabled, the Windows Server 2003 Setup Wizard screen appears. If it is not enabled, launch the Windows Server 2003 Setup Wizard by running the Setup.exe program from the Windows Server 2003 CD-ROM.

2. On the Welcome to Windows Server 2003 Family page, select Install Windows Server 2003 to begin upgrading the PDC to Windows Server 2003 and Active Directory. This step launches the Windows Setup Wizard.

3. On the Welcome to Windows Setup page, select the installation type of Upgrade (Recommended). This begins the upgrade of the Windows NT4 server operating system to Windows Server 2003 and Active Directory. Select Next to continue.

4. On the Licensing agreement page, use the scroll button to read the Microsoft licensing agreement. After reading the license page, select I Accept this agreement, and select Next to continue.

5. The copy of Windows Server 2003 should have a license key that came with the Windows Server 2003 CD-ROM software. Enter the 25-character product code and select Next.

The Setup Wizard begins the installation of Windows Server 2003 by copying necessary files to the PDC's hard drive. The upgrade progress can be monitored from the progress bar in the lower-left corner of the installation screen. When the Setup Wizard has completed copying files, the server automatically restarts.

Upgrading to Active Directory

When the Server Setup Wizard has completed upgrading the operating system to Windows Server 2003, the system restarts automatically and begins running the Active Directory Installation Wizard. To install Microsoft's Active Directory, follow these steps:

1. At the Welcome to the Active Directory Installation Wizard screen, select Next. This upgrades the existing Windows NT4 domain and domain security principles to Active Directory.

> **NOTE**
>
> Choosing this option maintains the existing NT 4 Domain and upgrades all domain security principles directly to Active Directory. All NT4 user accounts, domain groups, and computer accounts will automatically be upgraded into the new Active Directory domain.

   When the installation of Active Directory has completed, the next step is to review the Active Directory Users and Computers management console to ensure that all security principles have been upgraded properly.

2. Because this is an in-place upgrade, at the Create New Domain page, select the option to create a new Domain in a New Forest, and select Next.

3. As mentioned earlier, Active directory requires Domain Name System (DNS) to be installed before the Active Directory installation can continue. If the network has a DNS Server compatible with Windows Server 2003 and Active Directory, select Yes, I will configure the DNS client.

4. If there is no DNS Server on the network and this server is intended to be the first DNS Server within the new Active Directory Domain, select No, just install and configure DNS on this computer, and select Next to continue.

5. On the New Domain page, type the DNS name of the domain—for example, **companyabc.com**. Select Next to continue. Before completing the installation, use the scrollbar to review the server configuration summary page. Ensure that the configuration information is correct. If changes are required, use the Back button to modify the server configuration. If the installation summary is correct, click Next to continue.

6. Before choosing Finish to complete the in-place upgrade, review the Installation Wizard information. This information can identify whether any errors were experienced during setup.

> **NOTE**
>
> It is a good practice to review the server event and system logs upon completing any upgrade. Review each log and identify errors and warnings that can potentially affect the stability of the server that is being upgraded and cause problems with domain authentication.
>
> Also review the Active Directory Users and Computers snap-in to ensure that all security principles have been migrated successfully to Windows Server 2003 and Active Directory.

Migrating and Replacing Backup Domain Controllers

When the PDC upgrade has been completed, the next step is to either upgrade or replace the remaining network Backup Domain Controllers (BDCs). The preferred method of replacing BDC functionality is by promoting new servers to be Windows Server 2003 domain controllers via the DCPROMO process. However, there may be some instances where existing hardware should be preserved through direct upgrades of the BDCs. In these instances, a direct upgrade can take place.

When performing an upgrade of Windows NT4 BDCs, the Active Directory Installation Wizard offers the opportunity to change a server's domain membership type or server roles. For example, an exiting NT BDC can be migrated to Windows Server 2003 and Active Directory as a member server or a domain controller.

As a rule, upgrading BDCs hosting network services such as DHCP and WINS should be considered first. By migrating vital network services, network downtime and interruption of server-to-server communications are minimized.

Migrating Existing NT4 Domains to a New Windows Server 2003 Forest

In many instances, it might be more ideal to simply abandon a badly designed or inefficient NT domain structure and migrate the accounts into a new Active Directory forest. This process can be streamlined through the use of a tool included on the Windows Server 2003 CD: Microsoft Active Directory Migration Tool (ADMT) 2.0 (ADMT v2).

By installing and configuring a new Windows Server 2003 Active Directory domain with pre–Windows 2000 permissions and creating a domain trust between source and target domains, the ADMT can then be used to migrate any Windows NT4 security principle to Active Directory Domains and Organizational Units. By using this tool, organizations can then migrate security principles incrementally and still maintain shared resources located on each domain.

When using the ADMT to restructure domains, all NT4 security principles are copied or cloned from the Windows NT 4 domain and placed into Active Directory in the form of what is called **SIDHistory**. By cloning NT4 security principles, the source domain is left completely in place and uninterrupted, enabling administrators to easily roll back to the previous domain if required.

Installing and Configuring a New Windows Server 2003 Forest and Domain

Installing a new domain requires the installation of a new AD structure. One of the biggest advantages to this approach is that best-practice AD design can be used, and efficient, effective, and secure AD forests can be constructed. For more information on the best ways to design AD, specifically regarding deployment of Exchange Server 2003, refer to Chapters 4, "Exchange Server 2003 Design Concepts," and 5, "Designing an Enterprise Exchange Server 2003 Environment."

Configuring a Domain Trust Between Source Windows NT4 and Target Windows Server 2003 Domains

When migrating existing NT4 domains to a new Active Directory forest root or child domain, the trust relationships must be created between the existing Windows NT4 domains. The existing Windows NT4 domains are referred to as the **source domains**, and the newly created Windows Server 2003 Active Directory domains are the **target domains**. Follow these steps:

1. Begin by first configuring a trust on the target domain. On the Windows Server 2003 domain controller, open the administrator tools and launch Active Directory Domains and Trust Manager. From the Action menu option, open the Properties page for the Active Directory domain and select the Trust tab. This opens the Domain Trust configuration page.

2. Windows Server 2003 and Active Directory trusts are created using the New Trust Wizard. Select New Trust to start the wizard and be guided through the creation of a domain trust. Select Next at the Welcome to the New Trust page. On the Trust Name page, type the name of the Windows NT4 source domain. This enables Active Directory to establish connectivity with the source Windows NT4 domain. Select Next to continue.

> **NOTE**
>
> When configuring a domain trust, each domain must have the capability of resolving the domain name to a domain controller's TCP/IP Address. Install the Windows Internet Naming Service (WINS) on the target domain controller and configure the TCP/IP properties on the target and source domain controllers to use the newly installed WINS.

3. Select the type of trust to be established. On the Direction of Trust page, select Two-way, allowing connectivity and access to resources in both the target and source domains when migrating; select Next to continue.

4. To configure outgoing trust properties, select Allow authentication for all resources in the local domain. This option allows Windows NT4 security principles access to

all resources within the Active Directory target domain. Windows Server 2003 will automatically authenticate existing NT4 security principles within the target domain; this allows required administrator accounts access to each domain and domain group memberships. Select Next to continue.

5. The **trust password** is a password other than the domain administrator password. The trust password is unique to the trust being created and will be used by both the source and target domains to authenticate the trust. The same trust password must be used on both the Windows NT4 target domain and Windows Server 2003 source domain trust configurations. Enter a password for this trust to use and select Next to continue.

6. At this point, review the trust configuration; select Back to modify any setting that needs to be changed or select Next to complete creating the trust and view the configuration changes created by the Trust Wizard. Click the Next button to continue.

7. A dialog box will appear asking for confirmation of the ongoing trust. Before continuing, create and establish a trust relationship on the Windows NT4 source domain's Primary Domain Controller. At the Confirm Outgoing Trust page, select No, do not confirm the outgoing trust and click Next to continue.

8. Choose No, do not confirm the incoming trust option from the Confirm Incoming Trust page. Choose Next to complete the trust configuration. Review the trust configuration and select Finish to close the Trust Wizard.

9. To successfully establish a trust on the Windows NT source domain, the trusted domain must first be configured. To add the target domain to the Windows NT4 trusted domains, open the User Manager for Domains on the Windows NT4 Primary Domain Controller. Click Policies from the menu options and select Trust Relationships. This opens the Windows NT4 Trust Relationship page.

10. Begin by selecting the Add button under Trusted Domains. Enter the name of the target domain and a password that will be used by both domains to authenticate the trust. As mentioned earlier, this password is unique to the trust configuration and should be different from the domain administrator account password. This password will be used only to authenticate the domain trust between the source and target domains.

11. After the trusted domain has been established successfully, select Add under the Trusting Domain section of the page. Enter the name of the target domain and the password used to establish the trust. This adds the target domain to the Windows NT4 trusting domains and completes the configuration of the Windows NT4 trust. Click Close to close the Trust Relationships Dialog screen.

12. When the trust is created successfully, the New Trust Wizard can now confirm the trust settings. If choosing to validate the trust, use the administrator account name and password of the source domain to test access for both incoming and outgoing connectivity of the domain trust. Click OK to close the open dialog box.

Migrating Account and Resource NT Domains to Active Directory Domains

Using this option enables administrators to restructure existing Windows NT4 accounts and resources into newly created Windows Server 2003 Active Directory domains and organizational units (OUs).

Migrating account domains and resource domains to Active Directory Organizational Units allows enhanced security and ease of delegation within the Active Directory domain tree. When the Active Directory domain organizational unit (OU) structure is configured, the domain resources and security principles can be migrated by using the ADMT shown in Figure 14.2.

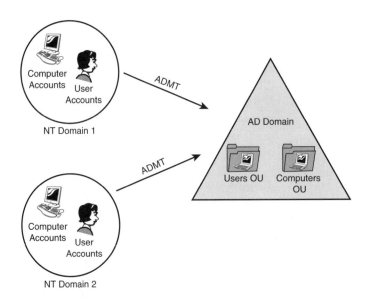

FIGURE 14.2   Consolidating NT domains into AD.

Implication of Migrating Security Principles

When security principles are created in a Windows NT4 domain, each individual object is assigned a unique security identifier or (SID). SIDHistory is a record of each security principle's previous Windows NT4 group and domain membership, and each SID is unique.

When these types of security principles are migrated to Windows Server 2003 and Active Directory, each security principle is assigned a new SID with information about its new domain and group membership. Because the new SID does not contain information about the security principle's previous domain membership, when a user or group accesses domain resources on the old Windows NT4 domain, such as files, users might find that they no longer have permission to specific resources.

To avoid these issues during and after the migration, use the Microsoft ADMT to migrate a security principle's SIDHistory. The ADMT can migrate the security principles SIDHistory for each object, maintaining previous information and avoiding permissions issues later in the migration.

Understanding and Using the Microsoft Active Directory Migration Tool 2.0 (ADMT v2)

The Active Directory Migration Tool (ADMT) is an effective way to migrate users, groups, and computers from one domain to another. It is robust enough to migrate security permissions and Exchange mailbox domain settings, and it supports a rollback procedure in the event of migration problems. ADMT is composed of several components and functions:

- **ADMT Migration Wizards**   ADMT includes a series of wizards, each specifically designed to migrate specific components. Different wizards exist for migrating Users, Groups, Computers, Service Accounts, and Trusts.

- **Low Client Impact**   ADMT automatically installs a service on source clients, which negates the need to manually install client software for the migration. In addition, after the migration is complete, these services are automatically uninstalled.

- **SIDHistory and Security Migrated**   Users will continue to maintain network access to file shares, applications, and other secured network services through migration of the SIDHistory attributes to the new domain. This preserves the extensive security structure of the source domain.

- **Test Migrations and Rollback Functionality**   An extremely useful feature in ADMT v2 is the ability to run a mock migration scenario with each migration wizard. This helps identify any issues that might exist prior to the actual migration work. In addition to this functionality, the most recently performed user, computer, or group migration can be "undone," providing rollback in the event of migration problems.

ADMT v2 installs very easily, but requires knowledge of the various wizards to properly use. In addition, a best-practice process should be used when migrating from one domain to another.

The migration example illustrated in the following sections describes the most common use of the ADMT, an inter-forest migration of domain users, groups, and computers into another domain. This procedure is by no means exclusive, and many other migration techniques can be used to achieve proper results. Matching the capabilities of ADMT with the migration needs of an organization are important.

Deploying ADMT in the Lab

ADMT v2 comes with unprecedented rollback capabilities. Not only can each wizard be tested first, the last wizard transaction can also be rolled back in the event of problems. In addition to this, however, you should reproduce an environment in a lab setting and test a migration in advance, to mitigate potential problems that might arise.

The most effective lab can be created by creating new domain controllers in the source and target domains, and then physically segregating them into a lab network, where they cannot contact the production domain environment. The Operations Master (OM) roles for each domain can then be seized for each domain using the `ntdsutil` utility, which creates exact replicas of all user, group, and computer accounts that can be tested with the ADMT.

Installing and Configuring ADMT

The installation of the ADMT component should be accomplished on a domain controller in the target domain to which the accounts will be migrated. To install, follow these steps:

1. Insert the Windows Server 2003 CD into the CD drive of a domain controller in the TARGET domain.

2. Select Start, Run, type **X:\i386\admt\admigration.msi** (where **X:** is the CD drive), and press Enter.

3. At the welcome screen, click Next to continue, as illustrated in Figure 14.3.

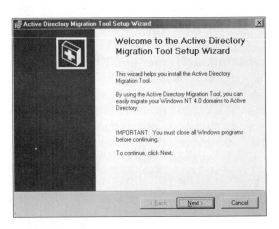

FIGURE 14.3   Installing ADMT v2.

4. Accept the EULA and click Next to continue.

5. Accept the default installation path and click Next to continue.

6. When ready to begin the installation, click Next at the next screen.

7. After installation, click Finish to end the Wizard.

Domain Migration Prerequisites

As previously mentioned, the most important prerequisite for migration with ADMT is lab verification. Testing as many aspects of a migration as possible helps establish the procedures required and identify potential problems before the procedures are done in the production environment.

There are several functional prerequisites that must be accomplished before the ADMT can function properly. Many of these requirements revolve around the migration of passwords and security objects, and are critical for this functionality.

Creating Two-Way Trusts Between Source and Target Domains

The source domain and the target domains must be able to communicate with each other and share security credentials. Consequently, it is important to establish trusts between the two domains before the ADMT can be run.

Assigning Proper Permissions on Source Domain and Source Domain Workstations

The account that will run the ADMT in the target domain must be added into the Builtin\Administrators group in the source domain. In addition, each workstation must include this user as a member of the local administrators group for the computer migration services to be able to function properly. Domain group changes can be easily accomplished, but a large workstation group change must be scripted, or manually accomplished, prior to migration.

Creating a Target OU Structure

The destination for user accounts from the source domain must be designated at several points during the ADMT migration process. Establishing an OU for the source domain accounts can help simplify and logically organize the new objects. These objects can be moved to other OUs after the migration and this OU can be collapsed, if desired.

Modifying Default Domain Policy on Target Domain

Unlike previous versions of Windows Operating Systems, Windows Server 2003 does not support anonymous users authenticating as the Everyone group. This functionality was designed to increase security. However, for ADMT to be able to migrate the accounts, this must be disabled. After the process is complete, the policies can be reset to the default levels. To change the policies, follow this procedure:

1. Open the Domain Security Policy (Start, All Programs, Administrative Tools, Domain Security Policy).

2. Navigate to Console Root, Default Domain Policy, Windows Settings, Security Settings, Local Policies, Security Options.

3. Double-click on Network access: Let Everyone permissions apply to anonymous users.

4. Check Define this policy setting and choose Enabled, as indicated in Figure 14.4. Click OK to finish.

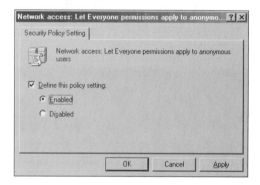

FIGURE 14.4   Allowing Anonymous Access for ADMT.

5. Repeat the procedure for the Domain Controller Security Policy Snap-In.

Exporting Password Key Information

If current passwords will be migrated, a 128-bit encrypted password key from the target domain should be installed on a server in the source domain. This key allows the migration of password and SIDHistory information from one domain to the next.

To create this key, perform the following procedure from the command prompt of a domain controller in the target domain where ADMT was installed:

1. Insert a floppy disk into the drive to store the key (the key can be directed to the network but, for security reasons, is better off directed to a floppy).

2. Change to the ADMT directory by typing `cd program files\active directory migration tool` and pressing Enter.

3. Type `admt key SOURCEDOMAINNAME a: password` and press Enter (where *SOURCEDOMAINNAME* is the NetBIOS name of the source domain, `a:` is the destination drive for the key, and *password* is a password that is used to secure the key). Refer to Figure 14.5 for an example.

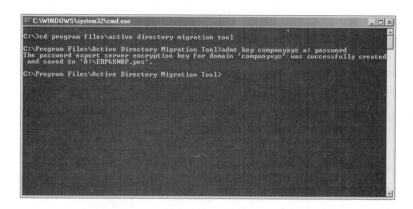

FIGURE 14.5   Creating a password export key.

4. Upon successful creation of the key, remove the floppy disk and keep it in a safe place.

Installing Password Migration DLL on Source Domain

A special Password Migration DLL should be installed on a domain controller in the source domain. This machine will become the Password Export Server for the source domain. The following procedure outlines this installation:

1. Insert the floppy disk with the exported key from the target domain into the disk drive of the server.

2. Insert the Windows Server 2003 CD into the CD drive of the domain controller in the source domain where the Registry change was enacted.

3. Start the Password Migration Utility by selecting Start, Run, and typing **X:\i386\ADMT\Pwdmig\Pwdmig.exe** (where **X:** is the drive letter for the CD).

4. At the welcome screen, click Next.

5. Enter the location of the key that was created on the target domain; normally this will be the A: drive, as indicated in Figure 14.6. Click Next to continue.

6. Enter the password twice that was set on the target domain and click Next.

7. At the Verification page, click Next to continue.

8. Click Finish after the installation is complete.

9. The system must be restarted; click Yes when prompted to automatically restart. Upon restart, the proper settings will be in place to make this server a Password Export Server.

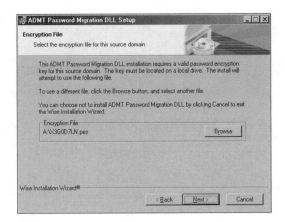

FIGURE 14.6 Accessing the password export key.

Setting Proper Registry Permissions on the Source Domain

The installation of the proper components creates special Registry keys, but leaves them disabled by default, for security reasons. A specific Registry key should be enabled to allow passwords to be exported from the Password Export Server. The following procedure outlines the use of the Registry Editor to perform this function:

1. On a domain controller in the source domain, open Registry Editor (Start, Run, Regedit).

2. Navigate to

   HKEY_LOCAL_MACHINE\SYSTEM\CurrentControlSet\Control\Lsa

3. Double-click on the AllowPasswordExport DWORD value.

4. Change the properties from 0 to 1 - Hexadecimal.

5. Click OK and close Registry Editor.

6. Reboot the machine for the Registry changes to be enacted.

At this point in the ADMT process, all prerequisites have been satisfied and both source and target domains are prepared for the migration.

Migrating Accounts Using the Active Directory Migration Tool

When the target domain structure has been finalized, built, and "burnt in" as part of a pilot, and ADMT has been installed, the process of migrating the user, computer, and other accounts can begin. As previously mentioned, the built-in wizards in ADMT stream-line the process and give a great deal of flexibility regarding migration options.

Migrating Groups Using ADMT

In most cases, the first objects to be migrated into a new domain should be groups. The reason for this suggestion is the fact that if users are migrated first, their group member-ship does not transfer. However, if the groups exist before the users are migrated, they automatically find their place in the group structure. To migrate groups using ADMT v2, use the Group Account Migration Wizard:

1. Open the ADMT MMC snap-in (Start, All Programs, Administrative Tools, Active Directory Migration Tool).

2. Right-click on Active Directory Migration Tool in the left pane and choose Group Account Migration Wizard.

3. Click Next to continue.

4. On the next screen, illustrated in Figure 14.7, the option to test the migration is available. As previously mentioned, the migration process should be thoroughly tested before actually being done in production. In this example, however, the migration will be done. Choose Migrate now and click Next to continue.

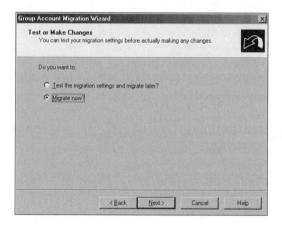

FIGURE 14.7   ADMT test run options.

5. Select the source and destination domains and click Next to continue.

6. The subsequent screen allows for the group accounts from the source domain to be selected. Select all required by using the Add button and selecting the objects manu-ally. After the groups have been selected, click Next to continue.

7. Enter the destination OU for the accounts from the source domain by clicking Browse and selecting the OU created in the prerequisite steps outlined above. Click Next to continue.

8. On the following screen, several options appear that will determine the nature of the migrated groups. Clicking the Help button details the nature of each setting. In the sample migration, the settings detailed in Figure 14.8 are chosen. After choosing the appropriate settings, click Next to continue.

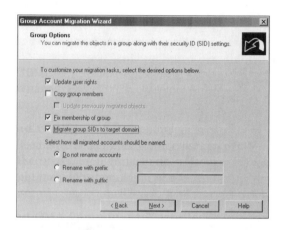

FIGURE 14.8   Group options in ADMT.

9. If auditing has not been enabled on the source domain, the prompt illustrated in Figure 14.9 will appear, which gives the option to enable auditing. This is required for migration of the SIDHistory. Click Yes to continue.

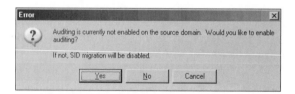

FIGURE 14.9   The enable auditing dialog box.

10. Another prompt might appear if auditing is not enabled on the target domain. Enabling auditing is required for migration of SIDHistory and can be disabled after the migration. Click Yes to enable and continue.

11. A local group named SOURCEDOMAIN$$$ is required on the source domain for migration of SIDHistory. A prompt asking to create this group will be displayed at this point, as illustrated in Figure 14.10, if it has not been created beforehand. Click Yes to continue.

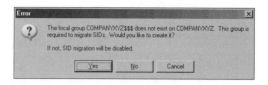

FIGURE 14.10   Local group creation for ADMT.

12. Another dialog box may appear asking to create a Registry key named `TcpipClientSupport` in the source domain. This is also required for SIDHistory migration. Click Yes to continue.

13. If the Registry key was created, an additional prompt is displayed asking whether the PDC in the source domain will require a reboot. In most cases, it will, so click Yes to continue.

14. The next prompt, illustrated in Figure 14.11, exists solely to stall the process while the reboot of the source PDC takes place. Wait until the PDC is back online and then click OK to continue.

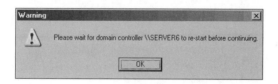

FIGURE 14.11   Waiting for the source domain PDC to reboot.

15. The subsequent screen allows for the exclusion of specific directory-level attributes from migration. If the need arises to exclude any attributes, they can be set here. In this example, no exclusions are set. Click Next to continue.

16. A user account with proper administrative rights on the source domain should now be entered in the screen shown in Figure 14.12. After it's entered, click Next to continue.

17. Naming conflicts often arise during domain migrations. In addition, different naming conventions may apply in the new environment. The screen illustrated in Figure 14.12 allows for these contingencies. In the example illustrated, any conflicting names have the `XYZ-` prefix attached to the account names. After the settings have been defined, click Next to continue.

18. The verification screen is the last wizard screen before any changes have been made. Ensure that the procedure has been tested before running it, because ADMT will henceforth write changes to the target Windows Server 2003 Active Directory environment. Click Finish when ready to begin group migration.

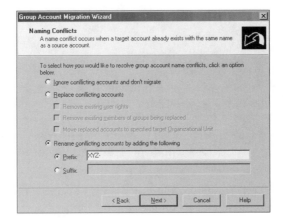

FIGURE 14.12   Naming conflict options.

19. The Group migration process will then commence. Changing the refresh rate, as illustrated in Figure 14.13, allows a quicker analysis of the current process. When the procedure is complete, the log can be viewed by clicking on View Log. After you complete these steps, click the Close button to end the procedure.

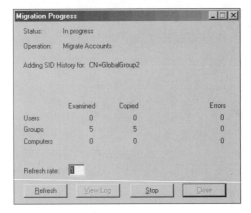

FIGURE 14.13   The group account migration process.

Migrating User Accounts Using ADMT

User accounts are the bread and butter of domain objects, and are one of the most important components. The biggest shortcoming of ADMT v1 was its inability to migrate passwords of user objects, which effectively limited its use. However, ADMT v2 does an excellent job of migrating users, their passwords, and the security associated with them. To migrate users, follow this procedure:

1. Open the ADMT MMC Console (Start, All Programs, Administrative Tools, Active Directory Migration Tool).

2. Right-click on Active Directory Migration Tool and choose User Account Migration Wizard, as indicated in Figure 14.14.

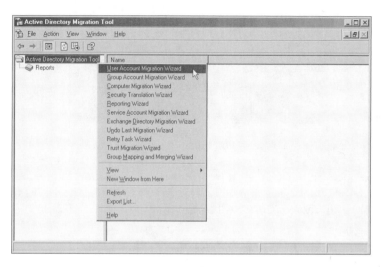

FIGURE 14.14   Starting the user account migration process.

3. Click Next at the welcome screen.

4. The next screen offers the option to test the migration before actually performing it. As previously mentioned, this is a recommended process; in this example, the full migration will be performed. Select Migrate Now and then click Next.

5. Select the source and target domains in the subsequent screen and click Next to continue.

6. The following screen enables you to choose user accounts for migration; click the Add button and select the user accounts to be migrated. After all user accounts have been selected, click Next to continue.

7. The next screen enables you to choose a target OU for all created users. Choose the OU by clicking the Browse button. After the OU has been selected, similar to what is shown in Figure 14.15, click Next to continue.

8. The new password migration functionality of ADMT v2 is enacted through the following screen. Select Migrate passwords and select the server in the source domain that had the Password Migration DLL installed in previous steps. Click Next to continue.

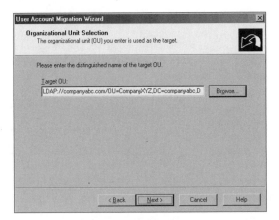

FIGURE 14.15   Selecting the organization unit in the migration wizard.

9. The subsequent screen deals with security settings in relation to the migrated users. Click Help for an overview of each option. In this example, the settings illustrated in Figure 14.16 are chosen. Click Next to continue.

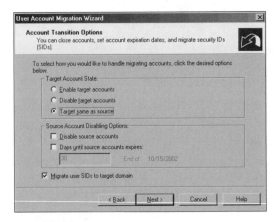

FIGURE 14.16   Account transition options.

10. Enter the username, password, and domain of an account that has Domain Admin rights in the source domain. Click Next to continue.

11. Several migration options are presented as part of the next screen. As before, press Help to learn more about some of these features. In this example, the options illustrated in Figure 14.17 are selected. Click Next to continue.

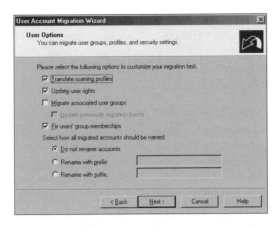

FIGURE 14.17 User options in ADMT.

12. The next screen is for setting exclusions. Any property of the user object that should not be migrated should be specified here. In this example, no exclusions are set. Click Next to continue.

13. Naming conflicts for user accounts are common. A procedure for dealing with duplicate accounts should be addressed in advance and can be designated in the next wizard screen, as illustrated in Figure 14.18. Select the appropriate options for duplicate accounts and click Next to continue.

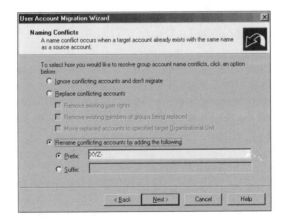

FIGURE 14.18 Naming conflict settings.

14. The following verification screen presents a summary of the procedure that will take place. This is the last screen before changes are written to the target domain. Verify the settings and click Next to continue.

15. The Migration Progress status box displays the migration process as it occurs, indicating the number of successful and unsuccessful accounts created. When the process is complete, review the log by clicking View Log and verify the integrity of the procedure. A sample log file from a user migration is illustrated in Figure 14.19. Click Close when finished.

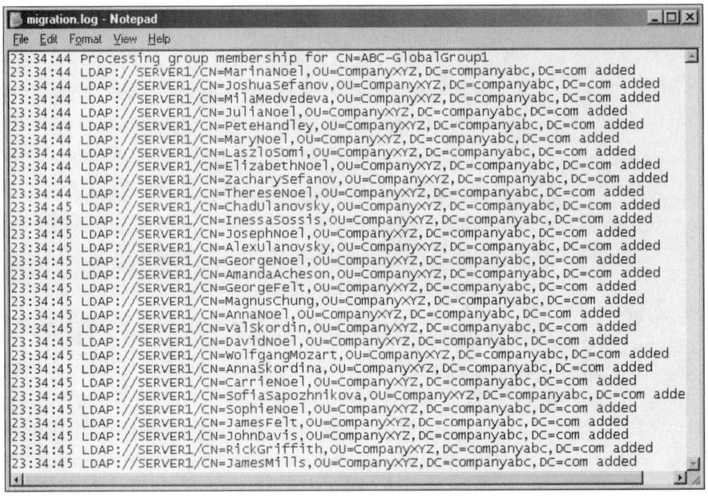

FIGURE 14.19   A sample user migration log.

Migrating Computer Accounts Using ADMT

Another important set of objects that must be migrated is also one of the trickier ones. Computer objects must not only be migrated in AD, they must also be updated at the workstations themselves so that users can log in effectively from their consoles. ADMT seamlessly installs agents on all migrated computer accounts and reboots them, forcing them into their new domain structures. This process is outlined in the following steps:

1. Open the ADMT MMC Console (Start, All Programs, Administrative Tools, Active Directory Migration Tool).

2. Right-click on Active Directory Migration Tool and choose Computer Migration Wizard.

3. Click Next at the welcome screen.

4. As in the previous wizards, the option for testing the migration is given at this point. It is highly recommended to test the process before migrating computer accounts. In this case, a full migration will take place and Migrate now is chosen. Click Next to continue.

5. Type the names of the source and destination domains in the drop-down boxes of the next screen and click Next to continue.

6. In the following screen, select the computer accounts that will be migrated by clicking the Add button and picking the appropriate accounts. Click Next to continue.

7. Select the OU to which the computer accounts will be migrated and click Next to continue.

8. The next screen enables for the specification of which settings on the local computers will be migrated. Click the Help button for a detailed description of each item. In the example, all items are checked, as illustrated in Figure 14.20. Click Next to continue.

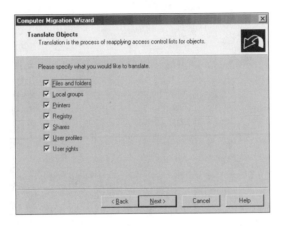

FIGURE 14.20   Specifying settings to be migrated.

9. The subsequent screen prompts you to choose whether existing security will be replaced, removed, or added on to. In this example, the security will be replaced. Click Next to continue.

10. A prompt is displayed informing you that the user rights translation will be performed in Add mode only. Click OK to continue.

11. The next screen is important. It enables an administrator to specify how many minutes a computer will wait before restarting itself. In addition, the naming convention for the computers can be defined, as illustrated in Figure 14.21. After choosing options, click Next to continue.

12. As in the previous wizards, exclusions for specific attributes may be set in the following wizard. Select any exclusions desired and click Next to continue.

13. Naming conflicts are addressed in the subsequent screen. If any specific naming conventions or conflict resolution settings are desired, enter them here. Click Next to continue.

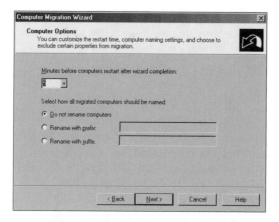

FIGURE 14.21   Computer timing options.

14. The completion screen lists a summary of the changes that will be made. Review the list and click Finish when ready. All clients that will be upgraded will subsequently be rebooted.

15. After the migration process has completed, the migration log will be available for viewing by clicking the View Log button. After all settings have been verified, click Close.

16. The client agents will be distributed to all clients that have been migrated. Each agent is installed automatically, and counts down until the designated time limit that was set during the configuration of the migration wizard. The dialog box illustrated in Figure 14.22 appears on each workstation.

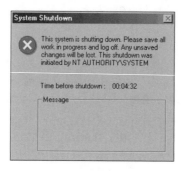

FIGURE 14.22   The automatic workstation restart.

17. Click Close on the Migration Console to end the wizard.

Migrating Service Accounts Using ADMT

With the combination of performing an in-place upgrade and the need to support applications that require service accounts—such as Microsoft Exchange and other third-party products—the ADMT Service Account Migration Wizard can assist in moving this account information to Active Directory. To migrate these service accounts, perform the following steps:

1. From the ADMT management console, launch the Service Account Migration Wizard by selecting Action.

2. Select the source domain from which the service accounts reside and the target domain where the service accounts will be migrated. Select the Next button when ready to continue.

3. The Update service account information page gathers service account information for the selected sources domain. If this is the first time you are using the Service Account Migration Wizard, select Yes, update the information.

4. The No, use previously collected information option is not available if the wizard has not been run previously. This option enables the migration of service accounts without collecting service account information each time the wizard is run.

5. On the Service Account Selection page, enter the computer that will host the service accounts that are being migrated. Click the Add button to enter and check the computer account names that host the services accounts being migrated. Click OK to continue.

6. The Active Directory Migration Tool Monitor will appear. Review the status as the ADMT installs the agent on the computers selected.

7. On the Service Account Information page, review the service account being migrated. Use the Skip/Include button to select or deselect accounts for this migration. The Update CSM now option updates the service control entry. After the proper accounts have been selected, choose Next to continue.

The Service Account Migration Wizard summary verifies the tasks and results of the migration. Use the scrollbar to review the tasks of the service account migration. Click Finish to close the Service Account Wizard.

The Active Directory Migration Tool can be used to migrate additional Windows NT4 Domain resources to Active Directory. Always review the results of each migration and test permissions and functionality before continuing with any of the migrations.

Migrating Other Domain Functionality

In addition to the group, user, and computer migration wizards, several other wizards exist that can migrate specific domain-critical components. These wizards operate using the same principles that the wizards previously presented use, and are as straightforward in their operation. The following is a list of the additional wizards included in ADMT v2:

- Security Translation Wizard

- Reporting Wizard

- Exchange Directory Migration Wizard

- Retry Task Wizard

- Trust Migration Wizard

- Group Mapping and Merging Wizard

Virtually all necessary functionality that needs to be replaced when migrating from one domain to another can be transferred by using ADMT v2. It has proven to be a valuable tool that gives administrators an additional option to consider when migrating and restructuring Active Directory environments.

Summary

Many organizations have been waiting for that "killer app" to justify an upgrade from an NT 4.0 domain structure to Active Directory. Exchange Server 2003 fits this role in many cases. Before deploying Exchange Server 2003, however, a migration from NT 4.0 to Windows Server 2003 AD must take place. The upgrade path to Windows Server 2003 can be accomplished via an in-place upgrade of each NT domain into AD, or via a migration from the old NT domain structure into a brand new AD forest via the ADMT v2. Each option has its pros and cons, and it is important to determine which option is the most ideal for each organization, because the benefits of Exchange Server 2003 cannot be achieved without this very important step.

Best Practices

The following are best practices from this chapter:

- Choose the in-place Upgrade method when looking for a speedier and more straight-forward upgrade process.

- Choose the Migration with ADMT method when it is preferable to create a new domain structure and consolidate existing domains.

- Test the hardware compatibility of any server that will be directly upgraded to Windows Server 2003 against the published Hardware Compatibility List from Microsoft.

- Migrate groups before users when using the Active Directory Migration Tool. This preserves the user's group membership.

- Use the Microsoft Compatibility Check Tool on the Windows Server 2003 CD to test application compatibility.

- Review the server event and system logs upon completing any upgrade.

- When possible, replace NT BDCs with new Windows Server 2003 DCs, as opposed to upgrading them.

- Test the ADMT migration process before performing the actual migration.

14

CHAPTER 15

Migrating from Exchange v5.5 to Exchange Server 2003

Understanding Exchange 5.5 Migration Options and Strategies

In the past, Microsoft has taken a great deal of heat over the complexity of its migration path from Exchange 5.5 to Exchange 2000. Because of these difficulties, special consideration was given to making the process of migration from Exchange 5.5 to Exchange Server 2003 a much more structured, risk-averse approach. Consequently, a set of very well-designed tools known as the Exchange Deployment Tools was created to assist administrators with the task of migrating off Exchange 5.5. In addition to these tools, specific knowledge of the architecture of both Exchange 5.5 and Exchange Server 2003, and how they interact in a migration process is recommended.

This chapter focuses on best-practice migration from Exchange 5.5 to Exchange Server 2003. It discusses the differences between Exchange 5.5 and Exchange Server 2003, and it then details specific steps required to migrate an environment. Close attention is given to new migration techniques made available with the Exchange Deployment Tools, in addition to the more "manual" approaches to migration.

Comparing Exchange 5.5 and Exchange Server 2003 Environments

Exchange 5.5 left a lot to be desired when it came to enterprise deployments. It was a fantastic product in small and medium-size companies and for collaboration at the department level. This section examines some of the ways that Exchange 5.5 was typically deployed and how its shortcomings are resolved in Exchange Server 2003. The idea behind this section is to give Exchange 5.5 architects and administrators some ideas of how they can leverage the capabilities of Exchange Server 2003. In most environments, upgrading all the Exchange 5.5 servers to Exchange Server 2003 will not be the best solution to leverage Exchange Server 2003. Some places in the environment could or should be consolidated or eliminated.

Detailing Design Limitations in Exchange 5.5

Exchange 5.5 environments generally followed a distributed deployment model in which Exchange servers were placed in each remote location, typically having more than 20–30 users. This was especially true for organizations that were deployed in early Exchange deployments. This was due to several factors in the product and in the network environment.

Combined Administration and Routing

Exchange 5.5 tied the hands of messaging architects by limiting Exchange designs around the site boundary. The Site in Exchange 5.5 was the boundary for administration as well as message routing. Exchange 5.5 directory replication occurs every 15 minutes within an Exchange site, and every server in a site communicates with every other server in that site. Messages also route within a site directly from the source to the destination server. Unless bandwidth was unlimited in the organization, architects had to draw site boundaries to control message routing and directory replication. Many organizations that chose a single-site design paid the price with frequent RPC message timeouts and eventually switched to a multisite design. Because message routing and administration are linked, a distributed administration model was automatically created that was an additional headache. Windows NT 4.0 didn't do a good job of providing granular administration. Anyone with administrative rights in the domain could add himself to the global group that was assigned rights in the Exchange Administrator program. This really meant that distributed message routing and centralized administration just was not possible if someone in the remote office needed to manage the Exchange server.

Lack of Scalability

In Exchange 5.5 environments, scalability was usually a cap that was set based on the size of the mail and public folder server database size or the number of users supported per server. When the cap was reached, users were moved from one server to another. Mailbox limits could vary widely between organizations, from a conservative 500 users to a less conservative number of about 2,500. Many organizations capped the database size or number of users per server due to the 16GB mail and public folder store limitation of the standard edition of the Exchange server software. Even after the limitation was removed in the enterprise edition, organizations were limited in the size of the database by the amount of time offline maintenance, backup, and restore operations took on the server. The cap was then set based on the organization's comfort level with the risk of losing the server and the amount of recovery time to get a failed server operational. Many organizations found that when they began to exceed about 30GB, the store became unmanageable.

Small Degree of Redundancy

In most Exchange 5.5 deployments, mail servers were distributed to locations that had more than 20–30 users, an arbitrary number of users that was selected on the size and availability of WAN bandwidth, whether backup links existed, and the organization's comfort with the level of risk. This was due to the desire to provide a decent level of performance with the capability to keep mail services running in the remote location online in case of WAN failure. Redundancy was also provided through the use of multiple connector servers for foreign mail, SMTP, and OWA. Having multiple connector servers allowed one connector server to fail or have a fault; another connector server would be available to service messaging routing needs.

Questionable Stability

In corporate locations, stability was achieved by keeping databases small and by separating public folders and message-routing services from mail-message services. Distributed services came in the form of dedicated public folder servers and connector servers such as cc:Mail connector servers, Outlook Web Access server, and SMTP bridgehead servers for Internet Mail.

How Exchange Server 2003 Addresses Exchange 5.5 Shortcomings

Exchange Server 2003 provides the features necessary to build a more robust messaging environment. It removes many of the boundaries that tied the hands of architects and administrators in Exchange 5.5. As Exchange Server 2003 matures, the messaging designs continue to centralize, with only a portion of the services still being distributed. Exchange Server 2003 improves upon the shortcomings of Exchange 5.5 in the following ways:

- **Separate administration and routing**   In Exchange Server 2003, separate routing and administration can be achieved through Routing and Administrative Groups. To fully use these new containers, the organization must be converted to Native Mode Exchange Server 2003. This requires all Exchange 5.5 servers to be converted to Exchange Server 2003 or be uninstalled from the organization. The combination of Administrative and Routing Groups with the granular permission of Active Directory helps messaging administrators better control access to the messaging services in the organization.

- **Increased degree of scalability**   Scalability is provided in multiple mail and public folder databases that can be used to keep the database performance high while keeping backup and restore times low. This means that the number of users supported per server can be increased, reducing the number of servers on the network. Each database can be mounted and dismounted individually, allowing the server to continue to function with a single database offline.

- **Improved redundancy**   Redundancy in Exchange Server 2003 is provided through full support of active-active clustering. Active-active clustering enables all nodes in the cluster to simultaneously service users so that organizations get the full benefit of their hardware investment while still getting the redundancy and high availability that clustering provides. Connectors in Exchange Server 2003 can also be redundant. By using SMTP for message delivery and a link-state routing algorithm, message-routing designs can be built to route messages efficiently and to take advantage of redundant links on the WAN.

- **Enhanced stability**   Stability is provided within the Windows Server 2003 operating system and at the core of Exchange Server 2003 in the Extensible Storage Environment (ESE) database. Small efficient databases, redundant connector designs, and clustering technology all increase the stability of Exchange Server 2003, improving the end-user experience and letting information technology groups create service level agreements that they can stand by.

Prerequisites for Migrating to Exchange Server 2003

Before moving the Exchange 5.5 organization to Exchange Server 2003, several items need to be addressed from a technical implementation and design standpoint. Refer to Chapter 4, "Exchange Server 2003 Design Concepts," and Chapter 5, "Designing an Enterprise Exchange Server 2003 Environment," for information on Exchange Server 2003 design concerns.

Checking Current Environment with the Exchange Server 2003 Deployment Tools

The Exchange Deployment Tools are an invaluable asset to any deployment team. They are straightforward and robust, and they cover a multitude of migration scenarios. Even die-hard Exchange upgrade enthusiasts with years of Exchange 2000 migration experience under their belt can benefit from the tactical advice and safeguards built into the tools.

The Exchange Deployment Tools guide administrators through the Exchange Server 2003 migration process in a step-by-step fashion. The tools themselves can be invoked by simply inserting the Exchange Server 2003 CD (or clicking Setup.exe if autorun is disabled) and then clicking on the Exchange Deployment Tools link. The tools, illustrated in Figure 15.1, initially lead the migration team through a series of prerequisite steps.

These prerequisite steps should be followed exactly as described in the tool. In fact, the entire migration process outlined in this chapter can be followed via the Exchange Deployment Tools. In addition to running through the prerequisite steps listed in the tools, you must take several key factors into account before deploying Exchange Server 2003.

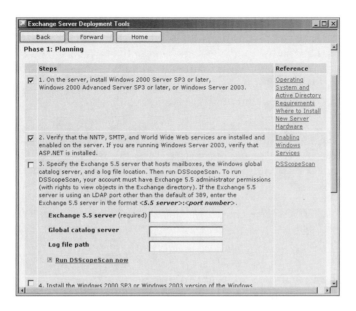

FIGURE 15.1   Exchange Deployment Tools.

Preparing the Exchange 5.5 Organization for the Migration

When moving to Exchange Server 2003, one of the biggest items that organizations should be concerned about is that Exchange Server 2003 is a one-to-one environment. This means that there is only one Exchange Server 2003 organization per Active Directory forest. Many organizations have one or more Exchange organizations in their environment. This type of installation can result from mergers and acquisitions that were never fully meshed or breakaway lines of business that established their own organization, or it could be done by design to create an SMTP relay routing hub. In any case, only one organization can remain in Exchange Server 2003, and this organization must be chosen before the start of the migration.

> **TIP**
>
> For organizations designed to support SMTP relay functions, continue to use them through the migration process and then replace them with Routing Groups. If the Exchange 5.5 relay servers are under the control of another group in the organization, place the Routing Group with the relay server in its own Administrative Group.

The second piece of the one-to-one environment that must be one-to-one is the number of mailboxes per Active Directory account. In Exchange 5.5, a Windows NT account could have an unlimited number of mailboxes associated with it. In Active Directory, the messaging components of the user account are just additional attributes of the user, so the mailbox is really part of the user account. It was quite common for Exchange 5.5

administrators to use a single account for multiple mailboxes, especially for administrative functions such as backup and virus-scanning products, and also for resources such as conference rooms. Linking the Active Directory accounts to the Exchange 5.5 mailboxes can be done either manually for a few mailboxes or for a large number of mailboxes by using the NTDSNoMatch utility, or by using the Resource Mailbox Wizard in the ADC Tools, described in more detail later in this chapter.

> **TIP**
>
> To view the Windows NT Accounts with multiple mailboxes, use the Exchange 5.5 Administrator program and run a directory export to a CSV file. In the Exchange Administrator program, select Tools, Directory Export and export all mailboxes from the Global Address List container. Open the export file in Excel and sort the spreadsheet by the Primary Windows NT account column. Scrolling through the Excel sheet reveals all of the Windows NT 4.0 accounts that were used on more than one mailbox.

Consolidating the Exchange 5.5 Organization

The more items that exist in Exchange 5.5, the more items must be migrated to Exchange Server 2003. It's a given that mail database and public folder servers need to be migrated, but all the connector servers might not be necessary in the Exchange Server 2003 environment. Now is the time to rethink the Exchange design. By consolidating servers and using features such as active-active clustering, it is now possible to locate all the Exchange installations at a few central hubs on the WAN where the administrators with the best Exchange skills reside. In addition, the enhanced remote client access capabilities introduced in Exchange Server 2003 allow for site consolidation, further reducing the number of servers that must be supported. Of course, the migrated Exchange Server 2003 environment can mirror the exact same configuration as Exchange v5.5. It's just an option (and opportunity) to rethink the best configuration for the organization.

Later revisions of Exchange 5.5 introduced a utility called the Move Server Wizard that allows for the consolidation of Exchange 5.5 organizations and sites. An organization's migration can be made simpler by consolidating the Exchange sites into a single site. If the organization must remain in Mixed Mode for an extended period of time, the organization should consider consolidating into a single site before the migration process. Having a single site allows the administrators of the organization to move mailboxes and still retain flexibility with message routing. To run the Move Server Wizard, the organization must be at Exchange 5.5 Service Pack 1 or higher.

> **CAUTION**
>
> You cannot run the Move Server Wizard after you begin migrating into a mixed Exchange v5.5/Exchange Server 2003 environment. You must be in full Exchange Server 2003 Native Mode before you have a chance to rearrange and configure your Exchange Server 2003 Administrative Groups; therefore if you want to make any Exchange Organization modifications, be sure to do them *before* you begin your migration to Exchange Server 2003.

Foreign Mail System Connectivity

One of the biggest changes for organizations moving from Exchange 5.5 to Exchange Server 2003 regarding foreign mail connectivity is that there is no Exchange Server 2003 version of the PROFS/SNADS connector. The easiest solution to this problem is to leave a single Exchange 5.5 site behind to handle the PROFS/SNADS connectivity. The downside to this solution is that it delays the organization's move to Exchange Server 2003 Native Mode until another solution is put into place. For a long-term solution, investigate using SMTP to connect the systems, or migrate the PROFS user to Exchange Server 2003.

A second issue regarding foreign mail connectivity is that organizations might have put so much effort into getting their connectors stable and configured properly that they might not want to move their foreign mail connectors to Exchange Server 2003. As long as the organization can remain in Mixed Mode, it's okay to leave the connectors in Exchange 5.5. As with the PROFS/SNADS connector, it's better to leave all Exchange 5.5 connectors in a single Exchange 5.5 site than multiple sites. If this means moving the connector anyway to consolidate to a single Exchange 5.5 site, or if a single Exchange site doesn't make sense because of geography or WAN issues, consider moving the connectors sooner rather than later to Exchange Server 2003.

Upgrading Service Pack Levels

To migrate from Exchange 5.5 to Exchange Server 2003, some or all of the Exchange 5.5 servers must be running at least Service Pack 3, and preferably Service Pack 4. Most organizations are already at that level, but those that are not should plan to perform the Service Pack 3 upgrade before starting the Exchange migration. Although it is wise to upgrade all, only one Exchange 5.5 server in the organization technically must run SP3—the one that the ADC replicates to.

If the organization is planning to consolidate services before migrating to Exchange Server 2003, it makes sense to postpone the Service Pack 3 upgrade until the consolidation through the Move Server Wizard is completed.

Structuring the Migration for Best Results

When structuring the migration, the end goal is to move to the new platform without disrupting current services or losing functionality. The only way to be sure that service and functionality will not be lost during the migration is to perform lab testing. Having a fallback plan and solid disaster-recovery processes are also essential when planning the Exchange Server 2003 deployment. By breaking the migration into sections, the organization can move cautiously through the migration without making too many changes at one time. The following best practices deploy Exchange Server 2003 by migrating each service type at a time. For many smaller remote locations, this might not be feasible and all services might have to be migrated at the same time. Migrating by service type is usually the best solution for corporate sites and large remote offices.

Single Site Exchange 5.5 Migrations

Within the same Exchange 5.5 site, administrators have the flexibility of moving users between servers. Single-site Exchange 5.5 installations become a single Administrative Group with a single Routing Group when converted to Exchange Server 2003. If granular message routing is needed, additional Routing Groups can be added and servers within the Administrative Group can be moved to new Routing Groups after the conversion to Native Mode.

Because servers cannot be moved between Administrative Groups even after the conversion to Native Mode, administrators need to examine whether a single Administrative Group will fulfill the organization's administrative needs. Additional Administrative Groups can be added to the organization, but only by installing new Exchange Server 2003 systems. Users can be moved between Administrative Groups by moving the mailbox from group to group, but only after the switch to Native Mode.

Multisite Exchange 5.5 Migrations

Multisite migrations are a bit more complex than single-site migrations because an Exchange Server 2003 system must be established in each Exchange 5.5 site. After the first Exchange server is installed, administrators can use the **Move Mailbox method** to migrate users to Exchange Server 2003.

After the migration, the organization will contain multiple Administrative Groups with a single Routing Group in each that matches the Exchange 5.5 configuration. Even after the conversion to Native Mode, the servers in each site cannot be moved between Administrative Groups, so administrators need to examine whether this design will still work for the organization.

Understanding why the multiple sites were established might help in deciding how to handle the multiple sites. If the decision to have multiple sites was to originally delegate control of administration, the multiple Administrative Groups might still be needed. If multiple sites were implemented to control message flow and directory replication, consolidating many of the Administrative Groups might be desired.

Multiorganization Exchange 5.5 Migrations

Multiorganization environments must consolidate to a single Exchange Server 2003 organization to migrate to Exchange Server 2003 unless the organization plans to support multiple Active Directory forests. Multiple organization environments have the following choices when moving to Exchange Server 2003:

- **Select one organization to be migrated to Exchange Server 2003**   Use the most heavily populated organization if it fits the company's standards. Create new Exchange Server 2003 mailboxes for users in the other organization. Use ExMerge to move user data from the abandoned organization to Exchange Server 2003.

- **Start with a clean Exchange Server 2003 organization and do not migrate either organization**   Both organizations feel equal pain that might be politically acceptable. Look at the ExMerge utility to migrate user data, or run both Exchange 5.5 organizations for a short period of time and allow users to forward mail to their Exchange Server 2003 mailbox.

- **Use the Move Server Wizard to collapse one organization into the other before migrating**   Use the company-standard organization for the organization to be migrated to Exchange Server 2003. Merge the other organization into it before migrating through the Move Server Wizard. No one loses mail during the migration, but it might be a hard sell politically.

Preparing the Active Directory Forest and Domain for Exchange Server 2003

After the prerequisite steps have been satisfied, the Exchange Deployment Tools prompt the administrator to run the Forestprep and Domainprep processes. These processes can be invoked manually via setup.exe switches (/forestprep and /domainprep), or they can simply be launched via the Exchange Deployment Tools, as illustrated in Figure 15.2.

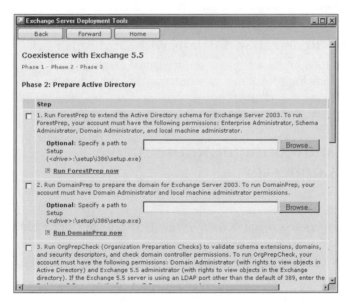

FIGURE 15.2   Launching Forestprep and Domainprep from the Exchange Deployment Tools.

A greater understanding of what tasks these two utilities perform is crucial to understanding the Exchange deployment process as a whole.

Extending the Active Directory Schema

To extend the Active Directory schema, Exchange Setup relies on the capabilities of the /forestprep switch, which can be invoked via the Exchange Deployment Tools. Running the Forestprep procedure requires that the account invoking the command have Schema Admin privileges in the schema root domain because the command extends the Active Directory schema to support the attributes that Exchange Server 2003 requires. The schema extension is quite extensive, and the changes are replicated to all domain controllers in the Active Directory forest. This might require special consideration into replication issues if the AD forest is large and spread out across slow replication links.

Preparing the Windows Server 2003 Domains to Support Exchange Server 2003

The Active Directory domains that will host Exchange servers or mailbox-enabled users must be prepared before installing the first Exchange Server 2003 system. Prepare the Windows Server 2003 domains using the /domainprep switch, also invoked via the Exchange Deployment Tools. The /domainprep process configures the Recipient Update Service parameters, which are responsible for keeping Exchange address lists up-to-date and for creating proxy addresses for users based on recipient policy addressing configuration. In addition, it creates the Exchange Server 2003–specific groups that allow Exchange services to run without a service account.

Verifying the Organization Settings with OrgPrepCheck

Exchange Server 2003 introduces a new utility named OrgPrepCheck to validate that the Forestprep and Domainprep utilities were functionally successful. The OrgPrepCheck utility is invoked via the Exchange Deployment Tools and is a recommended way of determining whether it is safe to proceed with the migration process.

Installing and Configuring the Active Directory Connector

Unlike in Exchange 2000, the Active Directory Connector (ADC) does not need to be installed until after the /forestprep command has run. This was designed so that only a single schema extension is required for upgrading to Exchange Server 2003, as opposed to the dual-extension of Exchange 2000.

After the prompt by the Exchange Deployment Tools, the ADC can be installed. The connection agreements in ADC are necessary to synchronize directory entries between the Exchange 5.5 and Exchange Server 2003 systems. Unlike in Exchange 2000, the Exchange Server 2003 ADC can be installed on a member server and is often installed on the first Exchange Server 2003 system in a site.

Organizations can choose to implement one or more Active Directory Connectors in the organization. Implementing additional ADC connectors and connection agreements should not be seen as a fault-tolerant solution for the ADC. The ADC should be seen as a temporary coexistence solution, with the migration being the intended end goal.

ADC installations are better off being left as simple as possible. A single ADC installed with one connection agreement to each Exchange 5.5 site is much easier to manage than multiple ADCs, all with their own connection agreements. This might or might not be possible based on the Exchange 5.5 site design and WAN layout. The ADC and its connection agreements should communicate with servers on the same network segment that will require multiple ADC installations.

Installing the ADC

Both the Active Directory domain controller and the Exchange 5.5 server that will be joined through the Active Directory Connector should be on the same physical network segment. Schema Admin and Enterprise Administrator rights are required to install the ADC.

Plan a few days to install and configure the ADC and the connection agreements. The initial installation and configuration take only a few hours, but it generally takes a few days to work out the kinks and resolve the errors in the Application Event Log. Problems in the ADC will show up later and complicate the migration, so don't rush the ADC installation. Microsoft recommends allocating 2 hours for replicating about 5,000 objects in a single direction, but the length of time for replication really varies on the number of connection agreements, recipient containers, and populated attributes on the actual directory objects.

The ADC has the capability to delete objects in both directories, so check whether the backup media and procedures have been recently verified before configuring the ADC. The organization should be familiar with how to perform an authoritative restore through NTDSUTIL for the Active Directory database.

The first step in installing the ADC is to create or choose a user account that will be used to run the ADC service and manage the connection agreements. This account does not have to be the same account that is used in each of the connection agreements configured later in the chapter. This account needs to be added to the Administrators group in the domain if the ADC is installed on a domain controller or to the local Administrators group if the ADC is installed on a member server.

To manually start the ADC installation, insert the Exchange Server 2003 CD and select ADC Setup from the autorun menu, or simply invoke the setup from the Exchange Deployment Tools. The ADC prompts for the component selection and allows just the MMC administration snap-in to be installed or the ADC service. Select both components when installing the ADC on the server. If the ADC will need to be remotely managed, the administration component can be installed later on the administrator's workstation.

Next, the installation prompts for the path to install the ADC and the ADC service account credentials. When the installation is complete, the next step is to configure the connection agreements to begin synchronizing the Active Directory and Exchange 5.5 directories.

Creating Connection Agreements

Configuring connection agreements (CAs) has been the bane of many an Exchange 2000 administrator. Improperly configured connection agreements can seriously corrupt an Active Directory or Exchange 5.5 database, so it is extremely important to properly configure CAs for the migration process. Luckily, Exchange Server 2003 includes a series of ADC Tools that streamline the process of creating CAs for migration, as illustrated in Figure 15.3. After installation, it is highly recommended that you use these wizards to install and configure the CAs.

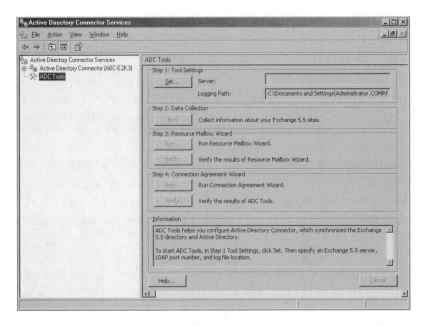

FIGURE 15.3   ADC Tools.

Two tools in particular are extremely helpful in the migration process. The first tool, the Resource Mailbox Wizard, illustrated in Figure 15.4, can help to identify users with multiple mailboxes and fix them in advance of the migration. This tool streamlines the process that the ntdsutil utility previously utilized.

The second tool, the Connection Agreement Wizard, walks an administrator through the tricky process of creating the connection agreements required to migrate from Exchange 5.5. The wizard helps to identify "gotchas" such as the AD domain being in Mixed Mode (it should be changed to Native Mode in advance of the migration) and other important factors. As illustrated in Figure 15.5, it automatically creates a recipient CA and a public folder CA, which can then be manually tweaked as necessary.

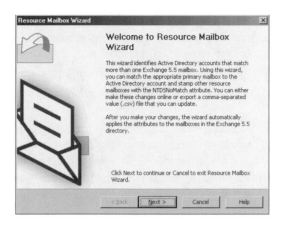

FIGURE 15.4   Resource Mailbox Wizard.

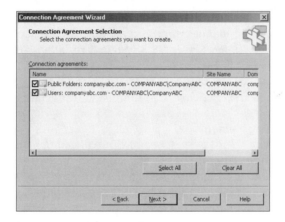

FIGURE 15.5 Connection Agreement Wizard.

After initial setup, several properties can be configured on the ADC to give the administrator more information and control over the ADC and its connection agreements. Attribute replication, account-matching rules, and diagnostic logging properties should all be configured before building the connection agreements and replicating directory entries. Even when using the default settings on the ADC, it is a best practice to prototype the ADC replication processes in a lab before attempting the synchronization on production systems.

Connection agreements are configured by an administrator who controls the type of objects that are replicated between Active Directory and Exchange 5.5. They also contain the credentials and connection information needed to connect to both systems and other attributes, such as handling deletion and what to do when there is no matching account for the mailbox in the destination directory. Connection agreements operate using two different approaches:

- **One way**   Information is synchronized only one way. The connection agreement can be from Windows or from Exchange, but not from both. After the direction is selected, the opposite system's tabs and controls are grayed out.

- **Two way**   Information is synchronized in both directions. This is generally the preferred method and keeps the configuration simple.

Connection agreements also need to be designated as primary or not. A primary connection agreement has the capability to create objects in the directory. A connection agreement that is not marked as primary cannot create new objects and can only update the attributes of existing objects. To ensure that objects are created, the ADC marks all connection agreements as primary by default.

Configuration Connection Agreements

Configuration connection agreements are used for coexistence between the Exchange 5.5 and Exchange 2003 servers, and they transfer information such as site addressing and routing information between the Exchange platforms. The configuration connection agreement cannot be created manually and is created by the Exchange Server 2003 set-up program when the first Exchange Server 2003 system is installed. After the replication of the configuration information, Exchange 5.5 sites are visible in the Exchange System Manager program and are represented as Administrative Groups. Exchange Server 2003 systems are also visible in the Exchange 5.5 Administrator program.

Recipient Connection Agreements

Recipient connection agreements are responsible for replicating mailbox, distribution list, and custom recipient information from the Exchange 5.5 directory to Active Directory. They are also used to send users, groups, and contacts from Active Directory to Exchange 5.5. Recipient Connection Agreements can be configured as one-way or two-way connection agreements. Most often a two-way connection agreement is used. Each connection agreement has its own schedule, so using one-way connection agreements might be preferred if the organization has specific requirements on when each side should be updated.

Public Folder Connection Agreements

Public folder connection agreements are responsible for replicating mail-enabled public folder information from and to Exchange 5.5 and Active Directory. Public folder connection agreements can be configured only as two-way connection agreements. It is a best practice to create one public folder connection agreement per Exchange 5.5 site. This is true even if the organization does not mail-enable public folders. Administrators might not be aware of some folders that are mail-enabled, and it is best to create the connection agreement for each Exchange 5.5 site, to reduce the likelihood of problems with the folders during the migration.

Configuring Connection Agreements

As previously mentioned, it is wise to allow the ADC Tools to create the necessary CAs for the migration process. If a manual CA will need to be configured, however, it can be done in the following fashion. Open the ADC MMC snap-in on the domain controller running the ADC by selecting Start, All Programs, Microsoft Exchange, Active Directory Connector. Right-click the Active Directory Connector service icon for the server and select New, Recipient Connection Agreement.

The following tabs must be populated:

- **General** Select the direction and the ADC server responsible for the connection agreement. It's usually best to select a two-way connection agreement for the primary connection agreement.

- **Connections** Enter the username and password combination that will be used to read and write to Active Directory. Next enter the server name and LDAP port number for the Exchange 5.5 server, and the username and password that will be used to read and write to the Exchange 5.5 directory. When entering the user credentials, use the format domain\user—that is, companyabc\administrator.

TIP

To locate the LDAP port number on the Exchange 5.5 server, open Exchange Administrator and access the LDAP protocol properties under the Protocols container beneath the server object.

- **Schedule** The directory synchronization process takes place between midnight and 6 a.m. daily under the default schedule. Use the grid to modify the schedule, or select Always, which replicates every five minutes. Remember to select the check box for Replicate the Entire Directory the Next Time the Agreement Is Run to perform a full synchronization on the first run.

- **From Exchange** Select all the recipient containers in the Exchange 5.5 site to synchronize with Active Directory. Remember to select any containers that might be used as import containers for foreign mail connectors. Next select the destination container in Active Directory where the ADC will search for matching accounts and create new accounts. Select the object types to replicate, such as mailboxes, distribution lists, and custom recipients.

- **From Windows** Select the Organizational Units in Active Directory to take updates from and the Exchange 5.5 container to place the updates in. The object types to replicate are selectable for users, groups, and contacts. The check boxes for Replicate Secured Active Directory Objects to the Exchange Directory and Create Objects in Location Specified by Exchange 5.5 DN are best left blank in most instances. Click Help while in the From Windows tab for more information on these options.

- **Deletion** The Deletion option controls whether deletions are processed or stored in a CSV or LDF file, depending on the platform. If this is a short-term connection

15

for migration, it's usually best to mark these options to not process the deletions and store the change in a file. The CSV and LDF files get created in the path that the ADC was installed into. Each connection agreement has its own subdirectory, and the output CSV and LDF files get created there.

- **Advanced**   The Advanced tab is set correctly for the first primary connection agreement and does not need to be modified. The settings on this tab should be modified when multiple connection agreements exist or when configuring the ADC to replicate between Exchange organizations. Leaving the Primary Connection Agreement check box selected on multiple connection agreements for the same containers creates duplicate directory entries. Never have the ADC create contacts unless the ADC is being used to link two Exchange organizations for collaboration purposes.

To configure a public folder connection agreement, right-click the Active Directory Connector service icon for the server and select New, Public Folder Connection Agreement.

- **General**   Select the ADC server responsible for the connection agreement. The direction can be only two-way on public folder connection agreements.

- **Connections**   Enter the username and password combination that will be used to read and write to Active Directory. Next enter the server name and LDAP port number for the Exchange 5.5 server, and the username and password that will be used to read and write to the Exchange 5.5 directory. When entering the user credentials, use the format domain\user—in this case, companyabc\administrator.

- **Schedule**   The directory-synchronization process will take place between midnight and 6 a.m. daily under the default schedule. Use the grid to modify the schedule. Select the check box for Replicate the Entire Directory the Next Time the Agreement Is Run to perform a full synchronization on the first run.

- **From Windows**   The only option available here is the check box for Replicate Secured Active Directory Objects to the Exchange Directory. This replicates objects that contain an explicit deny in the Access Control List to Exchange 5.5. Exchange 5.5 does not support explicit deny entries, so the objects are not replicated by default.

The final step is to force the connection agreement to replicate immediately. To force the replication, right-click the connection agreement and select Replicate Now. Be sure to check the Application Event Log in Event Viewer for errors during the replication process.

Installing the First Exchange Server 2003 System in an Exchange 5.5 Site

Because there are many prerequisite tasks and processes to run, getting to the point of the actual Exchange Server setup is a watershed event. The following section double-checks that the prerequisites have been fulfilled. When installing the first Exchange Server 2003 system, it is recommended that you use a server that has been wiped clean and has a fresh installation of Windows Server 2003. This is because the first server in Exchange holds many critical Exchange organizational management and routing master tables, and having a new, clean server ensures that the masters are created and stored on a solidly configured system.

Installing the First Exchange Server 2003 System

The actual Exchange Server 2003 installation of the first server is quite easy after the prerequisite conditions are met. The installation takes about 30 minutes on average.

One final step before running the Exchange Server 2003 setup is to run a tool called SetupPrep, as illustrated in Figure 15.6. This tool validates that all necessary prerequisites are in place for the installation of the first Exchange Server 2003 in the site.

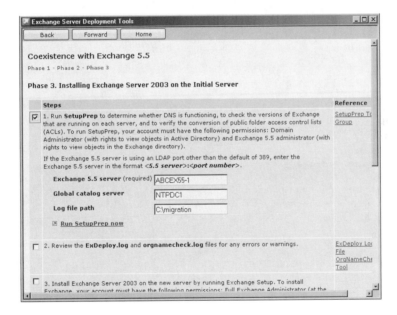

FIGURE 15.6   Running SetupPrep.

After SetupPrep has been run, the actual setup of the server can be invoked via the tools or simply by running the Setup.exe in the \setup\i386 folder. The following steps properly install Exchange Server 2003 on the system on which they are run:

1. Click Next at the Welcome Wizard.

2. Agree to the end-user licensing agreement and click Next.

3. Choose the installation path and ensure that Typical Installation is chosen. Click Next.

4. Select Join or Upgrade an Existing Exchange 5.5 Organization, as illustrated in Figure 15.7, and click Next.

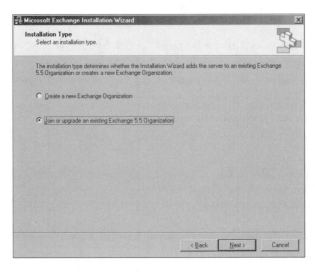

FIGURE 15.7   Joining an Exchange 5.5 organization.

> **NOTE**
>
> It is imperative that Join or Upgrade an Existing Exchange 5.5 Organization is chosen at this point. If Create a New Exchange Organization is chosen, connectivity will be lost to the Exchange 5.5 organization, and serious steps will be required to regain the functionality.

5. Enter the name of an Exchange 5.5 server in a site the Exchange Server 2003 system will join.

6. Click OK at the prompt to test prerequisite conditions.

7. Select I Agree to agree to the license agreement.

8. Enter the password of the Exchange 5.5 service account.

9. Verify the installation options, and click Next to start the installation.

10. When the installation is complete, click Finish.

To install additional Exchange Server 2003 systems, the installation process is almost identical, and the same procedure can be followed.

Understanding What Happens Behind the GUI During the Installation

Quite a few items are installed and configured during the installation. The following items describe some of the major components that are installed and configured during setup. The new terms and features are discussed more in depth in the next few sections.

- **Exchange Server 2003 binaries and services installed**   All the basic services for Exchange Server 2003 are installed and started. The SMTP and NNTP services from IIS are modified for Exchange Server 2003.

- **Changes to Active Directory Configuration container**   Information about the Exchange installation, such as Administrative and Routing Group configurations, are in the Services container.

- **Exchange Server added to Exchange Domain Servers security group**   The machine account for the server is added to the Exchange Domain Servers security group to let Exchange Server 2003 run under the local system account.

- **Configuration connection agreement created**   A new connection agreement is added to the ADC to replicate configuration and routing information between Exchange 5.5 and Exchange Server 2003.

- **Recipient Update Service created**   The RUS is created to update address lists and recipient policies in Active Directory.

- **Site Replication Service (SRS) installed**   The SRS is installed and synchronizes the directory with the Exchange 5.5 server in the site.

Configuration Connection Agreement

During the installation, a new connection agreement is added to the Active Directory Connector. The ConfigCA is responsible for replicating the configuration information between the Exchange platforms. The ConfigCA replicates items such as the Site Addressing Policies and the routing information in the Gateway Address Routing Table (GWART).

Site Replication Service

The Site Replication Service provides directory interoperability between the Exchange 5.5 and Exchange 2003 servers. The SRS runs as a service and is needed only during the migration period. SRS uses LDAP to communicate between directories, and to Exchange 5.5 servers it looks just like another Exchange 5.5 server. The SRS works in conjunction with the Active Directory Connector for directory synchronization.

Only one SRS is allowed per Exchange Server 2003 system. Additional SRSs can be added, as long as there are additional Exchange Server 2003 systems available to run the service. The SRS has no configuration parameters in the Exchange Server 2003 System Manager.

15

Synchronization can be forced through the SRS by accessing the SRS from the Exchange 5.5 Administrator program.

SRSs are created on all servers that house Exchange 5.5 Directory Replication Connectors. The Directory Replication Connector is replaced by the SRS to perform intersite replication with the remote Exchange 5.5 site; if an Exchange Server 2003 is configured to communicate with an Exchange 5.5 server, the Site Replication Service automatically is installed and configured at the time of Exchange Server 2003 installation.

> **TIP**
>
> To view the Directory Replication Connector endpoints in the SRS, open Exchange System Manger and expand the Tools icon. Next click the Site Replication Services icon and then select Directory Replication Connector View from the View menu. Each Exchange 5.5 site's Directory Replication Connector is now displayed under the Site Replication Service.

No Service Account in Exchange Server 2003

Exchange Server 2003 runs under the Local System account. This is a major change from Exchange 5.5, where the Exchange Service account had access to every user's mailbox. The benefit of the new architecture is that the service account was a single point of failure in case of a password change or if the account was deleted. When Exchange Server 2003 systems communicate between servers, they are authenticated by the server's machine account in Active Directory.

When the /domainprep option is run, it creates two groups called Exchange Domain Servers and Exchange Enterprise Servers. During Exchange setup, the Exchange server's machine account is added to a Global Security group called Exchange Domain Servers. The Exchange Domain Servers group is granted permissions on all Exchange objects to allow the Exchange Server 2003 services to access and update Active Directory. The Exchange Enterprise Servers group contains the Exchange Domain Servers groups from all domains in the forest and provides cross-domain access between all Exchange Server 2003 systems.

Recipient Update Service

The Recipient Update Service is responsible for updating address lists and email addresses in Active Directory. Two objects are contained in the Recipient Update Services container by default. The Recipient Update Service is responsible for updating the Enterprise Configuration information in Active Directory, such as Administrative and Routing Group information. The domain specified is responsible for updating the address lists and email addresses configured on objects in the Active Directory domain that the Exchange server resides in. The address list and email addresses are configured under the Recipient Policies and Address List icon, discussed previously in this section.

Understanding Exchange Server 2003 Mailbox-Migration Methods

Two methods exist for moving mailboxes to Exchange Server 2003, and each differs in hardware requirements and the amount of risk and interoperability during and after the migration. The following migration methods for mailboxes are covered in this section:

- Move Mailboxes
- ExMerge

Migrating Using the Move Mailbox Approach

Moving user mailboxes between servers is the safest migration method because the servers' databases are not in jeopardy if the migration fails. Moving the users also provides the opportunity to use new hardware with little or no downtime. In addition, moving users allows the organization to migrate users in sizeable chunks over time. Outlook profiles automatically are updated on the desktop, and users are redirected to the new Exchange Server 2003 systems when they log on. The limitation of moving users to a new server is that they can be moved only to an Exchange Server 2003 system in the same Administrative Group. Moving users can also slow the speed of the migration, which can be seen as a positive or negative, depending on the organization's goals.

The Exchange Server 2003 database is much more efficient than Exchange 5.5 was at storing messages. Even with full copies of all messages created by moving the users, administrators might actually see the database size shrink when comparing the size of the Exchange 5.5 and Exchange Server 2003 databases before and after migration. Quite a bit of empty space in the Exchange 5.5 database might also account for a portion of the reduced database size.

To move user mailboxes, open the Active Directory Users and Computers administrative tool and right-click the user to move; then select Exchange Tasks, as illustrated in Figure 15.8.

1. Click Next at the welcome screen.

2. Choose the option for Move Mailbox and click Next.

3. Select the destination server and mailbox store, and click Next.

4. At the next screen, choose either to create a failure report if corruption is detected or to skip corrupted items and continue the mailbox move. Click Next to continue.

5. At the next prompt, you can specify what time the Move Mailbox command should start and finish by. This is very useful when scheduling mailbox moves for off-hour periods. Click Next to continue.

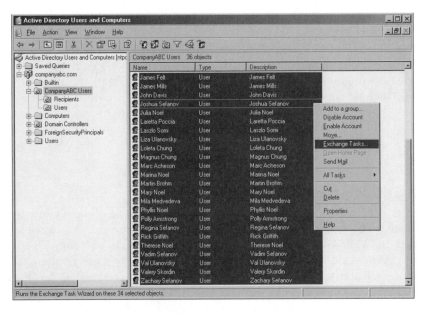

FIGURE 15.8   Selecting mailbox-enabled users to move.

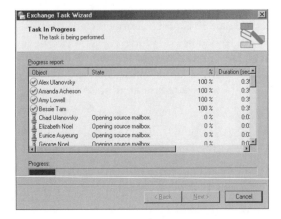

FIGURE 15.9   Moving mailboxes to Exchange Server 2003.

Connections are then made to the source and destination server, and the mailbox contents are moved four at a time, as illustrated in Figure 15.9. If the move is unsuccessful, the user's mailbox still is available on the source Exchange 5.5 server.

Leapfrogging Server Migrations to Reduce Costs

If server hardware or budget is a limiting factor in the project, the organization might want to consider using a leapfrog method (also called the swing upgrade method) to migrate the users to Exchange Server 2003. Using the leapfrog method, fewer servers need to be purchased to perform the migration through the move users method.

One server still needs to be installed into the Exchange 5.5 site to house the SRS. Users can then be moved to that server or a second Exchange Server 2003 system installed into the site. After all users, connectors, and public folders are moved off the Exchange 5.5 server, that server can be formatted and reinstalled as an Exchange Server 2003 system, allowing the next Exchange 5.5 server's users to be migrated to Exchange Server 2003.

This greatly reduces the speed of the migration process and also requires a Native Mode Windows Server 2003 domain to support the public folders if they are scattered across the Exchange 5.5 servers. Another option for public folders in this scenario is to consolidate the public folders by replicating all the folders to a single Exchange 5.5 server in the site if a Native Mode Windows Server 2003 domain is not available. Connectors could also pose a problem with this method and require a solution before starting the leapfrog process.

One problem with this leapfrog method to be aware of is to not remove the first Exchange 5.5 server in a site until it's the last remaining system in that site. The first Exchange server in the site hosts folders and other functions that are required by the Exchange 5.5 organization.

Using ExMerge to Migrate Mailboxes

Exmerge.exe is a Microsoft utility that can extract the contents of a user's mailbox to a personal store (PST) file. The PST file created by ExMerge can be added to a user's Outlook profile so the user can access the contents of his old mailbox. ExMerge can also import the PST file to a destination mailbox to another server, site, or organization. On the destination server, ExMerge can merge the imported PST file or overwrite data in the target mailbox.

ExMerge can be used in disaster recovery and in migration scenarios to move user data from point A to point B by selecting the source and destination Exchange servers. ExMerge can be used when an organization wants to start with a clean Exchange Server 2003 environment and wants to be able to move mailbox contents to the new Exchange Server 2003 mailbox or archive the contents of the Exchange 5.5 mailbox in case a user needs access to his old information. ExMerge can also be used to move mailbox contents in organization-naming hierarchies that are the same or different. This is beneficial to organizations that want to build a new naming context when converting to Active Directory and Exchange Server 2003.

A few issues should be considered when using ExMerge to move mailbox contents to a new organization. The biggest one is that the capability to reply to all recipients on old messages could be lost. At a minimum, end-users need to force the names on old messages to be resolved against the new directory by using Alt+K or the Check Name button on the toolbar. End-users might be confused and frustrated if the new system cannot locate all of the users. This can occur if all users have not been migrated from the old organization or if mail connectivity to foreign mail systems has not been re-established in the new Exchange organization. To avoid these problems, every migrated mailbox must have the X.500 address of the old organization added to it, either manually or via a third-party tool.

The second-biggest issue is that appointments on the user's calendar that contain other attendees are severed. The original appointments were resolved to the attendee's old addresses when they were created. This means that if the user deletes the appointment or makes a change to the time or location of the meeting, the other attendees will not be notified.

Even with these issues, ExMerge can be just the thing organizations are looking for, especially when they have survived multiple mergers and acquisitions and are looking to start over with Exchange Server 2003. If the organization plans to use ExMerge for the entire migration process, spend extensive time prototyping the merge process to catch other issues the organization might encounter.

ExMerge merges the following information:

- User folders
- User messages
- Outlook calendars
- Contacts
- Journal
- Notes
- Tasks
- Folder rules that were created in Exchange 5.0 or later

ExMerge does not support the following:

- Forms
- Views
- Schedule+ data
- Folder rules that were created in Exchange 4.0

ExMerge also supports advanced options such as extracting folder permissions. It can filter the messages for extraction from the source store by attachment name or subject that are accessible under the Options button on the source server selection screen.

ExMerge can be configured in either a one- or a two-step merge process. One-step merge processes copy the data from the source mailbox to a PST and then merge the data into the same mailbox on the destination server. The distinguished name of the mailbox and container path of the source and destination servers must be identical to perform a one-step merge.

When using ExMerge to move mailbox data from different organizations and sites, administrators need to be aware that ExMerge cannot create a mailbox on a destination server or set alternative recipient and forwarding rules on the source server. Another item that administrators should be aware of is that ExMerge runs only on Windows Server 2003. ExMerge needs to be able to access several Exchange Server 2003 DLL files. To run ExMerge, copy the `Exmerge.exe` and `Exmerge.ini` files to the Exchange \bin directory, or update the system path to include the Exchange \bin directory if ExMerge will run from another file location.

To run ExMerge using Exchange 5.5 as the source and Exchange Server 2003 as the destination, the credentials used for ExMerge must have Service Account Administrator privileges in Exchange 5.5 at the Organization, Site, and Configuration container levels. The credentials must also have at least Receive As permission on the destination Exchange 2003 mailbox.

Migrating Exchange 5.5 Public Folders to Exchange Server 2003

Exchange mailboxes on the new Exchange Server 2003 systems must be able to access system and public folders, and subsequently require copies of the information that existed in those folders. Previously, in Exchange 2000, this required a fairly manual process of marking top-level public folders for replication and then propagating those changes down to subfolders. With Exchange Server 2003, however, a utility called pfmigrate automates this functionality. The options for pfmigrate are illustrated in Figure 15.10.

The pfmigrate utility can be used in advance of a migration to make copies of public folders on the new servers; it then can be used later to remove the public folder copies from the old Exchange 5.5 servers.

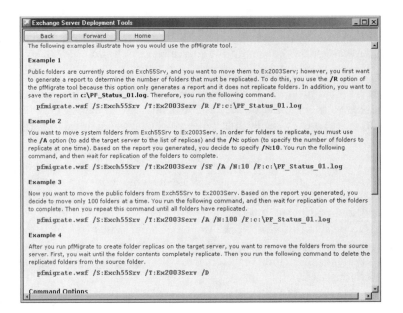

Figure 15.10   PFMigrate options.

Migrating Exchange 5.5 Connectors and Services to Exchange Server 2003

With connectors in general, the best migration path is to build parallel connectors on Exchange Server 2003 systems. This way, the Exchange 5.5 connectors can remain intact and continue to route mail and perform directory synchronization with the foreign mail system.

The benefits of running connectors on both systems are as follows:

- Involves less risk when migrating the connectors

- Enables administrators to view Exchange 5.5 connector configuration when configuring and administering the Exchange Server 2003 connector

- Allows for controlled mail flow testing

- Provides a fallback plan if software defects or configuration issues are encountered with the Exchange Server 2003 connector

While testing the Exchange Server 2003 connectors, configure the Exchange Server 2003 connector with a higher cost and limited address space. This enables administrators to perform controlled tests of mail flow. When the organization is comfortable with the test results, the address space can be configured to match that of the Exchange 5.5 connectors.

Also, the cost parameter on the connector can be dropped below that of the Exchange 5.5 connector, and the Exchange Server 2003 connector can begin routing all mail to the foreign system. The Exchange 5.5 connectors can remain in place until the organization is comfortable shutting them down.

Many Exchange 5.5 connectors also provide directory synchronization with foreign mail systems. Directory synchronization on the Exchange Server 2003 version of the connector should not be enabled until the mail flow through the connector works properly and the organization is ready to use the Exchange Server 2003 connector full-time. Most connectors such as GroupWise and Lotus Notes provide filtering options for directory synchronization. Marking the option Do Not Import Address Entries of This Type and using an asterisk (*) as a wildcard means that no entries will be imported and directory synchronization will remain on the Exchange 5.5 server. Also do not export address entries to the foreign mail system, to avoid duplicate address entries in the foreign mail system's address list.

> **TIP**
>
> Take screenshots of all connector configuration property pages before attempting to migrate any connector. A lost setting such as an address space entry that is not transferred to the Exchange Server 2003 connector can cause a major routing or directory synchronization disaster on both mail platforms.

Migrating the Internet Mail Service

The Internet Mail Service has been replaced by several components in Exchange Server 2003:

- SMTP Connector

- Internet Message Format

- Message Delivery Properties

The Internet Mail Service needs to be replaced by an equivalent SMTP Connector in Exchange Server 2003. After the migration, the new connector must be reconfigured to match the settings of the old IMS.

Migrating Site Connectors

Site Connectors in Exchange v5.5 are replaced by Routing Group Connectors in Exchange Server 2003. Routing Group Connectors that communicate with Exchange 5.5 server communicate over RPC. When Routing Group Connectors communicate between Exchange Server 2003 systems, they communicate over SMTP.

To build parallel connectors to Exchange 5.5 sites, create a Routing Group Connector to the remote Exchange 5.5 site and configure the local bridgehead server as the new Exchange Server 2003 connector server.

Migrating Foreign Mail Connectors

Exchange Server 2003 includes support for the following foreign mail connectors:

- GroupWise Connector
- Lotus Notes Connector
- X.400 Connector

The best strategy to migrating these connectors is to use a parallel connector strategy. The following configuration settings must be reconfigured after an upgrade is in place on the foreign mail connectors:

- Directory synchronization schedule
- Address spaces
- Import container and export container configurations
- Delivery restriction options, such as message size

Always prototype the configuration, mail transfer, and directory synchronization for foreign mail connectors in a lab environment before implementing them in production. Mistakes in foreign mail connector configuration are usually quite costly and require extensive clean-up on both sides of the connection.

Creating Support for Unsupported Connectors

To support unsupported connectors such as the PROFS/SNADS, cc:Mail, and MSMAil connectors, remain in Mixed Mode Exchange Server 2003 and leave an Exchange 5.5 site to handle the unsupported connector. For a long-term solution, consider an SMTP solution for mail transfer and LDAP for directory synchronization. Another solution is to locate a third-party replacement connector.

Completing the Migration to Exchange Server 2003

When all Exchange 5.5 servers are no longer required, the organization can convert to Native Mode Exchange Server 2003. This section covers the steps that need to be accomplished before the conversion to Native Mode can be executed. This section also covers some of the post-migration clean-up processes that need to be run in the Exchange Server 2003 organization. Not all of the clean-up processes need to be run in all environments; this depends on the method the organization used to populate Active Directory.

Converting to Native Mode

Converting to Native Mode provides the organization with the following benefits and flexibility:

- Multiple Routing Groups are supported.

- Routing Groups can contain servers from different Administrative Groups.

- Servers can move between Routing Groups.

- Mailboxes can be moved between Administrative Groups.

- SMTP becomes the default routing protocol.

There are very few reasons to keep an Exchange organization in Mixed Mode after all Exchange 5.5 servers have been removed. You should change your Exchange organization to Native Mode in the following scenarios:

- No more Exchange 5.5 servers exist in the organization.

- No plans exist to add Exchange Server 5.5 servers to the organization in the future—the likelihood for a merger or acquisition is low.

- No need exists for connectors or gateways that run only on Exchange 5.5.

To convert to Native Mode Exchange Server 2003, the following steps must be accomplished in the following order:

1. Delete all Directory Replication Connectors.

2. Delete all Exchange 5.5 servers from each remaining site.

3. Delete the recipient connection agreements and all other connection agreements for each Exchange 5.5 site.

4. Delete the Site Replication Service (SRS) from all Exchange Server 2003 systems.

5. Switch to Native Mode using the Change Mode button on the organization's properties.

Deleting All Directory Replication Connectors

For any remaining Exchange 5.5 site that will not be migrated to Exchange Server 2003, the Directory Replication Connectors must be deleted.

Use the Exchange System Manager to delete all Directory Replication Connectors. To delete the Directory Replication Connectors, click Tools to view Site Replication Service. Click the View menu and select Directory Replication Connector View. Click each Directory Replication Connector and press Delete.

Next force replication to propagate the deletion of the Directory Replication Connectors in the Active Directory Connector Manager by using the Replicate Now option on the connection agreements for the site. Verify the deletion of the Directory Replication Connectors by opening the Exchange System Manager on another Exchange Server 2003 system and viewing the Site Replication Service with the Directory Replication Connector view. When the Directory Replication Connector no longer appears, the deletion has been replicated.

Removing All Exchange 5.5 Servers from the Organization

When all the Exchange 5.5 servers are no longer needed, they should be uninstalled through the Exchange 5.5 setup program. The last server to be uninstalled should be the server that was the first server in the site or that contains the first server in the site components.

After all the servers have been uninstalled, the last server must be deleted manually from the Exchange hierarchy. To delete the server from the hierarchy, use the Exchange 5.5 Administrator program to connect to the Exchange Server 2003 system running the Site Replication Service and locate the list of servers in the site. Click the server to be removed and then click Edit, Delete. A warning appears if the server still contains mailboxes or connectors. Click Yes to continue the deletion. Another warning appears if there are still public folder replicas on the server. Click Yes to continue the deletion.

The next step is to force replication through the ADC for all connection agreements for the site by using the Replicate Now option. Verify that the server has been removed from Active Directory through the ADC before deleting the connection agreements and uninstalling the ADC. The server should no longer appear in the Exchange System Manager.

Removing the ADC

Open the Active Directory Connector Manager and delete all connection agreements. If the connection agreements are not deleted, the membership of distribution groups could be lost.

If the Active Directory Connector is no longer needed and all connection agreements have been removed, uninstall the Active Directory Connector through Control Panel, Add/Remove Programs. Also remember to disable or delete the service account used for the ADC if it's not used for any other services.

Deleting the SRS

The Site Replication Services are the last services to be deleted before the conversion to Native Mode can take place. To delete the Site Replication Service, open the Exchange System Manager and expand the Tools icon. Next expand the Site Replication Services icon, and then right-click each Site Replication Service and click Delete.

Throwing the Native Mode Switch

After the conversion to Native Mode, there is no way to return to mixed mode. The organization should be completely confident about the transition. When all the prerequisite steps have been accomplished, the Change Mode button on the organization properties in the Exchange System Manager should be available. Use the following steps to convert to Native Mode Exchange Server 2003:

1. Open the Exchange System Manager.

2. Right-click the organization and click Properties.

3. Click the General tab, and then click Change Mode under Change Operations Mode. Click Yes to permanently switch the organization's mode to Native Mode.

After the conversion to Exchange Server 2003 Native Mode, Administrative Groups are always displayed in the organization. Administrators have the choice of disabling the display of Routing Groups.

Performing Post-Migration Clean-Up

Depending on the method that was used to populate the Active Directory, the organization might have to use a utility called ADClean that merges duplicate Active Directory accounts created during the migration process to Exchange Server 2003. If the Active Directory Connector was used to populate the Active Directory from the Exchange 5.5 directory before the Windows NT 4.0 domain accounts were migrated to Active Directory, two entries will exist for each user. The two user account entries should be merged through ADClean to complete the migration and clean up Active Directory.

The most efficient method of migrating to Exchange Server 2003 is to migrate the Windows NT 4.0 user accounts to Active Directory before beginning the Exchange Server 2003 migration, either through an in-place upgrade of the Windows NT 4.0 Primary Domain Controller or by using a migration tool such as the Active Directory Migration Tool (ADMT) v2.0 or other third-party tool. This eliminates the need to run the ADClean utility because the ADC will automatically match the Active Directory account to the mailbox, as long as it's specified as the primary Windows NT account for the mailbox. The ADC will then add the attributes for the mailbox to the existing Active Directory user account.

Duplicate accounts in Active Directory can also occur if two ADC recipient connection agreements were created and marked as primary on a particular container. One account displays as disabled with a red x in the user icon and with a –1 appended to the display name. The other account displays normally. ADClean can also be used to merge these accounts. To merge accounts created due to duplicate connection agreements, run ADClean and select the container to search. On the next screen, verify the accounts to merge and then choose the option to begin the merge or export the merge to a file for import through ADClean later.

> **TIP**
>
> The Search Based on Exchange Mailboxes Only option allows ADClean to search for only duplicate accounts created by the ADC.

The ADClean utility is installed during setup in the \exchsrvr\bin directory. ADClean gives administrators the capability to manually select accounts to be merged or run the wizard to search for and suggest accounts to be merged. The merge can be executed immediately or exported to a .csv file to be reviewed by the administrator and then executed later through ADClean.

Summary

Migration from Exchange 5.5 to Exchange 2000 was a wild ride and required a great deal of planning and insight into the migration process to ensure success. Exchange Server 2003 greatly improves upon the migration capabilities, however, with the addition of the Exchange Deployment Tools. Using these tools, in addition to understanding best practices of the underlying procedures taking place, can do much to increase the reliability and success rate of an Exchange migration and more easily lead an Exchange 5.5 environment to the advanced feature set of Exchange Server 2003.

Best Practices

- Utilize the Exchange Deployment Tools for the entire migration process to streamline the deployment and reduce risk.

- Migrate using the Move Mailbox process whenever possible, and resort to the ExMerge process only if migrating between Exchange organizations.

- Install the Active Directory Connector on the first Exchange Server in the Site.

- Switch the AD domain to Native Mode in advance of the ADC setup and Exchange migration, to ensure proper replication of security groups.

- Use the site and server consolidation strategies in Exchange Server 2003 to significantly reduce the number of servers that will need to be supported.

- Rely on the ADC Tools to configure the connection agreements, and modify them only if there is a specific reason to do so.

- Leave an Exchange 5.5 Server in place only if it is needed to support connectors that are unsupported in Exchange Server 2003.

Migrating from Exchange 2000 to Exchange Server 2003

The differences between Exchange 2000 and Exchange Server 2003 are not monumental. In many ways, Exchange Server 2003 is more akin to a major service pack to Exchange 2000 than anything. With this in mind, upgrading an existing Exchange 2000 implementation to Exchange Server 2003 might not be high on many organizations' wish lists. However, the lack of major architectural differences between the two builds of Exchange can actually work to make an upgrade a more tempting prospect. The ease of upgrading from Exchange 2000 can bring the enhanced capabilities of Exchange Server 2003, particularly in the areas of remote connectivity and productivity, closer.

Ease of upgrade aside, due diligence should still be used when planning the deployment. A well-constructed prototype environment can help facilitate a smooth deployment of Exchange Server 2003, test design assumptions, and reduce the risk associated with any migration project. In addition, a migration to Exchange Server 2003 can also serve as a good opportunity to restructure an inefficient or ill-designed Exchange 2000 implementation.

This chapter focuses on best practice approaches to migrating from an existing Exchange 2000 implementation to Exchange Server 2003. Pros and cons of various migration approaches are presented, and sample step-by-step guides are detailed. In addition, special scenarios, such as multi-forest migrations, are discussed and illustrated.

Outlining Migration Options from Exchange 2000 to Exchange Server 2003

The upgrade process from Exchange 2000 to Exchange Server 2003 was sold by Microsoft to be something that even a manager could perform. The idea was that an upgrade could involve simply throwing in an Exchange Server 2003 CD and clicking a few buttons. In many situations, the upgrade process can truly be this simple. Other more complex migrations involve additional thought into the migration process, however, because there are some fundamental security differences between the two products that can affect a migration process.

Among the upgrade scenarios available for Exchange 2000 to 2003 migrations, the field can essentially be narrowed to two major options: migrations using the move mailbox approach, and migrations using the in-place upgrade method. Other migration scenarios typically use a combination of these approaches or involve a significant degree of complexity.

Understanding Exchange Server 2003 Migration Prerequisites

Because Exchange 2000 and Exchange Server 2003 are similar in many ways, there are fewer incompatibilities between them than one might think. A few functions performed by Exchange 2000 cannot be upgraded to Exchange Server 2003, however, and should be called out in advance of a migration. In addition, several prerequisites exist that need to be satisfied before the upgrade takes place.

The following is a list of prerequisites that an Exchange 2000 environment should accomplish before upgrading to Exchange Server 2003:

- **OS and Exchange Level**   Exchange Server 2003 must be installed on either Windows 2000 SP3 or greater, or Windows Server 2003. Exchange 2000 also must be running at Exchange SP3 or greater.

- **Hardware Level**   The minimum requirements for running Exchange Server 2003 are a 133MHz processor, 256MB of RAM, and 500MB of available disk space. That said, a production Exchange Server will run much more efficiently with faster equipment.

- **Applicable Services Installed on Exchange System**   An Exchange Server 2003 System requires that the SMTP, NNTP, and WWW Services be enabled. If running Windows Server 2003, ASP.NET must also be enabled.

- **Exchange Front-end Servers Upgraded First**   If front-end server architecture is deployed on Exchange 2000 servers, the front-end server or servers must be upgraded to Exchange Server 2003 first.

- **DNS and WINS**   DNS and WINS must be properly configured within the environment.

- **AD Requirements**   At least one, and preferably all, domain controllers in each AD site must be running with Windows 2000 SP3 or greater (or Windows Server 2003) to upgrade to deploy Exchange Server 2003 in the forest. In addition, a global catalog server must be located at no more than one AD site away, although preferably in the same site.

Identifying Exchange Server 2003 Migration Incompatibilities

The following services, which run on Exchange 2000, are incompatible and must either be removed or left on a running Exchange 2000 system:

- Exchange Conferencing Server

- Chat and Instant Messenger

- Key Management Server

- Mobile Information Server (MIS)

- cc:Mail and MS Mail connector

Any Exchange 2000 Server that is running these services and is marked for upgrade must remove these services before proceeding. If their functionality is required, a legacy Exchange 2000 Server can be left after the upgrade to run the components required. Mailboxes on Exchange Server 2003 systems will still be able to access their functionality in this scenario.

Understanding Exchange Server 2003 Deployment Enhancements

Many of the changes between Exchange 2000 and Exchange Server 2003 are in the realm of server deployment. The process of deploying Exchange servers has been streamlined and optimized over the process used in Exchange 2000. Unlike most Microsoft applications, the process to deploy Exchange 2000 was not straightforward, and involved a series of command-line setup options and counter-intuitive procedures. Although Exchange Server 2003 greatly improves upon this model, it also can make changes that affect current server functionality. It is important to note the major changes to the Exchange setup process, to more accurately scope an upgrade scenario. The following list is a breakdown of the changes made to the setup process:

- **Deployment Tools**   The CD for Exchange Server 2003 includes a powerful set of deployment tools, which walk an administrator through the process of deploying Exchange Server 2003 under multiple scenarios. The step-by-step technique employed by this utility helps eliminate common mistakes and reduces the risk associated with deploying Exchange.

- **Granular Permissions Improvements**   Exchange Server 2003 handles installation permissions more intelligently, by allowing Exchange Full Administrators at the

16

Admin Group level to install Exchange, and by not overwriting custom permissions each time a new server is set up. In addition, security improvements remove the ability of regular domain users to physically log in to Exchange Servers.

- **Intelligent Setup**   Exchange Server 2003 improves the intelligence of the setup process by monitoring for such common errors as the Exchange Groups having been moved or renamed, and combines the schema extensions necessary for both the ADC and Setup components into a single extension process. In addition, it is no longer required for the setup of an Exchange server to contact the schema master Operations Master (OM) Role.

- **Default Public Folder and Message Size Limits**   Exchange Server 2003 defaults all public folders to a 10MB limit, in addition to defaulting maximum message size to 10MB. Unless a custom setting is already applied in Exchange 2000, upgrading to Exchange Server 2003 will default to these values regardless of whether they are wanted.

- **IIS Secured and Configured**   When upgrading an Exchange 2000/Windows 2000 system to Exchange Server 2003/Windows Server 2003, the functionality of IIS is upgraded and secured. Through this process, however, functionality for other IIS applications might break. Examine IIS functionality in advance of the migration to ensure that the securing process will not affect current functionality.

- **ActiveSync and OMA Components Installed**   Exchange Server 2003 automatically installs the components required to support Outlook Mobile Access (OMA) and Exchange ActiveSync.

Migration Techniques Using the In-Place Upgrade Method

The in-place upgrade method is one of the simplest approaches to migration and can be an important tool if used effectively. In short, the in-place upgrade is composed of two steps: upgrading the Exchange 2000 component to Exchange Server 2003, and then upgrading the operating system from Windows 2000 to Windows Server 2003.

> **NOTE**
>
> Although the operating system upgrade is not technically required, it is desirable to run Exchange Server 2003 on IIS 6.0, which is available only with Windows Server 2003. IIS 6.0 provides a series of security and uptime enhancements for Exchange, and is subsequently highly recommended.

The in-place upgrade method has several advantages to its execution:

- **Design Simplicity**   When the design of the Exchange 2000 environment is already proven to be sound and reliable, the in-place upgrade approach enables a continuation of the elements of that design. The same servers contain the same mailboxes, and the overall design structure remains intact. The need for a long, drawn-out design process is reduced, and the focus shifts to simply scheduling the downtime for the server upgrade.

- **Hardware Reuse**   Existing hardware can be easily reused through the simple upgrade process. Organizations with an investment in current hardware can easily reallocate that hardware to the new environment through the upgrade process and eliminate the need to purchase new hardware.

- **Database Conversion Streamlined**   The in-place upgrade approach simply upgrades the Exchange 2000 databases in place, which is a faster procedure than the move mailbox method.

- **Eliminated Client-Reconfiguration**   By keeping the same servers and server names, non-Outlook clients, such as POP3 and IMAP clients, do not need to be reconfigured to point to a new set of servers. Although Outlook clients automatically reconfigure themselves if mailbox locations change, non-Outlook clients that may access Exchange normally have to be reconfigured to point to the new location. The in-place upgrade process eliminates this.

In general, this approach is useful for organizations with a solid existing Exchange 2000 design, who are simply interested in deploying Exchange Server 2003 for the increased productivity and security improvements. It is extremely useful for "quick and dirty" upgrades and can be successfully used for many organizations.

Understanding Migration Techniques Using the Move Mailbox Method

One of the most flexible, safe, and effective approaches to upgrading is the move mailbox method. This method involves the introduction of new Exchange Server 2003 systems into an existing environment, testing them out and "burning" them in, and then migrating the mailboxes from Exchange 2000 to Exchange Server 2003. After the mailboxes are migrated, the Exchange 2000 servers can be retired.

The flexibility of this approach stems from the following distinct advantages:

- **Simplified Rollback**   By not reformatting or removing the old servers, the rollback procedure is optimized. A simple restore of premigration databases to the old servers can have users back up and running in the event of a problem with the migration.

- **Hardware Replacement**   This approach is useful if the servers that host Exchange 2000 are on older or overused hardware, because the present mailboxes can be easily moved to newer or more robust servers.

- **System Burn-in Time**   By allowing the new servers to be deployed in advance of the migration, they can be preconfigured with all security settings, antivirus configuration, software updates, and other settings. In addition, the hardware itself, such as disk drives and power supplies, can be stress-tested in advance of the production move to the new servers. This helps eliminate the risk associated with moving to new hardware and software.

- **New OS Builds**   By building the Windows Server 2003 and Exchange Server 2003 systems from scratch, legacy issues with software on old systems can be avoided. Although the in-place upgrade procedures have been improving in recent years, it is still good practice to build a system from scratch rather than perform an upgrade.

- **New Database Structure**   Migrations using the move mailbox method create new Exchange databases for the migrated users. This can resolve some lingering database corruption issues and also serves to defragment existing Exchange 2000 databases.

- **Architecture Changes Facilitated**   Organizations that are not happy with their current Exchange 2000 database or server structure can use this technique to restructure their environment. For example, organizations that originally deployed Exchange 2000 Standard Edition and were limited to a single database, can use the move mailbox approach to move their mailboxes to a multidatabase system running with the Enterprise Edition of Exchange Server 2003.

- **Pilot Availability**   By deploying the new servers in advance of the migration, a small subset of users can be migrated in advance to test the functionality of the new system. These users can be members of a pilot group, which enables any bugs to be worked out of the system in advance of the migration.

The move mailbox method also enables a certain degree of flexibility in the execution of the approach. If the old hardware is still robust and is required to be recycled into Exchange Server 2003 servers, a leapfrog approach to the move mailbox process can be used by moving mailboxes from one server to the next, rebuilding the old server with new software, and then moving those mailboxes back. Combinations of this approach can also be used, which increases the flexibility of this option.

Understanding Complex and Combined Approach Migration Techniques

The larger the organization, the more potential for complexity in the existing Exchange 2000 design. Some Exchange deployments make use of multiple separate Exchange organizations running in separate Exchange forests. These types of environments can make use of advanced tools—such as Microsoft Identity Integration Services 2003 (MIIS 2003), InterOrg/PF, and dedicated Exchange forests—to achieve their migration goals.

Organizations may choose to migrate to Exchange Server 2003 using a combined approach, wherein some of the systems that are migrated are upgraded in place and other systems use the move mailbox approach. The strength in each of the two strategies is that they enable the flexibility to be used in conjunction with each other.

In the case of multiple Exchange 2000 organizations, the decision can be made to collapse those organizations and their corresponding AD forests into a single forest, or to synchronize the information between the organizations using MIIS 2003. A third option enables the creation of a dedicated Windows Server 2003 forest and Exchange Server 2003 organization that is used by the various existing forests in the environment. Domain trusts between the domains and the Exchange forest are used to grant rights for users' accounts to access Exchange data, as illustrated in Figure 16.1.

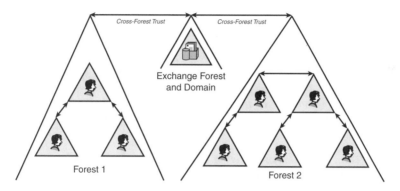

FIGURE 16.1   Dedicated Exchange organization.

Deploying a Prototype Lab for the Exchange Server 2003 Migration Process

Regardless of the method that is chosen to migrate Exchange, care should be taken to test design assumptions as part of a comprehensive prototype lab. A prototype environment can help simulate the conditions that will be experienced as part of the migration process. Establishing a functional prototype environment also can help reduce the risk associated with migrations. In addition to traditional approaches for creating a prototype lab, which involves restoring from backups, several techniques exist to replicate the current production environment to simulate migration.

Creating Temporary Prototype Domain Controllers to Simulate Migration

Construction of a prototype lab to simulate existing Exchange 2000 infrastructure is not particularly complicated, but requires thought in its implementation. Because an exact copy of the Active Directory is required, the most straightforward way of accomplishing this is by building a new domain controller in the production domain and then isolating that domain controller in the lab to create a mirror copy of the existing domain data. DNS and global catalog information should be transferred to the server when in production, to enable continuation of these services in the testing environment.

> **NOTE**
>
> There are several considerations to keep in mind if planning this type of duplication of the production environment. First, when the temporary domain controller is made into a global catalog server, the potential exists for Exchange 2000 to identify it as a working global catalog server and refer clients to it for directory lookups. When the server is brought offline, the clients would experience connectivity issues. For these reasons, it is good practice to create a temporary domain controller during off-hours.

A major caveat to this approach is that the system must be completely separate, with no way to communicate with the production environment. This is especially the case because the domain controllers in the prototype lab respond to requests made to the production domain, authenticating user and computer accounts and replicating information. Prototype domain controllers should never be added back into a production environment. Removing the domain controller from the production network topology can help to ensure that it does not communicate back changes as well.

Seizing Operations Master (OM) Roles in the Lab Environment

1. Because Active Directory is a multimaster directory, any one of the domain controllers can authenticate and replicate information. This factor is what makes it possible to segregate the domain controllers into a prototype environment easily. There are several different procedures that can be used to seize the OM roles. One approach uses the `ntdsutil` utility: Open a Command Prompt by selecting Start, Run and typing **cmd**. Press Enter.

2. Type **ntdsutil** and press Enter.

3. Type **roles** and press Enter.

4. Type **connections** and press Enter.

5. Type **connect to server** *SERVERNAME* (where *SERVERNAME* is the name of the target Windows Server 2003 domain controller that will hold the OM Roles) and press Enter.

6. Type **quit** and press Enter.

7. Type **seize schema master** and press Enter.

8. Click Yes at the prompt asking to confirm the OM change.

9. Type **seize domain naming master** and press Enter.

10. Click Yes at the prompt asking to confirm the OM change.

11. Type **seize pdc** and press Enter.

12. Click OK at the prompt asking to confirm the OM change.

13. Type **seize rid master** and press Enter.

14. Click OK at the prompt asking to confirm the OM change.

15. Type **seize infrastructure master** and press Enter.

16. Click OK at the prompt asking to confirm the OM change.

17. Exit the Command Prompt Window.

After these procedures have been run, the domain controllers in the prototype lab environment will control the OM roles for the forest and domain, which is necessary for additional migration testing.

> **NOTE**
>
> Although the temporary domain controller procedure just described can be very useful toward producing a copy of the AD environment for a prototype lab, it is not the only method that can accomplish this. The AD domain controllers can also be restored via the backup software's restore procedure. A third option—which is often easier to accomplish but is somewhat riskier—is to break the mirror on a production domain controller, take that hard drive into the prototype lab, and install it in an identical server. This procedure requires the production server to lose redundancy for a period of time while the mirror is rebuilt, but is a "quick and dirty" way to make a copy of the production environment.

Restoring the Exchange Environment for Prototype Purposes

After all forest and domain roles have been seized in the lab, the Exchange server or servers must be duplicated in the lab environment. Typically, this involves running a restore of the Exchange server on an equivalent piece of hardware. All of the major backup software implementations contain specific procedures for restoring an Exchange 2000 environment. Using these procedures is the most ideal way of duplicating the environment for the migration testing.

Validating and Documenting Design Decisions and Migration Procedures

The actual migration process in a prototype lab should follow, as closely as possible, any design decisions made regarding an Exchange Server 2003 implementation. It is ideal to document the steps involved in the process so that they can be used during the actual implementation to validate the process. The prototype lab is not only an extremely useful tool for validating the upgrade process, it can also be useful for testing new software and procedures for production servers.

The migration strategy chosen—whether it be an in-place upgrade, a move mailbox method, or another approach—can be effectively tested in the prototype lab at this point. Follow all migration steps as if they were happening in production.

16

Migrating to Exchange Server 2003 Using the In-Place Upgrade Approach

As previously mentioned, the in-place upgrade method is the most straightforward approach toward migration. Existing server architecture and database structure is maintained. In many ways, this type of upgrade simply involves throwing in the Exchange Server 2003 CD and performing the upgrade.

An upgrade to Exchange Server 2003 is a two-step process. The first step involves upgrading the Exchange application component to Exchange Server 2003. The second step involves upgrading the operating system from Windows 2000 to Windows Server 2003. Exchange Server 2003 supports upgrading only Exchange first, because Exchange 2000 cannot function on a Windows Server 2003 operating system. The OS does not *require* upgrading, but it is recommended to do so to take advantage of all the new Exchange Server 2003 features that tie into the new OS.

Making Use of the Exchange Server 2003 Deployment Tools

Microsoft has streamlined its Exchange deployment process by creating a set of deployment tools to assist with the Exchange installation process. With Exchange 2000, Microsoft found that the complexity of the upgrade process created confusion among the uninitiated, and led to some rather serious support calls. The Exchange deployment tools provide step-by-step checklists to ensure that the upgrade process is uneventful.

Using the Exchange Server 2003 Deployment tools is a straightforward process and is the first step toward upgrading an existing Exchange 2000 Server in place. To initiate the upgrade process, perform the following steps:

1. Insert the Exchange Server 2003 CD into the CD Drive.

2. Select Start, Run, and type *X*:**setup.exe** (where *X* is the CD drive).

3. At the welcome screen, click the Exchange Deployment Tools link.

4. Select Deploy the first Exchange 2003 server.

5. Select Upgrade from Exchange 2000 Native Mode.

6. Review and perform the tasks listed under the prerequisites list in Deployment Tools, as illustrated in Figure 16.2.

The prerequisite tasks listed should be performed in any situation, and can help ensure that everything is in place before beginning intrusive tasks, such as upgrading the AD schema. Microsoft included these tasks in the deployment tools to proactively identify potential issues with the Exchange server setup before they become major production incidents.

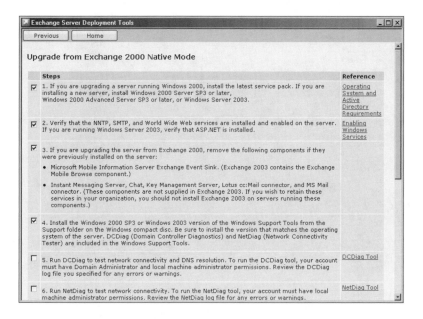

FIGURE 16.2   Exchange setup prerequisites.

Upgrading the Active Directory Schema with Exchange ForestPrep

Exchange Server 2003 requires that the Active Directory schema be modified to support the new enhancements in the product. The schema of Active Directory contains a list of all attributes and objects that can exist in the directory, and is the core framework around which Active Directory operates. It is a critical piece of an enterprise directory, and great care should be taken when examining changes to its structure, such as those enacted during Exchange Server setup. After the initial steps have been followed with the Exchange deployment tools, Exchange ForestPrep can be run on a domain controller in the schema root domain. It can be run manually or from the command line, or it can be invoked from the Exchange deployment tools, as follows:

1. While in Exchange Deployment Tools, ensure that all prerequisite steps have been completed.

2. Click the Run ForestPrep Now link.

3. After waiting for Setup to initialize, click Next at the welcome screen.

4. Select I agree and click Next.

5. Review and ensure that ForestPrep is selected for the Action, as illustrated in Figure 16.3, and click Next.

16

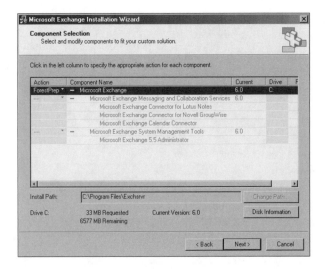

FIGURE 16.3   Exchange ForestPrep.

6. Enter the name of the account that will be used for subsequent installations of Exchange. This account will be granted Exchange Full Administrator rights at the Organization level. Click Next to continue.

7. Click Finish at the final screen for the ForestPrep procedure.

> **NOTE**
>
> The changes made to the AD schema can be viewed via low-level LDAP tools, such as ADSI Edit. This particular tool can be installed as part of the Windows Server 2003 Support Tools pack, which is located on the Windows Server 2003 CD in the `\Support\Tools` directory.

Preparing Each Domain for Exchange Server 2003 with DomainPrep

After the AD schema has been upgraded and the changes have propagated throughout the AD forest, each domain in the forest must be prepared for Exchange Server 2003 via the DomainPrep procedure. Although DomainPrep can be run via the command prompt (`setup /domainprep`), it can also be launched via the deployment tools as follows:

1. On a domain controller in the root domain, restart Deployment Tools and continue from the end of the ForestPrep procedure.

2. Click Run DomainPrep now to start the DomainPrep procedure.

3. Click Next at the welcome screen.

4. Select I agree and click Next.

5. Ensure that DomainPrep is selected under Action and click Next.

6. Click OK to any messages that appear about insecure groups that might exist in the domain. DomainPrep will run, as illustrated in Figure 16.4.

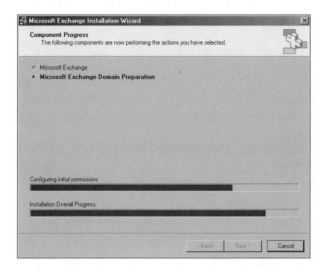

FIGURE 16.4   Exchange DomainPrep.

7. Click Finish when complete.

8. Repeat on a DC in each domain in the AD forest.

> **NOTE**
>
> DomainPrep must be run on each domain in a forest, even though it might have been run during the setup of Exchange 2000, because Exchange Server 2003 DomainPrep performs additional required tasks.

The DomainPrep procedure creates groups necessary for Exchange and sets appropriate permissions for the accounts required. The groups that it creates (Exchange Domain Servers and Exchange Enterprise Servers) must be kept in the default Users container in AD and must not be renamed to ensure functionality.

Running the In-Place Upgrade of an Exchange 2000 System to Exchange Server 2003

After all the prerequisites have been satisfied, ForestPrep has been run and replicated, and DomainPrep has created the appropriate groups and permissions in each domain, the actual upgrade procedure for Exchange Server 2003 can commence. The upgrade process should be run from the server that is to be upgraded, and can be manually initiated or invoked via the Deployment Tools, as follows:

1. Run Exchange Deployment Tools on the Exchange 2000 Server to be upgraded and verify that all tasks up to the DomainPrep have been completed.

2. Click Run Setup Now.

3. Click Next at the welcome screen.

4. Select I agree and click Next.

5. Ensure that Upgrade is listed under Action, as illustrated in Figure 16.5, and click Next.

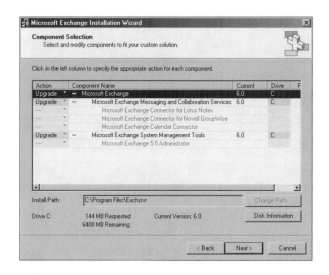

FIGURE 16.5   Exchange upgrade.

6. Review the final settings and click Next; Exchange will update.

7. When the installation is complete, click Finish.

At this point, Exchange is updated from Exchange 2000 to Exchange Server 2003. The new Exchange System Manager tool is installed, and the bulk of Exchange Server 2003 functionality is present for all mailboxes on the server.

Upgrading the Operating System from Windows 2000 to Windows Server 2003

The final piece of the puzzle, which makes an Exchange 2003 system complete, is the upgrade of the base operating system to Windows Server 2003. Certain functionality, especially regarding security, cannot be achieved until the base OS for Exchange Server 2003 is running the new OS. Fortunately, the upgrade from Windows 2000 to Windows Server 2003 is straightforward, and can be accomplished via the following steps:

1. Insert the Windows Server 2003 CD.

2. Run the appropriate `Setup.exe` (Enterprise or Standard Edition).

3. Select Install Windows Server 2003 (Enterprise Edition).

4. Verify the Installation Type to be Upgrade, as illustrated in Figure 16.6, and click Next.

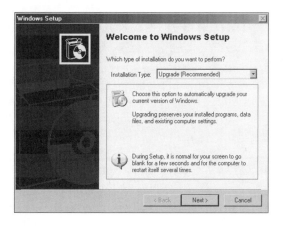

FIGURE 16.6   Upgrading to Windows Server 2003.

5. Select I accept this agreement and click Next.

6. Enter the appropriate License Key and click Next.

7. Select No, skip this step and continue installing Windows, when prompted to download update files.

8. Review any incompatibilities on the next screen and click Next. Setup will start copying files, reboot, and complete the installation.

Upon the successful completion of the steps outlined in this section, an Exchange 2000 system will be upgraded to Exchange Server 2003, using the in-place upgrade method. At this point, any additional servers that have been marked for upgrade can use this procedure.

16

Upgrading Additional Exchange 2000 Servers to Exchange Server 2003

Each additional server that is running Exchange 2000 can be upgraded using the same technique described in the previous sections. The prerequisite steps, ForestPrep and DomainPrep do not need to be repeated for each additional server, however. Unlike with Exchange 5.5, there is no functional difference between an all–Exchange 2003 or mixed Exchange 2000/2003 environment, so there is no Exchange Server 2003 Native Mode. Most of the differences will be noticeable at the client level, however, in the form of improvements to the client experience, such as OMA, ActiveSync, RPC over HTTP, and improved security.

Migrating to Exchange Server 2003 Using the Move Mailbox Method

As previously mentioned, the move mailbox method of migration can be ideal for organizations who require a new set of hardware for their Exchange servers or who desire to reconstruct some portions of their Exchange infrastructure. The move mailbox method is also an effective way of minimizing the risk associated with a migration to Exchange Server 2003.

Deploying Exchange 2003 Servers in Advance of the Move Mailbox Migration

The greatest advantage to the move mailbox approach lies in the ability to deploy a new system to function as an Exchange 2003 Server. The server can be set up and configured with all applicable settings and third-party utilities before a single mailbox is moved to it.

Just as the in-place upgrade process (described earlier) required AD to be upgraded, the move mailbox approach has the same requirements. This process involves running the ForestPrep and DomainPrep options before the first server is deployed. After these prerequisites are satisfied, the setup of the server can begin:

1. Insert the Exchange Server 2003 CD into the CD Drive.

2. Select Start, Run, and type **D:\setup.exe** (where **D** is the CD drive).

3. At the welcome screen, click the Exchange Deployment Tools link.

4. Select Deploy the first Exchange 2003 server, as illustrated in Figure 16.7.

5. Select Upgrade from Exchange 2000 Native Mode.

6. Review and check off the prerequisites list in the Deployment Tools.

7. Click the Run ForestPrep Now link.

8. After waiting for Setup to initialize, click Next at the welcome screen.

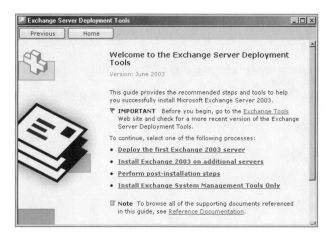

FIGURE 16.7   Using the Exchange Server Deployment Tools.

9. Select I agree and click Next.

10. Review and ensure that ForestPrep is selected for the Action and click Next.

11. Enter the name of the account that will be used for subsequent installations of Exchange, as illustrated in Figure 16.8, and click Next.

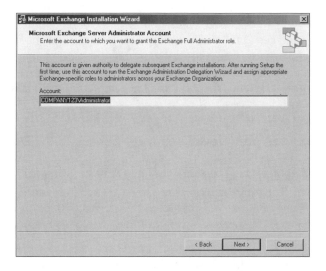

FIGURE 16.8   Selecting the Exchange Administrator during ForestPrep.

12. Click Finish at the final screen for the ForestPrep procedure.

13. Click Run DomainPrep now to start the DomainPrep procedure.

14. Click Next at the welcome screen.

15. Select I agree and click Next.

16. Ensure that DomainPrep is selected under Action and click Next.

17. Click OK to any messages that appear about insecure groups that might exist in the domain.

18. Click Finish when complete.

19. Click Run Setup Now from the Deployment Tools.

20. Click Next at the welcome screen.

21. Select I agree and click Next.

22. Ensure that Typical is listed under Action and click Next.

23. Review the final settings and click Next; Exchange will update.

24. When the installation is complete, click Finish.

All these steps are necessary to install the first Exchange Server 2003 system into an existing Exchange 2000 environment. Subsequent Exchange 2003 systems can also be set up at this point, via the post–DomainPrep procedures outlined earlier.

Enabling New Server "Burn-In" and Pilot Testing

One of the main advantages to the move mailbox approach is that the new systems can now be "burnt in" and tested without affecting production users. A small subset of mailboxes can also be migrated to the new system to test functionality and ensure compatibility with an organization's systems. After the pilot is complete, a full mailbox migration can then take place with less overall risk.

Moving Mailboxes to the New Exchange Server 2003 Databases

After all Exchange Server 2003 systems have been deployed and their configurations finalized, the actual migration process of moving mailboxes from Exchange 2000 to Exchange Server 2003 can begin. The move mailbox procedure in Exchange Server 2003 has been vastly improved over the one that was present in Exchange 2000. Features such as error detection, multiple migration streams, and scheduling enable a much-improved experience.

The move mailbox procedure should be scheduled to run during off-hours, because it effectively takes a user's mailbox out of service during the move operation. The mailbox is out of service for only the duration of the move, and is available again after the process is complete for that mailbox. Migration time varies, depending on network connectivity and hardware speed, but about 2GB/hr can be expected during the move operation.

To move mailboxes from an Exchange 2000 Server to one of the new Exchange 2003 systems previously set up, perform the following tasks:

1. From the new Exchange 2003 Server, select Start, All Programs, Microsoft Exchange, Active Directory Users and Computers.

2. Select the Mailbox-Enabled Users who are to be migrated. Right-click on them and choose Exchange Tasks.

3. At the welcome page, click Next.

4. Select Move Mailbox and click Next.

5. Select the Server and Information Store to move the mailboxes to and click Next.

6. Select Skip corrupted items and create a failure report, as illustrated in Figure 16.9, and click Next.

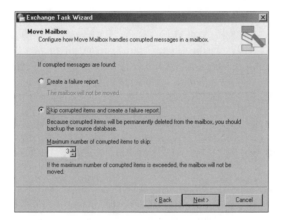

FIGURE 16.9   Move Mailbox corrupt item options.

7. Choose the time to begin migrating and the time to stop migrating and click Next. The wizard will begin moving mailboxes, four at a time, as illustrated in Figure 16.10.

8. Upon completion of the migration process, the migration dialog box will indicate the success or failure of each mailbox migrated, which can be reviewed.

After a mailbox is migrated, a user can then access it via Outlook or other clients. The Outlook client automatically detects the change in Exchange Home Server and updates itself, connecting to the new mailbox automatically. Other functionality—such as OWA for Exchange Server 2003 and ActiveSync with Pocet PC devices—also becomes available after the move and once Exchange is properly configured.

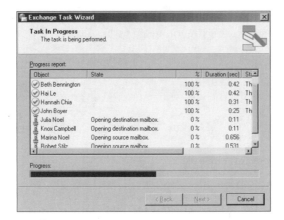

FIGURE 16.10   Moving mailboxes.

Replicating Public Folders from Exchange 2000 to Exchange Server 2003

Just as the mailboxes are migrated from one set of Exchange 2000 servers to another set of Exchange Server 2003 systems, the public folders should be replicated before retiring the old Exchange 2000 servers. Previously, this procedure involved a manual replication of folder hierarchy, which could prove to be a tedious process. Microsoft addressed this drawback with a new utility called PFMigrate, which is accessible via the Exchange Deployment Tools. PFMigrate can create public and system folder replicas on new systems, and remove them from old servers. The following procedure outlines how to use PFMigrate to migrate from an Exchange 2000 Server to an Exchange Server 2003 system:

1. Open a Command Prompt (select Start, Run; type **cmd**; and press Enter).

2. Type **cd D:\support\Exdeploy** and press Enter.

3. To create a report of current public folder replication, type the following:

    pfmigrate.wsf /S:*OLDSERVERNAME* **/T:***NEWSERVERNAME* **/R /F:c:\LOGNAME.log**

    This generates a report named LOGNAME.log on the C: drive. *OLDSERVERNAME* should be the name of the Exchange 2000 system, and *NEWSERVERNAME* should be the new Exchange Server 2003 system.

4. To replicate System Folders from the Exchange 2000 server to the Exchange 2003 server, type the following:

pfmigrate.wsf /S:*OLDSERVERNAME* /T:*NEWSERVERNAME* /SF /A /N:100
/F:c:\\LOGNAME.log

5. To replicate Public Folders from Exchange 2000 to Exchange Server 2003, type the following:

pfmigrate.wsf /S:*OLDSERVERNAME* /T:*NEWSERVERNAME* /A /N:100 /F:c:\\LOGNAME.log

6. After all public folders have replicated, the old replicas can be removed from the Exchange 2000 Servers by typing the following, as illustrated in Figure 16.11:

pfmigrate.wsf /S:*OLDSERVERNAME* /T:*NEWSERVERNAME* /D

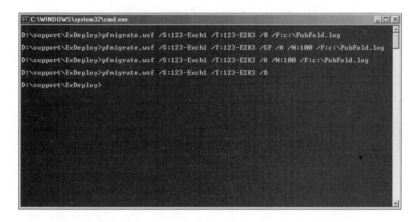

FIGURE 16.11   Command-line PFMigrate functionality.

7. The LOGNAME.log file can be reviewed to ensure that replication has occurred successfully and that a copy of each public folder exists on the new server. A sample log from this procedure is illustrated in Figure 16.12.

TIP

Become familiar with the command-line options that are available with the PFMigrate tool, because they can be useful for managing the replication of public folders across a newly deployed Exchange Server 2003 environment.

16

Moving Connectors from Exchange 2000 to Exchange Server 2003

If the eventual goal of the migration process involves retiring the Exchange 2000 infrastructure, it will be necessary to move all connectors from the Exchange 2000 servers to the new Exchange 2003 systems. The most important consideration when moving connectors is to ensure that no messages that use or flow through the connectors are lost.

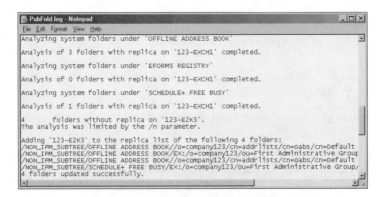

FIGURE 16.12   Sample PFMigrate log file.

In some cases, Exchange 2000 might have been deployed with specific SMTP connectors to provide outgoing mail flow through specific servers. These types of connectors should be rerouted to pass through Exchange 2003 systems and ensure the proper flow of outgoing mail.

As previously mentioned, there are some Exchange 2000 components that are not supported in Exchange Server 2003. This includes two connectors: the MS Mail connector and the cc:Mail connector. If these connectors are in use, an Exchange 2000 server must be left in the organization to support them, because they cannot be migrated over to Exchange 2003 Servers.

Changing the Recipient Update Service Server from Exchange 2000 to Exchange Server 2003

Before Exchange 2000 can be retired, an Exchange Server 2003 system must be designated as the Recipient Update Service (RUS) Exchange Server for the organization and for each domain. To do this, perform the following:

1. On the Exchange Server 2003 System, open Exchange System Manager (select Start, All Programs, Microsoft Exchange, System Manager).

2. Navigate to Recipients, Recipient Update Service.

3. Right-click Recipient Update Service (Enterprise Configuration) and choose Properties.

4. Under Exchange Server, click Browse.

5. Type the name of the Exchange 2003 Server that will become the RUS System and click OK.

6. Click OK when the new server is listed, as illustrated in Figure 16.13.

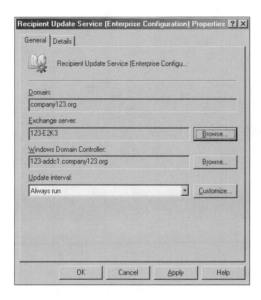

FIGURE 16.13   Changing RUS server settings.

7. Repeat for all domain Recipient Update Service settings.

Retiring Legacy Exchange 2000 Servers

After all mailboxes, public folder replicas, and connectors have been moved off the old Exchange 2000 infrastructure, the old Exchange servers can be retired and removed from service. The easiest and most straightforward approach to this is to uninstall the Exchange 2000 component via the Add-Remove Programs applet in Windows. To perform this operation, do the following:

1. On the Exchange 2000 Server, select Start, Settings, Control Panel.

2. Double-click Add/Remove Programs.

3. Select Microsoft Exchange 2000 and click Change/Remove.

4. Click Next at the welcome screen.

5. Under Action, select Remove from the drop-down box, as illustrated in Figure 16.14, and click Next to continue.

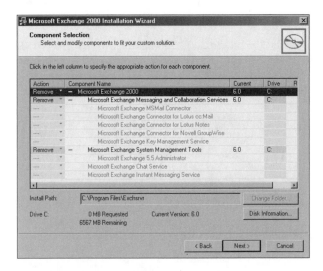

FIGURE 16.14   Removing an Exchange 2000 Server.

6. At the summary screen, click Next to continue. Exchange 2000 will then be uninstalled.

7. Repeat the process for any additional Exchange 2000 Servers.

Upon removal of the last Exchange 2000 system, the environment will then be completely upgraded to Exchange Server 2003, with all mailboxes, public folders, and connectors moved to the new environment.

> **NOTE**
>
> It might be wise to keep old Exchange 2000 Servers around for a few weeks after a move mailbox migration, because the old servers will be required to direct clients to their new mailbox locations. After all Outlook clients have connected to their new mailboxes, the old servers can then be safely retired.

Summary

A migration from Exchange 2000 to Exchange Server 2003 is more of an upgrade than an actual migration. The similarities between the two systems make it not as critical or desirable to migrate in many situations. On the other hand, these same similarities also make it very straightforward to migrate and take advantage of advanced Exchange Server 2003 functionality. With proper diligence, the techniques described in this chapter can be used to migrate an existing Exchange 2000 infrastructure to Exchange Server 2003 to realize this functionality.

Best Practices

The following are best practices from this chapter:

- Use the in-place upgrade procedure for "quick and dirty" upgrades or when server equipment is newer.

- Use the move mailbox procedure when deploying new server hardware or changing basic server architecture, or for risk-averse migrations.

- Create a prototype lab to test the migration process and validate design assumptions.

- Keep an Exchange 2000 Server in place to support legacy tools—such as Conferencing Server, KMS, Chat, and Instant Messenger Server—and other non-supported functionality if it is required in the migrated environment.

- Leave legacy Exchange 2000 Servers in place for a few weeks following a move mailbox migration to ensure that all clients are redirected to their new mailbox locations.

- Consider the use of advanced tools—such as MIIS 2003, InterOrg/PF, and dedicated Exchange forests—for complex situations involving multiple Exchange organizations.

- When using the move mailbox approach, allow time between the deployment of the new servers and the migration to enable the new servers to "burn in." This is also an ideal time to migrate a pilot set of users.

- Use the Exchange Deployment Tools to help minimize any issues associated with the migration process.

16

CHAPTER 17

Compatibility Testing for Exchange Server 2003

At this point in the book, the new features of Exchange Server 2003 have been presented and discussed in depth, as have the essential design considerations and migration processes. The goal of this chapter is to examine the process of testing the actual applications that rely on the Exchange Server infrastructure.

This chapter provides insight into the steps to take in gathering the information needed before the testing process, how to actually test the applications and document the results, and how to determine whether a more extensive prototype testing process is needed. It is vital to go through this process, rather than simply winging it to ensure the success of the project and avoid a displeased user community. The application testing process is intended as a quick way to validate the compatibility and functionality of the proposed end-state for the upgrade.

Currently many companies are seeking to "right-size" their network environment, and might be using the upgrade as a chance to actually reduce the number of servers that handle Exchange processes on the network. At the end of the process, fewer servers will handle the same tasks as before, and new functionality might have been added, making the configurations of the individual servers that much more complex, and making it even more important to thoroughly test the mission-critical messaging applications on the server. For example, with the improved ability of Exchange Server 2003 to manage databases and support more RAM, combined with Windows Server 2003's enhanced fault tolerance features, one Exchange Server 2003 might replace a handful of Exchange 5.5 servers. Thus it's even more important that this configuration be tested to ensure that the performance meets user expectations and that the features that are used every day by the employees to share knowledge and collaborate are in place.

The results of the application compatibility testing process will validate the goals of the project or reveal goals that need to be modified due to application incompatibility or instability. If one key application simply won't work reliably on Exchange Server 2003, an Exchange 5.5 Server might need to be kept as part of the messaging environment, which changes the overall design. As discussed in Part II of this book, "Microsoft Exchange Server 2003 Messaging," there is a variety of different combinations of Exchange server software that can be combined in the end configuration, so the chances are good that there will be a way to keep the troublesome applications working in the new environment.

The Importance of Compatibility Testing

The process presented in this chapter is an essential step to take in validating the design for the end-state of the migration or upgrade. The size of the organization and the breadth and scope of the upgrade are important factors to consider in determining the level of testing needed, and whether a full prototype should be conducted.

The differences between a prototype phase and an application testing phase can be dramatic or negligible based on the nature of the upgrade. A prototype phase replicates the end-state as completely as possible, often using the same hardware in the test lab that will be used in the production rollout.

> **CAUTION**
>
> Application testing can be performed on different hardware with different configurations than the end-state, but be aware that the more differences there are between the testing environment and the actual upgraded environment, the more risk for unexpected results there will be. Essentially you can do an application testing phase without a complete prototype phase, but you shouldn't do a prototype phase without a thorough application testing process.

Most network users don't know or care which server or how many servers perform which task or house which application, but they will be unhappy if the application that allows them to synchronize their Pocket PC, BlackBerry, or Palm device no longer works. If the ability to fax from the desktop suddenly disappears, instant messaging vanishes, or they can't access email from an Internet café, the Exchange administrator can expect emails with a lot of capital letters in them. Many companies have integrated voicemail with Exchange so that users simply click on a voicemail to listen to it, and changes to this functionality can harm the business processes of the company. New antispam software can inadvertently block messages from key customers, if they contain a word such as sale or act now.

If the organization already has Active Directory in place and is on Exchange 2000 Server, the risk of application incompatibility is likely to be less than if the organization is moving from an older operating system, such as NT 4 Server, or a competing operating system, such as Novell NetWare. The upgrade from Exchange 2000 might well use the existing server hardware and perform in-place upgrades, or in the case of an upgrade from Exchange 5.5, it may involve implementing entirely new server hardware and new server fault tolerance features, which further change the operating environment. If this is the case, a full prototype phase may not be needed, but applications testing should still take place.

Preparing for Compatibility Testing

Although the amount of preparation needed will vary based on a number of factors, certain steps should be followed in any organization: The scope of the testing should be identified (what's in and what's out), the goals of the testing process should be clarified, and the process should be mapped out.

A significant advantage of following a phased design methodology, as presented in Chapter 2, "Planning, Prototyping, Migrating, and Deploying Exchange Server 2003 Best Practices," is in the planning discussions that take place and in the resulting Statement of Work and Design and Migration documents that are created as deliverables. Often, companies contract messaging experts, who help companies avoid classic mistakes, to assist in the process. By the end of this planning process, it will be very clear why the project is happening, which departments need which features and capabilities, and what budget is available to perform the work. The timeline and key milestones also will be defined.

If a phased discovery and design process hasn't been followed, this information needs to be gathered to ensure that the testing process addresses the goals of the project stakeholders and that the right applications are in fact tested and verified by the appropriate people.

Determining the Scope for Application Testing

At this point in the process, a list should be put together that clarifies which Exchange Server 2003 version is to be used, which version of server software will be used, which add-in features are required, and which third-party applications are needed. As discussed previously, Exchange Server 2003 can be installed on either Windows 2000 Server or Windows Server 2003, and on the Standard or Enterprise versions of the NOS. Smaller companies might choose to use the Standard versions of Windows Server 2003 and Exchange Server 2003, while larger organizations might require the Enterprise versions of each.

A key issue to discuss at this point is whether it is acceptable to have multiple versions of the Windows Server operating system and of Exchange Server in the final solution. Some organizations want to control costs of both software and support services and require a single NOS and single version of Exchange Server. These organizations would rather choose a different messaging application than keep an older application in place that isn't compatible with the newest NOS and version of Exchange.

Besides the core Exchange Server 2003 software, additional components can be installed that extend the functionality of the software, such as Outlook Mobile Access (OMA), Mobile Information Server (MIS), or Live Communications Server (LCS).

> **NOTE**
>
> Although the Standard Edition of Exchange Server 2003 is significantly cheaper than the Enterprise Edition of the license, cost should not be the primary reason for choosing one version over another. It is not as simple to upgrade from the Standard to Enterprise Edition as just changing a software license key. It typically requires setting up a brand new server with the Exchange 2003 Enterprise Edition (on top of Windows Server 2003 Enterprise Edition) and migrating mailboxes from server to server. An organization should seriously consider whether it needs the functionality of the Enterprise Edition before choosing to buy and install the Standard Edition to upgrade easily later.

Third-party applications should be identified as well. The applications most often used include tape backup software modules or agents, antivirus software, fax software, and voicemail integration products. Additional third-party add-on products may include

- Administration
- Antispam
- Backup and storage
- Collaboration
- Customer Relationship Management (CRM)
- Content checking
- Disclaimers
- Email antivirus
- Fax connectors
- List server software
- Log monitoring
- Migration
- POP 3 downloaders
- Reporting
- Security and encryption
- SMS and paging

The hardware to be used should be listed as well, to ensure that it is available when needed. Ideally the exact hardware to be used in the upgrade will be ordered for the application testing process, but if that is not possible, hardware with specifications similar to that of the servers that will eventually be used should be allocated. Although processor speed and amount of RAM will most likely not make a difference to whether the application functions properly on the server platform, certain hardware devices should be as similar as possible. Tape drives, for example, should have the same features as the ones to be used in the production environment, since this is one of the most critical components. If an autoloader will be used in the production environment, one should be made available for the application testing process. If faxing from the Outlook in-box is required, the same faxing hardware should be allocated as well.

Some applications require clients to be present for the testing process, so at least one workstation class system should be available for this purpose. Connectivity to the Internet may also be needed for testing the functionality of remote access products and antivirus software.

A sample checklist of requirements for summarizing the scope of the application testing phase is shown in Table 17.1.

TABLE 17.1   Checklist for Application Testing

Server #1	Details (include version #s)
Server specs required:	
Processor	
RAM	
Hard drive configuration	
Other	
Network OS and service packs:	
Exchange version and service packs:	
Tape backup software version and agents:	
Antivirus software and related modules:	
Additional third-party apps required:	
Additional hardware required:	
SAN device	
Tape drive	
UPS	
Switch/hub	
Other	
Internet access required?	Yes / No

This process should not take a great deal of time if previous planning has taken place. If the planning phase was skipped, some brainstorming will be required to ensure that the scope includes all of the key ingredients required for the application testing. The goals for the application testing process will also affect the scope, which is covered in the following section.

Defining the Goals for Compatibility Testing

As with the previous step of defining the scope of the testing process, defining the goals might be a very quick process, or might require some discussions with the stakeholders involved in the project.

One useful way of looking at the goals for the project is to treat them as the checklist for successful completion of the testing. What conditions need to be met for the organization to confidently move forward with the next step in the Exchange upgrade? The next step might be a more complete prototype testing phase, or for smaller organizations it might be a pilot rollout, where the new messaging environment is offered to a select group of savvy users.

These goals are separate from the business goals the company may have, such as "more reliable messaging infrastructure," or "improved feature set of email client." A more complete prototype phase could seek to address these goals, while the application testing process stays focused on the performance of the specific combinations of operating system, Exchange Server 2003, and imbedded and connected applications.

A convenient way to differentiate the goals of the project is to split them into key areas, as described in the following sections.

Time Frame for Testing

This goal can be defined with the statement "The testing must be completed in X days/weeks."

If there is very little time available to perform the testing, this limits how much time can be spent on each application and how many end-users can put each through its paces. It also necessitates a lesser degree of documentation. Remember to include time for researching the applications' compatibility with the vendors as part of the timeline. A quick project plan might be useful in this process as a way of verifying the assumptions and selling the timeline to the decision-makers.

Estimating the Duration of the Application Testing Process

A good rule of thumb is to allow four hours per application for basic testing, and eight hours for a more thorough testing process. This allows time for the initial research with the vendors, configuration of the NOS and Exchange Server 2003 software, and testing of the applications. Of course the total time required will vary based on the types of applications to be tested.

For example, a Windows Server 2003 system with Exchange Server 2003, tape backup software, antivirus software, fax software, and voicemail connectivity (six total applications) would take an estimated three days to test for basic compatibility and functionality and six days for more rigorous testing.

If another system configuration is to be tested in the same lab—which has Windows 2000 Server SP3, tape backup software, antivirus software, fax software, and voicemail connectivity—allocate the same amount of time even though only one component is different: three to six days. Note that if more than one resource is available to perform the testing, these configurations can be tested in parallel, shortening the *duration* of the process, but not the *work effort*.

It's always better to have some extra time during the testing phase. This time can be used for more extensive user testing, training, or documentation.

Contingency time should ideally be built in to this goal. Resources assigned to the testing can get sick, or applications might require additional testing when problems are encountered. Vendors might not provide trial versions of the software as quickly as desired, or new versions of software or even the hardware itself can be delayed. With many companies seeking to consolidate the number of servers in use, it is not uncommon to see labs evolve through the testing process. Different versions of the Windows operating system are used, as are different versions of the Exchange Server 2003 software.

Budget for the Testing

This goal can be defined with the statement "The testing must be completed within a budget of $X."

Of course, there might be no budget allocated for testing, but it's better to know this as soon as possible. A lack of budget means that no new hardware can be ordered, that evaluation copies of the software (both Microsoft and the third-party applications) need to be used, and that no external resources will be brought in. If budget is available or can be accessed in advance of the production upgrade, a subset of the production hardware should be ordered for this phase. Testing on the exact hardware that will be used in the actual upgrade, rather than a cast-off server will yield more valuable results.

Resources to Be Used

This goal can be defined with the statement "The testing will be completed by in-house resources and/or external consultants."

Often, the internal Exchange Admin staff is too busy with daily tasks or tackling emergencies that spring up (which might be the reason for the upgrade in the first place), and staff personnel should not be expected to dedicate 100% of their time to the testing process.

If an outside consulting firm with expertise in Exchange Server 2003 is going to be used in the testing process, it can be a good leverage point to have already created and decided upon an internal budget for the testing process. This cuts down on the time it takes to debate the approaches from competing firms.

Extent of the Testing

The extent of compatibility testing can be defined with the statement "Each application will be tested for basic, mid-level, or complete compatibility and feature sets."

This goal might be different for different types of applications—for example, mission-critical applications need extensive testing, whereas less critical applications might have more basic testing performed. A short timeframe with a tightly limited budget won't allow extensive testing, so basic compatibility will most likely be the goal.

Defining the Different Levels of Compatibility Testing

Basic compatibility testing, as used in this chapter, essentially means that the mission-critical applications are tested to verify that they load without errors and perform their primary functions properly with Exchange Server 2003. Often the goal with basic testing is to simply see if the application works, without spending a lot of time or money on hardware and resources, and with a minimum amount of documentation and training. Note that this level of testing reduces but does not eliminate the risks involved in the production roll-out.

Mid-level testing is defined as a process whereby Exchange Server 2003 is configured with *all* of the applications that will be present in the eventual implementation, so that the test configuration matches the production configuration as closely as possible to reduce the chance of surprise behavior during the rollout. This level of testing requires more preparation to understand the configuration and more involvement from testing resources, and should include end-users. Some training should take place during the process, and documentation is created to record the server configurations and details of the testing process. Although this level of testing greatly reduces the risks of problems during the production migration or upgrade, the migration process of moving data between servers and training the resources on this process hasn't been covered, so some uncertainty still exists.

Complete testing adds additional resource training and possibly end-user training during the process, and should include testing of the actual migration process. Complete training requires more documentation to record the processes required to build or image servers and perform the migration steps. Complete testing is what is typically defined as a prototype phase.

Training Requirements During Testing

This goal can be defined with the statement "Company IT resources will/will not receive training during the application testing process."

Although the IT resources performing the testing will learn a great deal by going through the testing process, the organization might want to provide additional training to these individuals, especially if new functionality and applications are being tested. If external consultants are brought in, it is important that the organization's own resources are still involved in the testing process, for training and validation purposes. The application testing phase might be an excellent time to have helpdesk personnel or departmental managers in the user community learn more about new features that will soon be offered so they can help support the user community and generate excitement for the project.

Documentation Required

This goal can be defined with the statement "Documentation will/will not be generated to summarize the process and results."

Again, the budget and timeline for the testing will affect the answer to this question. Many organizations require a paper trail for all testing procedures, especially when the Exchange infrastructure will have an impact on the viability of the business itself. For other organizations, the messaging environment is not as critical, and less or no documentation may be required.

The application testing phase is a great opportunity to document the steps required for application installations or upgrades if time permits, and this level of instruction can greatly facilitate the production rollout of the upgraded messaging components.

Extent of User Community Involvement

This goal can be defined with the statement "End-users will be included/not included in the testing process."

If there are applications such as Customer Relationship Management (CRM), document routing, voicemail or paging add-ons, or connectivity to PDAs and mobile devices, a higher level of user testing (at least from the power users and Executives) should be considered.

Fate of the Testing Lab

This goal can be defined with the statement "The application testing lab will/will not remain in place after the testing is complete."

There are a number of reasons that organizations decide to keep labs in place after their primary purpose has been served. Whenever a patch or upgrade to Exchange Server 2003 or to a third-party application integrates with Windows Server 2003, it is advisable to test it in a nonproduction environment. Even seemingly innocent patches to antivirus products can crash a production Exchange Server. Other updates might require user testing to see whether they should be rolled out to the production servers. Databases can also be taken offline and copied to the lab for grooming and maintenance. So although this might seem like a trivial question, it is important to clarify at this stage.

Documenting the Compatibility Testing Plan

The information discussed and gathered through the previous exercises needs to be gathered and distributed to the stakeholders to assure that the members of the team are working toward the same goals. These components are the scope and the goals of the application testing process, and should include timeline, budget, extent of the testing (basic, mid-level, complete), training requirements, documentation requirements, and fate of the testing lab. This step is even more important if a formal discovery and design phase was not completed.

17

By taking the time to document these constraints the testing process will be more structured and less likely to miss a key step or get bogged down on one application. The individuals performing the testing will essentially have a checklist of the exact testing process so are less likely to spend an inordinate amount of time on one application, or "get creative" and try products that are not within the scope of work. Once the testing is complete the stakeholders will also have made it clear what is expected in terms of documentation so the results of the testing can be presented and reviewed efficiently.

This summary document should be presented to the stakeholders of the project for review and approval; then the organization will be ready to proceed with the research and testing process for Exchange Server 2003 compatibility.

Researching Products and Applications

Armed with a detailed list of the applications that will be tested, the application testing team can begin contacting the vendors of the products and validate whether the vendor certifies its product(s) to be compatible.

An inventory of the Exchange-related applications should be created, and this spreadsheet can then be expanded as compatibility information is gathered; if designed properly, it can be used throughout the testing process.

Creating an Inventory of the Messaging Applications

It is usually fairly obvious which applications are installed on the Exchange Server or connect to it and are considered to be part of the messaging infrastructure. If an application uses Exchange Server resources or is installed on an Exchange Server, it should be tested in the application testing phase. If a different messaging system is in place, it is more likely that the exact applications in use will require more significant upgrades or equivalent products will need to be identified.

As illustrated in Table 17.2, a spreadsheet can easily be created that lists the messaging servers currently in place and the software applications installed on each.

TABLE 17.2   Server Inventory List

Server Name	Server OS, SP#, Role	Messaging OS (w SPs)	Software Installed (w version #)
CAEX1	Windows 2000 Server SP3	Exchange 2000 Enterprise, SP3	Veritas BackUp Exec v.x Veritas Exchange Agent v.x Trend AntiVirus v.x RIM BlackBerry v.x
CAEX2	Windows 2000 Server SP3	Exchange 2000 Conferencing Server, SP3	Veritas BackUp Exec v.x

The key items that should be recorded are the names of the server, the versions of the operating system and messaging server software installed, the role of the device, and the names, manufacturers and versions of add-on software products.

Care should be taken to identify *all* applications running on each messaging server, including tape software, antivirus software, and network monitoring and management utilities, which are in addition to the more obvious database, email messaging, document routing, or other business applications.

If Microsoft Systems Management Server (SMS) or a similar management product capable of generating an inventory list of installed applications (along with hardware capabilities) is in use, it saves time by automatically detecting the software applications installed.

Prioritizing the Applications on the List

When the list is completed, it's a good idea to assign priorities to the applications. Departmental managers should be consulted for their opinions on which applications are essential and enable their users to perform their work on a day-to-day basis. Often there may be applications in place that are rarely used, and can be removed from the new environment.

Prioritization can occur based on the criticality of the application. Three basic levels, which are self-explanatory are critical, near-critical, and nice to have. After this first level of categorization has taken place, a rough order of installation can be assigned. This order may change based on the results of the application testing.

This additional set of information is helpful during the testing process because applications that are listed as nice-to-haves and are at the bottom of the list can be passed over if time and budget constraints are too tight, or if the application or utility proves problematic. Certain utilities should be considered critical, such as tape backup software and Exchange agents, antivirus software, and—in zero downtime environments—the network management tools required to monitor the performance of the servers.

Paging connectivity software was essential for many organizations, but in many cases has been replaced by newer technologies, such as the RIM BlackBerry. Faxing software was very popular several years ago but may not be needed any more, so it can be put at the bottom of the list.

Verifying Compatibility with Vendors

Armed with the full list of applications that need to be tested for compatibility, the application testing team can now start hitting the phones and delving into the vendors' Web sites for the compatibility information.

For early adopters of Exchange Server 2003, more research may be needed because vendors tend to lag behind in publishing statements of compatibility with new products. Past experience has shown that simply using the search feature on the vendor's site can be a frustrating process, so having an actual contact to call who has a vested interest in providing the latest and greatest information (such as the company's sales representative) can be a great time-saver.

> **NOTE**
>
> Experience has shown that the applications written by Microsoft that are to be upgraded to the new Exchange Server 2003 environment are not always compatible without updates or patches. Exchange add-ons—such as Instant Messenger, SharePoint Portal, or Conferencing Server—may have changed radically or not be yet upgraded to be compatible with Exchange Server 2003, so compatibility should not be assumed. Information is usually readily available on any such changes on the home pages for the specific products on Microsoft's Web site.

Each vendor tends to use its own terminology when discussing Exchange Server 2003 compatibility (especially when it isn't 100% tested); a functional way to define the level of compatibility is with the following four areas:

- Compatible

- Compatible with patches or updates

- Not compatible (requires version upgrade)

- Not compatible and no compatible version available (requires new product)

When possible, it is also a good practice to gather information about the specifics of the testing environment, such as the version and SP level of the Windows operating system the application was tested with, along with the hardware devices (if applicable, such as tape drives, specific PDAs, and so forth) tested.

Tracking Sheets for Application Compatibility Research

For organizational purposes, a tracking sheet should be created for each application to record the information discovered from the vendors. A sample product inventory sheet includes the following categories:

- Vendor name

- Product name and version number

- Vendor contact name and contact information

- Level of criticality: critical, near critical, nice to have

- Compatible with Exchange Server 2003: yes/no/did not say

- Vendor-stated requirements to upgrade or make application compatible

- Recommended action: None, patch/fix/update, version upgrade, replace with new product, stop using product, continue using product without vendor support

- Operating system compatibility: Windows Server 2003, Windows 2000 Server, Windows NT Server, other

- Notes (conversation notes, URLs used, copies of printed compatibility statements, or hard copy provided by vendor)

It is a matter of judgment as to the extent of the notes from discussions with the vendors and materials printed from Web sites that are retained and included with the inventory sheet and kept on file. Remember that URLs change frequently, so it makes sense to print the information when it is located.

In cases where product upgrades are required, information can be recorded on the part numbers, cost, and other pertinent information.

Six States of Compatibility

There are essentially six possible states of compatibility that can be defined, based on the input from the vendors, and that need to be verified during the testing process. These levels of compatibility roughly equate to levels of risk of unanticipated behavior and issues during the upgrade process:

1. The application version currently in use is Exchange Server 2003–compatible.

2. The application version currently in use is compatible with Exchange Server 2003, with a minor update or service patch.

3. The application currently in use is compatible with Exchange Server 2003, with a version upgrade of the application.

4. The application currently in use is not Exchange Server 2003–compatible and no upgrade is available, but it will be kept running as is on an older version of Exchange Server (or other messaging platform) in the upgraded Exchange Server 2003 messaging environment.

5. The application currently in use is not Exchange Server 2003–compatible, and will be phased out and not used after the upgrade is complete.

6. The application currently in use is not Exchange Server 2003–compatible per the vendor, or no information on compatibility was available, but it apparently runs on Exchange Server 2003 and will be run only on the new operating system.

Each of these states is discussed in more detail in the following sections.

Using an Exchange Server 2003–Compatible Application

Although most applications require some sort of upgrade, the vendor might simply state that the version currently in use will work properly with Exchange Server 2003 and provide supporting documentation or specify a URL with more information on the topic. This is more likely to be the case with applications that don't integrate with the Exchange Server components but interface with certain components and might even be installed on separate servers.

It is up to the organization to determine whether testing is needed to verify the vendor's compatibility statement. If the application in question is critical to the integrity or security of the Exchange data stores, or provides the users with features and capabilities that enhance their business activities and transactions, testing is definitely recommended. For upgrades that have short time frames and limited budgets available for testing (basic testing as defined earlier in the chapter), these applications may be demoted to the bottom of the list of priorities and would be tested only after the applications requiring updates or upgrades had been tested.

A clear benefit of the applications that the vendor verifies as being Exchange Server 2003–compatible is that the administrative staff will already know how to install and support the product and how it interfaces with Exchange and the helpdesk. End-users won't need to be trained or endure the learning curves required by new versions of the products.

> **NOTE**
>
> As mentioned previously, make sure to clarify what NOS and which specific version of Exchange Server 2003 was used in the testing process, because seemingly insignificant changes, such as security patches to the OS, can influence the product's performance in your upgraded environment. Tape backup software is notorious for being very sensitive to minor changes in the NOS or version of Exchange, and tape backups can appear to be working but might not be. If devices such as text pagers or PDAs are involved in the process, the specific operating systems tested and the details of the hardware models should be verified if possible to make sure that the vendor testing included the models in use by the organization.
>
> If a number of applications are being installed on one Exchange Server 2003 system, there can be conflicts that would not be predictable. So for mission-critical Exchange Server 2003 applications, testing is still recommended, even for applications the vendor asserts are fully compatible with Exchange Server 2003.

Requiring a Minor Update or Service Patch for Compatibility

When upgrading from Exchange 2000, many applications simply need a relatively minor service update or patch for compatibility with Exchange Server 2003. This is less likely to be the case when upgrading from Exchange 5.5 or a competing messaging product, such as Lotus Notes or Novell GroupWise.

During the testing process, the service updates and patches are typically quick and easy to install, are available over the Internet, and are often free of charge. It is important to read any notes or readme files that come with the update, because specific settings in the Exchange Server 2003 configuration might need to be modified for them to work. These updates and patches tend to change and be updated themselves after they are released, so it is worth checking periodically to see whether new revisions have become available.

These types of updates generally do not affect the core features or functionality of the products in most cases, although some new features may be introduced; so they have little training and support ramifications because the helpdesk and support staff will already be experienced in supporting the products.

Applications That Require a Version Upgrade for Compatibility

In other cases, especially when migrating from Exchange 5.5 or a competing messaging system, a product version upgrade is required, and this tends to be a more complex process than downloading a patch or installing a minor update to the product. The process will vary by product, with some allowing an in-place upgrade, where the software is not on the Exchange Server 2003 server itself, and others simply installing from scratch.

The amount of time required to install and test these upgrades is greater and the learning curve steeper, and the danger of technical complexities and issues increases. Thus additional time should be allowed for testing the installation process of the new products, configuring them for optimal Exchange connectivity, and fine tuning for performance factors. Training for the IT resources and helpdesk staff will be important because of the probability of significant differences between the new and old versions.

Compatibility with all hardware devices should not be taken for granted, whether it is the server itself, tape backup devices, or SAN hardware.

If a new version of the product is required, it can be difficult to avoid paying for the upgrade, so budget can become a factor. Some vendors can be persuaded to provide evaluation copies that expire after 30–120 days.

Noncompatible Applications That Will Be Used Anyway

As discussed earlier in this chapter, Exchange Server 2003 can coexist with previous versions of Exchange and of the Windows operating system, so an Exchange Server 2003 migration does not require that every messaging server be upgraded. In larger organizations, for example, smaller offices might choose to remain on Exchange 2000 for a period of time, if there are legitimate business reasons or cost concerns with upgrading expensive applications. If custom scripts or applications have been written that integrate and add functionality to Exchange 5.5 or Exchange 2000, it might make more sense to simply keep those servers intact on the network.

An example of this scenario could be a paging application that runs on Exchange 5.5 but is used by a few users and is being phased out, so it doesn't make financial sense to pay for an upgrade. Another example could be a faxing server where a number of proprietary fax boards were purchased and it continues to meet the needs of the company.

Although it might sound like an opportunity to skip any testing because the server configurations aren't changing, connectivity to the new Exchange Server 2003 configurations still needs to be tested, to ensure that the functionality between the servers is stable.

Again, in this scenario the application itself is not upgraded, modified, or changed, so there won't be a requirement for administrative or end-user training.

Noncompatible Applications That Will Be Eliminated and Applications That Are Not Compatible and Will Not Be Used

An organization might find that an application is not compatible with Exchange Server 2003, no upgrade is available, or the cost is prohibitive, so it decides to simply retire the application. Exchange Server 2003 includes a variety of new features, as discussed throughout the book, that might make certain utilities and management tools unnecessary. For example, a disaster recovery module for a tape backup product might no longer be needed after clustering is implemented. A VPN solution might be retired because OWA provides enhanced performance and provides the look and feel of the full Outlook client.

Care should be taken during the testing process to note the differences that the administrative, helpdesk and end-users will notice in the day-to-day interactions with the messaging system. If features are disappearing, a survey to assess the impact can be very helpful. Many users will raise a fuss if a feature suddenly goes away, even if it was rarely used, whereas if they were informed in advance the complaints could be avoided.

Noncompatible Applications That Seem to Work

The final category applies to situations where no information can be found about compatibility. Some vendors choose to provide no information and make no stance on compatibility with Exchange Server 2003. This puts the organization in a tricky situation, and it has to rely on internal testing results to make a decision. Even if the application seems to work properly, the decision might be made to phase out or retire the product if its failure could harm the business process. If the application performs a valuable function, it is probably time to look for, or create, a replacement, or at least to allocate time for this process at a later time.

If the organization chooses to keep the application, it might be kept in place on an older version of Exchange or moved to the new Exchange Server 2003 environment. In either case, the administrative staff, helpdesk, and end-users should be warned that the application is not officially supported or officially compatible and might behave erratically.

Creating an Upgrade Decision Matrix

Although each application will have its own inventory sheet, it is helpful to put together a brief summary document outlining the final results of the vendor research process and the ramifications to the messaging upgrade project.

Table 17.3 provides a sample format for the upgrade decision matrix.

TABLE 17.3   Upgrade Decision Matrix

Item #	Vendor	Product Name	Version	Exchange 2003 Compatibility Level	Decision
				1) Compatible as is	(N) No change
				2) Needs patches	(P) Patch/fix
				3) Needs upgrade	(U) Upgrade
				4) Not compatible	(R) Replace
1	Veritas	BackUp Exec	v.x	2	U
2	Veritas	Exchange Agent	v.x	3	U
3	Trend	ScanMail	v.x	3	U
4	RIM	BlackBerry	v.x	1	N

As with all documents that affect the scope and end-state of the messaging infrastructure, this document should be reviewed and approved by the project stakeholders.

This document can be expanded to summarize which applications will be installed on which messaging server if there are going to be multiple Exchange Server 2003 servers in the final configuration. In this way, the document can serve as a checklist to follow during the actual testing process.

Assessing the Effects of the Compatibility Results on the Compatibility Testing Plan

After all the data has been collected on the compatibility, lack of compatibility, or lack of information, the compatibility testing plan should be revisited to see whether changes need to be made. As discussed earlier in the chapter, the components of the compatibility testing plan are the scope of the application testing process, and the goals of the process (timeline, budget, extent of the testing, training requirements, documentation requirements, and fate of the testing lab).

Some of the goals might now be more difficult to meet, and might require additional budget, time, and resources. If essential messaging applications need to be replaced with version upgrades or a solution from a different vendor, additional time for testing and training might be required. Certain key end-users might also need to roll up their sleeves and perform hands-on testing to make sure that the new products perform to their expectations.

This might be the point in the application testing process that a decision is made that a more complete prototype testing phase is needed, and the lab would be expanded to more closely, or exactly, resemble the end-state of the migration.

17

Lab-Testing Existing Applications

With the preparation and research completed, and the compatibility testing plan verified as needed, the actual testing can begin. The testing process should be fairly anticlimactic at this point because the process has been discussed at length, and it will be clear what the testing goals are and which applications will be tested. Due diligence in terms of vendor research should be completed and now it is just a matter of building the test server or servers and documenting the results.

The testing process can yield results that are unforeseen, because the exact combination of hardware and software may affect the performance of a key application; but far better to have this occur in a nonproduction environment where failures won't affect the organization's ability to deliver its services.

During the testing process, valuable experience with the installation and upgrade process will be gained and will contribute to the success of the production migration. The migration team will be familiar with—or possibly experts at—the installation and application migration processes when it counts, and are more likely to avoid configuration mistakes and resolve technical issues.

Allocating and Configuring Hardware

Ideally, budget is available to purchase the same server hardware and related peripherals (such as tape drives, UPS, PDAs, text pagers) that will be used in the production migration. This is preferable to using a server machine that has been sitting in a closet for an undetermined period of time, which might respond differently than the eventual hardware that will be used. Using old hardware can actually generate more work in the long run and adds more variables to an already complex process.

If the testing process is to exactly mirror the production environment, this would be considered to be a prototype phase, which is generally broader in scope than compatibility testing, and requires additional hardware, software, and time to complete. A prototype phase is recommended for more complex networks in which the upgrade process is riskier and more involved and the budget, time, and resources are available.

Don't forget to allocate a representative workstation for each desktop operating system that is supported by the organization and a sample remote access system, such as a typical laptop or PDA that is used by the sales force or traveling executive.

Allocating and Configuring the NOS and Exchange Server 2003

By this point, the software has been ordered, allocated, downloaded, and set aside for easy access, along with any notes taken or installation procedures downloaded in the research phase. If some time has elapsed since the compatibility research with the vendors, it is worth checking to see whether any new patches have been released. The upgrade decision matrix discussed earlier in the chapter is an excellent checklist to have on hand during this process to make sure that nothing is missed that could cause delays during the testing process.

When configuring the servers with the appropriate operating systems, the company standards for configurations should be adhered to, if they have been documented. Standards can include the level of hard drive redundancy, separation of the application files and data files, naming conventions, roles of the servers, approved and tested security packs, and security configurations.

Next, Exchange Server 2003 should be configured to also meet company standards and then for the essential utilities that will protect the integrity of the data and the operating system, which typically include the backup software, antivirus software and management utilities and applications. After this base configuration is completed, it can be worth performing a complete backup of the system or using an application such as Ghost to take a snapshot of the server configuration in case the subsequent testing is problematic and a rollback is needed.

Loading the Remaining Applications

With the Exchange Server 2003 configured with the NOS, Exchange, and essential utilities, the value-added applications can be tested. Value-added applications enhance the functionality of Exchange and enable the users to perform their jobs more efficiently and drive the business more effectively. It's helpful to provide a calendar or schedule to the end-users who will be assisting in the testing process at this point so they know when their services will be needed.

There are so many different combinations of applications that might be installed and tested at this point that the different permutations can't all be covered in this chapter. As a basic guideline, first test the most essential applications and the applications that were not identified previously as being compatible. By tackling the applications that are more likely to be problematic early on in the process, the testing resources will be fresh and any flags can be raised to the stakeholders while there is still time left in the testing process for remediation.

Thorough testing by the end-users is recommended, as is inclusion of the helpdesk staff in the process. Notes taken during the testing process will be valuable in creating any configuration guides or migration processes for the production implementation.

17

> **NOTE**
>
> Beyond basic functionality, data entry, and access to application-specific data, some additional tests that indicate an application has been successfully installed in the test environment include printing to different standard printers, running standard reports, exporting and importing data, and exchanging information with other systems or devices. Testing should be done by end-users of the application and administrative IT staff who support, maintain, and manage the application. Notes should be taken on the process and the results because they can be very useful during the production migration.

Application Compatibility Testing Tool

Microsoft offers a tool called the Windows Application Compatibility toolkit (ACT), which is a collection of documents and tools that can help identify compatibility problems on applications that are installed on a Windows 2000 or 2003 Server. This tool isn't designed specifically for Exchange Server 2003 applications, but it can be very helpful in determining whether the application in question—especially an application where no information is provided by the vendor or a custom application—has obvious problems or potential security holes. This level of testing falls under the medium level or complete levels of testing, mentioned previously in this chapter, which is valuable to organizations with more complex Exchange messaging environments that need to be as stable as possible.

There are three components to this tool: the Microsoft Application Compatibility Analyzer, the Windows Application Verifier, and the Compatibility Administrator.

The Application Compatibility Analyzer, shown in Figure 17.1, gathers an inventory of all the applications running on the server and then cross references the results online with a database maintained by Microsoft to produce an assessment report.

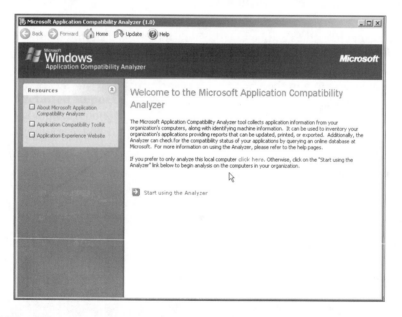

FIGURE 17.1   Windows Application Compatibility Analyzer.

For application development, Windows Applications Verifier then tests for potential compatibility errors caused by common programming mistakes, checks the application for memory-related issues, determines an application's compliance with requirements of the "Certified for Windows Server 2003" Logo Programs, and looks for potential security issues in an application.

At the time of this writing this application is available for download from
`http://www.microsoft.com/downloads` by performing a search for `application compatibility toolkit`.

Testing the Migration and Upgrade Process

This section touches on the next logical step in the testing process. After it has been veri-fied that the final configuration agreed upon in the planning process is stable and decided which applications and utilities will be installed on which server, the actual upgrade process can be tested. As discussed in Chapters 15, "Migrating from Exchange 5.5 to Exchange Server 2003," and 16, "Migrating from Exchange 2000 to Exchange Server 2003," Exchange Server 2003 comes with a number of built-in migration testing and facilitating utilities and tools.

Documenting the Results of the Compatibility Testing

A number of documents can be produced during the compatibility testing process. Understanding the expectations of the stakeholders and what the documents will be used for is important. For example, more detailed budgetary information might need to be compiled based on the information, or go/no go decisions might need to be reached. Thus a summary of the improvements offered by Exchange Server 2003 in the areas of reliabil-ity, performance visible to the user community, and features improved and added, might need to be presented in a convincing fashion.

At a minimum, a summary of the testing process should be created, and a final recom-mendation for the applications to be included in the production upgrade or migration should be provided to the stakeholders. This can be as simple as the upgrade decision matrix discussed earlier in the chapter, or it can be more thorough, including detailed notes of the exact testing procedures followed. Notes can be made available summarizing the results of end-users testing, validating the applications, and describing results—both positive and negative.

If the testing hardware is the same as the hardware that will be used in the production upgrade, server configuration documents that list the details of the hardware and software configurations can be created; they will ensure that the servers built in the production environment will have the same fundamental configuration as was tested in the lab.

A more detailed build document can be created that walks the technician through the exact steps required to build the Exchange Server 2003 system, in cases where many messaging servers need to be created in a short period of time.

The level of effort or the amount of time to actually perform the upgrade or the migration of a sample mailbox can be recorded as part of the documentation, and this information can be very helpful in planning the total amount of time that will be required to perform the upgrade or migration.

17

Determining Whether a Prototype Phase Is Required

The issue of whether a more complete prototype phase is needed or if a more limited application compatibility testing phase is sufficient has come up several times in this chapter. The essential difference between the two is that the prototype phase duplicates as exactly as possible the actual end-state of the upgrade, from server hardware to peripherals and software, so that the entire upgrade process can be tested to reduce the chance of surprises during the production upgrade. The application testing phase can be less extensive, involve a single server, and be designed to verify that the applications required will work reliably on the Exchange Server 2003 configuration. Compatibility testing can take as little time as a week—from goal definition, to research, to actual testing. A prototype phase takes considerably longer because of the additional steps required.

Following is a checklist that will help your organization make the decision:

- Is sufficient budget available for a subset of the actual hardware that will be used in the upgrade?

- Is sufficient time available for the configuration of the prototype lab and testing of the software?

- Are the internal resources available for a period of time long enough to finish the prototype testing? Or is budget available to pay for external consulting resources to complete the work?

- Is the Exchange Messaging Environment mission-critical to the business' ability to go about its daily activities and generate revenues, and will interruption of Exchange services cost the company an unacceptable amount of money?

- Does the actual migration process need to be tested and documented to ensure the success of the upgrade?

- Do resources need to be trained on the upgrade process (building the servers, configuring the NOS, Exchange Server 2003 software and related applications)?

If you find that the answers to more than half of these questions are yes, it's likely that a prototype phase will be required.

Summary

Exchange Server 2003 compatibility testing should be performed before any upgrade or migration. The process can be completed very quickly for smaller networks (basic testing) or for larger networks with fairly simple messaging environments.

The first steps include identifying the scope and goals of the project to make sure that the stakeholders are involved in determining the success factors for the project. Then research needs to be performed, internal to the company, on which applications are in place that are messaging-related. This includes not only Exchange Server, but tape backup software, antivirus software, network management and monitoring tools, add-ons (such as faxing, text messaging, paging, synchronization utilities for PDAs and remote users, and document routing software), and inventory sheets created summarizing this information. Decisions as to which applications are critical, near critical, or just nice to have should also be made. Research should then be performed with the vendors of the products, tracking sheets should be created to record this information, and the application should be categorized in one of six states of compatibility. Next the testing begins, with the configuration of the lab environment that is isolated from the production network, and the applications are loaded and tested by both administrative and end-user or helpdesk staff. The results are then documented, and the final decisions of whether to proceed are made.

With this process, the production upgrade or migration is smoother, and the likelihood of technical problems that can harm the business' ability to transact or provide its services is greatly reduced. The problems are identified beforehand and resolved, and the resources who will perform the work gain familiarity with all the products and processes involved.

Best Practices

The following are best practices from this chapter:

- Take the time to understand the goals of the project (What will the organization gain by doing the upgrade?) as well as the scope of the project (What is included and what is excluded from the project?).

- Understand all the applications that connect with Exchange Server 2003 and whether they are critical, near critical, or simply nice to have.

- Document the research process for each application, because this will prove to be very valuable if problems are encountered during the testing process

- Create a lab environment that is as close to the final end-state of the upgrade as possible. This reduces the variables that can cause problems at the least opportune time.

- Test applications for compatibility with both typical end-users of the application and application administrators who support, maintain, and manage the application.

17

PART VI

Microsoft Exchange Server 2003 Administration and Management

IN THIS PART

Exchange Server 2003 Mailbox, Distribution Group, and Administrative Group Administration

With Exchange Server 2003, there are new ways of accomplishing familiar tasks. This chapter guides Exchange administrators through the standard practices of managing basic Exchange Server 2003 Administrative Groups, User Mailbox administration, and Distribution Groups.

Exchange administrators can review new features of Exchange Server 2003 and common scenarios for implementing and managing Exchange Server 2003 permissions and features that assist in the day-to-day administrative tasks of Exchange.

Exchange Administration and the Delegation Wizard

As with previous versions of Exchange, administration is determined by permissions. With Exchange Server 2003, administrative rights and permissions are based on the new Exchange roles. Roles determine the level of permissions and rights to administrator Exchange objects within the Exchange organization.

In this section, we review each of these new Exchange administrative roles, how to use role-based administration within an Exchange Server 2003 organization, and the rights granted to each.

Also as part of managing Exchange permissions, we look at working with extended permissions, defining what extended permissions are used for and how to implement these into an Exchange Server 2003 environment using features such as the Exchange Server 2003 Delegation Wizard.

Implementing Role-Based Administration

Administration in Exchange Server 2003 has been simplified from the standard practice of applying permissions. As previously required, permissions were set by applying rights to Active Directory users and groups within the permission pages of Exchange objects. With Exchange Server 2003, assigning permissions has been simplified by implementing role-based administration within the Exchange hierarchy, which can be assigned using the Exchange Server 2003 Delegation Wizard. By assigning roles, delegation of permissions and administration throughout the organization can easily be set to accounts and groups at the organization and Administrative Group levels.

Depending on where in the Exchange organization roles are assigned, different levels of permissions can be applied to different Exchange server objects. Delegating permission in the Exchange organization, administrators can leverage each of these three Exchange server administrative roles to assign permissions at the Exchange Organization and Administrative Group levels:

- Exchange Full Administrator

- Exchange Administrator

- Exchange View Only Administrator

Permissions can be assigned allowing for different administrators at the organizational level and at the Administrative Group level. Separate roles can also be assigned to different Administrative Groups within the same Exchange organization. This can be very effective for larger organizations that want to decentralize Exchange administration.

Assigning Roles to Groups

When planning and assigning Exchange roles, it is simpler to manage and understand administrative permissions when roles are assigned to groups rather than individual user accounts. Create new Administrative Groups and use these groups to assign roles at the desired Exchange server levels.

When assigning Exchange roles to security groups, the account being used to manage or view Exchange objects must be a member of the security group that has been granted an Exchange role.

Exchange Full Administrator

The Exchange Full Administrator role is the least restrictive of all three Exchange Server 2003 roles. Similar to Full Control, using this role allows Exchange administrators to fully administer Exchange objects by giving them the capability to add, delete, and change Exchange permissions and objects. Assign the Exchange Full Administrator role to Exchange administrators who require complete access to Exchange for configuring and managing the entire Exchange organization.

Exchange Full and Administrator Requirements

To enable the Exchange Full Administrator or Administrator roles, the group or users object being assigned these roles must also maintain local administrator group membership to the Exchange server. This is required on any Exchange server on which these roles are being assigned.

Important!

Adding permissions to the local administrators group must be completed manually. When assigning roles, not having this set will not restrict roles from being assigned. However, it must be completed for the role-based administration to be effective.

Exchange Administrator

The Administrator role is ideal for assigning administrative privileges to users and groups that require rights to perform the daily administration to objects within Exchange. The Administrator role allows Exchange administrators to add, change, or modify objects only.

Exchange View Only Administrator

The Exchange View Only role is the most restrictive of all Exchange roles. The Exchange View Only role provides permissions to view Exchange objects only. There are no add and modify rights associated with this role, and it is most effectively implemented for groups and accounts that require the capability to view objects in the other Exchange organizations and Administrative Groups.

NOTE

The Exchange View Only role can be used to restrict administrative permissions between Exchange Administrative Groups. Assign the Exchange View Only role to allow Administrative Group administrators to view objects in other Administrative Groups without granting permissions to add and modify objects.

Understanding and Implementing Extended Permissions

Another method by which Exchange Server 2003 administrators can manage and controls administrative access to Exchange objects is to implement extended permissions. Extended permissions are Exchange-specific and allow for more granular security by giving administrators the capability to set permissions in addition to and beyond the standard Active Directory permissions. Extended permissions can be applied when roles and rights require

more granular configurations and can be applied to individual objects rather than at organizational and Administrative Group levels.

Exchange Server 2003 extended permissions can be applied to servers in the organization,
individual databases, public folders, address lists, and protocols.

To implement extended permissions, open the Security tab of an Exchange object. Each
Security tab contains both Active Directory–integrated Windows permissions and
Exchange extended permissions, as shown in Figure 18.1.

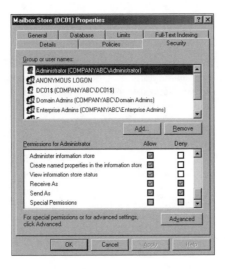

FIGURE 18.1   Public folder security and permissions.

Delegating Administrative Rights

With an understanding of what roles and permissions are available to administrators in
Exchange Server 2003, the task becomes determining which roles and permissions are
required for the specific needs in each area of Exchange Server 2003 and how to apply
them at the different levels of the organization.

For example, as the Exchange Server 2003 organization begins to expand, the Exchange
environment might require additional Administrative Groups to be configured. This

configuration might also be ideal for decentralizing administrative duties required to maintain each Administrative Group and Exchange objects belonging to them.

With multiple Administrative Groups, permission can be applied to individual Exchange Server 2003 administrators, granting them the capability to perform the day-to-day tasks required to manage users and objects in each Administrative Group. Also, individuals or groups can be granted extended permissions to provide an even more granular set of permissions on objects such as a mailbox store or a public folder tree within a specific Administrative Group.

To apply roles and permission, administrators must perform each separately and in different methods. Unlike applying extended permissions, applying Exchange roles can be accomplished by using the Delegation Wizard, which is included with the Exchange System Manager.

The Delegation Wizard is a tool built into the Exchange Server 2003 System Manager that allows administrators to assign Exchange roles only to objects at the organization and Administrative Group levels within the Exchange organization.

The application of extended permission must be performed by opening the property pages of the object where the permission will be applied and by selecting the Security tab.

Understanding the Scope of Roles Being Applied

When assigning Exchange roles using the Delegation Wizard, the level of permissions being assigned depends on the level of the Exchange organization in which permission roles are being assigned.

For example, if an administrator group called Admins is assigned Full Administrator rights on the Exchange organization, this group of accounts has full administrative rights to the entire Exchange organization and any Administrative Group within the organizational structure.

Imagine that an account is granted the Full Administrator role on an Administrative Group called Administrative Group 1 and is granted the View Only role to Administrative Group 2. This account can fully add, modify, and delete objects in Administrative Group 1 but can only traverse to Administrative Group 2 to view objects—it cannot add to or modify anything in Administrative Group 2.

Using the Delegation Wizard

To implement Exchange roles using the Delegation Wizard, begin by opening the Exchange System Manager and complete these steps:

1. On the Exchange server with the Exchange System Manager, select Start, All Programs, Microsoft Exchange, System Manager.

2. Select the Administrative Group to which the administrative roles are to be applied.

18

3. From the Action menu, select Action, Delegate Control. This launches the Welcome to the Exchange Administration Delegation Wizard, shown in Figure 18.2. Select Next to begin.

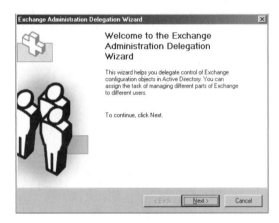

FIGURE 18.2   Welcome to the Exchange Administration Delegation Wizard.

4. On the Users and Groups page, click the Add button to select the group or account and the role that will be applied to the Administrative Group.

5. Select Browse and select the group or account to be used. Select OK when finished.

6. From the Role Selection tab, use the arrow to choose the role Full Administrator, and click OK.

7. Select Next to complete the Delegation Wizard. Review the configuration window to ensure that the selection is correct and that the proper role is being applied. Choose Finish to apply the role to the first Administrative Group.

> **NOTE**
>
> This procedure can be repeated to add accounts and groups to any role at the organization and Administrative Group levels within the Exchange System Manager.

Auditing Administrative Tasks in Exchange Server 2003

To help manage changes as roles and permissions are assigned to different groups and accounts, Exchange Server 2003 auditing can help administrators determine successful changes and failures based on groups or user accounts configured to be audited when performing tasks on Exchange containers and objects. Auditing features are available only when auditing Exchange containers and objects within any Administrative Group of the Exchange organization.

Auditing allows tracking of changes, reads, deletes; the creation of child objects; and send as, receive as, and other helpful tracking options to assist the administrator in monitoring roles and permissions as they are applied. Auditing can also be configured to be inherited to child objects and subcontainers, as well as applied to a single container with an Administrative Group.

As an example of how to enable auditing on an Exchange container or object, perform the following the steps to enable auditing on an object within the first Administrative Group in the Exchange organization.

1. Open the Exchange System Manager and select the first server in the first Administrative Group.

2. Select the properties of the server and select the Security tab.

3. Click the Advanced button in the lower-left corner to open the Advanced Security page for the server.

4. Click the Auditing tab to open the Auditing Configuration page.

5. Click the Add button and select the group or user account on which auditing will be enabled. Click OK when finished.

6. Select the Apply Onto options and select This Object, subcontainers, and children objects. This applies the audit setting to all server containers and objects.

7. Choose the auditing feature that will be applied by placing a check in the box under Access Options. For this scenario, select Create Children and then select Successful.

NOTE

This setting creates an entry in the event logs of the server when a child object is created.

Other settings, such as the Read option, automatically enable other auditing features. This is by design and allows Exchange to enable the proper permission to apply the auditing function.

Managing Mailboxes and Message Settings in Exchange Server 2003

The key function of Exchange is to provide mailbox functionality to end-user accounts within Active Directory. This section assists Exchange Server 2003 administrators in enabling and managing end-user mailboxes, mailbox options, and the information stores where they reside.

Also included are the step-by-step tasks to help administrators configure user mailbox options in the Exchange System Manager and tips for managing the new Exchange Server 2003 features, such as wireless browsing and user-initiated synchronization. We also cover methods and tools to use when administering and maintaining mailboxes within the information store.

Managing Exchange Mailboxes

Administrators can manage Exchange user mailboxes using two methods. The first and most common is using the Active Directory Users and Computers snap-in. Using Active Directory Users and Computers, administrators can mail-enable and manage mailboxes from an individual user account perspective as they reside in their perspective Organizational Unit.

The second option is using the Exchange System Manager to manage mailbox attributes and settings. Some user Exchange tasks can also be performed through the Exchange System Manager, but this method is most commonly used to set mailbox options such as message limits and storage limits on a global or storage container level for all mailboxes.

Mail-Enabling Active Directory Objects

When an account is mail-enabled, Exchange creates a mailbox for the Active Directory object and enables Exchange functionality based on the policies and settings on the Exchange store where the mailbox is created.

Windows Active Directory objects can be mail-enabled using two methods: doing so when the account object is originally created in Active Directory, and using the Exchange Tasks Wizard in the Active Directory Users and Computers snap-in.

To create a mailbox for an object when a new Active Directory account is created, select the Create an Exchange Mailbox option during the configuration of the account.

When this option is selected, administrators must also select an alias name for the Exchange user and the Exchange server and mailbox store where the mailbox will reside. This option creates a mail-enabled Active Directory account.

When accounts exist that were not mail-enabled during creation, objects can be mail-enabled individually or in bulk by using the Exchange Tasks Wizard in the Active Directory Users and Computers snap-in. To mail-enable Active Directory objects, complete these steps:

1. Open the Active Directory Users and Computers snap-in and select the account or account objects to be mail-enabled.

2. To open the Exchange Task Wizard, click the Action menu and select the Exchange Task option.

3. At the Welcome to Exchange Task Wizard, select Next.

4. On the Available Task screen, select the Create Mailbox option and click Next.

5. Choose the mail store and server where the mailbox will reside, and select Next.

6. Review the summary and select the Finished button when the mailbox has been created.

> **NOTE**
>
> After a mailbox has been created, the Back button cannot be used to change the options configured when the account is mail-enabled.

Implementing Message Limits and Storage Limits

Implementing message and storage limits is often considered when planning the installation of an Exchange Server 2003 server. Capacity planning and the total number of users planned per server can directly affect the decisions regarding the implementation of information storage limits.

Each can have considerable effects on an Exchange Server 2003 server as well as the network performance that Exchange Server 2003 installed.

Using storage limits can be beneficial to help manage the total amount of data being stored within a storage group. Given the total amount of users planned per storage group and the storage limits being implemented, administrators can determine the maximum storage size that any storage container can grow. This can effectively assist Exchange administrators in managing and maintaining information stores to a size that can easily be backed up in a timely manner. Managing the database sizes through storage limits can also assist in shortening the total amount of time needed to perform maintenance on a single Exchange database.

Limits can be implemented with Exchange Server 2003 in two ways. Limits can configured globally using the Exchange System Manager or can be applied on an individual basis from the properties of a mail-enabled object.

Understanding and Implementing User Mailbox Options

With each mail-enabled Active Directory object, administrators can configure multiple Exchange options to customize the Exchange mailbox. Each mail-enabled account in Active Directory contains Exchange pages with options specific to the individual account.

The Exchange options pages in the user's properties can be used and configured to override the storage container settings created through the Exchange System Manager. These options are often used when a member of a storage container requires message limits, delivery restrictions, and alternate email addresses that differ from the default setting placed on the container.

18

To set these options on a specific user object, refer to the following settings to determine
which best fits the needs being implemented.

Exchange General

The General Exchange tab is used to set restrictions and limits for a specific user mailbox.
These options and their definitions are listed here:

- **Mailbox Store**   The Mailbox Store tab cannot be modified from the User Option
  page. It is used to identify the mailbox store of which the account is a member.

- **Alias**   The alias name for a mailbox is used as an alternate logon name for the user
  account. The option is set when the object is mail-enabled and can be changed at
  any time from this tab.

- **Delivery Restrictions**   Select this option to configure the maximum size limits
  for outgoing and inbound mail. This option can also be used to specify specific
  email accounts that the mail-enabled object can and cannot send receive messages
  from.

- **Delivery Options**   The most common use for the delivery tab is to configure
  accounts and enable the send on behalf privileges options for the accounts, as well
  as limit the total number of addresses the object can send messages to.

- **Storage Limits**   Enabling storage limits sets the total size that a mail-enabled user
  can allow the mailbox to grow. As a defined mailbox limit is reached, the account is
  warned that it is reaching the limit set, requiring the user to remove mail objects
  from within the mailbox. This option also allows an administrator to configure
  deleted item retention. This determines how long deleted objects will remain hidden
  within a mailbox for recovery purposes before objects are permanently deleted.

Email Addresses

The Email options page allows administrators to configure additional addresses for a
specific user's account. This option contains addresses based on the recipient policy
configured through the Exchange System Manager. If a user requires additional mail
addresses, select the New tab to add any of the available Microsoft compatible addresses.

Managing New Mailbox Features

With Exchange Server 2003 are new mailbox features that were not available with previous versions of Exchange. With Exchange Server 2003, user wireless support is now
included in Exchange operating systems and greatly enhances the capability to provide
end-user support and compatibility with wireless devices such as cellphones and
pocket PCs.

Using Wireless support features, Microsoft Windows Pocket PC clients can now use
Microsoft Active Sync and Pocket Outlook to access Exchange server data and synchronize
Outlook information.

Using the Properties tab of a mail-enabled object or the Exchange Tasks Wizard, administrators can select features to enable and disable on an individual or multiple Exchange mailboxes.

Using Wireless Services

Exchange Server 2003 now supports advanced wireless cellular and 802.1X connectivity. This was not previously available in early versions of the Exchange server family. The advanced wireless features enable end-user remote access support and wireless synchronization to Exchange mail using built-in Exchange technology such as Outlook Web Access.

Located on the Exchange Features tab of a mail-enabled user's properties page, the Wireless Services option allows mail-enabled objects access to individual Exchange mailbox data using supported wireless 802.1X devices, Pocket PCs, and Internet-ready cellular phones.

Wireless Functionality

When Active Directory objects are mail-enabled, these features are in an enabled state by default. Each feature is managed and changed through the end-user properties pages by easily disabling and enabling the desired method of wireless access.

Review the wireless features (see Figure 18.3) and their descriptions to better understand Exchange Server 2003 wireless functionality and the options provided with each feature.

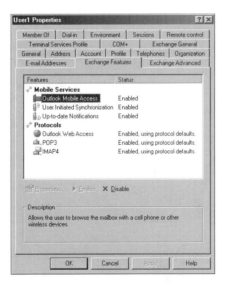

FIGURE 18.3   Users properties and Exchange features page.

- **Outlook Wireless Access**   With Outlook Wireless Access enabled, the user can browse mailbox information from wireless devices and cellular Internet-enabled phones.

- **User Initiated Synchronization**   When enabled, this option allows individual users to synchronize mail information with wireless devices. This option is not associated with active sync desktop synchronization and is enabled by default.

- **Always Up-to-Date Notification**   Enabled and used with user-initiated synchronization, this option notifies wireless users when changes have occurred requiring synchronization.

> **TIP**
>
> As a best practice, administrators should disable any features not required to enhance remote security to Exchange Server 2003 and control user access from remote locations.
>
> Additional information on enabling and configuring mobile synchronization can be found in Chapter 23, "Implementing Mobile Synchronization in Exchange Server 2003."

Managing User Protocols

Protocols allow individual mail-enabled users to access Exchange mail using different methods and functionality. Access control to Exchange Mail can be controlled from an individual mail account based on the type of access granted.

By default, Exchange Server 2003 features enable all users to access Exchange using the POP3, Outlook Web Access, and IMAP4 protocols. In most situations, all three of these features are not required for every mail-enabled user in the Exchange organization.

Each feature is fully configurable on an individual account basis and can also be modified by disabling the protocol from the Exchange System Manager. Protocols such as POP3 access cannot be enabled fully unless the Exchange Server 2003 server has been configured to support this protocol.

Changing the Status of Exchange Features

Any time an Active Directory object is mail-enabled, each of the Exchange features is enabled by default. To control or modify the status of any Exchange feature, use the individual user's Properties tab to change the status of the feature from Enabled to Disabled.

> **NOTE**
>
> Using the Exchange Features tab enables and disables only the functionality for the individual mail-enabled user. Each of these features requires additional configuration, such as the implementation of an Outlook Web Access front-end server or the configuration of a server and client to enable POP access to Exchange mail data.

Some additional firewall configuration might also be required for access to Outlook Web Access from Internet remote locations.

To change the status of one or more Exchange features for multiple mail-enabled objects in Exchange, use the Exchange Task Wizard.

For example, an organization can disable wireless features for multiple users in Active Directory by following these steps:

1. Open the Active Directory Users and Computers snap-in and select the accounts to be modified.

2. From the Exchange System Manager menu, select Action, select the Exchange tasks, and select Next at the welcome screen.

3. Select the Configure Exchange Features option and click Next to continue.

4. From the Configure Exchange Features selection, choose the feature to be modified. Select the Disable or Enable tab to change the feature for all users. Modify all options before continuing, and select Next to apply the changes.

5. Review the configured changes and the results of these changes on the Task Summary screen. Select the Back button to adjust any required changes. Select Next to complete the modification and fully apply the settings.

Moving Exchange User Mailboxes

When moving mailboxes in previous versions of Exchange, moves were completed through the Active Directory Users and Computers snap-in using the Mailbox Move Wizard. This tasks could become difficult when moving multiple mailboxes because administrators were required to locate each mail-enabled account in the Active Directory tree, regardless of where they resided.

These limitations of Exchange 2000 Server move tools have been eliminated in Exchange Server 2003. By including the Move mailbox functionality in the Exchange System Manager, administrators can select and move objects with much greater flexibility. Using the Exchange System Manager to move mailboxes now enables them to move multiple mailboxes easily and effectively.

Using the Mailbox Move tool through the Exchange System Manager, entire Exchange server mailbox stores or mailboxes within a store can be selected and moved from one location to another easily.

Simple Tasks to Prepare for Moving Mailboxes

Before moving a mailbox or multiple mailboxes, tasks can be completed in advance to avoid the loss of mail data and streamline the move process.

By backing up the Exchange information stores and eliminating unwanted mail data using the Mailbox Manager and mailbox recipient policies, administrators can perform moves in less time through eliminating unwanted data residing in the mailboxes being moved. This allows the newly moved mailboxes in the destination store to be populated only with information needed.

Backing Up Exchange Mailboxes

Before moving and removing mail data from mailboxes, it is always a good practice to back up the Exchange server from where mailboxes are being moved. Also, backing up the individual mailboxes before cleaning and moving allows for the recovery of any messages if mailbox owners identify messages that needed to be recovered.

To back up a mailbox or a group of mailboxes, administrators can effectively use any of the following methods if the recovery of mail information is required:

- **Full and brick-level backup**   Use a third-party backup product to back up and validate the backup of the Exchange information store or individual Exchange mailboxes.

- **Export mail data to PST files**   Use Exchange utilities such as the Microsoft Exchange Server 2003 Exchange Merge Wizard (Exmerge.exe) to export all user mail data to individual PST files. To obtain the Exchange Merge Wizard, download the tool from Microsoft by going to www.microsoft.com/exchange/tools/2003.asp.

Cleaning Unneeded Mailbox Data

Using the Mailbox Cleanup Wizard to remove unnecessary mailbox information such as deleted items and outdated calendar information shortens the total amount of time required to move mailboxes. Cleaning mailboxes before moving also ensures that the mailbox data being moved is only what is required and clean.

Use the Mailbox Cleanup Wizard to remove unwanted mailbox information before moving mailboxes. To open and schedule mailbox cleanup, see the section "Implementing Mailbox Recipient Policies," later in this chapter.

Moving Mailboxes Between Storage Groups and Servers

Limitations for moving mailboxes have been greatly reduced in Exchange Server 2003. When leveraging the Mailbox Move tool through the Exchange System Manager, administrators can move mailboxes or groups of mailboxes and can run multiple instances of moves at the same time.

Also, options can now be configured to address corrupted mail items and scheduling that previously interrupted the move process or caused it to fail.

Through the options available with the Mailbox Move tool in Exchange Server 2003, corrupted mailboxes and mailbox items can now be skipped and not moved instead of causing the entire move to fail. In addition, these corruptions are now written to a log file and can be retrieved to review and address issues with corrupted mailboxes.

View the Mailbox Move logs to troubleshoot failed item moves and resolve any issues with the move. Move logs can be retrieved by going to Documents and Settings, Profile, My Documents, Exchange Task Wizard Logs folder (where the drive letter is the drive of the Documents and Settings folder and profile represents the account being used).

Options can also be configured to determine the total number of corrupted items to be skipped. Using the Maximum Number of Corrupted Items to Be Skipped option, values can be configured manually between 3 and 100.

CAUTION

When using the Mailbox Move tool options, the default setting for skipping corrupted items is set to three items.

When corrupted items are skipped, items are deleted and not retained in the information store. Be sure to back up information to avoid the loss of any mail items not intended to be deleted.

Scheduling and Move Cut Off times are also now available and configurable for scheduled mailbox moves. For example, administrators can schedule moves of mailboxes to be run outside business hours. If the move has not completed by the specified cutoff time, the mailbox being moved and the remaining mailboxes are left in the original location.

Multiple Mailbox Move Tool

The Exchange Server 2003 version of the Move Mailbox tool allows administrators to run several instances of mailbox moves at the same time. Depending on level of hardware resources, such as memory and processor speed available, multiple instances of the Mailbox Move tool can be run in parallel with adequate performance.

TIP

Test a handful of mailbox moves using the Mailbox Move tool to ensure that the server performance is not affected when running multiple instances of the move function.

Moving Mailboxes Between Storage Groups

To move mailboxes between administrative storage groups, open the Exchange System Manager and select the Administrative Group where the mailboxes to be moved reside. Complete the following steps to move Exchange mailboxes between storage groups:

1. Highlight the mailboxes to be moved.

2. From the Action menu, select the Exchange Tasks option and click the Next button on the welcome screen.

3. At the Available Tasks page, select Move Mailbox and click the Next button to continue.

4. Select the destination mailbox store where the mailboxes will be moved. Click the Mailbox Store option and choose the destination store where the mailboxes will be moved. Select Next when complete.

5. Configure the options for addressing corruption, and set the desired limits for this move. Select the Next button to begin the mailbox move.

6. To continue moving the mailbox, on the Schedule Page, select Next to continue.

7. On the summary page, review the results of the mailbox move, and select Finish.

Moving Mailboxes to a Different Exchange Server

Moving mailboxes from one Exchange server to another is often done to assist administrators in load-balancing multiple Exchange server environments and even when replacing outdated hardware.

This task is accomplished in the same manner as moving mailboxes between storage groups. Using the Mailbox Move tool, mailboxes can be moved between servers with same options available when moving mailboxes on the same server. This can help administrators ensure that corrupted information is not moved to the new mailbox store, causing failures at a later time.

To move mailboxes between servers, follow these steps:

1. Select the mailbox store where the mailboxes reside. Select and highlight the mailboxes to be moved.

2. From the Action menu, select the Exchange Tasks option and click the Next button on the welcome screen.

3. At the Available Tasks page, select Move Mailbox and click the Next button.

4. Select the destination mailbox store where the mailboxes will be moved. Click the Server option and choose the destination server where the mailboxes will be moved to. Select Next when complete.

5. Configure the options for addressing corruption and set the desired limits for this move. Select the Next button to begin the mailbox move.

6. To continue moving the mailbox, on the Schedule page, select Next.

7. On the summary page, review the results of the mailbox move and select Finish to complete the move.

NOTE

Mailboxes can be moved between servers only when the servers are part of the same site. When servers are in different sites, the mailboxes cannot be moved using the Move Mailbox function. Moving mailboxes between servers in different sites requires the use of the ExMerge utility, covered in the section "Backing Up Exchange Mailboxes."

Creating and Managing Exchange Contacts

In many situations, organizations are required to communicate with non-native Microsoft mail systems, non-Exchange mail recipients, and external SMTP addresses. These situations are ideal for an Exchange Server 2003 recipient type called contacts.

Known as custom recipients in previous Exchange versions, contacts are created in Active Directory and viewed in the Global Catalog in the same manner as a mail-enabled user object. Each contact can be assigned an SMTP address in the domain where the contact resides. This allows the contact to receive internal and external mail using the same email domain as mail-enabled users.

Creating Exchange Contacts

To create a contact in Exchange Server 2003, begin by opening the Active Directory Users and Computers management console. Select the Organizational Unit where the contact will be created and follow these steps for creating a contacts list:

1. From the Action menu, select New and Contact.

2. Enter the information to identify the contact in Active Directory.

   For example:

   First name = John

   Middle initial = M

   Last name = Doe

   Display name = John Doe

3. Select Next to continue.

4. On the Email page, enter the alias name for the contact being created.

5. To create an email address for the contact, ensure that the Create an Exchange Email Address check box is selected.

6. Click the Modify button to begin creating an email address for the contact.

18

7. Select the SMTP Address option to create a contact address that will forward messages to an external Internet email account.

   Enter the fully qualified Internet email address to be use for the contact; for example: JohnDoe@CompanyABC.com.

   Use the Advanced tab to configure and override the default Internet mail message formats.

8. Click OK when done, validate the email address, and then select Next, Finish. This completes the process of creating a new contact.

Mail-Forwarding Options with Contacts

The primary function of contacts is to forward internal Exchange messages to external mail recipients. This function allows contacts to accept messages using the same domain name as all mail-enabled objects in Active Directory and to send these messages to a mail system outside the Exchange organization.

To create a contact to forward mail to an external SMTP email address, follow these steps:

1. Open the Active Directory Users and Computers management console, and select the Organizational Unit where the contact will be created.

2. From the Action menu, select New, Contact.

3. Enter the name of the contact and display name that will be used when viewing the contact in the Active Directory Global Catalog. Click the Next button to continue.

4. On the New Object page, ensure that Create an Exchange Email Address is selected. Click the Modify button to create the external SMTP email address where messages will be forwarded. Click Next when complete.

5. Review the information in the Summary page and click Finish when done.

Contact Email Address Types

Exchange contacts can be configured to communicate with multiple types of mail systems. Using the built-in address types of Exchange Server 2003 contacts, contacts and mail addresses can be configured to provide coexistence between mail systems or to communicate with other mail systems. Built into Exchange Server 2003, multiple email types are readily available as contact email options. In addition to the built-in mail address types shown in Table 18.1, other mail addresses types can be configured. Types can also be configured using the Custom Address option.

TABLE 18.1   Contact Address Types

X.400 Address	Microsoft Mail Address
SMTP Address	cc:Mail Address
Lotus Notes Address	Novell GroupWise Address

Additional Contact Address Types

In addition to these types of addresses, other contact addresses types can be configured using the Custom Address option. This option allows contacts to be mail-enabled with address types not listed in the New Email Address Type options tab.

Using Custom Email options can allow contacts to communicate with other types of mail systems when configuring other types of addresses for use with contacts; the administrator must configure the email address and mail system type. Additional configuration might be required when using this option, to allow Exchange Server 2003 to communicate with nonstandard mail system types.

Modifying and Adding Contact Email Addresses

When managing users and contacts, administrators are often required to modify addresses and address types. To accomplish this, administrators can simply modify the contact address by opening the Active Directory Users and Computers management console.

Select the contact that will be modified by expanding the domain tree and selecting the Organizational Unit where the contact resides.

Finding Contacts and Recipients

An additional method of finding contacts and other Active Directory objects is to use the Find Users, Contacts, and Groups tool built into the Active Directory Users and Computers management console. Properties of Active Directory objects can then be accessed by highlighting and right-clicking the Active Directory object.

Contact attributes can be modified by opening the properties page of the contact and modifying the desired attribute or email address.

Planning and Creating Distribution Groups

Distribution Groups are created when a collection of Active Directory Objects requires membership to a mail-enabled list in Exchange Server 2003. This allows the Distribution Group to receive messages to a single address in Exchange, which can then be distributed to all members of the group.

Also known as distribution lists in Microsoft Exchange 5.5, Distribution Groups can now be created to span domains. However, Distribution Groups posses no capability to be listed in the Active Directory Discretionary Access Control List (DACL) for purposes of assign permissions.

When working with Distribution Groups, functionality and replication depend on several domain and forest factors. Depending on the type of group—Universal, Global, or Local—and the Exchange server and domain functional levels where the group is created, each type of group can be configured to nest other groups or replicate across domains. In this section, we review the different Distribution Group scopes, the functionality of each scope, and how Distribution Groups are created.

> **NOTE**
>
> With Exchange Server 2003 and Active Directory, the scope of the Distribution Groups can easily be converted when the domain functional level is in Native Mode. Using the properties of the Distribution Group, administrators can select the scope and type that the Distribution Group can become.

Determining Distribution Group Scopes

Before creating Distribution Groups in Exchange Server 2003, it is important to understand what capabilities each scope enables. Distribution Groups can be created in one of the three following scopes: as a Universal Distribution Group, Domain Distribution Group, and Domain Local Distribution Group.

Each scope provides different functionality within the Active Directory domain and forest in which it reside. Depending on the scope of Distribution Group, other Distribution Groups, user accounts, and even contacts can be members of a single Distribution Group.

Review each type of group to assist in planning and creating the most appropriate Distribution Group for your organization.

- **Domain Local**   Best utilized in a single domain scenario, the Domain Local scope allows the following member types: account objects (user accounts, contacts), additional groups with the Domain Local scope, groups with the Global scope, and groups with the Universal scope. Each Domain Local group exists only within the domain it is created, and group membership is not present when viewing the Global Catalog.

- **Global**   Global Distribution Groups are configured when access to view the group is required in the Global Catalog. Although the Global Distribution Groups can be seen in the Global Catalog, membership of the group is not visible. Each Global group is present only within the domain it is created, and changes are not replicated outside to other domains.

- **Universal**   Universal groups allow administrators to nest nonreplication Global and Domain Local groups for ease of management. Use the Universal scope to consolidate Distribution Groups from multiple domains. All changes to universal groups are replicated to all Global Catalog servers in the forest. Nesting groups requires less replication traffic when changes occur to a member of the nested group.

Creating Distribution Groups

To create a Distribution Group, administrators must first determine the scope for the groups and the address name that the group will receive messages as. In this scenario, you will create a Distribution Group with the Global scope. This group will be mail-enabled to receive and distribute messages to all its members in the local domain.

To begin creating the Distribution Group, open the Active Directory Users and Computers management console and select the Organizational Unit where the Distribution Group will reside. Complete the following steps to add a Distribution Group to Active Directory:

1. From the Action menu tab, select New and then Group.

2. On the New Object Group tab, enter the name of the Distribution Group.

3. Make the scope for the distribution Global, and select the type of group as Distribution.

4. The Create In tab allows you to create the email address for the Distribution Group. Click the check box Create an Exchange Email address. This option mail-enables the Distribution Group.

5. If required, modify the alias name for the Distribution Group and select the Administrative Group that your group will be associated with. Click Next, Finish to finish creating the group.

> **NOTE**
>
> The Associated Administrative Group option is used to determine which default recipient policy and email address will be assigned to the Distribution Group.

Adding Distribution Group Membership

After the Distribution Group has been created, the administrator can add members to the group. To add members to the group, select the Distribution Group and open the properties of the group by selecting Action, Properties. Then complete the following steps:

1. From the Properties tab of the Distribution Group, select the Members tab.

2. Click the Add button to select the Active Directory accounts to be added to the group.

3. To show all the accounts in the domain, select the Advanced tab. Select the domain where the account resides and click Find Now. This searches Active Directory and displays all accounts and groups in the domain selected.

> **NOTE**
>
> To search for contacts, enable the contacts search function by selecting the Object Type tab and placing a check in the selection next to Contacts.

4. Select the account objects to be added as members to the Distribution Group. Select OK twice to return to the Members tab.

5. Repeat these steps until all members and objects have been added to the Distribution Group.

Creating Query-Based Distribution Groups

Query-based Distribution Groups are identical in functionality to a normal Distribution Group. The one benefit to the new Exchange Server 2003 feature is that query-based Distribution Groups assign group membership based on LDAP queries.

Available only in Exchange Server 2003 Native Mode, query-based Distribution Groups allow administrators to dynamically assign members to the group without having to perform the manual task of adding and removing account objects after the group is created.

For example, using the Filter option, if a query-based Distribution Group is created, membership can be defined by selecting all mail-enabled users within the Active Directory domain. This option adds all mail-enabled account objects to the Distribution Group membership; any new accounts also are added as they are mail-enabled in Active Directory.

Filter options for created query-based groups include the following:

- Users with Exchange Mailboxes
- Users with External Mail Addresses
- Mail-Enabled Groups
- Contacts with External Email Addresses
- Mail-Enabled Public Folders
- Customer Filters

To create a query-based Distribution Group, open the Active Directory Users and Computers management console, and select the Advanced Features option from the View menu.

1. Select the Organizational Unit where the query-based Distribution Group will be created. From the Action menu, select New, and Query-Based Distribution Group.

2. On the New Object tab, enter the name for the new query-based Distribution Group and select Next to continue.

3. For this exercise, click the Change button and select Domain.com, Users Organizational Unit. This option applies this filter to all users in the Users Organizational Unit. Next, select the Users with Exchange Mailbox option. This applies the option to all accounts in the User container with a mailbox.

4. Select Next to continue and Finish to finish creating the new query-based Distribution Group.

Managing and Maintaining Distribution Groups

As organizations grow and the Exchange Server 2003 tree becomes more complicated, administrators can find themselves faced with the task of managing and maintaining large numbers of Distribution Groups, as well as dealing with the effects of these groups when replicating across the network.

To simplify the day-to-day administrative tasks associated with adding and removing group memberships, administrators can now assign an Active Directory user account permissions to manage a Distribution Group. This account can be added to the Managed By tab of the Distribution Group properties, allowing the account to manage and update the membership list of the Distribution Group it is assigned.

Creating a Distribution Group Manager

To add an account to manage a Distribution Group, select the Distribution Group and open the properties pages of the Distribution Group by selecting File, Properties from the Active Directory Users and Computers management console. To add the account, complete the following steps:

1. Select the Managed By tab and click the Change button to add an account to manage the Distribution Group.

2. Click the Advanced tab and search Active Directory for the account to be added. Select the account and click the OK button when complete.

3. Select the Manager Can Update Membership List check box to enable permission for the account added, and click OK when complete.

The account added can now change and update the membership to the distribution list.

Managing Distribution Group Replication

Another area related to managing Distribution Groups is maintaining effective and seamless replication. In larger environments, changes to universal group memberships are replicated to all Global Catalog servers in the Active Directory forest and, in some cases, affect bandwidth availability over WAN links.

To avoid replication issues related to Distribution Groups, administrators can nest global groups and local groups with a single Universal group. By nesting groups, account changes and membership changes are completed at the domain level. Because these changes occur within the Global group and not the Universal group level, replication of changes to the Global Catalog server is not required.

Mail-Enabling Groups

With Exchange Server 2003, both distribution and security groups can be mail-enabled to receive messages for all members. Unlike a security group, a distribution group is strictly created for the association in Exchange to receive and distribute messages. When groups are converted from one type to another, they are not always automatically mail-enabled.

To mail-enable a group in Exchange Server 2003, first select the group in Active Directory Users and Computers and complete these steps:

1. From the Action menu, select Exchange Task.

2. On the Welcome to Exchange Task screen, select Next.

3. On the Available Task screen, select Establish Email Address on Groups and click Next.

4. Confirm the mail alias for the group and select Next.

5. Select Finish to finish adding an email address to the group.

It is always a good practice to open the properties page for the group and review the email addresses to ensure that they were added correctly.

Creating and Managing Exchange Server 2003 Administrative Groups

Exchange Server 2003 Administrative Groups are created to group and maintain Exchange objects for reasons of permissions management and administrative distribution. For example, if an organization is based in three locations worldwide with three groups of Exchange administrators in each location, three separate Administrative Groups can be created and managed by each location to maintain servers and policies in the separate Administrative Groups.

Exchange Server 2003 Administrative Groups are used to manage and maintain Routing Group containers, chat networks, public folder containers, and system policies. Each of these containers can house multiple objects and each can be managed individually.

Also, administrative Group functionality differs depending on the functional level of the Exchange Server 2003 organization, as well as the type of Administrative Group that is created.

> **Administrative Groups**
>
> By default, Administrative Groups are disabled in the Exchange Server 2003 System Manager. This is by design, to allow ease of viewing and management in the Exchange System Manager for smaller organizations. To enable Administrative Group functionality, select the properties page for the Exchange Server 2003 organization and select Display Administrative Groups.

Mixed Mode

When a new Exchange Server 2003 organization is installed, the Exchange organization is in Mixed Mode, by default. Mixed Mode facilitates interoperability between Exchange Server 2003 and Exchange 5.X servers. This also means that certain Administrative Group functionality is not available in a Mixed Mode environment.

When Exchange Server 2003 is in a Mixed Mode environment, the following is true:

- Exchange mailboxes cannot be moved between Administrative Groups.

- Routing Groups consist of only the server installed in the Administrative Group.

- Exchange 5.5 sites are mapped to Administrative Groups.

Native Mode

After an Exchange organization function level is raised to Native Mode, Exchange Administrative Group functionality is enhanced and limitations of a Mixed Mode environment are no longer a consideration. Administrative Group functionality in Native Mode includes the following:

- Exchange Mailboxes can be moved between Administrative Groups.

- Servers can be moved between Routing Groups.

- Routing Groups can contain servers from multiple Administrative Groups.

- Simple Mail Transport Protocol is enabled as the default routing protocol.

Administrative Groups Models

As we begin to grasp Administrative Groups and the purpose in both Native and Mixed Mode environments, the main design consideration is what model best fits your organizational needs.

In this section, we review two very simple concepts of Exchange Server 2003 Administrative Group management. The first is a centralized management model, and the second is a decentralized one. Because Exchange Administrative Groups are basically collections of objects grouped together for purposes of management, the structure and administrative topology of your organization could dictate the best administrative model for your organization.

Centralized

A centralized administrative model best fits an organization with fewer locations and a smaller centralized administrative staff. Because there is no need to distribute administrative permission, a centralized model is ideal for smaller organizations.

This model can also be effective in larger organizations. When a larger organization requires individual Exchange functionality to be managed by different groups or user accounts, a centralized model can still be implemented.

For example, CompanyABC is a larger organization with multiple Exchange servers and locations. However, the administrative model requires permissions to be configured for one group to manage the Routing Groups within the Administrative Group and another group of administrators to manage recipient policies.

Decentralized

A decentralized administrative model is very effective when larger organizations have multiple offices and require administration based on each location.

For example, CompanyABC has 40 Exchange servers with administrative staff in 10 separate locations. In this scenario, 10 Administrative Groups can be configured, and Exchange servers and recipient policies can be assigned to the appropriate Administrative Group for management.

Creating Administrative Groups in Exchange Server 2003

To create an Administrative Group in Exchange Server 2003, administrators must first enable the option to view Administrative Groups in the Exchange Systems Manager.

To enable viewing Administrative Groups, open the properties page of the Exchange organization and complete the following steps:

1. If the Administrative Groups are not visible in the Exchange System Manager, select the organization from the top of the Exchange tree. Select Action and Properties from the Exchange System Manager menu.

2. Check the Display Administrative Groups check box and click OK. This adds the Administrative Groups to the Exchange Systems Manager.

To add additional Administrative Groups in Exchange Server 2003, select the Administrative Groups container in the Exchange Systems Manager. Begin by following these steps:

1. From the Action menu, select New, Administrative Group.

2. On the Properties page, enter the name of the Administrative Group to be added. Click OK to continue.

3. After the Administrative Group is created, administrators can add system policy containers, Routing Group containers, and public folder containers.

Delegating Control over Administrative Groups

To manage and assign permission to Exchange Server 2003 Administrative Groups, administrators can leverage the Exchange Delegation Wizard.

Using the Delegation Wizard at the Administrative Group level assigns one of three roles to the account or group being assigned permissions over the Administrative Group. These three levels of permission are as follows:

- **Exchange View Only Administrator**   Allows administrators permissions to view objects of the Administrative Group but not change any properties of the Exchange object.

- **Exchange Full Administrator**   This role allows assign permissions to fully administer Exchange system objects and permissions.

- **Exchange Administrator**   The administrator role can fully administer Exchange system information only.

To assign roles and permissions over an Administrative Group using the Delegation Wizard, perform the following steps:

1. Select the Administrative Group where the delegation of roles will be assigned using the Delegation Wizard.

2. From the Action menu, select the Delegate Control options. On the Welcome to the Exchange Administration Delegation Wizard screen, select Next.

3. Click the Add button and select the Active Directory account or group being delegated control over the Administrative Group.

4. When the account or group has been selected, select the Exchange role to be assigned. Select OK to continue.

5. Select Next and Finish to finish delegating control over the Administrative Group.

Creating and Managing Routing Groups

In all but small single or multiple Exchange server organizations, there is a need for more complex configurations to connect multiple Exchange servers. In these scenarios, locations and Exchange servers are connected using Routing Groups and Routing Group connectors.

18

As multiple Routing Groups are created, each Routing Group can be connected by creating an Exchange Routing Group connector using multiple connection types:

- Routing Group Connector

- SMTP Connector

- X.400 Connector

Routing Groups are located in the Exchange System Manager and are located in each Administrative Group. A single Routing Group is self-sufficient and possesses certain limitations when in a Exchange Server 2003 Mixed Mode environment.

Understanding Exchange Server 2003 Routing Groups

A Routing Group is a collection of Exchange servers that communicate with each other directly over the same internal network or reliable connection.

When multiple Routing Groups must be created, each individual group must be connected using one of three available Exchange connection types:

- **Routing Group Connector**   This connector is the default connector type. It can be used to connect a single or multiple Exchange bridgehead server for load balancing of message traffic.

- **SMTP Connector**   The SMTP connector uses the Simple Mail Transport Protocol to connect and communicate with remote Routing Groups, non-Exchange mail systems, and the Internet mail host.

- **X.400 Mail Connector**   Limited to a single local and remote host, the X.400 connector is primarily designed for communications between Exchange Server 2003 and X.400 mail systems.

Mixed Mode
When Exchange Server 2003 is in a mixed environment, Routing Groups can consist of only servers that had been installed directly into the Administrative Group where the Routing Group resides. Additional servers from other Administrative Groups cannot be added to the Routing Group.

Native Mode
After the functional level has been raised to Native Mode, Exchange servers can be managed and moved between Routing Groups.

Also, Routing Groups in a single Administrative Group can contain servers from other Administrative Groups.

Installing Routing Groups

Depending on whether you are installing additional Routing Groups into the existing Administrative Group, different tasks must be performed to create new Routing Groups.

To create and establish Routing Groups within a new Exchange Administrative Group, the first step is to create the Routing Group container. The Routing Group container is similar to a folder in Windows Explorer and is used to house and organize one or more Routing Groups.

> **NOTE**
>
> The default first Administrative Group contains the default Routing Group container. Only one Routing Group container is allowed in each Administrative Group. Multiple Routing Groups can then be added to each Routing Group container.

When creating and configuring a new Routing Group into a new Administrative Group, the first step is to create the routing container. To install the Routing Group container, begin by selecting the new Administrative Group in the Exchange System Manager where the container will be located.

1. Select the Action menu from the Exchange System Manager and select New, Routing Group Container. This creates a container called Routing Groups.

2. To begin installing individual Routing Groups, from the Exchange System Manager, select the Routing Group container where the Routing Groups will reside.

3. From the Action menu, select New, Routing Group.

4. Enter the name of the new Routing Group, and enter any details or administrative descriptions in the Detail tab. Select OK when finished.

Moving Exchange Servers Between Routing Groups

After Administrative Groups have been populated with Exchange servers and Routing Groups, one task often completed is moving servers between Routing Groups. This task is usually performed as administrators begin to create a more complex Exchange organization and routing infrastructure.

With Exchange Server 2003, administrators can move Exchange server between Routing Groups. However, one limitation is that Exchange servers cannot be moved between Administrative Groups.

To move an Exchange server to a different Routing Group, begin by opening the Exchange System Manager. Expand the Routing Group folder where the Exchange server resided, and expand the Routing Group folder where the Exchange server will be placed. Simply drag and drop the Exchange server object from the source Routing Group to the destination Routing Group.

18

> **CAUTION**
>
> When using and configuring Routing Groups, ensure that new Exchange servers are installed in the proper Administrative Group where their Routing Group resides. Exchange Server 2003 systems cannot be moved between Administrative Groups in Exchange Server 2003.

Using Recipient Policies

Exchange Server 2003 contains two type of recipient policies. The first type of recipient policy deals with mail-enabled objects and how email addresses are created based on naming conventions defined in the policy. The second addresses management of end-user mailboxes and the limitation that can be applied to user mailboxes based on policy membership.

Recipient policies can be created to define how naming conventions will be applied to mail-enabled objects in Exchange. By creating a recipient policy, administrators can define how usernames of specific email address types will be viewed in Exchange when an object is mail-enabled.

Different from email-based policies, mailbox recipient policies deal with setting mailbox restrictions such as size limits and age limits; they are configured in the same location as email-based policies. Defining mailbox recipient policies can allow administrators to control and manage the total amount of data retained in the Exchange information store.

> **NOTE**
>
> For more information on mailbox recipient policies, see section "Using the Mailbox Manager Utility," later in this chapter.

When a policy is created, each type of recipient policy can be assigned to specific users and mail-enabled objects within Active Directory by defining policy membership during the creation of the policy.

For example, an SMTP mail recipient policy can be created to ensure that all users who belong to the Users Organizational Unit will be enabled with an SMTP email address using the following naming convention:

Username = Jill Summer

SMTP address = CompanyABC.com

SMTP email address = SummerJ@CompanyABC.com

Implementing Email Address Recipient Policies

When Exchange Server 2003 is installed, a default recipient policy is created to assign an SMTP address and X.400 address to be used for all mail-enabled Active Directory objects.

This recipient policy defines how all mail-enabled Active Directory objects will be assigned email addresses in Exchange. It is based on the Active Directory domain name where the Exchange server is installed.

When creating additional email-based recipient policies, administrators can define several attributes for each policy created. Beginning with policy membership, administrators can assign a recipient policy to a specified group of users only. Additional address types also can be assigned to specific groups of users.

Along with the default email address, other email types are preconfigured and available to be added as recipient policy email addresses. Additional email types are most often defined when creating coexistence between Exchange Server 2003 and other messaging systems. Exchange Server 2003 supports X.400, SMTP, Lotus Notes, Microsoft Mail, cc:Mail, and Novell GroupWise addressing, by default. Custom addresses can be defined for a message type that is not built into Exchange Server 2003.

Defining Recipient Policy Naming Standards

By default, email-based recipients use the default `UserName@domainname.com` naming standard. Administrators can define string values to change the default rules that determine how user naming conventions will be implemented. These are naming attributes or values that determine the way a user's name will be defined and displayed—for example, first name.last name or the first initial and then last name. Using the value strings listed here, administrators can modify the default recipient policy or create a new policy to customize the name convention based on specific organizational needs.

Use the following values to modify recipient email addresses and naming conventions:

> %g = Given name (first name).
>
> %s = Surname (last name).
>
> %i = Middle name.
>
> %d = Display name.
>
> %m = Exchange alias name.
>
> %r = Replace character x with the character y in the username—for example, in %rxy, if the character x = y, the character will be deleted in the user's name.

Naming conventions can also be defined by the total number of characters in the name, as well as additional characters such as periods between names.

For example, by placing a number in front of the naming value, administrators can define how many characters will be displayed for that name type. Notice the period between the naming values; this adds a period between the first initial and the last name.

Example:

```
%1g.%s@ComanyABC.com = J.Doe@ComanyABC.com
```

18

Defining Recipient Policy Membership Using Search Filters

Each recipient policy can be applied to Exchange mail-enabled objects by using filters to define policy memberships. As with defining other memberships, policy memberships are defined using the same Active Directory Search tool. The Active Directory Search tool allows membership to be defined in the following areas:

- Users with Exchange Mailboxes
- Users with External Mail Addresses
- Mail-Enabled Groups
- Contacts with External Email Addresses
- Mail Enabled Public Folders
- Query-Based Distribution Groups

Implementing Mailbox Recipient Policies

To create a recipient policy, you need to define the criteria based on the previous information used in this example:

1. Policy will be applied to Users with Exchange Mailboxes.
2. Domain name CompanyABC.com will be added as a primary SMTP address.
3. String values will be added to create a first initial and last name standard.

To begin creating the new recipient policy, open the Exchange Server System Manager and follow these steps.

1. Select the recipient container and then Recipient Policies.
2. Select the Action menu and choose New, Recipient Policy.
3. In the New Policy dialog box, check the Email Address options and click OK to continue.
4. On the Properties tab of the new recipient policy, enter the name for the new policy.
5. To define policy membership, select the Modify button under Filter Rules.
6. Ensure that the Users with Exchange Mailboxes is the only option selected and click OK.
7. When you select OK, the message shown in Figure 18.4 appears.

   This dialog box reminds administrators that changes must be applied before they become effective. Click OK to continue.

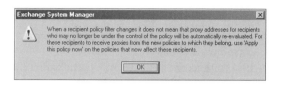

FIGURE 18.4   Exchange System Manager Proxy Address dialog box.

8. Now that the membership has been defined, select the Email Addresses (Policy) tab to define the email address and naming convention.

9. The default domain name and X.400 address appear in the Address Types dialog box. In this scenario, an additional SMTP address will be defined and added to the policy. Select New to begin adding the CompanyABC.com SMTP address.

10. Select the SMTP Address option, and click OK to continue.

11. On the SMTP Address Properties page, enter **n** the naming values and SMTP domain name defined earlier in the section (see Figure 18.5). Select Apply, OK to continue.

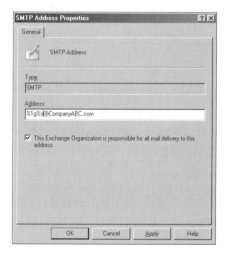

FIGURE 18.5   SMTP Address Properties page.

12. On the Email Address Properties page, the new address appears. To set the new address as the primary SMTP address, check the box next to the new address and select Set As Primary. The option sets the new address in bold and creates the address as the primary SMTP address for all policy members.

13. Select OK to continue. You are prompted to update all corresponding email addresses for the members of the new policy. Select Yes to apply the changes.

Editing and Changing Existing Recipient Policies

Each recipient policy can be modified simply by changing the listed values that already have been defined. When a policy is created in Exchange Server 2003, all attributes and addresses can be modified as long as the account has permissions to manage and change Exchange Server 2003 objects.

To modify existing policies or event default policy, the administrator can simply perform the following steps:

1. Open the policy to be modified for the recipient policy container by selecting the policy. Click the Action menu and select Properties.

2. Modify the desired values and properties of the policy.

3. Select OK from the Policy properties page. A dialog box is displayed. Click OK to apply the changes to all policy members.

WARNING

Clicking OK to apply the changes causes all receipt members to receive the policy change. Review the changes and make sure that no undesired modifications will be applied. Incorrect settings can disable email functionality for users who do not need the policy change.

Administering Recipient Update Services

Recipient Update Services, also known as RUS, are used to apply SMTP domains to recipients residing in domains where Exchange Server 2003 is not installed. The RUS is also responsible for managing and maintaining address list membership and updating address changes to ensure that accurate information is available at all times.

When installing Exchange Server 2003, each Exchange organization is installed with a default RUS. When installed, the default service contains two individual services. One is responsible for managing mail addresses and lists at the enterprise level, and the other is responsible for doing so at the domain level.

When working with multidomain environments, it is not always cost-effective or feasible to install multiple Exchange Server 2003 systems to support small amounts of users in each domain. RUS can assist in providing email functionality to accounts that belong to other domains in the Active Directory forest.

Understanding Recipient Update Services

The Recipient Update Services in Exchange Server 2003 are responsible for providing SMTP domain email functionality within and beyond the default domain where the Exchange server is installed. This means that administrators can now prepare and mail-enable accounts in additional domains without actually installing Exchange Server 2003 directly into the domain.

Managing Recipient Update Services

To create, modify, and delete a RUS, the administrator must posses the Exchange Full Administrator role in the Exchange organization where the service is being managed.

In addition, any Exchange server services in additional domains will be granted permission to modify Exchange properties in the domain being serviced by the RUS.

Another key function of RUS is to provide and replicate accurate and detailed address list information to other domains in the Active Directory forest.

Each RUS can also be configured to replicate information on a predefined schedule to provide optimal network performance and avoid bandwidth saturation when replicating changes across WAN links.

Deploying Recipient Update Services

Additional Recipient Update Services can be created to provide support in domains both with and without Exchange Server 2003. Most important, understanding the requirements for creating a RUS can avoid any problems when mail-enabling recipients in another domain.

To create a RUS to provide support in a domain where Exchange is not installed, the domain must first be prepped to provide Exchange Server 2003 support:

1. From a domain controller in the domain without Exchange, insert the Exchange Server 2003 CD-ROM into the CD drive.

2. Click Start, Run from the Start menu on the Windows domain controller.

3. The domain where email functionality will be enabled must be Domainprep before the RUS can be created. Using a domain administrator account, enter **D:\I386\Setup.exe /domainprep** in the Run command dialog box (D: represents the drive letter of the CD-ROM drive on the domain controller).

NOTE

For more information on the Domainprep task, see Chapter 3, "Installing Exchange Server 2003."

After the domain has been prepared for Exchange Server 2003, a RUS installation is the same for domains adding additional services and domains without Exchange Server 2003. To establish a RUS to provide email support to the domain members, create the service for the domain by following these steps:

18

1. Open the Exchange System Manager and select the RUS container.

2. On the Exchange System Manager menu, select the Action option and click New, Recipient Update Service.

3. On the New Object Recipient Update Service dialog box, click Browse. Select the domain where the recipient update service will function. Click OK when complete.

4. On the second New Object Recipient Update Service screen, select the Exchange server responsible for servicing the domain. Click the Browse button to open the Active Directory Search tool, and select the Exchange server providing the service. Click the OK button to return to the New Object screen, and select Next to continue.

5. Review the information provided to ensure that the configuration is correct, and select Finish.

Managing Recipient Update Services

RUS can be managed in multiple ways to help with server performance and network bandwidth. As an organization becomes larger and server performance, availability, and even replacement become a factor, services and communication can be modified on the RUS to use other domain controllers and Exchange servers in the forest and domain.

Service can also be scheduled to replicate at nonpeak network traffic hours, to avoid bandwidth issues and network performance issues. In addition to scheduled replication, changes and updates to the address list can be pushed manually by administrators to force update changes.

Performing a Manual Update with Recipient Update Services

Also, when applying changes to the address list, administrators can push changes and update directory information directly from the Exchange System Manager, ensuring that updates are processed immediately. To force a recipient update manually, complete the following steps:

1. From the Exchange System Manager, select the RUS responsible for providing the update needed.

2. On the Exchange System Manager menu, select Action, Update Now. This manually forces the system's update to other Global Catalogs and domains in the forest.

Setting and Configuring an Update Schedule

When a RUS is created, it must replicate changes with other domains to ensure that the address list and email addresses are applied and viewed correctly and that the information is accurate and always up-to-date. To accomplish this, each RUS is configured with an update schedule that is also created when the service is created.

By default, the replication schedule is set to run every hour. However, the replication schedule is fully configurable and can be changed to meet network and organizational needs.

Administrators might modify the default schedules for several reasons. For example, changes to the address list need to be replicated sooner than every hour in some cases.

Things to Know About Scheduling

When custom schedules are configured, each update is run at the beginning of the schedule block configured. Allow enough time for the address list to update before the next replication occurs.

Important: When the Never Run schedule option is selected, no changes or modifications to address lists and email addresses are applied. This is true even in the domain that the recipient update service is servicing.

Using the Update Interval Selections drop down box, preconfigured Exchange replication schedules can be selected and configured to provide accurate replication.

To modify the default schedule, open the Exchange System Manager and select the RUS where the schedule will be modified. To change the replication schedule, complete the following steps:

1. Scheduling options are located on the properties page of the RUS. To open the RUS properties, select the Action option from the Exchange System Manager menu and select Properties.

2. To configure a new update schedule, select a preconfigured schedule from the Update Interval drop-down menu or click Customize to create a custom schedule.

3. After the schedule has been configured, select Apply to save the changes and close the properties of the RUS.

Using the Mailbox Recovery Center Tool

One of the most exciting new features of Exchange Server 2003 is the Mailbox Recovery Center tool. Integrated into the Exchange System Manager, this tool allows administrators to automatically reconnect disassociated mailboxes back to Active Directory accounts. In addition, recovering individual mailboxes and multiple mailboxes can be completed simultaneously using the Exchange System Manager.

Mailbox conflicts between Active Directory accounts can now be identified and resolved using the Mailbox Recovery Center, and mailboxes can be merged as well.

Identifying Disconnected Mailboxes

When a mailbox is disassociated from the Active Directory account it was originally created for, it becomes a disconnected mailbox in Exchange. This can occur if an Active

Directory account is deleted and the mailbox was not marked for deletion, or if the account has somehow become corrupted and is no longer available.

These disconnected mailboxes are displayed in the Exchange Systems Manager by placing a large red X next to the mailbox name, indicating that the mailbox is in a disconnected state. In some instances these mailboxes are not marked as disconnected. When this occurs, the Mailbox Recovery Center tool can be used to identify these mailboxes when they are not visible as disconnected in the mailbox store.

To identify disconnected mailboxes using the Mailbox Recovery Center tool, begin by adding the mailbox store to the Mailbox Recovery Center in the Exchange Systems Manager. To do so, complete the following steps:

1. Open the Exchange System Manager and open the Tools container. From the Tools container, highlight the Mailbox Recovery Center.

2. From the Exchange System Manager menu, select Action, Add Mailbox Store. Enter the name of the mailbox store to be added, or select the Advanced function to perform a search for the mailbox store. When the appropriate mailbox store has been selected, choose OK to continue.

3. Now that the mailbox store has been added to the Recovery Center, any disconnected mailboxes residing in the mail store will appear in the right pane, as shown in Figure 18.6.

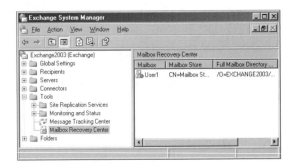

FIGURE 18.6   Recovery Center disconnected accounts.

TIP

When tasks are completed using the Mailbox Recovery Center tool, it is a best practice to remove the mail store from the tool.

Resolving Mailbox Conflicts

When mailboxes become disconnected or conflict with multiple Active Directory Accounts, the Mailbox Recovery Center tool provides a seamless method to resolve these conflicts and prepare the Exchange mailbox for reconnection.

To resolve a conflicting mailbox in Exchange Server 2003, open the Exchange System Manager. Begin by completing these steps:

1. From the Tools container, highlight the Mailbox Recovery Center tool.

2. From the Exchange System Manager menu, select Action, Add Mailbox Store. Enter the name of the mailbox store to be added, or select the Advanced function to perform a search. When the appropriate mailbox store has been selected, choose OK to continue.

3. In the Mailbox Recovery Center tool's right pane, select the mailbox or mailboxes to be resolved by highlighting each mailbox.

4. From the Exchange System Manager menu, select the Action menu and choose Resolve Conflicts.

5. On the Welcome to Exchange Mailbox Conflicts Resolution Wizard screen, select Next.

6. Using the User Matching screen, select the Active Directory account or account to be resolved. If the account is not present, click the Browse button to search Active Directory for the account that the mailbox was associated with.

7. When the account has been selected, choose Next to continue. On the final screen, you should see the message "Wizard has enough information to correct the problem and prepare the account for reconnection." Select Finish to complete the tasks.

Matching and Recovering Mailboxes

One advantage to using the Mailbox Recovery Center tool is that you can match mailboxes to non–mail-enabled accounts in Active Directory. For example, if an Active Directory account is deleted, administrators can create a new account with the same name and use the Mailbox Recovery Center tool to reassociate the mailbox to a new non–mail-enabled account. This option can be used even when the mailbox is marked for deletion.

To re-create an account and reconnect a mailbox, begin by doing the following:

1. Create the account or accounts in Active Directory Users and Computers using the same name or names as the mailboxes being recovered.

2. Open the Exchange System Manager and select the Tools container. Highlight the Mailbox Recovery Center tool.

3. On the Exchange System Manager menu, select Action, Add Mailbox Store. Enter the name of the mailbox store where the mailboxes being recovered reside, or select the

18

Advanced function to search for the mailbox store. When the appropriate mailbox store has been selected, choose OK to continue.

4. In the Mailbox Recovery Center tool's right pane, select the mailbox or mailboxes to be recovered by highlighting each mailbox.

5. From the Exchange System Manager menu, select the Action menu and choose Find Match. This begins the Mailbox Recovery Center tool's search for the correct Active Directory accounts.

6. At the Welcome to Microsoft Exchange Mailbox Matching Wizard, select Next, review the result of the match, and choose Finish to complete matching the mailbox to the Active Directory user account.

> **NOTE**
>
> If no match is found by the Match Wizard, perform the steps in the Resolving Mailbox Conflicts section to search for the mailbox and associate it to a user account. Then repeat the step to match the mailbox to the Active Directory account.

When the Match Wizard has completed, run the Reconnect tool to reconnect the mailboxes to the Active Directory account by performing the following steps:

1. In the Mailbox Recovery Center tool's right pane, select the mailbox or mailboxes to be reconnected by highlighting each mailbox.

2. From the Exchange System Manager menu, select the Action menu and choose Reconnect.

3. At the Welcome to the Exchange Mailbox Reconnect Wizard, select Next.

4. Review the information provided in the Ready to Proceed dialog box and select Next to continue.

5. Review the results of the reconnect, and click Finish when done.

Using the Mailbox Manager Utility

A familiar tool to Exchange 2000 administrators is the Mailbox Manager utility. This utility is now built into Exchange Server 2003 and is installed by default when the Exchange server is installed and configured.

In Exchange Server 2003, Mailbox Manager tasks are configured differently than in previous versions of Exchange. These tasks are now configured using the mailbox recipient policies. Mailbox recipient policies are used to manage and enforce email-retention policies and cleanup tasks in the same manner that these tasks were previously configured. The one benefit to using the policies in Exchange Server 2003 is that they are now replicated to all Exchange servers in the organization by the Recipient Update Service, eliminating the need to configure mailbox management on every server when performing mailbox-cleanup tasks.

These policies can be created and configured to move or delete mailbox items based on size and age limits, specific folders, and times when the Mailbox Manager should be run by the policy.

Accessing the Mailbox Manager

Mailbox recipient policies are created using the recipient policies container. Using the Exchange System Manager, administrators can add mailbox recipient policies via the same method used to add standard recipient policies.

By selecting the recipient policy container in the Exchange System Manager and choosing the Action menu, new recipient policies can be created to perform the mailbox-cleanup task.

When a policy is configured and created, the recipient policies container can be used on any Exchange server in the organization to view and modify the mailbox recipient policy.

Understanding Mailboxes Manager Options

When creating a policy for the Mailbox Manager to run, administrators need to understand the different tasks' options and the implications of using each option when it is added to a recipient policy.

When configuring options using the mailbox recipient policy, policies can easily be created by selecting the preconfigured tasks available. To understand the different options available, review the following descriptions of the preconfigured tasks.

Move to Deleted Items

Working with the limits configured in the policy, this option moves all items meeting the configured limits to the Deleted Items folder in the Exchange mailbox.

Move to System Cleanup

An effective way to move and keep items in case recovery is needed is to use the System Cleanup option. This creates a partial replica of the mailbox folders. Each item exceeding the policy limits is then moved to corresponding system folders and stored.

Using the System Folders

When the Move Messages to the System Folders option is configured using the Mailbox Manager, a replica of the user mailbox hierarchy is created and placed in a folder called System Cleanup. Deleted messages are then moved to the same folder where they resided in the user's mailbox, creating a partial replica of the user mailbox.

This option is often used as an alternative to placing aged messages in the Deleted Items folder. When the Deleted Items folder option is selected, if a user has selected to enable the option to empty deleted items when logging off, messages are deleted permanently, requiring a restore if a message needs to be recovered.

> The system folders can easily restore messages to the original location and archive information based on the recovery period configured through the Mailbox Manager.

Delete Immediately

The Delete Immediately option is the most aggressive of all cleanup task options. This option immediately deletes all items exceeding the configured policy limits.

Generate Report Only

When using this option, no messages are affected; this option is often best implemented to determine the total effect of actually running a policy that will delete or move items. The result can then be reviewed and evaluated by administrators before performing the actual tasks.

Reporting with Mailbox Manager

As a best practice, it is often a good idea to create a recipient policy in Generate Report Only mode to identify message totals and sizes that will be deleted when the actual tasks are performed. When this option is selected, a report can be generated in two methods:

- **Send Summary Report to Administrator**   This option provides administrators with the total size of all messages deleted or moved to other folders during the mailbox-cleanup process.

- **Send Detailed Report to Administrator**   This option provides administrators with a complete report, listing the policies, folders, and messages that the Mailbox Manager processed during cleanup.

To create a new report-only task, begin by opening the Exchange System Manager and selecting the recipient policies container. Begin configuring the new mailbox recipient policy in Report Only mode by completing the following steps:

1. Select Action from the Exchange System Manager menu, and select New, Recipient Policy.

2. Select the Mailbox Manager Settings option on the New Policy dialog box screen, and click OK to continue.

3. On the Properties page for the mailbox recipient policy, enter the name **Report Policy** in the Name field.

4. Select the Modify tab to assign policy membership for the mailbox policy. For this exercise, select Users with Exchange Mailboxes only and click OK to continue.

5. In the Recipient Policy Change dialog box, click OK.

6. Select the Mailbox Manager Setting (Policy) tab. From the Processing a Mailbox drop-down menu, select Generate Report Only.

7. For this exercise, leave all the default options in place and click the OK button to continue.

Configuring Mailbox-Cleanup Tasks

To configure an actual mailbox-cleanup task, administrators need to determine the message size limits and age limits before configuring the mailbox recipient policy. When a new policy is created, Exchange Server 2003 defaults the message limits to the following values:

> Message size limits = 1024KB.
>
> Message age limits = 30 days.
>
> All folders in the Exchange mailbox are selected.

In this scenario, the default values will be used when creating the new mailbox recipient policy. To create the recipient policy, begin by opening the Exchange System Manager and complete these steps:

1. Click the Recipients container and select the recipients policies container.

2. On the Exchange System Manager menu, select Action, New, Recipient policy.

3. Select the Mailbox Manager Settings option on the New Policy dialog box, and click the OK button to continue.

4. On the Properties page for the mailbox recipient policy, enter the name for the cleanup policy in the Name field.

5. Select the Modify tab to assign policy membership for the mailbox policy. For this exercise, select the Users with Exchange Mailboxes tab and click OK to continue.

6. On the Recipient Policy Change dialog box, click OK.

7. Select the Mailbox Manager Setting (Policy) tab to configure the cleanup tasks for this policy.

8. At the Mailbox Manager Setting page, select the options for the mailbox-cleanup tasks being configured. Review the selection, as shown in Figure 18.7, and select the folder for which the Mailbox Manager will perform the cleanup tasks.

Scheduling Mailbox Manager Tasks

After the Mailbox recipient policy has been created, the next step is to plan and configure the schedule to run the Mailbox Manager task. If no corresponding schedule is created for

the mailbox recipient policy, the policy configuration will not be implemented and the
tasks will not run.

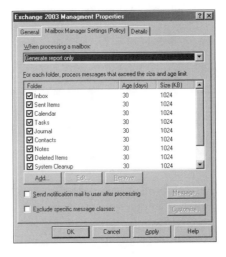

FIGURE 18.7   Mailbox Manager settings.

When planning and configuring a schedule, one important consideration is determining
when it is best to run the scheduled task. Because mailbox-cleanup tasks can be demanding on Exchange server resources and the information store, as a best practice, Exchange
administrators should plan and schedule cleanup tasks to occur during off-hours, when
the Exchange system is in less demand.

To begin configuring the schedule, follow these steps:

1. Open the Exchange System Manager and select the Exchange server where the tasks
   will run.

2. With the Exchange server highlighted, select the Action option for the Exchange
   System Manager and select Properties.

3. Click the Mailbox Management tab on the Exchange server to configure the schedule for the policy to run.

   • **Start Mailbox Management Process**   This option allows administrators
     to select a predefined schedule for the policy to use. Administrators also can
     select Custom to create a custom schedule by selecting the Customize tab.

   • **Reporting**   With this option, a detailed or summary report is sent to the
     administrator account defined in the Administrator tab.

   • **Administrator**   Use the Browse tab to select an administrator account that
     will receive the report when the task is run.

> **NOTE**
>
> Although each mailbox recipient policy is replicated to all Exchange servers, the administrator must configure the schedule for the policy to run on each server in the organization.

Summary

As validated by the length of this chapter, a lot of things can be done to administer an Exchange environment. Administration can be broken down into delegating administration in Exchange; administering mailboxes, contacts, and Distribution Groups; and managing Administrative Groups and Routing Groups.

The delegation of administration in Exchange Server 2003 gives the organization the capability to distribute administration across multiple Exchange administrators equally or with varying levels of delegated authority. The delegation task sets up the framework from which the task of managing and administering objects in Exchange can be conducted.

After delegation has been assigned, the various levels of administrators can manage mailboxes for creating mailboxes, setting default address settings, moving mail between servers, and even recovering mailboxes that were accidentally deleted. The mail and mailbox administrative tools included in Exchange Server 2003 give administrators a variety of rights and privileges to make administrative changes as necessary.

Beyond just dealing with users with mailboxes, Exchange Server 2003 provides administrative controls over Distribution Groups for mailing lists of users, as well as contacts that are associated with email addresses without mailboxes assigned. Managing these objects provides the administrator naming resources that simplify the addressing of mail users in the organization.

Finally, managing Administrative Groups and Routing Groups separates administrative boundaries as well as message-routing boundaries, to partition administration and management as appropriate for an organization.

All of these administrative functions might be complicated when viewed as a whole, but when trying to make an Exchange environment work in a fashion that suits the needs of an organization, the various tools and functions greatly help administrators with their tasks. After more than five generations in development, Exchange Server 2003 provides a variety of flexible administrative methods for managing the Exchange administrative environment.

Best Practices

- Most administrators of the Exchange environment should be set as Exchange Administrators, leaving the Exchange Full Administrator role only to one individual, who will have the authority to grant the Exchange Administrator right to others.

- Exchange View Only Administrators should be used for operations staff, network infrastructure staff, or other administrators who need to view the status of Exchange functions but who should not need to directly modify or make changes to the functions.

- Auditing should be enabled to track all administrative changes in Exchange. This ensures a trail for viewing modifications or changes to key Exchange settings.

- Message and storage limits give administrators the capability to control the size of messages sent or received, or the amount of message space a user may store for messages. An organization can set up different groups with different message and storage limits, thus setting an organization standard configuration while allowing certain users to exceed the standard.

- With wireless mobility built into Exchange Server 2003, an administrator can allow users to synchronize their Pocket PC–enabled device or view messages using their HTML-enabled mobile phones.

- The ExMerge utility not only provides administrators the capability to back up mailboxes for a migration, but it also allows administrators to move mailboxes from one server to another in case a user needs to move between Exchange sites.

- Moving mailboxes between databases or servers within an Exchange Site can be done by simply using the Mailbox Move tool built into the Exchange System Manager.

- Contacts are used in the Exchange System Manager to enable an address where mail messages can be forwarded to another address. This is commonly used to reroute or forward messages out of the Exchange environment into another messaging system, possibly during a migration or in a mixed-mail environment.

- Distribution Groups can be used to create internal mailing lists that might be different from security groups created within Windows. When possible, try to create a Windows security group and mail-enable the group rather than creating separate security groups and Distribution Groups that include the same list of users.

- Query-based Distribution Groups should be used when group membership might change. The use of query-based Distribution Groups can dynamically create a distribution list based on an Active Directory user's Object Properties information.

- Routing Groups should be created any time messages should be throttled between locations. This might be to manage communication between locations over a slow or unreliable communications line, or to provide redundancy between sites.

- Administrative Groups should be created to set up administrative boundaries in an organization. However, if all administrators will share administrative responsibilities (that is, every administrator is a member of each Administrative Group), the organization should seriously consider a single Administrative Group and simplify the process.

- The Mailbox Recovery Center tool can recover disconnected mailboxes or resolve mailbox conflicts. However, it does not fix corrupted mailboxes. An organization should leverage mailbox-recovery functions covered in Chapter 32, "Recovering from a Disaster," for mailbox recovery due to data corruption.

- The Mailbox Manager utility should be used to clean up an Exchange messaging system of unused objects, report on the status of Exchange mail transactions, and perform automated cleanup tasks on mailboxes.

CHAPTER 19

Exchange Server 2003 Management and Maintenance Practices

The messaging system in most environments has come to be considered a mission-critical application. People are reliant on messaging as a primary form of communication. As a direct result, messaging dependability is no longer just a good thing to have—it is a requirement.

An integral part of ensuring that any system is dependable or reliable is care and feeding. Take the classic car example for instance. You should change the oil every 3,000–6,000 miles, replace air filters, change fuel filters, and more. In fact, even when you buy a new car the car dealership recommends a maintenance schedule to keep your car healthy.

The same principles apply when you are trying to keep Exchange Server 2003 running as smoothly as possible. Proper management and maintenance minimizes downtime and other problems and keeps the system well tuned. The more Exchange Server 2003 management and maintenance processes and procedures are neglected, the higher your chances of the system slowing to a crawl, becoming corrupted, or even being unavailable for any extended period of time. This chapter focuses on the details and best practices necessary for a knowledgeable administrator or engineer to manage and maintain the Exchange Server 2003 messaging environment to keep it stable and reliable.

Managing Exchange Server 2003

Managing Exchange Server 2003 in this context is not about how to perform necessarily common tasks such as using the interface to add a database. Instead, managing Exchange

Server 2003 includes identifying and working with the server's functional roles in the network environment, auditing network activity and usage, and monitoring the environment.

Similarly with Windows Server 2003, Microsoft has come a long way with how servers can be managed. Exchange Server 2003 management can be done locally or remotely. Although local and remote management could be done in previous Exchange versions, Exchange Server 2003 supercedes that functionality with new and improved processes and tools that assist administrators in their management.

Managing by Server Roles and Responsibilities

Exchange Server 2003 systems can participate in various responsibilities in the messaging environment. Some of these responsibilities may be intertwined due to budget constraints, business requirements, or technical justifications. No matter how the roles and responsibilities play out in the environment, it's important to manage them appropriately based on the roles of the server. The management aspects for some of the roles that Exchange Server 2003 can undertake are listed in the following sections.

Mailbox Store Server

An Exchange Server 2003 mailbox store server, also known as a back-end server, is primarily responsible for safely storing a mail-enabled user's messages, attachments, files, folders, and other files. Messages sent to a user are stored in the user's mailbox, which is contained within a mailbox store.

For this reason, the mailbox store databases require attention using the Exchange System Manager (ESM) and frequent maintenance routines. Refer to "Best Practices for Performing Database Maintenance" for more information. Equally important, however, is managing user accounts.

Public Folder Server

Similar to the mailbox store server role, the public folder server role stores message postings and other messages in a hierarchical fashion. Although there isn't a user object specifically associated with a public folder, an entire public folder database is dedicated to a single public folder hierarchy. When the system has multiple public folders, there will be multiple databases to manage and maintain.

Front-end Server

Front-end (FE) servers are Exchange Server 2003 servers that do not contain mailbox or public folder stores. In fact, FE servers typically serve as proxy servers to back-end (mailbox or public folder) servers. FE servers are possible because Internet Information Server (IIS) manages messaging-related protocols, such as Internet Message Access Protocol version 4 (IMAP4), Post Office Protocol version 3 (POP3), Network News Transfer Protocol (NNTP), and Messaging Application Programming Interface (MAPI). One of the most common roles of an FE server is to provide Web access to back-end mailbox or public folder stores using Outlook Web Access (OWA).

Although there aren't any databases to manage or maintain on an FE server, keep the following important considerations in mind:

- **Connections**   Users connect to FE servers using HTTP. They may also connect via Secure Sockets Layer (SSL) for encrypted communications if the server is configured for increased protection. These connections are important to monitor, especially when the FE server is on the perimeter network (also known as the DMZ) or otherwise facing the Internet. Another management and maintenance aspect to keep in mind is authentication and access controls. Periodically review the event logs to review security issues.

- **IIS Metabase**   Because IIS is one of the driving forces behind an FE server, it is critical to manage the IIS metabase to maximize the server's health. This can involve keeping the metabase backed up, reviewing IIS logs, and reviewing security.

Bridgehead Server

An Exchange Server 2003 bridgehead server is a connection point among other Exchange servers either inside or outside the organization. It connects other servers that use the same communications protocols. The most notable examples are bridgehead servers connecting routing groups and connecting dissimilar mail systems. These systems require special attention to their specific functionality and often require an administrator to keep closer watch on the server for a given period of time. For instance, a bridgehead server hosting connectors to foreign messaging systems requires an administrator to monitor connections to the server, the specific connectors, and other messaging systems with which it interacts.

SMTP Relay Server

SMTP relay servers are similar to bridgehead servers in that they both can route messages from one system to another. They serve as mail gateways that relay mail. Mail systems facing the Internet can route mail to internal mail systems or to other external systems. It is not recommended however to allow your SMTP relay server to route messages between two external hosts on the Internet, because your system can then be used for spamming. When managing SMTP relay servers, keep track of how the system is being used and periodically check whether it is routing between external hosts on the Internet.

Auditing the Environment

Auditing gathers and keeps track of activity on the network, devices, and entire systems. By default, Windows Server 2003 enables some auditing, although many other auditing functions must be manually turned on. Windows Server 2003 should be used with Exchange Server 2003 auditing to customize your auditing requirements and provide comprehensive amounts of information that can be analyzed.

Auditing is typically used for identifying security breaches or suspicious activity. However, auditing is also important to gain insight into how the Exchange Server 2003 systems are performing and how they are accessed. Exchange Server 2003 offers three types of auditing: audit logging, protocol logging, and message tracking.

Audit Logging

Exchange Server 2003 uses Windows Server 2003 audit policies to audit how users access and use Exchange servers, as shown in Figure 19.1. Audit policies are the basis for auditing events on a Windows Server 2003 system. Depending on the policies set, auditing might require a substantial amount of server resources in addition to those resources supporting the server's functionality. Otherwise, it could potentially slow server performance. Also, collecting lots of information is only as good as the evaluation of the audit logs. In other words, if a lot of information is captured and it takes a significant amount of effort to evaluate those audit logs, the whole purpose of auditing is not as effective. As a result, it's important to take the time to properly plan how the system will be audited. This enables you to determine what needs to be audited, and why, without creating an abundance of overhead.

> **NOTE**
>
> To audit Exchange Server 2003 uses, enable object access auditing. You can audit both successful and unsuccessful events.

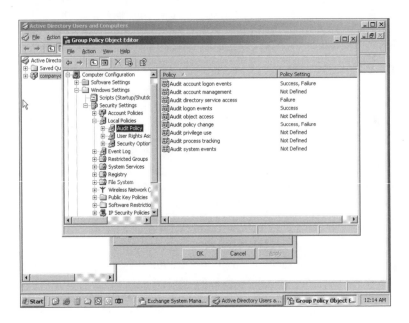

FIGURE 19.1   Windows Server 2003 audit policies.

Protocol Logging

Protocol logging is great for troubleshooting issues with the mail system protocols SMTP, NNTP, or HTTP. It can give you information regarding messaging commands that a user sends to the Exchange Server 2003 server. This includes, but isn't limited to, IP address, bytes sent, data, time, protocol, and domain name.

With the exception of auditing HTTP, which is performed using the IIS snap-in, SMTP and NNTP auditing is enabled through the ESM. To enable protocol logging, follow these steps:

1. Start the ESM by selecting Start, All Programs, Microsoft Exchange, System Manager.

2. In the left pane, expand Servers, Server Name, Protocols and find the protocol to enable logging.

3. In the right pane, right-click on the protocol's virtual server and select Properties.

4. On the General tab, select Enable logging check box.

5. From the drop-down list that appears, select the logging format for auditing the protocol. You can choose from Microsoft IIS Log File Format, NCSA Common Log File Format, ODBC Logging, and W3C Extended Log File Format.

Message Tracking

Out of the three auditing techniques that you can use specifically with Exchange Server 2003, message tracking is by far the least resource-intensive. For this reason, it's more than just a troubleshooting tool. You can use message tracking also for statistical analysis, reporting, and deducing where a message is located in the system.

Message tracking is enabled within the ESM. Simply expand servers and then select properties of the Exchange Server 2003 server for which you want to enable message tracking. Select Enable message tracking within the General tab, as shown in Figure 19.2. Click OK when the information window displays. Optionally, you can select Enable subject logging and display.

The information captured by message tracking is kept in the Exchsrvr\<servername>.log file—for example, %SystemDrive%\Program Files\Exchsrvr\server2.log. You can configure Exchange to remove the log file after it is so many days old to conserve disk space. As you can see in Figure 19.3, at first glance the log file might appear somewhat cryptic. It is full of useful information, however, that can be used to track down messages.

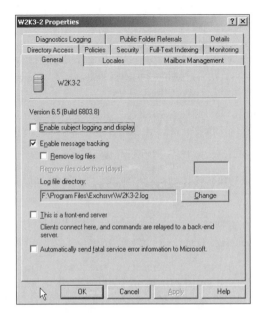

FIGURE 19.2 Enabling message tracking.

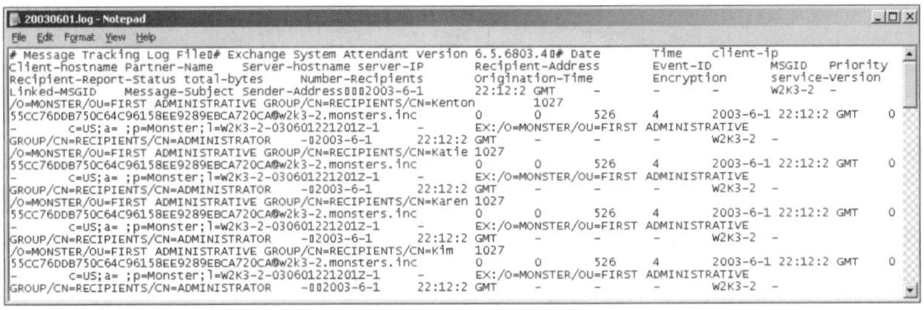

FIGURE 19.3 Viewing the message tracking log.

Managing Exchange Server 2003 Remotely

Windows Server 2003's built-in feature set enables it to be easily managed remotely. This same feature set can be used to manage Exchange Server 2003, which can significantly reduce administration time, expenses, and effort by enabling administrators to manage systems from remote locations rather than having to be physically at the system.

The most common tools available to remotely manage a system are

- **Microsoft Management Console (MMC)**   The MMC not only provides a unified interface for most, if not all, graphical interface utilities, it also can be used to connect and manage remote systems. For example, administrators can use the ESM or Active Directory Users and Computers to manage the local computer and a remote system.

- **Remote Desktop for Administration**   This empowers administrators to log onto a remote system as if they were logging onto the system locally. The desktop and all functions are at the administrators' disposal.

- **Scripting with Windows Script Host (WSH)**   Scripting on Windows Server 2003 can permit administrators to automate tasks locally or remotely. These scripts can be written using common scripting languages. There are many scripts that come bundled with Exchange Server 2003 that can perform a myriad of tasks, such as configuring recipient policies, newsgroups, virtual servers, and much more.

- **Command-line Utilities**   Many command-line utilities are capable of managing systems remotely.

- **Telnet**   Telnet is a gateway type of service through which an administrator or client can connect and log on to a server running the Telnet Server service. It is not exactly the most flexible or best tool to use for either Windows Server 2003 or Exchange Server 2003 but it can be easily used to test SMTP functionality. By entering

   ```
   telnet <servername or server IP address> 25
   ```

   you can test whether Exchange Server 2003 is responding to SMTP requests.

CAUTION

By default, Telnet sends usernames and passwords across the network in plain text.

Maintenance Tools for Exchange Server 2003

To effectively and appropriately administer Exchange Server 2003, you must use several tools. These tools include MMC snap-ins that get installed with Exchange Server 2003, tools native to the Windows Server 2003 operating system, and tools you must install separately from the Exchange Server 2003 CD-ROM.

Managing Exchange with the Exchange System Manager

The ESM shown in Figure 19.4 is one of the primary tools provided with Exchange Server 2003 that you will use to manage the Exchange messaging environment. The ESM is an MMC snap-in that is installed, along with the correct DLL files and Registry entries, from the Exchange Server 2003 CD-ROM. The installation of the ESM is the default and is under Microsoft Exchange System Management Tools.

19

You can manage the entire Exchange Server 2003 organization from within ESM, assuming that you have the proper access privileges. All the Exchange configurations will be made within this snap-in.

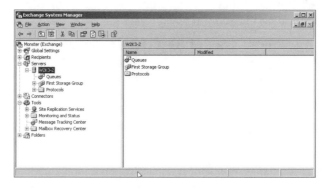

FIGURE 19.4   Exchange Server 2003 ESM.

The ESM can also be installed on a client computer or another server and manage the Exchange Server 2003 servers remotely. This provides flexibility for administrators in networks of all sizes.

Active Directory Users and Computers

Active Directory Users and Computers is an MMC snap-in that is used to manage users, groups, computers, contacts, organizational units, and group policy. It is installed on all domain controllers, but can also be used by installing the Windows Server 2003 Admin Pak (adminpak.msi) located in the i386 directory on the Windows Server 2003 CD-ROM. It is also installed automatically when you install the Exchange System Management Tools from the Exchange Server 2003 CD-ROM.

Active Directory Users and Computers is used instead of the ESM snap-in for managing Active Directory mail-enabled objects, because Exchange Server 2003 uses and stores information in AD rather than its own directory. This tool is the only graphical user interface (GUI) where an administrator can make email-related configuration changes to users, groups, and contacts. The exception to this is moving or deleting mailboxes, which can be done using the ESM.

Common mail-enabled object attributes are readily available in Active Directory Users and Computers, such as delivery restrictions, storage limits, wireless services, protocols, and much more. However, there are several other mail-related fields that can be configured when you select the Advanced Features view mode in the Active Directory Users and Computers snap-in. To enable this mode, simply choose the Advance Features from the view menu from within this snap-in.

The following options are visible with Advanced Features:

- **Exchange Advanced tab**   The Exchange Advanced tab, shown in Figure 19.5, presents options to choose a simple display name, hide the recipient from Exchange address lists, view and modify Exchange custom attributes, configure server and account information for the Internet locator service, and modify mailbox rights.

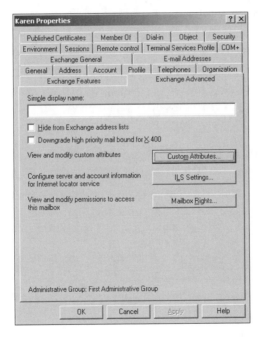

FIGURE 19.5   Exchange Advanced tab options.

- **Microsoft Exchange System Objects Container**   This visible container displays Exchange system objects, such as the offline address book, schema-root, SystemMailbox, and more.

Windows Server 2003 Backup

The Windows Server 2003 backup utility (`ntbackup.exe`) is installed by default on any Windows Server 2003 system and is located under the Start, All Programs, Accessories, System Tools menu. Out of the box, this utility can back up and restore the entire system, including the system state and data.

In order to properly back up and restore Exchange Server 2003 databases and log files using `ntbackup.exe`, the Exchange administrator should either run the backup locally or from another Exchange Server 2003 server. Local and remote Exchange storage groups and databases can be backed up and restored from any Exchange 2003 server, but not from any other server.

Third-party software vendors, such as Legato and Veritas, produce Exchange Server 2003 backup and restore agents for the purpose of remote Exchange database backup.

Exchange Maintenance with the `ntdsutil` Utility

Exchange Server 2003 uses Windows Server 2003 AD to store all its directory information. As a result, it is important to keep AD as healthy as possible in order to ensure that Exchange Server 2003 remains reliable and stable.

Windows Server 2003 automatically performs maintenance on AD by cleaning up the AD database on a nightly basis. The process occurs on domain controllers approximately every 12 hours. An example of the data that is removed would be tombstones. **Tombstones** represent the markers for previously deleted objects. The process deletes unnecessary log files and reclaims free space.

The automatic cleanup process does not perform all the maintenance required. The maintenance processes that the automatic cleanup does not perform are compression and defragmentation of the Active Directory database file. To perform this function, use the `ntdsutil` command-line utility to defragment and compress the database.

> **CAUTION**
>
> To avoid possible adverse affects with the AD database, run `ntdsutil` in Directory Service Repair Mode. Reboot the server, press the F8 key, and then select this mode of operation.

Integrity Checking with the `isinteg` Utility

`isinteg.exe` is an Exchange database integrity checker utility used for maintaining, testing, and repairing database table integrity. The utility is bundled with Exchange Server 2003 and is located in the `Exchsrvr\bin` directory.

> **CAUTION**
>
> Using this utility for anything other than test mode can result in irreversible changes to the database. This utility is not usually used in anything other than test mode, unless there is a specific problem reported.
>
> Therefore, if there is a specific problem to be addressed and corrected, perform the maintenance on a restored copy of the database(s) in a lab environment before attempting to use this utility on a production system.

Dismount the Exchange databases that you plan to perform maintenance on and stop the Microsoft Exchange Information Store prior to running this utility. Keep in mind that this makes the databases unavailable to users before maintenance or problems are corrected.

Database table integrity problems are caused by corruption, which can occur if the server is shut down improperly, if the drive or controller fails, and so forth. To determine whether there are integrity problems with the database, you can do the following:

1. Run isinteg in test mode.

2. View recorded errors in the Event Viewer.

3. Run eseutil /g.

The following is an example of isinteg:

```
isinteg -s ServerName [-fix] [-verbose] [-l logfilename] -test testname[[,
testname]...]
    -s              ServerName
    -fix            check and fix (default - check only)
    -verbose        report verbosely
    -l filename     log file name (default - .\isinteg.pri/pub)
    -t refdblocation (default - the location of the store)
    -test testname,...
        folder message aclitem mailbox(pri only) delfld acllist
        rcvfld(pri only) timedev rowcounts attach morefld ooflist(pri only)
        global searchq dlvrto
        peruser artidx(pub only) search newsfeed(pub only) dumpsterprops
        Ref count tests: msgref msgsoftref attachref acllistref aclitemref
        newsfeedref(pub only) fldrcv(pri only) fldsub dumpsterref
        Groups tests: allfoldertests allacltests
 isinteg -dump [-l logfilename] (verbose dump of store data)
```

Database Maintenance with the eseutil Utility

Although isinteg, an Exchange-specific utility, is used for maintaining, testing, and repairing database table integrity, eseutil is a database-level utility that is not application-specific. For instance, it can be used to maintain, test, and repair AD and Exchange databases. More specifically, `eseutil` is used to maintain database-level integrity, perform defragmentation and compaction, and repair even the most severely corrupt databases. It is also the utility to use when maintaining Exchange Server 2003 transaction log files to see which transaction logs you need to replay or which log file the `Edb.chk` file points to.

CAUTION

Have either a tape backup or other media backup copy of the databases and an offline copy of the database files prior to using the `eseutil` utility, This utility can produce irreversible changes within the database and should be used with extreme caution.

NOTE

While `isinteg` identifies and fixes database table integrity, ESEUTIL investigates the data that resides in the table for any corruption or errors. This is why it is called a database-level utility. The `eseutil` options are shown in Table 19.1.

TABLE 19.1   `eseutil` Syntax

Mode of Operation	Syntax
Defragmentation	`eseutil /d <database name> [options]`
File dump	`eseutil /m[mode-modifier] <filename>`
Recovery	`eseutil /r <logfile base name> [options]`
Integrity	`eseutil /g <database name> [options]`
Repair	`eseutil /p <database name> [options]`
Restore	`eseutil /c [mode-modifier] <path name> [options]`

Exchange Message Tracking

As mentioned earlier, Exchange Server 2003 has a feature called message tracking that gives an administrator the ability to track a message from when it arrives in the Exchange organization until message delivery is complete. Message tracking can also inform the administrator of where a message was delayed or got stuck on the way out of the Exchange organization. This tool is primarily used for finding out where lost messages ended up and to verify which route a message takes for delivery.

Exchange Queue Viewer

Exchange Queue Viewer is used to view the contents of the queues for each particular protocol on a server. Although this tool is more of a troubleshooting tool, it is important to periodically check protocol queues (for example, SMTP or X.400 queues) to ensure that there are no delivery problems.

Best Practices for Performing Database Maintenance

Database maintenance is an easy task to put off because it is one of the most involved maintenance practices you will perform with any version of Exchange. It is also, however, one of the most important maintenance tasks to perform, and it is recommended that administrators run database maintenance routinely. Doing so keeps the Exchange Server 2003 system healthy, prevents downtime, helps maintain service levels, minimizes corruption, and reduces chances for data loss.

If your organization requires a reliable and stable messaging environment—and most organizations do—periodic database maintenance can be used to achieve these goals. The primary reason why Exchange systems at some point become less reliable or less stable is that any database that is not maintained suffers from at least a certain level of corruption. There are also other reasons why databases get corrupted:

- Improper shutting down of the system

- Poorly managed systems

- A poorly maintained disk subsystem

- Hardware failures

- Databases exceeding a manageable size

- Failure to use or review systems or operational management tools

- Manual modification of Exchange databases

- Deletion of Exchange transaction logs

- Assumption that Exchange Server 2003 performs all the database maintenance that is required

- Neglect

Database maintenance consists of both online and offline maintenance processes and procedures. Online maintenance is performed automatically by default, and offline maintenance is more involved. It requires dismounting the specific database within a given storage group and running the appropriate utilities against it. It is the offline maintenance that is most often overlooked.

> **CAUTION**
>
> Exchange Server 2003 databases and transaction log files should never be manually modified. Use only the utilities meant to be used for Exchange Server 2003.

Online Database Maintenance

Similar to AD's automatic maintenance schedule, Exchange Server 2003 out of the box provides general database cleanup maintenance on each of the databases. During the automatic Exchange Server 2003 database cleanup, the following five tasks are performed:

- **Tombstone Maintenance**   Deleted messages are compacted for both user mailboxes and public folders. This process looks for deleted messages and makes sure they have been deleted from the databases, and any references to the delete messages (including the data space the message actually took up) are cleared from the database.

- **Index Aging**   Index aging cleans up user-defined views that are created within the Outlook client and that have not been accessed or used within the predefined timeframe set in the Aging Keep Time Registry entry.

- **Age Folder Tombstones**   This task applies only to the public folder storage area of the messaging system. All folder tombstone entries that are older than the default 180 days are permanently removed from the list. This event helps control the size of the folder tombstone list.

- **Update Server Versions**   The Exchange public store uses the server's version information to establish and maintain the functionality between different versions of Exchange that might be in use throughout an enterprise.

- **Message Expiration**   Messages in the public folders that have exceeded the predefined time value for remaining on the server are deleted from the system.

Automatic online database maintenance performs approximately 60% of the regular functions needed to maintain integrity of the Exchange databases. These maintenance tasks are all performed while the entire system is online. Another 10–20% of maintenance can be accomplished by refreshing the Exchange-related services within the Services MMC snap-in.

> **NOTE**
>
> Online database maintenance also reclaims unused whitespace in the database, but it does not compact or defragment it.

Unfortunately, even performing up to 70% or 80% of maintenance is not enough to ensure maximum use of the Exchange Server 2003 production environment. In fact, the remaining percentage of Exchange Server 2003 maintenance is vital to the overall health and integrity of the Exchange databases. Offline maintenance picks up where online maintenance left off.

Performing Offline Database Maintenance

As mentioned earlier, and as the name implies, offline database maintenance prevents users from accessing the particular database that you are servicing. For this very reason, it is important to perform offline database maintenance during non-business hours. Equally important, it is a good idea to schedule this downtime to minimize its effects on end-users.

Offline database maintenance is useful for repairing, recovering, and defragmenting Exchange Server 2003 databases. The `eseutil` and `isinteg` utilities are used to perform the maintenance. The most common maintenance procedure is defragmenting the databases, and you do not want to repair or recover databases more than you absolutely have to. These maintenance functions are built into `eseutil`. To minimize having to repair or recover a database, include offline database defragmentation maintenance routines in the company's maintenance schedule. A best practice for defragmenting the database is on a quarterly basis. However, this depends on the size of the database, the issues that are being experienced, and scheduling considerations.

> **NOTE**
>
> The following steps to perform offline database maintenance assume that the database has been copied offline to another volume.

To perform offline database maintenance, follow these steps:

1. Log on using an account that has Exchange Full Administrator privileges to the Exchange server that houses the databases that will be maintained.

2. Open the ESM by selecting Start, All Programs, Microsoft Exchange.

3. Expand the Administrative Groups, First Administrative Group, Servers, <ServerName>, <StorageGroupName> in the left pane.

4. Right-click the database that will be maintained and select Dismount Store.

5. Select Yes to continue to dismount the store.

6. Open a Command Prompt by typing **cmd** from the Start, Run dialog box and clicking OK.

7. Change the drives and directory to where `isinteg` resides (the default is `%SystemDrive%\Program Files\Exchsrvr\Bin\`).

8. Type

   isinteg.exe -s <ServerName> -test allfoldertests

   and then press Enter. At this point you will see a list of the databases on the server, indicating which ones are online or offline, as shown in Figure 19.6.

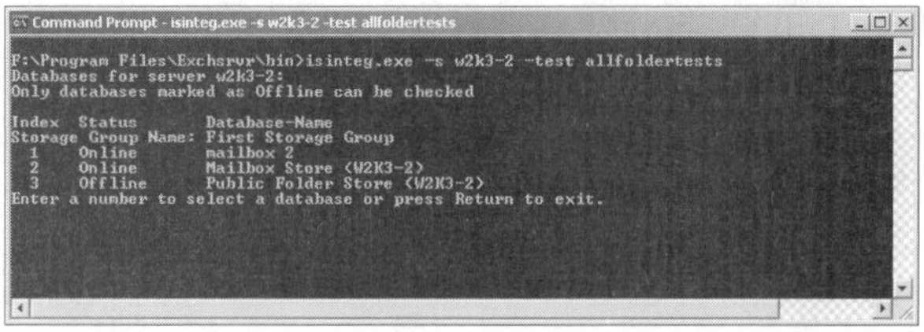

FIGURE 19.6   Performing maintenance using `isinteg`.

9. Choose to run maintenance on the offline database by typing the appropriate number. Press Enter, then choose Y, and finally Enter again to confirm.

   If `isinteg` finds errors, run the appropriate fix as recommended and displayed within the command prompt. The same error and recommended fix is recorded in the Application Event log. If necessary, repeat the `isinteg` integrity check until no errors are reported. When no errors are reported continue to the next step.

Preparing to Use `eseutil`

The `eseutil` utility requires the administrator to enter the full path and name of the EDB database file. It assumes that the streaming database file (STM) is located in the same directory as its corresponding database and it has the same prefix for the database filename. For example, the database `mailbox store 2` has the following 2 files:

`D:\Program Files\Exchsrvr\MDBDATA\mailboxstore2.edb`

`D:\Program Files\Exchsrvr\MDBDATA\mailboxstore2.stm`

If the filenames or paths are different for the two database files, refer to the online help for `eseutil` to add the switch to specify the path to the STM file.

---

10. At the command prompt, type the following command to perform a database-level integrity check:

    `Eseutil.exe /g "D:\Program Files\Exchsrvr\MDBDATA\mailboxstore2.edb"`

    and press Enter. The double quotes are necessary for paths with spaces in the names. If errors are reported, refer to Chapter 32, "Recovering from a Disaster."

11. At the command prompt, type the following command to defragment the database:

    `Eseutil.exe /d "D:\Program Files\Exchsrvr\MDBDATA\mailboxstore2.edb"`

    and press Enter. Again, the double quotes are necessary for paths with spaces in the names.

> **TIP**
>
> Although it is always a good practice to perform offline database maintenance, including defragmentation, on a quarterly basis, it is necessary only when the amount of free space in the database is greater than 15% of the total database size.
>
> To calculate the percentage of free space, take the total free space recorded in the Application Log (Event ID 1221) and divide that by the total database size (the size of the EDB file plus the size of the STM file).

12. When the database compaction completes, mount the database using the ESM.

13. Using Windows Backup or a third-party product, perform a backup of the database.

Database Maintenance Through Mailbox Moves

When you consider what it means to do database maintenance, it is easy to think about the online and offline maintenance routines mentioned previously. Online and offline database maintenance each have their purposes with offline maintenance routines capable of performing the most thorough maintenance. Offline maintenance though requires some downtime and the exact downtime duration depends not only on the size of the database but also on the condition that it is in. For example, offline maintenance of a 40GB database can possibly take well over a day or more to perform defragmentation or corrections on the database.

Another less intrusive method to periodically performing database maintenance that also does not require nearly as much downtime is moving mailboxes to another mailbox store. An Exchange administrator can create a new mailbox store either on the same Exchange Server 2003 server or on a separate server altogether. Once the new mailbox store is created, the administrator can move mailboxes over to the new mailbox store. By moving the mailboxes over to the new mailbox store, the database is in optimal condition.

> **NOTE**
>
> As with any maintenance processes or procedures, it is important to perform backups of Exchange prior to performing the maintenance tasks. Also, moving mailboxes for maintenance reasons should be performed during non-business hours to avoid interrupting users.

In some cases where the 40GB database is experiencing many corruptions, not all mailboxes will be able to be moved without generating errors. For instance, there may be roughly 5-10 percent of the mailboxes still on the original mailbox store that generated errors and did not move over to the new mailbox store. If this occurs, the administrator can perform offline maintenance routines mentioned in the section entitled "Performing Offline Database Maintenance." The benefit is that instead of performing a long and arduous offline maintenance routines on a 40GB database, the routines will be run on a

19

much smaller database and consequently will not require a significant amount of down-time. Instead of taking possibly over a day to perform offline maintenance, the routines only require a few hours.

Prioritizing and Scheduling Maintenance Best Practices

Exchange Server 2003, even without its scheduled maintenance routines, is a very efficient messaging system. However, as mailboxes and public folders are used, there is still logical corruption. Natural wear and tear occurs, as it does in any other system. For this reason, it is important to implement a maintenance plan and schedule to minimize the impact that corruption to these databases has on the overall messaging system.

Scheduled tasks need to be performed daily, monthly, and quarterly. These recommended best practices also are intended to keep administrators informed of the status of the Exchange Server 2003 messaging environment. They can save an abundant amount of time in the long run by minimizing or even avoiding issues that can grow into bigger problems.

> **TIP**
>
> Document the Exchange Server 2003 messaging environment configuration and create a change log to document changes and maintenance procedures.

Daily Maintenance

Daily maintenance routines require the most frequent attention of an Exchange adminis-trator. However, these tasks should not take a significant amount of time to perform.

Verify the Online Backup

Daily, online backups should verify that the previous night's backup was successful. The actual verification process depends on the backup solution that is being used. In general, review the backup program's log file to determine whether the backup has successfully completed. If there are errors reported or the backup job set does not complete success-fully, identify the cause of the error and take the appropriate steps to resolve the problem.

In addition, it is also a best practice to do the following to back up an Exchange Server 2003 server:

- Include System State data to protect against system failure.

- Keep note of how long the backup process is taking to complete. This time should match any service level agreements that may be in place.

- Verify that transaction logs are deleted if circular logging is disabled. If not, perform a full backup.

Check Free Disk Space

All volumes that Exchange Server 2003 resides on (Exchange system files, databases, transaction logs, and so forth) should be checked on a daily basis to ensure that ample free space is available. If the volume or partition runs out of disk space, no more information can be written to the disk. Without disk space to write to, the Exchange services stop running.

Review Message Queues

Message queues should be checked daily to ensure that there are no messages stuck in the queue. Use Queue Viewer to view and manage SMTP, MTA, and connector messaging queues to keep messages flowing.

Check Event Viewer Logs

On Exchange Server 2003 servers, check the Application Log within the Event Viewer for Warning and Stop error messages. These error messages might directly lead you to an issue on the server, or some error messages may be symptomatic of other issues. Filtering for these event types can save a lot of time evaluating whether one of these events has occurred within the last 24 hours. If you are using a systems or operational management solution, this process and more can be automated. In addition, these solutions can also provide enhanced reporting functionality.

Weekly Maintenance

Tasks that do not require daily maintenance, but still require frequent attention, are categorized in the weekly maintenance routines. These routines are described in the following sections.

Document Database File Sizes

Unless you set mailbox storage limitations, the size of the mailbox databases can quickly become overwhelmingly large. If the volume housing the databases is not large enough to accommodate the database growth beyond a certain capacity, services can stop, databases can get corrupted, performance can get sluggish, or the system can halt. Even when you do set mailbox size limitations, you should know the size of the databases and the growth rate. By documenting the database size(s), you can better understand system usage and capacity requirements.

Verify Public Folders Replication

Many environments rely on public folders to share information, and the public folder configurations (for example, multiple hierarchies, multiple replicas, and more) vary widely from environment to environment. With environments that replicate public folder information among different Exchange Server 2003 servers, keep abreast of whether the information contained within those folders is kept up to date.

There are several ways to perform quick tests to see whether information is replicating correctly, including manually testing replication, using the Exchange Server 2003 Resource

Kit's Public Folder Administration tool (`PFAdmin.exe`), and reviewing the `Ex00yymmdd.log` and `Ex01yymmdd.log` files. If problems exist, you can use the logs just mentioned to troubleshoot.

Verify Online Maintenance Tasks

Exchange Server 2003 records information in the Application Log about online maintenance that occurs automatically. Check this event log to verify that all the online maintenance tasks and other scheduled tasks are being performed and that no problems are occurring. Using the common event IDs given in the following list, you can easily search by the ID number to review online maintenance and other scheduled tasks. In the right pane of the Event Viewer, click on the Event column to sort events by their ID number:

- **Event ID 1221** This event reveals how much free space there is in a database. This information is also useful in determining when offline database defragmentation may be necessary.

- **Event ID 1206 and 1207** Both IDs inform about deleted item retention processing.

- **Event ID 700 and 701** These IDs indicate the start and stop times of the online database defragmentation process. Check to make sure that the process does not conflict with Exchange database backups, and make sure the process completes without interruptions.

- **Event IDs 9531–9535** All these IDs are about deleted mailbox retention processing.

Analyze Resource Utilization

With any system—and Exchange Server 2003 is no different—it is important to know how well the overall system is performing. At a minimum, you should monitor system resources at least once a week. Concentrate on monitoring the four common contributors to bottlenecks: memory, processor, disk subsystem, and network subsystem.

Check Offline Address Book Generation

An Offline Address Book (OAB), also known as an Offline Address List (OAL), is routinely generated for remote users to download and view address lists while offline. By default, the OAL is generated daily if there are changes. Use the ESM to determine the last time it was generated to make sure that remote users can obtain an updated copy. This is performed by viewing the Property pages of the OAL located under the Recipients, Offline Address List container.

> **NOTE**
>
> If you are experiencing problems with OAL generation, enable diagnostic logging and review the Application Log for any OAL Generator category events.

Monthly Maintenance

Recommended monthly maintenance practices for Exchange Server 2003 do not require the frequency of daily or weekly tasks, but they are nonetheless important to maintaining the overall health of the system. Some general monthly maintenance tasks can be quickly summarized; others are explained in more detail in the following sections.

General tasks include

- Refresh the Exchange Server 2003 services to free up memory resources and kick-start online maintenance routines.

- Install approved and tested service packs and updates.

- Schedule and perform, as necessary, any major server configuration changes, including hardware upgrades.

Test Uninterruptible Power Supply

Uninterruptible Power Supply (UPS) equipment is commonly used to protect the server from sudden loss of power. Most UPS solutions include supporting management software to assure that the server is gracefully shut down in the event of power failure, thus preserving the integrity of the system. Each manufacturer has a specific recommendation for testing, and its procedure should be followed. However, it should occur no less than once a month, and it is advantageous to schedule the test for the same time as the server reboot.

Analyze Database Free Space

As mentioned earlier in "Performing Offline Database Maintenance," an approximation of a database's fragmentation can be made using the database size and the amount of free space. The amount of free space that can be recovered from a defragmentation and compaction is provided within Event ID 1221 entries.

Quarterly Maintenance

Although quarterly maintenance tasks are infrequent, some might require downtime and are more likely to cause serious problems with Exchange Server 2003 if not properly planned or maintained. Therefore proceed cautiously with these tasks.

General quarterly maintenance tasks include the following:

- Check mailbox and public folder stores' Property pages to verify configuration parameters, review usage statistics, determine mailbox sizes, and more.

- Check storage limits to ensure that data storage requirements will not exceed capacity, given the current rate of growth (stemming from the information taken from the weekly maintenance task).

Perform Offline Maintenance

As mentioned earlier, offline maintenance is one of the most important maintenance tasks to perform, but it can be time consuming and hazardous. Remember to properly plan, schedule during off-hours, and perform both an online and offline backup of the information stores prior to beginning the tasks. A little extra care up front can save you lots of time troubleshooting. For more information on this process, refer to "Performing Offline Database Maintenance," earlier in this chapter.

Validate Information Store Backups

At first glance, you might consider the process of validating database backups as simply checking the backup logs to see whether they were successful. On the contrary, validating the backups involves performing a full restore onto a test server in a lab environment. This not only ensures that Exchange Server 2003 can be easily recovered in times of disaster but it also irons out any issues in the restore process and keeps administrators in practice for recovering the system; when disaster strikes, they are adequately prepared.

> **TIP**
>
> Document the process of restoring Exchange Server 2003 databases. If documentation already exists, verify that the existing process has not changed. If it has changed, update the documentation.

Post-Maintenance Procedures

Post-maintenance procedures are designed to quickly and efficiently restore Exchange operations to the environment following maintenance procedures that have required downtime. Devising a checklist for these procedures ensures that there is not unnecessary messaging disruption. The following is a sample checklist for maintenance procedures:

1. Start all the remaining Exchange services.

2. Test email connectivity from Outlook and Outlook Web Access.

3. Perform a full backup of the Exchange Server 2003 server(s).

4. Closely review backup and server event logs over the next few days to ensure that no errors are reported on the server.

Reducing Management and Maintenance Efforts

As you have seen throughout the chapter, there are numerous utilities available with Exchange Server 2003 for managing, maintaining, and monitoring the messaging system. These utilities can save enormous amounts of time and energy if properly used.

On the other hand, as messaging systems grow in size and complexity, so do the responsibilities of the administrators who work with them on a daily basis.

In any messaging environment, an administrator must consider opportunities for reducing maintenance efforts to maximize effectiveness and efficiency (that is, doing the right jobs or tasks correctly). Besides, management and maintenance that are streamlined or automated can be tied directly to significant cost savings for the company. Equally important, it keeps you one step ahead of the system so that you are proactively managing and maintaining rather than reacting to the problems.

Using Microsoft Operations Manager

Microsoft Operations Manager (MOM) is one tool that can be used to streamline and automate many of an administrator's messaging responsibilities. More specifically, the MOM Application Management Pack provides the key features required to manage, maintain, and monitor the Exchange Server 2003 environment.

Key features to consider evaluating include, but are not limited to, the following:

- Alerting when various thresholds are met, such as resource utilization statistics or capacity

- Performance baselining and continuous monitoring of system resources and protocols (for example, SMTP, POP3, and IMAP4)

- Trend analysis of usage and performance

- A full knowledgebase of Exchange-specific solutions tied directly to over 1700 events

- Reporting on usage, problems, security-related events, and much more

Summary

Messaging is considered a mission-critical application, and it should be well managed and maintained. With proper care and feeding, Exchange Server 2003 can stay healthy and optimized to handle your environment's business and technical requirements.

Best Practices

The following are best practices from this chapter:

- Manage Exchange Server 2003 based on server roles and responsibilities.

- Audit the messaging environment, using Windows Server 2003 auditing.

- Use Exchange Server 2003's protocol logging and diagnostic logging for troubleshooting purposes.

- Install the ESM on a client computer to remotely administer Exchange Server 2003. Use the same version of Exchange Server 2003 and service pack level of the servers being managed.

19

- Keep AD well-tuned using `ntdsutil`, because Exchange Server 2003 directly relies on it.

- Avoid possible adverse affects with the AD database by running `ntdsutil` in Directory Service Repair mode.

- Perform an online and offline copy of the information stores prior to running offline maintenance tasks.

- Use `isinteg` in test mode unless there is a specific problem reported.

- Never manually modify Exchange Server 2003 databases and transaction log files.

- Document the Exchange Server 2003 messaging environment configuration and create a change log to document changes and maintenance procedures.

- If you are experiencing problems with OAL generation, enable diagnostic logging and review the Application Log for any OAL Generator category events.

- Document the process of restoring Exchange Server 2003 databases. If documentation already exists, verify that the existing process has not changed. If it has changed, update the documentation.

- Create post-maintenance procedures to minimize time needed for restoration.

- Include the System State data in daily backup routines.

- Reduce management and maintenance efforts, using the MOM Application Management Pack.

CHAPTER 20

Documenting an Exchange Server 2003 Environment

Documentation is not only an integral part of the installation or design of an Exchange Server 2003 environment, it is also important for the maintenance, support, and recovery of new or existing environments.

Documentation serves several purposes throughout the life cycle of Exchange Server 2003 and is especially critical on a per-project basis. In the initial stages of a project, it serves to provide a historical record of the options and decisions made during the design process. During the testing and implementation phases, documents such as step-by-step procedures and checklists guide project team members and help ensure that all steps are completed. When the implementation portion of the project is complete, support documentation can play a key role in maintaining the health of the new environment. Support documents include administration and maintenance procedures, checklists, detailed configuration settings, and monitoring procedures.

This chapter is dedicated to providing the breadth and scope of documentation for an Exchange Server 2003 environment. Equally important, it provides considerations and best practices for keeping your messaging environment well documented, maintained, and manageable.

Planning Exchange Server 2003 Documentation

When planning Exchange Server 2003 documentation (whether for general purposes, specific aspects such as disaster recovery, or a particular project), several factors should be considered:

- The business requirements of the organization

- The technical requirements of the organization

- The audience that will be using the documents

- How and when the documents will be produced

The extent of the documentation depends on the business and technical requirements of the organization. Some organizations require that each step be documented, and other organizations require that only the configuration be recorded. Careful consideration should be given to any regulatory requirements or existing internal organization policies.

After the specific documentation requirements have been determined, it is important to consider who the audience for each document will be. Who will use each document, in what setting, and for what purpose? It would be impractical to develop a 300-page user guide when all the user wants to do is log on to the messaging system. In that case, all that would be required is a quick reference guide. Properly analyzing the purpose and goals of each document aids in the development of clear and useful documentation.

Planning the schedule for document production often requires a separate project timeline or plan. The plan should include checkpoints, sponsorship or management review, and a clear schedule. Tools such as Microsoft Project facilitate the creation of a documentation project plan (see "Design and Planning Documentation," later in this chapter). The project plan can also provide an initial estimate of the number of hours required and the associated costs. For instance, based on previous documentation projects, there is an estimate that 1–2 pages per hour will be produced.

Benefits of Documentation

Although many of the benefits of Exchange Server 2003 documentation are obvious and tangible, others can be harder to identify. A key benefit to documentation is that the process of putting the information down on paper encourages a higher level of analysis and review of the topic at hand. The process also encourages teamwork and collaboration within an organization and interdepartmental exchange of ideas.

Documentation that is developed with specific goals, and goes through a review or approval process, is typically well organized and complete, and contributes to the overall professionalism of the organization and its knowledgebase. The following sections examine some of the other benefits of professional documentation in the Exchange Server 2003 environment.

Knowledge Sharing and Knowledge Management

The right documentation enables an organization to organize and manage its data and intellectual property. Company policies and procedures are typically located throughout multiple locations that include individual files for various departments. Consolidating this information into logical groupings can be beneficial.

> **TIP**
>
> Place documentation in various locations where it is easily accessible for authorized users, such as on the intranet, in a public folder, or in hard-copy format.

A complete design document consolidates and summarizes key discussions and decisions, budgetary concerns, and timing issues. This consolidation provides a single source of information for questions that might emerge at a later date. In addition, a document that describes the specific configuration details of the Exchange server might prove very valuable to a manager in another company office when making a purchasing decision.

All of the documents should be readily available at all times. This is especially critical regarding disaster recovery documents. Centralizing the documentation and communicating the location helps reduce the use of out-of-date documentation and reduce confusion during a disaster recovery. It is also recommended that they be available in a number of formats, such as hard copy, the appropriate place on the network, and even via an intranet.

Financial Benefits of Documentation

Proper Exchange Server 2003 documentation can be time consuming and adds to the cost of the environment and project. In lean economic times for a company or organization, it is often difficult to justify the expense of project documentation. However, when looking at documents, such as in maintenance or disaster recovery scenarios, it is easy to determine that creating this documentation makes financial sense. For example, in an organization where downtime can cost thousands of dollars per minute, the return on investment (ROI) in disaster recovery and maintenance documentation is easy to calculate. In a company that is growing rapidly and adding staff and new servers on a regular basis, tested documentation on server builds and administration training can also have immediate and visible benefits.

Financial benefits are not limited to maintenance and disaster recovery documentation. Well-developed and professional design and planning documentation helps the organization avoid costly mistakes in the implementation or migration process, such as buying too many server licenses or purchasing too many servers.

Baselining Records for Documentation Comparisons

Baselining is a process of recording the state of an Exchange Server 2003 system so that any changes in its performance can be identified at a later date. Complete baselining also pertains to the overall network performance, including WAN links, but in those cases it might require special software and tools (such as sniffers) to record the information.

20

An Exchange Server 2003 system baseline document records the state of the server after it is implemented in a production environment and can include statistics such as memory use, paging, disk subsystem throughput, and more. This information then allows the administrator or appropriate IT resource to determine at a later date how the system is performing in comparison to initial operation.

Using Documentation for Troubleshooting Purposes

Troubleshooting documentation is a record of identified system issues and the associated resolution. This documentation is helpful both in terms of the processes that the company recommends for resolving technical issues and a documented record of the results of actual troubleshooting challenges. Researching and troubleshooting an issue is time consuming. Documenting the process followed and the results provides a valuable resource for other company administrators that might experience the same issue.

Design and Planning Documentation

Parts I, "Microsoft Exchange Server 2003 Overview," and II, "Microsoft Exchange Server 2003 Messaging," of this book focus on many planning and designing aspects for Exchange Server 2003. Whether you're planning a migration, an entirely new environment, or a specific project, design and planning documentation is critical. All projects, regardless of size, are more successful if they have a well-developed design and migration plan.

Documenting the Design

As outlined in Chapters 4, "Exchange Server 2003 Design Concepts," and 5 "Designing an Enterprise Exchange Server 2003 Environment," the first step in the implementation of an Exchange Server 2003 environment is the development and approval of a design. Documenting this design contributes to the success of the project. The design document records the decisions made during the design process and provides a reference for testing, implementation, and support. Typically, a design document includes the following components:

- The goals and objectives of the project

- A summary of the existing environment and the background that led to the project

- The details of the new Exchange Server 2003 environment

- The details of the migration process

Documenting the goals and objectives of the project helps ensure that the project team and stakeholder interests are in alignment. The goals and objectives of the project should be as specific as possible, because after the goals are defined, they help shape design decisions.

Summarizing the existing environment creates a snapshot of the preimplementation environment, which provides a reference point for development of the new design and a historical record should a rollback be required. Including the background behind the decision to implement Exchange Server 2003 further defines the historical record and supports the goals and objectives.

The following is an example of a table of contents for a design document:

```
Exchange Server 2003 Design Document
Project Overview
Design and Planning Process
Existing Environment
        Network Infrastructure
        Active Directory Infrastructure
        Exchange Topology
        Backup and Restore
        Administrative Model
        Client Systems
Exchange Server 2003 Architecture
        Goals and Objectives
        Exchange Server 2003 Mailbox Server Placement
        Public Folder Servers
        Connector Servers
        Front-end Servers/Outlook Web Access
        Global Catalog Placement
        Administrative Groups
        Server Sizing and Loading
        Active Directory Connector
        Administrative Model
        Application Considerations and Integration
        Exchange Server 2003 Clients
Appendix A: Existing Environment Diagrams
```

Exchange Server 2003 Design

The Exchange Server 2003 design details the decisions made with regard to the end-state of the Exchange Server 2003 environment. These decisions include server configuration information, database design, messaging policies, and more.

The level of detail included in the document, high-level or more specific configurations of each server, depends on the document's audience. However, the design document should not include step-by-step procedures or other details of how the process will be accomplished. This level of detail is better handled, in most cases, in dedicated configuration or training documents.

20

Creating the Migration Plan

After the end-state or design is developed and documented, the plan on how this state will be implemented can be developed. A migration plan outlines the high-level tasks required to test and implement the design. The development of a well-constructed migration plan helps avoid mistakes and keeps the project on track.

> **NOTE**
>
> The results of testing the design in a prototype or pilot might alter the actual migration steps and procedures. In this case, the migration plan document should be modified to take these changes into account.

The following is a table of contents for an Exchange Server 2003 migration plan:

```
Exchange Server 2003 Migration Plan
Goals and Objectives
Approach
Roles
Process
        Phase I - Design and Planning
        Phase II - Prototype
        Phase III - Pilot
        Phase IV - Implementation
        Phase V - Support
Migration Process
        Active Directory Preparation
        Exchange Server 2003
Summary of Migration Resources
Project Scheduling
Exchange Server 2003 Training
Administration and Maintenance
```

Outlining the Project Plan

A project plan is essential for more complex migrations and can be useful for managing smaller projects, even single server migrations. Developed from the high-level tasks and outlined in the migration plan, detailed tasks and subtasks are identified in the order in which they occur. The duration of these tasks will vary but it is recommended that they be no less than a half-day duration, because a project plan that tries to track a project hour by hour can be hard to keep up to date. Of course, the size of the project also dictates the project plan's level of detail.

Tools such as Microsoft Project facilitate the creation of project plans (see Figure 20.1). Using Microsoft Project enables the assignment of one or more resources per task and the assignment of duration and links to key predecessor tasks. The project plan can also provide an initial estimate of the number of hours required from each resource and the associated costs if outside resources are to be used. What-if scenarios are easy to create by simply adding resources or cutting out optional steps to determine the effect on the budget and resources.

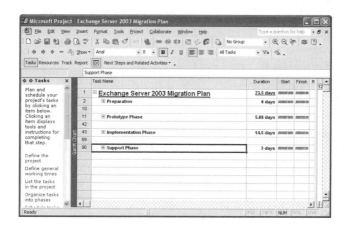

FIGURE 20.1   A sample project plan.

Developing the Test Plan

Thorough testing is critical in the success of any implementation project. A test plan details the resources required for testing (hardware, software, and lab personnel), the tests or procedures to perform, and the purpose of the test or procedure.

It is important to include representatives of every aspect of the network in the development of the test plan. This ensures that all aspects of the Exchange Server 2003 environment or project and its impact will be included in the test plan.

Test plans, although they will vary within each environment, should consider using a framework such as this:

```
Summary
➡The purpose of this document is to outline the testing strategy for the migration
➡to Exchange Server 2003. Before Exchange Server 2003 is deployed, the design must
➡be tested in an environment that simulates and protects the production
➡environment. Devising and conducting tests that reflect conditions in the target
➡environment verify the design.

Exchange Server 2003 Testing Methodology
        Testing Phases
        Documentation
```

Developing the Migration Documentation

Migration documentation is typically created during the testing or prototype phase of the project. Migration documentation, comprised of a combination of procedures and check-lists, provides a roadmap of the Exchange Server 2003 migration. The documents might need updating after the initial or pilot implementation to more accurately reflect the migration process.

Server Migration Procedures

Server migration tasks should be decided on during a design and planning process. Detailed procedures associated with those tasks are then developed and confirmed during a prototype/testing phase. It is also important to validate the documents each time a server is rebuilt to ensure that critical steps are not left out. When complete, this information can save a great deal of time during the implementation.

> **TIP**
>
> Server migration procedures should be written in such a way so that even less-experienced resources are able to use the procedures for the actual migrations.

The procedures covered can include, but are not limited to, the following:

- Server hardware configuration details

- Service pack (SP) and hotfixes to install on each server

- Services (such as DNS and DHCP) to enable or disable (including any appropriate settings)

- Applications (for example, antivirus) to install and appropriate settings

- Security settings

- Steps required to migrate mail to the new server(s)

- Steps required to test the new configuration to ensure full functionality

- Steps required to remove old servers from production

Desktop Client Configuration Procedures

Desktop configurations might change during the migration to, the implementation of, or the configuration change of Exchange Server 2003. If the Outlook client is already in use, server configuration changes might affect only the Outlook profile. All changes and the change procedure should be documented to ensure that there is a uniform user experience after the implementation.

> **NOTE**
>
> The desktop configuration change process should be discussed in the design and planning phase.

Mail Migration Procedures

One of the most frequently identified messaging systems implementation goals is to migrate all the existing mail, contacts, mailing lists, calendar items, and more without losing any data. Developing complete and accurate messaging migration procedures during the testing phase helps migrate existing production messaging data and prevents data loss.

Checklists

The migration process, based on the amount of data that must be migrated, can often be a long process. It is very helpful to develop both high-level and detailed checklists to guide the migration process. High-level checklists determine the status of the migration at any given point in the process. Detailed checklists ensure that all steps are performed in a consistent manner. This is extremely important if the process is being repeated for multiple sites.

The following is an example of an Exchange Server 2003 server build checklist:

```
Task:                                              Initials
Notes
Verify BIOS and Firmware Revs
Verify RAID Configuration
Install Windows Server 2003 Enterprise Edition
Configure Windows Server 2003 Enterprise Edition
Install Security Patches
Install Support Tools
```

20

```
Install System Recovery Console
Add Server to Domain
Install Antivirus
Install Exchange Server 2003 Enterprise
Configure Exchange
Install and Configure Backup Agent on Exchange
Apply Rights For XX-Sysadmins
Set up and Configure Smart UPS
```

Sign off: Date:

Exchange Server 2003 Environment Documentation

As the business and network infrastructure changes, it's not uncommon for the messaging infrastructure to change as well. Keep track of these changes as they progress through baselines (how the Exchange Server 2003 environment was built) and other forms of documentation, such as the configuration settings and connectivity diagrams of the environment.

Server Build Procedures

The server build procedure is a detailed set of instructions for building the Exchange Server 2003 system. This document can be used for troubleshooting and adding new servers, and is a critical resource in the event of a disaster.

The following is an example of a table of contents from a server build procedure document:

```
Windows Server 2003 Build Procedures
        System Configuration Parameters
        Configure the Server Hardware
                Install Vendor Drivers
                Configure RAID
        Install and Configure Windows Server 2003
                Using Images
                Scripted Installations
        Applying Windows Server 2003 Security
                Using a Security Template
                Using GPOs
                Configuring Antivirus
                Installing Service Packs and Critical Updates
        Backup Client Configuration
Exchange Server 2003 Build Procedures
```

```
      System Configuration Parameters
      Configuring Exchange as a Mailbox Server
            Creating Storage Groups
            Creating Databases
      Configuring Exchange as a Public Folder Server
            Creating a Public Folder Database
      Configuring Front-end Functionality
            Configuring SSL
```

Configuration (As-Built) Documentation

The configuration document, often referred to as an as-built, details a snapshot configuration of the Exchange Server 2003 system as it is built. This document contains essential information required to rebuild a server.

The following is an Exchange Server 2003 server as-built document template:

```
Introduction
➥The purpose of this Exchange Server 2003 as-built document is to assist an
➥experienced network administrator or engineer in restoring the server in the event
➥of a hardware failure. This document contains screen shots and configuration
➥settings for the server at the time it was built. If settings are not implicitly
➥defined in this document, they are assumed to be set to defaults. It is not
➥intended to be a comprehensive disaster recovery with step-by-step procedures for
➥rebuilding the server. In order for this document to remain useful as a recovery
➥aid, it must be updated as configuration settings change.

System Configuration
      Hardware Summary
      Disk Configuration
            Logical Disk Configuration
      System Summary
      Device Manager
      RAID Configuration
      Windows Server 2003 TCP/IP Configuration
      Network Adapter Local Area Connections
Security Configuration
      Services
      Lockdown Procedures (Checklist)
      Antivirus Configuration
Share List
Applications and Configurations
```

20

Topology Diagrams

Network configuration diagrams, such as the one shown in Figure 20.2, and related documentation generally include local area network (LAN) connectivity, wide area network (WAN) infrastructure connectivity, IP subnet information, critical servers, network devices, and more. Having accurate diagrams of the new environment can be invaluable when troubleshooting connectivity issues. For topology diagrams that can be used for troubleshooting connectivity issues, consider documenting the following:

- Internet service provider contact names, including technical support contact information

- Connection type (such as frame relay, ISDN, OC-12)

- Link speed

- Committed Information Rate (CIR)

- Endpoint configurations, including routers used

- Message flow and routing

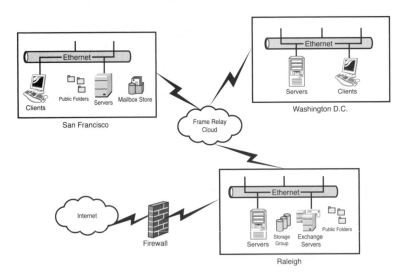

FIGURE 20.2   A sample network diagram.

Administration and Maintenance Documentation

Planning and implementing an Exchange Server 2003 environment is just the beginning of documentation possibilities. Proper documentation can also be critical in maintaining a reliable network. Administration and maintenance documentation helps an administrator organize and keep track of the different steps required to ensure the health of the Exchange environment like the management and maintenance best practices described in

Chapter 19, "Exchange Server 2003 Management and Maintenance Practices." This documentation can also facilitate the training of new resources and reduce the variables and risks involved in these transitions.

One key component to administration or maintenance documentation is a timeline detailing when certain procedures should be followed. To properly maintain an Exchange environment, certain daily, weekly, monthly, and quarterly procedures should be followed. These procedures, such as database maintenance and mailbox deletion, should be documented to make sure that the procedures are clearly defined and the frequency in which they should be performed is outlined.

Step-by-Step Procedure Documents

Administration and maintenance documentation contains a significant amount of procedural documentation. These documents can be very helpful for complex processes or for processes that are not performed on a regular basis. Procedures range from technical processes that outline each step to administrative processes that help clarify roles and responsibilities.

Organizational Policy Documents

When it comes to messaging, there are a number of system, recipient, and management policies that can and should be established (for example, message size limits, message retention policies, and naming conventions). Establishing clear policies helps establish user expectation and limit database size. In addition, with maintenance and administration policies it helps to have a well-developed, complete, and approved policy document that makes it clear who is responsible for what in specific situations.

Documented Checklists

Administration and maintenance documentation can be extensive, and checklists can be quick reminders for those processes and procedures. Develop comprehensive checklists that will help administrators perform their scheduled and unscheduled tasks. A timeline checklist highlighting the daily, weekly, monthly, and quarterly tasks helps keep the Exchange environment healthy. In addition, these checklists function as excellent auditing tools.

Disaster Recovery Documentation

Disaster recovery documentation should be a requirement for every project. Regardless of size, an organization should go through the process of contemplating various disaster scenarios and determining what its needs would be in the event of a disaster. A disaster can range from a hard disk failure to a fire that destroys the entire site. Each type of disaster can pose a different threat to the day-to-day functioning of an organization. Therefore, it's important to determine every possible scenario and begin planning ways to minimize the impact of those disasters.

20

Planning for a disaster can be time consuming and expensive. However, generally speaking this does not outweigh the benefits of creating such documentation. Even a quick analysis showing how downtime resulting from a disaster might affect the company with regard to reputation, time, productivity, expenses, and loss in profit or revenue versus how much time it takes to create documentation can show the advantages of documenting and being prepared. The true purpose for the evaluation, though, is to assist an organization in determining how much should be invested in remedies to avoid or minimize the impact of a disaster.

A number of different components comprise disaster recovery documentation. Without this documentation, full recovery is difficult at best. The following is a table of contents for the areas to consider when documenting disaster recovery procedures:

```
Executive Summary or Introduction
Disaster Recovery Scenarios
Disaster Recovery Best Practices
        Planning and Designing for Disaster
Business Continuity and Response
        Business Hours Response to Emergencies
        Recovery Team Members
        Recovery Team Responsibilities
        Damage Assessment
        Off-Hours Response to an Emergency
        Recovery Team Responsibilities
        Recovery Strategy
        Coordinate Equipment Needs
Disaster Recovery Decision Tree
Software Recovery
Hardware Recovery
Server Disaster Recovery
Preparation
        Documentation
        Software Management
        Knowledge Management
Server Backup with NetBackup
        Client Software Configuration
Restoring the Server
        Build the Server Hardware
        Post Restore
Exchange Disaster Recovery
        Disaster Recovery Service Level Agreements
        Exchange Disaster Recovery Plan
        Exchange Message / Mailbox Restore Scenario
        Complete RAID 5 Failure
```

```
    Complete RAID 1 Failure
    NOS Partition Failure
    Complete System Failure
    NIC, RAID Controller Failures
Train Personnel and Practice Disaster Recovery
```

Disaster Recovery Planning

The first step of the disaster recovery process is to develop a formal disaster recovery plan. This plan, while time consuming to develop, serves as a guide for the entire organization in the event of an emergency. Disaster scenarios, such as power outages, hard drive failures, and even earthquakes, should be addressed. Although it is impossible to develop a scenario for every potential disaster, it is still helpful to develop a plan to recover from different levels of disaster. It is recommended that organizations encourage open discussions of possible scenarios and the steps required to recover from each one. Include representatives from each department, because each department will have its own priorities in the event of a disaster. The disaster recovery plan should encompass the organization as a whole and focus on determining what it will take to resume normal business function after a disaster.

Backup and Recovery Development

Another important component of a disaster recovery development process is the evaluation of the organization's current backup policies and procedures. Without sound backup policies and procedures, a disaster recovery plan is useless. It is not possible to recover a system if the backup is not valid.

A backup plan does not just encompass backing up data to tape or other medium. It is an overarching plan that outlines other tasks, including advanced system recovery, offsite storage, testing procedures, and retention policies. These tasks should be carefully documented to accurately represent each backup methodology and how it's carried out. Full documentation of the backup process includes step-by-step procedures, guidelines, policies, and checklists.

Periodically, the backup systems should be reviewed and tested, especially after any configuration changes. Any changes to the system should be reflected in the documentation. Otherwise, backup documents can become stale and can add to the problems during recovery attempts.

Recovery documentation complements backup documentation. The primary purpose of the documented backup process is to provide the ability to recover that backup in the event of an emergency. Recovery documentation should outline where the backup data resides and how to recover from various types of failures, such as hard drive failure, system failure, and natural disasters. Just like backup documentation, recovery documentation takes the form of step-by-step procedures, guidelines, policies, and checklists.

20

Exchange System Failover Documentation

Many organizations use clustering in their Exchange environment to provide failover and redundancy capabilities for their messaging systems. When a system fails over, having fully tested and documented procedures helps get the system back up and running quickly. Because these procedures are not used often, they must be thoroughly tested and reviewed in a lab setting so that they accurately reflect the steps required to recover each system.

Performance Documentation

Performance documentation helps monitor the health and status of the Exchange environment. It is a continuous process that begins by aligning the goals, existing policies, and service level agreements of the organization. When these areas are clearly defined and detailed, baseline performance values can be established, using tools such as the System Monitor, Microsoft Operations Manager (MOM), or third-party tools (such as PerfMon or BMC Patrol). These tools capture baseline performance-related metrics that can include indicators such as how much memory is being used, average processor use, and more. They also can illustrate how the Exchange Server 2003 environment is performing under various workloads.

After the baseline performance values are documented, performance-related information gathered by the monitoring solution should be analyzed periodically. Pattern and trend analysis reports need to be examined at least on a weekly basis. This analysis can uncover current and potential bottlenecks and proactively ensure that the system operates as efficiently and effectively as possible. These reports can range from routine reports generated by the monitoring solution to complex technical reports that provide detail to engineering staff.

Routine Reporting

Although built-in system monitoring tools log performance data that can be used in reports in conjunction with products such as Microsoft Excel, it is recommended that administrators use products such as MOM for monitoring and reporting functionality. MOM can manage and monitor the Exchange systems and provide preconfigured graphical reports with customizable levels of detail. MOM also provides the framework to generate customized reports that meet the needs of the organization.

Management-Level Reporting

Routine reporting typically provides a significant amount of technical information. Although helpful for the administrator, it can be too much information for management. Management-level performance reporting should be concise and direct. Stakeholders do not require the specifics of performance data, but it's important to take those specifics and show trends, patterns, and any potential problem areas. This extremely useful and factual information provides insight to management so that decisions can be made to determine proactive solutions for keeping systems operating in top-notch condition.

For instance, during routine reporting, administrators identify and report to management that Exchange Server processor use is on the rise. What does this mean? This information by itself does not give management any specifics on what the problem is. However, if the administrator presents graphical reports that indicate that if the current trends on Exchange Server processor use continue at the rate of a 5% increase per month, an additional processor will be required in 10 months or less. Management can then take this report, follow the issue more closely over the next few months, and determine whether to allocate funds to purchase additional processors. If the decision is made to buy more processors, management has more time to negotiate quantity, processing power, and cost instead of having to pay higher costs for the processors on short notice.

Technical Reporting

Technical performance information reporting is much more detailed than management-level reporting. It goes beyond the routine reporting to provide specific details on many different components and facets of the system. For example, specific counter values might be given to determine disk subsystem use. This type of information is useful in monitoring the health of the entire Exchange environment. Trend and pattern analysis should also be included in the technical reporting process to not only reflect the current status, but to allow comparison to historical information and determine how to plan for future requirements.

Security Documentation

Just as with any other aspect of the Exchange environment, security documentation also includes policies, configurations and settings, and procedures. Administrators can easily feel that although documenting security settings and other configurations are important, it might lessen security mechanisms established in the Exchange Server 2003 environment. However, documenting security mechanisms and corresponding configurations are vital to administration, maintenance, and any potential security compromise. Security documentation, along with other forms of documentation—including network diagrams and configurations—should be well guarded to minimize any potential security risk.

A network environment might have many security mechanisms in place, but if the information—such as logs and events obtained from them—isn't reviewed, security is more relaxed. Monitoring and management solutions, described in the performance documentation section, can help consolidate this information into reports that can be generated on a periodic basis. These reports are essential to the process of continuously evaluating the network's security.

In addition, management should be informed of any unauthorized access or attempts to compromise security. Business policy can then be made to strengthen the environment's security.

Change Control

Although the documentation of policies and procedures to protect the system from external security risks is of utmost importance, internal procedures and documents should also be established. Developing, documenting, and enforcing a change control process helps protect the system from well-intentioned internal changes.

In environments where there are multiple administrators, it is very common to have the interests of one administrator affect those of another. For instance, an administrator might make a configuration change to limit mailbox size for a specific department. If this change is not documented, a second administrator might spend a significant amount of time trying to troubleshoot a user complaint from that department. Establishing a change control process that documents these types of changes eliminates confusion and wasted resources. The change control process should include an extensive testing process to reduce the risk of production problems.

Procedures

Although security policies and guidelines comprise the majority of security documentation, procedures are equally as important. Procedures include not only the initial configuration steps, but also maintenance procedures and more important procedures that are to be followed in the event of a security breech.

Additional areas regarding security that can be documented include, but are not limited to, the following:

- Auditing policies including review
- Service packs (SPs) and hotfixes
- Certificates and certificates of authority
- Antivirus configurations
- Encrypting File System (EFS)
- Password policies (such as length, strength, age)
- GPO security-related policies
- Registry security
- Lockdown procedures

Training Documentation

Training documentation for a project can be extensive and ranges from user training to technical training. The most important aspect of training documentation is to make sure that it meets the needs of the individual being trained. The two key documents created and used in organizations are focused for the benefit of end-users, and technical documents are focused toward administrators.

End-User

Proper end-user training is critical to the acceptance of any new application. Developing clear and concise documentation that addresses the user's needs is key in providing proper training. As discussed earlier, developing specific documentation goals and conducting an audience analysis are especially important to the development of useful training materials.

Technical

Administrators and engineers are responsible for the upkeep and management of the Exchange environment. As a result, they must be technically prepared to address a variety of issues, such as maintenance and troubleshooting. Training documentation should address why the technologies are being taught and how the technologies pertain to the Exchange environment. In addition, the training documentation should be easy to use and function as a reference resource in the future.

Summary

The development of documentation for the Exchange Server 2003 environment is important not only to establishing the environment, but to the health, maintenance, and ongoing support of the system. After this documentation is developed, it must be thoroughly tested—preferably by a disinterested party—and maintained. Every change that is made to the environment should be changed in the documentation.

Best Practices

The following are best practices from this chapter:

- Determine the business needs for documentation.

- Determine the goals of each document.

- Determine the audience and the need for each document.

- Validate and test the documentation.

- Develop audience-level specific training materials.

- Establish a documentation update process.

20

CHAPTER 21

Using Terminal Services to Manage Exchange Servers

To keep maintenance and administration costs down and promote efficiency in any Exchange Server 2003 messaging environment, you must have a secure and reliable means of managing the servers remotely. Windows Server 2003 and Exchange Server 2003 have these capabilities built in so that you do not have to rely on third-party solutions.

You can manage Exchange Server 2003 systems remotely in different ways, and it is important to understand not only what these options are but also which one is best for your particular environment. This chapter complements Chapter 19, "Exchange Server 2003 Management and Maintenance Practices," and expands on the different remote management capabilities and when to use them.

Terminal Services Modes of Operation

There are two Terminal Services functions within Windows Server 2003: Remote Desktop for Administration and Terminal Services (formerly known as Terminal Services Application Mode). Remote Desktop for Administration mode is installed (but not enabled) by default; Terminal Services must be manually installed and configured.

Remote Desktop for Administration

As mentioned earlier, Remote Desktop for Administration is included and installed with the Windows Server 2003 operating system and needs only to be enabled. This eases automated and unattended server deployment by enabling an administrator to deploy servers that can be managed remotely after the operating systems have completed installation. This mode can also be used to manage a headless server, which can reduce the amount of space needed in any server rack. More space can be dedicated to servers instead of switch boxes, monitors, keyboards, and mouse devices.

Remote Desktop for Administration limits the number of terminal sessions to two, with only one Remote Desktop Protocol (RDP) or Secure Sockets Layer (SSL) for remote administration connection per network interface. Only administrators can connect to these sessions. No additional licenses are needed to run a server in this Terminal Services mode, which enables an administrator to perform almost all the server management duties remotely.

Even though Remote Desktop for Administration is installed by default, this mode does not have to be enabled. Some organizations might see Remote Desktop for Administration as an unneeded security risk and choose to keep it disabled. This function can easily be disabled throughout the entire Active Directory (AD) forest by using a Group Policy setting to disable administrators from connecting through Remote Desktop for Administration.

Planning for Remote Desktop for Administration Mode

Unless Remote Desktop for Administration is viewed as a security risk, you should enable it on all internal servers to allow remote administration. For servers that are on the Internet or for DMZ networks, Remote Desktop for Administration may be used, but access should be even more restricted. For example, consider limiting access to a predefined IP address or set of IP addresses, using firewall ACLs to eliminate unauthorized attempts to log on to the server. Another option is to limit connections to the server based on protocol.

> **NOTE**
>
> The level of encryption for remote sessions by default is 128-bit (bidirectional). It is also important to note that some older Terminal Services Clients might not support that level of encryption.

Enabling Remote Desktop for Administration

Remote Desktop for Administration mode is installed on all Windows Server 2003 servers by default and needs only to be enabled. To manually enable this feature, follow these steps:

1. Log on to the desired server with Administrator privileges.

2. Click Start, right-click the My Computer shortcut, and then click Properties.

3. Select the Remote tab, and under the Remote Desktop section, check the Allow users to connect remotely to your computer box, as shown in Figure 21.1.

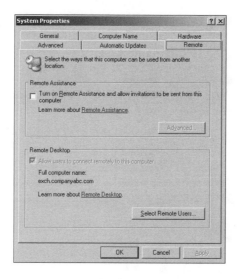

FIGURE 21.1   Enabling users to connect to the system remotely.

4. Click OK in the Systems Properties page to complete this process.

Remote Administration (HTML)

Formerly known as the Terminal Services Advanced Client (TSAC) in Windows 2000, the Remote Administration (HTML) tool can also be used to manage Exchange Server 2003. The primary intention of this tool is to provide basic remote administration capabilities for Internet Information Services 6.0 Web servers, as shown in Figure 21.2. However, there are capabilities built in that enable administrators to not only check server status, logs, and IIS functionality, but also to manage server network configurations and email alerts, and use the Exchange System Manager (ESM) through Remote Desktop, as shown in Figure 21.3.

Installing and Enabling Remote Administration (HTML)

As hinted at in the last section, Remote Administration (HTML) is a Windows Server 2003 IIS component, and it cannot be used to manage earlier versions of IIS. It is also not enabled by default. This does not mean that using this tool creates unnecessary security risks. Instead it keeps Windows Server 2003 security in a more consistent, locked-down state, and you need to manually install and configure its settings to meet the security requirements of your company.

To install Remote Administration (HTML), do the following:

1. Select Add or Remove Programs from the Start, Control Panel menu.

2. Choose Add/Remove Windows Components and then highlight Application Server in the Windows Components Wizard window.

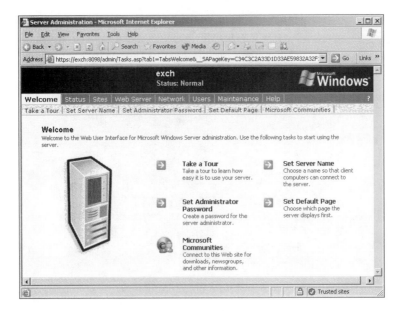

FIGURE 21.2   Remote Administration (HTML) tool options.

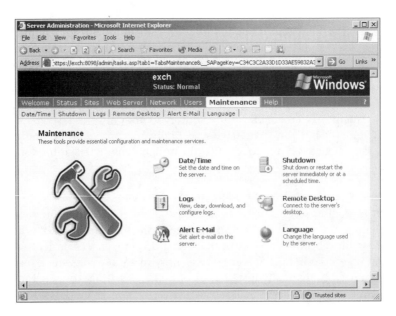

FIGURE 21.3   Remote Desktop access from the Remote Administration tool.

3. Click Details and then highlight Internet Information Services (IIS) in the Application Server window.

4. Click Details again and highlight World Wide Web Services. Click Details one more time in order to view the Remote Administration (HTML) option, as shown in Figure 21.4.

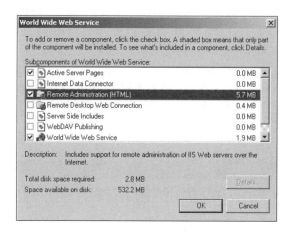

FIGURE 21.4   Installing the Remote Administration (HTML) tool.

5. Click OK three times to return to the Windows Components Wizard window and then click Next.

6. When installation completes, click Finish.

To enable Remote Administration (HTML), perform the following steps:

1. Select the Internet Information Services Manager from the Start, Administrative Tools menu.

2. Expand the server and also the Web Site folder to display a list of Web sites hosted on the Exchange Server 2003 server.

3. Right-click the Administration Web site and then select Properties.

4. Within the Web site identification section, record the port numbers that are displayed for the TCP and SSL ports. The defaults are 8099 and 8098.

5. Select the Directory Security tab and then click the Edit button under IP address and domain name restrictions section. You can select restrictions either by IP address, a group of IP addresses, or by domain name.

CAUTION

Although you can grant access to all computers, all computers in an IP address subnet, or all computers in a domain, you should limit the number of computers that may have access using Remote Administration (HTML) to Exchange Server 2003. Otherwise, unnecessary security vulnerabilities can be introduced on the Exchange Server 2003 server.

6. In the IP Address and Domain Name Restrictions window select Denied Access, and then click the Add button. Note that you can optionally click DNS Lookup to verify the name of the server to which you are granting access.

7. In the Grant Access window, click Single computer and then enter in the IP address of the computer to which you want to grant access.

8. Click OK twice and then close the IIS Manager.

To remotely administer the Exchange Server 2003 Server from the computer that has been granted access, open Internet Explorer and type **https://*servername*:8098** where *servername* is the name of the server. You will be prompted to provide username and password credentials in order to log onto the server.

NOTE

As mentioned earlier, Remote Administration (HTML) provides the necessary tools for managing essential IIS components and basic Windows Server 2003 features, but it also provides a link for the Remote Desktop. The Remote Desktop is the Web-based equivalent of Remote Desktop for Administration. This link must be used if you are to manage an Exchange Server 2003 server. Therefore, the Remote Administration (HTML) tool is useful on older or non-Windows computers that need access for remote Exchange Server 2003 management purposes. Otherwise, if the computer accessing Exchange Server 2003 remotely via the Remote Administration (HTML) tool also has the Remote Desktop Connection tool (for the client side), it begs the question of why the Remote Desktop for Administration tool is not being used in the first place. Unless a security policy dictates that the RDP port should not be open on the firewall, the Remote Desktop for Administration tool is recommended.

Remote Desktop Administration Tips and Tricks

There are several key points to consider before using either Remote Desktop for Administration or Remote Administration (HTML), including, but not limited to, the following:

- **Make sure resources are available.** What IT personnel resources, if any, are available at the remote location or at the Exchange Server 2003 server's location? If a problem arises with the connection to the remote Exchange Server 2003 server or the server itself (for example, a disconnection) there should be contingency plans available to recover and continue to remotely manage the system. Generally speaking it is a good idea to have someone in the vicinity that can assist the administrator in some form or fashion.

- **Use care when modifying network configurations.** With any remote administration tool, you are dependent upon the connectivity between the client computer and the Exchange Server 2003 server that is being remotely managed. If network configuration settings must be modified remotely, consider having alternative methods of access. For instance, dial-up or a separate network connection might minimize downtime or other issues stemming from loss of connectivity.

- **Use disconnect and reset timeout values.**   Anytime a connection is accidentally broken or an administrator disconnects, the remote session is placed into a disconnected state that can later be reconnected and used to manage a server remotely. Disconnect and reset timeouts are not configured by default for remote desktop administration tools. These values can be used to ensure that administrators are not unintentionally locked out (for example, when there are two remote sessions that are active but in a disconnected state). Generally speaking, using 10–20-minute timeout values allows enough time for administrators to reconnect if they were accidentally disconnected. Moreover, it helps minimize the number of sessions that are disconnected and not being used.

- **Coordinate remote administration efforts.**   The number of remote administration connections is limited to a precious two. Therefore, plan and coordinate efforts to reduce the number of attempts to access Exchange Server 2003 servers remotely. This also helps ensure that remote administration activities do not conflict with other administrators and sessions—or, in the worst of cases, corrupt information or data on the server.

Terminal Services

Terminal Services mode is available in all editions of Windows Server 2003 (that is, Standard, Enterprise, and DataCenter) except the Web edition. It enables any authorized user to connect to the server and run a single application or a complete desktop session from the client workstation. Because the applications are loaded and running on the Terminal Services server, client desktop resources are barely used; all the application processing is performed by the Terminal Services server. This enables companies to extend the life of old, less-powerful workstations by running applications only from a Terminal Services server session.

Terminal Services is generally not considered a viable technology to manage Exchange Server 2003 remotely. Although it is possible to use Terminal Services to manage Exchange Server 2003, there are several planning considerations that must be addressed to determine whether Terminal Services is suitable in your environment.

Planning Considerations for Using Terminal Services

Terminal Services can require a lot of planning, especially when you're considering whether to use it to manage Exchange Server 2003 remotely. Because Terminal Services is intended to make applications available to end-users rather than serve as a remote management service, security, server performance, and licensing are key components to consider before using it in a production environment.

Terminal Services Security

Terminal Services servers should be secured following standard security guidelines defined in company security policies and as recommended by hardware and software vendors. Some basic security configurations include removing all unnecessary services from the Terminal Services nodes and applying security patches for known vulnerabilities on services or applications that are running on the Terminal server.

An administrator can use Group Policy to limit client functionality as needed to enhance server security, and if increased network security is a requirement, can consider requiring clients to run sessions in 128-bit high-encryption mode.

Windows Server 2003 Terminal Services can be run in either Full Security or Relaxed Security Permission compatibility mode to meet an organization's security policy and application requirements. Permission compatibility mode was created to help lock down the Terminal server environment to reduce the risk of users mistakenly installing software or inadvertently disabling the Terminal Services server by moving directories or deleting Registry keys. This mode can be used for most certified Terminal server applications. Relaxed Security mode was created to support legacy applications that require extended access into the server system directory and System Registry.

In addition to all the more common security precautions that are recommended for Terminal Services, you must also consider how running Terminal Services on an Exchange Server 2003 server affects security. Using a server with both Terminal Services and Exchange Server 2003 roles and responsibilities can be a dangerous combination and should be considered only in the smallest of environments with very relaxed security requirements. In any circumstance, the combination is not recommended.

Combining the two services and configuring Terminal Services to remotely manage Exchange Server 2003 can result in many security-related hazards, including the following:

- A single misconfiguration or setting can enable users to change specific Exchange Server 2003 settings or parameters.

- Users authorized to shut down or restart the system might inadvertently do so, causing messaging downtime.

- Application-specific security might conflict or in some cases unintentionally allow or restrict access to messaging components on the server.

Terminal Server Licensing

Terminal Services requires the purchase of client access licenses (CALs) for each client device or session. A Terminal Services License Server also must be available on the network to allocate and manage these CALs. When a Terminal Services server is establishing a session with a client, it checks with the Terminal Services License Server to verify whether this client has a license. A license is allocated if the client does not already have one.

> **NOTE**
>
> Using Terminal Services to connect to and remotely manage an Exchange Server 2003 server does not exempt you from needing a Terminal Services CAL. This adds to the overall cost of supporting Exchange Server 2003.

To install licenses on the TS License server, the Terminal Services License server must first be installed and then activated online. The TS License server requires Internet access or dial-up modem access to activate the client access licenses added to the server.

When a Terminal Services server cannot locate a Terminal Services License Server on the network, it still allows unlicensed clients to connect. This can go on for 120 days without contacting a license server, and then the server stops serving Terminal Services sessions. It is imperative to get a license server installed on the network as soon as possible—before Terminal Services servers are deployed to production.

Using Terminal Services on Pocket Devices

Many mobile devices, such as pocket PCs, have Terminal Services Client components built in to the device's operating system, as shown in Figure 21.5. The Terminal Services Client connects to the server as a client computer would connect, using Remote Desktop for Administration. After it's connected, as shown in Figure 21.6, administrators can manage the Exchange Server 2003 server from the mobile device the same way they would if they were logged in locally. The obvious downside to using a mobile device is the screen size. Although some mobile devices can resize the screen to accommodate the entire desktop on it, the screen size and resolution is limited.

Locking Down PDA Terminal Services

Securing mobile devices, such as the Pocet PC illustrated in the figure, is often more challenging than securing a client computer or another server. Because the device is designed for mobility, it opens up the possibility of losing the device or having it stolen. Then an unauthorized person could use it to gain access to the network environment.

An obvious deterrent is securing access to the mobile device's useability. For instance, a person has to use a password in order to use the mobile device. If the mobile device were stolen or found, the person with the device would have to figure out the password before gaining access to the mobile device. Pocket PC 2002 and higher support four-digit PIN numbers (similar to a bank ATM card) and strong, alphanumeric passwords. In addition, each time the wrong password is entered, a timed delay increases before the person can attempt to reenter a PIN or password. The time delay increases exponentially after each unsuccessful logon attempt.

Another important aspect to secure is mobile device communications with the rest of the world. The type of security that can be used depends on how the mobile device is configured to communicate. Most devices, however, support using SSL or Wired Equivalent Protocol (WEP).

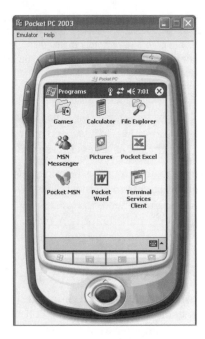

FIGURE 21.5   The Terminal Services Client component on a Pocket PC device.

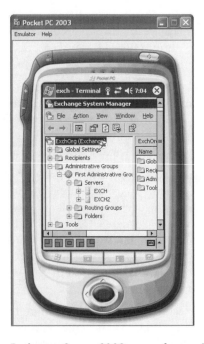

FIGURE 21.6   Managing an Exchange Server 2003 server from a Pocket PC device.

> **NOTE**
>
> Although viruses for mobile devices are rare, it is important to implement virus protection software. Antivirus software can also help prevent tracing or monitoring applications from being installed that could record everything that is entered into the mobile device, including passwords.

Using Exchange System Manager to Remotely Manage Exchange Server 2003

Throughout this book there have been references to using the EESM to perform Exchange-related tasks, such as setting Exchange Server 2003 configuration parameters, monitoring queues, and managing mailboxes. Almost every Exchange-related task that can be done is performed through the ESM. The exceptions include, but are not limited to, those tasks related to AD and offline maintenance of the Exchange databases.

This primary tool for Exchange, shown in Figure 21.7, is a Microsoft Management Console (MMC) snap-in (Exchange System Manager.msc) and it gets installed by default on all Exchange Server 2003 servers. The ESM can also be installed on a client computer so that you can manage Exchange from any location from which you have connectivity to the servers.

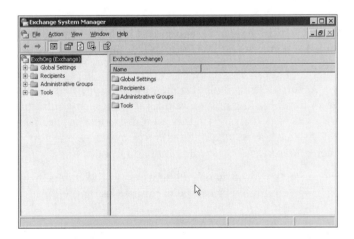

FIGURE 21.7   The Exchange System Manager interface.

> **TIP**
>
> Figure 21.7 shows a more advanced view of the ESM, which displays routing and administrative groups. This view can be selected by right-clicking on the Exchange organization within the ESM and selecting Properties. In the Properties window within the General tab, check the routing and administrative group views that you want displayed.

The ESM can be used to manage a single server or groups of servers. As a result, you can manage any of the Exchange servers in your environment, no matter where they are physically located. If you use Remote Desktop for Administration for Exchange management and troubleshooting, it will more than likely still require you to use the ESM. Many tasks for managing Exchange Server 2003 servers, such as monitoring Event Viewer logs and analyzing performance statistics, are related more directly to the operating system and can be managed and maintained through Terminal Services or Remote Desktop for Administration. Other tasks, such as enabling message tracking or configuring front-end server functionality, should be managed through the ESM.

> **CAUTION**
>
> The ESM communicates with servers using Remote Procedure Calls (RPCs). This method of communication is not considered secure by default when traversing over public networks such as the Internet.

Benefits of Remote Management Using the ESM

There are many inherent benefits of using the ESM to manage and maintain Exchange Server 2003 remotely, including the following four primary advantages:

- **Extensibility**   The ESM snap-in provides the foundation or framework for the Exchange Server 2003 related tasks that can be performed locally and remotely.

- **Convenience**   Given the proper access rights, Exchange administrators can manage multiple Exchange Server 2003 servers, routing groups, and administrative groups from a single, unified interface.

- **Consistency**   As the previous bullet implies, the ESM provides a consistent interface for everyone administering or maintaining the messaging infrastructure. The same snap-in is used, regardless of whether administration has been delegated or different functions—such as public folder administration, connectors, or messaging policies—are being maintained by specific individuals or groups.

- **Mixed Environments**   Most management aspects of Exchange management even in a mixed Exchange environment can be performed using the ESM.

Managing a Mixed Exchange Environment with ESM

Some network environments, especially large, enterprise networks, might have a period of time where coexistence with previous Exchange versions is necessary or unavoidable. For instance, Exchange 2000 might be kept in the environment for extended periods of time because it is providing functionality, such as Instant Messaging.

In these circumstances it is important to minimize versions of the ESM that are being used to manage the messaging infrastructure; otherwise, compatibility issues might arise. Microsoft does not recommend or support managing Exchange Server 2003 features using the Exchange 5.5 or Exchange 2000 version of the ESM. There are only a few exceptions to this advisory:

- Use the Exchange 2000 ESM to manage specific Exchange 2000 features that are no longer included with Exchange Server 2003 (for example, Key Management Service or Instant Messaging). Otherwise, use the Exchange Server 2003 ESM.

- Exchange 5.5 servers should be managed using the Exchange 5.5 ESM, except when moving or migrating mailboxes to an Exchange Server 2003 server.

- When you manage connection agreements (for example, during an upgrade to Exchange Server 2003), manage the connection agreements on a per server basis. In other words, manage connection agreements on an Exchange 2000 server using the Exchange 2000 ESM.

Summary

Many messaging environments today require an easy and effective way of remotely managing and maintaining systems. Both Windows Server 2003 and Exchange Server 2003 have tools built in that administrators can use to securely manage and maintain Exchange Server 2003 from any location. This chapter examined the most common remote management tools and highlighted which ones are more appropriate in various real-world circumstances.

Best Practices

The following are best practices from this chapter:

- Carefully plan which Exchange Server 2003 servers should use Remote Desktop for Administration or Remote Administration (HTML) for remote management.

- Restrict Remote Desktop for Administration or Remote Administration (HTML) access on Exchange Server 2003 servers that are facing the Internet (for example, limiting access to a predefined IP address or set of IP addresses).

- Have a person in the vicinity of the server that is being managed remotely assist the administrator in case network connectivity is lost.

- Use care when modifying network configurations over a Remote Desktop for Administration connection.

- Use disconnect and reset timeout values for Remote Desktop for Administration connections.

- Plan and coordinate remote administration efforts to reduce the number of attempts to access Exchange Server 2003 servers remotely.

- Do not implement Terminal Services on an Exchange server solely to manage Exchange Server 2003 remotely.

- Use the advanced view of the ESM when using multiple routing and administrative groups.

- Use RPC over HTTPS or Remote Desktop for Administration with high encryption when managing Exchange Server 2003 servers remotely over public networks using ESM.

PART VII

New Mobility Functionality in Microsoft Exchange Server 2003

IN THIS PART

CHAPTER 22

Designing Mobility in Exchange Server 2003

With previous versions of Microsoft's Exchange product, mobility either meant setting up a dial-up or VPN connection to a full Outlook client on a laptop or ending up being drastically limited in features with a partially featured Outlook Web client, or purchasing a third-party product and integrating it into Exchange. With Exchange 2003, however, mobility now includes several options that provide full access to mail, calendars, and contacts, plus varying built-in methods to access information using mobile phones or PDA devices.

Microsoft's strategy on mobility is to provide the ability to have access to email, calendar, contacts, and other important information virtually anywhere. The various mobile access methods to Exchange include

- Full Outlook client access over VPN
- Full Outlook client access using HTTP Proxy
- Outlook Web Access from a browser
- Pocket PC access updated by Exchange ActiveSync
- Mobile phone access using mobile Web
- Accessing Exchange by non-Windows systems

Accessing Outlook Using VPN Connectivity

One of the long-supported methods of mobile connectivity to Exchange has been to set up a VPN client on the remote system and synchronize content between client and server. Exchange 2003 continues to support this method, and improvements in the Outlook 2003 client provide improvements in synchronization.

Outlook VPN synchronization enables users, typically with laptop computers, to access the same Outlook information whether they are connected to the LAN or working remotely from the network. When connected remotely, the user works offline and synchronizes his or her client content to the Exchange server.

VPN connectivity for Outlook is covered in depth in Chapter 25, "Getting the Most Out of the Microsoft Outlook Client," which provides best practices on how organizations implement remote access connectivity to Outlook and procedures for installing and configuring the client for synchronization.

Connecting Outlook over HTTP Proxy

New to Outlook 2003 and Exchange 2003 is the capability of synchronizing between the Exchange server and Outlook client without setting up a VPN connection. This new functionality is commonly referred to as MAPI over HTTP, RPC over HTTP, or HTTP Proxy. Effectively this functionality, which is new to Windows 2003, enables a user to establish a secured connection over HTTP for data synchronization. Rather than simply allowing secured browser access using SSL, HTTP Proxy provides an Outlook client to connect to an Exchange server for full Outlook synchronization.

Using HTTP Proxy eliminates the challenge of establishing a VPN connection that might otherwise have traditional VPN ports blocked by firewalls. HTTP Proxy is covered in depth in Chapter 25.

Using Outlook Web Access As a Remote Client

For mobile access to Exchange without the need of transporting mail with a laptop computer, Microsoft Exchange 2003 continues its support of a browser-based client with Outlook Web Access (OWA, pronounced "oh-wah"). Microsoft has drastically improved the OWA client with significant feature enhancements in the Web client, such as spell checker, rules, and preview mode. Many organizations have chosen to implement Outlook Web Access in Exchange Server 2003 as the primary client for users of Exchange because of the full features of the new OWA client.

OWA is good for home access because an IT organization does not have to arrange to install and support the full Outlook client on home systems, and OWA is a good solution for kiosk or Internet café usage. Because OWA uses a standard browser over http port 80 or https port 443, there are few restrictions or limitations on client access to Exchange using OWA.

Implementing OWA in a server environment is covered in Chapter 10, "Outlook Web Access 2003," and the client piece of OWA is covered in Chapter 26, "Everything You Need to Know About Outlook Web Access Client."

Using Exchange ActiveSync for PDA Connectivity

New to Exchange is the capability of extending mobility from the user property page in
Active Directory Users and Computers to enable more than just laptop synchronization
and browser access and to include mobile synchronization with devices such as pocket
PCs. In previous versions of Exchange, an organization that wanted to synchronize a Pocet
PC device would either have users install ActiveSync software on their desktop and
synchronize their Pocet PC devices individually, or purchase a third-party or add-on
gateway product, such as Microsoft Mobile Information Server.

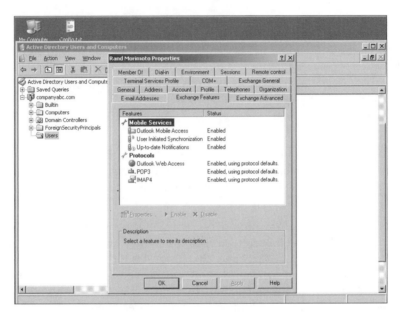

FIGURE 22.1   User property page for mobile configuration.

Exchange ActiveSync is built in to Exchange 2003 and supports the synchronization of
Pocet PC PDAs, Pocet PC-enabled mobile phones, and SmartPhone devices. Pocket devices
that have network connectivity—whether Ethernet, wireless LAN, or mobile public
network—can securely synchronize to Exchange 2003. The synchronization connects mail,
calendar, contacts, notes, and files linked between Exchange 2003 and the mobile device.

Exchange ActiveSync functionality is covered in more detail in the section "Leveraging
Exchange ActiveSync for PDA Mobile Communications," later in this chapter.

Using Mobile Web Access for Wireless Phone Access

For mobile devices that are not operating under the Windows CE operating system for
Pocet PC Exchange ActiveSync synchronization—such as mobile phones—Exchange 2003
supports mobile Web access by these devices. Mobile Web support in Exchange 2003

includes xHTML used in WAP 2.x devices, cHTML, and HTML browser-based device support. With the capability for HTML-type devices to access Exchange client information—such as mail, calendar, contact, and other folder information—users who rely on their mobile phone device can send and receive information directly with Exchange.

Chapter 24, "Configuring Client Systems for Mobility," covers the setup of mobile devices to access mobile Web information in Exchange. The basics of mobile Web access is covered in more detail in the section "Using Outlook Mobile Access for Browser-based Devices," later in this chapter.

Using Non-Windows Systems to Access Exchange

When mobile access to Exchange is required that does not fit any of the categories covered so far in this section, see Chapter 27, "Outlook for Non-Windows Systems," which provides alternatives. Mobile system access by non-Windows devices includes Apple Macintosh systems or Unix-based system access to Exchange.

Automatic Update on Mobile Devices

Key to Microsoft's strategy and offerings for mobile access is the ability for remote users to have access to all of their mail, calendar, contact, and Exchange information, regardless of where they are and what type of device they have available. Part of the strategy is to make sure that Exchange information is always up to date.

Rather than synchronizing information once a day and then working off a cached version for several hours, with the high likelihood that information will be grossly out of date by the next synchronization period, Exchange 2003 provides the ability to keep devices automatically updated throughout the day. In addition to enabling the user to pull down or request a synchronization of information at any time, technology has been built in to Exchange 2003 that pushes updated information to devices, even "waking up" the device—using the Short Message Service (SMS)—to accept updates that can keep important information readily available to the mobile user.

Leveraging Exchange ActiveSync for PDA Mobile Communications

Pocket PC devices have become more popular over the past couple of years, not only because more devices now include mobile Windows, but also because the ability to fully synchronize calendar, contacts, and other Outlook information makes the functionality more useable. Instead of having to convert contacts, appointments, or messages between disparate applications or learning new tools, a Pocet PC device uses a similar interface to natively synchronize content.

Additionally, because the interface and content remain in native formats, not only do users have the ability to access their email, calendar, and contact information, but they also have full access to other Outlook folder content, such as subfolders and attachments.

22

So if users have managed their Outlook folders with custom containers—organizing information by client, project, or chronological date, or other method—those folders also can be accessed and synchronized.

Additional improvements in the Exchange ActiveSync with Exchange 2003 include the ability to prevent users from pushing everything, but customizing information synchronization by preventing the sync of nonessential messages, attachments, or content. This offers the ability to create filters and define characteristics on message downloads, decreasing the traffic between the mobile device and the server. Although information can be filtered to prevent the automatic synchronization of this content, Exchange 2003 does provide the ability for the user to manually request the attachment or other filtered information to be transmitted. So the user has the ability to focus bandwidth and information access as effectively as possible.

Flexibility of Information Synchronization

When synchronizing information between Exchange 2003 and a Pocet PC-enabled device, the device can be connected by a variety of different connectivity methods. The device can be connected through a traditional cradle using the network connectivity of the host system to synchronize with Exchange. A Pocet PC-enabled device can be directly connected to a network using an Ethernet adapter in the device. Through the Ethernet adapter, the device can communicate with the Exchange 2003 server.

A Pocet PC-enabled device can also communicate over wireless methods, and can have a wireless LAN adapter using 802.11b, 802.11a, 802.1x, Bluetooth, or infrared. A wireless LAN connection truly disconnects the user from a cradle or physical connection to the network. This provides mobility for the user to access Exchange content anywhere within an office or campus facility. With wireless mobility, the user can keep calendar appointments, email messages, and other up-to-date information accurate and accessible.

When the device is not within the range of a local area network wireless connection, more mobile public network connectivity can extend real-time synchronization regionally, nationally, or globally. Using cellular phone, PCS, GPRS, 1xRTT, GSM, and other public network systems, a properly equipped Pocet PC device can enable users to synchronize their mail, calendar, contact, and other information anytime and anywhere.

Customizing Synchronization Characteristics

Pocket PC-enabled devices can synchronize folders and subfolders with Exchange and have the capability of filtering and truncating information that is sent and received by the device. Customization of sync characteristics also includes the ability to delete messages or information on the device and have those changes synchronized up to the Exchange server to be deleted on the server copy of the information. The same applies to information that might be deleted using Outlook Web Access, using the full Outlook client software, or by other Exchange client applications that replicate the changes back down to the Pocet PC device. Having full control over the synchronization characteristics, along with the ability to delete in one place what is replicated to all user devices, drastically improves the ability of users to control information regardless of what device they use to access their Exchange information.

Improving Mobile Performance

As a user accesses Exchange using a variety of different mobile devices, there are times that the bandwidth availability between the Exchange server and the device is grossly limited. Although local area network connections have commonly relied on 100MB, speeds and thus the opening and accessing of large 2MB attachments or 10MB files go unnoticed. However, when a mobile user tries to synchronize a 2MB file over a 9600 baud mobile connection, the file could take 20–30 minutes to transfer, preventing the user from getting urgent emails or other messages during the transfer. Also, many wireless service providers charge based on packets transferred, so the automatic sending and receiving of large attachments could be very expensive. Exchange ActiveSync, included with Exchange 2003, enables the user to choose whether to synchronize attachments.

With Exchange ActiveSync, there is also a smart reply and smart forward function that prevents the need to have an attachment received or sent to the mobile device in order for the user to reply or forward the attachment. For example, a user might receive a large Word document to review. Rather than receiving the document, reviewing it, and then forwarding it to someone where the large attachment would be received and then sent by the mobile device, Exchange ActiveSync enables the user to reply and forward the attachment without the attachment ever being received by the mobile device. The user simply forwards the message to another user. Exchange ActiveSync knows to grab the attachment off the Exchange server and forward it to the user, and not require the mobile device to retransmit the same attachment across the network.

Additional performance-improving features of Exchange ActiveSync are the ability for a user to define peak and nonpeak times to synchronize information and the ability to change those synchronization scheduling options when roaming. By specifying peak time for sending and receiving information, a user can specify higher priority and more frequent transmission of messages. During nonpeak times, the user can specify to have large attachments sent, because message receipt and sending might not be as critical.

Another performance-improving function in Exchange 2003 is the ability for a user to mix the function of ActiveSync with Outlook Mobile Access; this is covered in more detail in the next section, "Using Outlook Mobile Access for Browser-Based Devices." Rather than sending or receiving a large attachment, an HTML Web view of the attachment can be done, enabling the user to view the attachment over a Web browser.

Improving Mobile Security

Although Exchange 2003 supports sophisticated methods for sending and receiving messages and attachments, organizations must ensure the security and integrity of the information. Exchange ActiveSync supports S/MIME encrypted attachments and 128-bit encryption on transmissions between server and client devices. With support for encryption and encrypted attachments, security of information can be improved.

Using Outlook Mobile Access for Browser-Based Devices

As mentioned at the start of this chapter, for devices that are not Pocet PC-enabled, Microsoft Exchange 2003 supports HTML Web browser view of content. This functionality is built in to the Outlook Mobile Access function of Exchange and supports xHTML devices, such as WAP 2.x markup devices, cHTML devices, and standard HTML Web devices. These devices include mobile phones and Web-enabled Palm OS type devices in addition to other mobile wireless devices.

Simplified Browser-Centric Commands

Outlook Mobile Access, or OMA, provides simple browser-based commands that enable users to manage their email, calendars, contacts, and tasks. Because many of these HTML-based mobile devices do not have large screens or large memories, it is important to minimize the type of information transmitted or sent between the mobile device and Exchange. Because users who send mail to an Exchange 2003 recipient do not know that the recipient is using a mobile phone device for receipt of mail or other information, it is important for the Exchange Outlook Mobile Access tool to do appropriate conversion and modification of content sent to the mobile device.

Some of the browser-centric commands that are part of Outlook Mobile Access include

- **Managing Email**   OMA enables users to have inbox messages, calendar appointment information, and contact data displayed in single-line text that can be more easily read by limited-lined mobile devices. Additionally, OMA enables users to compose, reply, and forward messages using a single button command of a mobile device. Users also can access other folders within Exchange, search the Global Address List, and search contacts.

- **Managing Calendars**   Outlook Mobile Access enables a user to view and create appointments in Exchange, to accept and decline appointments, and to accept appointments as tentative. Through simplified single button commands, a user can reply to a meeting request.

- **Managing Contacts**   The Outlook Mobile Access client enables users to create, delete, and modify contacts in Exchange. In addition to being able to dynamically query the contacts and the Global Address List, users can also add addresses to their personal contacts in the Exchange Global Address List. Contacts can also be used to begin an email message or to initiate a phone call to the contact.

- **Managing Tasks**   Outlook Mobile Access also enables a user to update tasks, mark tasks as complete, and create notes that can be read, reviewed, and accessed not only by the OMA client but also by other Outlook client systems.

Minimizing Downloads Through Enhanced Features

As mentioned earlier in this section, because the transmission bandwidth to an HTML Web model device typically is done with limited bandwidth, any ability of the messaging client to decrease information transmission drastically improves the user experience. OMA provides the ability for a user to simply and quickly delete a message without having the contents of the message transmitted to the device, and users can mark a message as unread so that they would be reminded to look at the message at a later date.

Additional OMA functions provide the ability to flag a message for follow-up at a later date, similar to a reminder on a message that may require more attention. And OMA provides the ability for users to have only a portion of information sent to their device, with the option to download more if necessary. Many times, after reading the first few words of a document, a user determines that the content of the message is not urgent and then marks the message for view and access at a later time.

Designing the Appropriate Use of Exchange 2003 Mobility Capabilities

When implementing Exchange 2003 with the expectation of using the Exchange ActiveSync and Outlook Mobile Access functionality, an Exchange design architect needs to determine the best way to take advantage of the technology. Fortunately, the ActiveSync and Outlook Mobile Access functions are relatively low in bandwidth and processing demands on the Exchange environment, so a single server can typically scale to the initial needs of most organizations. Design and scalability of Exchange 2003 mobility do not necessarily require a lot of performance planning, but you do need the right technology for the expected use.

Identifying Mobile Devices in Use

In defining the organization's use of mobile devices, such as PDAs and mobile phones, it's helpful to start with understanding what type of devices are currently used in the organization. Because there's been neither industry standardization nor support for common gateway or integration products, most organizations have one of every type of mobile device available in their organization. When trying to support one of every device, the organization is challenged with trying to meet the integration and education needs of several different types of devices, and in many cases trying to support devices that do not necessarily meet the needs of the user(s) in the first place.

So rather than trying to support every type of device in the organization, the initial inventory should be intended at understanding the devices in use. To determine the type of devices used and the basic connectivity, ask users to fill out a questionnaire similar to the one in Table 22.1.

TABLE 22.1   Identifying Mobile Devices in Use

Type of Device in Use	Wireless or WAN Connection?	Cradle or Standalone Connection?
Pocket PC PDA device		
Pocket PC-enabled mobile phone		
Palm pilot device		
Palm OS-enabled device		
Palm OS-enabled mobile phone		
xHTML, cHTML, or other browser-supported mobile phone		

Users who are determined to have mobile devices should be asked questions to determine their current use of email, calendaring, or other synchronization of information. Ask users questions similar to the ones shown in Table 22.2.

TABLE 22.2   Identifying Mobile Device Features

Feature	Yes	No
Do you use your mobile device to check email?		
Do you use your mobile device to send email?		
Do you use your mobile device to view and enter contacts?		
Do you use the calendaring function on your mobile device?		
Do you use notes or to-do lists on your mobile device?		

Other questions, such as those in Table 22.3, help determine whether the mobile device should be prioritized for integration to Exchange 2003.

TABLE 22.3   Identifying Exchange 2003 Integration Potential

Task	Description
How often do you synchronize your mobile device with your desktop system (once a day, once a week, every hour, continuously)?	
If you had the ability to synchronize your device more often, would you?	
If you do not synchronize your device regularly, is there an impact on information accuracy or business-critical issues?	
Does your mobile device meet your mobile information access needs, or do you want additional functionality?	

Frequently determined from the answers to these various questionnaires is that most users have minimal mobile information access needs and use their current mobile device for a limited set of features. So rather than trying to integrate every mobile device in the organization to Exchange 2003 initially, identify the users who have the most need and the most functional use of their mobile device now, and add those users to the first round of Exchange 2003–integrated devices. Then add additional users in waves, based on need and anticipated value received from the integration.

Quite commonly, users aren't happy with the device they are using, and connecting their device to Exchange 2003 will still not improve the device or how they use it. So rather than integrating devices that do not meet the need of the users, wait until other users get functional use out of Exchange 2003, and consider recommending a standardization of future mobile devices throughout the organization, based on the successful use by the first few waves of users.

Choosing the Right Mobile Solution

After interviewing users in the organization about their use of mobile devices, you might find that certain devices meet user needs and other devices do not. There are frequently two types of users: those that are heavy email users and those that are heavy phone users. Trying to make a phone user into a mobile email user, or vice versa, usually does not result in improved user satisfaction.

A mobile phone with 3–4 8-character lines and a numeric phone keyboard is not a device that best suits someone that needs extensive email capabilities. A Pocet PC device that has full Outlook capabilities but does not have public mobile wireless access also lacks appropriate functionality.

Exchange 2003 has the tools and the functionality to meet the needs of organizations, so it's up to the organization to match users with appropriate devices that can then connect to the fully equipped Exchange 2003 environment.

Understanding Exchange ActiveSync and OMA

An easy way to understand how Exchange 2003 works for mobile users is to leverage the mobile device emulators and software developer's kits for Pocet PC and HTML-based mobile phone units. It's a lot easier and a lot cheaper to download the emulation tools than to buy hardware, set up mobile services, and do initial feature and function testing on real devices.

For Pocet PC functionality testing, Microsoft has a Pocet PC developer's kit that comes with a full functioning Pocet PC emulator. You can download the emulator from Microsoft's homepage at

http://www.microsoft.com/windowsmobile/information/devprograms/default.mspx

The software developer's kit, also known as the Windows Mobile 2003 SDK, comes with an emulation program, similar to the one shown in Figure 22.2, that enables you to connect to a network, establish an Exchange ActiveSync connection to Exchange 2003, and synchronize email, calendar, contacts, and other information between Exchange 2003 and this Pocet PC-emulated device.

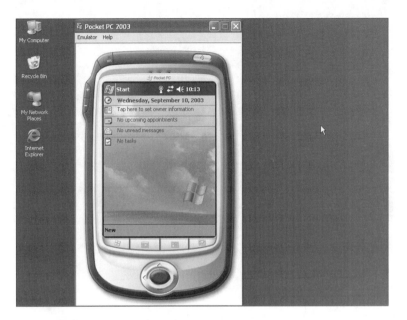

FIGURE 22.2   Microsoft Pocet PC emulator.

The Pocet PC emulator requires the installation of eMbedded Visual C++ 4 along with eMbedded Visual C++ Service Pack 2 or higher to run. The emulator can be installed on any workstation connected to the network that the Exchange 2003 server is connected to, or the emulator can be set to VPN from another segment into a RRAS server on the network where the Exchange 2003 server resides.

Similar functionality can be emulated for a mobile phone. Openwave makes a mobile phone simulator, shown in Figure 22.3, that can be downloaded free from its Website:

`http://www.openwave.com/products/developer_products/omdt/client_sdk.html`

This emulator enables the testing of mobile phone access to Exchange 2003. An organization can get familiar with how a mobile phone works with Exchange 2003—relative to screens, menu commands, message reply, attachment handling, and other functionality—which might take several weeks with a physical mobile phone.

With an emulator on a workstation, basic connectivity, wireless phone connectivity, and other infrastructure testing is eliminated, thus enabling the Exchange administrator to focus on features and functionality. After the basic features and functions of HTML-based Exchange access are understood, the organization can then make the decision to rent, purchase, and evaluate mobile phone connectivity to Exchange.

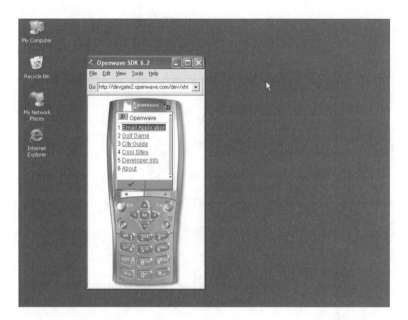

FIGURE 22.3 Openwave mobile phone simulator.

Active Prototype and Pilot Testing of Exchange Mobility

The active prototype and pilot testing phase of Exchange mobility involves actual testing of mobile devices to an Exchange 2003 server. Because basic features and functionality were tested with the emulators, the knowledge learned from software emulation enables the evaluator to better translate the basic functionality knowledge into the specific phone or PDA device. This minimizes the fumbling around of device features and enables the individual to better test the true functionality of the device.

The challenge introduced at this phase is physical connectivity of the device to the local area network or to the public network. Whereas the emulators were typically tested right on the network backbone, from a system such as a desktop or laptop already successfully communicating on the network, a real-world test of a device is usually over some wireless network connection. A number of challenges can prevent a user from successfully testing the system: IP address allocation, proper routing of information between device to server, and routing from server to device. Even firewalls and other security devices can prevent a newly connected mobile device from successfully sending and receiving information over the network. In time, the administrator will isolate the problem; fortunately with some testing of the emulators, the tester will at least know the basics of what to try and what to test after the physical connections are established.

Organizational Scalability of Exchange Mobility

The testing of an emulator—or even a couple of devices—does not necessarily test the full functionality or scalability of the Exchange 2003 network environment. As noted earlier in this chapter, the use of these mobile devices generates very low network and server performance bandwidth demands, and it is actually not too difficult to leverage dozens, if not hundreds, of mobile users off a single Exchange 2003 server, which usually far exceeds the initial prototype testing and pilot phase of most organizations.

For most organizations, the initial phase involves just a handful of users. Even when 5–10 users are involved in a pilot phase, their usage and traffic demands on the Exchange environment is negligible. The level that an organization must start considering performance and bandwidth demands is when the organization exceeds 200–300 simultaneous mobile connections. When the potential server access demand exceeds around 200 simultaneous mobile connections, an additional server should be considered. An additional server may be needed when there is fewer than 200–300 simultaneous mobile connections when the server is also acting as a Global Catalog look-up server, voicemail integration server, private and public folder access server, or an Outlook Web Access server. When additional server services are added to a system, an organization might need to consider moving the Outlook mobile functionality to another server system.

Using Exchange Mobility for the Mobile Executive

When looking at various scenarios for mobile user access, the mobile executive frequently comes to mind as an individual that can benefit from real-time access to calendar, contacts, and office communications. Prior to Exchange 2003, many executives carried around a mobile phone or a PDA; however, the devices were rarely synchronized on a regular basis, causing calendars on the PDA to be drastically different from the executive's real calendar.

By having Exchange 2003 provide real-time synchronization of information, executives can always look at the most current version of their calendar, and the assistant back at the office has to spend less time adjusting appointments after conflicts are determined.

Technologies Used by Mobile Executives

Frequently a mobile executive uses a mobile phone to keep in contact with the office or to communicate with other managers or clients. The executive also needs access to up-to-date calendar information and contact information. Some executives add to basic email, calendar, contact, and office communications with real-time email access, using devices such as Research in Motion's Blackberry device, or with a pager and accessible mobile phone. All this functionality leads the executive to have to carry around 2–3 different devices, none of which have the most current information.

Achieved Benefits by Executives

The benefit of leveraging the mobile capabilities of Exchange is the ability for executives to have the most up-to-date information on their Pocet PC devices without the need to contact their assistant or make last-minute changes to avoid conflicts. Exchange 2003 mobility simplifies the process organizations must go through to connect users to the office network. These benefits improve time to implement and cross-training turnaround, which ensures a more reasonable expectation for accessing the information.

Replacing Laptops with Mobile Pocket Devices

Many users in organizations have a laptop computer for the sole purpose of checking emails, contacts, and calendars; however, they find it time-consuming to turn on the computer, wait for it to boot up, and then launch Outlook to finally check their calendar. Although a laptop is relatively easy to set up and provides full mobile access to information, laptops are rarely connected on a full-time basis. Users still need to plug in to a phone line to dial up and synchronize their system, or find a high-speed Ethernet or wireless LAN connection to link to their network.

Technologies Used for Mobile Laptop Users

Pocket PC devices with mobile LAN or WAN connections can provide these types of users with access to their email, calendar, contacts, and other business-critical information with a much smaller device to carry around and at a fraction of the cost. With the instant-on capabilities of the Pocet PC devices and the ability to connect to a public wireless network similar to those used by mobile phones, a Pocet PC device can provide even better access and connectivity to information.

Of course, every organization still has its power users who want or need a full laptop computer with their files and other information. With the ability to read emails, use Word documents, easily make minor edits to documents, view or play PowerPoint presentations, watch or display videos, listen to MP3 files, and other tasks on a Pocet PC device, however, the small instant-on wireless connected devices might be a perfect replacement for many laptop users.

Achieved Benefits by Mobile Laptop Users

Users who find the functionality of the Pocet PC device meets their needs can frequently eliminate their need for a laptop computer, pager, PDA, cell phone, and wireless email device—such as a Blackberry—and consolidate all the tasks into a simple Pocet PC-enabled mobile phone.

Leveraging a Low-Cost PDA Instead of an Expensive Tablet

With the release of the tablet PC in the past several years, many organizations have been reconsidering the use of pen-based technology for business applications. Although pen technologies have been used for years in hospitals, warehouses, and freighting companies, the devices have been focused at very specific tasks in a limited number of industries. However with tablet PCs, an organization can build forms in Microsoft Word or Access and can easily have users fill them in using a pen input device without complicated programming and application development.

Unfortunately, tablet PCs are typically more expensive than normal laptop computers, increasing the cost of input device computing. So the lowering of application cost is transferred to a higher cost per unit of the devices placed in the field.

Technologies Used for Pocket PC Mobility

Because the Pocet PC device includes Pocket Word, Pocket Access, and Pocket Excel, and has other full application functionality, the pen input function of the Pocet PC can be leveraged for many functions for which dedicated pen-based systems or expensive tablet PC systems have been considered. A form created in Microsoft Word can be transferred to a Pocet PC device, and a user can use the pen to fill in the form and write in comments. Through integrated wireless LAN and WAN connections on the Pocet PC, a user can transmit information from the Pocet PC over simple Exchange 2003 messaging to a central depository of information.

Achieved Benefits of Pocket Device Use

Using a Pocet PC device instead of a more expensive laptop, tablet PC, or proprietary pen system, an organization can get a low-cost input system, wireless mobility, easy access to information, and simple mobile data entry. Faster application-creation time and lower-cost input translates to a faster return on investment and a easier way for the organization to leverage the technology into meeting its business needs.

Summary

Microsoft's strategy on mobility has drastically improved with the release of Exchange 2003, because organizations can now provide several different ways for users to access Exchange information rather than a single Outlook client method, as has been the case in the past. However, because users can access Exchange using a variety of different methods and protocols is not a good reason for all the methods to be activated and used.

Exchange ActiveSync, built in to Exchange 2003, provides an organization the ability to eliminate having their desktop computer systems on all the time. By centralizing synchronization to a server-based component, an organization can now eliminate the need for individual systems with cradles attached to an environment where users can connect to Exchange ActiveSync through Ethernet connections, wireless LAN connections, wireless public access network connections, or even over VPN from another network location.

Exchange 2003 also integrates full support for HTML-Web–based access to Exchange content, thus enabling users with mobile phones to access their Exchange information. Although a mobile phone is not the best device for large extensive emails, by connecting the mobile phone to Exchange mobile access, an organization can simplify its support for email access if users want access only to their contacts, calendar, or other basic information.

In many cases, there is no additional hardware needed to begin using the mobility functions of Exchange 2003, and as the organization needs to scale its use of Exchange mobility, it can add another server to the environment.

Best Practices

The following are best practices from this chapter:

- Choose the right mobile solution for the right user. No one solution fits all.

- Organizations where users might need extensive email and attachment viewing might consider using a Pocet PC-enabled device.

- Emulators, such as the Pocet PC or the Openwave mobile phone, are easy to set up and can test the functionality of Exchange 2003 mobility without the addition of specialized hardware devices.

- When choosing a mobile access method, a user who frequently uses a mobile phone for communications and wants to limit the number of devices carried around should consider the HTML-Web–based access to Exchange 2003 information.

- Organizations might find that users who currently carry around three to four devices, such as a mobile phone, pager, PDA, and wireless email system, can consolidate to a single Pocet PC mobile phone device that satisfies several needs.

- An organization should not open the pilot testing use of Exchange 2003 mobility devices to all employees, but rather test the functionality with a handful of employees who can then build on best practices of the organization and implement the mobile solution immediately throughout the organization.

- Use Pocet PC devices to replace more expensive tablet PC devices or proprietary pen-based systems that require custom programming. Pocket PC devices can leverage standard Microsoft Word forms and Microsoft Access data entry systems.

- Users who have a mobile phone, PDA, pager, and wireless email device, such as Blackberry, might find that a Pocet PC device can provide at least as much functionality.

CHAPTER 23

Implementing Mobile Synchronization in Exchange Server 2003

Preparing for Mobility in an Exchange 2003 Environment

The ability to synchronize Pocet PC devices and access Exchange information from a mobile phone no longer needs to be a planned and budgeted decision. It can be just the decision to enable mobile access for mobile devices. Exchange 2003, both the Standard Edition and Enterprise Edition of the server software, fully support the connectivity and synchronization of Pocet PC–enabled devices and access by mobile phone devices. As with any technology that comes free and built in, the key is not how to install the software, but rather how to configure it properly and optimize the configuration to meet the needs of the organization.

Understanding ActiveSync Versus Outlook Mobile Access

Exchange 2003 mobility includes two separate components, Exchange ActiveSync and Outlook Mobile Access. Exchange ActiveSync is used to synchronize Pocet PC–enabled devices with Exchange data such as email messages, calendar appointments, and contacts. Normally when users with a Pocet PC device want to synchronize their information, they have to place their device in a cradle connected to their desktop computer. Not only does the cradle minimize the user's ability to truly be mobile, it usually means that the calendar and information on the device is not in sync with the information being managed and accessed by others in the organization. Many users of Palm PDAs and early Pocet PC devices complained that they received dozens of appointment conflicts and missed critical information because their mobile device was not updated to the server at the office. For many mobile users, the ability to have an up-to-date calendar or to receive email messages wirelessly required the purchase and use of yet another mobile device, such as a Research in Motion (RIM) Blackberry. However, with full mobile synchronization capabilities of using Exchange 2003 ActiveSync, a mobile Pocet PC user can have real-time synchronization to Exchange data.

The Outlook Mobile Access component built in to Exchange 2003 provides the capability of a mobile phone to access Exchange information using real-time access. With a wireless phone that supports the Wireless Application Protocol (WAP) 2.x or a device that supports XHTML browser access, a mobile phone user can request access to an Exchange 2003 server to view email messages, calendar appointments, and contacts. With Outlook Mobile Access supporting full HTML browsers and i-Mode devices built in to mobile phones and personal digital assistants (PDA), users have flexibility in choosing the type of device they use to access their Exchange information.

> **NOTE**
>
> Users in Japan using Compact HTML (CHTML) can also access Exchange 2003 Outlook Mobile Access to view emails, calendar appointments, and contacts.

Functionality in Exchange 2003

The mobile functionality for support for Pocet PC synchronization and mobile phone access used to require an organization to purchase the Microsoft Mobile Information Server (MMIS) product as an add-in to Exchange 2000. However, all of the mobile functionality of MMIS is now built directly into Exchange 2003, and the functions have been enhanced.

Simply by installing Exchange 2003, Pocet PC users can immediately configure their Pocet PC device to specify the Exchange 2003 Server as the host server, and the Pocet PC will begin synchronizing mail, calendar, and contacts.

Designing and Planning a Mobile Access Exchange Environment

The designing and planning process for mobility in Exchange Server 2003 is dependent on the number of servers, location of servers, and security desired in the configuration. In its simplest configuration, a single Exchange 2003 server can act as the mailboxes server, also known as the **back-end server functions**, and as the interface to client systems, known as the **front-end server functions**.

For a small organization with fewer than 50 users all located in a single site, the organization can easily have a single Exchange 2003 server act as the front-end and back-end server. The server can host the mailboxes and be the connection point where users log on and access their mail.

When an organization has multiple locations that span across a wide distance, which could cause degrading, the organization may choose to have one or more Exchange servers in each location. This enables users in one site to access the server closest to their site, and users in another site to access the server closest to them. The two servers can be connected to flow mail between the two locations; however, the users effectively connect to the server closest to them. In this particular case, the organization could have one server in one site acting as the front-end and back-end server, and another server in another site acting as the front-end and back-end server for that site.

An organization may choose to split the front-end services from the back-end services, thus having two separate servers for a single site. The decision to have a dedicated front-end server from a back-end server is a choice of security and scalability. From a security perspective, the organization would expose the front-end server to the Internet for remote mobile access. The organization would secure and protect the back-end server because it has the mailboxes that hold data that might be confidential or require access restrictions. This splitting of the front-end and back-end servers creates a barrier between the two servers that can enable better management of information.

The other reason for having a separate front-end server is to enable scalability for front-end connectivity. If an organization has hundreds of users with very small mailboxes, the organization might *need* only a single back-end mailbox server, but might *choose* to have two to three front-end servers to host the client-to-server connectivity. An organization can load-balance the front-end servers so that the messaging administrators can manage the incoming access to the server in a way that optimizes the connection between users and servers.

In the end, an organization can have one server acting as both the front-end and back-end server, or the organization might choose to have multiple front-end/back-end combination servers for users, which might span several sites in the organization. An organization that wants to optimize the performance of front-end communications might choose to split the front-end from the back-end server, and then have several front-end servers available to load-balance incoming user connectivity.

Optimizing the Number of Front-end Servers

The correct number of front-end and back-end servers varies based on the size, number of locations, and access demands of each organization. If the decision on the number of locations and placement of servers based on the number of sites has already been made, the decision about how to scale front-end servers for mobility becomes the resulting decision. Exchange 2003 mobility connections to Pocet PC and mobile Web devices is a function of concurrent access. Even though an organization has 500 users—all with mobile devices— the likelihood that all 500 devices are simultaneously accessing the server is minimal. Even if all 500 devices happen to be connected at the same time, the amount of data transacted by the front-end server is limited.

By using the counters in the MMC performance monitoring tool, an administrator can calculate the load being placed on a server. For monitoring Outlook Mobile Access statistics, Exchange 2003 has the following counters:

- Average Response Time
- Browse Count
- Browse Rate
- Calendar Request Rate
- Contact Request Rate
- Cumulative Time for All Requests
- Cumulative Simultaneous Browses
- HTTP status 100 count
- HTTP status 200 count
- HTTP status 300 count
- HTTP status 400 count
- HTTP status 500 count
- Inbox Request Rate
- Last Response Time
- Maximum Simultaneous Browses
- Task Request Rate
- Total Calendar Requests
- Total Contact Requests
- Total Inbox Requests
- Total Number of Task Requests

Of these counters, the ones to monitor include Average Response Time, Cumulative Simultaneous Browses, Maximum Simultaneous Browses, and Late Response Time.

The Average Response Time and Last Response Time indicates how quickly a request is being served by the Exchange 2003 server, and whether any of the requests are being delayed—typically due to congestion on the server. The Cumulative Simultaneous Browses and Maximum Simultaneous Browses provide comparative information about the number of users accessing the system, both on an ongoing basis and at any given time. With the four counters enabled, the performance tool looks similar to Figure 23.1. By understanding

the traffic demands, late requests, and the number of users accessing the system simultaneously, an administrator can provide a basic level of assessment about whether the
current server is adequate for the organization or whether an additional server is needed.

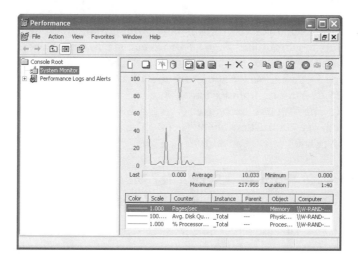

FIGURE 23.1   Equivalent site costs on multiple site links.

Trying Mobility Before Making a True Investment

One of the challenges organizations face in trying to test and evaluate new technologies is
the cost of purchasing the devices needed to test the configuration. There are relatively
easy ways for an organization to set up and test Pocet PC functionality and mobile phone
functionality without having to purchase physical mobile devices.

Microsoft has available a Pocet PC emulator. The emulator provides a fully working Pocet
PC 2003 device that can be configured for mobile connections to an Exchange 2003
server. The Pocet PC emulator can be downloaded from Microsoft at
http://www.microsoft.com, using the keyword pocketpc emulator.

For mobile phone testing, the same requirement applies; most organizations need to have
a mobile phone purchased to test the functionality of the technology. Unlike the purchase
of many devices, mobile phone services typically require the contracting of at least one
year of services. Even if an organization tests the mobility function and does not like how
it works, it is obligated to pay for a full year of service or pay an early cancellation penalty.
The best way around this is to download mobile phone emulator software, such as the one
from OpenWave (http://www.openwave.com). OpenWave provides an emulation tool that
enables users to establish a connection to Windows 2003.

Installing an Exchange Server 2003 Server for Mobile Access

The installation of an Exchange 2003 server for mobile connectivity does not require the installation of any special server, software, update, or gateway product. Exchange 2003 has mobility built in to the Exchange 2003 software. By simply installing Exchange 2003 on a server as part of an upgrade from Exchange 5.5 or Exchange 2000, or as part of a completely clean installation, the mobility functions are automatically included. See Chapter 3, "Installing Exchange Server 2003," for the installation of Exchange Server 2003, or Chapters 15, "Migrating from Exchange v5.5 to Exchange Server 2003," and 16, "Migrating from Exchange 2000 to Exchange Server 2003," on the migration from Exchange 5.5 or Exchange 2000. These chapters cover the process of installing or migrating the basic Exchange 2003 server software.

Creating a Separate Front-end Server for Mobile Connections

As noted in the section "Preparing for Mobility in an Exchange 2003 Environment," earlier in this chapter, an organization may choose to split the front-end client access server from the back-end database server functions. To separate the front-end and back-end server functions

1. Install a new Exchange Server 2003 into an existing Exchange site.

2. Set the properties of the new Exchange server to be a front-end server only.

3. Clean up nonessential components on the new front-end server to prepare it to be just a front-end server.

Setting an Exchange Server to Be a Front-end Server Only

To be configured as a front-end server to an existing Exchange 2003 site, the server should be configured to be a front-end server only. By default, an Exchange server is activated to be both a front-end and a back-end server. To make a server into a dedicated front-end server, do the following:

1. On an Exchange 2003 server that has already been joined to the site, open the Exchange System Manager.

2. Traverse through the Exchange System Manager through Administrative Groups, Administrative Group Name, Servers.

3. Right-click on the server and select Properties.

4. Click on This is a front-end server, as shown in Figure 23.2.

5. Select OK.

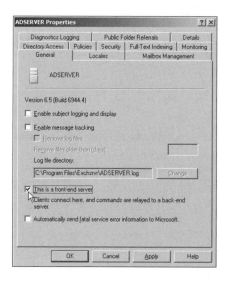

FIGURE 23.2 Selecting a server as a front-end server.

Removing Information Stores

After a server is set to be a front-end server, certain unneeded functions can be deleted from the server. This not only makes the server run more efficiently, but it also makes the server more secure. One of the tasks of cleaning up an Exchange front-end server is to remove the information store and databases.

To delete the information stores on a front-end server, do the following:

1. Click on Start, Programs, Microsoft Exchange, System Manager.

2. Navigate to Administrative Groups, Administrative Group Name, Servers, Server Name, Storage Groups.

3. Right-click on Mailbox Store and choose Delete.

4. Click Yes.

5. Click OK.

6. Using Windows Explorer, navigate to the directory where the databases are stored and manually delete the database files.

> **CAUTION**
>
> Before deleting any database or information store, unless you are positive the database or infor-
> mation store is completely empty and unused, you might want to do a full backup of the data-
> base, store, and system, in case a user's mailbox was inadvertently hosted on the system.
> Sometimes during an early implementation of Exchange, an organization might start with one or

two servers in a pilot test environment. A mailbox stored on one of the test servers might have eventually become the front-end server for the organization. It's always safer to back up a system than to make assumptions and regret the decision later. Using the NTBackup utility covered in Chapter 31, "Backing Up the Exchange Server 2003 Environment," is a quick way to back up a system.

Adding Additional Front-end Servers for Scalability

After the first dedicated Exchange 2003 front-end server has been added to the site, additional servers can be added by following the same procedure as noted in the section "Installing an Exchange Server 2003 Server for Mobile Access," earlier in this chapter. The addition of front-end servers provides better scalability for client systems to connect to their Exchange mailboxes. The front-end server by default can host any Exchange client, not just Pocet PC and Outlook Mobile Access clients. The front-end servers are also full hosts for Outlook Web Access clients, full Outlook clients, and POP3 and IMAP clients. This provides the organization with the ability to add and remove front-end servers as the client demand increases or decreases in the organization. Because front-end servers do not host mailbox or information routing functions, they are much easier to add and remove than full Exchange servers participating in a site.

Configuring Firewall Ports to Secure Communications

There are several ways a mobile client can connect to a dedicated Exchange front-end server or Exchange server acting as both the front-end and back-end server. The client system can connect to the Exchange server in the following ways:

- Securely over Port 443, using Secure Sockets Layer (SSL)

- Unsecured over Port 80

- Connected through a VPN client

Of these three methods, the preferred method is to use a secured SSL connection over Port 443. The SSL connection provides both security and the fastest performance. An unsecured connection minimizes the configuration task of installing a certificate on the Exchange server for SSL communications and is simpler to configure; however, without encrypted communications, traffic between the mobile device and the Exchange server is being transmitted in a format that can be intercepted and deciphered by any individual with a radio frequency packet analyzer.

A VPN connection from a mobile device to an Exchange server can leverage existing VPN technologies implemented in an organization; however, the overhead of the VPN client can reduce performance by 5–15%. Because many of the public wireless services transmit at rates less than 30–50 Kbps, the 5–15% degradation in performance caused by a VPN client can impact the user experience.

By enabling SSL and using SSL encryption between the mobile device and Exchange 2003, an organization can optimize performance while maintaining a secured connection.

If SSL is used, Port 443 should be enabled through the firewall to the Exchange front-end server. If no encryption will be enabled, only standard Port 80 is enabled. If a VPN connection is created, that establishes a connection from the client to the Microsoft Routing and Remote Access (RRAS) server that will then enable the VPN client to route to the Exchange 2003 server for client access.

Migrating from Microsoft Mobile Information Server

If an organization already has the Microsoft Mobile Information Server (MMIS) installed as part of an Exchange 2000 mobile-enabled environment, the migration path to Exchange 2003 is pretty clear: There is no migration path. The organization has two options to replace Microsoft Mobile Information Server with Exchange 2003. One option is to install Exchange 2003 on a new server and migrate mailboxes from the old MMIS-enabled Exchange 2000 server to the new Exchange 2003 server. Or the organization can uninstall MMIS from the Exchange 2000 server and then do an in-place upgrade to Exchange 2003 on that server.

Installing Exchange 2003 Mobility from Scratch

The more dependable and preferred method of migrating off Microsoft Mobile Information Server to Exchange 2003 is to just start from scratch with a new server, the non-upgrade approach. In this scenario, the existing Exchange 2000 server with MMIS installed remains in the Exchange site. A new Exchange 2003 is installed and joined to the existing Exchange site. Mailboxes are then moved, using the Mailbox Move function in the Exchange Services Manager tool to move mailboxes off the old Exchange 2000 server with MMIS to the new Exchange 2003 server.

This non-upgrade approach of moving mailboxes from an Exchange 2000 server with MMIS to Exchange 2003 enables the administrators of an organization to simply move users' mailboxes off an old server to the new server. There are no conversions of mail, and the mailboxes are migrated in real time with little or no interruption of service to users because mailboxes can be migrated in the middle of a production day.

NOTE

Although mailboxes can be migrated in the middle of a production day, the Mailbox Move process will not move a mailbox in use. Move mailboxes when users are not logged in to the system. This can be done at a time when a user is out to lunch or otherwise not expecting to use Outlook for a period of time. If you attempt to move a mailbox while the mailbox is in use, the Exchange server will wait until the user exits his or her mail client (such as Outlook) and then automatically begin the mailbox move process from the old server to the new server.

Any time a server is added to an Exchange site, or mailboxes are moved from server to server, the Exchange environment should be properly backed up and information validated to ensure that a clean backup has been secured.

23

After a user's mailbox has been migrated from the old Exchange 2000 server running MMIS to the new Exchange 2003 server, the user now has full mobile access through the Exchange 2003 mobility functions rather than the older MMIS mobility functions. All sequences and processes for the client remain the same; however, because of improvements in compression and algorithms that prioritize the replication of information more effectively in Exchange 2003, the user will experience much better performance. More details on performing a server-to-server migration using the move-mailbox method of migration is covered in Chapter 16.

Replacing an Existing Mobile Information Server

The other method of replacing the Microsoft Mobile Information Server on an Exchange 2000 server with Exchange 2003 is to do an in-place upgrade from Exchange 2000 to Exchange 2003. This process requires the MMIS software to be uninstalled from the Exchange 2000 server before proceeding with the Exchange 2003 in-place upgrade. To uninstall MMIS, after conducting a full backup for normal best-practice safety purposes, select Start, Settings, Control Panel, Add/Remove Program. Select the Microsoft Mobile Information Server application and click on Remove. This removes the MMIS from the server.

After the MMIS is uninstalled, a server can then be upgraded in place to Exchange 2003. The step-by-step procedure for performing an in-place upgrade from Exchange 2000 to Exchange 2003 is covered in Chapter 16.

> **NOTE**
>
> When a server is being upgraded in place, a full backup should be conducted on the server. This ensures that a safe backup copy is available in the event of a catastrophic failure during the migration process. Because the in-place upgrade provides no easy rollback in the event of a failed upgrade attempt, the Move Mailbox method described in the section "Installing Exchange 2003 Mobility from Scratch," earlier in this chapter, is the preferred method for improving the integrity of the migration process.

Configuring Mobile Exchange Features

After an Exchange 2003 server has been installed on the network, the services needed to support mobility are also already installed. By going into the Active Directory Users and Computer utility, an administrator can view the mobility options automatically enabled for a user.

Viewing Mobile Services

The mobile services are controlled on a user-by-user basis so that an organization can choose to enable or disable mobility on a selected basis. By default, mobility services are enabled for all users. To view the mobile services options available for a user, do the following:

1. Open the Active Directory Users and Computers management tool.

2. Traverse the directory to the user you want and right-click Properties on the user.

3. Click on the Exchange Features tab and a screen similar to the one shown in Figure 23.3 appears.

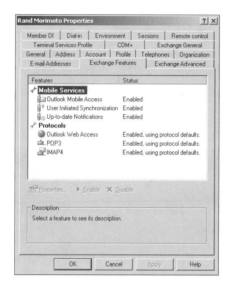

FIGURE 23.3   Exchange Features tab in Active Directory Users and Computers.

Notice that on the Exchange Features tab Outlook Mobile Access, User Initiated Synchronization, and Up-to-Date Notifications are automatically enabled. These functions enable users to have access to their mail immediately from a mobile device.

Configuring Mobile Services

To change the configuration of the mobile services for users, an Exchange administrator can disable the services functions. There are two ways the services can be disabled.

The first way of disabling mobile services is to select the mobile service to be disabled and click on the disable button below the Mobile Services and Protocols window. This method requires the administrator to select each user, select properties, and make the setting changes one setting at a time.

The other way of disabling mobile services that can work for a single user—but also can be used to select multiple users to do a mass disabling of the mobile services—is to use the Exchange Tasks Wizard. To initiate the Exchange Tasks Wizard, do the following:

1. Select the user or users from the Active Directory Users and Computers management tool by holding down the Ctrl key and clicking on the names for which certain mobility functions should be disabled.

2. Right-click and select Exchange Tasks.

3. Click Next on the initial Welcome to the Exchange Task Wizard screen.

4. Select the Configure Exchange Features task and select Next.

5. Select the exchange features and choose to either enable or disable based on the requirements you want (see Figure 23.4). Select Next to execute the task modifications.

6. Click Finish when done.

This process modifies the Exchange Tasks for the selected users.

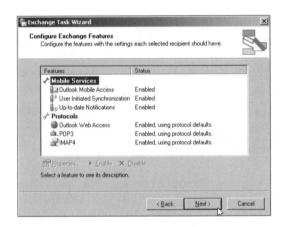

FIGURE 23.4   Selecting Exchange task items to modify the settings.

Configuring Mobile Services Properties for ActiveSync

Besides configuring the mobile services features for each user, the Exchange ActiveSync function can be globally enabled or disabled as a function on the entire Exchange environment. This is done in the Exchange System Manager utility.

The options can be viewed by doing the following:

1. Launch the Exchange System Manager tool.

2. Expand the Global Settings container.

3. Right-click and select Properties on the Mobile Services option. A Mobile Services Properties page is displayed, as shown in Figure 23.5.

4. Select the option for Exchange ActiveSync to enable or disable the function, and then click OK.

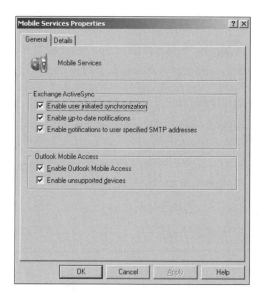

FIGURE 23.5   Viewing the Exchange Mobile Services Properties page.

The three Mobile Services Properties options are

- **Enable User-Initiated Synchronization**   This option, when enabled, allows a Pocet PC device to synchronize with mailboxes on Exchange. If this option is deselected, users with Pocet PC devices will not be able to synchronize with their mailboxes.

- **Enable Up-to-Date Notifications**   This option uses the new feature in Exchange 2003 that enables an Exchange 2003 server to wake up a Pocet PC device and have the device autoinitiate a synchronization. Because ActiveSync synchronization is a client-initiated task, technically the only way to synchronize with Exchange would be to have a user manually synchronize his or her device, or to create a set schedule where the device autosynchronizes. However, when users are charged for connection time by their service provider, they do not necessarily want to—or should not—synchronize their device unless there is something to synchronize. The up-to-date notifications process initiates the synchronization from a server function when a message or other information needs to be updated with the mobile device.

- **Enable Notifications to User-Specified SMTP Addresses**   By enabling this function, users can use their existing wireless service provider for notifications of changes or updates, rather than having the user autoinitiate synchronization tasks.

These mobility property changes can effectively enable the Exchange administrator(s) to disable mobility functions for all users.

Configuring Mobile Services Properties for OMA

Outlook Mobile Access can also be enabled to allow the Exchange administrator(s) to enable support for the access by OMA devices to Exchange 2003. The two options to enable or disable for Outlook Mobile Access are

- **Enable Outlook Mobile Access**   This option, when enabled, provides access by OMA-supported devices to view their email, calendar, and contact information.

- **Enable Unsupported Devices**   When a device is not directly supported by Exchange 2003 OMA, this option provides best-effort support for nonsupported devices.

By selecting to enable or disable the mobile services properties for OMA, the Outlook Mobile Access functionality can be allowed or disallowed for the entire organization.

Summary

With mobility built in to Exchange Server 2003, an organization no longer needs to decide whether it wants to add mobility. There are no special servers that need to be added to the network and no special add-ins to load on the servers. Exchange administrators choose whether they want to enable the Pocet PC and the Outlook Mobile Access capabilities for the organization, or to disable the functionality organizationwide for a future date.

The other key decision when rolling out mobility functions across an organization is the infrastructure to support the users connecting to the mobile servers. Front-end servers can be set up and dedicated to enable better scalability and isolation of security to a limited-scope server. For a smaller organization, combining front-end and back-end functions into a single server is frequently more economical and makes a simpler messaging environment. Fortunately with Exchange 2003, an organization can start with a combination front-end/back-end server configuration, and then split off the front-end to a separate server at a later date if the organization wants separate server functions.

The task of providing mobility to users is a relatively simple process, with much of the setup and configuration focused on the mobile devices, covered in Chapter 24.

Best Practices

The following are best practices from this chapter:

- If mobility functions are not used in the organization, the Exchange administrator should disable the Pocet PC and the Outlook Mobile Access mobility services from the Exchange Service Manager utility.

- To create a secured mobile connection from mobile devices to the Exchange 2003 server, SSL should be enabled and used rather than the simple Port 80 unsecured access.

- Although a VPN connection can be used to create a secured connection from a mobile device to an Exchange 2003 server, the overhead of the VPN on a relatively low mobile wireless connection could greatly degrade performance. Using SSL for the mobile connection can provide security without all the overhead.

- Organizations with only a few users, or a large organization with a small remote site, may choose to set up Exchange mobility on a single server that hosts both the Exchange mailboxes and acts as the front-end server where users with mobile devices connect for mobile mail, calendar, and contact access.

- Organizations that have a lot of users connecting to their Exchange server(s) should consider splitting off the front-end server functions to a dedicated server. This enables better scalability for user connections to Exchange, and also provides an additional layer of security between user-connected servers and the back-end database housing information.

- Using the Pocet PC 2003 Emulator that is available to be downloaded from Microsoft can help an organization evaluate the functions of Pocet PC mobility and creates a simple way for the organization to test whether mobility and mailbox synchronization is working properly, thus isolating any phone carrier or public wireless network problems that might be preventing successful operations.

- The Pocet PC Emulator can also help an organization train its workforce on how to use mobility functions of the Pocet PC device. The full functions of the mobile device can be run on a workstation or server and displayed on a projection system, or screen shots can be taken for documentation.

- Mobile phone emulators that can be downloaded off the Internet from companies such as OpenWave.com can also simplify the testing process of mobile access. Running OMA functions from an emulator can also simplify the testing, training, and documentation process of validating mobility.

- The simplest way to migrate from Microsoft Mobile Information Server on Exchange 2000 to Exchange 2003 mobility is to add an Exchange 2003 server to an existing Exchange 2000 site and move mailboxes over to the new server. This minimizes the risk of failure of uninstalling MMIS from a server and conducting an in-place upgrade on a production server.

CHAPTER 24

Configuring Client Systems for Mobility

Chapter 22, "Designing Mobility in Exchange Server 2003," provided an overview of the mobility options for Exchange 2003, and Chapter 23, "Implementing Mobile Synchronization in Exchange Server 2003," focused on the server setup for mobile devices. This chapter keys in on the client components for mobility, namely the configuration and operation of Pocet PC–enabled devices using Exchange 2003 ActiveSync and mobile phone devices using Outlook Mobile Access.

Identifying Mobile Devices to Be Supported

With the release of Exchange 2003, organizations no longer have to purchase add-on products to support access of emails, calendars, contacts, and other Exchange information from Pocet PC or mobile phone devices. As long as a mobile device is supported by Exchange 2003, it just needs to be configured properly and the device will connect to Exchange.

Over the past few years, however, there have been many different versions of the Windows CE and Pocket PC operating system and dozens of different mobile phone/mobile Web access standards. Those supported by Exchange 2003 and highlighted in this chapter include

- Pocket PC 2002 (using ActiveSync)

- Pocket PC 2003 (using ActiveSync)

- Smartphone 2003 (using ActiveSync)

- xHTML used in WAP 2.x devices (using Outlook Mobile Access)

- cHTML (using Outlook Mobile Access)

- HTML browser-based (using Outlook Mobile Access or Outlook Web Access)

Windows CE 2.0 or CE 3.0 devices supported Outlook synchronization, but the operating system supported only cradle-based synchronization. An option that was added in the Pocket PC 2002 and Pocket PC 2003 operating system was a tab that enabled the user to enter the IP address or DNS name of an Exchange server to access. Windows CE 2.0 and 3.0 devices associated with only a PC connection. A user who has an Internet-connected Windows CE device or a CE device that has network or wireless connectivity, however, *can* access Exchange 2003 using the HTML browser-based access. The user with those devices performs a real-time lookup and view of email messages, calendar appointments, contacts, and other Exchange information. The difference is in the ability to synchronize the information for offline access that is built in to the Pocket PC 2002 and 2003 versions of the operating system.

Other organizations might have devices running on the Palm operating system, such as Palm PDAs, Sony Clie, or Handspring devices. The Palm OS devices do not directly synchronize with Exchange 2003, although third-party gateway products have existed since Exchange 5.5 and Exchange 2000; these gateway products connect to an Exchange 2003 environment for synchronization of the Palm OS devices. Just like the support for the Windows CE 2.0 and 3.0 devices, Palm OS devices can access Exchange 2003 email, calendar, and contacts using the Outlook Mobile Access or Outlook Web Access functionality. Using the Web access–based methods to communicate, a Palm OS device can have real-time access to Outlook information; however, the information is not synchronized for offline access.

Supporting the Pocket PC 2002 Synchronization with Microsoft Exchange 2003

The Pocket PC 2002 operating system was one of the first Windows CE family of products that supported mobile communications. The hardware devices, such as the Compaq iPaq, had either PCMCIA wireless adapters or built-in 802.11 and Bluetooth wireless communications to the devices. Later versions of the Pocket PC 2002 devices came with mobile phone connections for a combination of mobile phone and wireless LAN connectivity.

A three-step process enabled a Pocket PC 2002 device to synchronize information between the device and Exchange 2003:

1. Configure the Pocket PC 2002 network connection.

2. Configure the Pocket PC 2002 ActiveSync parameters.

3. Choose to synchronize the Pocket PC 2002 device to Exchange.

For network or Exchange administrators who want to test out the functionality of Pocket PC 2002 mobility to Exchange, there is a Pocket PC 2002 emulator that is freely downloadable from Microsoft and that has all the functions of the standard Pocket PC 2002 device. The emulator helps an administrator get familiar with setup and configuration without having to actually buy a device or work through unique driver download configurations for mobile connections or wireless adapters.

Installing the Pocket PC 2002 Emulator

For administrators who want to test the functionality of Pocket PC 2002 emulation, this section focuses on the download and installation of the emulator on a standard Windows workstation. After it's installed on a Windows workstation, the emulator can then be configured and tested against the Exchange 2003 environment.

Requirements to Run the Pocket PC 2002 Emulator

To install the eMbedded Visual Tools 3.0, Microsoft states that its requirement is a system running Windows 98 Second Edition or higher, 150MHz or faster, 32MB or more of available memory, 720MB of available disk space, network adapter, VGA video, and a mouse. The emulator is a pretty basic tool and does not require a high processing system; however, it does load a fair amount of code into memory, so typically a P3 or faster Windows 2000 or XP workstation with 192MB RAM is recommended. The host workstation also needs a network adapter connected to a network connection that will access the Exchange 2003 server.

It is typically recommended to first test the Pocket PC emulation on an internal backbone segment to make sure the connection to the Exchange server is not blocked by external firewalls, routers, or other external perimeter devices. The host workstation needs network connectivity, and although it's not a requirement to run the Pocket PC 2002 emulator, the system should be able to connect to the Exchange server using Outlook Web Access or from an Outlook client. This ensures that the host workstation has the appropriate network connectivity for the emulator to connect to the server.

> **NOTE**
>
> The Pocket PC 2002 emulator does not require its own IP address on the network, and there is no network connectivity configuration required on the emulator. The emulator simply passes through the existing LAN connection of the host workstation. If the workstation has connectivity to Exchange for Outlook or Outlook Web Access, that same connection is used by the emulator.

Downloading the Pocket PC 2002 Emulator

The Pocket PC 2002 emulator, also known as the Pocket PC 2002 Software Development Kit (SDK) is a free download from Microsoft. It is included in the eMbedded Visual Tools 3.0—2002 Edition. When the eMbedded Tools 3.0 is installed, the SDK emulator for both Pocket PC 2002 and Smartphone 2002 are also installed, with the core driver and libraries needed to run the software development kit. You will find the eMbedded Tools 3.0 on http://www.microsoft.com (search on **embedded tools 3.0**); the evt2002web_min.exe file is 210MB.

> **NOTE**
>
> If you already have the eMbedded Visual Tools 3.0 on your host workstation, you can just download and install the Pocket PC 2002 emulator. Go to http://www.microsoft.com, search on the words **Pocket 2002 SDK**, and download the ppc2002_sdk.exe file (66MB).

Installing eMbedded Visual Tools 3.0 and the Pocket PC 2002 Emulator

After downloading the eMbedded Visual Tools 3.0, install the Embedded Visual Tools application. Use the following steps:

1. Launch the evt2002web_min.exe executable for the eMbedded Visual Tools 3.0 to install it on the host workstation. This extracts the files to a temporary directory and launches the installation wizard.

2. The installation wizard displays a welcome screen; click Next to continue.

3. After reading the end-user license agreement and agreeing to the information, click I accept the agreement and then click Next.

4. When prompted for the product license number and user ID, enter the evaluation ID that is noted on the main Web page where you downloaded the eMbedded Visual Tools. The product ID noted is TRT7H-KD36T-FRH8D-6QH8P-VFJHQ. Enter your name and company name so the screen looks similar to Figure 24.1, and then click Next.

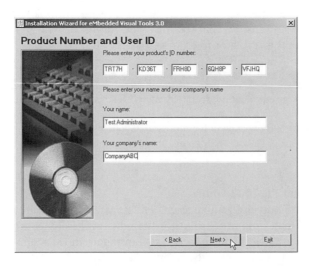

FIGURE 24.1   Entering the product ID and username.

5. When prompted, select to install all of the eMbedded tools and then click Next.

> **NOTE**
>
> When installing the eMbedded Visual Tools 3.0, the Pocket PC 2002 and the Smartphone 2002 SDKs are installed by default. This minimizes the need to download and install the emulators separately.

6. Choose a folder you want to install the software in (the default is `c:\Windows CE Tools`) and then click Next.

7. Click OK to pass by the eMbedded tools setup product ID information.

8. Click on Continue when prompted to confirm the installation of the Tools Setup, which includes the eMbedded Visual Basic 3.0, eMbedded Visual C++ 3.0, and Common Components.

9. After the installation of the eMbedded tools, the Pocket PC SDK begins to extract and install. Click on Next at the InstallShield welcome page.

10. Read and accept the license agreement and then click on Next.

11. Enter your name and company name and then click on Next.

12. Select to have a Complete Install and click on Next.

13. Choose to install in the default destination folder and click on Next.

14. Click on Install to complete the installation of the Pocket PC 2002 SDK.

15. When the Pocket PC 2002 SDK has completed its installation, click on Finish, and then the Smartphone 2002 SDK installation begins to extract and install.

16. Click on Next at the InstallShield for the Smartphone 2002 SDK screen.

17. Read and accept the license agreement and then click on Next.

18. Enter your name and company name and then click on Next.

19. Select to have a Complete Install and click on Next.

20. Choose to install in the default destination folder and click on Next.

21. Click on Install to complete the installation of the Smartphone 2002 SDK.

22. When the Smartphone 2002 SDK has completed its installation, click on Finish.

Launching the Pocket PC 2002 Emulator

After the installation is complete, the Pocket PC 2002 emulator can be launched. Because this is a Software Development Kit, the launch of the Pocket PC 2002 emulator is done from within the eMbedded Visual Basic 3.0 program. Before the emulator can be launched, the binary emulation image for the proper SDK needs to be selected. To select the binary emulator, use the following steps:

1. Select Start, Programs, Microsoft Windows SDK for Smartphone 2002, Emulator Binary Switch.

2. In the Select SDK window, choose Pocket PC 2002, and then click on OK.

3. When prompted to choose the emulation image, go to

   `c:\Windows CE Tools\wce300\Pocket PC 2002\emulation\English-No Radio`

   Select the `wwenoril.bin` file and click on OK.

After the binary emulation has been selected, the Pocket PC 2002 emulator can be loaded by launching the eMbedded Visual Basic 3.0 program. To launch the emulator, use the following steps:

1. Select Start, Programs, Microsoft eMbedded Visual Tools, eMbedded Visual Basic 3.0.

2. When eMbedded Visual Basic 3.0 loads, from the New Project screen, choose the Windows CE for Pocket PC 2002 icon, as shown in Figure 24.2; then click on Open.

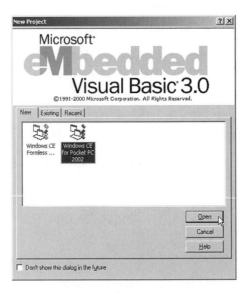

FIGURE 24.2   Selecting to open the Pocket PC 2002 emulator.

3. When the Pocket PC 2002 emulator is opened within eMbedded Visual Basic 3.0, select Run, Execute. This launches the emulator, and a screen similar to the one shown in Figure 24.3 appears.

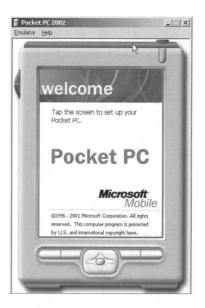

FIGURE 24.3   The initial Pocket PC 2002 emulator screen.

The Pocket PC 2002 emulator is now ready to be configured.

Configuring a Pocket PC 2002 Device for Network Connectivity

After the Pocket PC 2002 emulator has been installed, or for administrators that have a Pocket PC device in front of them, the first thing to do is configure the device for network connectivity. Network connectivity comes in a variety of forms, including the following:

- Pocket PC with an Ethernet adapter or wireless adapter

- Pocket PC with a mobile phone connection to the Internet

- Pocket PC emulator connected to a host workstation

Each configuration is slightly different and is individually highlighted in the next section.

Configuring a Pocket PC 2002 Device with an Internal Network Adapter

To configure a Pocket PC 2002 device with an internal Ethernet or wireless network adapter, follow these steps:

1. On the Pocket PC device, select Start, Settings, Connections, and then click on the Network Adapters option.

2. Choose the network adapter you want to configure. Figure 24.4 shows the selection of an NE2000 Compatible Ethernet driver.

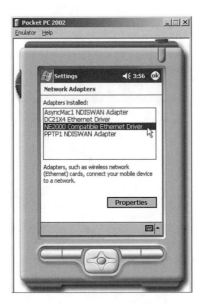

FIGURE 24.4   Choosing a network adapter to configure.

3. Click on properties to configure the adapter.

4. Select Use server-assigned IP address if DHCP is available on the network that this device will be connecting to, or choose Use specific IP address and enter a static IP address for the device.

5. If the device is DHCP-configured, skip to step 6; otherwise, click on the Name Servers tab and enter the address for the DNS (and optionally the WINS) servers on the network.

6. Click on OK in the upper-right corner; a notice appears informing you that the adapter will be used. Remove and reinsert the adapter to activate it with the new settings. Click OK to continue.

7. Click OK, and then click on the X in the upper-right corner to complete the network adapter setting.

After the hardware settings on the network adapter have been selected, select the adapter as the default outbound connection. To choose the adapter as the default, use the following steps:

1. Select Start, Settings, Connections, and click on the Connections icon.

2. Make sure that the first option, When needed, automatically connect to The Internet using these settings, is set to Work Settings. On the same screen, make sure that the option When needed, automatically connect to Work using these settings and the option My network card connects to are set to Work, as shown in Figure 24.5.

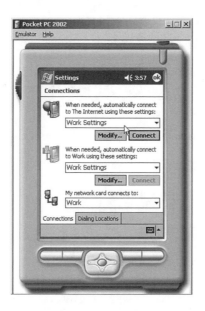

FIGURE 24.5   Choosing the work settings for network connectivity.

  3. If a proxy server is used, click on the Modify button to open the Work Settings page.

  4. Click on the Proxy Settings tab and click on the This network uses a proxy server to connect to the Internet check box. Then enter the name of the proxy server.

  5. Click on OK and then on OK again. Click on X in the upper-right corner.

The Pocket PC 2002 device is now configured for network connectivity.

To test whether the Pocket PC 2002 device is working properly, launch Pocket Internet Explorer and confirm whether network connectivity to the Internet is available. To test Internet Explorer, use the following steps:

  1. Select Start, Internet Explorer.

  2. On the main Internet Explorer home screen, click on the PocketPC.com graphic and then click on the Go to PocketPC.com link toward the bottom of the page.

  3. Internet Explorer should traverse the network and provide a Windows Mobile page, assuming the host computer has connectivity to the Internet. If the network segment that the Pocket PC device is on does not have connectivity to the Internet, the Pocket PC device will not have Internet connectivity. Possibly choose an Internet Intranet Web server or other system to check whether the device is communicating properly on the network segment to which it is connected.

Configuring a Pocket PC 2002 Device with a Mobile Phone Connection

If the Pocket PC 2002 device is a Pocet PC–enabled mobile phone, the service provider of the phone will typically have a GSM or GPRS Internet connection service included with the phone. Follow the instructions provided with the phone to connect the phone to the Internet so that you can effectively surf the Internet with the mobile phone.

Usually the process requires following these steps:

1. Select Start, Settings, Connections, and then click on the Connections icon.

2. For the setting When needed, automatically connect to The Internet using these settings, there usually is a pull-down option that says ISP Connection or Internet Provider or GPRS Provider. This varies between mobile phone providers; however, it will likely note that the connection is to the Internet using the mobile phone Internet service connection.

3. Click on OK and then click on the X in the upper-right corner to set the device for Internet connectivity.

To test whether the Pocket PC 2002–enabled mobile phone is working properly, launch Pocket Internet Explorer and confirm whether network connectivity to the Internet is available. To test Internet Explorer, use the following steps:

1. Select Start, Internet Explorer.

2. On the main Internet Explorer home screen, click on the PocketPC.com graphic and then click on the Go to PocketPC.com link toward the bottom of the page.

3. Internet Explorer should traverse the network and provide a Windows Mobile page, assuming the host computer has connectivity to the Internet. If the Pocket PC–enabled mobile phone does not have connectivity to the Internet, check the manual or contact the technical support for the mobile phone to get assistance on connecting the mobile phone to the Internet.

Configuring a Pocket PC 2002 Emulator

Because the Pocket PC 2002 emulator uses the IP settings built in to the host computer, as long as the host computer has network connectivity, the emulator will have network connectivity. To validate the configuration, use the following steps:

1. Select Start, Settings, Connections, and click on the Connections icon.

2. Make sure that the first option, When needed, automatically connect to The Internet using these settings, is set to Work Settings. Additionally, make sure the option When needed, automatically connect to Work using these settings and the option My network card connects to are set to Work.

> **NOTE**
>
> No proxy settings should be set on the Pocket PC 2002 emulator, because any proxy settings, DNS settings, or other hardware device settings are taken directly from the host workstation.

3. Click on OK and then on OK again. Click on X in the upper-right corner.

The Pocket PC 2002 emulator is now configured for network connectivity.

To test whether the Pocket PC 2002 emulator is working properly, launch Pocket Internet Explorer and confirm whether network connectivity to the Internet is available. To test Internet Explorer, use the following steps:

1. Select Start, Internet Explorer.

2. On the main Internet Explorer home screen, click on the PocketPC.com graphic and then click on the Go to PocketPC.com link toward the bottom of the page.

3. Internet Explorer should traverse the network and provide a Windows Mobile page, assuming the host computer has connectivity to the Internet. If the host computer does not have network connectivity to the Internet, the Pocket PC emulator will not have Internet connectivity either. Possibly choose an Internet Intranet Web server or other system to check whether the device is communicating properly on the network segment to which it is connected.

Establishing a Connection Between the Pocket PC 2002 and Exchange 2003

After the Pocket PC device has network connectivity, a connection between the device and the Microsoft Exchange server needs to be established. To create the connection, use the following steps:

1. Select Start, ActiveSync to launch the Pocket PC ActiveSync program.

2. Click on Tools at the bottom of the screen, and then click on Options.

3. Click on the Server tab, and for server, enter the DNS name or the IP address of the Exchange server.

4. Click on the Advanced button and enter the logon name, password, and domain of the Outlook/Exchange user account that the Pocket PC device will use to synchronize information. Click to select the Save Password box as the information the password needs to be enabled.

5. Click on OK to go back to the Server screen and choose the options you want to synchronize—such as the Inbox, Calendar, or Contacts—by clicking on the box.

6. Click on OK, and then click on the X in the upper-right corner to save the Exchange server settings.

24

Synchronizing Data Between Pocket PC 2002 and Exchange 2003

To synchronize information between the Pocket PC 2002 device and the Exchange 2003 server, use the following steps:

1. Select Start, ActiveSync to launch the ActiveSync program.

2. Click on the Sync button to begin synchronization, as shown in Figure 24.6.

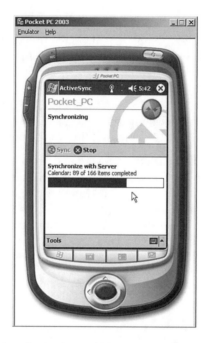

FIGURE 24.6   Synchronizing the Pocket PC 2002 device with Exchange 2003.

Supporting Pocket PC 2003 Synchronization with Exchange 2003

When Exchange 2003 started to ship, the Pocket PC 2003 operating system also just started to become available on the market. If an organization has the choice of the Pocket PC 2002 or the Pocket PC 2003 operating system, it should select the Pocket PC 2003 operating system and gain the following advantages:

- Exchange 2003 initiates a sync of information when information becomes available on the Exchange server, such as a new email message or calendar appointment request.

NOTE

The Pocket PC 2002 operation does not support the Exchange 2003 SMS initiation of a synchronization, so Pocket PC 2002 users need to either initiate the sync themselves each time they want to update their information, or schedule the update to occur on a regular basis. Dependent on the frequency of the sync and the service plan with the mobile Internet provider, this continuous synchronization of information can either wear down the battery of the unit or incur connection charges with the Internet provider.

- The Pocket PC 2003 operating system supports the ability to synchronize information without SSL for organizations that might choose to run synchronization unencrypted. The default on the Pocket PC 2002 is always SSL-encrypted.

- The Pocket PC 2003 operating system provides better support for instant messenger, Microsoft Passports, and other network and security functions that are frequently leveraged in mobile communication environments.

The installation and configuration of the Pocket PC 2003–enabled device is similar to that of the Pocket PC 2002 device. Some of the configuration options are slightly different, however, so the following sections cover the installation, configuration, and synchronization specific to Pocket PC 2003 devices.

For network or Exchange administrators who want to test the functionality of Pocket PC 2003 mobility to Exchange, a Pocket PC 2003 emulator is freely downloadable from Microsoft that has all of the functions of the standard Pocket PC 2003 device. The emulator helps an administrator get familiar with setup and configuration without having to actually buy a device or work through unique driver download configurations for mobile connections or wireless adapters.

NOTE

The eMbedded Visual C++ 4.0 for the Pocket PC 2003 emulator and the eMbedded Visual Tools 3.0 used for the Pocket PC 2002 emulator conflict with each other. Effectively, the 4.0 tool overwrites key components of the 3.0 tool that run the Pocket PC 2002 emulator, and the Pocket PC 2002 emulator will not run with the 4.0 tools installed. If you plan to test both Pocket PC 2002 and Pocket PC 2003 emulation, install the eMbedded tools and emulators on separate systems.

Installing the Pocket PC 2003 Emulator

For administrators who want to test the functionality of Pocket PC 2003 emulation, this section focuses on the download and installation of the emulator on a standard Windows workstation. When installed on a Windows workstation, the emulator can then be configured and tested against the Exchange 2003 environment.

Downloading the Pocket PC 2003 Emulator

The Pocket PC 2003 emulator is a free download from Microsoft. Go to
http://www.microsoft.com, search on the words **Pocket 2003 SDK**, and download the
ppc2003_sdk.exe file (86MB).

In addition to downloading the Pocket PC 2003 emulator, you also need to download a
copy of the eMbedded Visual C++ 4.0 and the eMbedded Visual C++ 4.0 Service Pack 2 or
higher. The eMbedded Visual C++ 4.0 and Service Pack need to be installed before the SDK
emulator to provide the core driver and libraries needed to run the SDK. The eMbedded
Visual C++ 4.0 and Service Pack can be found at

http://msdn.microsoft.com/vstudio/device/embedded/download.aspx

The file eVC4.exe is 333MB, and evc4sp2.exe (Service Pack 2) is 42MB.

Requirements to Run the Pocket PC 2003 Emulator

To install eMbedded Visual C++ 4.0, Microsoft states its requirement is a system running
Windows 2000 or Windows XP, a 450MHz or faster Pentium-II class system, 128–192MB or
more of available memory, 200MB of available disk space, network adapter, VGA video,
and a mouse. The host workstation needs a network adapter connected to a network
connection that will access the Exchange 2003 server.

It is typically recommended to first test the Pocket PC emulation on an internal backbone
segment to make sure the connection to the Exchange server is not blocked by external
firewalls, routers, or other external perimeter devices. The host workstation needs network
connectivity, and although it's not a requirement to run the Pocket PC 2003 emulator, the
system should be able to connect to the Exchange server using Outlook Web Access or
from an Outlook client. This ensures that the host workstation has the appropriate
network connectivity for the emulator to connect to the server.

> **NOTE**
>
> The Pocket PC 2003 emulator does not require its own IP address on the network and there is no
> network connectivity configuration required on the emulator. The emulator simply passes
> through the existing LAN connection of the host workstation. If the workstation has connectivity
> to Exchange for Outlook or Outlook Web Access, that same connection is used by the emulator.

Installing eMbedded Visual C++ 4.0

After downloading the eMbedded Visual C++ 4.0 and Pocket PC 2003 SDK, the two applications should be installed. To do so, use the following steps:

1. Launch the eVC4.exe executable for the eMbedded Visual C++ 4.0 to install it on the
   host workstation. This extracts the files to a temporary directory (for example,
   c:\evc4\) and launches the installation wizard.

2. Go into the temporary directory and run `setup.exe`. The installation wizard displays a welcome screen; click Next to continue.

3. After reading the end-user license agreement and agreeing to the information, click I accept the agreement and then click Next.

4. When prompted for the product license number and user ID, enter the evaluation ID that is noted on the main Web page where you downloaded the eMbedded Visual Tools. The product ID noted is TRT7H-KD36T-FRH8D-6QH8P-VFJHQ.

5. When prompted, select to install all the eMbedded tools and then click Next.

> **NOTE**
>
> Unlike with the eMbedded Visual Tools 3.0 that also installed the Pocket PC 2002 and the Smartphone 2002 SDKs, the eMbedded Visual C++ 4.0 installs only the eMbedded Visual C++ 4.0 tools. Install the Pocket PC 2003 emulator and the Smartphone 2003 emulators separately.

6. Choose a folder you want to install the software in (the default is `c:\Windows CE Tools`) and then click Next. The Windows CE Platform Manager 4.0 will begin to install.

7. Click OK at the eMbedded tools setup product ID information screen.

8. Click on Continue when prompted to confirm the installation of the eMbedded Visual C++ 4.0 Setup that includes the eMbedded Visual C++ 4.0 and Common Components.

9. After the installation of the eMbedded Visual C++ 4.0 tools, click OK when the setup notes it was completed successfully.

10. The installation wizard for the Standard SDK for Windows CE .NET setup begins to extract and install. Click on Next at the welcome page, and then read and accept the license agreement. Click on Next.

11. Enter your name and company name and then click on Next.

12. Select to have a Complete Install and click on Next.

13. Choose to install in the default destination folder and click on Next.

14. Click on Install to complete the installation of the Standard SDK for Windows CE .NET.

15. When the installation of the Standard SDK for Windows CE .NET has completed its installation, click on Finish.

After the base eMbedded Visual C++ 4.0 has been installed, install eMbedded Visual C++ 4.0 Service Pack 2 or higher. Use the following steps:

1. Run `evc4sp2.exe`. Choose a directory where you want to expand the files (for example, `c:\evcsp2\`).

2. Go to the directory you selected, open the DISK1 directory, and run the `setup.exe` program.

3. At the eMbedded Visual C++ 4.0 SP2 setup welcome screen, click Next.

4. Read and accept the end-user license agreement and click on Next.

5. Click on Install to begin the installation of the Service Pack.

6. When the Service Pack has completed installation, click on Finish.

Installing the Pocket PC 2003 Emulator

After the eMbedded Visual C++ 4.0 and Service Pack have been installed, install the Pocket PC 2003 SDK. Use the following steps:

1. Launch the Microsoft Pocket PC 2003 SDK.MSI script that you downloaded, which will begin the installation process on your host workstation.

2. At the welcome screen, click on Next.

3. Read the license agreement, select I accept the terms in the License Agreement, and click on Next.

4. Confirm your customer information (name and organization name) and then click Next.

5. Select a Complete Installation and then click Next.

6. Click on Next to choose the default destination folders.

7. Click on Install to begin the installation of the Pocket PC 2003 SDK.

8. Click on Finish when completed.

Launching the Pocket PC 2003 Emulator

After the installation has been completed, the Pocket PC 2003 emulator can now be launched. To launch the Pocket PC 2003 emulator, select Start, Programs, Microsoft Pocket PC 2003 SDK, Pocket PC 2003 Emulator.

> **NOTE**
>
> When you select Start, Programs, Microsoft Pocket PC 2003 SDK, and you do not see a Pocket PC 2003 Emulator icon, as shown in Figure 24.7, confirm that you installed the eMbedded Visual C++ 4.0 Service Pack before installing the Pocket PC 2003 SDK. Missing that step is a common problem with all of the downloads that need to be installed. If the icon does not exist, uninstall the Pocket PC 2003 SDK (from the Start, Settings, Control Panel, Add/Remove Programs tool), reinstall the eMbedded Visual C++ 4.0 Service Pack 2 or higher, and then reinstall the Pocket PC 2003 SDK.

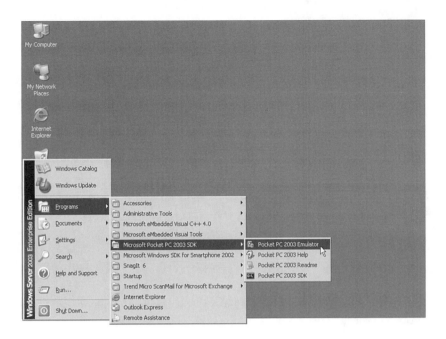

FIGURE 24.7   Choosing the Pocket PC.

Wait a few seconds and the Pocket PC 2003 emulator will automatically start. The Pocket PC 2003 emulator is now ready to be configured.

Configuring a Pocket PC 2003 Device for Network Connectivity

After the Pocket PC 2003 emulator has been installed, or for administrators that have a Pocket PC device in front of them, the first thing to do is configure the device for network connectivity. Network connectivity comes in a variety of forms, including:

- Pocket PC with an Ethernet adapter or Wireless adapter

- Pocket PC with a mobile phone connection to the Internet

- Pocket PC emulator connected to a host workstation

Each configuration is slightly different and is individually highlighted in the next section.

Configuring a Pocket PC 2003 Device with an Internal Network Adapter

To configure a Pocket PC 2003 device with an internal Ethernet or wireless network adapter, follow these steps:

1. On the Pocket PC device, select Start, Settings, Connections. Click on the Connections Icon and then on the Advanced tab.

2. Click on the Network Card button and choose the network adapter you want to configure.

3. Select Use server-assigned IP address if DHCP is available on the network that this device will be connecting to, or choose Use specific IP address and enter a static IP address for the device.

4. If the device is DHCP-configured, skip to step 5; otherwise, click on the Name Servers tab and enter the address for the DNS (and optionally the WINS) servers on the network.

5. Click on OK in the upper-right corner and a notice appears notifying you that the adapter will be used. Remove and reinsert the adapter to activate it with the new settings. Click OK after reading the notice.

6. Click OK and then click on the X in the upper-right corner to complete the network adapter setting.

After the hardware settings on the network adapter have been selected, select the adapter as the default outbound connection. To choose the adapter as the default, use the following steps:

1. Select Start, Settings, Connections. Click on the Connections icon, on Advanced, and on the Select Networks button.

2. Make sure that the first option, Programs that automatically connect to the Internet should connect using, is set to My Work Network. Additionally, make sure the option Programs that automatically connect to a private network should connect using is set to My Work Network.

3. If a proxy server is used, click on the Edit button under the first My Work Network option to open the My Work Network page.

4. Click on the Proxy Settings tab and then on the This network uses a proxy server to connect to the Internet check box. Then enter the name of the proxy server.

5. Click on OK three times, and then on X in the upper-right corner.

The Pocket PC 2003 device is now configured for network connectivity.

To test whether the Pocket PC 2003 device is working properly, launch Pocket Internet Explorer and confirm whether network connectivity to the Internet is available. To test Internet Explorer, use the following steps:

1. Select Start, Internet Explorer.

2. On the main Internet Explorer home screen, click on the PocketPC.com graphic.

3. Internet Explorer should traverse the network and provide a Windows Mobile page, assuming the host computer had connectivity to the Internet. If the network segment that the Pocket PC device is on does not have connectivity to the Internet, the Pocket PC device will also not have Internet connectivity. Possibly choose an Internet Intranet Web server or other system to check whether the device is communicating properly on the network segment it is connected.

Configuring a Pocket PC 2003 Device with a Mobile Phone Connection

If the Pocket PC 2003 device is a Pocket PC enabled mobile phone, the service provider of the phone will typically have a GSM or GPRS Internet connection service included with the phone. Follow the instructions provided with the phone to connect the phone to the Internet so that you can effectively surf the Internet with the mobile phone.

Usually the process is as follows:

1. Select Start, Settings, Connections. Click on the Connections icon, on the Advanced tab, and on the Select Networks button.

2. The first option, Programs that automatically connect to the Internet should connect using, usually has a pull-down box that says ISP Connection, Internet Provider, or GPRS Provider. This varies between mobile phone providers; however, it likely notes that the connection is to the Internet. The option commonly refers to using the mobile phone Internet service connection.

3. Click on OK, and then on OK again. Click on X and again on X in the upper-right corner.

The Pocket PC 2003 device is now configured for network connectivity.

To test whether the Pocket PC 2003–enabled mobile phone is working properly, launch Pocket Internet Explorer and confirm whether network connectivity to the Internet is available. To test Internet Explorer, use the following steps:

1. Select Start, Internet Explorer.

2. On the main Internet Explorer home screen, click on the PocketPC.com graphic.

3. Internet Explorer should traverse the network and provide a Windows Mobile page, assuming the host computer had connectivity to the Internet. If the Pocket PC–enabled mobile phone does not have connectivity to the Internet, check the manual or contact the technical support for the mobile phone to get assistance on connecting the mobile phone to the Internet.

Configuring a Pocket PC 2003 Emulator

To configure the Pocket PC 2003 emulator for network connectivity, because the device uses the IP settings built in to the host computer, as long as the host computer has network connectivity, the emulator will have network connectivity. To validate the configuration, use the following steps:

1. Select Start, Settings, Connections. Click on the Connections icon, on the Advanced tab, and then on the Select Networks button.

2. Make sure that the first option, Programs that automatically connect to the Internet should connect using, is set to My Work Network. Additionally, make sure the option Programs that automatically connect to a private network should connect using is set to My Work Network, as shown in Figure 24.8.

24

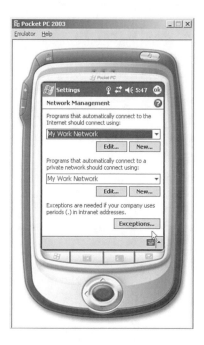

FIGURE 24.8   Configuring the network settings for connectivity.

> **NOTE**
>
> No proxy settings should be set on the Pocket PC 2003 emulator, because any proxy settings, DNS settings, or other hardware device settings are taken directly from the host workstation.

3. Click on OK, again on OK, and then on the X in the upper-right corner.

The Pocket PC 2003 emulator is now configured for network connectivity.

To test whether the Pocket PC 2003 emulator is working properly, launch Pocket Internet Explorer and confirm whether network connectivity to the Internet is available. To test Internet Explorer, use the following steps:

1. Select Start, Internet Explorer.

2. On the main Internet Explorer home screen, click on the PocketPC.com graphic.

3. Internet Explorer should traverse the network and provide a Windows Mobile page assuming the host computer had connectivity to the Internet. If the host computer does not have network connectivity to the Internet, the Pocket PC emulator will not have Internet connectivity either. Possibly choose an Internet Intranet Web server or other system to check whether the device is communicating properly on the network segment to which it is connected.

Establishing a Connection Between the Pocket PC 2003 and Exchange 2003

After the Pocket PC device has network connectivity, establish a connection between the device and the Microsoft Exchange server. To create the connection, use the following steps:

1. Select Start, ActiveSync to launch the Pocket PC ActiveSync program.

2. Click on Tools at the bottom of the screen and then click on Options.

3. Click on the Server tab and for server, enter the DNS name or the IP address of the Exchange server.

4. Click on the Options button and enter the logon name, password, and domain of the Outlook/Exchange user account that the Pocket PC device will use to synchronize information. Click to select the Save Password box as the information the password needs to be enabled.

5. Click on OK to go back to the Server screen and choose the options you want to synchronize—such as Inbox, Calendar, or Contacts—by clicking on the box.

6. Click on OK, and then click on the X in the upper-right corner to save the Exchange server settings.

Synchronizing Data Between Pocket PC 2003 and Exchange 2003

To synchronize information between the Pocket PC 2003 device and the Exchange 2003 server, use the following steps:

1. Select Start, ActiveSync to launch the ActiveSync program.

2. Click on the Sync button to begin synchronization.

Using the Pocket PC 2002 and Pocket PC 2003

After connectivity has been established on the Pocket PC device and information has been synchronized, the Pocket PC has Outlook inbox, calendar, and contact information stored in the non-volatile memory of the device. Users can look at their information; queue up messages to be sent; create and accept calendar appointments; and view, add, and edit contact information. Because the Pocket PC 2002 and Pocket PC 2003 interfaces are similar, the function of using the Pocket PC device is consolidated into a common section.

> **NOTE**
>
> Although the Pocket PC device stores email, calendar, and contact information in non-volatile memory, the devices are known to lose all memory and configuration settings if the battery is drained and the device is left uncharged for a few days. It's important that users keep their Pocket PC device charged or at least see that the device is not left uncharged for an extended period of time.

Viewing Inbox Information

Users can access their inbox, select other folders to synchronize, queue up messages to be sent, and manage their mailbox Outlook information. To access the Outlook email information, select Start, Inbox.

While in the Inbox, a user can open an email message by clicking twice on a mail message. The message can be read. If the user wants to view an attachment, by default, attachments are not sent to the Pocket PC. By clicking on an attachment, the arrow for the attachment turns from grey to green noting that the attachment is flagged for download. The next time the device is synchronized, the attachment will be downloaded.

To create a new mail message, click on New at the bottom of the Inbox screen and a blank email message will appear. Enter the email address and subject, and write the message. Click on Send to have the message queued up to be sent.

To download more than just the Inbox information, select Tools, Manage Folders and then select the folders, as shown in Figure 24.9, that are to be synchronized and managed. Click on OK and then go to ActiveSync and sync the device. Information from the folders will automatically be downloaded.

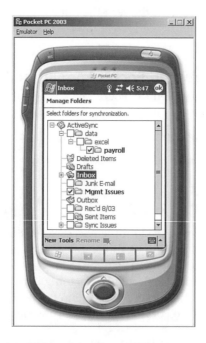

FIGURE 24.9   Choosing other folders to synchronize.

After the managed folders information has been downloaded, within the Inbox, click on the Inbox option in the upper left of the Inbox program to show the Outlook folders.

Select a different folder and view the messages that are now managed along with the Inbox.

Viewing Calendar and Contacts Information

Calendar and contacts information is also common for mobile users to access information remotely. To access the Outlook Calendar or Contacts information, select Start, Calendar or Start, Contacts, respectively.

When viewing calendar appointments, a user can select a day, a week, or a month view. Depending on the option selected, the user sees more detail (such as in a daily view), as shown in Figure 24.10, or less detail (such as in a monthly view).

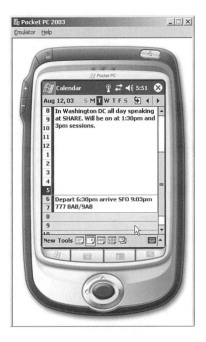

FIGURE 24.10   Viewing a detailed day view.

To add a new appointment, selecting New brings up a page that enables the user to enter details of the appointment. Appointments that are created on the Pocket PC device can note date, time, reminder, and categories; invite other attendees; show status information and sensitivity information; and contain notes about the appointment.

For contacts, a person in the address book can be viewed and edited, or an email or phone call can be initiated from the Pocket PC device from within the contacts. Contacts can be added, deleted, or even beamed from one Pocket PC device to another Pocket PC device.

Working with Smartphones

Another type of mobile device is a hybrid Windows CE device and mobile phone. Unlike a Pocket PC device that has a touch screen display and looks more like a PDA than a telephone, the Smartphone is a mobile phone that has a Windows interface for viewing inbox messages, calendar appointments, contacts, and other Outlook information.

As with Pocket PC devices, an organization can purchase a Smartphone and test the functionality, or it can download a Smartphone emulator and test the functionality of the Smartphone device to Exchange 2003.

Using a Smartphone Wireless Device

There are several vendors that have adopted the Smartphone technology into their mobile phone device. The benefit to Exchange administrators is that a Smartphone by definition comes with mobile connectivity, so the device is Internet-ready from the time the device is powered on. Besides being able to use the phone as a mobile phone, a user can also access the Internet using the built-in Internet Explorer browser.

If users have problems with Internet connectivity with a Smartphone, they contact the wireless phone carrier for support. The carrier typically has technical support that helps users connect the Smartphone to the Internet for general browsing. When they can browse the Internet, the Smartphone can be configured to access Exchange 2003 for synchronization of email, contacts, calendar appointments, and other Outlook information.

Using a Smartphone Emulator

The Smartphone 2003 emulator (the SDK) is a free download from Microsoft. Go to `http://www.microsoft.com`, search on the words **Smartphone 2003 SDK**, and download the `Microsoft Smartphone 2003 SDK.msi` file (55MB).

In addition to downloading the Smartphone 2003 emulator, you also need to download a copy of the eMbedded Visual C++ 4.0 and the eMbedded Visual C++ 4.0 Service Pack 2 or higher—unless you installed the eMbedded Visual C++ 4.0 and Service Pack when you installed the Pocket PC 2003 SDK. The eMbedded Visual C++ 4.0 and Service Pack should be installed before the SDK emulator to provide the core driver and libraries needed to run the software development kit. The eMbedded Visual C++ 4.0 and Service Pack can be found at

`http://msdn.microsoft.com/vstudio/device/embedded/download.aspx`.

The `eVC4.exe` is 333MB and the `evc4sp2.exe` (Service Pack 2) is 42MB.

Requirements to Run the Smartphone 2003 Emulator

To install eMbedded Visual C++ 4.0, Microsoft states its requirement is a system running Windows 2000 or Windows XP, 450MHz or faster Pentium-II class system, 128MB–192MB or more of available memory, 200MB of available disk space, network adapter, VGA video, and a mouse. The host workstation also needs a network adapter connected to a network connection that will access the Exchange 2003 server.

It is typically recommended to first test the Smartphone emulation on an internal backbone segment to make sure the connection to the Exchange server is not blocked by external firewalls, routers, or other external perimeter devices. The host workstation needs network connectivity, and although it's not a requirement to run the Smartphone emulator, the system should be able to connect to the Exchange server using Outlook Web Access or from an Outlook client. This ensures that the host workstation has the appropriate network connectivity for the emulator to connect to the server.

> **NOTE**
>
> The Smartphone 2003 emulator does not require its own IP address on the network, and there is no network connectivity configuration required on the emulator. The emulator simply passes through the existing LAN connection of the host workstation. If the workstation has connectivity to Exchange for Outlook or Outlook Web Access, that same connection is used by the emulator.

Installing eMbedded Visual C++ 4.0

After downloading the eMbedded Visual C++ 4.0 and Smartphone 2003 SDK, install the two applications using the following steps:

1. Launch the eVC4.exe executable for the eMbedded Visual C++ 4.0 to install it on the host workstation. This extracts the files to a temporary directory (for example, c:\evc4\) and launches the installation wizard.

2. Go into the temporary directory and run setup.exe. The installation wizard displays a welcome screen; click Next to continue.

3. After reading the end-user license agreement and agreeing to the information, click I accept the agreement and then click Next.

4. When prompted for the product license number and user ID, enter the evaluation ID that is noted on the main Web page where you downloaded the eMbedded Visual Tools. The product ID noted is TRT7H-KD36T-FRH8D-6QH8P-VFJHQ.

5. When prompted, select to install all the eMbedded tools and then click Next.

> **NOTE**
>
> Unlike with the eMbedded Visual Tools 3.0 that also installed the Pocket PC 2002 and the Smartphone 2002 SDKs, the eMbedded Visual C++ 4.0 installs only the eMbedded Visual C++ 4.0 tools. Install the Pocket PC 2003 emulator and the Smartphone 2003 emulators separately.

6. Choose a folder you want to install the software in (the default is `c:\Windows CE Tools`) and then click Next. The Windows CE Platform Manager 4.0 will begin to install.

7. Click OK past the eMbedded tools setup product ID information.

8. Click on Continue when prompted to confirm the installation of the eMbedded Visual C++ 4.0 Setup, which includes the eMbedded Visual C++ 4.0 and Common Components.

9. After the installation of the eMbedded Visual C++ 4.0 tools, click OK when the setup notes it was completed successfully.

10. The installation wizard for the Standard SDK for Windows CE .NET setup begins to extract and install. Click on Next past the welcome page, read and accept the license agreement, and then click on Next.

11. Enter your name and company name and click on Next.

12. Select to have a Complete Install and click on Next.

13. Choose to install in the default destination folder and click on Next.

14. Click on Install to complete the installation of the Standard SDK for Windows CE .NET.

15. When the installation of the Standard SDK for Windows CE .NET has completed its installation, click on Finish.

After the base eMbedded Visual C++ 4.0 has been installed, install eMbedded Visual C++ 4.0 Service Pack 2 or higher using the following steps:

1. Run `evc4sp2.exe`. Choose a directory where you want to expand the files (for example, `c:\evcsp2\`).

2. Go to the directory you selected, go into the DISK1 directory, and run the `setup.exe` program.

3. At the eMbedded Visual C++ 4.0 SP2 setup welcome screen, click Next.

4. Read and accept the end-user license agreement and click on Next.

5. Click on Install to begin the installation of the Service Pack.

6. When the Service Pack has completed installation, click on Finish.

Installing the Smartphone 2003 Emulator

After the eMbedded Visual C++ 4.0 and Service Pack have been installed, install the Smartphone 2003 SDK using the following steps:

1. Launch the Microsoft Smartphone 2003 SDK.msi package.

2. At the welcome screen, click on Next.

3. Read the end-user license agreement, select I accept the terms in the License Agreement, and click on Next.

4. Enter your name and organization and click on Next.

5. Click on Complete for the type of installation.

6. Click on Next to select the default destination folder information.

7. Click on Install to initiate the installation.

8. When the installation has completed, click on Finish.

Launching the Smartphone 2003 Emulator

After the Smartphone 2003 SDK has been installed, launch the emulator by selecting Start, Programs, Microsoft Smartphone 2003 SDK, and the Smartphone 2003 Emulator. By default, the Smartphone emulator establishes a link to the Internet as long as the host workstation that the emulator is installed on has Internet connectivity.

Synchronizing Data Between the Smartphone and Exchange 2003

A user's Outlook information can be synchronized between Exchange 2003 and a Smartphone device. The user can choose to synchronize email, calendar, and contact information. To synchronize information between the Pocket PC 2003 device and the Exchange 2003 server, use the following steps:

1. Configure ActiveSync by selecting Options in the ActiveSync window.

2. Select Server Settings, Connection, and enter the username, password, and domain. Enable the Save password setting and server name, and then select Done.

3. Select Inbox and enable the check box to synchronize the Inbox with the server.

4. Select Calendar and enable the check box to synchronize the Calendar with the server.

5. Select Contacts and enable the check box to synchronize the Contacts with the server.

6. Select the Sync option to begin synchronization, as shown in Figure 24.11.

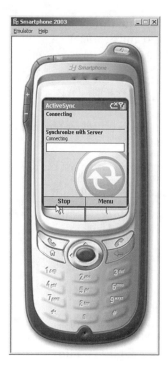

FIGURE 24.11   Synchronizing Smartphone with Exchange 2003.

Establishing a Link from a Mobile Phone to Exchange 2003

Exchange 2003 also supports the access of information from mobile phones that are not Pocket PC–enabled devices. Web-enabled phones offer you the ability to view email messages, calendar appointments, contact information, and other Outlook/Exchange information. Unlike the Pocket PC device that downloads and synchronizes information, the Web-enabled device offers a real-time view and information lookup.

The Web-enabled device uses the Outlook Mobile Access capability of Exchange 2003. Outlook Web Access assumes users access their Outlook information from a full-screen desktop computer, but Outlook Mobile Access (OMA) assumes users access their Outlook information from a much smaller screen. In some cases, the OMA screen may be only 8–10 characters wide and 4–5 lines deep, and the device might communicate at speeds equivalent to less than 9600 baud. With limited bandwidth and limited screen view size, the transfer of OMA information must be extremely efficient.

Establishing Connectivity for a Mobile Phone Device

To connect a mobile phone to Exchange 2003, you first establish network connectivity for the device. Two types of mobile phone devices are addressed in this section. One device is a physical wireless Web-enabled phone, and the other device is a Web-enabled emulator.

Connectivity of a Web-enabled Wireless Phone

Fortunately, the nature of a mobile phone is that it has connectivity to some service, typically a mobile phone carrier. The mobile phones that are Web-enabled have HTML, WAP, cHTML, or other wireless Web access and typically are configured from the factory to provide Internet Web access capabilities. To establish Internet connectivity, the best thing to do is read the instructions for the device. The technical support for the phone or carrier vendor will provide assistance on Internet connection.

After the mobile phone has the capability of accessing Web pages on the Internet, the device is ready to be configured for connection to Outlook Mobile Access (covered in the section "Using Outlook Mobile Access to Exchange 2003," later in this chapter).

Connectivity Using a Web-enabled Phone Emulator

For administrators who want to test Web-enabled Outlook Mobile Access but are not ready to commit to purchasing a mobile phone, a Web-enabled phone emulator is a great way to set up and test the OMA functionality. Openwave Systems Inc. (http://www.openwave.com) provides a mobile phone emulator that can be used with Exchange 2003. The emulator can be set up on a network-connected Windows workstation that can host the emulator. As with the Pocket PC 2002, Pocket PC 2003, and the Smartphone emulators, the system should have connectivity to the Exchange 2003 server that will be tested.

Downloading the Web-enabled Emulator

To download the Openwave Mobile SDK, go to

```
http://developer.openwave.com/omdt/select_component.html
```

From that page, select to download the Complete Mobile SDK (54MB).

Installing the Web-enabled Emulator

After the Openwave Mobile SDK has been successfully downloaded, install the Web-enabled mobile phone emulator by expanding the OpenwaveMobileSDK.zip file and then launching the Openwave_SDK_622.exe file in the client\SDK directory. This installs the emulator on the host workstation.

Using Outlook Mobile Access to Exchange Server 2003

With either a Web-enabled mobile phone or the Openwave Mobile SDK emulator in front of you, you can now begin to navigate the OMA interface to Exchange 2003. As noted earlier, because OMA is a real-time Web-access tool and not a synchronization tool, the only prerequisite to running the OMA is to have a mobile phone or emulator that has Internet connectivity.

With Internet connectivity, a user enters the Web URL **http://{servername}/OMA**. When OMA is accessed on the Exchange server, the user sees a screen similar to the one shown in Figure 24.12. The user can move around the menu and select to view a message in the Inbox, Calendar, Contacts, or Tasks; search the directory; compose a new message; or change preferences.

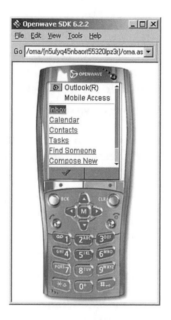

FIGURE 24.12   The Outlook Mobile Access screen.

When a user selects the Inbox, the mobile phone establishes a connection with the Exchange 2003 server and displays a list of inbox mail headers. The user can select a message and choose to open it. The mobile phone establishes a connection to the Exchange 2003 server and downloads the message.

Users can also choose to open the calendar and select a day they wish to view calendar appointments. When a day is selected, the phone makes a call to the Internet, and OMA retrieves the calendar appointments for the given day and displays it on the screen, as shown in Figure 24.13.

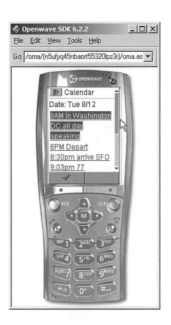

FIGURE 24.13   Viewing a calendar day of appointments in OMA.

Summary

Mobility in Exchange 2003 through the use of Pocket PC devices, Smartphones, and Web-enabled mobile phones provides organizations the ability to extend Exchange to users that might otherwise not have regular connectivity to their messages, calendar appointments, contacts, and other information. With mobile access built in to Exchange 2003, an organization sets up the mobile device and enables users to connect to the Internet and then access their information.

Through the implementation of SSL encryption on information transfers, the data sent and received is secured, and all information remains on the Exchange Server should users lose their mobile device. Mobility has been greatly extended with Exchange 2003 to provide more ways for users to access Outlook and Exchange information.

Best Practices

The following are best practices from this chapter:

- When evaluating the functions of mobile connectivity, download the emulators for Pocket PC, Smartphone, and Web-enabled mobile phone instead of buying physical devices.

- When testing mobile connectivity, test connectivity internally to a network before testing it externally to minimize any firewall, router, or external communication challenges that might prevent successful communication with an Exchange 2003 server.

- Always use SSL encryption when establishing connectivity between mobile devices and Exchange 2003.

- If you have a choice, get the Pocket PC 2003 version of a device instead of the Pocket PC 2002 version to provide Exchange Server–initiated updates and communications with remote devices as opposed to relying on device-initiated downloads and synchronization.

- Although Pocket PC devices store information in non-volatile memory, sometimes when a Pocket PC device's battery is completely drained and the device is left uncharged for a period of time, it loses information. Therefore, keep the device charged—or at least make sure to synchronize the device to keep an active copy of all information up on Exchange.

PART VIII

Client Access to Microsoft Exchange Server 2003

IN THIS PART

CHAPTER 25

Getting the Most Out of the Microsoft Outlook Client

What's Common Across All Versions of Outlook

Outlook has "come a long way" since Outlook 97. When Outlook 97 was being designed, the Outlook team worked without any real communication with the Exchange team, the team that was building the servers to run their application! As a result, the collaborative tools didn't really exist in Outlook 97, and although operability between Exchange and Outlook existed, it was lacking. However, starting with Outlook 98, the integration of the two teams has become tighter. This culminates in the release of Outlook 2003, which, not by chance, is being released at the same time as Exchange Server 2003. This sends a clear message that the two teams now work very closely with each other. During the design process, the Outlook team received user input of desired features and implemented what it could; the team also communicated with the Exchange team to implement what the Outlook team couldn't or what would work better on the server side. The results are greater integration of products, better solutions for the end user, and improved collaborative tools.

Comparing Outlook 97, Outlook 98, Outlook 2000, Outlook XP/2002, and Outlook 2003

Many features currently available in Outlook 2003 have been around for many generations of Outlook. However, with each generation, a concerted effort has been made to make things better, faster, more streamlined, and more integrated. In the beginning in Outlook 97, the focus of Outlook was almost strictly messaging and calendaring. In subsequent generations of Outlook, the focus turned more toward automated functions such as forms and rules, as well as application integration with Instant Messenger and Internet Explorer, and integration with Exchange.

The last few versions have focused more on security than past versions, especially in Outlook XP and Outlook 2003. A focus on views, the user interface, and easier ways for the end user to flag and organize mail items have also become a major focus, evident the most in XP and Outlook 2003. Throughout all Outlook versions, the focus has always been to streamline the new version, add new functionality, and make Outlook faster. With Outlook 2003, a major focus is on collaborative tools. With the use of Microsoft's Sharepoint Portal in tandem with Exchange Server 2003, the collaborative functionality of Outlook is far superior than that of Outlook 2003 without Sharepoint Portal. However, the collaborative functionality is still enhanced in the latest version of Outlook.

The Basic Outlook Features

As mentioned earlier, the basic outlook features (such as the Calendar, messaging, and tasks) have been around since Outlook 97. However, throughout the versions, changes have been made to enhance their ease of use and navigation, and to include new application integration such as Instant Messenger and Netmeeting.

With regard to messaging, each new version strives to make enhancements to sending and receiving email, such as addressing changes, address book changes, and other sending/receiving functionality improvements. Additionally, enhancements to the user dictionaries make it easier to view sizes of email messages, arrange messages to make them easier to organize and view, and generally streamline the end user experience.

Security

Security enhancements have also been included in each Outlook iteration. For example, as spam has become more of an issue, the newer versions of Outlook have included client-configurable antispam options. All versions have improved upon the S/MIME support.

Collaboration

Collaboration is a major reason companies use Outlook as their end user messaging product. With each new version, the collaborative power of Outlook has increased. Although many tools are available for an Outlook 2003 user with just Exchange on the back-end, with the addition of Microsoft's new Sharepoint Portal product, the possibilities for collaboration with Outlook 2003 and Exchange Server 2003 have reached impressive new levels. The section on collaboration later in this chapter focuses only on the collaborative tools available to users who aren't using Sharepoint. However, if collaboration is of major importance in an enterprise, the administrator should investigate implementing Sharepoint Portal for the full collaborative possibilities.

Other Enhancements

With each new release of the Outlook client, Microsoft added new features to enhance the functionality of the product. Whether making it faster, sleeker, or more user-friendly, or adding/removing features and functionality, each new iteration is better than the previous version and integrates better with Exchange as well as other applications. Outlook 2003 is no exception to this rule. This chapter covers many of the most useful new features, as well as some of the older ones. However, with all the improvements and changes, a full book could be written on the new Outlook 2003 client alone.

What's New in Outlook 2003

As stated previously, with each new version of Outlook, new features are added, in addition to enhancements to already existing features. Following are some of the new features that users might find most beneficial.

Understanding the New Outlook 2003 Interface

The new Outlook interface incorporates many changes that were requested by users. The new four-pane view is much more user-friendly, and the Preview pane allows for a great deal more space for previewing email than was available previously. The buttons in the Shortcut pane below the Folder pane provide a quick new way to access the different features of Outlook. Additionally, new features provide better ways to quickly view and organize email.

Similarities with OWA

The new Outlook 2003 GUI is extremely similar to the GUI that Outlook Web Access users using Exchange Server 2003 experience. Outlook 2003 provides many more features than OWA does, but the similarities between the two provide the end user with a much greater comfort level; they also lessen the need for end user training in OWA usage. The similarities between the two products are the result of the close work between the two teams. Outlook Web Access is discussed in great detail in Chapter 26, "Everything You Need to Know About the Outlook Web Access Client."

Methods for Highlighting Outlook Items

As stated before, with each iteration of Outlook, the methods for organizing and finding messages have been enhanced. This is because mail has become more of a way of sharing information, and the pure volume of mail that end users receive has increased. The newest version of Outlook provides even more methods for highlighting, flagging, alerting, and organizing mail than were available previously.

Using Quick Flags

Quick flags have been enhanced in Outlook 2003. Now the end user can right-click on a message and assign a colored flag to a message, making it stand out from other messages and making grouping easier by arranging messages by flag color. Because the flag colors have no predetermined meaning, the user can then assign importance or categorization to each flag color. To assign a quick flag, do the following:

1. Right-click on the gray flag icon on the far-right side of the email message in the Inbox to access the flag options.

2. Right-click once on the flag color desired, choose Flag Complete to mark the flag completed and change the colored flag to a check mark.

Another option is to configure a reminder on the flag. The options for the reminder include these:

1. Flag the message.

2. Right-click on the flag and choose Add Reminder.

3. Choose the reason to flag the message and then a due date (Figure 25.1).

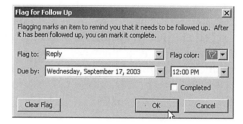

FIGURE 25.1   Adding a reminder to a flag.

4. Click OK when completed. The user receives a standard pop-up reminder when the flag comes due.

After a message is flagged, the messages can be arranged by clicking on the arrow on the top of the flag column in the Inbox to arrange messages by flagging.

Making Key Appointments Stand Out with Color

Within the Calendar, this new feature allows the customization of appointments with colors, to make them stand out from their brethren.

To choose a color and a label, follow these steps:

1. Open the appointment in the Calendar.

2. Click on the drop-down box next to Label, to the right of the Location box.

3. Choose the color and label that best apply to the message.

4. Click Save, Close.

> **TIP**
>
> The Calendar colors can also be accessed while in the Calendar area by clicking on the Calendar Colors button in the toolbar, or by right-clicking on the Calendar object before opening it and choosing Label.

Viewing Information About Email Quickly

Outlook 2003 includes a quick pop-up box that provides information about the email, such as sender name, the size of the file, and the date/time the message was received. To view the quick summary, simply hold the mouse over a message; the pop-up box that provides this information appears.

Proposing a New Meeting Time

A new feature for the Calendar is for meeting invitees, not just the meeting organizer, to be able to propose a new meeting time when they receive a meeting invitation. To propose a new time for a meeting, do the following:

1. Open the meeting invitation.

2. Click on the Propose New Time button to the right of the Accept/Tentative/Decline boxes.

3. Choose the new time using any of the standard ways of choosing a meeting time, as shown in Figure 25.2.

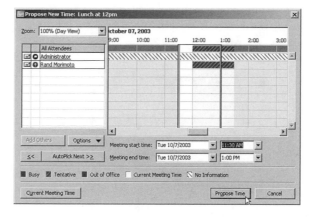

FIGURE 25.2   Proposing a new time for a meeting.

4. Click the Propose Time button when done.

5. Click Send when completed.

Using the New Search Functionality

Outlook 2003 greatly enhanced the searching functionality within Outlook. The user can now save searches: If they frequently complete the same search, they can save time by saving the search for future use. Additionally, the Search In functionality from the toolbar makes accessing the search capability even faster.

Using the Search In Functionality

The Search In functionality is easily accessible from the top of the toolbar above the main panes. To perform a search, do the following:

1. Enter the word(s) to search for in the Look For box, or click on the Find button in the toolbar.

2. Click the drop-down arrow next to Search In to choose the part of Outlook in which to search.

3. Click Find Now to begin the search. The results are shown in the window below the search.

Saving Searches

To save a search, the search must be started from within the Folder list under Search Folders. The following steps should be followed:

1. Right-click on Search Folders and choose New Search Folder.

2. Within the New Search Folder pop-up box, shown in Figure 25.3, choose the search folder and criteria. Depending on what is picked in the top, the user might be presented with more options to fill out before commencing the search. Choose also what part of Outlook to search.

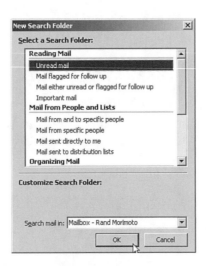

FIGURE 25.3   Creating new search folder criteria.

3. Click OK when completed.

4. The search completes and the results are displayed in the center pane. Additionally, the search is saved under the Search Folders area in the Folder list.

5. To delete the saved search, click on it and choose Delete.

> **TIP**
>
> For saved searches to be accessed via Outlook Web Access (OWA), they must be created in Outlook 2003 first and then saved.

Associating Items with Specific Contacts

Any Microsoft Office document, as well as a mail message, Calendar item, or task, can be linked to a contact and then appears in the Activities tab of the contact. This is useful to keep track of all correspondence and information regarding the contact.

To link an item to the contact, do the following:

1. Open the contact.

2. Go to Actions, Link, Items to link an item within Exchange, as shown in Figure 25.4.

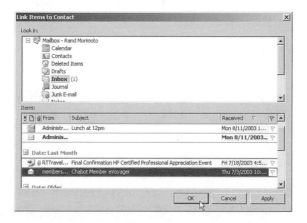

FIGURE 25.4   Linking an item to an Outlook contact.

3. Or, go to Actions, Link, File to browse the network or the local hard drive to link a file.

4. Click on Item to choose an Outlook item to link, including items from public folders.

25

Outlook maintains links in the Activities tab until they are removed manually by the end user.

To remove a link to a contact, there is a different method, for an Outlook component and for a document. To remove a link for an Outlook component, do the following:

- Double-click on the message for which the link should be removed.

- When it's open, go to View, Options.

- To the right of the Contacts button, delete the contact listed there.

- Close the object.

To remove a link for a document, do the following:

- Double-click on the document for which the link should be removed.

- Delete the message that was created with the document included in it.

Managing Multiple Email Accounts from One Place

Outlook 2003 allows the end user to access multiple email accounts from one Outlook box, including IMAP, POP3, and HTTP mail accounts.

To configure Outlook to access multiple mailboxes, do the following:

1. Go to Tools, Email Accounts.

2. Choose Add a New Email Account.

3. Click Next.

4. Select the correct email server for the account, depending on the type of email account (POP3, HTTP, Exchange, IMAP).

5. Click Next.

6. Enter the appropriate information for the email account so that it can be properly connected.

> **TIP**
>
> For an Exchange Server account, click Check Names. Verify that the Exchange server successfully verified the name entered; it becomes underlined after this happens.
>
> For an MSN Hotmail subscriber, enter the hotmail email address and password only.
>
> For a POP3 server, verify that it is properly configured by clicking Test Account Settings.

7. Click Next.

8. Click Finish.

> **TIP**
>
> Additional mailboxes in user profiles can be enabled automatically upon installation by using the Custom Installation Wizard, which is discussed in the next section, "Customizing the End user Experience."

Customizing the End User Experience

The Custom Installation Wizard can be used to change the user interface and options, at least with the initial rollout of Outlook. However, Group Policy can also be used after the installation is complete to change the user experience. This section goes into detail only about using the Custom Installation Wizard.

Using the Custom Installation Wizard

The Custom Installation Wizard (CIW) is part of the Office 2003 Resource Kit and can be found in the core tool set that is installed by default when the kit is installed. The Resource Kit can be downloaded from `www.microsoft.com/downloads`. The CIW is an extremely handy tool to customize the installation choices in Microsoft Office products.

In Outlook, it allows for specifying what previous Office versions will be upgraded or removed, as well as configuring features such as Search Folder options, integration with Instant Messenger, how the messages appear in the Outlook notification area, and the order in which items appear in the navigation pane. Almost anything that is an option or behavior in Outlook can be controlled by the CIW.

Creating a PRF File Using the Custom Installation Wizard

This section does not present detailed directions on how to use the CIW; it only touches on the choices available for Outlook customization.

To use the Custom Installation Wizard, follow these steps:

1. Download and install the Office 2003 Resource Kit.

2. Launch the Custom Installation Wizard. You'll see an initial screen like Figure 25.5.

3. Go through the first few screens until you reach the Set Feature Installation screen that determines what Office product to customize.

4. Make sure that Outlook is selected for installation. Use the drop-down boxes to choose what installation features to install for Outlook. Click Next when done.

5. Continue clicking Next until you reach the Change Office User Settings screen. At this screen, configure the Outlook features to behave as the enterprise requires by enabling or disabling the choices available for Outlook. (The interface is very similar to that of Group Policy.)

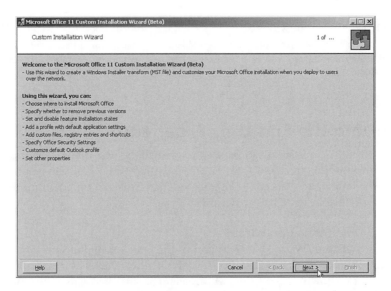

FIGURE 25.5   Custom Installation Wizard initial screen.

6. Continue through the pages by clicking Next until the Outlook: Customize Default Profile page is reached. Here, choose one of the following.

- **Use Existing Profile**   Outlook will use the existing user Outlook profile. If none exists, it will use the new one.

- **Modify Profile**   Change the existing profile. If none exists, it will use the new one.

- **New Profile**   Use this new profile for all users, whether or not one already exists.

- **Apply PRF**   Apply the profile changes that are configured in the PRF file. Specify the PRF to apply to the users.

7. Click Next when completed.

8. The next screen, Outlook: Specify Exchange Settings, allows for customization of the Exchange settings. Determine the Exchange server, the username, and whether to use the Cached Mode (Configure an Exchange Local Mailbox). Click Next when completed.

9. The next screen, Outlook: Add Accounts, allows for the addition of POP3, IMAP, Internet accounts, PST files, OAB, PABs, and other mailbox options to be included in the Outlook profile automatically.

10. The next screen, Outlook: Remove Accounts and Export Settings, allows the administrator to determine whether other email accounts (MS Mail or Lotus cc:Mail) should be removed, as well as whether to export the PRF for manual text editing. Click Next when done.

11. The next screen, Outlook: Customize Default Settings, allows for the customization of converting the Personal Address Book (PAB) to an Outlook Address Book (OAB) and handles the configuration of the default email editor (such as Wordmail) and default email format (such as HTML). Click Next when done.

12. Continue clicking Next until you reach the final screen, which states "You have completed the Custom Installation Wizard" and tells the name and location of the Custom Installer Transform file.

13. Click Exit.

The PRF file is now created and available for deployment in the enterprise.

Configuring Registry Keys During Installation

The CIW also allows for the configuration of other Registry entries to be included in the installation of Outlook. Registry entries can be created and added, as well as removed, via the CIW. Being able to add these Registry entries greatly increases the customizability of Outlook 2003. Changes to the Registry are done in the Add/Remove Registry Entries page (about page 12) in the Custom Installation Wizard.

To do this, the administrator must know the following information and enter it on the Add/Remove Registry Entries page:

1. The root Registry key (such as HKEY_LOCAL_MACHINE or HKEY_CURRENT_USER)

2. The data type value (such as DWORD)

3. The actual Registry key (without the root Registry key at the beginning of it) (such as Software/Microsoft/Office/10.0/etc)

4. The Value name (the name of the key value in the Registry to which the Registry value gets assigned)

5. The value data (such as 1 or 0—whatever is correct for the value name and the configuration desired)

This data must be inputted correctly into the CIW and saved while in the CIW. Then it will become part of the custom installation of Outlook for the enterprise.

Using PRF Files

Customized Outlook Profile Files (PRF files) are not new to Outlook 2003. In fact, the Outlook 2003 PRF format is the same as it was in Outlook 2000. However, the methods formerly used to create the PRF files (Newprof.exe and Modprof.exe) are no longer used in Outlook 2003. Using the Custom Installation Wizard, an administrator can make the required Outlook interface changes that are desired and then save those changes to a PRF file. The PRF file can then be pushed to the users in many different ways, updating or creating an Outlook profile that is different from the default Outlook profiles.

Older Outlook 98 and Outlook 2000 PRF files can be used and updated. To update older PRF files that include corporate or workgroup settings only, import the file into the Custom Installation Wizard, update it as necessary, and save it through the Custom Installation Wizard. For older PRF files that don't have the corporate and workgroup setting configured—for example, a file that has only Internet mail settings—a new PRF file should be created using the Custom Installation Wizard.

It is possible to add further customization beyond what is available in the CIW by manually editing the PRF file using Notepad.

Applying PRF files

Additionally, when a new PRF file is invoked, Outlook checks to make sure that no services are duplicated and that all accounts have unique names. Many different methods can be used to push the PRF files to the users:

- PRF files are executables, so they can be easily updated by the users by double-clicking on them.

- You can import the PRF file into the Custom Installation Wizard or Custom Maintenance Wizard as a transform. Then use the transform when Outlook is updated or deployed.

- You can configure a Registry key to run the PRF file when Outlook starts up. This key can be included in a transform.

- To specify the PRF as a command-line option for Outlook.exe to import automatically, use the following command:

```
Outlook.exe /importprf \\servername\sharename\outlook.prf
```

Security Enhancements in Outlook 2003

Microsoft announced its Secure Computing initiative in 2002. For Outlook 2003, this means a great increase in the number of security and antispam features within Outlook 2003 and Exchange Server 2003.

Support for Secured Messaging

As a result of Microsoft's security initiatives, as well as the standard increases in security functionality in Outlook that occur with every Outlook iteration, Outlook 2003 expanded its support for secured messaging, including S/MIME V3 and smart card support.

S/Mime Support, Digital Signatures, and Email Encryption

S/MIME support has been around in Outlook 2003 for a few versions. However, with Outlook 2003, S/MIME V3 is now supported. Email messages are encrypted by the sender's public key and can be accessed, opened, and decrypted only with the recipient's private key. This private/public key exchange is critical for secure email correspondence.

Use of S/MIME support requires that the user has a certificate for cryptography on the user's computer (and is stored locally either in the Microsoft Windows Certificate Store or on a smart card), but this can be pushed through Registry settings or via Group Policy to easily implement S/MIME throughout an organization. Outlook 2003 also provides support for the X.509v3 standard, which requires third-party encryption keys, such as ones created by digital security companies such as Verisign. By using S/MIME, the sender ensures that the email is encrypted and is read only by the intended recipient.

S/MIME V3 support also includes support for digital signing. Digital signing allows for security labels and signed secure message receipts. Outlook 2003 allows for enterprise-wide enforced security labels such as "For internal use only" or labeling messages to restrict the forwarding or printing of messages. Additionally, the user can now request S/MIME affirmation of receipt of a message. By requesting a receipt, the sender confirms that the recipient recognized and verified the digital signature because no receipt is received unless the recipient, who should have received the message, actually did receive the message. Only then does the sender receive the digitally signed read receipt.

> **TIP**
>
> The security features mentioned in this entire Security section can also be configured by the administrator via Group Policy, using the `outlk11.adm` Group Policy template. Open the Group policy that will have the template applied (usually on the domain level), import the template, and go to the following location to view the Group Policy choices for Security Settings: `User Configuration\Administrative Templates\Microsoft Outlook 2003\ Tools | Options\Security`.

Setting Email Security on a Specific Message

Security such as cryptography can be set for an individual email in the options of the open email message. Clicking on the Options button opens the Message Options dialog box. There, the end user clicks on Security Properties to set the security settings for the message. The user can choose to encrypt the message and/or add a digital signature, request S/MIME receipt, and configure the security settings.

To do this, follow these steps:

1. Open a new message.

2. Click on Options.

3. Click the Security Settings button.

25

4. Add security settings as desired, similar to the ones shown in Figure 25.6.

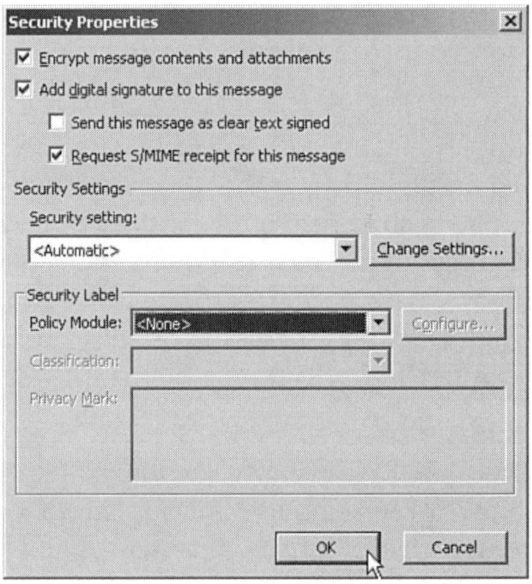

FIGURE 25.6   Setting security settings for Outlook mail.

5. Click OK when completed.

Setting Email Security on the Entire Mailbox

Security settings can also be configured for the whole user mailbox so that they apply at all times.

To do this, follow these steps:

1. Go to Tools, Options.

2. Click on the Security tab.

3. Enable the choices desired for security for the entire mailbox:

    • A. Encrypt Contents and Attachments for Outgoing Message

    • B. Add Digital Signature to Outgoing Messages

    • C. Send Clear Text Signed Messages When Sending Signed Messages (picked by default) (This allows users who don't have S/MIME security to read the message.)

    • D. Request S/MIME Receipt for All S/MIME Signed Messages

4. For all choices (except choice C) to work properly, the user must get a digital certificate provided by the administrator. This can be imported by clicking on the

Import/Export button at the bottom of the window beneath Digital IDs (Certificates) or by clicking on Get a Digital ID.

5. After you import the digital certificate, the security functionality is complete.

6. Click OK when completed.

Attaching Security Labels

Security labels are a feature in Outlook 2003 that are configured by the administrator and used by the users to add security messages to headings of email messages. Security labels require digital certificates. They denote the sensitivity and security of the email and can include headers such as "Do not forward outside of the company" or "Confidential." They can be configured on a message-by-message basis or for the entire mailbox.

To configure a security label for a single message, follow these steps:

1. Open a new message.

2. Click Options.

3. Click Security settings.

4. Click the check box marked Add Digital Signature to This Message.

5. Choose the security label, classification, and privacy mark that apply to the message.

6. Click OK when completed.

To configure a security label for all messages in the mailbox, follow these steps:

1. Go to Tools, Options.

2. Click the Security tab.

3. Click Settings.

4. Click Security Labels.

5. Choose the policy module, classification, and privacy mark that will apply to all messages.

6. Click OK when completed.

Using Junk Email Filters

Improved antispam features have now been integrated into both Outlook 2003 and Exchange Server 2003. The end user can configure the level of antispam filtering desired and control it. The Junk Email filter determines whether a message should be treated as junk or legitimate email. The filter analyzes each message to determine whether it's likely to be considered a junk email message by the end user. The default setting is Low, which catches only the most obvious junk email. However, the end user can throttle the sensitivity of the junk email feature to catch more junk email. Messages that the filter determines to be junk are moved to a Junk Email folder, where the end user can check for emails that were accidentally specified as junk. However, the user can also configure it to permanently delete junk email messages as they arrive and not move them to the folder at all.

To configure junk email filtering, follow these steps:

1. In Outlook 2003, go to Tools, Options, Preferences tab.

2. Under Email, click on the Junk Email button.

3. On the Options tab, choose the level of blockage desired, as shown in Figure 25.7. Outlook 2003 is configured for Low blockage by default.

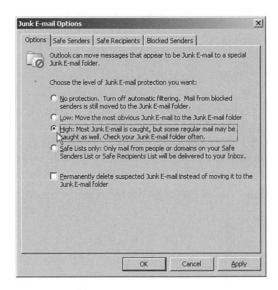

FIGURE 25.7   Setting junk mail protection level.

4. Click OK when completed, unless the sender lists will be utilized. The additional tabs are the Safe Senders, Safe Recipients, and Blocked Senders tabs.

The Safe Senders List

If the filter determines that a message is junk, the end user can add the sender's email address to the end user's Safe Senders, thereby preventing the filter from determining any later emails from that sender as junk. Both email addresses and domains can be added to the safe sender list. Entries in the end user's contacts list are automatically included in the Safe Senders list, as are any names in the GAL. Finally, for the most aggressive antispam throttling, the end user can configure mail to receive only from the safe sender list. However, this is obviously a very aggressive policy and could result in many lost emails.

The Safe Recipients List

The Safe Recipients list basically does the same thing as the Safe Sender list, but it is for email lists or groups that the end user is a member of. Any messages sent from that group automatically are considered "safe."

The Blocked Senders List

The opposite of the Safe Senders list is the Blocked Senders list. Again, domain names and specific email addresses can be entered into this list; thereby, the end user never receives email from those senders. The junk email then is handled as other junk email is handled (either deleted immediately or shunted to a junk email folder.)

To add users to the Safe Senders, Safe Recipients, and Blocked Senders lists, do the following:

1. Select Tools, Options and go to the Preference List tab. Select the Junk Email button.

2. Choose one of the tabs (Safe Senders, Safe Recipients, or Blocked Senders), and then click on Add to insert the user to the appropriate list, as shown in Figure 25.8.

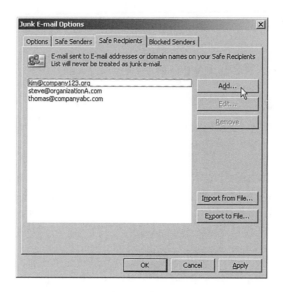

FIGURE 25.8   Adding names to one of the Blocked Senders lists.

3. Type in the SMTP email address of the user, group, or domain (such as jdoe@companyabc.com or companyabc.com).

4. Click OK when finished.

> **TIP**
>
> Some third-party companies provide lists of junk senders. If your company wants to provide the end users with a list of trusted or junk senders, the end user can easily import the list by clicking on the Import from File button.

Preventing Spam Beaconing

Junk mail senders might send HTML messages that include inline references to external content, such as pictures or sounds. When the end user opens the message or views it in the Preview pane, his computer retrieves this external content, thus verifying the end user as a "live" address to the sender. This technique is known as a Web beacon. If left unblocked, it can make the end users more of a target for junk mail.

To enable spam beacon filtering, from Outlook 2003, do the following:

1. Click Tools, Options and select the Security tab.

2. Under Download Pictures, click the Change Automatic Download Settings button.

3. Configure the necessary security settings. The default is to disallow any pictures or other HTML content.

4. Click OK when finished.

Understanding RPC over HTTP

RPC over HTTP allows remote users to connect to Exchange Server 2003 using the Outlook 2003 MAPI client via the Internet, but without the need for a VPN or other tunneling software, smart cards, or other security tokens. It gives these remote users secure communication access to Outlook features found only in the MAPI client.

Installing and Configuring RPC over HTTP on the Server End

RPC over HTTP requires configuration on the Exchange Server to support HTTP Proxy. Two items must be configured on the server operating as the front-end server for the remote connection:

- Install RPC over HTTP Windows component
- Configure IIS to support RPC over HTTP secured communications

Installing the RPC over HTTP Windows Component

To be able to run RPC over HTTP, the RPC over HTTP Windows component needs to be installed. To install the component, do the following:

1. From the Windows 2003 front-end server that will host the RPC over HTTP client connections, run Start, Settings, Control Panel, Add or Remove Programs.

2. Select Add/Remove Windows Components.

3. Highlight the Network Services component and then click Details.

4. Select the RPC over HTTP Proxy option, as shown in Figure 25.9. Then click OK.

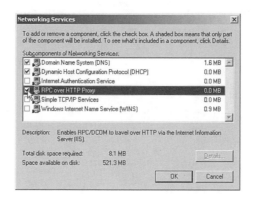

FIGURE 25.9   Selecting the RPC over HTTP Proxy Windows component.

5. Click Next to begin installation, and then click Finished when done.

Configuring IIS to Support RPC over HTTP

After the RPC over HTTP Proxy Windows component has been installed, IIS needs to be configured to support RPC secured communications. To do so, do the following:

1. Select Start, Programs, Administrative Tools, Internet Information Services (IIS) Manager.

2. Traverse the IIS tree past the server, Web Sites, Rpc. Right-click on the Rpc container and select Properties.

3. Select the Directory Services tab and click on Edit.

4. Deselect the Enable Anonymous Access option.

5. Select the Basic Authentication option (the Integrated Windows Authentication option should also be selected by default). Click OK.

6. Click on Edit and select both Require Secure Channel (SSL) and Require 128-Bit Encryption. Click OK.

Installing and Configuring RPC over HTTP on the End user Workstation

After HTTP over RPC is configured on the server end, the end user's workstation systems need to be configured for security end-to-end communications.

The end user must be running Windows XP with SP1 or higher, as well as Outlook 2003. In addition, the end user needs to install a hotfix to enable RPC over HTTP.

The hotfix can be found at `http://support.microsoft.com/default.aspx?scid=KB; EN-US;331320`.

1. Install the patch.

2. Reboot the PC.

After the hotfix is installed, launch Outlook 2003:

1. Go to Tools, Email Accounts.

2. Choose View or Change Existing Email Accounts.

3. Click Next.

4. Select the Microsoft Exchange Server account and click Change.

5. Click the More Settings button on the Exchange Server Settings page.

6. Click the Connection tab.

7. Click the Connect to My Exchange Mailbox Using HTTP check box, as shown in Figure 25.10.

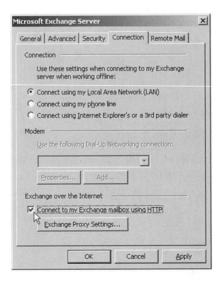

FIGURE 25.10   Selecting the connection to Exchange using HTTP.

8. Click on the Exchange Proxy Settings button.

On the Exchange Proxy Settings screen, configure the following:

1. For Connection Settings, enter the URL of the Exchange server that has been configured as the RPC proxy server.

2. Click Connect Using SSL Only.

3. Click Mutually Authenticate the Session When Connecting with SSL.

4. Enter the URL for the proxy server.

5. If the user is located on a fast network, leave the default of connecting via TCP/IP first and then HTTP. If the user is on a slow network, connect using HTTP first and then TCP/IP.

6. For Proxy Authentication Settings, choose the method that works best for the enterprise:

   The default method is Password Authentication (NTLM).

   Basic Authentication will prompt a user for a username and password each time the user connects to the exchange server. If SSL is not being used, the password will be sent in clear text.

7. Click OK twice.

8. Click Next.

9. Click Finish.

The most secure method of user connection uses the following settings, which are also the default settings when RPC over HTTP is first configured:

- Connect with SSL Only
- Mutually Authenticate the Session When Connecting with SSL
- Password Authentication is NTLM

Using Outlook 2003 Collaboratively

Outlook 2003 expands the collaborative tools of previous versions and includes some new features as well. This section covers some of the collaborative features included in Outlook 2003.

Viewing Shared Calendars in Multiple Panes

Outlook 2003 now allows a user to view an additional Calendar in a shared pane. In previous versions, if an additional Calendar was opened, it was opened in a new window. Now a user can open multiple Calendars that they have permissions to view and can line them up side by side and view or compare them.

To open more Calendars, do the following:

1. Choose File, Open, Other User's Folder.

2. Choose the name of the user and select Folder Type: Calendar. The Calendar opens in the main window and automatically removes the mailbox owner's Calendar.

3. To view both the end user Calendar and the additional Calendar, go to the Folder pane. There is an area under the monthly Calendar that provides check boxes for what Calendars the end user wants to view. Click on the My Calendar box to view both the end-user Calendar and the additional Calendar.

> **TIP**
>
> Note that each additional Calendar is a different color, and the corresponding check box on the left is the same color.

4. Continue to add the Calendars desired and click on the check boxes to remove or add Calendars to view.

5. When completed, click on the My Calendar check box and deselect all the additional Calendars.

> **TIP**
>
> Viewing shared Calendars can also be accessed from the Calendar area by clicking on the Open a Shared Calendar hyperlink in the Folder List pane. Enter the name and click OK. This automatically shows both the mailbox owner's Calendar and the new Calendar(s).

Enabling Calendar Sharing

For security reasons, Calendars are not shared by default. The end user must specify users with whom to share a Calendar.

To enable the mailbox owner's Calendar to be shared, follow these steps:

1. Click on the hyperlink Share My Calendar, in the Folder List area in Calendars.

2. The Calendar Properties box appears.

3. Click on Add.

4. Browse or enter the name or group to get access to the Calendar (see Figure 25.11).

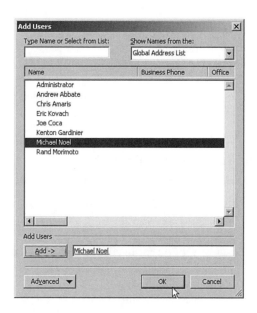

FIGURE 25.11   Sharing a Calendar with another user.

5. Click OK.

6. The end user must now assign the permissions for other users to have to the Calendar. Outlook provides predefined roles for permissions that appear in the Permission Level box. Clicking the drop-down menu and choosing a predefined permission level shows what permissions are being granted, making it easy to chose desired permissions. To create a unique set of permissions, choose an initial Permissions level and then check the boxes and radio buttons to assign the unique permissions.

7. Click OK when completed. The user(s) specified will have those rights to the end user's Calendar until the end user specifically removes them by going through the same process mentioned, and then clicking on the user or group with permissions to the Calendar and choosing Remove.

Sharing Other Personal Information

Outlook also enables an end user to share other personal information, such as the Inbox, contacts, and tasks. This is all done through the same method listed previously (except that the user must be in the Contacts or Tasks areas to access the proper hyperlink to share that component of Outlook). The exception is enabling mail sharing, which doesn't provide a hyperlink.

To enable mail sharing, follow these steps:

1. Right-click on the Inbox in the Folder view.

2. Choose Sharing.

3. Enter the users or groups and permissions levels, as described previously in the "Enabling Calendar Sharing" section.

Delegating Rights to Send Email "On Behalf Of"

To enable a user to send email on someone's behalf, follow these steps:

1. Go to Tools, Options and select the Delegates tab.

2. Click Add.

3. Add the name of the user or group that needs the rights.

4. Click OK.

5. Choose the permission level for each component of Outlook.

6. Click OK when completed.

7. To send the delegates a summary message of their rights, click on the check box next to Automatically Send a Message to Delegate Summarizing These Permissions before clicking OK.

8. To enable the delegates to see private items, click on the box next to Delegate Can See My Private Items before clicking OK.

> **TIP**
>
> The Delegates tab under Tools, Options is also an easy place where the end user can assign permissions to view Outlook components from one place rather than having to configure the option individually. However, the permissions provided are less numerous and customizable than if done through the methods listed in the previous two sections.

Sharing Information with Users Outside the Company

Throughout the different Outlook versions, collaborative functionality has constantly increased with each version. Outlook 2003 provides some additional collaborative features, as well as some of the old tried-and-true features that have been around for many versions.

Configuring Free/Busy Time to Be Viewed via the Internet

End users can publish their free/busy information outside of the company, if desired, by either using a company-provided Web site for publishing the information or using a free service provided by Microsoft called the Microsoft Office Internet Free/Busy Service (both users must have a Microsoft Passport account to use the Microsoft Service). Via either method, users outside of the company can view another's free/busy information via the Web from a shared location and can use the Web site to schedule meetings with each other. This is available for users of Outlook 2002 or later.

To configure free/busy time to be displayed on the Internet, follow these steps:

1. Go to Tools, Options, Calendar Options.

2. Click Free/Busy Options.

3. Choose the number of months of free/busy data to publish to the service, as shown in Figure 25.12.

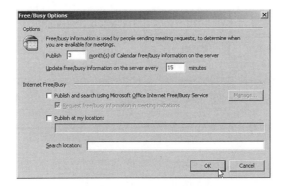

FIGURE 25.12   Providing three months of free/busy data publishing.

4. To also update how often Outlook updates the free/busy service with new information, under Options, type a number from 1 to 99 in the box Update Free/Busy Information on the Server Every X Minutes.

To configure which service will publish the free/busy information, follow these steps:

1. To use a locally provided Web site, click Publish at My Location and enter the URL to the location. Go to step 10.

2. To use the Microsoft Office Free/Busy service, click the check box next to it and click the Manage button.

3. The user is directed to log into the site using a Microsoft Passport username and password.

4. Agree to the terms of use by clicking on Yes, I Agree.

5. Click Continue.

6. Enter the email addresses of the users allowed to access the free/busy data.

7. Include a message to nonmembers that will be sent to them telling them that they have been authorized to view the free/busy information.

8. Click OK.

9. Close the Internet window after noting that the authorization process is complete.

10. Back in Outlook, click OK.

11. The user might be prompted to install some files to complete the installation of the added functionality.

12. Click Yes to install. The Outlook feature then is installed.

13. Click OK two more times.

Viewing Free/Busy Time via the Internet

If permitted by the end user of the free/busy information, another end user can view that information from the Web site. The user can send meeting requests, add the user to a group schedule, and see free/busy time. To do this, the end user must access the free/busy time Web site, click on View Free/Busy Times on the Web, and enter the email address of the user whose free/busy time is to be viewed.

Using iCalendar and vCalendar

iCalendar and vCalendar are RFC-compliant features of the Outlook 2003 Calendar that support communication between different Calendar clients. This allows a Calendar event created in one technology to be imported into another Calendar technology.

vCalendar is the older version of the two Calendar features. It is widely supported by many different mail programs; when in doubt, it is best to use the vCalendar feature. However, recurring appointments cannot be saved in the vCalendar format.

The iCalendar is built on the vCalendar technology, but it provides added journal entries and additional free/busy information. However, because it's built on the vCalendar technology, mail services set up to support iCalendar support vCalendar as well. iCalendar also supports recurring appointments.

To send an iCalendar or vCalendar meeting request, first create the Calendar event. Then save it in the proper format and add it as an attachment to an email message; send it to the recipient, who can then import the iCalendar or vCalendar attachment.

To create an iCalendar entry, follow these steps:

1. Open or create the appointment that will become the iCalendar.

2. Choose File, Save As.

3. Click iCalendar Format, as shown in Figure 25.13, and then click on Save.

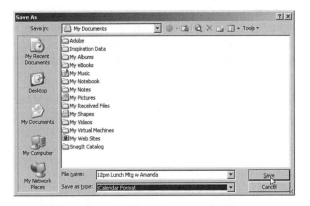

FIGURE 25.13   Saving an appointment as an iCalendar file.

4. Send the newly created .ics attachment in an email message to the recipient. The recipient will then import the attachment into his Calendar program.

To create a vCalendar entry, follow these steps:

1. Open or create the appointment that will become the vCalendar.

2. Choose File, Save As.

3. Click vCalendar Format (*.vcs) in the Save As box.

4. Send the newly created .vcs attachment in an email message to the recipient. The recipient will then import the attachment into his Calendar program.

Outlook 2003 can be also configured to always use the iCalendar format when meeting requests are sent directly over the Internet.

To enable the iCalendar functionality, follow these steps:

1. Go to the Calendar.

2. Go to Tools, Options, Calendar Options.

3. Click on Advanced Options.

4. Click the check box When Sending Meeting Requests over the Internet, Use iCalendar Format.

Now the end user can send a meeting request as he would normally, but it will function across the Internet.

To turn off iCalendar, clear the check box mentioned in step 4.

Sending Contact Information to Others

Another collaborative feature that isn't new to Outlook 2003 but that is very useful is the Virtual Business Cards, or vCards. These enable the user to send Outlook contact information to others outside the company, to be imported into the contact list program.

vCards can be emailed as attachments, can be included in auto signatures, can be saved to a file elsewhere, and can be imported and saved as contacts when received.

To email a vCard, follow these steps:

1. Open the contact that will become the vCard.

2. Go to Actions, Forward as vCard, as shown in Figure 25.14.

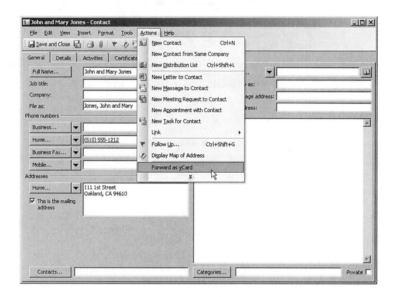

FIGURE 25.14   Forwarding a contact as a vCard.

3. Input information into the email and send the email.

When the user receives the card, he can open it and Save and Close into his own contacts area.

To include a vCard in an auto signature, follow these steps:

1. Edit an existing auto signature or create a new one.

2. In the box below where the auto signature is entered, there is a vCard Options box. Choose an existing vCard.

3. If one doesn't exit, click on New vCard from Contact and choose the contact to create a vCard for.

4. Click Add.

5. Click OK.

Using Public Folders to Share Information

Although using public folders to work collaboratively is not a concept new to Outlook 2003, it's worth mentioning its usefulness in collaborative work. Public folders can be shared between different groups of users, across sites and servers. Folders can be replicated across servers for fast receipt of information or can be downloaded locally to users' workstations for easy access while offline. The folders can be repositories for email, documents of all types, group contact lists, or shared Calendars. They can be monitored so that posting is okayed through a folder monitor before it happens, and they can be mail-enabled as well. They are very useful for collaborative working.

Using Group Schedules

Group Schedules are a new feature to Outlook 2003. These enable the user to create groups of users and to quickly view their Calendars. The Group Schedules features also allows a user to send all the members of the Group Schedule an email or to schedule a meeting request.

Configuring Group Schedules

Before anything can be done with a group schedule, one must be created by the end user.

To create a new group schedule, follow these steps:

1. Select Action, View Group Schedules. The Group Schedules dialog box appears.

2. Click New.

3. Name the Group Schedule.

4. Click OK.

5. The Customized Group Schedules dialog box appears.

6. Click Add Others.

7. Type the name of the user(s) in the Type Name or Select from List box, and click To after the user has been selected (see Figure 25.15). Note that more than one user at a time can be selected and added to the To area.

8. When all users are selected, click OK.

9. Click Save and Close.

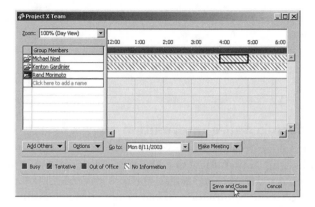

FIGURE 25.15   Adding usernames to the Group Schedules.

After the Group Schedule has been created, to view it and work with it, follow these steps:

1. Click on the View Group Schedules button.

2. Select the group schedule to view.

3. Click Open.

Sending Email or Meeting Requests to Group Schedules

After a group schedule is created, it is possible to send emails and meeting requests to the group from within the Group Schedule view.

To schedule a meeting, follow these steps:

1. Click on the Make Meeting button from within the Group Schedule view for the specific group.

2. Choose New Meeting to just send the meeting request to one member.

3. Choose New Meeting with All to send the meeting request to all members of the group schedule.

4. Fill out the meeting request as you would normally do.

To send an email, follow these steps:

1. Click on Make Meeting.

2. Choose New Mail Message to send to an individual member of the group.

3. Choose New Mail Message to All to send to the whole group.

4. Fill out the email message as you would normally do, and send the message.

Using Synchronized Home Page Views

Through Group Policy or the Custom Installation Wizard, Outlook can be configured to point to specific Web pages when the end user clicks on any of the root folders in Outlook (Inbox, Calendar, Notes, and so on). These Web pages can be used to share information in a collaborative way.

To configure shared Web home page views, do the following:

1. Open the Group Policy Object Editor (GPEdit.exe) using Start, Programs, Administrative Tools, Group Policy Object Editor.

2. Go to User Configuration, Administrative Tools. Right-click on Administrative Tools and select Add, Remote Templates.

3. Add the outlk11.adm template into Group Policy. Then click Close.

> **NOTE**
>
> outlk11.adm is installed in the \windows\inf directory when Office 2003 Resource Kit is installed on a system. outlk11.adm can be copied to the hard drive of the system being used to configure Group Policies, or the Office 2003 Resource Kit can be installed on the system.

4. Go to User Configuration, Administrative Tools, Microsoft Outlook 2003, Folder Home Pages for Outlook special folders, as shown in Figure 25.16.

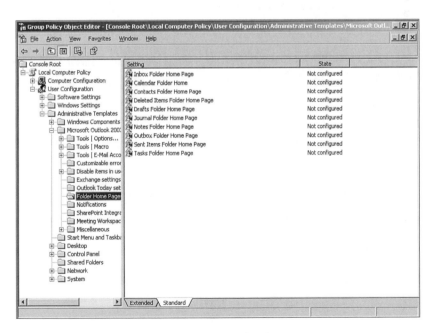

FIGURE 25.16   Configuring default folder locations for OWA.

25

5. Double-click on the Outlook home page to configure (for example, Inbox Folder home page, Calendar Folder home page, and so on).

6. Click Enabled.

7. Click Show Associated Web Page, and enter the URL of the Web page.

8. Choose any other options and edit the default setting.

9. Click OK when completed.

Using Outlook Cached Mode for Remote Connectivity

Outlook 2003 has new features to enhance the end user experience of those who access Outlook remotely. With the new Cached Mode, the OST and OAB are more seamlessly intertwined and easier to configure and use, and the experience should be faster for the end user than it was previously.

The core idea behind Cached Mode is that offline users have a full copy of their mailbox stored locally (in an OST) that automatically updates while online without user intervention. While using Cached Mode, the user should be able to be online, should receive email and synchronize the mailbox, and should be able to disconnect from the network and reconnect to the network without exiting from Outlook—without experiencing any delays or the application hanging. The cached mailbox eliminates the constant need for a user to be connected to the Exchange server and the network.

The cached Exchange Mode is very useful in networks where network and server connectivity are an issue (slow links as well as disconnections), as well as for a user who frequently goes off and on the network during the day. It keeps the user from being interrupted by network disconnectivity or slowness.

The User Experience in Cached Mode

When the user is connected to the Exchange server, the word Connected appears in the lower-right corner of the Outlook window. The message "All folders are up-to-date" also should be displayed.

When connectivity is lost, the message will say "Disconnected" and will give the date and time the folder was last updated.

When connectivity is first restored, the message will say "Trying to connect." When connectivity is re-established, the word Connected reappears; to the left of that are updates telling the user what is automatically occurring to get the mailbox up-to-date. These messages could be "Waiting to update the full items in Inbox," "Sending Complete," or "All folders are up-to-date."

While the user is offline, some slowing when using Outlook might occur. However, the whole application will not hang as it would have previously.

Deploying Cached Exchange Mode

Cached mode can be deployed by using custom Outlook deployment and the Custom Installation Wizard or by using Group Policy.

Deploying Cached Mode Manually

When configuring a user's Outlook Profile manually, it's possible to configure Cached Mode at that time.

To configure Cached Mode manually, do the following:

1. Begin configuring a user profile in the standard manner.

2. When the Email Accounts page is reached, make sure the Use Cached Exchange Mode box is checked.

3. Finish configuring the Outlook profile.

Deploying Cached Mode Using the Custom Installation Wizard

To deploy Cached Mode in Outlook 2003, one method is to use the Custom Installation Wizard to create a custom profile. The custom profile can be used to push out the custom profiles to multiple users when Outlook is distributed to the users.

> **NOTE**
>
> This section refers to the Custom Installation Wizard. This can be found in the Office 2003 Resource Kit in the core tool set.

To customize the Custom Installation Wizard, do the following:

1. While in the Custom Installation Wizard, go to the Outlook: Specify Exchange Settings page.

2. Click Configure an Exchange Server Connection.

3. Configure the following options:

   - To specify a new location for OST files (one method to change to Unicode OST files):

     1. Click on More Settings.

     2. Click Configure Cached Exchange Mode on the Outlook: Specify Exchange Settings page.

- To configure a default behavior for downloading messages, do the following:

    1. Go to the Outlook: Specify Exchange Settings page.

    2. Click Configure New or Existing Profiles to Use a Local Copy of the Exchange Mailbox.

    3. Click the check box Configure an Exchange Local Mailbox.

    4. Click Use Local Copy of Mailbox.

    5. Choose the default download option desired for the default behavior: Download Only Headers, Download Headers Followed by the Full Item, or Download Full Items.

Deploying Cached Mode Using Group Policy

Another method for configuring Cached mode is to use Group Policy to push the new policy. If the Cached Mode Group Policy is assigned on a group-by-group basis (rather than to the whole domain at once), a phased approach to deployment will be achieved.

To access the Cached Mode Outlook configuration option (and any Outlook configuration options), the administrator must install the Outlook 2003 Group Policy template (outlk11.adm) first. The process for accessing the outlk11.adm in Group Policies is covered in the earlier section "Using Synchronized Home Page Views."

1. Open the Group Policy that has the Outlook administrative template installed. Go to User Configuration, Administrative Templates, Microsoft Outlook 2003, Tools, Email Accounts, Cached Exchange Mode.

2. Double-click on Disable Cached Exchange Mode on New Profiles.

3. Enable the policy.

4. Uncheck the box Check to Disable Cached Exchange Mode on New Profiles, as shown in Figure 25.17.

5. Click OK.

6. Double-click the Cached Exchange Mode (File, Cached Exchange Mode) object.

7. Enable the policy.

8. In the drop-down list Select Cached Exchange Mode for New Profiles, choose a download option (either Full Items, Headers Only, or Headers Followed By the Full Item).

9. Close the Group Policy.

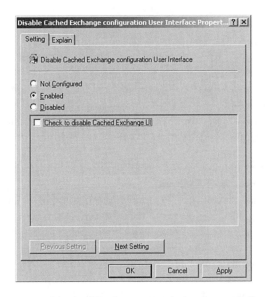

FIGURE 25.17   Enabling the Cached Exchange mode by Group Policy.

Deployment Considerations

Because enabling cached exchange mode forces the end users to synchronize a full copy of their mailbox to their local OST file as well as a full copy of the OAB, the drain on an Exchange server can be very substantial if many users are initially configured to use Cached Mode at one time. The best choices for configuring Cached Mode initially are these:

- Continue to allow the users to use their current OST files. Then the full mailbox isn't downloaded; only the changes are. To do this, when deploying Outlook, clear the Replace Existing Accounts check box in the Outlook profiles. Alternatively, do not specify a new Exchange server in the MAPI profile because this creates a new OST file.

- Deploy Cached Mode to groups of users at a time rather than the whole enterprise. Combined with the next point in this list, the effect on the Exchange server will be the least.

- Initially deploy Outlook 2003 without Cached Mode enabled. Provide users who will be receiving the Cached Mode with an initial "seed" OST file that captures their mailbox, as well as a full OAB download on a CD and instructions on how to configure the OST and OAB. Then, when Cached Mode is turned on, the users already have an OST file and the OAB, so downloading from the server is minimized.

Using Cached Exchange Mode

Cached mode changes the user experience, and an administrator might consider some additional user training for those who are using Cached Mode to let users know of the differences. Some of these differences are mentioned next.

The Send/Receive Button

It's important to let Cached Mode users know that it is unnecessary to click the Send/Receive messages button with the new Cached Mode functionality. This now happens automatically.

RPC over HTTP and the Cached Exchange Mode

It is recommended that users running RPC over HTTP also be users of cached Exchange mode. This is because this mode allows for "fluky" connections to Exchange, which also might occur while the RPC over HTTP user is accessing Exchange via the Internet.

Slow-Link Connection Awareness

Cached mode is configured to consider any link below 128Kbps to be "slow." It automatically implements the following email-synchronization behaviors:

- OAB is not downloaded (neither partial nor full download).

- Mail headers only are downloaded.

- The rest of the mail message and attachments are downloaded when the user clicks on the message or attachment to open it.

To change the slow link configuration, click on the On Slow Connection, Download Only Headers check box in Outlook 2003. This can be configured via Group Policy or custom Outlook installation files.

Cached Exchange Mode and OSTs and OABs

Cached mode downloads a full copy of the user's mail to the OST file stored locally on the user's hard drive. However, administrators need to be aware of some considerations regarding OSTs and Cached Mode to make their configurations of the cache more efficient.

Cached Mode OST Considerations

When configuring cached mode for users with large mailboxes, the new Outlook 2003 Unicode-formatted OST file should be enabled instead of using the older ANSI OST file method. This is because the Unicode OST files are capable of holding up to 20GB of data, whereas the old ANSI OST files have a limit of 2GB of data. If the use of Unicode is enabled through Group Policy and Outlook checks the file format on an OST and determines that a user is using ANSI, Outlook automatically creates a new Unicode OST and synchronizes it with Exchange. The policy can also be configured to prompt or not prompt the user before taking this action. (However, it will not automatically create a new Unicode PST file—only OST files.)

To specify Unicode for new Outlook OST files through Group Policy, follow these steps:

1. Add the `outlk11.adm` template in Group Policy. The process for accessing `outlk11.adm` in Group Policy is covered in the previous section "Using Synchronized Home Page Views."

2. Go to User Configuration, Administrative Templates, Microsoft Outlook 2003, Miscellaneous, PST Settings.

3. Click on Preferred PST Mode (Unicode/ANSI).

4. Enable the policy.

5. Choose the new default type for PST to be Enforce Unicode PST.

6. Click OK.

OST files can increase the size of the mailbox stated on the Exchange server by up to 50–80%. This is because of the less efficient storage method used in OST files. The administrator might want to consider doing the following to decrease the size of mailboxes for users who are using Cached Mode:

- Encouraging the use of autoarchiving of Exchange data for users with large mailboxes

- Not configuring synchronization of public folder Favorites unless absolutely necessary

It is imperative that the OST and OAB be stored locally on a drive that has sufficient space to hold the OST, however large it might grow. If the user's computer doesn't have enough space, errors will occur when Cached Mode tries to download the mailbox locally. For example, it might be best to not configure the OST to reside on the system drive and instead to configure it on a data drive, if possible.

Caching mode works best when the OST isn't close to its capacity. It is faster if only 5–10% of the OST size is being used. Generally, it's best if the OST doesn't grow to be bigger than 1GB because then performance degrades.

Cached Mode and Outlook Address Book (OAB) Implications

It is possible to download a No Details Outlook address book, but users using cached mode should download the Full Details OAB because they can experience significant delays when they access the OAB and the full details are not locally accessible. When this occurs, the user's workstation must make a call to the Exchange server for the full data, which can cause delays for the user experience.

It's also a good idea for users running Cached Mode to download the Unicode OAB rather than the older ANSI OAB. This is because the Unicode OAB has more details held locally than the ANSI format, which decreases the number of server calls needed when a user accesses the OAB.

The OAB is synchronized every 24 hours, by default, down to the offline OAB. If there are no updates to the server OAB, there will be no updates to the offline OAB.

Outlook Features That Decrease Cached Mode's Effectiveness

Cached Exchange mode is easy to configure, but many Outlook 2003 features can decrease its effectiveness. The features discussed next all cause Outlook 2003 to send calls to the Exchange server for information. For users using Cached Mode, these calls to the server can greatly decrease the effectiveness and speed of the Cached Mode and thus should be avoided.

Delegate Access and Accessing Shared Folders or Calendars

These both require access to the Exchange server to view other users' Outlook items. Cached mode won't download another user's data to the local OST, so this nullifies the use of Cached Mode.

Outlook Add-ins

Outlook add-ins such as Activesync can result in Outlook not utilizing important items, such as the Download Headers Only functionality that makes Cached Mode work so well. They also can cause excessive calls to the Exchange server or network. Avoid Outlook add-ins, if possible.

Instant Messaging Integration

Instant Messenger requires network connectivity. Thus, with Cached Mode, it is not a good idea to enable this functionality.

Digital Signatures

Verification of digital signatures requires Outlook to check for a valid signature for messages, requiring a server call as well.

Noncached Public Folders

This, too, requires a call to the server. Consider synchronizing the user's frequently used public folders to the OST (keeping an eye on the mailbox size as well).

Including Additional Searchable Address Books

If the enterprise includes custom address books and contact lists, and has enabled them to be searchable and useable for email addressing, this results in the client calling the server. Consider not using these if your users use Cached Mode.

Customizing the User Object Properties

If the enterprise has created customized items on the General tab of the properties box of a user, this always requires a call to the server: When user properties are displayed, the General tab always is displayed first. Therefore, if these are necessary, consider placing the customized fields on a different tab in the user properties that will be called only when that tab is accessed, not every time the user properties are accessed.

Summary

The Outlook client is a very versatile client that most people use just for opening email messages, creating Calendar appointments, and sending messages. However, the Outlook client provides a whole lot more for organizations looking to expand the capabilities of the client and to provide group Calendar sharing, secure remote communications, and better information-management functionality with Outlook and Exchange.

Although hundreds of features were built into previous versions of the Outlook client, the new Outlook 2003 client adds several new ones regarding user productivity and group communications in an Exchange Server 2003 environment. Some of the new features include quick flags, the capability to propose new meeting times, the capability to associate items with a specific contact, and new message search capabilities.

Also new with Outlook 2003 are the tools that come with the Office 2003 Resource Kit. The new Resource Kit tools provide custom installation capabilities to automate the installation of Outlook either through Group Policies or as integrated through other scripted installation tools.

Security is another major enhancement to Outlook 2003, with several new improvements for encrypted client-to-server communications using RPC over HTTP, the capability to add security to specific messages, and the capability to set security for an entire mailbox. Also part of the secured client function in Outlook 2003 is the capability to set up junk mail filters that allow or deny incoming and outgoing messages between users.

Finally, a new Cached Mode method of access enables a user to manage mail, Calendar appointments, and other content within Outlook, regardless of whether that user is connected to Exchange. Cached mode access provides managed connectivity for unreliable remote access connections and improves the user experience when connection to an Exchange server is interrupted by either network failures or a temporary connection interruption.

All of the new capabilities of Outlook 2003, as well as the capability to leverage existing features in earlier versions of Outlook, provide an improved user experience within an Exchange Server 2003 environment.

Best Practices

- Previous versions of the Outlook client are sufficient for most email users, but those who want to get the most out of Exchange Server 2003 should upgrade to Outlook 2003.

- Quick flags should be used to draw attention to messages that require follow-up or other attention.

- Key appointments can be flagged with colors to draw attention to appointments in user Calendars.

- Using the new search capabilities of Outlook 2003 can drastically improve the time it takes for a user to find messages or information within Outlook.

- The Custom Installation Wizard in the Office 2003 Resource Kit should be downloaded and used to help deploy Outlook configurations and manage Outlook settings either by script or through Group Policy.

- Instead of establishing a VPN before accessing an Exchange server from a remote Outlook 2003 client, the RPC over HTTP should be enabled to provide SSL-based 128-bit encrypted end-to-end communication from client to server.

- Calendars can be set up in group schedules to provide a side-by-side view of appointment Calendars for individuals or groups of users.

- Free/busy times can be configured to be viewable from the Internet, to provide nonconnected users access and views to appointment schedules.

- Outlook supports standard iCalendar, vCard, and vCalendar formats for the exchange of information across Exchange systems and cross-platforms.

- Cached mode for the Outlook client can improve performance for remote users across slow, unreliable, or failed client-to-server connections.

CHAPTER 26

Everything You Need to Know About Outlook Web Access Client

Many users found previous versions of the Outlook Web Access (OWA) client a good client substitute when they didn't have access to the full Outlook client. With OWA in Exchange 2003, however, many organizations are finding the Web client to have all the features needed to make OWA a primary messaging client for many users in an organization.

With this new version, Microsoft successfully incorporated some of the most frequent customer requests for changes to OWA. This chapter focuses on helping Exchange 2003 administrators and OWA users get to know how to leverage the capabilities of Outlook Web Access. It is written with both new users and users familiar with OWA in mind and therefore includes both basic instructions for how to use OWA and directions for how to use the new and advanced features of OWA. Descriptions of the new features are discussed throughout, so to fully discover all the new features, read the chapter from start to finish.

Understanding Microsoft's Direction on OWA

Outlook Web Access in Exchange 2003 provides a much more robust client interface, available via the Web. Additionally, OWA leverages newer technology, such as XML and the .NET framework, to make it more powerful and useful. Arguably, OWA has changed the most of any aspect of Exchange 2003 from previous versions.

Creating a Common Interface

A tremendous change in the 2003 OWA and previous versions of OWA is its look and feel and its similarity to the full Outlook 2003, which is covered in Chapter 25, "Getting the Most Out of the Microsoft Office Client." Although there are still differences between Outlook 2003 and OWA (including those inherent in using Web-based access and standard access), the look and feel and many of the features are exactly the same. Elements such as spell checker, keyboard shortcuts, the ability to configure rules, reading panes, and other improvements help it feel familiar and therefore easier and friendlier to use, even for the least savvy end-user.

Making a Full-Feature Web Client

The offshoot of creating OWA in this manner is that clients feel more comfortable using OWA as their only mail client, secure in the knowledge that they do so without losing many features or much functionality! OWA is no longer regarded as only a remote access mail client, but can be used day in and day out by users both in the office and out of it. Some organizations might even decide not to deploy the full Outlook 2003 at all, and use OWA exclusively as the standard Exchange client for their users. However, it should be noted that Outlook 2003 does provide additional features that OWA doesn't provide, but the more robust OWA certainly makes it an attractive alternative.

Integrating XML in the Client Interface

Microsoft has taken the major step of integrating XML into the client interface of OWA, because the integration of XML into all Microsoft products that use the Web is a major push for Microsoft. This means that OWA can better integrate data, and a similar code is used throughout Exchange and other Microsoft products that are served on the Web, such as Outlook Mobile Access (OMA) devices. The inclusion of XML and IIS 6 means that OWA is more secure and better locked down than previous versions.

Leveraging the .NET framework

OWA uses the new .NET framework and Internet-centric technology that enables applications to more easily integrate with each other. It sits on top of XML Web services but enables XML to be used by OWA. It uses the powerful .NET framework to be more compatible with other technologies to a deeper level—to exchange data on a Web-based communications layer. The .NET framework also enables a user to access OWA using IE 6 (SP1 or higher) to use the Microsoft Passport functionality to access OWA and the MapPoint functionality in contacts discussed later in this chapter. The .NET framework makes OWA a better Web interface and application.

Using the Basics of OWA/2003

OWA, like most Outlook client software, is basically used for sending and receiving email via the Web. Basic email messaging has been the focus for the Exchange client software programs and will continue to be, with added features providing even more functionality for collaboration and communications. There are some organizations that either don't want their employees to be bothered with all the features or are using older or different browsers. To accommodate all users, Microsoft created user modes in Outlook Web Access 2003 that provide differing levels of feature availability. Some of the improvements and functionality changes in OWA 2003 are available only while using the premium user mode, and not the basic user mode.

Understanding User Modes

OWA's login now uses forms-based authentication, which provides the end-user with two modes of use, depending on the application used to access OWA. Users with Internet Explorer 5.01 or above have the option of choosing the premium mode (or Premium Client Version) of OWA or the basic user mode (or Basic Client Version). Users with Netscape-or-older versions of Internet Explorer or other Internet Access methods must use the basic mode for viewing OWA.

The Premium Mode

The premium mode provides users with the full OWA experience. All available enhancements, views, and features are available using the premium mode, as shown in Figure 26.1. However, the premium mode is more bandwidth-intensive, so that must be accounted for when choosing the access mode.

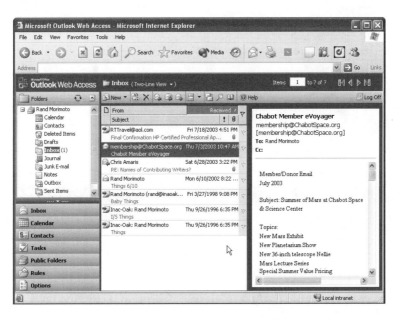

FIGURE 26.1   Premium mode Outlook Web Access.

The Basic Mode

Significantly fewer options and features are available to the user accessing OWA through the basic mode, as shown in Figure 26.2. However, the basic mode provides any user with the ability to access OWA by any Internet application. It also provides an alternative method for those with slow dial-up links to gain basic functionality without employing all the bells and whistles available to them via the premium mode.

Depending on the configuration of the Exchange server, the choice of whether to access OWA via the premium or basic mode may be presented at the user OWA logon screen. When users input their credentials, they also must choose the mode to use. The features presented are dependent on that choice.

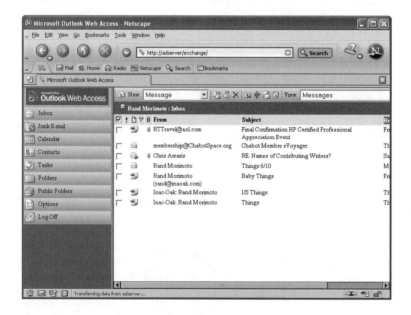

FIGURE 26.2   Basic mode Outlook Web Access.

> **NOTE**
>
> This chapter is written from the viewpoint of a user who is accessing OWA via the premium mode. The experience for a user accessing OWA via the basic mode will vary from the descriptions in this chapter.

What's New in the OWA Client (Since Exchange 2000)

There are many new features in OWA 2003. This section discusses old and new features. Table 26.1 details the new features and indicates which are available in both basic and premium modes, and which are available only in the premium mode. The table does not include a full list of OWA features.

TABLE 26.1   Features of OWA

Feature	New Feature	Premium Mode *Only*	Basic and Premium Mode
User interface			
New user interface	X		X
Resize panes	X	X	
Public folders open in own window	X	X	
Last window size remembered	X	X	
Split screen view	X	X	
Logoff on toolbar	X	X	
Deferred View Update	X	X	
General Functionality			
Keyboard shortcuts	X	X	
Saved searches	X	X	
Items per page	X		X
Search folders shown in folder tree	X	X	
GAL property sheets	More Information in the sheets		X (but only in received items and draft items)
Server-side rules	X	X	
Spell Checker	X	X	
Context menus/right-click functionality	X	X	
Notifications of new email and reminder in Navigation pane	X	X	
Mail Functionality			
Send/receive email			X
Two-line view	X	X	
Preview pane	X	X	
New message notification		X	
Quick flags	X	X	
Auto signature	X		X
Mark message read/unread	X	X	
Message sensitivity Infobar	X		X
Mail icons	X		X
Find names from messages	X	X	
Customizable font in email editor	X	X	
Reply/forward in Infobar	X		X

26

TABLE 26.1 Continued

Feature	New Feature	Premium Mode *Only*	Basic and Premium Mode
Calendar Functionality			
Reply to/forward meeting requests	X		X
Preferred reminder time changes	X	X	
Launch invitation in own window	X	X	
Receive reminders			**X**
Set default reminder time	X		
View calendar from meeting request	X	X	
Contact Functionality			
Create contacts			X
Add recipients to contacts	X	X	
Send mail from find names	X	X	
Tasks Functionality			
Create tasks	X		X (but no reminders)
Set default reminder time	X		
Security Upgrades			
S/MIME support	X	X	
Clearing credentials at logoff	X	X	
IE 6 SP1 or later			
Cookie authentication time-out	X	X	
Block external content—spam beacon blocking	X		X
Timed logoff	X		X
Attachment blocking (basic OK)	X		X

Logging In

The login interface might appear different from the older versions of OWA, depending on the configuration of the Exchange server.

Logon Screens

If the Exchange server is configured to use forms-based authentication, users can choose basic or premium mode upon logon if they are using Internet Explorer 5.01 or greater, as shown in Figure 26.3.

If the Exchange server is configured for forms-based authentication but you are using an older version of IE or another application, such as Netscape, you receive the authentication screen, but not the choice of basic or premium mode.

If the server isn't configured to use forms-based authentication, you receive a basic logon screen and when logged in, receive premium or basic mode, depending on what application was used to access OWA.

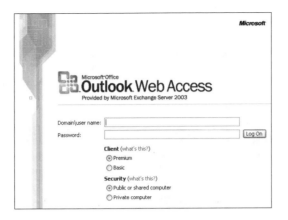

FIGURE 26.3   Prompt for Premium or Basic authentication.

Login Credentials

Also depending on how the administrator has configured OWA, users might have to enter their domain name, and then their username—for example, companyabc\Amanda. The user may use the fully qualified name, such as Amanda@companyabc.com. Users also might be able to omit the domain name and enter just a username—for example, Amanda. After successfully logging in, the user is presented with the default OWA screen.

Security Options on Logon

When presented with the basic/premium logon window, there are also options available regarding security. Users can choose whether they are on a public or shared computer or a private computer.

If the Private Computer option is clicked, the time before OWA automatically logs off after inactivity is longer than if the Public or shared computer option is selected.

Getting to Know the Look and Feel of OWA/2003

As stated previously, the user interface (UI) of the new OWA client looks almost exactly like the Outlook 2003 client. It has the same basic pane structure, same blue color scheme, the full folder tree, and the ability to change the widths of the columns, and it includes many of the similar elements in Outlook 2003. This familiar look and feel will make even the most tentative user feel more comfortable using OWA and should lessen the amount of additional user training for the OWA client users. In addition to similar look and feel, it incorporates many of the same features that are included in Outlook 2003 into the premium version (and some in the basic version) of OWA.

26

Using Multiple Panes

By default, when you initially open OWA, you are presented with four basic panes, as shown in Figure 26.4. These panes were designed to help you cope with information overload by using better organization of data and better use of space.

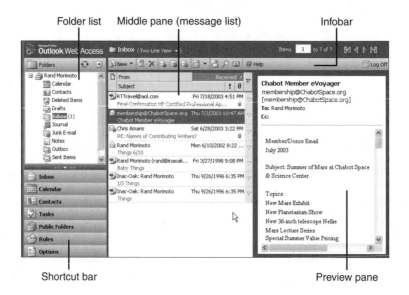

FIGURE 26.4   Outlook Web Access panes.

The folder list is the upper-left pane, which lists all the folders available to the user mailbox (Calendars, Journal, Inbox, Folders, Sync Issues, Sent Items, Junk Email, and so forth).

Below the folder list is the Outlook or shortcut bar that lists all the shortcuts to Inbox, Calendar, Contacts, Tasks, Public Folders, Rules, and Options. Additionally, when new mail appears, a new vertical button appears that states You have new mail. You can then click that button to refresh OWA and receive the new message.

The middle pane lists the contents of whatever Exchange feature is chosen in the folder list or the shortcut bar. For example, if Inbox is highlighted in the folder list, the middle pane displays the messages in your Inbox. For other options, such as the Calendar, you might have only one pane in the middle, not a split screen as you do when the inbox is highlighted.

The far-right pane is optional and is called the reading pane. The reading pane is turned on by default. This shows the content of the email message highlighted in the center pane.

The toolbar across the top is called the Infobar. It provides choices that are available while you view the information in the middle pane. The choices change depending on what is being viewed (Inbox, Calendar, and so forth) and therefore what choices are available.

Changing the Size of the Panes

You can easily configure the width or height of the panes. OWA saves the pane sizing when you log out and remembers the pane size and restores it when you log back into OWA.

- To change the size, hold the mouse over the borders between the panes and wait for the double arrow or horizontal double arrow to appear.

- When the arrow appears, continue holding down the left mouse key and move the border right/left or up/down to create the size you want.

- When the pane is in the proper place, release the left mouse button, and the pane will maintain the created size.

Using Pull-Down Menus

Icons designate pull-down menus with an arrow next to them. To view the choices, click the arrow to the right of the icon or the icon to see a menu similar to the one in Figure 26.5. To choose an option, move the mouse down the list and the choices are highlighted. To choose an option, highlight the option and click once while it's highlighted.

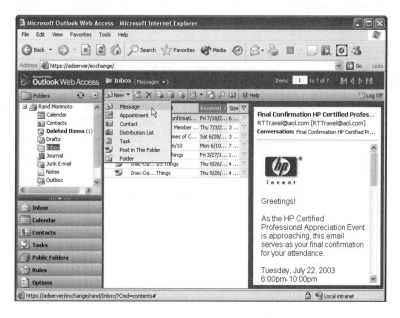

FIGURE 26.5 Pull-down menu in Outlook Web Access.

If there is no arrow next to the icon, the icon provides only a single choice, by clicking it.

Moving Through the OWA features

There are a couple of ways to move through the different OWA features. The first is by clicking the buttons that represent the feature you would like to access. For example, the shortcut bar presents you with labeled buttons for options, such as the Contacts or Inbox. Clicking once on the button accesses the feature and opens it in the center pane.

Another option is to click the icon in the folder tree in the folder pane in the upper-left corner. Clicking the Inbox or Contacts icon opens that feature in the center pane.

Moving Through Email Pages

You can configure how many email messages are displayed on the screen; yet despite the number configured, only a limited number of messages can fit in the middle pane and thus can appear at a time.

To scroll through the pages of email messages, click the arrows above the Infobar. Clicking the left- or right-arrow button moves you to the next page of email. To go to the end or beginning, click the arrow with the vertical line next to it. The arrow pointing left displays the beginning of the email pages; the arrow to the right displays the end. You also can type the page of email you want to view in the area that says Items X to # of #. However, this can be an inexact method to find an email, because it's tough to know exactly what page holds the email message you need, especially if you have a great many pages of emails.

Changing the Viewing Order and Using the Two-Line View

Users can change the viewing order of email messages in the Inbox or other email folders. The default initial configuration is to display the most recent messages at the top of the list using the Two-Line View and separated by Day and Date headings. To change the view so the new messages go to the bottom of the list, click the word *received* in the middle pane with an arrow pointing downward next to it. This rearranges the messages so the oldest is at the top.

Users can also choose to turn off the two-line view. The two-line view enables the user to view not just the email title but also the first line of the message. Combined with the reading pane, it gives users quicker access to view their email without having to open the message.

The two-line view is configured on by default. To change the two-line view to a different view, click the drop-down menu next to the word Inbox above the Infobar and choose any other option. The choices are Messages, Unread Messages, By Sender, By Subject, By Conversation Topic, Unread By Conversation Topic, and Sent To:

- **Messages**   The Messages option removes the double-line view and shows the subject bars of the messages, ordered by date and time received.

- **Unread Messages**   The Unread Messages option shows only the messages that are unread. All other messages are hidden from view until another view is picked.

- **By Sender**   The By Sender option groups the messages by the sender's name. It creates an alphabetical list of those who have sent messages. Each sender has his or her own header with a plus sign next to the name. To show the messages sent by the senders, either double-click the sender name title bar or click the plus sign next to the name. The messages are then displayed, with the most recent at the top of the list.

- **By Subject**   The By Subject option displays the messages by the subject line of the messages and then displays all messages that share that heading (for example, replied-to emails) in a hierarchy below the initial subject heading message. This view can be useful when you're trying to find a particular message with a title and want to see all the corresponding/following messages. It lists all the empty subject headers and the reply messages first in a single group for each, however, which can be difficult to manage.

- **Unread by Conversation Topic**   The By Conversation Topic groups messages by emails that have been replied to; this combines them as a type of discussion. This choice displays messages in the same type of hierarchy as the By Subject selection.

- **Unread by Conversation Topic**   The Unread by Conversation Topic option also groups messages by topic, but hides all messages except those that are unread.

- **Sent To**   The Sent To option groups the messages by recipient. This view shows groups as well as users to whom the messages were sent.

Using the Reading Pane

As with previous versions of the Outlook Web Access client, the reading pane is an optional feature. Turning on the reading pane opens a vertical pane on the far-right side of the OWA user interface, which shows the content of the message. The ability to scroll through the contents in the reading pane enables you to view the whole message without having to physically open it. Even the location of the reading pane is customizable and can be located on the right vertical pane, or as a horizontal pane at the bottom of the page, or removed entirely.

To configure the reading pane

1. Click the reading pane icon. The drop-down menu provides choices as to where to put the reading pane (the default location is the right side of the OWA UI).

2. Choose Right to configure the vertical pane on the right side; choose Bottom to configure the horizontal pane.

3. Choose Off to turn the reading pane off. When the reading pane is removed, the middle pane will expand to take up the space the reading pane used.

Attachments can now be accessed via the reading pane, using the methods discussed later in this chapter in the section "Using OWA Mail Features."

Additionally, if the message has been viewed in the reading pane and another message in the message list is clicked, the previous message is no longer bold and is marked as read, even if it hasn't been physically opened. Even though you might have read the message, a read receipt does not go back to the requestor unless the message is actually opened. You can click on Click here to send a receipt in the far-right pane to send a read receipt without opening the message. If you open the message and click on Click here to send a receipt just below the toolbar at the top of the message, the read receipt also is sent.

Creating New Folders

You can easily create many different types of additional folders that will appear in the folders view:

1. To create a new folder, click anywhere in the folders view (not the shortcuts view) in the left pane.

2. Right-click the mouse on any folder in the folders pane to see the menu shown in Figure 26.6.

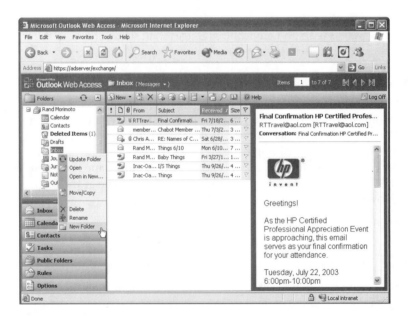

FIGURE 26.6   Adding a new folder to Outlook.

3. Choose New Folder.

4. Name the folder.

5. Choose the location where it should be created by clicking the folder in which the new folder will reside.

6. Choose what type of folder to create:

   - Appointment Items creates a calendar container.

   - Contact Items creates a new contact list.

   - Journal Items creates a new journal folder.

   - Mail Items creates a new repository to hold email messages.

   - Note Items creates a new Note folder.

   - Task Items creates a new repository for task items.

7. Click OK when the folder is properly named and in the right location.

The folder is immediately accessible for use and appears in the folder list.

Displaying Public Folders in Their Own Windows

You can view public folders by clicking the Public Folders button in the shortcuts pane. The public folders open in their own new Internet window. This gives you a great deal more space in which to work. When you finish using public folders, close the public folders window by clicking the X in the upper-right corner.

Using OWA Help

Help is available by clicking Help in the toolbar. The Help feature does not enable searching or viewing by index. However, Help topics are segregated into groups according to the topic headings. For example, if your question deals with contacts, you can navigate to the contacts area, and all the topics dealing with contacts are listed there. By clicking the plus sign (+), you expand all the topics under the contact heading that become available. When you click a subheading, the Help information appears in the right pane.

Logging Off OWA/2003

The logoff button is located on the right of the Infobar. With the logoff functionality being easily available at all times, it makes it much easier to securely log out of OWA and close your session than it was in previous versions of Outlook. Click the Logoff button to log off from OWA.

If the Exchange server is not configured to use Forms Based Authentication, you are forced to close the Internet browser window to finalize logging out. If the Exchange Server is configured to use Forms Based Authentication, click Logoff; you are presented with the login window again and are not forced to close the Internet browser window.

26

Using OWA Mail Features

Although there are many features available in OWA, the primary reason people use it is for the ability to access their email quickly and efficiently via the Internet. The new version of OWA makes using the email functionality portion of OWA easier and more robust than it has been. The next sections cover how to create and send email messages, including new features in OWA 2003 and advanced features dealing with sending and receiving email.

Creating an Email

There are many different methods for creating a new email. The first is by clicking the drop-down arrow next to New and choosing Message. The second is available while you are in the Inbox or other mail folder in the folder list. Click the envelope icon with the word New next to it. This pulls up a New Message window, used to create email messages.

Addressing an Email

There are also many methods to addressing an OWA email message. When the message is open, the To, CC, and BCC boxes appear and are blank. The recipient names go in these areas.

Primary recipients' names go into the To box. Secondary recipients—those to whom the message is not primarily targeted—go in the CC (carbon copy) box. BCC box stands for blind carbon copy, which means that the BCC recipient is invisible to all other recipients. Additionally, if you reply to all, the recipient in the BCC box will not receive the reply.

To address an email, type a name (for example, **Jane Doe**) or an email address (for example, **jdoe@companyabc.com**) into one of the three boxes. Note that multiple names should be separated by a semicolon (;).

> **NOTE**
>
> When a name is entered and before it has been checked by Exchange and verified, it appears as a single line of text and not underlined. After Exchange has checked the name—either against the Global Address List or contact list—or has confirmed that it is a legitimate formatted email address, the name becomes underlined and the box in which the name resides becomes a double-lined box. Any subsequent unchecked names go into the bottom of the box until they are checked, and then they are placed in the upper box.

Alternatively, use Find Names:

1. Click the To button to the left of the box area. This causes the Find Names dialog box to appear.

2. Enter the partial or full name of the recipient (for example, **Jane**).

3. Choose to find the names in the GAL or in the Contacts lists, and then click OK. OWA lists all the *Janes* in the Global Address List (GAL) or the Contacts List, whichever was searched.

4. Click the recipient to highlight the name.

5. Click To, CC, or BCC.

6. Click Close.

The final method is to use the Address Book (see the section "Using the Address Book," later in this chapter).

Removing a User from the TO, CC, or BCC Field in a Message

OWA 2003 makes it easier to remove a user from the address list in a message. To remove a user, right-click the recipient name or email address that needs to be removed and click Remove. There is no confirmation pop-up box; the name is immediately removed.

Adding Attachments

Attachments can be added to emails sent via OWA. To add an attachment, the email being composed must be open:

1. Click the paper clip icon in the toolbar on top of the message or click the Attachments button below the Subject line of the message. The Attachment dialog box appears.

2. Browse to the file to be attached and click it.

3. Click Attach, when completed, to attach the file to the email.

4. To add more attachments, click the Attachment icon again. Note that the same email size and attachment size limits apply in OWA as they do while in Outlook 2003, so be sure the attachments don't exceed those limits specified in Exchange.

5. Click Close when all attachments have been selected.

As shown in Figure 26.7, notice that all the attachments are listed below the Subject line, and the word Attachments is shown as an icon and the attachment name.

Sending an Email

To send the email, click the Send button with the envelope on it. At this time, if there are any issues with the names in the To, CC, or BCC boxes, OWA presents a dialog box highlighting the problem addressee. You can either Delete this recipient from the list or choose a different user from a list by clicking Change to. If neither option is helpful, click Cancel and remove the user manually, using the method listed previously for removing a user from the address list in a message.

When the changes are made, click OK and the message is immediately sent.

26

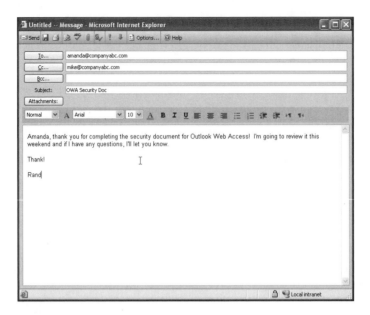

FIGURE 26.7   Attachments in Outlook Web Access.

Reading an Email

When an inbox receives a new email message, a notification box appears in two places. A message window appears in the lower-right of the screen, and a message box appears in the Shortcut menu. Both contain the message You have new mail.

To force OWA to look for new email, click the Send/Receive email button in the Infobar.

To read an email, double-click the message in the message list. This opens the email message in its own window, enabling you to view the contents.

Reading Attachments

If there is an attachment to the email, it is indicated in numerous places—in the message list, as a paper clip.

In the reading pane or in an opened email, an attachment will be listed below the Subject line and below the word "Attachment." The attachment will be underlined. To read the attachment, there are three options:

- The first option is to right-click the mouse on the underlined attachment name and choose Open. If allowed, the attachment opens in a new window.

- The second option is to right-click the mouse on the underlined attachment and choose Save target as. Choose a target location to which to save the file. After the file has been saved, browse to that location outside of OWA and open the attachment there.

- The third option is to double-click the underlined attachment, and if allowed, the attachment opens in a new window.

Some attachments that are at a high risk of containing viruses (such as executables) must be saved to a hard drive first, and cannot be opened directly from OWA. This is a security feature built into OWA to keep users from inadvertently opening a spamming virus that uses OWA/Outlook to send viruses to all entries in the user's Address Book. Saving the file to disk provides another level of virus protection, because generally, saving a file to a hard disk brings the machine's antivirus software into play, providing yet another assurance that the attachment isn't a virus. If the attachment is considered a high risk, OWA notifies the user that the attachment cannot be opened directly. The user then has to choose Save target as.

Replying or Forwarding an Email

Just as in the full Outlook 2003 client, OWA provides many options for emails to be replied to or forwarded. There are three methods to choose to reply or forward an email.

When a message is open, three buttons are available in the message dialog box toolbar. To reply to just the sender, click Reply to sender and then click OK. To reply to all the recipients in the list, click Reply to all. Note that this will not reply to any recipient in the BCC box. To forward the message to a different user not in the current recipient list, click Forward, and then enter the new recipient in the To box, using one of the addressing methods listed previously for addressing an email. When the message is properly addressed, click Send.

Another option is to right-click a message in the message list and choose Reply, Reply to all, or Forward from the context menu list, as shown in Figure 26.8.

The final method is to click a message once in the message list to highlight it and click one of the three envelope icons in the Infobar. The left button is the Reply option, the middle is the Reply to All option, and the right button is the Forward button.

Deleting Email

To delete a message while it's not open, highlight the email to be deleted and either press the Delete key or click the black X button in the toolbar.

To delete more than one message at a time, hold the Ctrl key down and click with the mouse on each message to be deleted to highlight it. After all are chosen, click the X button or press Delete.

To choose multiple messages in a row, hold down the Shift key and click the top message; while still holding down the Shift key, click the bottom message of the group. When all are highlighted, delete the message, using one of the two methods listed previously.

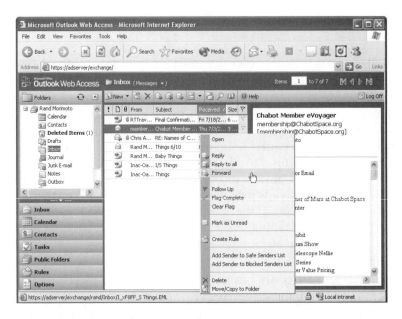

FIGURE 26.8   Reply, Reply to all, and Forward menu options.

To delete an email while it's open, click the black X button in the email dialog box.

Configuring Message Options: Importance, Sensitivity, and Tracking Options

Certain options are available that can be applied to the current email message being created.

To access the options while the message is open, click the Options button in the toolbar of the message. The Options dialog box appears, as shown in Figure 26.9. Here, message sensitivity and tracking options for this particular message can be configured. Click Close when the options for the message are completed.

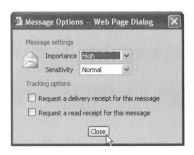

FIGURE 26.9   Message Options box.

Importance

Importance can be configured as low, medium, or high. By default, messages are marked as Medium. Configuring a message as low importance causes a downward-pointing blue arrow to appear to the left of the message when the recipient receives it.

Configuring an email message as high importance attaches a red exclamation mark (!) to the message that appears in the message list when the user receives the message. These choices don't actually speed up the delivery of the message, but provide a visual clue as to the message importance.

Sensitivity

Setting sensitivity adds no security to the email message. A visual clue appears at the top of the message (above the To and From boxes), suggesting the extra security assigned by the sender. The sensitivity setting also appears in the reading pane when the message is highlighted and is displayed in the Infobar when highlighted.

The choices for sensitivity settings are Normal, Personal, Private, and Confidential:

- **Normal**   Normal is the default setting for sensitivity: No message appears.

- **Personal**   The message reads: Please treat this as Personal.

- **Private**   The message reads: Please treat this as Private.

- **Confidential**   The message reads: Please treat this as Confidential.

Figure 26.10 is an example of a message that was marked Confidential and received.

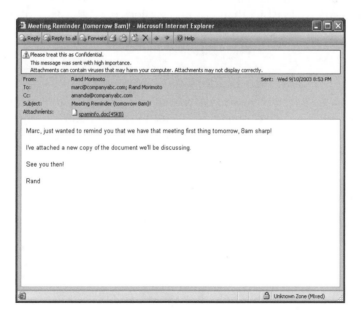

FIGURE 26.10   Treat-as-confidential notice on an email message.

Tracking Options

Tracking options enable you to track when the message has been delivered to a mailbox (which usually happens immediately) and request a read receipt when the recipient(s) has read the message. If you enable these options, you receive a message when each recipient receives and/or opens the message.

However, the recipient has the choice of whether to send a read receipt confirmation message. If the recipient chooses not to send the receipt, you do not receive a notification.

Additionally, if the recipient deletes an email configured with a read receipt without opening it, you receive a message stating that the message was deleted without being read.

Changing the Look of the Text in an Email Message

The look of the text in an email can be easily changed and formatted. The choices for manipulating text include changing the font, font size, and font color; applying formatting, such as spacing, indentation and bullets, paragraph left/right, show paragraph markers, indent, and underline; and applying styles, such as headers and address.

To manipulate the text while the create message box is open, highlight the text to be changed. Choose any of the options in the formatting toolbar below the Attachments area. There is no need to click an Apply or OK button—the changes are immediately made.

Taking Advantage of Advanced OWA Features

There are many advanced features in OWA that make finding users and user information and manipulating messages easier than previous versions of OWA. Many of the features listed in this section are not available in the basic mode. To check whether the feature is available, see Table 26.1 in the beginning of this chapter.

Moving Email Messages to Folders

You have the same visual folder view in OWA available in Outlook 2003, meaning that all your folders are available in OWA that are available in Outlook 2003. To move a message, click the message once to highlight it and drag it into the folder. There will be no confirmation message that the message moved successfully. However, clicking the folder to view the contents can be used to confirm the message was moved into the folder properly.

Using the Address Book

The Address Book is a search Address Book feature, which is new to OWA 2003. The Address Book is reached by clicking the open book icon in the Infobar.

After clicking the icon, the Find Names dialog box appears. You can enter searches by many different criteria:

- Display Name

- Last Name

- First name

- Title

- Alias

- Company

- Department

- Office

- City

When you input information in any of the search fields and click Find, as shown in Figure 26.11, OWA searches whatever list is configured in the Find Names In box atop the dialog box and returns all the matches to the search found in the list.

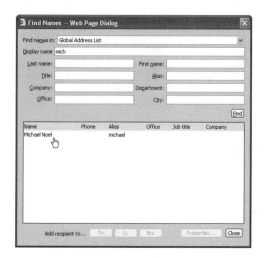

FIGURE 26.11   Finding a name in Outlook Web Access.

To search a contact list or other list in the GAL, click the drop-down menu next to Find Names In and choose the list from which to search. To see the properties of a user, click the user and click the Properties button.

To begin an email message to the user directly out of a user found in the Address Book, click the New Message button also at the bottom of the dialog box. When completed, click Close.

Marking Messages Read/Unread

To mark a message read/unread (bold/not bold), right-click the message once to highlight it and choose Mark as Unread, or Mark as Read, as shown in Figure 26.12.

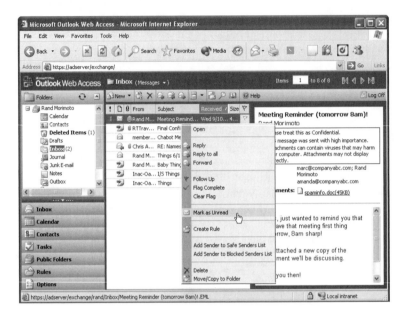

FIGURE 26.12 Marking a message as unread.

Viewing User Property Sheets

You can view a great deal of information about user entries in the GAL by accessing the user property sheets. Limited information is also available for senders from other organizations via the same method.

To view property sheets, a username must be visually apparent. This can be done by opening an email message so the sender or recipients are displayed in the window or by finding the user in the Address Book. This functionality is not available by viewing a user through the reading pane.

In the Address book, click the name of the user to view and choose Properties. If the user is in an email message, double-click the username in the sender or recipients list.

The Properties page opens, which lists the following information about the user:

- Name (first and last)
- Initials
- Alias

- Display name

- Address

- Title

- Company

- Phone numbers

- Office

This data is pulled from Active Directory if the user is in the GAL. If the user is viewing a user object in his Contacts list, the data is pulled from the Contact list.

Note that user information in the Contacts list can be modified by clicking the Add to Contacts button while the properties sheet is open. Clicking Add to Contacts opens an Untitled Contact sheet, which enables the user to add/change any additional information.

Click Save and Close when completed. When the contact closes, the Properties box must be closed by clicking Close. When completed, click Close again.

Using the OWA/2003 Spell Checker

One of the most anticipated features of the new OWA 2003 is the Spell Check feature. It is very similar to the spell checker feature in all Microsoft products, and should feel very familiar to users:

1. To enable Spell Check while creating a message in an untitled message box, click the Spell Check icon in the toolbar.

2. The first time Spell Check is used, a dialog box appears requesting a language selection. Choose the language by clicking the drop-down box.

3. When completed, click the Check Document button.

4. Spell Check then checks the message. If it finds any errors, it highlights the error in the main text box, as shown in Figure 26.13. In the Suggestions box, it provides suggestions of what OWA thinks the word should be.

5. Ignore the word and move to the next one, by clicking the Ignore button.

6. Manually change the word to a different spelling by entering the change in the Change To box. Then click the Change button.

7. Click a suggested word and click the Change button.

8. Spell Check will continue until it has checked the whole message. When completed, the Spelling dialog box disappears.

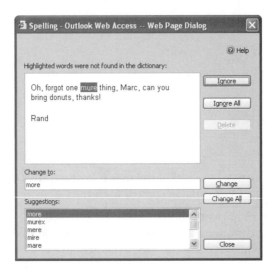

FIGURE 26.13   Spell-checking a message.

Specific configuration options are available regarding the functionality of the Spell Check feature (for example, configuring Spell Check to automatically occur before sending a message). Those options are discussed in the section "Customizing OWA Options/Spell Options," later in this chapter.

Configuring Rules Using the Rules Editor

OWA now enables the configuration of server-based rules to improve mail management. Whatever rules are created in OWA also appear in Outlook 2003, and vice versa.

To create a rule, click the Rules button in the shortcut bar. The Rules Pane appears in the right pane. Any existing rules are listed in the Rules pane.

The rules are applied from top down, in the order in which they reside in the list. Sometimes the effectiveness of the rule depends on its place in the list; therefore, move the rules up and down the list by clicking the Move Up or Move Down buttons to the right of the list of rules. Click the New button to create a new rule. The Edit Rule dialog box appears, as shown in Figure 26.14. There are many criteria available to complete a rule.

Specifying Rule Criteria

The first section in the Edit Rule dialog box specifies the criteria used to put a rule into effect. When you configure one of the options in the When a message arrives section, the rule parses all incoming email messages to look for the criteria. If the criteria match the rule, the actions in the Then section are put into effect.

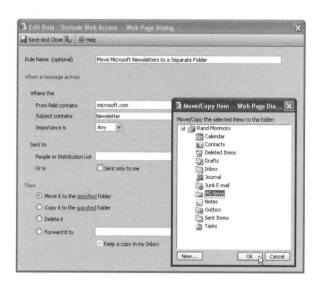

FIGURE 26.14   Edit Rule dialog.

In the Where The area, specify a specific sender of the email message. If an email comes from that sender, the rule goes into effect.

In the Subject Contains area, specify any specific text to search for. However, the text must match exactly or the rule won't consider it a match. The Importance setting can also be configured as a criterion.

In the Sent To area, the rule searches names or lists in the recipients list. If the Sent only to me choice is selected, the rule looks for messages sent only to the user, not to a distribution list or an email sent to the user if there are other recipients in the email.

The Then section is the crux of the rule. It specifies what to do with the messages that are found via the criteria listed previously:

- To move a message to a specific folder, click the Move it to the specified folder radio button. When this is configured, specify a folder to which to move the message. Note that a folder can be created from the folder choice dialog box by clicking the New button and clicking OK after the folder is created.

- To copy the message to a specific folder, thereby leaving a copy in the inbox and putting a copy elsewhere, click Keep a copy in my inbox.

- To configure the rule to delete the message, click the Delete It radio button.

- To forward the message to a specific user or a distribution group, click the Forward it to radio button and choose a user or group to receive the email.

- To keep a copy in the inbox, make sure the Keep a copy in my inbox check box is checked.

26

As always, when completed, click Save and Close; the new rule is then added to the list of rules in the Rules pane.

Displaying Context Menus

Message context menus are a new feature in OWA 2003. The context menus are available by right-clicking a message in the message list in the middle pane. The context list then provides the following choices:

- Open
- Reply
- Reply to All
- Forward
- Follow Up
- Flag Complete
- Clear Flag
- Mark as Unread
- Create Rule
- Delete
- Move/Copy to folder

When you move the mouse over the choice desired and click once, the action is then taken. Each of these options is discussed in this chapter.

There also are folder context menu items available, which appear when the user right-clicks on a folder in the folder list. The choices presented to the user are

- Update Folder
- Open
- Open in New
- Move/Copy
- Delete
- Rename
- New Folder

Enabling Quick Flags for Easier Reminders

Quick flags are an easy way to configure reminders to follow up on emails and specify the importance of them, by using one of six flag colors. The flags can also be cleared and marked Complete.

Quick flags can be configured on email messages in two methods. The first method is by accessing the context menu by right-clicking a message and choosing Follow Up. The other is to double-click the flag icon to the right of a message displayed in the middle-pane message list (under the word Received).

When a flag is configured on, right-clicking the flag gives you color options. Choose what color flag to apply to the specific message by highlighting a flag on the list and clicking it.

In a full mailbox, this feature can be very helpful to identify follow-up emails and emails you need to track. Additionally, when you click the flag icon at the top of the message list, the messages are arranged by flag color making finding them even easier.

> **NOTE**
>
> The colors used for flags have no assigned significance within Outlook. Each organization can choose to designate certain colors for different levels of importance or priority. The color flags merely designate similarities or differences between messages, not specific priority.

When a flagged message no longer needs to be flagged, right-click the message and choose Clear Flag, which returns it to a grayed out flag, or Flag Complete, which displays it as a check mark.

Performing Searches with Outlook

Outlook 2003 makes it possible to save frequently used searches so the user doesn't have to re-input all the search criteria multiple times. The searches are saved in a folder in the folder list called Search Folder. However, the search folders and searches must be created in Outlook 2003 (not OWA) for users of OWA to be able to use them.

To use already created searches, go to the folder list, click the Search Folder, and access the previously used searches to run them again.

Search functionality is available in OWA throughout the whole mailbox—in every folder—the searches just can't be saved in OWA. To search, follow these steps:

1. Click the highest folder in the folder hierarchy to search, and then click the Search icon in the Infobar. The Search dialog box appears, as shown in Figure 26.15.

2. To search subfolders of the folder listed in the You are searching this folder: line, click Search Subfolders.

26

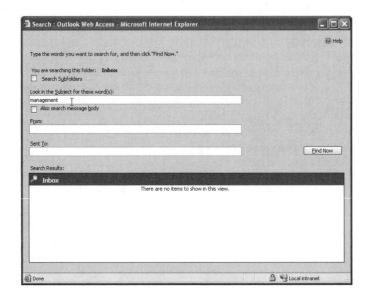

FIGURE 26.15   Search dialog.

3. Input the search criteria in the Look in the Subject for these words, if the text is in the subject line.

4. Click the Also search message body, if the search should also include the message body and not just the subject line.

5. To search for an email, narrow the search even further by choosing from whom the email was sent and/or to whom it was sent in the From and Sent to boxes.

6. After you input all the criteria, click Find Now. The results are then listed in the Search Results box.

7. To open the results, double-click a result in the Search Results box.

You cannot save a search in OWA. Click on the X in the upper-right corner when completed, which deletes the search.

Using Keyboard Shortcuts to Save Time

A significant improvement, which makes many sophisticated typists happy, is that now many of the familiar keyboard shortcuts used in Office now work while in OWA. Table 26.2 lists the keyboard shortcuts that can now be used in the OWA client.

TABLE 26.2 Keyboard Shortcuts Available in the OWA Client

Shortcut	Option
In Inbox View	
Ctrl+N	Open a new message window
Ctrl+Q	Mark message as read
Ctrl+U	Mark message as unread
Ctrl+R	Reply to message
Ctrl+Shift+R	Reply to all selected messages
Ctrl+Shift+F	Forward the selected message
In Message View	
Ctrl+>	View the next message in the list
Ctrl+<	View the previous message in the list
In Opened Message, While Creating a Message	
Ctrl+S	Save the message
Ctrl+Enter or Alt+S	Send the message
[F7]	Activate Spell Checker
Ctrl+K	Check names in the address boxes
Alt+T or Alt+C or Alt+B	Find names (look in Address Book)
In Contacts View	
Ctrl+Shift+L	Create a new contact distribution list
In Public Folders View	
Ctrl+N	Create a new posting in public folders
Ctrl+R	Reply to the posting
In Task View	
Ctrl+N	Create a new task

26

Understanding the Deferred View Update

To improve the speed of OWA, the new version includes a feature called Deferred View Update. This feature specifies how many changes to the window are enabled before the full OWA window refreshes. Changes can be things such as moving, copying, or deleting a message. In OWA 2003, the refresh is deferred until 20% of the window has changed. Until that threshold has been reached, the removed or moved items disappear but no additional or new items appear. The 20% is based not on the number of messages in the inbox, but on the number of items set to display per page (which is configured in the Options area and discussed in the section "Configuring Items per Page," later in the chapter). If you don't refresh the entire screen with every change, the bandwidth and expense of OWA decreases.

Customizing OWA Options

OWA enables you to customize and configure certain features universally for your OWA inbox. When the options are saved, they apply until they are changed, whether you are in OWA or in Outlook 2003. To access the options area, click the Options button in the shortcut bar. A list of options becomes available for customization and configuration. To save the configuration changes, click Save and Close in the toolbar on the top of the Options page; otherwise, the options are discarded when the options page is exited.

Configuring the Out of Office Assistant

The Out of Office Assistant, shown in Figure 26.16, enables you to create a message that will be automatically and instantly sent to any message senders who have configured the Assistant for their mailbox. The Out of Office assistant remains on until you turn it off. If the feature is turned on in Outlook 2003, it can be turned off in OWA, and vice versa:

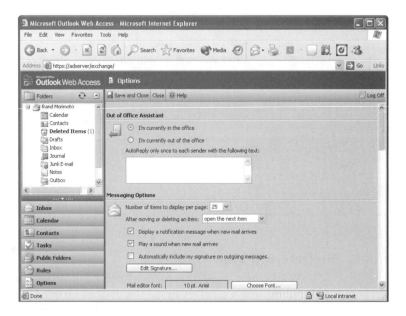

FIGURE 26.16   Out of Office Options page.

- To enable the Out of Office assistant, click I am currently out of the office. Then enter the text that will form the reply email back to the senders—for example, **Jane Doe will be out of the office until Jan 2, 2005.**

- To disable the Out of Office assistant, click I am currently in the office. OWA maintains the text from previous emails in the I am currently out of the office box until it is deleted manually or new text is entered.

- When completed, click Save and Close.

If a sender sends an email to a recipient with Out of Office Assistant configured, the sender receives the Out of Office notification only once, even if he sends repeated messages or sends to a distribution list of which the out-of-office recipient is a member.

Configuring Items per Page

You can control how many items per page are shown. By default, you are shown 25 items, but this can be changed to show up to 100 objects per page, making visual searching for messages much easier. You must click the drop-down menu to the right of Number of items to display per page and choose one of the provided numbers.

Setting Default Signatures

Another option in the Messaging Options is the creation of an Automatic Signature. The signature is text that you compose that will appear at the bottom of new email messages. Signatures usually provide personal information about the sender—such as name, company, title, and phone number—enabling you to preconfigure the information so it doesn't have to be typed every time. You can configure the signature to be automatically included in every message you send or to be added on a message-by-message basis:

- To configure the signature, click the Edit Signature button under Messaging Options.

- Enter the text that composes the signature.

- After entering the text, choose to configure the font, font size, and color; to use bullets; or to use styles. There are many other configuration choices available.

- When completed, click Save and Close.

When an initial signature is saved, its font size, choice of font, color, and choices such as bold, italic, and underline can be changed without opening the signature. Click the Choose Font button under Messaging Options. Choose the options desired and click OK when completed.

If the Automatically include my signature on outgoing messages, is checked, the signature will appear on any messages you create from scratch, forward, or reply to. If that option is not checked, you can add the signature on a message-by-message basis from within an open message you compose. To add the signature manually, click the icon in the New Message toolbar with the paper and hand with a pen. It automatically inserts the signature after the button is clicked.

Reading Pane Options

The Reading Pane options, shown in Figure 26.17, deal with the message list when Auto Preview is enabled. You must determine how long to wait with a message being previewed before it is marked as read. Choose from among the following options:

26

- **Mark item displayed in reading pane as read**   After a specified amount of time that the message is viewed in the reading pane, the message becomes marked as read.

- **Mark item as read when the selection changes**   This option marks the message as read when the user clicks on a new message, no matter how long it was in the reading pane.

- **Do not automatically mark items as read**   If configured, the messages are marked as read only when they are physically clicked on and opened.

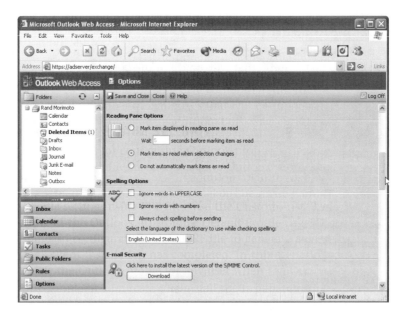

FIGURE 26.17   Reading pane Options page.

Spelling Options

The Spelling Options section provides configuration options for the Spell Check feature. If you check the Always check spelling before sending choice, the spell checker automatically launches after Sent is clicked on a message and before it is sent.

A default language can also be configured in this location. OWA supports the following 10 language groups: English (Aus, UK, US, Canada), French, German (pre- and post-reform), Italian, Korean, and Spanish.

Email Security

If S/MIME capabilities/compatibility is required, you must click the Download button to download and install the latest S/MIME version before OWA will be compatible with

S/MIME functionality. See the section "Understanding OWA Security," later in this chapter for more detailed information about S/MIME support. To download S/MIME support

1. Click the Download button.

2. When presented with a security warning, click Yes to Trust content from Microsoft. It will download some data and then present the security warning again. The download box disappears when the process has completed.

3. After the S/MIME capability is downloaded, several options appear. Choose which encryption options you want, or click the Re-Install button to reinstall the S/MIME support.

Privacy and Junk Email Prevention

OWA gives you many choices as to what to do with junk email, as shown in Figure 26.18, and provides default options, which are the minimum configuration suggested by Microsoft for spam control.

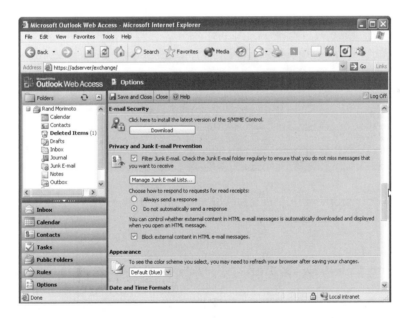

FIGURE 26.18   Privacy and junk email Options page.

To filter junk email, click the check box next to Filter Junk Email. When configured, Exchange moves any mail it considers junk to your Junk Email Folder in the folder list. When checked, you also must specify what is considered junk email by filling out the Manage Junk Email Lists dialog box. Specify Safe Senders, Safe Recipients, or Blocked Senders by adding their names or email addresses in the proper list.

The option to always trust email from contacts from your personal contact list is checked by default.

> **NOTE**
>
> Users in the GAL will not be considered as coming from junk email addresses; therefore, there is no reason to manage addresses from the Global Address List unless you specifically want to flag messages from an individual or individuals.

The final option in the junk email area is whether to block external content, the implications of which are discussed in the section "Spam Beacon Blocking," later in this chapter.

Appearance

The color scheme of OWA is configurable as well. The default is blue, but numerous choices are available. To choose a scheme, click the drop-down menu to the right of the 8-ball icon and choose the color scheme desired. Note that the color won't change until Save and Close is clicked.

Configuring Date & Time Formats

The Date & Time Formats options enable you to configure the time zone, time style, long date style, and short date style:

- The short date style appears in areas such as the right side of the Inbox pane where it lists the time messages were received, in the appointment start/end times, or in the due date on a task.

- The long date style appears in areas such as in the calendar at the top of a single day view.

Changing the time zone can be useful if you move to a different time zone and want OWA to reflect the new zone. To configure the time zone, click the drop-down and choose the proper time zone.

Configuring Calendar Options

The calendar options enable you to choose the day and times that describe a week in the Calendar. By default, the weeks begin on Sunday, the day start time is 8:00 a.m., and the end time is 5:00 p.m. This can be changed by clicking the drop-down menus to the right of the titles in the Calendar Options area in the Options menu.

The First Week of the Year choice specifies when the calendar should consider the first week of the year.

Configuring Reminder Options

Reminder options specify the default time of how soon before meetings, appointments, and task dates you are reminded. By default, all the configuration boxes are checked, and the default reminder time, which appears when you create a calendar or task item with a reminder, is 15 minutes. Configure any changes to reminders in this area by un-checking or checking the boxes or changing the reminder time by clicking the drop-down box.

Configuring Contact Options

Configuring Contact Options enables you to determine where OWA checks first for resolution of addresses in the address boxes in emails. By default, OWA checks the GAL first. To configure OWA to check your contacts first before the GAL, click the Contacts radio button.

Recovering Deleted Items

OWA also enables you to recover deleted Outlook items that have been purged from the Deleted Items folder. However, if the purge date configured on the Exchange server has passed, you cannot recover the expired deleted item. You have to contact your administrator to retrieve the item or have the item restored from tape. To recover a deleted item:

1. Access the Outlook Options area and go to the Recover Deleted Items area.

2. Click View Items. The Recover Deleted Items dialog box appears, as shown in Figure 26.19, presenting a list of available files to be recovered.

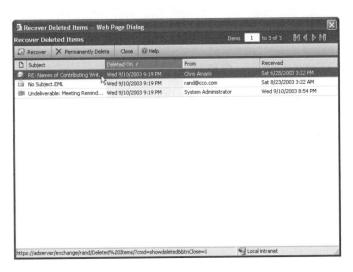

FIGURE 26.19   Recover Deleted Items dialog.

3. Click the item(s) to recover.

4. Click Recover.

5. Click Close. After they're recovered, the item(s) will reappear in the location from which they were deleted.

6. Click Permanently Delete to purge the items completely. This makes them unavailable to be recovered through the Recover deleted items dialog box.

7. Click OK at the confirmation box.

8. Click Close to clear the dialog box from the screen.

Changing the Active Directory Password

You can change your Active Directory password via OWA. This is extremely useful for mobile users who rarely come into the office. If you are on the road and your password expires, OWA enables you to access OWA and then forces you to change your password immediately. To change the password before prompted

1. Access the Outlook options area and then click the Change Password button.

2. Enter the old password.

3. Enter the new password.

4. Confirm the new password.

5. Click OK when completed.

Using the Calendar in OWA

Outlook Web Access 2003 provides a fully functional calendar for personal meeting appointments, group appointments, and reoccurring events. The calendar feature in Outlook Web Access includes the same functionality as the full Outlook client, including appointment views, creation, and changes.

Using Views

You can view your calendar in many different ways, either by day, week, or month. Then choose the view, and click the icons in the Infobar that show Today, 1, 7, and 31:

- **Today View**   The Today view goes to today's date in the single day view.

- **Day View**   The Day view displays a day at a time. Users can move from day to day by clicking the day they want on the calendar in the right pane.

- **Week View**   The Week view displays a week at a time in seven split panes in the middle pane. Brief descriptions of the day's appointments are shown in the seven panes.

- **Month View**   The Month view displays a month calendar, with brief titles for events in the calendar.

Creating an Appointment in Calendar

In OWA, all calendar objects are initially called Appointments, whether they are meeting requests with multiple invitees or appointments meant only for the individual user. To create a new appointment

1. Click the New button in the toolbar and choose Appointment to see a screen similar to the one in Figure 26.20.

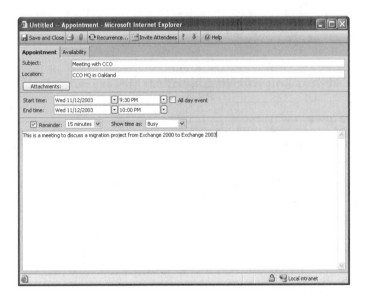

FIGURE 26.20   New calendar Appointment page.

2. To maintain the appointment as an appointment and not a meeting request (meaning no one else is invited), use the default Appointments dialog box that appears. Enter the subject of the appointment in the Subject box.

3. Enter the location of the appointment in the Location box.

To specify a start time, there are two choices:

- To manually enter the time, type the time in the Start time and End time boxes.

- To use the OWA calendar, click the drop-down menu boxes to the right of Start time and End time. From the calendar that is presented, click the date in the calendar to choose the date of the appointment.

To configure the time in a similar way

1. Click the drop-down menu to the right of Start time and End time and choose the start and end times.

2. It is optional to add text in the text area and to add attachments using the method discussed earlier in this chapter. If you want to do so, make these additions now.

3. To mark the appointment as important, click the ! icon in the toolbar.

4. When completed, click Save and Close.

Creating a Meeting Request in Calendar

To create a meeting, the same Appointment dialog box is used, but is changed in order to add the ability to invite others:

- To create a new meeting request, click the New button in the toolbar and choose Appointment. Input the subject of the meeting.

- To invite attendees, click the Invite Attendees button to display a page similar to Figure 26.21. The Appointment dialog box then changes appearance to add the Required, Optional, and Resources boxes.

Inviting Attendees

Adding attendees to the meeting requires some extra steps. To add attendees, there are two choices:

- Enter the names directly into the Required or Optional boxes. If inviting multiple attendees, put a semicolon (;) between the usernames.

- Click the Required or Optional buttons to use the Find Names OWA functionality. If using the Find Names functionality, locate the attendees using the methods listed earlier in this chapter and click the Required, Optional, or Resources buttons at the bottom of the Find Names dialog box to choose the box in which to put the invitees.

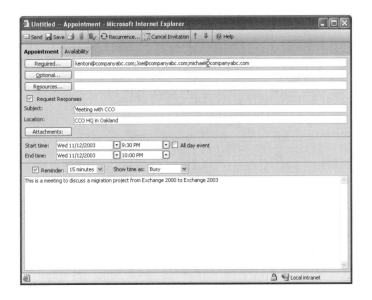

FIGURE 26.21   Calendar appointment invitation page.

To use the attendees calendars to view their availability, click the Availability tab. The Availability tab shows the schedules of the attendees by showing free time, busy time, or out-of-office time (not the details of what the attendees will be doing during those times, but whether they're available or not). If the attendees are busy at the specified time, you can choose a new time while viewing attendee availability.

To enter the new start and end times while viewing attendee availability, click the drop-down menus to the right of Start and End times and date and choose a new time. Another option is to click the actual calendar and move the start times and date by clicking and dragging the green and red vertical lines. The green line shows the start time, and the red line shows the end time.

Click the Appointment tab to complete the rest of the meeting request. Click Save and Close to close the meeting request and send it to the attendees.

Setting Recurring Appointments/Meetings

If a meeting or appointment occurs with regularity, OWA enables the creation of multiple appointments with a single meeting request or appointment. To enable recurring appointments, while the appointment dialog box is open, click the Recurrence button. The Recurrence pattern dialog box appears, as shown in Figure 26.22.

To set the recurrence pattern, choose whether the meeting is Daily, Weekly, Monthly, or Yearly by clicking the radio button to the left of the appropriate choice.

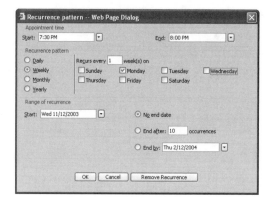

FIGURE 26.22   Recurrence pattern dialog.

Depending on which of those buttons is clicked, the items to the right will change. In the picture shown below, the Weekly recurrence gives the options of what days the appointment occurs upon, as well as how often—for example, Every X Week(s). If Daily is chosen, the options display daily choices, such as Every X days, or Every Week day.

Range of recurrence enables the configuration of an end date for the recurrences. A specific end date can be specified, or the recurrence can be configured with No end date or to End after X occurrences, where X is the number of times the event will occur.

When completed, click OK. To exit the recurrence box without saving the recurrence configuration, click Remove Recurrence. The Appointment dialog box reappears. Complete the Appointment or Meeting request as needed and Save and Close when completed.

Gaining Functionality from the Meeting Invitation Functions

The meeting invitation function enables you to forward a meeting request to others, reply to the meeting request, set reminder times, launch an invitation, or receive task and calendar reminders.

Forwarding and Replying To Meeting Requests

To forward or reply to a meeting request without accepting or rejecting the meeting, click the Forward To or Reply to, context menus or the buttons on the Infobar. If the request is opened normally, the recipient will not be able to reply to or forward the meeting request without accepting or rejecting the request. By forwarding or replying to a request, you can create a discussion of the invitation or share its information without accepting or rejecting the invitation.

Setting Preferred Reminder Time Changes

By default, the preferred reminder time is 15 minutes. This means that if you create a new outlook item that uses a reminder time, the default time will be 15 minutes. This is a configurable option and can be changed in the Options section of OWA discussed previously in the chapter.

To change the reminder time provided by a meeting invitation, open the event and click in the drop-down menu that displays the reminder time. Choose the desired reminder time.

Launching an Invitation in Its Own Window

To accept or deny a meeting request, the request must be opened. To open it, double-click the invitation that arrives in the inbox.

The invitation then opens in its own window, enabling the invitees to Accept the meeting, Tentatively accept the meeting, or Deny the request. This can be done by clicking the corresponding buttons in the toolbar in the meeting request box. Click the Send button when completed.

Accepting the meeting request automatically puts the request into your calendar with a dark blue heading on the left side of the meeting title in the Calendar view. Tentatively accepting the request also puts the meeting in your calendar, but it appears in a light blue heading. Denying the request doesn't alter your calendar. All three choices result in an email being sent back to the sender of the meeting request, stating the accepted status of each attendee.

Receiving Task and Calendar Reminders

When reminders occur in tasks or your calendar, a message similar to the one shown in Figure 26.23 appears in the shortcut bar and appears as a dialog box listing the reminders on your screen. You then can launch the task or appointment by clicking Open Item. You have three options:

- To dismiss all reminders at one time by clicking Dismiss All.

- To dismiss items individually by clicking once on the item and clicking Dismiss.

- To snooze the reminder, and choose the amount of time to snooze by highlighting the reminder and clicking Snooze. In the time specified in the snooze time, the reminder will appear again.

To view any reminders at any time, click the alarm icon button in the Infobar while in Calendar. The Reminder box appears after the button has been clicked.

26

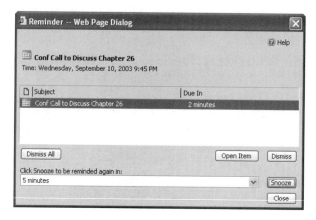

FIGURE 26.23   Calendar Reminder dialog.

Using Tasks in OWA

The Tasks option in Outlook Web Access is similar to a to-do list. Tasks can be created, viewed, and organized.

Creating Tasks

You can create tasks in OWA 2003 as you do in Outlook 2003. Tasks are used to remind yourself of jobs that must be completed by certain dates or times. It also enables you to set due dates and reminders and to follow the percent the task has been completed and its status. Tasks can be thought of as works in progress, because all criteria inside them can be easily changed when the task is saved, enabling frequent updates to the task's status or other specifics.

The Subject, Due date, and Completion status criteria can be sorted in the middle pane view while accessing tasks, making it easy to sort and view tasks.

To access tasks, click the Tasks button in the shortcut bar, or click New, Task in the Infobar. The New Task dialog box appears.

The methods used to input the subject, set the due dates and start dates, set a reminder, add attachments, complete text in the text box, and configure the task as recurring have been discussed earlier in the chapter and are applicable to configure tasks.

When the task has been configured, click Save and Close to finish the task and save it to your task list. The task will then appear on the list of tasks. The default order of the tasks is by due date, and tasks with no due date appear first.

Task Views

Like other OWA functions, tasks provide you with multiple views that can make the organization and viewing of tasks easier:

- **Simple List**   The simple list provides a one-line list by subject and due date, and indicates whether the task is completed.

- **Detailed List**   The detailed list provides the same criteria as the simple list, but indicates percentage completed, status, attachments, and importance.

- **Active Tasks**   Active tasks include the same criteria as the detailed view, but don't show any tasks that are 100% completed.

- **Next 7 Days**   This view includes only the tasks that are due in the next seven days.

- **Overdue Tasks**   Overdue tasks are all the tasks that are overdue and aren't marked as completed.

- **Taskpad**   The Taskpad view shows only the subject and due date for all tasks, with the status of in progress, not started, or waiting on someone else.

Using Contacts in OWA

Contacts enable you to create your own lists of users that might not be within the GAL. By entering them into Contacts, you can easily send emails and appointments to those contacts and create distribution lists made up of users in the GAL and those in your personal contact lists.

Creating Contacts

Creating contacts is a simple three-step process:

1. Click New/Contact in the Infobar. The New Contact dialog box appears, as shown in Figure 26.24.

2. Enter all pertinent information about the contact. The details tab enables even more details to be entered about the contact, such as nickname, manager, and even spouse name.

3. When completed, click Save and Close to save the contact in the contact list.

Editing Contacts

To edit an already created contact, double-click the contact. Edit the contact sheet as needed, and then click Save and Close when completed.

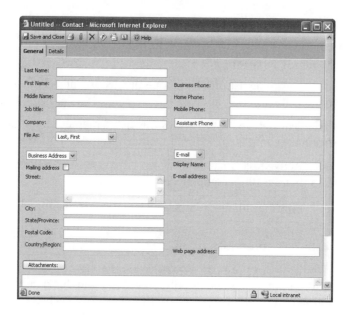

FIGURE 26.24   New Contact dialog.

Mapping Addresses from Contacts

When you click the Mapping button icon, if you have access to the Internet, OWA contacts mappoint.msn.com and pulls up a map of the location stated in the Address portion of the Contacts sheet.

Changing Contact Views

Just as the Inbox provides you with multiple views for email, Contacts provides six views for contacts:

- **Address Cards View**   Address cards are the standard, default view. The contacts look like Rolodex cards in the view, showing limited amounts of information about the contact.

- **Detailed Address Cards View**   Detailed Address Cards shows a few more fields than the standard Address Card view, but in the same format.

- **Phone List View**   Phone List view shows the contacts by name, company, and phone information in a single line per contact.

- **By Company View**   By Company view shows the contacts listed by company name headings. Contacts in the same company are listed below the company name heading.

- **By Location View**   By Location shows the contacts in the same format as the By Company view, but by location (regions) rather than by company name.

- **By Follow-up Flag View**   Follow-up Flag displays the contacts that require attention or need to be distinguished from other Contacts.

Deleting Contacts

To delete a contact, click the contact to highlight it and click the Delete button in the
Infobar or press the Delete key.

Finding Names

To find names in contacts, click the Address Book icon. When the familiar Find Names
dialog box appears, click Contacts in the Look in box to search contacts instead of the
GAL. This feature can be configured to always search Contacts rather than the GAL in the
OWA options area in OWA.

Sending Mail from Contacts

If a contact sheet is open, email can be sent directly to the contact if a correct email
address is configured for the contact. To send an email directly, click the Send email to
Contact button in the toolbar.

OWA then opens a new email dialog box with the addressee information already
completed, listing the contact as the intended recipient. Complete the email and send it.

Creating New Distribution Lists

From Contacts, you can create custom distribution lists. All distribution lists are then
saved in Contacts and differentiated from a standard contact with the group icon after it.

TIP
Contact Distribution lists can include only recipients from the GAL, not from the user's contact list.

To create a new distribution list, enter Contacts and do the following:

1. Click New, Distribution List. The New Distribution List box appears.

2. Enter the List Name (for example, **Local System Administrators**). To enter
   members of the list

   - Type the name of the users in the box under Add to Distribution List and click
     Add. The users must be entered one at a time. This method looks only in the
     GAL.

   - Click Find Names and find and enter names via the find name functionality
     discussed previously in this chapter.

3. When the names have been found, click the name and click the Distribution list button at the bottom of the Find Names dialog box. Then click Close to close the Find Names dialog box.

4. When the list is completed, click Save and Close.

Understanding OWA Security Features

Outlook Web Access has several enhancements for security, including support for S/MIME attachments, spam beacon blocking, attachment blocking, cookie authentication, and clearing user credentials during the logoff process.

S/MIME: Sending and Receiving Digitally Signed and Encrypted Messages

OWA 2003 now supports S/MIME functionality, giving you the ability to send and receive digitally signed messages using encryption. However, an ActiveX control must be loaded on each client. To download the ActiveX component manually, go to the OWA Options page. Configuration and loading of the S/MIME functionality was covered in the section "Email Security," earlier in the chapter.

Understanding Spam Beacon Blocking

OWA 2003 provides additional security against spam. If configured, OWA does not enable spam beaconing technology to function in OWA; it blocks links to external content on the Internet from being accessed from OWA. This greatly increases the antispam features of OWA by disabling the spammer's ability to hide beacons in spam messages. Those spam beacons automatically contact the spammers when the email messages are opened, letting the spammers know they have reached a live email address. By blocking this functionality, one more method of finding live addresses is eliminated from the spammer's arsenal.

Understanding Attachment Blocking

OWA also provides configurable functionality to block Internet attachments, such as links to Web sites, music, and other Internet technologies available only outside the firewall (on the Internet). Only administrators not on the OWA client can configure these options. Users are sent a message notifying them that the attachment is blocked.

Understanding Cookie Authentication Timeout and Timed Logoff

OWA 2003 uses cookies to hold the user authentication information. When a user logs out of OWA 2003, the cookie automatically expires, so a hacker can't use the cookie to gain authentication. Additionally, the cookie is configured to automatically expire—after 20 minutes of inactivity in OWA if the user specified a private computer, or 10 minutes if the user specified a shared or public computer.

After timed logoff has occurred and a user tries to reaccess OWA, he has to reenter user credentials.

The amount of time to wait before automatic logoff is configurable via the Registry by editing the Registry on the front-end Exchange Server.

Clearing User Credentials at Logoff

For users who access OWA 2003 via Internet Explorer 6.0 SP1 or greater and Forms Based Authentication, the user's logon credentials cache automatically clears when the user logs off from OWA 2003. It is no longer necessary to close the browser window to clear the cache. For users accessing OWA via other Internet browsers or via OWA servers that aren't configured to use Forms Based Authentication, users must still close the browser window to clear the cache and will be prompted to do so.

Tips for OWA Users with Slow Access

Some users might need to access OWA through a slow dial-up connection. OWA provides them with many ways to improve and speed up their OWA experience and access to mail. There are options that can be configured from the server and through group policy to improve access speeds, but users can help speed up their access whether or not the server-side improvements are implemented. Major options are

- Choose basic mode when logging into OWA

- Set low number of messages to be displayed on the page

- Turn off the reading pane

- Turn on two-line viewing

- Enable the blocking of Internet content

Summary

Outlook Web Access in Exchange 2003 is more than just a secondary email client when the user does not have full client access. Because of significant enhancements added to Outlook Web Access 2003, many organizations are finding the features of the premium Outlook Web Access client robust enough for users to use OWA as their primary client. Features such as a spell checker, preview mode, filters, and Address Book lookup provide the majority of the features users leverage on a regular basis. Outlook Web Access deserves much more attention by IT organizations to leverage OWA as a primary messaging client solution.

26

Best Practices

The following are best practices from this chapter:

- Use the basic mode OWA client when client bandwidth access is limited.

- Use the premium mode OWA client when full functionality is desired.

- Change pane size to customize the OWA view and meet your needs.

- Use Ctrl or Shift when selecting emails for deletion; this speeds up the process of deleting several messages at the same time.

- Use quick flags to create reminders or to bring attention to a message for Outlook users.

- Use keyboard shortcuts to simplify menu button tasks or functions.

- Customize task views to give a user the ability to see pertinent task information.

- Send mail to an email contact by selecting the contact and choosing to send the email to the contact.

- In Contact Distribution lists, include only recipients from the GAL, not from the user's contact list.

- Because S/MIME attachments are supported by OWA, use them to extend encryption and digitally signed messages for enhanced security.

CHAPTER 27

Outlook for Non-Windows Systems

With a variety of compatibility needs in today's mixed-platform business networks, administrators and IT managers are challenged with the complexities of providing client access to corporate mail systems for a variety of different clients, including those running non–Windows-based client operating systems.

When administrators need to meet these specific requirements, many of the challenges involved with connecting non-Windows–based clients to Exchange Server 2003 mail information are overcome. By providing compatibility through alternative messaging clients and Internet solutions, Exchange 2003 is an effective all-in-one corporate mail solution to support non–Windows-based client operating systems, such as Apple's Mac platform and Unix-based platforms.

Using the information in this chapter, administrators will learn the options available for connecting these non–Windows-based client systems and the applications available to provide access to Microsoft Exchange 2003 mailbox information.

This chapter discusses applications—such as Outlook for Macintosh, Web Access, and Entourage X—which provide connectivity for non–Windows-based clients to Exchange 2003 mail data. Each option is reviewed and discussed in detail to determine the different functions available with each solution and the compatibility when being used to connect to Exchange 2003 with the different alternative operating systems.

In addition to functionality and the conventional client server connectivity methods, this chapter also provides systems administrators with the step-by-step instructions to configure access to Exchange 2003, using concepts such as remote desktop and Windows 2003 Terminal Services.

Understanding Non–Windows-Based Mail Client Options

When enterprise network environments support non–Microsoft Windows-client operating systems, administrators must plan and support alternative means of access to Exchange mail information.

To accomplish this goal, administrators can use several options available to enable support to Exchange data and calendaring information for a variety of alternative non–Windows-based clients systems. Leveraging the built-in compatibility and functionality of Exchange Server 2003, access can be accomplished using multiple familiar client options, depending on the operating system being used and the functionality needed by the individual client.

Using client options such as Outlook for Macintosh, Outlook Web Access and the others listed later in this chapter, administrators can determine which method best fits the corporate mail needs of the organization, based on the operating system being used and compatibility of each solution.

Because these types of clients are usually the minority in most Microsoft Exchange environments, administrators can evaluate the functionality of these client solutions and implement each based on the requirements of the nonWindows based client requiring access to Exchange Information.

Supporting Mac Clients with Microsoft Outlook

When determining which client is best for supporting Mac users and desktops, the most important consideration is the required functionality of the client and the limitations involved with each available option.

To support Mac desktops with Exchange 2003, Microsoft provides the Outlook and Outlook Express clients for the Macintosh desktop operating system. Administrators can use the clients to support internal access and remote access using protocols such as Post Office Protocol (POP) and using these clients' options as is when supporting their Windows-based Outlook client cousins.

> **Supporting Outlook Options**
>
> For additional information on Outlook, Entourage, and supporting Mac clients in an Exchange environment, Microsoft provides comprehensive support information and instructions through the Mactopia support Web page at www.Microsoft.com/Mactopia.

In addition to Outlook and Outlook Express, Microsoft also provides another option for connecting Macintosh clients to Exchange 2003. Using the Entourage and Entourage X clients, Mac users can access mail and calendaring information with the look and feel more familiar to Macintosh users. Not the Outlook client, this alternative to Outlook is built on a separate platform and provides access to mail and calendaring information as well as contact management.

Providing Full Functionality with Remote Desktop for Mac

One of the most popular options when supporting Mac clients in a predominantly Windows-based environment is the remote desktop for Mac. When Mac clients require the full functionality of the Windows Outlook client, the one option that can easily provide this is the remote desktop client for Mac.

Using this option, administrators can not only provide access to Windows Outlook, but they can also provide full functionality of a Windows desktop to a Mac client. Through the remote desktop client, Mac users can access a Windows session using Terminal Services functionality, which enables the Mac client to see and use Windows through a remote connection. This function also gives Mac clients the ability to cut and paste information from the Remote Desktop Connection to the Mac operating system as well as full printing functionality to local connected Mac printers. One other benefit to the Remote Desktop Connection functionality is the ability to provide network access to all shared Windows resources without the need to support additional Mac services in the enterprise.

Using the Internet for Exchange Connectivity

One effective option available when you need only to provide access to Exchange information is leveraging the Outlook Web Access (OWA) functionality built in to the Exchange Server 2003 operating system. Because using this option is enabled through Internet Information Services, users can access OWA as they access a Web page from both the internal network and the Internet.

By using Web-based access to provide Exchange 2003 client functionality, administrators can consider this solution for a variety of different non–Windows-based client systems with Internet browsing enabled. Outlook Web Access provides a limited set of Outlook functions and requires no additional client software to be installed.

> **NOTE**
>
> Enabling Web Access to support non–Windows-based clients for both internal network access and access from the Internet requires additional configuration of the Exchange 2003 server and network firewall.
>
> For detailed information on how to design and enable Outlook Web services with Exchange 2003, see Chapter 10, "Outlook Web Access 2003."

Comparing Client Functionality and Compatibility

With each option and method of access to Exchange 2003, there are different options and functionality. As mentioned in the review of each method of access, some methods enable full functionality and others are limited.

27

Review the operating system requirements in Table 27.1 to determine whether the Mac operating systems meet the required revision for the method of access being considered.

TABLE 27.1   Client Compatibility

Outlook 2001	Outlook Express	Remote Desktop	Entourage X	OWA
OS 8.X	OS 8.1	OS X 10.1	OS X 10.1	N/A
OS 9.X	OS 9.X	or	or	
OS X Classic		higher	higher	

> **NOTE**
>
> The Mac Operating System OS X Classic is the additional software component that enables application compatibility for Mac OS 9 and earlier versions.

Determine the required functionality by using Table 27.2 to compare the features of each client access method. Review the functionality of each method and compare the result with the Mac OS you are working with.

TABLE 27.2   Client Functionality

Requirement	Outlook	Outlook Express	Remote Desktop	Entourage X w/Exchange Support	OWA
Email	x	x	x	x	x
Calendaring	x	No	x	x	x
Contacts	x	x	x	x	x
Directory Search	x	x	x	x	Limited
Offline Access	x	x	x	x	No
PST Archive	x	No	x	No	No

Outlook for Macintosh

The most functional of all available client options for Microsoft Exchange 2003, Outlook 2001 for Mac can easily provide the same functionality as its Windows-based cousin.

Review the compatibility information in the next section for each client access method to ensure that the client operating system you're planning to deploy meets the minimum hardware and operating systems requirements for installation.

Outlook Options for Macintosh

With the Outlook 2001 client for Mac, Mac users can access and share information with Windows-based users with the same functionality as any Windows client. In addition to the standard email and calendaring functions of Outlook, Mac users can also access information through the Exchange 2003 Public Folders.

Functionality using the Outlook 2001 client for Mac includes

- **Email Support**   With fully enabled email support for Exchange Server 2003, Outlook 2001 also includes message rules and the ability to enable message priority and message tracking.

- **Calendaring**   Mac users can use the calendaring feature of Outlook 2001 to create and send meeting requests and manage group calendaring functions.

- **Contacts**   Contact management is fully enabled and allows Mac users to access mail contacts and create a contact address list.

- **Public Folders Access**   Mac users can leverage Outlook 2001 to fully collaborate with Windows-based users through Exchange Public Folders.

- **Sharing Panel**   Users can enable access to calendaring information to other Exchange users, send on-behalf permissions, and have the ability to allow other users to view private items.

- **Single Sign-On**   Using Keychain from Apple, users can configure and enable this feature to provide single sign-on functionality when opening Outlook 2001.

- **Offline Folders**   As with Windows Outlook, offline synchronization is fully enabled in Outlook 2001 for Mac enabling users to synchronize email, calendars, contacts, and Public Folders.

- **Offline Address Book**   When Offline Synchronization is enabled, Mac users can also download the offline address book, enabling the email creation functionality when offline.

Configuring Support for Mac Clients

Before installing the Mac Outlook client for Exchange 2003, administrators must configure support from the client to connect to the network. In addition, the Apple Mac hardware must be evaluated to ensure that it meets the minimum required hardware specifications to support the Outlook 2001 client.

To enable TCP/IP support on the Mac operating system, complete these steps:

1. From the Apple menu, select Control, TCP/IP properties.

2. In the TCP/IP dialog Box, configure the TCP/IP properties as shown in Figure 27.1.

3. In this scenario, configure the TCP/IP Properties using a Static setting. Select the Connect Via option and then select Ethernet.

4. From the Configure tab, select Manually.

27

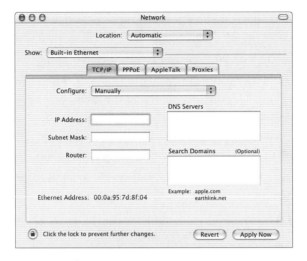

FIGURE 27.1   Mac client TCP/IP properties.

5. Enter the TCP/IP properties and DNS address being used on your network.

6. Close the TCP/IP properties and reboot the Mac system.

> **TIP**
>
> To enhance and ensure optimal performance when using Outlook 2001 for Mac, turn on the Virtual Memory of the Mac client through the Memory Control panel.

Before installing the Outlook 2001 client, ensure that the hardware being installed can meet the minimum requirement for supporting the Outlook client, as shown in Table 27.3.

TABLE 27.3   Outlook 2001 Hardware Requirements

Processor	Memory	Hard Disk Space
Mac PowerPC	32MB	20MB available disk space

> **TIP**
>
> If you are not sure which Mac platform and hardware you are using, use the Mac System Profiler tool available with the Mac operating system. To launch the Profiler Tool, select the Apple Menu and click the Apple System Profiler.

Configuring Outlook for Macintosh

After all requirements have been met, you can install and configure the Outlook 2001 client for connectivity to Exchange 2003. To accomplish this, follow the steps in the next section and review the resources to troubleshoot any issues you might encounter.

Installing Outlook 2001

To begin installing Outlook 2001, download or place the Outlook 2001 installation file in a folder on the Mac client. To begin the installation follow these steps:

1. Select and click the installation file to expand it.

2. Start the setup of Outlook by clicking twice on the `Outlook 2001.smi` file.

3. From the desktop, click twice on the Outlook 2001 file.

4. In the Outlook 2001 window, select and move the Outlook 2001 file to a location on the Mac local disk.

> **Downloading and Installing**
>
> When downloading the installation file from Microsoft, problems might occur if Stuffit Expander is installed on the Mac client. Use Stuffit Expander 5.5 or later when installing from a download.
>
> The Outlook 2001 client does not have an uninstall feature, as with standard Windows installations. Remove the installation files from the download location when the installation is complete.

Creating an Outlook Profile

After the installation of Outlook, you are prepared to configure the Outlook profile for the account that will be using the client. To create the first profile in a new installation of Outlook 2001, administrators can use the Run-First feature, which is launched the first time Outlook is opened.

To create the first profile in Outlook after the Run-First feature is launched, complete the following steps:

1. On the Create New Profile dialog box, enter the name for the new profile.

2. Enter the name of the account that the profile is being created for.

3. Enter the Name of the Exchange 2003 server being used to house the client mailbox being configured.

4. Select the Yes option to enable the Is This Computer Always Connected to a Network option.

5. To test the configuration, select the Test Settings option to verify the Exchange server and account name.

27

6. After connectivity and the account information have been verified, select the Create Profile options to continue.

7. Test access to Exchange by launching Outlook 2001; enter the account name, password, and domain when prompted.

Configuring the Profile to Use When Starting Outlook

Often when Mac desktops are shared, administrators can create multiple profiles to enable access to Exchange for multiple Mac users by repeating the steps in the last section. To enable the prompt to choose which profile to use when starting Outlook, open the Control Panel and follow these steps:

1. From the Apple, Control panel menu, select Outlook Settings.

2. To select the default profile, select the desired profile from the When Starting Outlook Use this Profile selection.

3. From the Outlook menu, select Edit, Preferences.

4. From the preferences selection, click the General tab.

5. Click the Prompt for a Profile to be used under the setting When Starting Microsoft Outlook, and select OK to complete the task.

Supporting Macintosh Clients

Administrators, in supporting Mac clients and Outlook for Mac, face some common issues when troubleshooting Mac clients, and tools are available to assist them. In addition, Microsoft provides links to support pages for Mac and Outlook for Mac.

One of the most common problems when dealing with Outlook connectivity is the TCP/IP configuration or functionality of the Mac client. Because there is no `ping` functionality with Mac, administrators can configure a static TCP/IP address on the client for testing connectivity.

By configuring a static TCP/IP address on the Mac client, administrators can perform a `ping` back to the client from a Windows server or workstation.

For more information on troubleshooting common issues with Outlook 2001, see the following links and references:

- For more information and downloads for Outlook 2001:

    `www.microsoft.com/mac/otherproducts/outlookformac/outlookformac.aspx?pid=`
    `outlookformac`

- To troubleshoot common Outlook issues and find support:

    `http://support.microsoft.com/default.aspx?ID=FH;EN-US;outmac&SD=GN&LN=EN-US`

Outlook Express

To support Remote Macintosh users, administrators can leverage the basic functionality of Outlook Express 5 for Mac. Using Outlook Express is an effective solution because remote users or mobile users can be supported using the limited functionality when emailing and working with address lists.

Although Outlook express for Mac is not a full-function client like Outlook for Mac, Outlook Express still offers comprehensive support in the following areas:

- **Email Support**   Access to Exchange email using the Simple Mail Transport Protocol (SMTP) and Post Office Protocol (POP).

> **NOTE**
>
> Messages accessed through Outlook Express are downloaded to the local client and removed from the local server. All client messages using this option are stored on the local Mac client after accessed and downloaded.
>
> To avoid large Outlook Express file sizes over time, the Empty Deleted Item is enabled by default.

- **Contact Address List**   Outlook Express supports contacts and address lists, which can be used to select addresses when creating and sending messages and to store personal contact information.

- **LDAP Support**   Lightweight Directory Access Protocol (LDAP) support enables an Outlook Express client's access to view information such as the Global Address List of an Exchange 2003 organization.

- **POP Support**   POP is the primary method of supporting Express clients when accessing Exchange from the Internet. This option requires the POP protocol to be enabled on Exchange 2003 and might require addition configuration of the firewall to enable passthrough of the POP protocol.

- **Password Support**   Usernames and passwords can be configured in advance, enabling users to open Outlook Express and access mail with a preconfigured account name and password.

Compatibility with Non-Windows Systems

Before installing Outlook Express 5 for Mac, use the Mac System Profiler tool to determine whether the hardware being installed meets the minimum Microsoft requirements for installing the Mac client. See Table 27.4 for a list of Mac requirements.

TABLE 27.4   Outlook Express for Mac Hardware Requirements

Processor	Memory	Hard Disk Space
Mac PowerPC	7MB	15MB available disk space

Installing and Enabling Support for Outlook Express 5

This section reviews the tasks required to configure the Mac client to support communication with Exchange 2003 from the internal network location and the Internet. After the network configuration has been completed, you will walk through the steps to install Outlook Express 5 onto the Mac operating system.

One common task when enabling support for Outlook Express 5 is to enable support for the client to use the TCP/IP protocol to communicate with and access Exchange mail. To enable support for TCP/IP, complete the following steps:

1. From the Apple menu, select the Control Panel and then TCP/IP properties.

2. On the TCP/IP dialog Box, configure the TCP/IP properties.

3. Select the Connect Via option and then select Ethernet.

4. From the Configure tab, select the method by which the address will be assigned—in this case, Manual.

5. Enter the TCP/IP properties and DNS address being used on your network.

6. Close the TCP/IP properties and reboot the Mac system.

> **NOTE**
>
> Using the TCP/IP Protocol enables client access from the internal network and from the Internet. This configuration is not the same as the protocol that will be used to access Exchange 2003 mail.

When installing Outlook Express for Mac, the installation file can be downloaded free from the Microsoft Web Site at

```
http://www.microsoft.com/mac/downloads.aspx?pid=download&location=/mac/DOWNLOAD/OE/
oe5.xml&secid=40&ssid=6&flgnosysreq=True
```

To begin installing Outlook Express 5, download the installation file to the Mac client and use the following steps:

1. Select and click the Download installation file to expand it.

2. In the Outlook Express 5 window, select and move the Outlook folder to a location on the Mac local disk.

Configuring POP Access with Outlook Express 5 for Mac

In this scenario, we configure the Mac Outlook Express client to connect to Exchange 2003 through an Internet connection using the POP protocol. This enables Outlook Express to access the Exchange 2003 server and authenticate downloading messages.

> **NOTE**
>
> Before configuring client connectivity to Exchange 2003 using the POP protocol, additional configuration of the Exchange server to enable the protocol is required. In addition, if accessing with POP from the Internet, the network firewall should be configured to enable POP access and the domain name for the Exchange 2003 POP server populated to the Internet.
>
> For more information on DNS, see Chapter 7, "Domain Name System Impact on Exchange Server 2003."
>
> For information on configuring your firewall and security best practices when enabling support with POP, consult the firewall manufacturer's product information.

To configure Outlook Express to connect an Exchange 2003 server using POP, begin by opening Outlook Express and follow these steps:

1. From the Tools menu, select Accounts.

2. On the Internet Accounts tab, click the Mail tab and select New.

3. To create a new email account, enter the name for the account in the Display Name dialog box, enter the name for the account being created, and select Next.

4. On the email screen, select the I already have an email address that I'd like to use, and enter the email address for the user being configured. Select Next to continue.

5. At the Email server information page, type **POP** under the My Incoming Mail Server selection.

6. Enter the fully qualified mail server name as listed in the next example. Then select Next to continues.

   Example:

   Incoming Mail Server = **Mail.CompanyABC.com**

   Outgoing Mail Server = **SMTP.CompanyABC.com**

> **NOTE**
>
> The Incoming and Outgoing Mail Server names should be added and populated to the Internet for proper DNS name resolution.
>
> When configuring this option for Internet access, the Outgoing mail server might need to be configured to point to the Outgoing Mail Server of the Internet service provider (ISP) being used.

7. At the authentication screen, enter the Logon Name and password for the account accessing the Exchange 2003 POP server, as shown in the next example.

   Example:

   Account Name = **MSoto@CompanyABC.com**

   Password = **************

27

8. To enhance security and limit the ability for others to access the Exchange POP account, uncheck the Save Password option and select Next to continue.

Password and Best Practices

To enhance security, leave the password entry blank; this requires users to enter the password each time they access Exchange.

In addition, when accessing Exchange through the POP protocol, it is best practice to use strong passwords to enhance security. Use the Active Directory Users and Computers management console to create a strong password for accounts using this method of access.

---

9. Complete the installation by entering the Account Name for the account being used and click Next to complete the installation.

10. Test accessing the Exchange 2003 POP services by selecting Send/Receive on the Outlook Express 5 toolbar.

Migrating and Backing Up Personal Address Books

One of the most common tasks when managing Outlook Express clients is backing up the contacts from the Outlook Express 5 for Mac client. When performing this task, administrators can export contact information and create comma-separated files for import into other mail programs and Outlook clients.

To complete the export of contact information for backup and migration reasons, follow the example in the next section. In this scenario, you back up the Outlook Express 5 for Mac Contacts to a comma-delimited CSV file. After it is backed up, the contacts are then imported in the full version of Outlook 2001 for Mac.

Backing Up Outlook Express Contacts

To begin, open the Outlook Express 5 for Mac client and follow the steps below to create a full backup of all the contact information.

1. From the File menu, select the option Export Contact.

2. In the Save dialog box, select the location where the export file will be saved by modifying the default Desktop location, as shown in Figure 27.2.

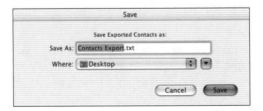

FIGURE 27.2   Exporting contacts.

3. In the Name dialog box, enter the name for the Export file to create.

> **NOTE**
>
> By default, export files are created as tab-delimited files only and are placed on the desktop.
>
> To convert the Export File to a CSV, use the steps in the next section, "Importing Contacts from Outlook Express 5 to Outlook 2001," to both convert the file and import contacts into other Outlook versions.

4. Click the Save button to create the export file and back up the Outlook Express contacts.

Importing Contacts from Outlook Express 5 to Outlook 2001

To import files into Outlook 2001 for Mac from Outlook Express 5, administrators must first convert the Export file to a CSV format using Microsoft Excel for Mac.

> **NOTE**
>
> To complete converting Outlook Express contact export files to CSVs, you must have Microsoft Office for Mac installed on the system being used.

To convert the export file to a CSV, launch the Excel for Mac application and follow these steps to create a CSV that will be used to import contacts into Outlook 2001 for Mac:

1. From the File menu, select Open.

2. Select the location and export file created in the previous steps and click Open.

3. When the Import Wizard begins, select Delimited in the original data type and select Next to continue.

4. Select the Tab option as the delimiter and click Next to continue.

5. On the data format tab, select General as the format and click Finish.

6. To save the new CSV file, from the File menu, select Save As. In the Save as dialog box, modify the file type to CSV Comma Delimited.

7. Enter the name for the new CSV file and select Save. This step creates a fully compatible CSV file for import into Outlook 2001.

> **TIP**
>
> To import the newly created CSV file into Outlook 2001 for Mac, select the Import option from the file menu and select the CSV file created in the previous steps. Selecting Open imports the CSV contacts into Outlook 2001.

27

Configuring and Implementing Entourage X for Mac

As an alternative to the Outlook options, Microsoft also provides the Entourages client platform for the Mac operating system. This option is very effective for Mac users because it provides both the same look and feel that Mac users are familiar with and the functionality of Outlook and Exchange.

The most compatible platform with the Mac operating system, Entourage X provides support for email, calendaring, and contact management when combined with software that enables support from Exchange 2003. Administrators can leverage the Entourage client to provide a compatible look and feel to Mac users while still providing full integration with the Windows client and enabling access to Exchange 2003 data.

Features and Functionality

The Entourage X client software combined with the Exchange Update provides enhanced functionality of the Entourage client and integration with the Exchange platform.

> **CAUTION**
>
> The Entourage X client and Exchange Update software available from Apple has been certified only for the Microsoft Exchange 2000 platform. Test all components and functionality of each in a lab environment before connecting any Entourage X clients to the Exchange 2003 organization.

When combined with the Exchange Update, Entourage X provides extensive support and enhanced functionality in the following areas:

- **HTML Email Support**   With the Exchange Update for Entourage X, HTML email format is fully supported, providing seamless integration with Windows-based Outlook clients.

- **Outlook Functions**   As with Outlook, Entourage X provides full support for calendaring, contacts, and scheduled tasks, integrated fully with Exchange 2003.

- **Offline Address Book**   Entourage X provides full synchronization of the Exchange 2003 offline address book.

- **LDAP Support**   Using the Entourage client, Mac users can now access the Global Address List.

- **Palm Support**   With Exchange Update from Entourage X, users can synchronize Exchange data with Palm handheld devices.

Deploying Entourage X

Requirements for installing Entourage X vary slightly from the requirements of Outlook and other Exchange solutions. Before installing and configuring Entourage X clients, administrators must ensure that minimum hardware requirements and the Exchange prerequisites have been configured. In addition, the client must be updated and installed with the required updates and software to support connectivity to Exchange.

Before installing Entourage, ensure that the following requirements and configurations have been enabled on the Exchange server:

- Microsoft Exchange 2000 Service Pack 2 or later

- IMAP/HTTP DAV/SMTP/LDAP

- Outlook Web Access

After the Exchange server has been configured, address the hardware and software requirements for installing Entourage by reviewing Table 27.5 and the software prerequisites.

Test the Mac client desktop hardware to ensure that it meets the minimum hardware requirements to install Entourage X, as listed in Table 27.5. If you do not know what hardware is installed on the Mac client, use the Mac System Profiler available on the Tools menu of the Mac client to display and evaluate the hardware of the Mac desktop.

TABLE 27.5   Entourage X for Mac Hardware Requirements

Processor	Memory	Hard Disk Space
G3, Mac OS X–compatible	128MB	196MB available disk space

After the Exchange server has been prepared and the hardware requirement for Entourage addressed, the next components to support Entourage are the updates and software requirements for the Mac client. Before the installation of Entourage X can be completed, the following components must be installed or updated in the Mac client:

- **Microsoft Office for Mac Update**   To support Entourage, the Microsoft Office installation on the Mac client must be updated to version 10.1.2 or higher.

- **Microsoft Exchange Update**   When connecting Entourage X to Exchange, the next component to be installed is the Exchange Update for Entourage X. Download this update from the Microsoft Mactopia Web site at:

  ```
  http://www.microsoft.com/mac/downloads.aspx?pid=download&location=/mac/
  DOWNLOAD/OFFICEX/exchangeupdate.xml&secid=5&ssid=14&flgnosysreq=True
  ```

After all updates have been completed and requirements met, the installation of Entourage X can be completed and the Entourage client connected to Exchange. To configure the Entourage client for Exchange support, follow these steps:

Enhancing Authentication with NTLM V2

To further leverage the available features of Windows and Exchange, administrators can enable NTLM version 2 for authentication of Mac users when connecting with Entourage clients.

To encrypt a password using NTLM V2, select the properties of the Exchange mail account and select the Advance Features tab. Enable password encryption by selecting the Always use secure passwords option.

---

1. Launch the Entourage X client, and select Tools, Accounts.

2. Select the Exchange service from the New drop-down box.

3. Enter the user information for the account connecting to Exchange with the client:

   - **Account Name**   This is the name on the account created in Active Directory for the Mac user.

   - **Password**   Provide the password for the Active Directory account or leave this entry blank to prompt the user to log in when connecting to Exchange.

   - **Domain Name**   Enter the name of the Active Directory domain where the account is a member.

Terminal Services Client for Mac

The Terminal Services Client for Mac can be considered and planned in the same manner as its Windows counterpart. When the prerequisites are met, administrators can use the Terminal Services Client to provide full Windows and application functionality to Mac users requiring Exchange services.

Through Terminal Services technology, Mac users are able to fully access the Windows client and Outlook application with all the features and functionality of Windows-based users.

Compatibility, Features, and Functionality

Because this remote desktop connection for Mac uses Windows Terminal Services, the only compatibility concern to be considered is the actual connection manager. All applications, when being run, are executed remotely and do not require additional compatibility between Windows-based applications, such as Outlook and the Mac client.

The Remote Desktop Connection manager is compatible with the Mac OS X 10.1 version or later. If required on an earlier version of the Mac client, upgrade the Mac operating system to meet the operating system requirements. Also ensure that the Mac client hardware meets the minimum hardware requirements for installing the Remote Desktop Connection for Mac, as shown in Table 27.6.

TABLE 27.6   Remote Desktop Hardware Requirements

Processor	Memory	Hard Disk Space
Mac PowerPC	128MB	3MB for installation 1.1MB after installation

One of the biggest benefits to the Remote Desktop Connection client from Mac is its integration with Windows and Mac clients. Because of this compatibility, Mac users are able to leverage the functionality and features of Windows Outlook when accessing exchange information and also leverage some of the following enhanced features when integrating Mac clients into a Windows Terminal Services environment:

- **Access to Windows**   The Remote Desktop Connection for Mac provides full access for Mac users into the Windows environment. This connection can be configured to the Windows desktop or restricted to an application such as Outlook.

- **Printing**   Through the Terminal Services connection, Mac users can access network printing and print information from applications to a networked Windows printer. To further enhance this feature, Mac users can print Windows information to the local Mac printer.

- **Access to Data**   Through the copy feature, Mac users are fully enabled to copy and paste data between the Mac client and the Windows Terminal Services session.

Before beginning any installation of the Remote Desktop Connection for Mac, Microsoft Windows Terminal Services and remote access must be enabled for supporting a remote connection with one or more of the following Microsoft Windows operating systems:

- **Windows XP**   Supported only through the Remote Desktop Connections feature of Windows XP, this method is limited to one concurrent connection.

- **Windows 2003**   Supported in all versions of Windows Server 2003, Terminal Services can be enabled to support remote access for multiple simultaneous connections.

- **Windows 2000**   Included in Windows 2000 Enterprise, Standard, and Datacenter Editions, the Terminal Service Application mode component must be enabled and will support multiple, simultaneous connections.

- **Windows NT 4.0 Terminal Server Edition**   This operation system enables support for multiple connections for both Windows sessions and application sessions.

27

TIP

When using Terminal Services for multiple client connections from Mac and Windows users, performance is dependent on the total amount of simultaneous connections and the total amount of available hardware resources installed in the server.

Installing the Terminal Services Client

To install and configure the Remote Desktop Connection for Mac, let's begin with a simple scenario of creating a one-to-one connection. In this scenario, you configure a Windows XP desktop and a Mac client to provide remote desktop connectivity to Microsoft Outlook.

To begin, enable the remote desktop feature of the Windows XP client by following these steps:

1. From the Windows XP desktop, select Start, My Computer and open the Properties page by right-clicking the mouse and selecting Properties.

2. Select the Remote tab and check the Allow users to connect remotely to this computer option, as shown in Figure 27.3.

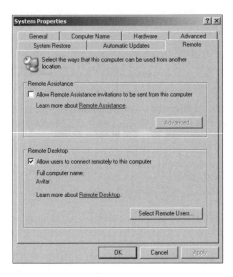

FIGURE 27.3   Remote desktop properties page.

3. Next, assign the account that may access the desktop remotely by clicking the Select the Remote Users button. Assign or create an account for the Mac users to authenticate with when accessing the Windows XP system remotely.

After the remote desktop configuration is complete and the client permissions to access Windows remotely have been configured, begin the installation of the Remote Desktop Connection for Mac by ensuring that the Mac client can communicate via TCP/IP on the network. Follow these steps to configure TCP/IP on the Mac client.

1. From the Apple menu, select Control, TCP/IP properties.

2. In the TCP/IP dialog box, configure the TCP/IP properties. In this scenario, configure the TCP/IP properties using a Static setting. Select Connect Via option and select Ethernet.

3. From the Configure tab, select Manual.

4. Enter the TCP/IP properties for the client and Domain Name System address being used on your network.

5. Close the TCP/IP properties and reboot the Mac system.

To install the Remote Desktop Connection for Mac, download the installation file from Microsoft and place the file on the local Mac client where it will be installed.

To install the client, complete the following steps:

1. Expand the downloaded installation file by clicking on the file twice.

2. Go to the Mac desktop and open the Remote Desktop Connection volume. Copy the Remote Desktop Connection folder into the local disk of the Mac client.

3. Remove the Remote Desktop Connection Volume and the original installation file by placing them in the Desktop Trash.

4. Launch the Remote Desktop Connection from the Remote Desktop Folder and enter the name of the system you are connecting to, as shown in Figure 27.4. Click Connect to establish the remote connection.

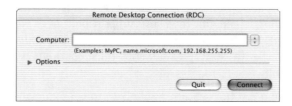

FIGURE 27.4 Remote Desktop Connection.

5. When prompted, enter the name and password of the account you configured to allow remote access to this desktop system.

Understanding Other Non-Windows Client Access Methods

In addition to the Mac operating systems, Exchange e2003 can support a variety of clients by enabling support for Internet Message Access Protocol (IMAP), SMTP, and POP. Using these protocols, Exchange administrators can provide imitated email functionality and support a variety of clients throughout the Exchange environment for email and communication purposes.

POP3 Access to Exchange

POP3 is one of the most popular methods of providing mail services on the Internet today. POP is highly reliable but has limited functionality. Users who access email with POP3 download all messages to the local client and send and receive messages only when a connection is established with the POP server.

When enabled with Exchange 2003, the POP protocol can be leveraged to provide email support to additional non–Windows-based clients' platforms. Through the common method of sending mail, multiple client platforms can communicate over email regardless of the actual desktop operating system and client mail software being used.

The POP3 functionality of Exchange Server 2003 can support multiclient environments, including the Eudora Mail client, the Netscape Mail client, and other POP-compatible nonspecific client platforms. This protocol is best used when supporting single client systems that download mail and store mail information locally.

IMAP Access to Exchange

IMAP is an additional method that can be used to support non–Windows-based client access to Exchange 2003 information. Designed to allow access to information stores located on a remote system, IMAP can also be used to support the Linux-based Netscape Mail clients.

Using the Netscape Mail client, Netscape users can access, collaborate, and store information on the Exchange 2003 server with the IMAP support built in to Netscape Communicator. With this functionality, networks can now incorporate additional operating systems, such as Linux with Netscape Mail, and still support email functionality between all Network users.

Use the preferences option on the Netscape Mail client to configure and enable support for IMAP communication with Exchange 2003.

Pocket PC Access

New to Exchange Server 2003, client mobile access is now fully integrated and supported when the Exchange 2003 server is installed.

Remote and mobile users can use the Outlook Pocket PC version to send, receive, and synchronize mail, calendaring, and task information, using the Windows Pocket PC 2003 platform over mobile information services built in to Exchange 2003.

For more information regarding the options and configuration to support Pcket PC access to Exchange 2003, see Chapter 24, "Configuring Client Systems for Mobility."

HTML Access

Another new feature with Exchange 2003 is HTML access. With this feature, administrators can use Internet-ready cellular telephones to provide HTML access to Exchange information for mobile users regardless of where they might be.

By providing additional mobile services and client permissions through Active Directory, alternate access can be granted to email and Exchange using Internet-ready mobile phone devices over HTML access.

For more information regarding HTML access options and configurations, see Chapter 24.

Outlook Web Access

One of the most effective methods of allowing access to Exchange information is OWA. Enhanced greatly in Exchange 2003, OWA can be used to provide HTML browser access to Exchange mailboxes from inside the network as well as the Internet.

Probably the biggest benefit to using the OWA solution to support non–Windows-based clients is that it is nondiscretionary as to which type of Internet browser can access it. Effective in functionality, Linux-based users and others using non–Windows-based systems can access OWA for email and calendar management in the same fashion as any Windows-based users.

For more information regarding OWA and enabling support, see Chapter 26, "Everything You Need to Know About the Outlook Web Access Client."

Summary

In a Microsoft-centric environment, administrators of networks often focus solely on Windows-based connections to Exchange and spend little time on options for non–Windows-based users. There are many options for non-Windows users, including a whole suite of clients for the Macintosh—such as Entourage, Outlook Express, Outlook for the Mac, and the Remote Desktop Connection. Additionally, Outlook Express is available on other non-Windows platforms, and Exchange can be accessed using industry-standard POP3 and IMAP protocols.

By choosing any of a variety of client applications to access Exchange, an organization can leverage the capabilities of Exchange beyond Windows users and provide messaging communications throughout an enterprise. Depending on the client application selected, some options provide just email communications and others provide the full suite of Outlook and Exchange business productivity functions, such as calendaring, contacts, notes, to-do lists, journals, public folders, and more.

An organization should not be limited in its ability to extend Exchange 2003 to all users within an enterprise, and with the leveraging of new client access capabilities, an organization can greatly improve its reach to all users in an organization.

27

Best Practices

The following are best practices from this chapter:

- When choosing a client configuration for Exchange, an organization should evaluate the different solutions available for non-Windows client connectivity.

- Outlook 2001 for the Macintosh will run on OS9 as well as OS X; however, on OS X, the Outlook client runs in OS9 emulation mode, so OS X users might consider using Entourage X or the Remote Desktop Connection client for access.

- To achieve the full Outlook functionality of Windows users, a non-Windows client might consider using a Terminal Services session, which provides full support for the full Windows client that is identical to the one Windows users access.

- Users who want calendar integration access tend not to want to use Outlook Express, which lacks calendar support, and should consider one of the other client applications that support calendaring.

- For POP3 to work, the function should be enabled on the Exchange server. However, if POP3 will not be used, the service should be disabled on Exchange to minimize any security risk caused by an unused service.

- To improve security, leave the password entry on the Outlook Express configuration page blank so that the user will be prompted for a password every time.

- Because different versions of the client software for the Macintosh have different support for various versions of the Mac OS, make sure to check compatibility before installing the client software.

- To enhance logon security, NTLM v2 should be enabled for Entourage clients to access an Exchange server.

PART IX

Client Administration and Management

IN THIS PART

Deploying the Client for Microsoft Exchange

Whether you are implementing Exchange 2003 Server for the first time, or upgrading an organization from previous versions of Microsoft Exchange Server, client deployments are always a major component when planning and implementing Exchange messaging functionality to client systems in the enterprise.

With many options available for deploying the Microsoft Exchange Outlook client, administrators can plan and leverage multiple options and technologies when configuring and pushing the Exchange 2003 Server Outlook client.

To assist in the planning and deploying of the Outlook client, this chapter provides information about the different options and the best practices when using them to deploy clients to the desktop, how to automate and configure the Exchange client profile, and how to work with automated configuration files—that is, Microsoft Outlook Profile (PRF) files. In addition, the basic tools are available for managing and administering the deployment of Exchange 2003 Server clients to the desktop.

Understanding Deployment Options

To centralize Exchange management, there are standard tools and enhancements in technologies that are part of the Windows Server family operating systems, enabling Exchange administrators to leverage their flexibility when deploying the Exchange 2003 Outlook client. Organizations can now use a variety of deployment methods and preconfiguration options to configure and deploy, as well as support, Exchange Outlook clients and remote and mobile systems.

As organizations begin the planning process, administrators and planners can adopt different deployment methods and execute client installations based on the type of client and the specific need for each type of client desktop. This section explores the different options available to deploy the Exchange 2003 Outlook client software to desktops in the enterprise and options and steps to configure the Outlook client options and methods for generating Exchange client profiles.

Available Methods of Deployment

With multiple options available, client deployments can be performed on many levels not previously available when installing the Outlook desktop client software. With integration between Windows 2003 and Exchange as well as new tools available to administrators, Outlook 2003 can be pushed to the desktop using any of the following methods:

- **Manual Installation**   Standard Installation enables administrators to incorporate configuration files with the installation process, define baseline settings and manually test the installation when complete.

- **Windows 2003 Group Policy**   Leveraging Group Policy Software Installation technologies and Microsoft Office 2003 Security Templates, Outlook clients can be pushed to desktop systems on the network. Using Group Policy, administrators can centrally configure Outlook Security and user options and enforce a baseline configuration of Outlook to all client systems.

- **Imaging Technologies**   When upgrading to Outlook or deploying new installations, organizations can image the Outlook client to the desktop or refresh the desktop image.

- **Systems Management Server**   Using Microsoft Systems Management Server, you can centrally deploy and push the Outlook client to large numbers of desktop systems through multiple locations in the enterprise. This option also enables tracking and information to manage a full Exchange Outlook client deployment.

Outlook Profile Generation

Most likely one of the biggest challenges to Exchange administrators is configuring Outlook profiles to communicate with Exchange 2003 Server. To automate this task, profiles can be scripted using tools available with the Office 2003 Resource Kit (ORK) from Microsoft.

Along with pushing clients using the methods described earlier, Outlook client profiles and Outlook Exchange server settings can be configured using the Custom Installation Wizard (CIW) and configuration files created with Outlook option settings.

Use the Office 2003 Custom Installation Wizard to create a PRF file setting that can be specified to configure the Outlook client profile and Outlook mail services options that set up the user profile.

With older versions Outlook, the NewProf.exe executable file is used to automatically generate Outlook user profiles after the installation of the client software is completed. Used in conjunction with a PRF file, this tool can also be used to specify user Outlook profile information and settings on a new Outlook client installation.

Configuring Outlook Client Options

Another enhanced functionality available to administrators when installing the Exchange 2003 Outlook client is the ability to predefine and set configuration options dynamically after the installation of the Outlook client software has finished.

Custom Installation Wizard

To deploy the Outlook client to desktops on the network with configuration options predefined, powerful tools such as the CIW, along with Office configuration files OSP and PRF, can be leveraged to define Outlook client options for large deployments with the need to specify client user options.

Windows Server Group Policy

An effective configuration option is the centralized management available through the Security Template for Outlook 2003. With the Group Policy feature of Windows Server 2003, standard and advanced options can be configured and established after the client is deployed. This option is effective because the options are configured after all clients with the setting are applied.

Transforms

The final option for defining Outlook client setting and configuration options is the Office Transforms. Transforms are configuration files used with the Windows Installer that contain information and modifications that will be applied to the Outlook client during installation.

This option is also created using the CIW and using the MST file extension.

28

Deploying Non–Windows-Based Options

With a variety of client systems to support, one other area to understand is how to deploy the Microsoft Outlook client for non–Windows-based systems, such as Macintosh desktops. To understand the installation process and configuration options for the types of clients, see Chapter 27, "Outlook for Non-Windows Systems."

Planning Considerations and Best Practices

Before deploying the Exchange 2003 Outlook client, organizations should consider all the details involved with the Outlook client deployment. Because most organizations support different types of clients and can have complicated messaging environments in multiple locations, client deployments should be reviewed and planned in detail to avoid any unforeseen potential issues.

Identifying the types of client needs involved in each deployment and reviewing the overall network topology can greatly enhance the performance of each deployment and assist with the transparent client installation.

Network Topology Bandwidth Consideration

In any situation, administrators must plan Outlook client deployments in a manner that avoids client network disruptions and bandwidth saturation when deploying to remote locations.

Evaluating the network environment and determining the needs of remote location for each deployment can help ensure a transparent deployment of the Outlook client. In a single-location network environment, planning the deployment can be accomplished by evaluating the bandwidth availability of the network to avoid network problems when pushing or deploying the Outlook client with Group Policy. Because the installation can be pushed over the network, deployments should be planned and pushed in smaller groups.

With multisite organizations, administrators must also plan and deploy the Outlook client without causing network disruptions. One larger factor in this scenario is Wide Area Network (WAN) links. Because these types of connections are generally much slower than local network connections, it is difficult to complete multiple Outlook client deployments without possibly causing communication issues over the WAN links.

With shares called Administrative Distribution Points in each remote location, deployments can still be centrally managed while deploying client installation from each local share. Using these Administrative Distribution Points can avoid bandwidth saturation over WAN links and enhance the overall time required to deploy the Outlook client in remote locations.

Planning Best Practices

To assist in the planning process involved with deploying the Outlook client, study the following common considerations and best practices:

- Deploying the Outlook client with the Microsoft Office suite provides enhanced functionality, such as using Microsoft Word for the Outlook client email editor.

- Documenting all profile settings and configuration options for each Transform, PRF, and custom installation file.

- Testing deployment options and profile generations in a test environment before deployment to network desktops.

- Deploying to a smaller pilot group first.

- Performing deployments in small groups and phases for ease of management.

- Creating and naming configuration files based on the group or configuration options they will apply. For example, create a file called **Public.PRF** to configure options for group workstations called Public Relations.

Addressing Remote and Mobile Client Systems

Addressing remote and mobile Exchange Outlook client needs presents an entirely different challenge for administrators when planning the Outlook client deployment. With remote and mobile users accessing the network in many different ways, administrators should consider the impact on the installation when clients access the network over low bandwidth links.

Scheduling remote and mobile users to come into a location where administrators can perform the installation manually can often be easier than deploying over slow network connections. If required to deploy Outlook for these types of clients, use the Installation State options page to install only the required components needed to support the Outlook client, reducing the overall size of the installation package. Leverage Administrative Installation Points located closest to the remote or mobile user's access point to deploy the Outlook client.

Managing the Outlook Deployment

It is difficult to manage the deployment of Outlook clients without additional software, such as Microsoft Systems Management Server (SMS). With Microsoft Systems Management Server, deployments can be tracked and managed down to the desktop level, enabling administrators to identify desktops needing the Outlook client, deploy Outlook, and even indemnify failed installations in a single report.

When options such as SMS are not available, it can be difficult to determine how the deployment of the Outlook client is progressing, because all evidence of the Outlook

28

client installation is not remotely present through the standard tool available in the ORK and Windows 2003. Administrators must use other methods to determine whether a software installation was successful:

- Look for MSI Installer events that are written into the Application Event Logs.

- On the local machine, view Add/Remove programs to see whether the Outlook update package is listed.

Preparing the Deployment

As the planning phase of the deployment comes to a close, administrators can focus on preparing the different areas of the Outlook client deployment.

For deploying the Outlook client successfully to desktop on the network, administrators can also use this time to prepare and test configurations that will be used for the actual Outlook client deployment.

Outlook Systems Requirements

Before pushing an Outlook client to desktop systems on the network, the desktop hardware must be evaluated to determine whether it meets the recommended Microsoft hardware and software requirements for installing Outlook.

> **TIP**
>
> With Microsoft Systems Management Server (SMS), inventories can be conducted on network desktop systems to identify hardware and software installed on each.

Ensure that the desktop systems meet the installation requirements needed by reviewing Table 28.1.

TABLE 28.1   System Requirements

Requirement	Outlook 2003	Outlook 2002
Processor speed	P233MHz	P133MHz
Memory	128MB	136MB w/Windows XP
		72MB w/Windows 2000
Hard disk space	400MB	135MB

> **TIP**
>
> The installation of Outlook 2003 also requires Microsoft Internet Explorer 5.01 or higher.

Planning Predefined Configuration Options

With a broad understanding of how the Outlook client can be deployed, another area to understand is which options can be configured when using the Custom Installation Wizard and Transform configuration files. Understanding the options available to administrators for configuring the Exchange Outlook client with PRF files, Transforms, and so forth enables administrators to create a baseline understanding of what options will be used prior to actually creating the individual configuration file.

Using the Custom Installation Wizard, you can configure the following features:

- **Outlook User Profile Settings** Administrators can specify how users' profiles will be created. Using this option, administrators can set new profiles, modify existing profiles, and add additional user profiles.

- **Exchange Server Settings** Settings defining Exchange server names and specific options, such as Exchange 2003 connection options, can also be defined.

- **Installation States for Outlook and Features** Using the installation options, you can define installation states to make features either available, available at first use, or not available.

- **Mail Options** Options such as PST and OST settings and synchronization options can be defined using the Custom Installation Wizard.

- **Settings and Options** Many of the options available when configuring Outlook through the Tool, Options tab of the Outlook client can also be defined when creating custom installation files.

- **Installation Path** Ensure that the installation directory path on the client desktop where the Outlook client will be installed contains enough free disk space to complete the installation.

Creating Administrative Installation Points

If the deployment requires Administrative Installation Points, administrators can create them using the Setup.exe program of the Outlook or Office installation software.

Using the Setup.exe program with Outlook or Office 2003, you can create Administrative Installation Points by running the installation with the /a switch.

To create the Administrative Installation Point, complete these steps:

NOTE

In the following example, the Administrative Installation Point is created using the Microsoft Office 2003 installation media.

1. Insert the Installation CD-ROM into the systems where the Installation Point will be created. Open a Run command dialog box by selecting Start, Run.

2. At the Installation screen, enter the product key that came with the Office 2003 installation software and select Next to continue.

> **NOTE**
>
> Use the Install location option on this screen to change the installation path that Outlook will use when being deployed.

3. Accept the End User License Agreement (EULA) and select Install; this begins the installation process.

4. Select the Installation state for Outlook and Outlook options; select Next to continue.

Automating Outlook Profile Settings

There are multiple options for configuring Outlook profiles when deploying. Most commonly used are the PRF files used to generate Outlook profiles and apply Outlook settings.

To configure profile settings using PRF files, use the Custom Installation Wizard. Define the profile setting in the Outlook: Customize Default Profile page. This section walks you through the standard configuration of the PRF file to generate a user's profile dynamically after the Outlook client installation has completed. In this scenario, you configure a single PRF file and create the Outlook profile for any user when the Outlook client is launched for the first time.

To create a new profile, open the CIW by selecting Start, Run, Microsoft Office, Microsoft Office Tools, Microsoft Office ORK, Custom Installation Wizard. Then follow these steps:

1. Select the default options until the Outlook: Customize Default Profile page appears. Select the New Profile option, enter **Outlook** for the profile name, and click Next.

> **TIP**
>
> To configure the PRF file to run when Outlook is launched for the first time, use the Add/Remove Registry Entries page of the Custom Installation Wizard.
>
> To enable the run-once option, make the following Registry changes:
>
> Delete the following key:
>
> `HKEY_CURRENT_USER\Software\Microsoft\Office\10.0\Outlook\Setup\First-Run`

Expand the Registry tree to the following:

`HKEY_CURRENT_USER\Software\Microsoft\Office\10.0\Outlook\Setup`

Add the String Value and enter the path of the PRF file share created earlier.

2. To configure the PRF file to dynamically configure each user profile, enter the **%UserName%** syntax in the User Name field. Also, enter the name of your Exchange 2003 Server, as shown in Figure 28.1.

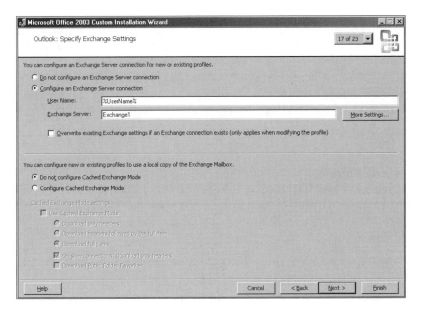

FIGURE 28.1   Exchange Server PRF file settings.

3. Because this PRF file is a default profile configuration file, select Next at the Add Accounts screen.

4. From the Remove Accounts and Export Settings screen, click the Export Profile settings. Enter the name **Outlook** for the name of the new PRF file and save the file to the desired location. Select Finish to complete the PRF file creation.

> **TIP**
>
> Microsoft PRF files can also be configured with additional Outlook profile settings, such as Personal folders and Outlook option settings. To understand more about configuring PRF files, go to www.microsoft.com/office/ork and search for .PRF.

Creating Transforms and Profile Files

There are several different types of configuration files that can be used to deploy Outlook client configuration to the desktop. In this section, you complete the steps needed to configure Outlook 2003 using the CIW to create Transforms and Profile files (PRF).

Creating Transforms

Transform (MST) files are created using the Office CIW available in the Office 2003 Resource Kit. Transforms can be used to create detailed custom settings when installing and configuring the Outlook client.

TIP

Use the Transform option when extensive settings are required for the Outlook deployment and when deploying Outlook with the Office application suite. Transforms can be configured with custom settings and Outlook profile information making this option the most comprehensive of all configuration options when deploying.

Be sure to document all settings expected to be used when creating configuration Transform files.

Configuring Transforms

To create a Transform file, download and install the Office 2003 Resource Kit (ORK) and launch the Custom Installation Wizard by selecting Start, Run, Microsoft Office, Microsoft Office Tools, Microsoft Office ORK, Custom Installation Wizard.
Then follow these steps:

1. From the Welcome to Microsoft Office Custom Installation Wizard Screen, select Next.

2. On the Open the MSI File page, enter the path and filename for the Outlook MSI Installation package, as shown in Figure 28.2. Use the Browse button to locate the MSI installation package being used for this Microsoft Transform file. Click the Next button to continue.

3. Because this scenario is creating a new Transform file, on the Open the MST File page, select the Create a New MST File option and select Next.

4. Select the location where the new MST file will be created and click Next.

5. Enter the location where the Outlook installation will be placed on the desktop when the client is deployed. Then enter the name of the organization that will be used for registration information.

6. If previous installations of Outlook and Microsoft Office exist on the desktop, select which installation version to remove.

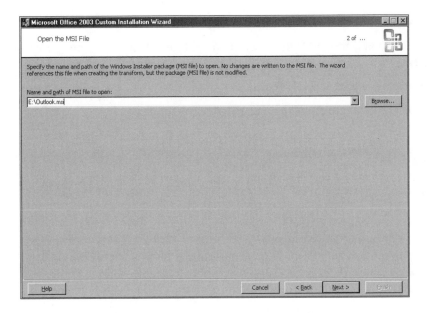

FIGURE 28.2 MSI selection page.

> **NOTE**
>
> This option removes any selected version and component of Microsoft Office prior to installation of the Outlook client.

7. On the Set Feature Installation States page, select the Outlook components that will be installed. Click the Microsoft Outlook for Windows and click the Run from my Computer option.

8. Use the Custom Default Application Settings page to define and add an Office Application Settings (OSP) file.

   If upgrading, select the Migrate User's Settings check box to maintain the existing user-defined options after the upgrade.

9. Use the Change the Office User Settings page to define the setting and options to be applied to Outlook after the installation is finished.

10. Use the Options pages to modify the Outlook installation; continue through the configuration pages to create the Transform files.

    Continue through the installation and configure the following:

    Add/Remove additional custom installation files.

    Add/Remove custom Registry Entries.

28

Modify Shortcuts and Outlook Icons.

If deploying across WAN links, select an additional installation point for the deployment.

Establish Outlook Security Settings.

Add additional programs to be installed with Outlook.

NOTE

For more information regarding options on each page and additional settings, use the help option on each page to review the Microsoft Custom Installation Wizard help file.

Configuring Profiles with Transforms

Customizing the configuration of the profile during the installation can be done on the Customize Default Profiles page. Using the options available, administrators can select the method in which to create the client profile with the Outlook Deployment tool.

For this Transform, select Apply PRF file and select the PRF file created in the previous section or select one of the following options, as shown in Figure 28.3:

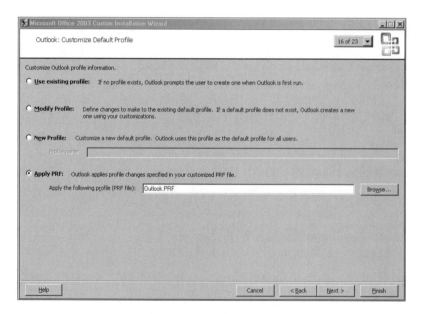

FIGURE 28.3   CIW profile options.

- **Use Existing Profile**   Used when upgrading the Outlook client, this option maintains the existing setting.

> **NOTE**
>
> When Use Existing Profile is selected and no profile is found on the client desktop, this option prompts the user to create the profile.

- **Modify Profile**   Select this option to customize profile information and Exchange Outlook Options.
- **New Profile**   Use this option to create a single new profile and configure connection settings.

Additional options are available, such as Send and Receive Options and Mail settings; continue through the configuration screens by choosing the options you want. The creation of the PRF file can be completed at any time by selecting the Finish button on any setup screen.

After the Custom Installation Wizard has completed, document the command syntax for running the Outlook `Setup.exe` with the Transform just created, as in the example in Figure 28.4.

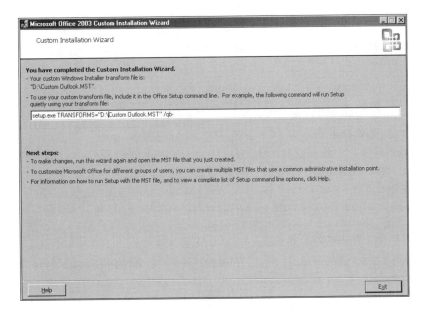

FIGURE 28.4   Completing the Custom Installation Wizard.

Installing the Exchange Client

The option that requires the most administrative attention—manually installing the Outlook client—is often required as an option when deploying the Outlook client. When considering these options, administrators must determine which option best fits the deployment needs by determining the overall number of manual tasks required for the installation.

All the options can be used together, but they can also be incorporated into the deployment individually to enhance the options available when installing clients manually and configuring settings. In this section, you review the basic steps for installing the Outlook client to desktop systems using Transforms, PRF files, and the switches available when using these options.

Using Transforms and PRF Files When Installing Outlook

When the options are not available to push the installation to client systems, administrators can still install the Outlook client and save valuable keystrokes and time by predefining profile information. Using these options with a manual installation scenario can greatly reduce the overall amount of time normally required to install the Outlook client manually. Administrators can now incorporate the manual installation process with preconfiguration files, such as PRFs and Transforms, and save time for each installation by not being required to manually configure each installation after completion.

When the required functionality is the client profile configuration setting and limited configuration options, the manual installation can easily be completed by using a simple PRF file. PRF files are simple to incorporate into the installation and require only the addition of a command-line switch with the Setup.exe installation program to deploy.

With more complex installation needs, administrators can create MST files to define Outlook settings, security profiles, and user options. This option is most effective and enables administrators to continue with installations rather than manually configure each client setting individually.

Installing the Outlook Clients with PRF Files

Using the steps in the last section to create the PRF file, administrators can then copy the file to the installation share for use when manually installing Outlook. This option prevents administrators from having to manually configure each client Outlook profile after the installation is complete.

To understand more about using PRF files when using the Windows installation program, complete these steps:

1. Create a folder share and place the Outlook.PRF file in the folder where it can be accessed from any location on the network.

When creating shares for PRF file access, provide the account being used to install Outlook Full Control to the PRF folder share.

2. To open a command prompt and begin an installation in Outlook using PRF files, begin by selecting Start, Run, and enter **command**.

3. From the command prompt, type

`d:\setup.exe /ImportPRF \\Outlook Files\Outlook.PRF`

where **d:** represents the location of the Outlook installation files and **Outlook Files** is the name of the folder share created to host the PRF configuration files.

When errors occur or it appears that the Outlook profile has not been set correctly, the PRF file can be run by using the Open command and manually installing the configuration information.

Manually Installing Outlook with Transforms

As stated earlier, Transforms offer the most functionality when predefining Outlook settings and profile information. Using Transforms, administrators can leverage multiple options and even multiple Transforms for configuring Outlook clients. To understand the command lines and syntax used when installing the Microsoft Outlook client with MST files, review the examples listed in the following sections.

Applying Transforms with the Outlook Setup.exe

In these examples, you use the OutlookSet1.MST Transform filename to customize the Outlook Installation. To incorporate Transforms into the Outlook installation, use the following command:

`Example: D:\setup.exe TRANSFORMS=OutlookSet1.mst`

Transforms can also be chained together for the application of more than one Transform to be applied when installing Outlook. When organizations create individual Transforms to specify different settings for individual groups or user types, the option to install multiple Transforms on a single installation is still possible. For example, an organization creates a baseline Transform defining settings that will be applied to all user and individual Transforms for specific groups. These files can be chained, making the Outlook settings easily manageable. Using a Setup.ini file with the proper syntax, you can link and apply Transforms in a very effective manner.

28

Pushing Client Software with Windows 2003 Group Policies

Using Windows Server 2003 Group Policy management tools, administrators can easily and inexpensively deploy the Outlook client to desktops using Group Policy software installation functionality. Using Group Policy to deploy the Outlook client, administrators can centralize many of the duties and support tasks requiring administrative overhead and resources when working with other options.

Group policies can provide extremely powerful administration and management options when deploying the Outlook client. Use the information provided in this section to set up and deploy the Outlook.MSI package.

For more detailed information regarding using Group Policy in the Exchange Server 2003 environment, see Chapter 29, "Group Policy Management for Exchange Clients."

Deploying Outlook with Group Policy Overview

Using Group Policy to deploy the Outlook client is one of the most effective and flexible options administrators can leverage.

However, before creating deployment packages, administrators should understand the basic functionality of Group Policy and Windows Server 2003. Review the information and overview provided in the next sections before planning and setting up Windows Server 2003 Group Policy to support the Outlook client deployment.

Administrative Options

Delegating the proper rights for administrators to manage and manipulate Group Policy when deploying Outlook clients is important. With the Delegation Wizard available with the Windows Group Policy snap-in, administrative rights can be assigned to Exchange administrators to manage and control the deployment Outlook to the desktop without interfering with the day-to-day options of the Windows systems. Using the Delegation Wizard to assign rights, administrators can grant permissions to individual accounts, groups, and Exchange server administrators.

Deployment Options

With Group Policy, the Outlook client can be deployed to the desktop using any of the following deployment methods:

- **Assigned to Computers**   This method of installation creates an Outlook installation package that is applied to workstations when a user logs onto the desktop. Using this option, all users have access to the Exchange client software after it's installed.

- **Assigned to Users**   When the installation package is assigned to users, application shortcuts are placed on the desktop of the user's profiles and in the Start menu of the individual user's profile. When these shortcuts are selected, the application installation is launched and completed.

- **Publishing the Installation**   When Outlook client software packages are published, the installation package is displayed in the Add/Remove Programs Group in the local desktop system control panel. Users can then initiate the installation by selecting the Install option.

With each method, Exchange 2003 administrators use the MSI installation file format to push the Outlook client's software packages from a central location or from Administrative Installation Points to the workstation or users on the network.

CAUTION

When deploying Outlook software using Group Policy, do not assign the option Install to users and computers at the same time. Assigning both options can create conflicts when installing Outlook and possibly corrupt the installation of the Outlook client when applying the update.

Best Practices for Deploying Outlook Clients

As with all aspects of Group Policy, the choices and configuration options of Outlook client deployment are numerous. Regardless of what method of Group Policy deployment is being used, some basic best practices apply to assist in avoiding unforeseen issues when deploying Outlook clients:

- Software packages must be in the format of an MSI package. Any other format type cannot be pushed using Group Policy.

- Always plan and configure Software Pushes at the highest levels possible in the domain tree. If the push is going out to more than one group or organizational unit, the software update should be configured to be pushed at the domain level. If the software update is being pushed to only a few groups or one organizational unit or multiple update packages are being pushed, configure the push at the group or organizational unit level.

- Deploy the Outlook client to the Computers Configuration rather than the User Configuration. Doing so avoids the installation from being applied more than once when a user logs on a different desktop system.

- When pushing updates in multiple locations, use Administrative Installation Points and Windows Distributed File System (DFS). This enables software installations to be installed from packages located closest to the client being installed.

Pushing Outlook Client

The steps in this scenario enable administrators to push the Exchange 2003 Outlook client package to workstations on the domain.

> **TIP**
>
> To enhance functionality when using Windows Server 2003 Group Policy, download and install the Microsoft Group Policy Management Console (GPMC) from Microsoft.

Open the Group Policy Management Console by selecting Start, All Programs, Administrative Tools, Group Policy Management. To create Outlook client software Group Policy Objects:

1. Select the Default Domain Policy for your domain by expanding `Forest/Domains/YourCompanyDomain/Group Policy Objects`.

2. Select the Default Domain Policy, click Action, and then click Edit. This opens the Group Policy Editor to create the Software Push.

3. Select Computer Configuration and then Software Installation.

4. From the Action menu, select New/Package.

5. Navigate the Open dialog to the network share where the `Outlook.MSI` was placed and select the MSI package being applied. Select Open to continue.

> **TIP**
>
> If prompted that the Group Policy editor cannot verify the network location, ensure that the share created to store the installation files has permission to allow users access to the share. Select Yes to continue when confirmed.

6. At the Deploy Software dialog, select Advance and click OK to continue. Windows Server 2003 will verify the installation package; wait for the verification to complete before continuing to the next step.

7. After the package is visible in the right pane of the software installation properties, highlight the install package and click Action/Properties.

8. On the Package properties page, select the Deployment tab. Review the configuration, click Assign, and ensure that the Install this Package at Logon option is selected, as shown in Figure 28.5. Select OK when complete.

When the new package is ready to deploy, test the update by logging on to a workstation and verifying that the package has installed using the steps listed in the section "Configuring the SMS Package for an Unattended Installation," later in this chapter. If problems exist, redeploy the package by selecting the software update; click Action, All Tasks, Redeploy Application to force the deployment.

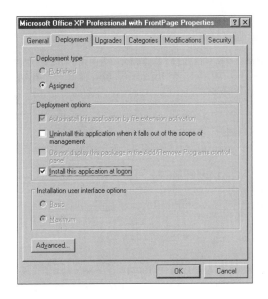

FIGURE 28.5   Outlook update properties.

Testing the Outlook Client Deployment

Using Group Policy, administrators cannot determine whether a software package was pushed successfully without additional management software such as Microsoft Systems Management Server. When viewing installations and managing deployments, all evidence of client installation using Group Policy can be seen only at the client desktop. Using the following two areas on the client desktop, administrators can determine whether a software installation was successful, and view the following manually:

- Look for MSI Installer events that are written into the Application Event Logs.

- On the local machine, view Add/Remove programs to see whether the Outlook update package is listed.

Deploying with Microsoft Systems Management Server

The most comprehensive option to deploy the Outlook client is Microsoft Systems Management Server (SMS). With the powerful software deployment functionality and management tools incorporated with SMS, this method becomes the best solution for deploying the Outlook client software to medium and large organizations.

Planning and Preparing Outlook Deployments with SMS

To prepare the Outlook client installation for use with Microsoft Systems Management Server, administrators must plan and prepare the deployment in many of the same ways as when using other options.

This section reviews and outlines the following options and deployment preparation tasks involved with using Microsoft Systems Management Server (SMS):

- **Software Distribution**   Plan and create administrative installation points to support software pushes in remote locations and separate subnets. SMS site server can be used in remote locations to support software distribution without requiring pushes over WAN links.

- **Evaluate Client Needs**   Determine the specific client installation needs and document the deployment plan and order in which SMS will push the Outlook client.

- **Inventory Using SMS Collections**   Leveraging the powerful functionality of SMS collections, administrators can perform detailed inventories of desktop client's hardware and software from evaluating and determining Outlook requirements prior to deploying.

Deploying with Systems Management Server 2.0

When deploying the Outlook client with Microsoft Systems Management Server, SMS leverages the Windows Installer to enhance the functionality of the deployment and add options and functionality to recover from failed installations.

When leveraging Windows Installer and SMS to push client software, the following options are available:

- **Pre-Defined Configuration Support**   Administrators can incorporate Transforms and PRF files with the distribution of the MSI package.

- **Per System Pushes**   Users can establish a connection to the Web site without providing credentials.

- **Unattended Installation**   Using the /qb option with the installation syntax for the MSI package, administrators can force an unattended installation to the Outlook client.

- **Administrative Installation Points**   As with other options, remote location and alternate location can be defined to support client pushes over slower connections.

Configuring the SMS Package for an Unattended Installation

Using the property pages of the MSI package file used with Systems Management Server to deploy Outlook clients, administrators can define the options to be used and how the package will be installed.

In this scenario, you configure the basic installation package for an unattended installation with Microsoft Systems Management Server:

1. Select the Outlook MSI file and open the Programs property page. Modify the Installer package properties by adding the command-line switch /**qn**, as shown in Figure 28.6.

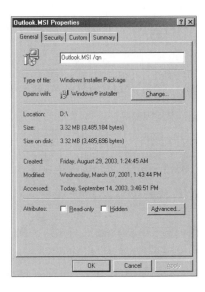

FIGURE 28.6   MSI general properties.

2. To complete configuring the unattended installation for the MSI package, click the Environment tab and uncheck the User Input Required option.

NOTE

To add a PRF file for use the with the SMS package, add this command:

`/ImportPRF \\`*`Outlook Files`*`\Outlook.PRF`

after the /qn switch (where *Outlook Files* represents the share location where the packages can be found).

Now that the installation package has been prepared, Microsoft Systems Management Server can be configured to push Microsoft Outlook clients to the desktop.

Managing Post-Deployment Tasks

Overall, without deployment and management software such as Systems Management Server, administrators are very limited in options for managing and validating Outlook client deployments. In this section, you review methods and functionality of Exchange

28

Server 2003 that can be leveraged to help determine the overall success of the deployment and troubleshoot common deployment issues.

Validating Successful Installations

When SMS is not available for managing and determining the success of the Outlook client deployments, administrators must use the standard tools and functionality available with Windows Server and Exchange Server 2003. Administrators can use several methods to review and validate client installation and ensure that the client can authenticate after the Outlook client is deployed into the production environment.

Review the following options to determine methods and tricks that can assist in validating Outlook client functionality after the deployment is complete:

- Installations can be validated by reviewing the Application Event Logs of the client systems and identifying MSI Installer events that are written into the Event Logs.

- On the local machine, view Add/Remove programs to see whether the Outlook update package is listed.

- Use the Logon page of the Exchange Mail Store to view and document Successful Client Logons and access to Exchange 2003 Mailboxes.

- Enable Diagnostic Logging on the Exchange 2003 server properties page to monitor MSExchangeIS events at the Mailbox activity when deploying clients.

Summary

When planning the deployment of Outlook clients, organizations can leverage different options depending on the type of client and the specific client needs identified during the discovery. If you use manual installation or Windows Server 2003 Group Policy and Systems Management Server, extensive planning and testing of Outlook client Transforms and Outlook profiles should be performed prior to deploying clients to the production environment.

Regardless of the deployment method, configuration settings and procedures should be documented and deployments of the Outlook client staged for manageability.

Best Practices

The following are best practices from this chapter:

- Use the Group Policy Management Console (GPMC) to plan and test policies prior to installation, as well as to debug policy problems after implementation.

- The Resultant Set of Policies (RSoP) should be used to analyze policy enforcement.

- Administrators should delegate rights to distribute the management and enforcement of group policies.

- Document configuration settings being applied to Outlook Transform and PRF files.

- With Microsoft Systems Management Server (SMS), inventories can be conducted on network desktop systems to identify hardware and software installed on each.

- The installation of Outlook 2003 also requires Microsoft Internet Explorer 5.01 or higher.

- To enhance functionality when using Windows Server 2003 Group Policy, download and install the Microsoft Group Policy Management Console (GPMC) from Microsoft.

- Use the Logon page of the Exchange Mail Store to view and document Successful Client Logons and access to Exchange 2003 Mailboxes.

- Enable Diagnostic Logging on the Exchange 2003 server properties page to monitor `MSExchangeIS` events at the Mailbox activity when deploying clients.

28

Group Policy Management for Exchange Clients

To further enhance the management features and options available with Exchange 2003 clients, Microsoft has developed new features and tools. These new enhancements enable client configuration and options to be managed and pushed to client systems using Windows Group Policies.

Using Windows Group Policy management tools, administrators can easily and inexpensively centralize many of the duties and support tasks previously demanding time and resources when working with Exchange clients. With Windows Group Policies, tools and resources available on the Office 2003 Resource Kit (ORK), Exchange client settings— and more—can be configured centrally and applied to Exchange clients in the enterprise using the Domain Group Policy functionality.

Group policies can provide extremely powerful administration and management support methods to desktops and Exchange clients. This chapter provides insight to the resources, available options, and best practices, as well as the techniques available to minimize administrative overhead and support Exchange 2003 client systems.

Administrators can leverage the information in this chapter to support the day-to-day tasks involved with managing Exchange 2003 client systems and users using Windows Group Policy. The new tools enable administrators to centrally manage Outlook and Outlook preferences, and customize the look and feel of Outlook and additional options by using only Windows Group Policy and policy security templates.

Understanding Group Policy Management with Outlook

One of the most powerful tools administrators have—Group Policy with Windows Server 2000 and now Windows Server 2003—has become an even more comprehensive part of the network environment and enterprise management strategy.

Group Policy functionality is used to deliver a standard set of security, controls, rules, and options to a user and workstation when authenticating to the domain. In addition, it can be used to configure everything from login scripts and folder redirection to enabling desktop features and preventing users from installing software on network workstations. With Exchange Server 2003 and the Outlook client, Group Policy can be used to control the preferences and options available when configuring and customizing the Outlook client.

This section helps Exchange administrators understand Group Policy and its functionality and characteristics when they manage the enforcement of policies.

Managing Group Policies

To manage Group Policy, administrators must understand that group policies apply only to Windows 2000 Professional, Windows XP, Windows Server 2000, and Windows Server 2003 server machines.

To access and manage Windows group policies, administrators can use the Group Policy snap-in available in the Administrative Tools program group of the Windows domain controller. Another, more powerful option for managing group policies with Windows Server is the additional tool available from Microsoft called the Group Policy Management Console GPMC for Windows Server 2003.

With the basic Group Policy Management snap-in, administrators are provided a standard management console through the built-in administrative tools of Windows server. Through the standard method of accessing Group Policy, administrators are provided a single interface to access, manage and configure policies with the standard options and functionality available in the built-in Windows tools.

The second option, the GPMC is the new tool available from Microsoft for configuring and using Group Policy with Windows Server 2003. Using the GPMC, administrators are provided with a handy tool to manage group policies with all the standard options available with the Administrative Tools built-in Management snap-in. In addition, the GPMC provides enhanced functionality and options for planning and testing Group Policy implementations prior to deploying and enforcing them on the Windows domain.

GPMC in Windows 2000 Domains

To manage Group Policy using the GPMC tool in a Windows 2000 domain, the GPMC must be installed on a Windows XP desktop on the domain being managed.

The GPMC must be installed on Windows Server 2003 or Windows XP. The `GPMC.msi` package can be downloaded from the `http://www.microsoft.com/Windowsserver2003/downloads/featurepacks/default.mspx` Web site. Search for `GPMC.msi` and download the tools. After it is installed, it can be found in the Start menu in the Administrative Tools program group by selecting the Group Policy Management option.

> **CAUTION**
>
> Because Group Policy can cause tremendous impact on users, any Group Policy implementation should be tested with the Using Resultant Set of Policies (RSoP) tool in planning mode. See the section entitled "Working with Resultant Set of Policies (RSoP)" later in this chapter to learn more about testing Group Policy and using the Group Policy Management tool in Simulation mode.

Understanding Policies and Preferences

When working with group policies, you have two methods for making changes on the local workstations: using preferences and using policies. With both preferences and policies, changes are applied and enforced using the local Registry of the machine where they are being applied.

With preferences, changes to options such as wallpaper or screensavers and software settings are applied locally. With policies, changes to the Registry are applied that affect security and Registry keys, which are protected by Access Control Lists (ACLs).

Although Group Policy overrides preference settings when working with applications, the policy does not overwrite the preference keys when preferences are set on the local system by the workstation users. This means that if a policy is created and configured, the policy is removed, and the preferences that were set by the local user before the policy was applied will return.

This makes policies a powerful tool when a network's administrator wants to control certain aspects of a client application or wants something the user accesses to remain static. Policies can be used to disable end-users from changing the appearance, configuration, or functionality of the item to which the policy was applied.

Group Policy Templates

One of the most important features for minimizing administration when working with Group Policy is leveraging security templates. Security templates are a powerful predefined set of security options available from Microsoft for applying group policy to a specific area or software component available to users on the network. Based on the type of users and environment needed, these templates can be a handy tool to create and enforce configuration settings on components already predefined in the template.

Not available with the standard installation of Windows Server 2000 and Windows Server 2003, these templates can be downloaded and imported into Group Policy Objects (GPOs)

29

where they can then either be implemented as is, or modified to meet the specific needs of the area in which the template applies. However templates are used, they are a great starting point for network administrators to obtain a base-level configuration of a client workstation's software components or security settings.

Templates can also be used to configure settings such as account policies, event log settings, local policies, Registry permissions, file and folder permissions, and Exchange Server 2003 client settings.

Defining the Order of Application

When applying Group Policy, each policy object is applied in a specific order. Computers and users whose accounts are lower in the AD tree may inherit policies applied at different levels within the Active Directory. Policies should be applied to Active Directory in the following order:

1. Local Security Policy

2. Site GPOs

3. Domain GPOs

4. OU GPOs

5. Nested OU GPOs on down until the OU at which the computer or user is a member has been reached

If multiple GPOs are applied to a specific AD object—such as a site or OU—they are applied in the reverse order from which they are listed. This means that the last GPO listed is applied first and if conflicts exist, settings in higher GPOs override those in lower ones.

Group Policy Refresh Intervals

When Group Policy is applied, the policy is refreshed and enforced at regularly scheduled intervals after a computer has been booted and a user has logged onto the domain. By default, Group Policy is refreshed every 90 minutes on workstation and member servers within the domain.

When you need to better control the refresh interval of a group policy, the refresh interval can be configured for each group policy by changing its time in the policy configuration. Using the GPMC, refresh intervals can be configured by going to domain policy and selecting the following:

- Computer Configuration, Administrative Templates, System, Group Policy (to change the interval for computer policies and domain controllers)

- User Configuration, Administrative Templates, System, Group Policy (to change the interval for user policies)

Changes made to existing GPOs or new GPOs being created are enforced when the refresh cycle runs. However, with the following settings, policies are enforced only at login or when booting a workstation to the domain, depending on the GPO configuration settings:

- Software installation configured in the Computer Policies

- Software installation configured in the User Policies

> **NOTE**
>
> When working with application settings, refresh intervals can be configured and customized to fit the environment needs. You should leave the refresh interval as the default, however, unless requirements call them to be modified.

Baseline Administration for Group Policy Deployment

Now that you have a base understanding of functionality and terminology of Group Policy, you can look at usage and how the configuration of group policies can vary greatly with each individual implementation.

Administrators can use this information to understand the more common methods of applying permissions to Group Policy for management purposes and the tools for testing Group Policy implementations prior to deployment in the production environment.

> **NOTE**
>
> In this section, some best practices for managing Group Policy are covered. For more information and details regarding Group Policy management, view the help information for managing Group Policy with Windows Server 2000 and Windows Server 2003.

Delegating GP Management Rights

It is important to delegate the proper rights for administrators to manage and manipulate Group Policy. For example, in larger organizations a very small group of users normally has permission to edit policies at the domain level. However, when specific requirements are needed to administer applications such as the Exchange client, permissions can be granted to specific areas with the Group Policy Management Console.

When creating specific permissions with the GPMC, administrators can delegate control for other administrators to manage the following areas within Group Policy:

- Create GPOs

- Create WMI filters

- Permissions on WMI filters

- Permissions to read and edit an individual GPO

- Permissions on individual locations to which the GPO is linked, called the scope of management (SOM)

To easily assign permissions to GPOs, administrators can use the Delegation Wizard.

Working with Resultant Set of Policies (RSoP)

The new GPMC provides administrators with a powerful tool for planning and testing Group Policy implementations prior to enforcing them on domain workstations and users. Using the RSoP tool in planning mode, administrators can simulate the deployment of a specified group policy, evaluate the results of the test, make changes as needed, and then test the deployment again. After RSoP shows that the GPO is correct, the administrator can then back up the GPO configuration and import it into production.

To run RSoP in simulation mode, right-click on Group Policy Modeling in the forest that will be simulated, and choose Group Policy Modeling Wizard. The wizard enables you to input slow links, loop-back configuration, WMI filters, and other configuration choices. Each model is presented in its own report as a subnode under the Group Policy Modeling node.

> **TIP**
>
> Because errors in Group Policy settings can impact users and client server connectivity, any Group Policy implementation should be tested using the RSoP tool in planning mode before applying the policy.

Managing Group Policy Inheritance

In order to maximize the inheritance feature of Group Policy, keep the following in mind:

- Isolate the servers in their own OU: Create descriptive Server OUs and place all the non–domain controller servers in those OUs under a common Server OU. If software pushes are applied through Group Policy on the domain level or on a level above the Server OU and do not have the Enforcement option checked, the Server OU can be configured with Block Policy Inheritance checked. As a result, the servers won't receive software pushes applied at levels above their OU.

- Use Block Policy Inheritance and Enforcement sparingly to make troubleshooting Group Policy less complex.

Group Policy Backup, Restore, Copy, and Import

One new major improvement to Group Policy management offers the ability to back-up (or export) the Group Policy data to a file. Using the backup functionality of the GPMC, any policy can be tested in a lab environment and then exported to a file for deployment in the production domain.

When backing up Group Policy, you back up only data specific to that GP itself. Other Active Directory objects that can be linked to GPOs, such as individual WMI filters and TCP/IP security policies, are not backed up, because of complications with restores when working with these specific areas. When backup is completed, administrators can restore the Group Policy data in the same location, restoring proper functionality to misconfigured and accidentally deleted group policies.

The import functionality of the GPMC also enables administrators to take an exported Group Policy file and import the Group Policy data into a different location from its original one. This functionality is true even in scenarios where no trust exists between domains.

Imports of Group Policy files can be completed using files from different domains, across forest domains, or within the same domain. This functionality is most powerful when you move a GPO from a test lab into production without having to manually re-create the policy setting tested in the lab environment.

Another helpful function of Group Policy Management is copying GPOs. If the administrator has configured a complex group policy and applied the setting to a specific organizational unit (OU) in the domain, the group policy can be copied and duplicated for application to another OU. When using the copy function, a new group policy is created. This new policy can then be placed and applied to the new location.

Outlook Client Group Policies

With a baseline understanding of how Group Policy functions in a Windows Active Directory Domain environment, Microsoft Exchange 2003 administrators can look at how Group Policy, GPOs, and security templates can be leveraged to enhance the ability of Management Exchange Outlook 2003 clients in the enterprise.

An all-in-one solution, Exchange administrators can also use the Group Policy function to create Administrative Distribution Points for pushing client software to the desktops. Working with predefined Group Policy templates available from Microsoft, administrators can now manage areas and control access and changes, ranging from restrictions and preventing configuration modifications to controlling the look and feel that affects the overall user experience when working with the Exchange Outlook 2003 client software.

In this section, you review the tools and options for managing the Exchange Outlook 2003 clients, specifically using Group Policy and predefined templates. You explore the options available with Group Policy when deploying and working with the Outlook client, Outlook Group Policy templates, and the steps for configuring administration privileges for managing the Exchange client through Group Policy.

29

Exchange Client Policy Options

To further enhance the management functionality when working with Exchange Outlook 2003 clients, the ORK now provides a predefined security template for managing Outlook clients using the Group Policy functionality of Windows domains.

Called Outlk11.adm, this template enables administrators to centrally manage and configure many of the security functions and preferences normally required to be configured at each individual Outlook client. Using Outlk11.adm, administrators can fully manage and configure the following areas:

- **Outlook Preferences**   The preferences options available with the security templates can be defined in the same manner as using the Options tab available in the Tools menu of the Outlook client. When defining preferences, administrators can control the standard look and feel of each component available with Outlook. Options include areas for enforcing items such as spell check and email format, calendaring views, and contacts options.

- **Exchange Settings**   Configuration items, such as profile configurations and auto archiving, can now be centrally configured.

- **SharePoint Portal Server Settings**   In addition to the Outlook client settings, using the templates enables administrators to configure access to SharePoint Portal server resources through the Outlook client.

Though the Outlk11.adm template enables you to configure many import options and preferences with the Outlook 2003 Exchange clients, not all areas are available with the template.

Adding the Outlook Administrative Template

Because the additional administrative templates are not configured by default when Windows Server 2003 is installed, administrators must download or install the Administrative Outlook Template manually. Available on the ORK, the Outlk11.adm is placed on the local drive of the systems where the ORK is installed.

To begin setting up the Outlook security template Outlk11.adm, start by installing the GPMC on the domain controller where the policy will be administered.

Next install the Microsoft ORK on a system where the template can be accessed from a domain controller for import into the Domain Group Policy.

> **TIP**
>
> To download the GPMC from Microsoft, go to
>
> http://www.microsoft.com/windowsserver2003/downloads/default.mspx
>
> The Office 2003 Resource Kit (ORK) can be downloaded from the Microsoft Office Web site at
>
> http://www.office.microsoft.com/home/default.aspx

After the ORK is installed, the `Outlk11.adm` file is automatically extracted and placed in the `C:\Windows\Inf` directory (where `C:` represents the drive where the Windows installation resides) on the local system drive where the ORK was installed.

To import the Outlook security template `Outlk11.adm` into the Domain Group Policy using the Group Policy Management Tool, use the following steps:

> **TIP**
>
> When importing the `Outlk11.adm` security template, it is best practice to import the template to the Default Domain Group Policy.

1. From a domain controller in the domain where the policy will be applied, open the Group Policy snap-in by selecting Start, All Programs, Administrative Tools, Group Policy Management.

2. Select the location Default Domain Policy where `Outlk11.adm` will be imported to, as shown in Figure 29.1.

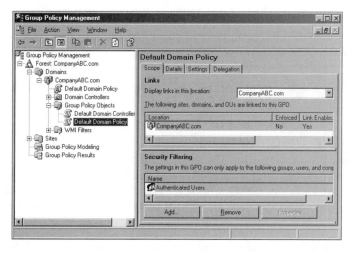

FIGURE 29.1   Group Policy Management Console.

3. From the Action menu select Edit; this opens the Group Policy Object Editor window.

4. On the Group Policy Object Editor, select Administrative Templates under the User Configuration option and right-click to choose Add/Remove Templates, as shown in Figure 29.2.

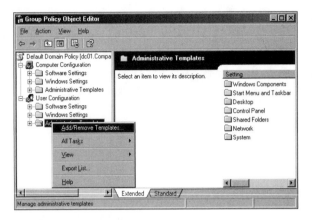

FIGURE 29.2   Group Policy Object Editor.

5. From the Add/Remove Templates dialog box, click the Add button.

6. Navigate to the location where `Outlk11.adm` was placed, as noted in step 2. Select the template to import OUTLK11.ADM and click the Open button.

7. Ensure that the OUTLK11 template has added the Add/Remove Templates dialog box, and click Close to continue.

You should now see the Microsoft Outlook 2003 template under the Administrative Templates folder in the Group Policy Editor.

Assigning Group Policy Delegates

Although Group Policy has traditionally been the management task of Windows domain administrators, with delegation, permissions can be assigned to additional resources and accounts to manage Exchange 2003 Outlook clients. Using the Delegation Wizard of the GPMC, accounts can assign and delegate rights to add, modify, and delete Group Policy Objects.

It is important to delegate the proper rights for administrators to manipulate the Microsoft Outlook 2003 Group Policy. Using the delegation option of the GPMC, administrators can assign a very small group of users permission to edit Outlook policies at the domain level. To enhance this functionality, it is also possible to allow diverse groups of administrators to configure group policies at lower levels of the Active Directory domain tree.

When assigning permissions, administrators can delegate the following rights:

- Create GPO
- Create WMI filters
- Permissions on WMI filters

- Permissions to read, edit, and so forth an individual GPO

- Permissions on individual locations to which the GPO is linked (SOM)

Using the Group Policy Delegation Wizard makes it easy to give the appropriate groups of administrators the rights they need to do their job and continue to administer Windows Server 2003 in the most secure way possible.

How to Delegate Rights over GPOs

To understand the steps required to assign rights over GPOs, let's look at the following scenario to assign one Active Directory account permission at the domain level. The rights that will be assigned to the account will be the Edit Group Policy Objects Only permissions.

To begin, open the GPMC by selecting Start, All Programs, Administrative Tool, Group Policy Management. Then follow these steps:

1. On the GPMC, select Domain Folder, Your Domain, Group Policy Objects, Default Domain Policy.

2. Select the Delegation tab in the right pane of the Domain Group Policy Object.

3. To add an account, select the Add button, enter the name of the account to be added, and click the OK button.

4. Select the rights to be assigned to the account by selecting the permission Edit in the drop-down box, as shown in Figure 29.3; select OK to continue.

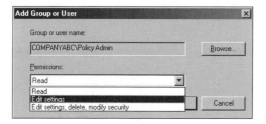

FIGURE 29.3   Add Group or User permissions.

The account has now been assigned rights to edit the domain-level GPO. Review the information and test settings to ensure that the permissions have been applied correctly.

Managing Group Policy Configurations

Through Group Policy, Outlook configuration settings can be configured and applied differently depending on how the GPO is applied.

Exchange administrators can not only centrally manage one group of Exchange 2003 Outlook clients, but they can configure and apply a completely different set of options enforced on a different group or OU in the domain by following these steps:

1. Open the GPMC and select the organizational unit to which to apply the GPO.

2. Select Action from the menu bar and select Link an Existing GPO.

3. From the Select GPO dialog box, choose the domain policy and click OK to link the domain policy to the desired organizational unit.

> **TIP**
>
> When linking the GPOs, access to the GPMC can be obtained through the Active Directory Users and Computers (ADUC) snap-in. Select the properties of the domain you are working with and select the Group Policy tab.

Administering Outlook Through Group Policy

One option not available with previous Outlook versions is the ability to centrally manage Outlook options and preferences. With the new Outlook Group Policy security template, administrators can centrally manage Outlook configuration and settings through group policies that require a visit to each Outlook client desktop in the past.

> **Configuring Profiles**
>
> Though there are many options and configuration choices using the Outlk11.ADM security template, one option not available is setting the profile information for Exchange 2003 Outlook clients.
>
> To configure client profile information and settings, see Chapter 28, "Deploying the Client for Microsoft Exchange."

Defining Baseline Outlook Preferences

One option that group policies enable organizations to accomplish when managing Exchange 2003 Outlook client is the ability to design, develop, and implement a baseline configuration for every Outlook client to use. Often this was not an option because of the exhaustive amount of administration involved, along with the inability to secure configurations from being modified.

With the option of standardizing configuration for all Outlook client systems, administrators must wonder which options can be configured to improve the productivity and functionality of the Exchange client for every user. Using the Group Policy Object settings to define simple Outlook configuration settings—such as Saving Sent Items, Spell Checking

Messages Before Sending, and Auto Archive Settings can not only improve the functionality of the Outlook client, but can also reduce administrative management overhead when supporting workstations and users.

Email Options

Some of the most useful email options available when configuring settings using Group Policy include

- **HTML/Microsoft Word Message Format**   The most enhanced of all Outlook Email Options is the HTML/Microsoft Word format. This option can be enabled to provide a robust email editor.

- **Junk Email Filtering**   Enabling the Junk Email option allows the configuration of filtering email at the client level.

- **OST/PST Creation**   Disabling or enabling the OST and PST options can provide control of network traffic and local system disk space utilization.

- **Empty Deleted Items Folder**   Controlling the total amount of space each user mailbox can grow helps control storage limits; administrators can enable this option.

- **Auto Archiving**   One area often requiring administrative overhead, the Auto Archive option can now be toggled via GPO settings.

- **Email Accounts**   Using this option, users can be prevented from adding additional account types.

Calendaring Options

In addition to the Email Option available, the following calendaring options can be defined to establish a base functionality for all Domain Outlook users;

- **Reminders Display Options**   Calendar Reminders can be disabled and enabled.

- **Working Hours and Work Week**   These options can be defined and set for all calendar views.

Contact Options

One interesting setting is the option in the Outlook security template for contacts. Administrators can define how each contact will be filed and displayed. For example, the Display Name can be set as First, [Middle], Last Name, and the File As option for the contact as Last, First.

There are many options available when configuring the Outlook client. Review the options and descriptions for each before applying settings and changes to the Outlook Group Policy Objects.

29

Managing the Look and Feel of the Exchange Client

Another powerful function of using group policies is the ability for an administrator to define the look and feel of the Outlook client. Administrators can now configure options to create a specific look and feel when using Outlook.

Group Policy preferences can be defined to customize the look of the Exchange 2003 Outlook Client. Options can be set to allow users access to information Web sites and SharePoint Portal Server Sites, providing an enhanced user experience and data access option not previously available.

Web Options Overview

Using the Preferences options of the GPO, settings can be defined to integrate and redirect Outlook users to valuable Web data using technologies such as Microsoft SharePoint Portal and Internet Information Services:

- **Custom Outlook Today**   Administrators can use the URL for Custom Outlook Today Properties settings to define a Web page that will be viewed when users access the Outlook Today home page.

- **Folder Home Pages Settings**   Each Outlook folder can now be redirected to a predefined Web page.

- **Share Point Portal Server**   With Outlook 2003 and Group Policy preferences, support to integrate SharePoint with Outlook can easily be enabled and disabled.

Configuring and Applying Outlook Group Policy Settings

With all the information gathered in the previous sections, administrators can now apply settings and configuration options using the GPMC and Outlook 2003 security template. To better understand the settings for applying a group policy, review the following mock installation scenario.

In this scenario, you create and apply a standard set of preferences to create an Exchange 2003 Outlook client baseline configuration for one OU in the Active Directory domain. As described earlier, one additional setting is applied to redirect the client's Outlook Today setting and direct users to a company Internet home page.

To begin, open the GPMC by selecting Start, All Programs, Administrative Tools, Group Policy Management; then follow these steps:

1. Select the Default Domain Policy by selecting Forest, Domains, YourCompanydomain, Group Policy Objects.

2. Select the Default Domain Policy, click Action from the GPMC menu, and click Edit. This opens the Group Policy Editor.

3. Select Administrative Templates under the User Configuration and select the Microsoft Outlook 2003 folder.

From this point, you can begin to enable options and apply preferences to the GPO. After options are enabled, they appear in the GPMC to be tested through RSoP and applied to the OU. In this scenario, you apply the HTML/Microsoft Word email editor options and redirect the Outlook Today page to point to a Web page called www.CompanyABC.com. To apply these settings, complete these steps:

1. Select the Microsoft Outlook 2003 folder and select Tools, Options, Mail Format, Message Format.

2. Double-click Message Format Editor in the right pane to open and configure the Message Format Policy settings.

3. As shown in Figure 29.4, select Enabled Option and click HTML/Microsoft Word in the drop-down box. Select OK to continue.

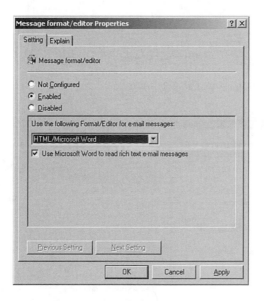

FIGURE 29.4   Message Format Editor properties.

4. Next, select the Outlook Today folder by selecting Microsoft Outlook 2003, Outlook Today.

5. Double-click URL for Custom Outlook Today Properties in the right pane.

6. To enable the redirection of the Outlook Today Home Page, click the Enable button and enter the URL to be displayed, as shown in Figure 29.5. Click OK when finished.

7. Open the GPMC and confirm that the settings are ready to be applied. From the GPMC, select Default Domain Policy and ensure that the Outlook settings appear as shown in Figure 29.6.

29

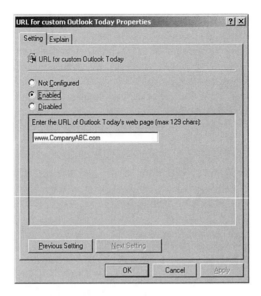

FIGURE 29.5   Custom Outlook Today properties.

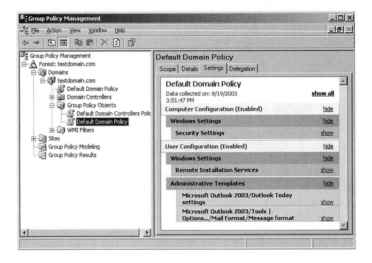

FIGURE 29.6   GPMC Outlook settings.

Now that the Group Policy options have been configured, you apply the settings to a group of users in the domain by following these steps:

1. To apply the settings to a group, click the Add button under Security Filtering in the right pane of the Default Domain Policy.

2. From the Select Users, Computers, or Groups search page, enter the name of the group the settings will be applied to and click OK.

3. Check to see whether the group has been added to the Security Filtering pane.

When the configuration is completed, it is good practice to back up the configuration and ensure that all the settings are enabled on the GPO by selecting Action/GPO Status.

Updates and Patch Management with Group Policies

One other advantage to group policies is the centralized deployment options available to distribute the Exchange 2003 Outlook client updates and patches. With Group Policy and the Microsoft MSI installation package format available with most updates, the Microsoft Outlook 2003 client installation software updates can be deployed from the centralized administrative distribution point to a predefined set of workstations configured in the GPO settings.

Deployment Options When Updating Exchange Clients

Using Group Policy, the Outlook client can be upgraded and patched using one of the three following deployment methods:

- **Assigned to Computers** This method of installation uses the Outlook Installation package on the workstation and is available when the workstation is restarted. Using this option, all users have access to the Exchange client software after it is installed.

- **Assigned to Users** When the installation package is assigned to users, Application Shortcuts are placed on the desktop of the user's profile and on the Start menu. When these shortcuts are selected, the application installation will be completed.

> **TIP**
>
> When using the Assigned Application options for both users and computers only, when a package is uninstalled, Group Policy automatically reassigns the installation to the user or computer.

- **Publishing the Installation** This is the most common method of deploying software updates to client systems. When a software package is published, the installation package is displayed in the Add/Remove Programs Group in the local desktop system control panel. Users can then initiate the installation by selecting the update.

Each method enables Exchange 2003 administrators to push MSI software update packages to the Outlook 2003 client from a central location or Administrative Installation Point, to the workstation or users on the network.

29

> **CAUTION**
>
> Do not assign the option to install updates to Users and Computers at the same time. Assigning both options can create conflict to how updates are installed and possibly corrupt the installation of the Outlook client when applying the update.

Deploying Client Updates

As with all aspects of Group Policy, the choices and configuration options of deployment updates are numerous. Regardless of which type of update package is being pushed, some basic best practices apply and can help make updates easier and less troublesome:

- Software packages must be in the format of an MSI package. Any other format type than an MSI cannot be pushed using Group Policy. Using third-party applications can help the administrator create customized MSI packages to deploy any type of software as well as software with predefined installation choices.

- Configure software pushes at the highest levels possible in the domain. If the push is going out to more than one group or organizational unit, the software update should be configured to be pushed at the domain level. If the software update is being pushed to only a few groups or one organizational unit, or if multiple update packages are being pushed, configure the push at the group or organizational unit level.

- Configure software pushes to the Computers Configuration rather than the User Configuration. This way, if users log into multiple computer systems, updates are not applied more than once.

- When pushing updates in multiple locations, use a technology such as Distributed File System (DFS) so software installations are installed from packages and sources close to the client being updated.

Pushing Client Updates

With the options available and a good understanding of the best practices for deploying software, the next step is to configure a GPO to push an update to the Outlook client. The steps in this scenario enable administrators to push a small update package to the Exchange 2003 Outlook client workstations on the domain.

Begin by downloading the update and creating a share on the folder where the update will be placed. Open the GPMC by selecting Start, All Programs, Administrative Tools, Group Policy Management. Then to create an Outlook Client software update Group Policy Object, follow these steps:

1. Select the Default Domain Policy for your domain by selecting Forest, Domains, YourCompanydomain, Group Policy Objects.

2. Select Default Domain Policy, click Action, and click Edit. This opens the Group Policy Editor to create the software push.

3. Select Computer Configuration and select Software settings, Software Installation.

4. From the Action menu, select New, Package.

5. Navigate the Open dialog to the network share where the MSI was placed and select the MSI package being applied. Select Open to continue.

> **TIP**
>
> If prompted that the Group Policy Editor cannot verify the network location, ensure that the share created earlier in these steps has permissions allowing users access to the share. Select Yes to continue after confirmed.

6. At the Deploy Software dialog box, select Advance and click OK to continue. Windows will verify the installation package; wait for the verification to complete before continuing to the next step.

7. When the Package is visible in the right window of the software installation properties, highlight the install package and click Action, Properties.

8. On the Package properties page, select the Deployment tab. Review the configuration, click Assign, and ensure that the Install this Package at Logon option is selected, as shown in Figure 29.7. Select OK when complete.

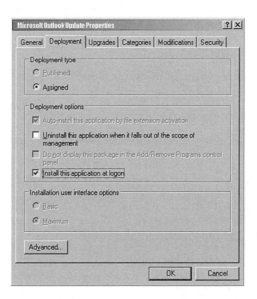

FIGURE 29.7 Outlook Update properties.

The new package is ready to deploy; test the update by logging on to a workstation and verifying that the packaged has installed. If problems exist, redeploy the package by selecting the software update and clicking Action, All Tasks, Redeploy Application to force the deployment.

Determining the Success of a Push

Without additional management software, administrators cannot determine whether a software package was pushed successfully, because all evidence of software pushes are seen locally on the client machines. On the local machines, there are two areas to check to determine whether a software installation was successful:

- Look for MSI Installer events that are written into the Application Event Logs.

- On the local machine, view Add/Remove programs to see whether the Outlook update package is listed.

Summary

Group policies can be leveraged to help Exchange administrators manage client connections and configurations to Exchange. Rather than accessing every user profile, configuration, or Outlook property, group policies can be enabled that centralize the administration and management of the client software. With new tools in Windows Server 2003 that provide better management of group policies, administrators can simplify their tasks while expanding on the capabilities of the client access to Exchange. From simple Outlook client preference changes to performing client software installation and patch management, group policies can be of significant help to administrators of organizations of any size.

Best Practices

The following are best practices from this chapter:

- Use the Group Policy Management Console (GPMC) to plan and test policies prior to installation, as well as to debug policy problems after implementation.

- Use the Resultant Set of Policies (RSoP) to analyze policy enforcement.

- Administrators should delegate rights to distribute the management and enforcement of group policies.

- Limit the use of the Block Policy Inheritance option to minimize the administrative tasks of group policy management.

- Use the Outlk11.adm template file from the Office 2003 Resource Kit (ORK) to improve administrative capabilities of Office 2003.

- When importing the Outlk11.adm security template, import the template to the Default Domain Group Policy.

- Use group policies to manage the look and feel of the Outlook client.

- Do not assign the option to install updates to Users and Computers at the same time. Assigning both options can create conflict about how updates are installed and corrupt the installation of the Outlook client when applying the update.

PART X

Fault Tolerance and Optimization Technologies

IN THIS PART

CHAPTER 30

System-level Fault Tolerance (Clustering/Network Load Balancing)

Using Microsoft Windows 2003 Cluster Service (MSCS) and Network Load Balancing (NLB) technologies, organizations can provide Exchange 2003 Server messaging systems with high-level availability and performance to improve network reliability in areas such as system uptime, Quality of Service (QOS), and recovery speed.

Using clustering, load balancing, and the Automatic System Recovery (ASR) functionality of Windows Server 2003, administrators can effectively provide enhanced reliability for Exchange Server 2003 in areas such as recovering from CPU failures, memory problems, hardware controller failures, and entire Exchange 2003 server failures.

In addition, clustering technologies, when used with Exchange Server 2003, can also be used to detect problems in the Exchange server application configurations and might be able to recover from them by restarting the application or failing over the application to another node in the cluster.

In this chapter, administrators can review and understand the options available for designing and implementing system-level fault tolerance using Windows 2003 clusters and Windows 2003 NLB with Exchange Server 2003.

Clustering and Load Balancing with Exchange 2003 Server

Supported only with the Microsoft Windows 2003 Enterprise Server and DataCenter Editions, Windows 2003 fault-tolerant options such as clustering and load balancing provide Exchange mailbox clients with high availability and performance when accessing Exchange 2003 messaging systems.

This section provides information to assist administrators in understanding the functionality of Exchange 2003 in Windows 2003 clusters and NLB, environment features available with each, and best practices for determining which solution best fits your Exchange 2003 server needs.

Clustering Terminology

Before deciding which fault-tolerant option is best, here are a few terms used to describe the way clustered Exchange 2003 servers operate:

- **Active/Active**   In Active/Active clustering, all servers in the cluster are servicing clients at the same time. Active/Active is also referred to as **shared everything architecture**.

- **Active/Passive**   In Active/Passive clustering, only one server in the cluster can service end-users per application while the other server(s) wait until a failure occurs before they begin to service clients. Active/Passive clustering is also referred to as **shared nothing architecture**.

- **Exchange Virtual Server**   An Exchange virtual server is the resource group that contains all resources for Exchange to operate on the cluster. This includes the Exchange Services, IP Address, and NetBIOS name of the server. To enable Active/Active clustering on a 2-node cluster, one Exchange virtual server is created per node in the cluster. If only one Exchange virtual server was installed then the server would be operating in Active/Passive mode. The NetBIOS name and IP address of the cluster form the virtual server. When failover occurs, the entire Exchange virtual server fails over to the surviving node in the cluster.

- **Resource DLL or `Exres.dll`**   Exres.dll is the gateway that handles the communication from the cluster service to the Exchange services. It is responsible for reporting failures and bringing resources online and offline.

- **Heartbeat**   A single UDP packet sent every 500 milliseconds between nodes in the cluster across the private network relays information on the health of the nodes in the cluster and on the health of the application. If there is no response, the cluster will begin a failover.

- **Failover**   Failover is the process of a node in the cluster taking over responsibility for the applications on another node.

- **Failback**   Failback is the process of moving applications that failed over to another node in the cluster back to the original node.

- **Quorum Resource**   This is the shared disk that holds the cluster server's configuration information. All servers must be able to contact the quorum resource to join the cluster.

- **Resource Group**   A resource group is a collection of Cluster Resources. A resource group defines which items fail over to a surviving server during failover. This includes Cluster Resource items such as IP address and Net BIOS name. A resource group is owned by only one node in the cluster at a time. The resource group Cluster Group is the first resource group created on the server and contains the IP Address and Net BIOS name of the cluster.

- **Cluster Resource**   Cluster Resources are IP Addresses, Net BIOS name, disks, or services—such as the Exchange System Attendant. Cluster Resources are added to Cluster Groups to form Exchange virtual servers.

- **Dependency**   Dependencies are specified when creating the Cluster Resources. A Cluster Resource that is specified as a dependency means that before a cluster Resource is brought online, whatever resources it's dependent on must be brought online first. For instance, a Net BIOS name is dependent on the IP Address; therefore, the IP Address must be brought online before the Net BIOS name can be brought online.

Fault-Tolerance Options

MSCS and NLB services support Exchange 2003 messaging by establishing QOS when supporting server availability with back-end Exchange 2003 servers and high performance when supporting Outlook Web Access front-end systems. For these fault-tolerant clustering technologies to be truly effective, administrators must understand the characteristics of each in order to choose which technology and configuration best fits their Exchange 2003 Server design and messaging application service needs.

Microsoft Cluster Service

The Microsoft Windows 2003 Cluster Service (MSCS) is a clustering technology that provides system-level fault tolerance by using failover. In Microsoft Exchange 2003 Server environments, cluster services are best used to provide access to mailbox information, Exchange 2003 resources such as public folders, and add-on applications such as virus wall systems and Internet mail bridgehead servers.

When a problem is encountered with a Cluster Resource, the cluster service attempts to fix the problem before failing it completely. The cluster node running the failing resource attempts to restart the resource on the same node first. If the resource cannot be restarted, the cluster fails the resource, takes the cluster group offline, and moves it to another available node, where it can then be restarted.

Several conditions can cause a cluster group to fail over. Failover can occur when an active node in the cluster loses power or network connectivity or suffers a hardware failure. When a Cluster Resource cannot remain available on an active node, the resource's group is moved to an available node, where it can then be restarted.

30

> **NOTE**
>
> In most cases, client communications can be affected by the failover process causing a short disruption in client/server communications. In some cases there may be no disruption.

Cluster nodes can monitor the status of resources running on their local system, and they can also keep track of other nodes in the cluster through private network communication messages (heartbeats). The heartbeats are used to determine the status of a node and send updates of cluster configuration changes to the cluster quorum resource.

The quorum resource contains the cluster configuration data necessary to restore a cluster to a working state. Each node in the cluster needs to have access to the quorum resource; otherwise, it will not be able to participate in the cluster. Windows Server 2003 provides three types of quorum resources, one for each cluster configuration model.

To avoid unwanted failover, power management should be disabled on each of the cluster nodes, both in the motherboard BIOS and in the Power applet in the operating system's Control Panel. Power settings that enable a monitor to shut off are okay, but the administrator must make sure that the disks are configured to never go into standby mode.

Network Load Balancing (NLB)

The second clustering technology provided with the Windows Server 2003 Enterprise and DataCenter server platforms is Network Load Balancing (NLB).)NLB clusters provide high network performance and availability by balancing client requests across several server systems. When the client load increases, NLB clusters can easily be scaled out by adding more nodes to the cluster, to maintain or provide better response time to client requests.

Network load balancing offers two great features: No proprietary hardware is needed to use load balancing, and an NLB cluster can be implemented and configured fairly easily and quickly.

NLB clusters are most effectively used to provide front-end support for Web applications. In addition they are very effective solutions when used for application functionality, such as Outlook Web Access and Terminal servers.

NLB clusters can grow to 32 nodes, and if larger cluster farms are necessary, the Microsoft Application Center server should be considered as an option for server platform support, along with technologies such as Domain Name System round-robin to meet this larger demand.

> **NOTE**
>
> When NLB clusters are configured, each server's configuration must be updated independently. The NLB administrator is responsible for making sure that configuration and information changes on each Exchange 2003 server are kept consistent across each node.

For more information on installing load balancing with Exchange 2003 Server, refer to the section "Configuring Network Load Balancing with OWA," later in this chapter.

Cluster Permissions with Exchange 2003 Environments

Unlike previous versions of Exchange server in clustered environments, Exchange Server 2003 does not require the cluster server account to be a Full Exchange Administrator at the Exchange organization or administrative group levels. With Exchange 2003, the account logon permissions are used to establish rights for the Cluster Administrator to manage the Exchange 2003 cluster configurations. Using logon permission, the Cluster Administrator can create, delete, or modify Exchange virtual server configuration, depending on the level in which the permissions are applied and the mode (Mixed or Native) in which clustered Exchange 2003 organization is running.

When working with Exchange 2003 Mixed and Native Mode cluster environments and multidomain models, some common best practices can be applied to help administrators understand how to set permissions to manage the Exchange cluster.

With Windows 2003 multidomain models and child domain configurations, Cluster Administrator accounts require a minimum of Administrator Only permissions at the Exchange organizational level. This permission configuration is required to configure and apply Recipient Policies and configure the responsible server for providing the organization with the proper Recipient Update Services.

In addition, when the Exchange 2003 organization is in Native Mode, if Exchange virtual servers are configured in routing groups and span multiple administrative groups, the Cluster Administrator must have Exchange Full Administrator permissions. This allows the account permissions to manage each administrative group and its Exchange virtual server members.

Management Options with Exchange Server 2003

When running Microsoft Exchange Server 2003 in clustered environments, administrators must implement clusters and load balancing technologies through Windows Server 2003. Microsoft Exchange Server 2003 does not provide any clustering technologies and management options for administering load balancing technologies.

> **Managing Clustering with Exchange**
>
> There are no options for managing clusters and load balancing with Exchange Server 2003. Administrators can leverage the Exchange Server 2003 Windows Management Instrumentation (WMI) to monitor the state of the Exchange Server 2003 Cluster Resources.

Administrators can manage and configure clusters and load balancing options through the Windows 2003 Cluster Administrator snap-in. For more information regarding cluster

30

management and configuration options, see the section "Managing Exchange 2003 Clusters," later in this chapter.

Clusters and Load Balancing Requirements

When installing Exchange Server 2003 in a Windows 2003 clustered configuration, Exchange Server 2003 checks to determine whether the hardware and software prerequisites for installation are met. For a better understanding of the hardware and software requirements involved with installing Exchange Server 2003 in fault-tolerant environments, review the information provided in this section and ensure that the basic requirements are met before attempting to install the Exchange cluster.

Cluster Node Hardware Requirements

When determining the hardware requirements for a cluster server node, administrators must meet the same hardware requirements as are needed for installing Windows 2003 Advanced Server or Windows 2003 DataCenter Server. Each server node to be incorporated in the cluster must meet the minimum hardware requirements for installing the Windows server platform and must also be listed in the Cluster Service Hardware Compatibility List (HCL). To verify that the proposed hardware meets these requirements, go to http:// www.microsoft.com/wwindowsserver2003/technologies/clustering/default.mspx.

When implementing fault-tolerant servers, hardware and hardware configurations on each server should be identical. For example, when installing PCI network cards, each card should be installed in the same slot on each server and have the same settings in the server's configuration properties. This minimizes configuration errors and troubleshooting confusion when the server is implemented as a node in the cluster.

When working with clustering, a single external disk storage cabinet is also required, which will be used to house the shared disks and quorum resource. It's best practice to configure these drives using a RAID level that provides fault tolerance.

The following are requirements for *both nodes* in the cluster:

- A local boot drive containing the Windows 2000 OS, which should be installed on a disk controller that is *not* connected to the shared storage

- Either a SCSI or Fiber Channel PCI host adapter connected to the shared storage

- Two PCI network adapters

Software Requirements

As mentioned earlier, Microsoft Windows 2003 cluster services require either Windows 2003 Enterprise Server or Windows 2003 DataCenter Server Editions. With the Enterprise Server Edition, support from 4-node clusters are provided as is with Windows with DataCenter ServerEdition.

Networking Requirements

Clusters with Windows Server 2003 require five static TCP/IP addresses to be dedicated to the cluster. Two TCP/IP addresses are used for the network adapters on the private network that control communication between the clustered Exchange server nodes, and an additional two are required for the network adapters on the public LAN. An additional IP address is used for the initial Windows 2003 cluster itself, which is the TCP/IP address to which clients connect.

> **NOTE**
>
> An additional IP address is required per Exchange virtual server on the Windows 2003 cluster. Running Exchange server in Active/Active mode requires two Exchange virtual servers. A 2-node Active/Active Exchange Server 2003 cluster requires a total of seven static TCP/IP addresses. For more information about Exchange 2003 virtual servers, review the section "Installing Exchange Server 2003 Clusters," later in this chapter.

As is with servers on the network, the Windows 2003 cluster also requires a NetBIOS name. This is the name that Exchange clients use to connect to the Exchange cluster and the cluster. In addition, each server node must also be configured as members in the same domain; however, they are not required to be members of the same domain from which clients are connecting.

> **CAUTION**
>
> When clustering with Exchange 2003 servers, each node must have two network adapters or NICs. When using clustered configurations like this, do not attempt to assign both the private and public TCP/IP addresses for the cluster nodes to the same network adapter. This configuration can cause instability in the cluster because of the possible disruption of the heartbeat communication between the clustered nodes, and is therefore unsupported by Microsoft technical support.

Shared Storage and Disks Requirements

Review the following information to understand the disk storage requirements, some best practice requirements, and some common best practices when working with clustered disk storage:

- All shared disks must be visible from both nodes. Check with the hardware vendor for known issues when using disk subsystem hardware in fault-tolerant environments and always install the latest BIOS revisions and support packs before setting up the cluster. Getting both servers to recognize the shared storage is usually the trickiest part of configuring the cluster.

- Any logical disk in the shared storage system must be configured as a Windows 2003 basic disk. Do not configure a dynamic disk in shared storage systems.

30

- All disk partitions used in the storage system must be formatted as NTFS.

- As best practice, use hardware-based fault-tolerant RAID sets on physical drive configurations to optimize performance and redundancy.

- Separate transaction logs and databases. Use hardware RAID 1 or 0+1 for the Exchange Server transaction log drives and RAID 5 or 0+1 for database storage.

- When creating the drive arrays on the shared storage device, be sure to create logical partitions in the RAID drive array utility so that Windows will see more than one hard drive. Five logical drives is usually optimum, to provide one drive for the quorum resource and two drives for each Exchange virtual server. Use one Exchange virtual server drive for the databases and the other for the transaction logs.

Implementing Fault-Tolerant Exchange Systems

Exchange administrators must design and implement Exchange messaging environments that can support the demanding uptime needs. Leveraging Windows Server 2003 clustering features, organizations can implement Exchange messaging systems with fault tolerance.

> **NOTE**
>
> When installing Exchange Server 2003 on a clustered Windows 2003 node, the Exchange 2003 installation automatically installs the cluster-aware Exchange 2003 version.

Preparing to Install Exchange 2003 Clusters

With a good understanding of the functionality and options of clustering with Exchange 2003 environments, administrators can begin implementing Windows 2003 in a cluster and place Exchange 2003 virtual servers in the cluster in multiple ways:

- **New Installation**   All Exchange 2003 preparation tasks, including ForestPrep and DomainPrep, are performed prior to implementing Exchange 2003 into the clustered environment.

> **NOTE**
>
> For more information regarding preparing, planning and deploying Exchange 2003, see Chapter 2, "Planning, Prototyping, Migrating, and Deploying Exchange Server 2003."

- **Post First Server**   Clusters can be used to add functionality to an already prepped and functional Exchange 2003 environment and Active Directory forest, allowing services' and users' mailbox information to be migrated to the Exchange 2003 and clustered virtual servers.

- **Coexistence**   Leveraging coexistence and compatibility, Exchange 2003 clusters can be implemented in the same environment as an existing Exchange 2003 server, providing additional functionality such as Outlook Web Access (OWA) services and load-balanced mailboxes during large organizationwide growth periods.

This section introduces the features available with the cluster version of Exchange 2003—what it is and how it is installed. In addition, you explore the steps administrators are required to perform when implementing and configuring Windows 2003 server clusters to support the Exchange 2003 platform.

General Features Overview

Although there are no management tools installed with the Exchange installation to configure and manage the Windows 2003 cluster, the cluster-aware version of Exchange 2003 introduces new features and functionality not available with the Standard version of Exchange 2003.

Review the following list to learn more about the features and behavior of the Exchange 2003 cluster-aware version:

- **Prerequisites Checking**   During installation of Exchange 2003 cluster-aware version, Exchange performs a prerequisite test to determine and validate that all requirements are met in the cluster before continuing the installation process.

- **Shared Nothing Architecture**   With Exchange 2003, Windows clustering behaves in a Shared Nothing Architecture when nodes are in a cluster. In this behavior, nodes in the cluster can all access the same shared data; however, no node in the cluster can access the same data at the same time. What this means is, if node 1 of the cluster is accessed as a shared resource on a disk, node 2 cannot access the resource until node 1 is either manually taken offline or is failed over.

- **Support for Eight Node Clusters**   Using Windows 2003 server clustering, organizations can build clusters with up to eight nodes.

- **Kerberos Authentication**   Exchange 2003 clusters use Kerberos authentication to enhance security; it is enabled by default.

- **Volume Mount Points**   New in Exchange 2003, support for volume mount points has been enabled for use with Windows 2003 clusters.

Planning Exchange 2000 Clusters

When planning clustering for Exchange Server 2003, there are several issues involving the network, software, storage, and load balancing that must be considered and planned.

30

Planning Network Resources

Exchange clusters require one TCP/IP address per virtual server in addition to the five TCP/IP addresses that were required to set up the Windows 2003 cluster environment. To run a 2-node Exchange cluster server in Active/Active mode, administrators are required to have two additional TCP/IP addresses to support the Exchange virtual servers. For example, a 2-node Active/Active cluster requires a total of seven static TCP/IP addresses.

Planning Cluster Disk Space

Storage space is another important factor when planning the Exchange cluster. As with the standard installation of any Exchange environment, administrators must consider the disk space requirements based on the expected growth of the Exchange server mailbox and data population.

To plan database drives and drive size requirements, calculate the expected size limit per mailbox and multiply the total by the number of expected mailboxes to calculate the disk space starting point. Also, factor in using deleted item retention, the company's growth rate, and the maximum number of mailboxes that will be supported on the cluster over its lifetime. To plan effectively, include an additional disk space in the final calculation to allow maintenance, unforeseen growth, and buffer space.

When planning drives to store Exchange server logs, plan enough disk space to support the overall operation of Exchange 2003. In addition, plan to include additional drive space for managing and maintaining logs, should backups be missed and files not flushed.

Software Requirements

To implement clustering technology with the Exchange Server 2003, administrators must use the Exchange Server 2003 Enterprise Edition. To install Exchange 2003 Enterprise in the cluster, administrators must install the installation files on the local disk of node in the cluster. For example, if administrators install the installation on node 1 in the C:\Exchsrvr directory, each node should also have the Exchange installation performed to C:\exchsrvr.

Load Balancing Mailboxes and Exchange Data

Load-balancing Exchange 2003 mailboxes and public folder information is important and can greatly improve the stability and performance of the Exchange 2003 cluster. When considering how to load-balance Exchange 2003 resources, it's up to the administrator to properly determine the total number of mailboxes per node in the cluster. Whether the cluster is configured for Active/Active or Active/Passive configuration, the bottom line is whether the surviving server will be able to handle the load should another server in the cluster be taken offline.

Validating Design Decisions and Testing

A front-end/back-end configuration can help reduce the load felt on the surviving node if there are a substantial number of Exchange 2003 server clients. Be sure to prototype cluster installations and configurations and execute detailed performance testing to calculate the most effective hardware and software configuration to support the load each node is expected to handle should the cluster fail over.

When load-testing to evaluate performance, perform tests on each node as it is online with other nodes at the same time. Validate functionality and performance and conduct the same set of tests on the cluster in a failover condition.

Installing Exchange Server 2003 Clusters

With all the information provided and a good solid plan in place, administrators can begin to install and configure Windows 2003 clusters for support Exchange 2003. The following section assists you in setting up Windows 2003 clusters and assumes that all hardware has been configured correctly and is compatible with clustering in the Windows 2003 Enterprise Edition.

On the cluster systems, install the Windows 2003 Enterprise Edition software and configure the following:

1. Configure the network TCP/IP address setting for both network adapters in the server.

2. In the domain where the server resides, create an administrative account for the cluster service.

3. If additional disks have been created, format additional drives with NTFS and validate the disk configurations, ensuring that there are no dynamic disks configured. If dynamic disks were created, modify to Basic and format using NTFS.

4. Review the server event logs and validate server functionality and domain membership.

Setting Up Windows 2003 Clusters

When the installation of Windows 2003 Enterprise server is complete, it is time to set up and configure the Windows 2003 cluster. Unlike previous versions of Windows clustering services, Windows 2003 clustering is installed by default when the server software is installed; it does not require additional steps to add the functionality to the server installation.

With the server installed and configured, set up the cluster and nodes by performing the following steps:

1. Launch the Cluster Administrator by selecting Start, All Programs, Administrator Tools, Cluster Administrator.

2. Because this scenario is a new installation, when the Cluster Administrator snap-in is launched, you are prompted to select the type of connection. To create a new cluster, select Create New Cluster from the connection tab, as shown in Figure 30.1.

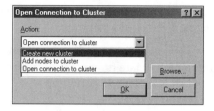

FIGURE 30.1   Choosing the connection type.

3. Selecting OK after choosing the connection type launches the New Server Cluster Wizard; at the welcome screen select Next.

4. From the Cluster Name and Domain screen, enter the name of the cluster and validate that the domain where the cluster is to be installed is selected.

5. Select the server where you are installing the cluster and select Next to continue.

6. Run the analyzer to validate the configuration and environment where the cluster will be installed. Identify any warnings and view the logs to correct problems, should the analyzer identify any problems before continuing.

7. Enter the cluster TCP/IP address and click Next.

8. Enter the Cluster Service account name and password created earlier and choose the correct domain. Click Next to continue.

> **NOTE**
>
> When the cluster service account was created, it was specified as a normal domain user. When you specify this account as the Cluster Service, the account is granted Local Administrator privileges on the cluster node and also delegates user rights to act as a part of the operating system and add computers to the domain.

9. On the Proposed Cluster Configuration page, review the configuration and choose the correct quorum type by clicking the Quorum button.

   Review the following information and select the proper quorum type for your installation:

   - To create a Majority Node Set (MNS) cluster, click the Quorum button on the Proposed Cluster Configuration page, choose Majority Node Set, and click OK.

   - If a SAN is connected to the cluster node, the Cluster Administrator automatically chooses the smallest basic NTFS volume on the shared storage device. Make sure the correct disk has been chosen and click OK.

   - If you're configuring a single node cluster with no shared storage, choose the local quorum resource and click OK.

10. Click Next to complete the cluster installation.

11. After the cluster is created, click Next and then Finish to close the New Server Cluster Wizard and return to the Cluster Administrator screen.

Adding Additional Nodes to a Cluster

With the cluster created and configured properly, it is time to add all the nodes to the cluster that will be used to support Exchange 2003. After the cluster is configured, the first server is installed as a node in a cluster. Additional nodes can be added to the cluster by completing the following steps:

1. Log on to the desired cluster node using the Cluster Administrator account.

2. Open the Cluster Administrator and choose Add Nodes to a Cluster. Enter the name of the cluster in the Cluster Name text box. Click OK to continue.

3. When the Add Nodes Wizard appears, click Next to continue.

4. Enter the server name of the new cluster node and click Add. Repeat these steps until all the additional nodes have been added in the Selected Computer text box. When complete, select Next to continue.

> **NOTE**
>
> The cluster analyzer then analyzes the additional nodes for functionality and cluster requirements. Review the results of the test and make any changes to correct any potential issues, as shown in Figure 30.2.
>
> To test the configuration again, click Re-analyze at any time.

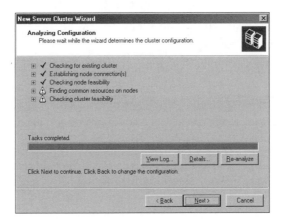

FIGURE 30.2   Node wizard analyzer.

30

5. When all testing is completed, enter the Cluster Service account password and click Next to continue.

6. Review the configuration on the Proposed Cluster Configuration page and click Next and Finish to complete the additional node installation.

Installing the Cluster-Aware Version of Exchange 2003

When performing the installation of the Exchange 2003 server, the Microsoft Exchange installation is cluster-aware. When the installation program from Exchange 2003 is installed into a clustered Windows 2003 server configuration, the Windows installer detects the presence of the cluster environment and begins the installation of the cluster-aware version of Exchange 2003. Through its process, administrators can confirm the installation of the cluster-aware installation by accepting the Exchange dialog prompt confirming the presence of the cluster and installation of the cluster-aware version. Use the following steps:

> **NOTE**
>
> In this scenario, the installation of Exchange 2003 and the configuration of the Exchange cluster is based on the post–first server environment. This scenario assumes that the Active Directory forest has already been prepared and the Exchange 2003 server is already in place servicing domain client systems.

1. Log on to the first node to be installed with the account that is a member of the Domain Admins and Exchange Admins security groups.

2. Install Exchange 2003 Enterprise Edition on the first node in the cluster from the Exchange 2000 Enterprise Edition installation CD-ROM.

3. Select to install Microsoft Messaging and Collaboration and Microsoft Exchange System Management Tools.

4. Install Exchange to a local drive in the clustered node, such as `C:\exchsrvr`.

> **NOTE**
>
> This location also is the same installation path used for each node in the cluster.

5. A dialog box should appear saying that setup has detected it is on a cluster and will install a cluster-aware version. Select OK to continue.

If no dialog prompts appear to confirm the installation of the cluster-aware version of Exchange 2003, check the configuration of the Windows 2003 cluster and ensure that the cluster is functioning correctly. Validate that each server in the cluster is aware of every other one and that all shared resources are available.

6. Install the Exchange server as you would any normal server. Place the new Exchange 2003 server into the proper administrative group and routing group and complete installation.

Configuring Exchange 2003 in a Cluster

When the installation is completed, launch the Cluster Administrator MMC snap–in and use the Application Wizard to create a new resource group and virtual server for use with Exchange 2003. Complete the following steps to set up Exchange 2003 in a clustered environment:

1. From the Cluster Administrator, select the first node created earlier and select File, Configure application to launch the Cluster Application Wizard.

2. On the welcome screen, click Next.

3. In the Create new Virtual Server page, select Create New Virtual Server and click Next.

4. On the Resource Group page, select Create New Resource and click Next, enter the name and description to be used for the new resource group, and click Next.

5. Enter the TCP/IP address to be used for the Virtual Exchange Server, as shown in Figure 30.3.

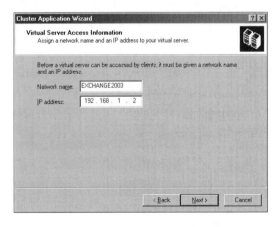

FIGURE 30.3   Virtual Server Access Information page.

30

6. Use the Advance Properties page to configure the properties and thresholds for the Exchange virtual server; click Next when completed.

7. On the Create Application Cluster Resource page, click No and then click Next.

8. Open the Exchange Virtual Server Resource properties page, and configure all nodes as possible owners by clicking the Modify button under possible owners.

9. Next create the Network Name resource for the Exchange Virtual Server Resource and configure both nodes as possible owners. Select the Exchange virtual server and select File, New, Resource.

10. Create the new Network Name resource and, when prompted, configure the dependencies, TCP/IP Address, and DNS information for the resource.

11. Bring the IP Address and Network Name resources online through Cluster Administrator by right-clicking the Exchange virtual server and selecting Bring Online, as shown in Figure 30.4.

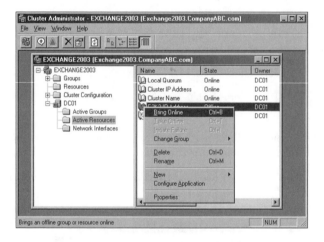

FIGURE 30.4   Bringing the cluster resources online.

12. Add disk resources to the Exchange virtual server resource group by dragging the disks to the Exchange virtual server resource group or right-clicking the disk in Cluster Groups and selecting Change Group.

> **NOTE**
>
> A disk can belong to only one Exchange virtual server resource group. Configure both nodes as possible owners for each disk.

13. Create the Exchange 2003 System Attendant in the Exchange virtual server resource group by selecting File, New, Resource and selecting Microsoft Exchange System Attendant under the resource type.

14. Set the Network Name and Disk resources as dependencies for the Exchange System Attendant, as done earlier by completing the wizard steps.

15. Select the same administrative group and routing group for the Exchange 2003 server. Use the same configuration information that was selected when the Exchange 2003 server was installed.

16. Enter the path to the data directory. Separate the paths for each by placing the logs and databases on separate shared disks, which were added to the Exchange virtual server resource group.

17. The remaining services are added automatically to the Exchange virtual server resource group.

Repeat these steps for each server in the cluster; when you are finished, configure the server cluster in an Active/Active configuration.

Managing Exchange 2003 Clusters

After Exchange 2003 clusters have been established and are functional on the network environment, administrators can use the built-in Windows 2003 Cluster Administrator to manage and modify the overall configuration of the Exchange cluster. In addition to the basic management, administrators must also understand the basic options for backing up Exchange 2003 cluster databases and restore options for recovering from failures. The next sections present basic management options and best practices when working with Windows 2003 cluster administration.

Configuration and Management Options

Overall, the only management option for configuring and modifying the Cluster Administrator is the Windows 2003 Cluster Administrator snap-in. When working with Exchange 2003 and Windows clustering, Windows Management Instrumentation (WMI) can be used to monitor the overall status of the Exchange 2003 cluster.

Another option for managing Windows 2003 cluster is the Cluster.exe command-line utility. The Cluster.exe utility can be used to access a cluster and manage cluster properties when the Cluster Administrator snap-in is not available.

Backing Up and Restoring Exchange 2003 Clusters

Administrators can leverage the built-in backup and disaster recovery functionality of Windows 2003 Server to back up and restore Exchange 2003 cluster configurations on local cluster nodes or all nodes configured in the cluster.

30

An ASR backup of a cluster node contains a disk signature or signatures and volume information, and the current system state, which includes Registry information, the cluster quorum, Windows boot files, COM+ class registration databases, and system services. A backup of all local disks containing operating system files also includes boot partitions and Exchange data.

Using the ASR utility, administrators can leverage the new built-in functionality of Windows 2003 ASR cluster restoration to perform complete restores of the cluster and nodes in the cluster.

Cluster Backups with Automated System Recovery

To perform an ASR backup, an administrator needs a blank floppy disk and a backup device—a tape device or disk storage, either locally to the server or a network share.

Keep in mind the total amount of required disk space to back up cluster service. Because ASR backs up all drives and data as well as applications, you should plan enough disk space to host backup in excess of 1GB.

To create an ASR backup, perform the following steps:

1. Log on to the cluster node with an account that has the right to back up the system. (Any Local Administrator, Domain Administrator, or Cluster Service account has the necessary permissions to complete the operation.)

2. Select Start, All Programs, Accessories, System Tools, Backup.

3. If this is the first time you've run Backup, it will open in Wizard Mode. Choose to run it in Advanced Mode by clicking the Advanced Mode hyperlink. After you change to Advanced Mode, the window should look similar to Figure 30.5.

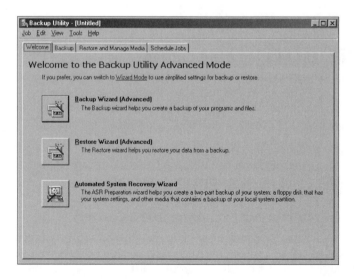

FIGURE 30.5   Windows Backup in Advanced mode.

4. Click the Automated System Recovery Wizard button to start the Automated System Recovery Preparation Wizard.

5. Click Next after reading the Automated System Recovery Preparation Wizard Welcome screen.

6. Choose your backup media type and choose the correct media tape or file. If you're creating a new file, specify the complete path to the file; the backup creates the file automatically. Click Next to continue.

7. If the file you specified resides on a network drive, click OK at the warning message to continue.

8. Click Finish to complete the Automated System Recovery Preparation Wizard and to start the backup.

9. After the tape or file backup portion completes, the ASR backup prompts you to insert a floppy disk that will contain the recovery information. Insert the disk and click OK to continue.

10. Remove the floppy disk as requested and label the disk with the appropriate ASR backup information. Click OK to continue.

11. When the ASR backup is complete, click Close on the Backup Progress window to return to the backup program or click Report to examine the backup report.

ASR backups should be performed periodically and immediately following any hardware changes to Exchange 2003 Server cluster nodes, including changes on a shared storage device or local disk configuration.

Restoring Cluster Nodes After a Failure

Cluster nodes can be restored after a cluster failure using a combination of restore methods. When one or all nodes in the cluster are nonoperational and the cluster node requires rebuilding from scratch, administrators can complete the following steps using the ASR to recover the lost Exchange 2003 cluster:

1. Shut down the failed cluster node.

2. On an available cluster node, log in using a Cluster Administrator account.

3. Select Start, Administrative Tools, Cluster Administrator.

4. If the Cluster Administrator does not connect to the cluster or connects to a different cluster, choose File, Open Connection.

5. From the Active drop-down box, choose Open Connection to Cluster. Then, in the Cluster or Server Name drop-down box, type a period (.) and click OK to connect.

6. Within each cluster group, make sure to disable failback to prevent these groups from failing over to a cluster node that is not completely restored. Close the Cluster Administrator.

30

7. Locate the ASR floppy created for the failed node or create the floppy from the files saved in the ASR backup media. For information on creating the ASR floppy from the ASR backup media, refer to Windows Server 2003 Help and Support tools.

8. Insert the operating system CD in the failed server and start the server.

9. If necessary, when prompted, press F6 to install any third-party storage device drivers. This includes any third-party disk or tape controllers that Windows Server 2003 will not recognize.

10. Press F2 when prompted to perform an Automated System Recovery.

11. When prompted, insert the ASR floppy disk and press Enter.

12. The operating system installation proceeds by restoring disk volume information and reformatting the volumes associated with the operating system. When this process is complete, restart the server as requested by pressing F3, and then click Enter in the next window.

13. After the system restarts, press a key if necessary to restart the CD installation.

14. If necessary, when prompted, press F6 to install any third-party storage device drivers. This includes any third-party disk or tape controllers that Windows Server 2003 will not recognize.

15. Press F2 when prompted to perform an Automated System Recovery.

16. When prompted, insert the ASR floppy disk and press Enter.

17. This time, the disks can be properly identified and will be formatted, and the system files will be copied to the respective disk volumes. When this process is complete, remove the ASR floppy when the ASR restore automatically reboots the server.

18. If necessary, specify the network location of the backup media using a UNC path and enter authentication information if prompted. The ASR backup will attempt to reconnect to the backup media automatically, but will be unable to if the backup media is on a network drive.

19. When the media is located, open the media and click Next. Finish recovering the remaining ASR data.

20. When the ASR restore is complete, if any local disk data was not restored with the ASR restore, restore missing information using the Windows NT Backup or a standard backup method being used in your organization.

Failover and Failback

Clusters that contain two or more Exchange nodes automatically have failover configured and enabled for each defined cluster group. When a node in a group becomes unavailable, the remaining server automatically becomes the available server. This server now inherits the role to service all Exchange 2003 clients accessing the cluster. By manually adding additional Exchange nodes to existing clusters, the administrator can add and modify the failover functionality to every node in the cluster.

Unlike failover, the failback functionality of Exchange 2003 clusters is not configured by default and needs to be manually configured to allow a designated preferred server to always run a particular cluster group when it is available. Administrators can modify these settings to define the thresholds and expected characteristics when in a failover or failback mode.

Cluster Group Failover Configuration

To create a failover and failback process, the cluster group failover configuration should be set up properly. Follow these steps to configure cluster group failover:

1. Select Start, Administrative Tools, Cluster Administrator.

2. When the Cluster Administrator opens, choose Open Connection to Cluster and type the name of the Exchange 2003 cluster to be configured.

3. Right-click the appropriate cluster group and select Properties.

4. Select the Failover tab and set the maximum number of failovers allowed during a predefined period of time. When the number of failovers is exceeded within the period interval, shown as a threshold of 10 in Figure 30.6, the cluster service changes the group to a failed state.

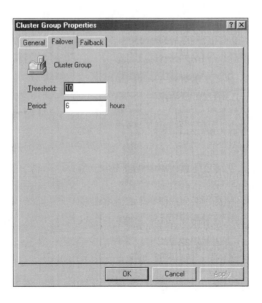

FIGURE 30.6   Failover Properties page.

30

5. Click Next and then Finish to complete the failover configuration.

6. Close the Cluster Administrator page to complete the configuration.

Outlook Web Access Front-end Server and Load Balancing Clusters

To provide even more enhanced performance and functionality when working with Exchange Server 2003, organizations can leverage the Windows 2003 NLB options available with the Windows 2003 server platform. Windows Server 2003 NLB is a separate functionality with clusters, and works by establishing a cluster of two or more systems using a single TCP/IP address.

This functionality is often effective when load-balancing front-end Exchange mail servers and Outlook Web Access with Exchange Server 2003. In this section, you explore NLB and Outlook Web Access, the steps to configure front-end Outlook Web Access servers using NLB options, and best practices.

Using Network Load Balancing

Because NLB is used to distribute network connections to create fault tolerance between servers and applications, using this feature is an exceptionally effective solution to provide high-level availability and quality of service to users accessing Exchange 2003 Outlook Web Access services.

To simplify the decision even more with NLB, no additional software and utilities are required other than the built-in functionality of Windows Server 2003 and the network interface cards configured in each server. After Exchange Outlook Web Access front-end servers have been configured, administrators can enable load balancing functionality through the NLB Manager available in the Windows Server 2003 administrative tools.

When configuring NLB, servers are established in clusters. Other areas to consider when configuring NLB services are modes in which the NLB service will be configured and the configuration of network interface cards.

NLB Modes and Port Configuration Overview

In the Unicast mode, clients and servers maintain a one-to-one relationship when communicating. In the multicast mode, servers respond by broadcasting a single multicast address, which clients attach when accessing information such as Web sites.

Another option when configuring NLB with Outlook Web Access is the ability to define the ports in which NLB cluster members will respond to client requests. This option is effective for the scenario because administrators can restrict and allow access to ports such as HTTP port 80 and Secure Socket Layer (SSL) port 443.

NLB Network Card Configurations

One of the first steps when configuring NLB cluster nodes is the configuration of the network interface cards in each server. A configuration of network cards can be completed using the NLB Manager and the TCP/IP properties of each node's network interface. One other option for configuring network interface cards is the command-line tool `nlb.exe`. This utility enables administrators to configure TCP/IP properties on NLB cluster nodes remotely and through the command line.

Configuring Network Load Balancing with OWA

Using the NLB Manager is the simplest method in configuring Outlook Web Access servers into a load balanced cluster configuration. When using the Network Load Balancing Manager, all information regarding the NLB cluster and load balancing TCP/IP addresses are added dynamically to each cluster node when configured. Using the NLB Manager also simplifies the tasks of adding and removing nodes by enabling administrators to use the NetBIOS name or TCP/IP address to identify nodes.

> **TIP**
>
> To effectively manage NLB clusters on remote servers, install and configure two network interface cards on the local NLB Manager system.
>
> For more information regarding Network Load Balancing services with Windows Server 2003, go to `www.microsoft.com/windowsserver2003/techinfo/overview/clustering.mspx`.

In the following example, NLB services will be implemented to provide support with two separate Outlook Web Access servers. This scenario assumes that each Outlook Web Access Server has already been installed and configured and is functioning.

To begin, configure the network cards for each Outlook Web Access system that you plan to configure in the NLB cluster:

1. Log on to the local console of a cluster node using an account with Local Administrator privileges.

2. Select Start, Control Panel, and select the properties of the Network Connections icon.

3. Open the properties of each network card to modify the properties by binding the appropriate cluster and dedicated IP addresses to each node's network card; use the advanced pages accessed through the General tab of the TCP/IP property page.

> **TIP**
>
> It is a good practice to rename each network card so you can easily identify it when configuring interfaces and troubleshooting problems.

30

After the TCP/IP properties of the network card for the two OWA servers have been configured and tested, you configure the NLB cluster through the NLB Manager. To begin, open
the NLB Manager and complete the following steps:

1. From the NLB Manager menu, select Cluster, New.

2. Enter the cluster IP address and subnet mask of the new cluster that will be used for
   both OWA servers' cluster members. Configure the following additional information,
   as shown in Figure 30.7:

   - Enter the fully qualified domain name for the cluster in the Full Internet name
     text box.

   - Enter the mode of operation (Multicast, since this is a Web functional configu-
     ration).

   - Configure a remote control password if you will be using the command-line
     utility (`nlb.exe`) to remotely manage the NLB cluster.

     Click Next to continue.

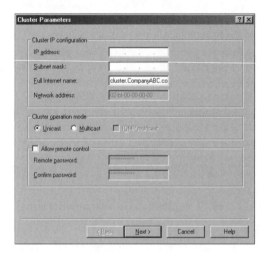

FIGURE 30.7   NLB Cluster Parameters page.

3. Enter any additional TCP/IP addresses that will be load-balanced and click Next to
   continue.

4. Configure the appropriate port rules for each IP address in the cluster. For OWA
   services being accessed from the Internet only, click the Edit tab and configure the
   port range to be 80, allowing HTTP traffic between cluster NLB servers.

5. On the Connect page, type the name of the server you want to add to the cluster in the Host text box and click Connect. Review the server information and highlight the network interface to be used for the server; click Next to continue.

6. On the Host Parameters page, set the cluster node priority. Each node requires a unique host priority, and because this is the first node in the cluster, leave the default of 1; click the Finish option when complete.

Add the additional OWA server to the NLB cluster by repeating these steps. Validate that the state of the clustered NLB system is listed in the NLB Manager as Started and close the Manager to complete the configuration.

> **TIP**
>
> Use the NLB Manager when performing maintenance on the NLB clustered members. When maintenance is necessary, you can change the default state of a particular NLB cluster node by placing it in a Stopped or Suspended state. This enables administrators to perform maintenance, such as security updates and service pack updates, and keep the server from joining the cluster following a reboot.
>
> For more information regarding Load Balancing and Exchange 2003 go to
>
> `www.microsoft.com/windowsserver2003/techinfo/overview/clustering.mspx`.

Summary

Administrators should carefully review the information in this chapter to understand the basic configuration options when working with Exchange Server 2003 and Microsoft clustering technologies. Information in this chapter provides insight to set up tasks and basic management options available with Exchange 2003 clustering environments and Network Load Balancing. Before implementing any of the technologies and configurations listed in this chapter, test and validate functionality in a non-production network environment to ensure proper functionality and avoid unforeseen issues when implementation occurs in the production environment.

Best Practices

The following are best practices from this chapter:

- Purchasing quality server and network hardware is a good start to building a fault-tolerant system, but the proper configuration of this hardware is equally important.

- Create disk subsystem redundancy using RAID technologies.

- Plan for a sufficient amount of TCP/IP addresses to support current and future cluster needs.

30

- Do not run both MSCS and NLB on the same computer; it is unsupported by Microsoft because of potential hardware sharing conflicts between MSCS and NLB.

- Active/Passive mode is easiest to manage and maintain, and the licensing costs are generally lower.

- To avoid unwanted failover, power management should be disabled on each of the cluster nodes, both in the motherboard BIOS and in the power applet in the control panel of the operating system.

- Carefully choose whether to use a shared disk or a non-shared approach to clustering.

- Use multiple network cards in each node so that one card can be dedicated to internal cluster communication.

- To reduce the chance of having a group failback to a node during regular business hours after a failure, configure the failback schedule to allow failback only during non-peak times.

- Thoroughly test failover and failback mechanisms.

- Do not change the cluster service account password using the Active Directory Users and Computers tool or the Windows security box if logged in with that account.

- Perform ASR backups periodically and immediately following any hardware changes to a cluster node, including changes on a shared storage device or local disk configuration.

- Create a port rule that allows only specific ports to the clustered IP address, and an additional rule blocking all other ports and ranges.

CHAPTER 31

Backing Up the Exchange Server 2003 Environment

Network and messaging system administrators know they're supposed to back up their networks on a regular basis, and almost every organization goes through the process of inserting tapes into a tape backup system to back up its network. Unfortunately far too many organizations merely put tapes into their tape drives and put little thought into both the process and purpose of backing up a system and the validation of assumptions that a backup really did successfully occur when expected.

Typically the only time administrators worry about a backup is when a catastrophic problem has occurred and a restoral is necessary. At that point, it is far too common for a tape restoral to not be successful due to improper backup procedures and tape media that has not been validated.

This chapter focuses on the creation of a successful backup and backup validation plan and process that will drastically improve an organization's ability to successfully restore from a catastrophe.

Using Backup to Solve Department Challenges

Before a backup plan can be created, administrators must understand what types of failures or disasters they need to plan for and the recovery requirements for each of these failures. Because there are several different types of recovery situations, you must ensure that the organization has a process in place to address specific recovery events.

As an example, although a full tape backup of the entire Exchange database can enable an organization to restore the databases from a catastrophic failure, a full image of the database does not help the organization easily restore a single mailbox or a single message. To restore a single mailbox or message from a full image of the entire Exchange databases requires a full restoral of the entire database, and then a manual extraction of the mailbox or message from the restored backup. So if an organization has a need to restore a single message or a single mailbox, there are best practice procedures to supplement a full image backup for the sole purpose of restoring just a single message or a single mailbox. These other methods or procedures include using a third-party tape backup utility to do a mailbox-by-mailbox backup, or to leverage the Mailbox Recovery Center utility built in to Exchange 2003 that is covered in detail in Chapter 32, "Recovering from a Disaster."

Understanding What Should Be Ready for Restoral

Learning what is necessary for a recovery gives administrators a list of all the elements they might need to back up for recovery when a particular failure is encountered. When they know what needs to be backed up, they can then create the backup plan. So it is recommended that administrators research each server service and application to understand what is necessary for recovery so that their backup plan will target the correct information.

There are several reasons an organization should have a backup of its Exchange information. The reasons an Exchange administrator might need to restore Exchange include the following:

- In case of a system crash

- In the event that the databases get corrupt and need to be recovered

- In a situation where an individual message, folder, or mailbox needs to be restored

- For the purpose of restoring Exchange in a lab for test purposes

Protecting Data in the Event of a System Failure

Server failures are the type of problem most organizations plan for, because a complete system failure creates the ultimate scenario where data needs to be restored from backup tape. Server hardware failures include failed motherboards, processors, memory, network interface cards, disk controllers, power supplies, and, of course, hard disks. Each of these failures can be minimized through the implementation of RAID hard drives, error correcting memory, redundant power supplies, or redundant controller adapters. In a catastrophic system failure, however, it is likely that the entire data backup would have to be restored to a new system.

Because data is read and written to hard drives on a constant basis, hard drives are frequently singled out as the most possible cause of a server hardware failure. Windows Server 2003 supports hot-swappable hard drives, but only if the server chassis and disk controllers support such a change. Windows Server 2003 supports two types of disks: basic disks, which provide backward compatibility; and dynamic disks, which enable software-level disk arrays to be configured without a separate disk controller. Both basic and dynamic disks, when used as data disks, can be moved to other servers easily. This provides data or disk capacity elsewhere if a system hardware failure occurs and the data on these disks needs to be made available as soon as possible.

> **NOTE**
>
> If hardware-level RAID is configured, the controller card configuration should be backed up using a special vendor utility; or it may need to be re-created from scratch if the disks are moved to a new machine.

To protect against a system failure, an organization needs to have a full image backup that can then be restored in entirety to a new or repaired server system.

Protecting Data in the Event of a Database Corruption

Data recovery also is needed in the event of a database corruption in Exchange. Unlike a catastrophic system failure, which can be restored from the last tape backup, data corruption creates a more challenging situation for information recovery. If data is corrupt on the system server, a restoral from the last backup might still have the corrupt database, so a data restoral needs to predate the point of corruption. This typically requires the ability to restore the database from an old tape and then recover incremental data since the clean database restoral.

Providing the Ability to Restore a Message, Folder, or Mailbox

In other situations, an organization might need to recover a single message, folder, or mailbox rather than a full database. With most full backups of an Exchange server, the restoral process requires a full restoral of all messages, folders, and mailboxes. If an administrator has to work with only a full image backup, typically a full restoral must be performed on a spare server and information extracted from the full restoral as necessary.

If message, folder, or mailbox recovery is required on a regular basis, the organization may elect to back up information in a format or process that provides an easier method of information recovery. This may involve the purchase and use of a third-party tape backup system, or a combination of various utilities available in Exchange 2003 to restore individual sets of information.

Preparing a Backup for a Test Lab Restoral

The last scenario where a restoral is performed is the situation wherein an organization wants to re-create an Exchange server for the purpose of testing the server in a lab. In this situation, a full restoral is conducted in an isolated environment. Because Exchange 2003 requires Active Directory for the user address list and distribution list, a recovery of an Exchange server for this purpose requires the restoral of a Global Catalog server and potentially other support servers, such as front-end servers or bridgehead servers.

Instead of just restoring a single server into a production environment, the lab restoral for testing purposes requires the restoral of several dependency server systems. The process of restoral also requires certain servers to be restored in a logical sequence so that the right persons are in place, like domain controllers, before member servers are restored. This sequence provides a more structured restoral that spans more than just the recovery of a system, but rather an entire system environment.

Maintaining Documentation on the Exchange Environment

When performing system backups, many administrators merely back-up servers and store tapes in-house or offsite, believing that the backup tape is the end goal of the backup process. Unfortunately the backup tape is only part of the necessary process involved in creating a successful recovery process. As identified in the last section, there are many different scenarios that require a data restoral, and in many cases, a full image restoral of an Exchange server is not the best solution to meet all situations.

A complete restoral of information presumes that the server the information being restored to is identical to the server that was backed up. If identical hard drive controller, network adapter, system board, and other server components do not exist, a full image restoral of a server will likely fail to recover from a server reboot—loaded drivers fail to enable. In these situations, the organization may choose to install the core Windows 2003 operating system on a new server with all the appropriate drivers for the new system, and then just restore the data.

To successfully restore just the Exchange data to a server, however, the server name, the domain the server is attached to, and the drive mappings must be identical to the server that was backed up. If the information is unknown, the ability for the organization to restore the information becomes a challenge.

This section covers the process of documenting key sets of information about each server, the server configuration, and the network information that can be used in the future as a server system requires recovery.

Server Configuration Documentation

Server configuration documentation is essential for any environment regardless of size, number of servers, or disaster recovery budget. A server configuration document contains a server's name, network configuration information, hardware and driver information, disk and volume configuration, or information about the applications installed. A complete server configuration document contains all the necessary configuration information a qualified administrator would need if the server needed to be restored and the operating system could not be restored efficiently. A server configuration document also can be used as a reference when server information needs to be collected.

31

The Server Build Document

A server build document contains step-by-step instructions on how to build a particular type of server for an organization. The details of this document should be tailored to the skill of the person intended to rebuild the server. For example, if this document was created for disaster recovery purposes, it may be detailed enough that anyone with basic computer skills could rebuild the server. This type of information could also be used to help IT staff follow a particular server build process to ensure that when new servers are added to the network, they all meet company server standards.

Hardware Inventory

Documenting the hardware inventory on an entire network might not be necessary. If the entire network does need to be inventoried, and if the organization is large, the Microsoft Systems Management Server can help automate the hardware inventory task. If the entire network does not need to be inventoried, hardware inventory can be collected for all the production and lab servers and networking hardware, including specifications such as serial numbers, amount of memory, disk space, processor speed, and possibly operating system platform and version.

Network Configurations

Network configuration documentation is essential when network outages occur. Current, accurate network configuration documentation and network diagrams can help simplify and isolate network troubleshooting when a failure occurs.

WAN Connection

WAN connectivity should be documented for enterprise networks that contain many sites to help IT staff understand the enterprise network topology. This document is very helpful when a server is restored and data should be synchronized enterprisewide after the restoral. Knowing the link performance between sites helps administrators understand how long an update made in Site A will take to reach Site B. This document should contain information about each WAN link, including circuit numbers, ISP contact names, ISP tech support phone numbers, and the network configuration on each end of the connection, and can be used to troubleshoot and isolate WAN connectivity issues.

Router, Switch, and Firewall Configurations

Firewalls, routers, and sometimes switches can run proprietary operating systems with a configuration that is exclusive to the device. During a system recovery, certain gateway connections, configuration routing information, routing table data, and other information might need to be reset on the restored server. Information should be collected from these devices, including logon passwords and current configurations. When a configuration change is planned for any of these devices, the newly proposed configuration should be created using a text or graphical editor, but the change should be approved before it is made on the production device. A rollback plan should be created first to ensure that the device can be restored to the original state if the change does not deliver the desired results.

Recovery Documentation

Recovery documentation, such as the server build document mentioned previously, can become reasonably complex and focused on a particular task. Recovery documentation aids an administrator in recovering from a failure for a particular server, server platform, specific service, or application. Recovery documentation is covered in Chapter 32.

Updating Documentation

One of the most important, yet sometimes overlooked, tasks concerning documentation is updating the documentation. Documentation is tedious, but outdated documentation can be worthless if many changes have occurred since the document was created. For example, if a server configuration document was used to re-create a server from scratch but many changes were applied to the server after the document was created, the correct security patches might not be applied, applications might be configured incorrectly, or data restore attempts could be unsuccessful. Whenever a change will be made to a network device, printer, or server, documentation outlining the previous configuration, proposed changes, and rollback plan should be created before the change is approved and carried out on the production device. After the change is carried out and the device is functioning as desired, the documentation associated with that device or server should be updated.

Developing a Backup Strategy

Developing the backup strategy involves planning the logistics of backing up the necessary information or data either via backup software and media or documentation, but usually as a combination of both. Other aspects of a backup strategy include assigning specific tasks to individual IT staff members so that the best person is in charge of backing up a particular service or server and ensuring that documentation is accurate and current.

Creating a Master Account List

Creating a master account list is a controversial subject because it contradicts what some security organizations call a best practice; however, many organizations follow this procedure. A master account list contains all the usernames and passwords with root privileges or top-level administrator privileges for network devices, servers, printers, and workstations. Not to be morbid, but a server restore may be required because of a disaster in a site that removed the server and the server administrator from accessibility. Without knowing the organizational-level password, site-level password, or server-level password on a system, an organization might be prevented from recovering server information.

The master account list can be printed and stored in a sealed envelope in a safe at the office or in an electronically encrypted copy. This list should be used only when the assigned IT staff members are not available, recovering from a failure is necessary, and only one of the accounts on the list has the necessary access. After the list is used, depending on who needed the temporary access, all the passwords on the list should be changed for security purposes, and another sealed list should be created.

Assigning Tasks and Designating Team Members

Each particular server or network device in the enterprise has specific requirements for backing up and documenting the device and the service it provides. To make sure that a critical system is being backed up properly, IT staff should designate a single individual to monitor that device and ensure the backup is completed and documentation is accurate and current. Assigning a secondary staff member who has the same set of skills to act as a backup if the primary staff member is unavailable is a wise decision, to ensure that there is no point of failure among IT staff.

Assigning only primary and secondary resources to specific devices or services helps improve the overall security and reliability of the device. By limiting who can back up and restore data—and even who can manage the device—to just the primary and secondary qualified staff members, the organization can rest assured that only competent individuals are working on systems they are trained to manage. Even though the backup and restore responsibilities lie with the primary and secondary resources, the backup and recovery plans should still be documented and available to the remaining IT staff.

Creating Regular Backup Procedures

Creating a regular backup procedure helps ensure that the entire enterprise is backed up consistently and properly. When a regular procedure is created, the assigned staff members soon become accustomed to the procedure. If there is no documented procedure, certain items might be overlooked and not be backed up, which can be a major problem if a failure occurs. For example, a regular backup procedure for an Exchange 2003 server could back up the Exchange databases on the local drives every night, and perform an Automated System Recovery (ASR) backup once a month and whenever a hardware change is made to a server.

Creating a Service-Level Agreement for Each Critical Service

A service-level agreement (SLA) defines the availability and performance of a particular device or service. This is usually linked to a failure. For example, a generic SLA could state that for the Exchange server EX01, if a failure occurs, it can be recovered and available on the network in four hours or less. SLAs are commonly defined specifically within disaster recovery solutions; sometimes the SLA is the *basis* for the disaster recovery solution. For example, if a company cannot be without its database for more than one hour, a disaster recovery solution must be created to meet that SLA.

Before an SLA can be defined, the IT staff member responsible for a device must understand what is necessary to recover that device from any type of failure. That person also must limit the SLA to only the failure types planned for in the approved disaster recovery solution. For example, suppose there is no plan for a site outage. The SLA might state that, if the device fails, it can be recovered using spare hardware and be back online in two hours or less. On the other hand, if a site failure occurs, there is no estimated recovery time because offsite backup media might need to be collected from an outside storage provider and hardware might need to be purchased or reallocated to re-create the device. The more specific the SLA is, the better chance of covering every angle.

Determining a Reasonable SLA

An SLA cannot be created until an IT staff member performs test backups and restores to verify that disaster recovery procedures are correct and that the data can be restored in the desired time frame. When an SLA is defined before the disaster recovery solution, the IT staff member needs to see whether a standard recovery procedure will meet the SLA; otherwise, a creative, sometimes expensive, custom solution might be necessary.

Selecting Devices to Back Up

Each device could have specific backup requirements. The assigned IT staff members are responsible for researching and learning the backup and recovery requirements to ensure that the backup will have everything that is necessary to recover from a device failure. As a rule of thumb for network devices, the device configuration should be backed up; on servers, local and shared storage data, operating system files, and operating system configurations should be backed up. Some backups consist of documentation and a few settings in a text file.

Creating a Windows Server 2003 Boot Floppy

In previous versions of Windows, if RAID 1 volumes were created using the operating system, instead of a hardware-based RAID volume, the administrator needed to create a specific boot disk. This disk pointed to the remaining disk to boot the server if the primary disk in the volume failed. Windows Server 2003 removes this dependency because it adds an additional line in the boot.ini file that points to the second disk's volume, enabling the server to boot properly using the remaining disk. The only caveat is that the administrator needs to select the correct option when the boot.ini file displays the boot options on the screen. The mirrored volume is referred to as **a secondary subsystem** secondary plex in the following boot.ini file information:

```
[boot loader]
timeout=30
default=multi(0)disk(0)rdisk(0)partition(1)\WINDOWS
[operating systems]
multi(0)disk(0)rdisk(0)partition(1)\WINDOWS="C: Microsoft Windows Server _
 2003 Enterprise Server" /fastdetect
multi(0)disk(0)rdisk(1)partition(1)\WINDOWS="Boot Mirror C: - secondary plex"
```

The preceding example is taken directly from a boot.ini file on a Windows Server 2003 system using software-level RAID 1 arrays for the system partition. The secondary subsystem is just a reference, but the disk controller and disk volume information point the boot loader to connect to the correct remaining partition.

Sometimes a boot floppy is necessary, especially if the boot and system volumes are different and the boot files are inaccessible. In a situation like this, a boot floppy is priceless. To create a boot floppy, format a floppy disk. From the local server console, copy the boot.ini, NTLDR, and NTDETECT files to the floppy disk. When the BIOS cannot locate the boot loader files, this floppy can be used to boot the system and point the system to the correct volume containing the operating system files.

Backing Up the Windows Server 2003 and Exchange Server 2003

The Windows Server 2003 operating system and the Exchange Server 2003 messaging system contain several features to enhance operating system stability, provide data and service redundancy, and deliver feature-rich client services. To provide the most disaster recovery options, many services have their own backup tools and might require additional attention. This section discusses ways to back up a Windows Server 2003 system, including key components needed to make an Exchange 2003 server operate. By preparing for a complete server failure, an organization is more likely to be able to recover to a previous state. This section also outlines specific Windows Server 2003 services that have tools to aid in the backup recovery process.

Backing Up Boot and System Volumes

A backup strategy for every Exchange 2003 system should always include the boot and system disk volumes. On many installations, the boot and system volume are the same, but sometimes they are located on completely separate volumes—usually on dual-boot computers. For the rest of this section, assume that they are both on the same partition, referred to as the system volume. This volume contains all the files necessary to start the core operating system. It should be backed up before and after a change is made to the operating system and once every 24 hours if possible.

When Exchange is installed on a Windows 2003 server, the installation will, by default, install on the system partition unless a different partition is specified during installation. On average, the amount of information stored on the system volume, with applications and services installed, is typically less than 1GB.

> **NOTE**
>
> When system volumes are backed up, the system state should be backed up at the same time to simplify recovery if a server needs to be rebuilt from scratch.

Backing Up Exchange Data Volumes

Having the Exchange databases written to a completely separate data drive from the operating system is typically recommended; this improves overall system and user data access performance. When systems are built with this recommendation in mind, backing up just the system volume does not back up the Exchange databases. Backing up the Exchange databases that are stored on a separate drive set frequently requires the backup administrator to specifically back up *both* the boot drive and the data drive. In far too many instances, organizations find out the hard way that they have been diligently backing up the Exchange server's C: drive, but have failed to back up the server's E: drive, which hosted the Exchange databases. Without a database backup, there is no data to be restored and recovered.

It is also important to note that the database volume usually has the most data needed for backup and recovery. This creates longer backup intervals and might require more than one tape depending on the size of the Exchange databases. For many organizations, a full backup of data volumes can be run only once a week, but to capture all new and modified data, incremental or differential backups can be run every day.

Backing Up Windows Server 2003 Services

Many Windows Server 2003 services store configuration and status data in separate files or databases located in various locations on the system volume. If the service is native to Windows Server 2003, performing a complete server backup on all drives and the system state, the critical data is almost certainly being backed up. A few services provide alternative backup and restore options. The procedures for backing up these services are outlined in the section titled "Backing Up Specific Windows Services," later in this chapter.

Backing Up the System State

The system state of a Windows Server 2003 system contains, at a minimum, the System Registry, boot files, and the COM+ class registration database. Backing up the system state creates a point-in-time backup that can be used to restore a server to a previous working state. Having a copy of the system state is essential if a server restore is necessary.

How the server is configured determines what will be contained in the system state, other than the three items listed previously. On a domain controller, the system state also contains the Active Directory database and the SYSVOL share. On a cluster, it contains the cluster quorum data. When services such as Certificate Server and Internet Information Services, which contain their own service-specific data, are installed, these databases are not listed separately but are backed up with the system state.

Even though the system state contains many subcomponents, using the programs included with Windows Server 2003, the entire system state can be backed up only as a whole. When recovery is necessary, however, there are several different options. Recovering data using a system state backup is covered in Chapter 32.

The system state should be backed up every night to prepare for several server-related failures. A restore of a system state is very powerful and can return a system to a previous working state if a change needs to be rolled back or if the operating system needs to be restored from scratch after a complete server failure.

Using the Active Directory Restore Mode Password

When a Windows Server 2003 system is promoted to a domain controller, one of the configurations is to create an Active Directory Restore mode password. This password is used only when booting into Active Directory Restore mode. Restore mode is used when the Active Directory database is in need of maintenance or needs to be restored from backup. Many administrators have found themselves without the ability to log in to Restore mode when necessary and have been forced to rebuild systems from scratch to restore the system state data. Many hours can be saved if this password is stored in a safe place, where it can be accessed by the correct administrators.

The Restore mode password is server-specific and created on each domain controller. If the password is forgotten, and the domain controller is still functional, it can be changed using the command-line tool ntdsutil.exe, as shown in Figure 31.1. The example in Figure 31.1 changes the password on the remote domain controller named adserver.companyabc.com.

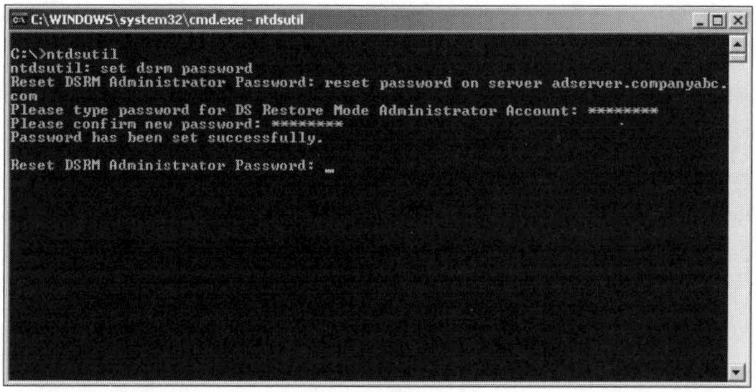

FIGURE 31.1 Changing the Active Directory Restore mode password (using ntdsutil.exe).

Using the Windows Backup Utility (Ntbackup.exe)

Windows Server 2003 includes several tools and services to back up and archive user data, but when it comes to backing up the entire operating system and disk volumes, Windows Server 2003 Backup is the program to use. Windows Server 2003 Backup is included on all the different versions of the platform. Some Windows Server 2003 services provide alternative backup utilities, but they still can be backed up using Ntbackup.exe.

Windows Server 2003 Backup provides all the necessary functions to completely back up and restore a single file or the entire Windows Server 2003 system. Third-party, or even other Microsoft, applications installed on a Windows 2003 server system should be researched to ensure that no special backup requirements or add-ons are necessary to back up the application data and configuration.

Windows Server 2003 Backup has been developed, or limited, to primarily backing up the local server, but it can back up remote server volumes as well. In the case of backing up remote server volumes, open files are skipped, and the system state can be backed up only from the local server.

Modes of Operation

The Windows Backup utility can run in two separate modes: Wizard and Advanced. Wizard mode provides a simple interface that enables a backup to be created in just a few easy steps:

1. Choose to back up or restore files and settings.

2. Choose to back up everything or specify what to back up.

3. Choose what data to back up only if you do not choose the option to back up everything.

4. Specify the backup media, tape, or file.

That is all it takes to use Wizard mode, but features such as creating a scheduled backup or choosing to disable Volume Shadow Copy can be performed only using Advanced mode.

Advanced mode provides greater granularity when it comes to scheduling and controlling backup media security and other backup options. In the following sections concerning Windows Server 2003 Backup, you use Advanced mode.

Using the Windows Backup Advanced Mode

Running the Windows Server 2003 Backup utility in Advanced mode enables administrators to configure all the available options for backups. Scheduled backups can be created; specific wizards can be started; and advanced backup options can be configured, such as verifying backup, using volume shadow copies, backing up data in remote storage, and automatically backing up system-protected files.

To create a backup in Advanced mode, use the following steps:

1. Click Start, All Programs, Accessories, System Tools, Backup.

2. If this is the first time you've run Backup, it will open in Wizard mode. Choose to run it in Advanced mode by clicking the Advanced Mode hyperlink.

3. Click the Backup Wizard (Advanced) button to start the Backup Wizard.

4. Click Next on the Backup Wizard Welcome screen to continue.

5. On the What to Back Up page, select Back Up Selected Files, Drives, or Network Data and click Next to continue.

6. On the Items to Back Up page, expand Desktop, My Computer in the left pane and choose each of the local drives and the system state, as shown in Figure 31.2. Then click Next to continue.

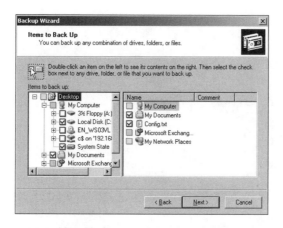

FIGURE 31.2   Selecting items to back up.

7. Choose your backup media type and choose the correct media tape or file. If you're creating a new file, specify the complete path to the file, and the backup will create the file automatically. Click Next to continue.

8. If the file you specified resides on a network drive, click OK at the warning message to continue.

9. If you chose tape for the backup, choose the media for the backup and choose to use a new tape.

10. Click the Advanced button on the Completing the Backup Wizard page to configure advanced options.

11. Choose the backup type and choose whether to back up migrated remote storage data. The default settings on this page will fit most backups, so click Next to continue.

12. Choose whether a verify operation will be run on the backup media and click Next. Disabling Volume Shadow Copy would be an option if a backup were just backing up local volumes, not the system state.

13. Choose the Media Overwrite option of appending or replacing the data on the media and click Next.

14. On the When to Back Up page, choose to run the backup now or to create a schedule for the backup. If you chose Now, skip to step 18.

15. If a schedule will be created, enter a job name and click the Set Schedule button.

16. On the Schedule Job page, select the frequency of the backup, start time, and start date, as shown in Figure 31.3, and click OK when completed. You can set additional configurations using the Settings tab.

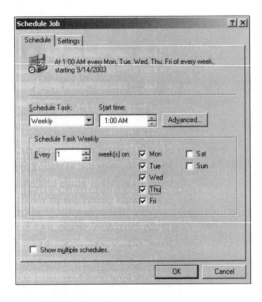

FIGURE 31.3   Creating a schedule for a backup.

17. On the Set Account Information page, enter the user account name and password that should be used to run the scheduled backup and click OK when completed.

18. Back on the When to Back Up page, click Next to continue.

19. Click Finish to save the scheduled backup or immediately start the backup job.

20. When the backup is complete, review the backup log for detailed information and click Close on the Backup Progress window when finished.

Automated System Recovery

Automated System Recovery (ASR) is a backup option that is used to back up a system to prepare for a complete server failure. An ASR backup contains disk volume information and a copy of all the data on the boot and system volumes, along with the current system state. ASR can be used to restore a system from scratch, and it will even re-create disk volumes and format them as previously recorded during the ASR backup. ASR does not back up the data stored on volumes that are solely used for data storage.

To perform an ASR backup, an administrator needs a blank floppy disk and a backup device; either a tape device or disk will suffice. One point to keep in mind is that an ASR backup will back up each local drive that contains the operating system and any applications installed. For instance, if the operating system is installed on drive C: and MS Office is installed on drive D:, both of these drives will be completely backed up because the Registry has references to files on the D: drive. Although this can greatly simplify restore procedures, it requires additional storage and increases backup time for an ASR backup.

ASR backups should be created for a server before and after any hardware changes are performed or when a major configuration change occurs with the system. ASR backups contain disk information, including basic or dynamic configuration and volume set type. They save volume or partition data so that when an ASR restore is complete, only the data stored on storage volumes needs to be recovered.

Creating an ASR Backup

An ASR backup can currently be created only from the local server console using the graphical user interface version of the Windows Server 2003 Backup utility.

To create an ASR backup, follow these steps:

1. Log on to the server using an account that has the right to back up the system. (Any Local Administrator or Domain Administrator has the necessary permissions to complete the operation.)

2. Click Start, All Programs, Accessories, System Tools, Backup.

3. If this is the first time you've run Backup, it will open in Wizard mode. Choose to run it in Advanced mode by clicking the Advanced mode hyperlink.

4. Click the Automated System Recovery Wizard button to start the Automated System Recovery Preparation Wizard.

5. Click Next after reading the Automated System Recovery Preparation Wizard welcome screen.

6. Choose your backup media type and choose the correct media tape or file. If you're creating a new file, specify the complete path to the file, and the backup will create the file automatically. Click Next to continue.

7. If you specified a file as the backup media and it resides on a network drive, click OK at the warning message to continue.

8. If you chose tape for the backup, choose the media for the backup and choose to use a new tape.

9. Click Finish to complete the Automated System Recovery Preparation Wizard and start the backup. As the ASR backup process begins, you will see the `ntbackup` utility processing the backup similar to what is shown in Figure 31.4.

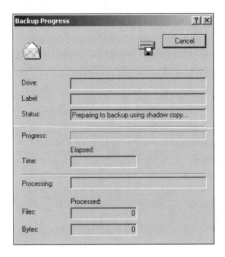

FIGURE 31.4   ASR backup in process.

10. After the tape or file backup portion completes, the ASR backup prompts you to insert a floppy disk to hold the recovery information. Insert the disk and click OK to continue.

11. Remove the floppy disk as requested and label the disk with the appropriate ASR backup information. Click OK to continue.

12. When the ASR backup is complete, click Close on the Backup Progress window to return to the backup program or click Report to examine the backup report.

> **NOTE**
>
> The information contained on the ASR floppy disk is also stored on the backup media. The ASR floppy contains only two files, `asr.sif` and `asrpnp.sif`, which can be restored from the backup media and copied to a floppy disk if the original ASR floppy cannot be located.

Tips on Using ASR

Tip on using ASR to ensure proper operations include performing an ASR backup after the server is built, updated, configured, and secured. Also, an ASR backup should be performed when hardware configurations change and periodically otherwise. On domain controllers, this period should be less than 60 days to ensure that the domain can be up and running again if an Active Directory authoritative restore is necessary.

ASR backs up only the system and boot partitions. ASR will not back up the Exchange databases if they are installed on a separate drive. A normal tape backup of the drive(s) storing the Exchange databases or any other drive volume with critical data should be backed up separately. ASR backups, on average, are 1.3GB–5GB. To prevent ASR backups from getting too large, user data and file shares should be kept off the system and boot volumes.

Backing Up Specific Windows Services

Most Windows Server 2003 services that contain a database or local files are backed up with the system state but also provide alternate backup and restore options. Because the system state restore is usually an all-or-nothing proposition, except when it comes to cluster nodes and domain controllers, restoring an entire system state might deliver undesired results if only a specific service database restore is required. This section outlines services that either have separate backup/restore utilities or require special attention to ensure a successful backup.

Disk Configuration (Software RAID Sets)

Disk configuration is not a service but should be backed up to ensure that proper partition assignments can be restored. When dynamic disks are used to create complex volumes—such as mirrored, striped, spanned, or RAID 5 volumes—the disk configuration should be saved. This way, if the operating system is corrupt and needs to be rebuilt from scratch, the complex volumes need to have only their configuration restored, which could greatly reduce the recovery time. Only an ASR backup can back up disk and volume configuration.

Certificate Services

Installing Certificate Services creates a Certificate Authority (CA) on the Windows Server 2003 system. The CA is used to manage and allocate certificates to users, servers, and workstations when files, folders, email, or network communication needs to be secured or encrypted. In many cases, the CA is a completely separate secured CA server; however, many organizations use their Exchange server as a CA server. This might be because of a limited number of servers with several services installed on a single server, or because the organization wants to use SSL for secured Outlook Web Access and installs Certificate Services on the Exchange server. Whatever the case, the CA needs to be backed up whether on the Exchange server or on a different server; if the CA server crashes and needs to be restored, it can be restored so users can continue to access the system after recovery.

> **CAUTION**
>
> For security purposes, it is highly recommended that the certificate services be enabled on a server other than the Exchange server. Definitely do not have the CA services on an Outlook Web Access server that is exposed to the Internet. The integrity of certificate-authenticated access depends on ensuring that certificates are issued only by a trusted authority. Any compromise to the CA server invalidates an organization's ability to secure its communications.

When the CA allocates a certificate to a machine or user, that information is recorded in the certificate database on the local drive of the CA. If this database is corrupted or deleted, all certificates allocated from this server become invalid or unuseable. To avoid this problem, the certificates and Certificate Services database should be backed up frequently. Even if certificates are rarely allocated to new users or machines, backups should still be performed regularly.

Certificate Services can be backed up in three ways: backing up the CA server's system state, using the CA Microsoft Management Console (MMC) snap-in, or using the command-line utility `Certutil.exe`. Backing up Certificate Services by backing up the system state is the preferred method because it can be easily automated and scheduled. But using the graphic console or command-line utility adds the benefit of being able to restore Certificate Services to a previous state without restoring the entire server system state or taking down the entire server for the restore.

To create a backup of the Certificate Authority using the graphic console, follow these steps:

1. Log on to the Certificate Authority server using an account with Local Administrator rights.

2. Open Windows Explorer and create a folder named **CaBackup** on the C: drive.

3. Select Administrative Tools, Certificate Authority.

4. Expand the Certificate Authority server and select the correct CA.

5. Select Actions, All Tasks, Back Up CA.

6. Click Next on the Certification Authority Backup Wizard Welcome screen.

7. On the Items to Back Up page, check the Private Key and CA Certificate box and the Certificate Database and Certificate Database Log box, as shown in Figure 31.5.

8. Specify the location to store the CA backup files. Use the folder created in the beginning of this process. Click Next to continue.

9. When the CA certificate and private key are backed up, this data file must be protected with a password. Enter a password for this file, confirm it, and click Next to continue.

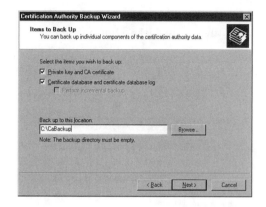

FIGURE 31.5   Selecting items for the Certificate Authority backup.

10. Click Finish to create the CA backup.

Internet Information Services

Internet Information Services (IIS) is Windows Server 2003's Web and FTP server. It is included on every version of the Windows Server 2003 platform. IIS stores configuration information for Web and FTP site configurations and security in the IIS metabase. The IIS metabase can be backed up by performing a system state backup of the server running IIS, but it can also be backed up using the IIS console. The IIS metabase should be backed up separately before and after an IIS configuration change is made to ensure a successful rollback and to have the latest IIS configuration data backed up after the update.

To back up the IIS metabase using the IIS console, use the following steps:

1. Log on to the IIS server using an account with Local Administrator access.

2. Click Start, All Programs, Administrative Tools, Internet Information Services (IIS).

3. If the local IIS server does not appear in the window, right-click Internet Information Services in the left pane and select Connect.

4. Type in the fully qualified domain name for the IIS server and click OK.

5. Right-click the IIS server in the left pane and select All Tasks, Backup/Restore Configuration.

6. The Configuration Backup/Restore window lists all the automatic IIS backups that have been created. Click the Create Backup button.

7. Enter the backup name and, if necessary, check the Encrypt Backup Using Password box, enter and confirm the password, and click OK when you're finished, as shown in Figure 31.6.

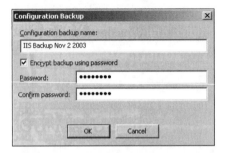

FIGURE 31.6   Creating an IIS configuration backup.

8. When the backup is complete, it is listed in the Configuration Backup/Restore window. Click Close to return to the IIS console.

Before a change is made to the IIS configuration, a backup should be manually created. When the change is completed, the administrator should either perform another backup or choose the option to save the configuration to disk. The administrator can save new IIS configuration changes to disk by right-clicking the IIS server, selecting All Tasks, and then choosing Save Configuration to Disk. This option works correctly only after a change has been made that has not yet been recorded in the IIS metabase.

Managing Media in a Structured Backup Strategy

Windows Server 2003 Backup uses the Removable Storage service to allocate and deallocate media. The media can be managed using the Removable Storage console in the Computer Management Administrative Tools, as shown in Figure 31.7. The Removable Storage service allocates and deallocates media for these services by enabling each service to access media in media sets created for the respective program.

Media Pools

The Windows Server 2003 Removable Storage service organizes media within **media pools** so that policies and permissions can be applied and different functions can be performed. For example, the backup media pool is allocated for media created using Windows Server 2003 Backup. Only users granted the privilege to back up or restore the system, or administer the removable media service, have access to this media pool.

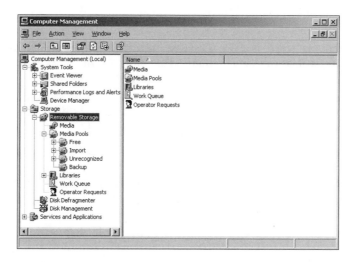

FIGURE 31.7   Removable storage console.

Free Pool

The **free pool** contains media that can be used by any backup or archiving software that uses the Windows Server 2003 Removable Storage service. Media in this pool are usually blank media or media marked as clean, and can be overwritten and reallocated.

Remote Storage Pool

The **remote storage poo**l is used on a server only if the Remote Storage server has been installed. This pool stores media allocated for the Remote Storage service. If no tape is found, the device reallocates media from the free pool.

Imported Pool

When media are inserted into a tape device and inventory is run, if the media are not blank and not already allocated to the remote storage pool or backup media pool, they are stored in the **imported media pool**. If the media are known to have been created with Windows Server 2003 Backup, opening the backup program and performing a catalog should be sufficient to reallocate this media to the backup pool set.

Backup Pool

The **backup pool** contains all the media allocated to the Windows Server 2003 Backup program.

Custom Media Pools

Custom media pools can be created if special removable media options are required. Media pool options are very limited in Windows Server 2003, and there should be no compelling reason to create a custom media pool.

Summary

Backing up an Exchange server is more than just putting in a tape every night and storing the tapes, but rather should follow very methodical processes. If a data restoral becomes necessary, the administrator of the messaging system wants to ensure that the information on the tape has been properly backed up and that the recovery goes as expected. The successful backup and restoral of key information is rarely successful by accident or by chance, and requires planning, testing, and documentation.

Additionally, a backup of a system is not satisfied solely by a full image backup of a server. Although a full image backup provides an organization the ability to restore from a complete disaster, it does not address the ability of the organization to restore portions of an Exchange environment, such as a specific message, folder, or mailbox. A full backup of an Exchange server also does not necessarily back up support functions of a fully operational Exchange environment, which includes the directory in Active Directory, certificates for secured Exchange access, or Web services needed to complete the operational restoral of a server.

Because a successful restoral is so important to an organization after a system failure, take steps to ensure that a server restore will be successful.

Best Practices

The following are best practices from this chapter:

- A successful backup and restoral plan includes backing up not only the Exchange server, but also any support servers, such as Global Catalog server, Certificate of Authority server, or front-end Web servers.

- Identify the different services and technologies, points of failure, and critical areas; prioritize in order of importance; and ensure all points of operation are backed up.

- Server configuration documentation is essential for any environment, regardless of size, number of servers, or disaster recovery budget. When restoring just the Exchange databases, other configuration information on Exchange, such as the server name, must be identical to the name of the backed up server; otherwise, the data will not successfully restore.

- Update documentation of an Exchange environment any time changes occur to ensure that core server and Exchange information is available should a component level restoral be needed.

- When backing up system volumes, the system state should be backed up at the same time to simplify recovery if a server needs to be rebuilt from scratch.

- Perform an ASR backup after a server is built, updated, configured, and secured. Also, perform an ASR backup when hardware configurations change.

- Perform an ASR backup on domain controllers on a regular basis to ensure that if an Active Directory authoritative restore is necessary, you can get the domain up and running again.

- Consider using the remote storage management functions built in to Windows Server 2003 to better manage historical backup information and backup media.

31

Recovering from a Disaster

When an Exchange server or environment isn't working properly, possibly due to database corruption, hardware failure, or just unknown reasons, there's an urgent need to get the Exchange system back up and running as quickly as possible. Several approaches can be used to recover from a disaster of a failed server. One approach is to follow the procedures recommended in Chapter 30, "System-Level Fault Tolerance (Clustering/Network Load Balancing)," and Chapter 31, "Backing Up the Exchange Server 2003 Environment," and then following the recovery procedures of a properly backed-up environment. However, in reality, most organizations do not proactively create an environment with disaster-recovery processes in place. This chapter has several recommendations on how to recover from a disaster, ranging from recovery from a proactively backed-up environment to an environment that has not been actively prepared for simple recovery. The recovery processes include a tape restore and procedures to repair and recover data from corrupt databases.

Identifying the Extent of the Problem

Before a successful recovery can be conducted, the extent of the problem must be determined. Different recovery strategies exist for recovering a lost mail message or folder than for recovering an entire mailbox. There are different recovery strategies for recovering a corrupt mailbox and for recovering an entire failed server. Using the right recovery process to solve the right problem requires the problem-resolution process to minimize the recovery time and the chance that a simple recovery will create bigger problems in the process.

In case of a system failure, many organizations try to recover the entire server. Depending on the amount of data, this could take several hours to get the system completely operational. Before beginning the process of restoring the entire server, it is important to analyze the amount of data that needs to be recovered, as well as the existing conditions of recovery methods. There is no need to restore from tape if the Recovery Storage Group option has been enabled on Exchange and can be used as part of the recovery process. Also, a full restore of a corrupt database on tape does not resolve the problem of a corrupt database on the server hard drive. Identifying what the problem is provides the best method for restoration.

Mailbox Content Was Deleted, Use the Undelete Function of Exchange

When information is deleted from a user's mailbox, whether it is an email message, a Calendar appointment, a contact, or a task, the information is not permanently deleted from the Exchange server. Deleted items go into the Deleted Items folder in the user's Outlook mailbox. The information is actually retained on the Exchange server for 30 days after deletion, even when it is supposedly permanently deleted from the Deleted Items folder.

> **NOTE**
>
> The Mail Retention feature needs to be enabled on the Exchange Server for Outlook information to be retained on the Exchange server.

Data Is Lost, Must Restore from Backup

If data is lost and the undelete function will not recover the information, the information needs to be restored from a backup. Depending on how much information was lost, this might involve a full recovery of the Exchange server from tape, or it might involve restoring just a single mailbox, folder, or message. Key to restoring information is determining what needs to be restored. If just a single message needs to be restored, there is no reason to recover the entire server in production. In many cases, when full tape backups have been conducted of an Exchange server, a full restore must be completed offline and then a specific mailbox, folder, or mail message must be extracted from the offline restored server to the production server. The restore process needs to take in account the restoration of the information desired without the restoration of the entire server, which might overwrite valid data.

The process of restoring all or partial data from tape is covered in the sections "Recovering from a Complete Server Failure" and "Recovering from Database Corruption," later in this chapter.

Data Is Okay, Server Just Doesn't Come Up

The failure of a server does not necessarily mean that the data needs to be restored completely from tape. In fact, if the hard drives on a dead server are still operational, the hard drives should be moved to an operational server or, at the very least, the data should be transferred to a different server. By preserving the data on the drives, an organization can minimize the need to perform more complicated data reconstruction from a tape restore, which could result in the loss of data from the time of the last backup.

The process of recovering data from a drive and recovering a failed server is covered in the section "Performing a Restore of Only Exchange Database Files," later in this chapter.

Data Is Corrupt—Some Mailboxes Are Accessible, Some Are Not

Data corruption commonly occurs on Exchange servers, not because Exchange is particularly an unreliable system, but because Exchange data is stored in a database that requires periodic maintenance. Without periodic maintenance, covered in Chapter 19, "Exchange Server 2003 Management and Maintenance Practices," the databases in Exchange become corrupt. Exchange database corruption that is not repaired can make portions of mailboxes stored on an Exchange server inaccessible.

When recovering from data corruption on an Exchange server, it is important to not only recover lost or inaccessible data, but also to also repair the database, to prevent existing data corruption from causing more problems on an Exchange server in the future.

When a mailbox or multiple mailboxes are corrupt, the good data in the mailboxes can be extracted with minimal data loss. By isolating the corruption and extracting good data, an organization that might not need to recover the lost data can typically continue to operate with minimal downtime.

The process of extracting mail from an Exchange database is covered in the section "Recovering from Database Corruption," later in this chapter.

Data Is Corrupt, No Mailboxes Are Accessible

Depending on the condition of an Exchange database, the information might be so corrupt that none of the mailboxes are accessible. Recovering data from a corrupt database that cannot be accessed is a two-step process. The first step is to conduct maintenance to attempt to get the database operational; the second step is to extract as much information from the database as possible.

The process of performing maintenance and extracting data from a corrupt database is covered in the section "Recovering from Database Corruption," later in this chapter.

Exchange Server Is Okay, Something Else Is Preventing Exchange from Working

If you know that the Exchange server and databases are operational and something else is preventing Exchange from working, the process of recovery focuses on looking at things such as Active Directory, Internet Information Server (IIS), the Domain Name System (DNS), and the network infrastructure, as with site-to-site connectivity for replication.

The process of analyzing the operation of other services is covered in the sections "Recovering Windows Server 2003 Domain Controllers" and "Recovering Active Directory," later in this chapter.

What to Do Before Performing Any Server-Recovery Process

If a full server recovery will be conducted, or if a number of different procedures will be taken to install service packs, patches, updates, or other server-recovery attempts as an attempt to recover the server, a full backup should be performed on the server.

It might seem silly backing up a server that isn't working properly, but during the problem-solving and debugging process, it is quite common for a server to end up being in even worse shape after a few updates and fixes have been applied. The initial problem might have been that a single mailbox couldn't be accessed, and after some problem-solving efforts, the entire server might be inaccessible. Having a full backup of the server in its current state provides a rollback to the point of the initial problem state. When the backup is complete, verify that the backup is valid, ensuring that no open files are skipped during the backup process or that, if the files are skipped, they are backed up in other open file backup processes.

> **CAUTION**
>
> When performing any recovery of an Exchange server or resource, be careful what you delete, modify, or change. As a rule of thumb, *never* delete objects that are known throughout the directory; otherwise, you will not be able to restore the object due to the uniqueness of each object. As an example, if you plan to restore an entire server from tape, you do not want to first delete the server and then add the server back during the restoration process. The restoration process requires the existence of the old server in the directory. Deleting the server object and then adding the object again later gives the object a completely different globally unique identifier (GUID). Even though you restore the entire Exchange server from tape, the ID of the server and all of the objects in the server will be different, making it more difficult to recover the server. Other replicable objects that should not be deleted include public folders, public folder trees, groups, and distribution lists.

Validating Backup Data and Procedures

Another very important task that should be done before doing any maintenance, service, or repairs on an Exchange server is to validate that a full backup exists on the server, test the condition of the backup, and then secure the backup so that it is safe. Far too many organizations proceed with risky recovery procedures, believing that they have a fallback position by restoring from tape, only to realize that the tape backup is corrupt or that a complete backup does not exist.

If the administrators of the network realize that there is no clean backup, the procedures taken to recover the system might be different than if a backup had existed. If a full backup exists and is verified to be in good condition, the organization has an opportunity to restore from tape if a full restore is necessary.

Preparing for a More Easily Recoverable Environment

Steps can be taken to help an organization more easily prepare for a recoverable environment. This involves documenting server states and conditions, performing specific backup procedures, and setting up new features in Exchange Server 2003 that provide for a more simplified restoration process.

Documenting the Exchange Environment

Key to the success of recovering an Exchange server or an entire Exchange environment is having documentation on the server configurations. Having specific server configuration information documented helps to identify which server is not operational, the routing of information between servers, and ultimately the impact that a server failure or server recovery will have on the rest of the Exchange environment.

Some of the items that should be documented include these:

- Server name
- Version of Windows on servers (including Service Pack)
- Version of Exchange on servers (including Service Pack)
- Organization name in Exchange
- Site names
- Storage group names
- Database names
- Location of databases
- Size of databases
- Public folder tree name
- Replication process of public folders
- Security delegation and administrative rights
- Names and locations of Global Catalog servers

Documenting the Backup Process

Important in simplifying a restore of an Exchange environment is to start with a clean backup to restore from. A clean backup is performed when the proper backup process is followed. Create a backup process that works, document the step-by-step procedures to back up the server, follow the procedures regularly, and then validate that the backups have been completed successfully.

Also, when configurations change, the backup process as well as system configurations should be documented and validated again, to make sure that the backups are being completed properly.

Documenting the Recovery Process

An important aspect of recovery feasibility is knowing how to recover from a disaster. Just knowing what to back up and what scenarios to plan for is not enough. Restore processes should be created and tested to ensure that a restore can meet service level agreements (SLAs) and that the staff members understand all the necessary steps.

When a process is determined, it should be documented, and the documentation should be written to make sense to the desired audience. For example, if a failure occurs in a satellite office that has only marketing employees and one of them is forced to recover a server, the documentation needs to be written so that it can be understood by just about anyone. If the IT staff will be performing the restore, the documentation can be less detailed, but it assumes a certain level of knowledge and expertise with the server product. The first paragraph of any document related to backup and recovery should be a summary of what the document is used for and the level of skill necessary to perform the task and understand the document.

The recovery process involved in resolving an Exchange problem should also be focused not only on the goal of getting the entire Exchange server back up and operational, but also on considering smaller steps that might help minimize downtime. As an example, if an Exchange server has failed, instead of trying to restore 100GB of mail back to the server, which can take hours, if not days, to complete, an organization can choose to restore just the user inboxes, Calendars, and contacts. After a faster system recovery of core information on a server, the balance of the information can be restored over the next several hours.

Including Test Restores in the Scheduled Maintenance

Part of a successful disaster-recovery plan involves periodically testing the restore procedures to verify accuracy and to test the backup media to ensure that data can actually be recovered. Most organizations or administrators assume that if the backup software reports "Successful," the backup is good and data can be recovered. If special backup consideration is not addressed, the successful backup might not contain everything necessary to restore a server if data loss or software corruption occurs.

Restores of file data, application data, and configurations should be performed as part of a regular maintenance schedule to ensure that the backup method is correct and that disaster-recovery procedures and documentation are current. Such tests also should verify that the backup media can be read from and used to restore data. Adding periodic test restores to regular maintenance intervals ensures that backups are successful and familiarizes the administrators with the procedures necessary to recover so that when a real disaster occurs, the recovery can be performed correctly and efficiently the first time.

Recovering from a Site Failure

When a site becomes unavailable due to a physical access limitation or a disaster such as a fire or earthquake, steps must be taken to provide the recovery of the Exchange server in the site. Exchange does not have a single-step method of merging information from the failed site server into another server, so the process involves recovering the lost server in its entirety.

To prepare for the recovery of a failed site, an organization can create redundancy in a failover site. With redundancy built into a remote site, the recovery and restore process can be minimized if a recovery needs to performed.

Creating Redundant and Failover Sites

Redundant sites are created for a couple of different reasons. First, a redundant site can have a secondary Internet connection and bridgehead routing server so that if the primary site is down, the secondary site can be the focus for inbound and outbound email communications. This redundancy can be built, configured, and set to automatically provide failover in case of a site failure. See Chapter 3, "Installing Exchange Server 2003," for details on creating Routing Group connectors and bridgehead servers.

The other reason for redundant site preparation is to provide a warm spare server site so that a company will be prepared to perform a server restore of a site server in case of a site failure. The site recovery can simply be having server documentation available in another site or having a full image of server information stored in another site. The more preparatory work is conducted up front, the faster the organization will be able to recover from a system failure.

Creating the Failover Site

When an organization decides to plan for site failures as part of a disaster-recovery solution, many areas need to be addressed and many options exist. For organizations looking for redundancy, network connectivity is a priority, along with spare servers that can accommodate the user load. The spare servers need to have enough disk space to accommodate a complete restore. As a best practice, to ensure a smooth transition, the following list of recommendations provides a starting point:

- Allocate the appropriate hardware devices, including servers with enough processing power and disk space to accommodate the restored machines' resources.

- Host the organization's DNS zones and records using primary DNS servers located at an Internet service provider (ISP) collocation facility, or have redundant DNS servers registered for the domain and located at both physical locations.

- Ensure that DNS record-changing procedures are documented and available at the remote site or at an offsite data storage location.

- For the Exchange servers, ensure that the host records in the DNS tables are set to low Time to Live (TTL) values so that DNS changes do not take extended periods to propagate across the Internet. The Microsoft Windows Server 2003 default TTL is 1 hour.

- Ensure that network connectivity is already established and stable between sites and between each site and the Internet.

- Create at least one copy of backup tape medium for each site. One copy should remain at one location, and a second copy should be stored with an offsite data storage company. An optional third copy could be stored at another site location and can be used to restore the file to spare hardware on a regular basis, to restore Windows if a site failover is necessary.

- Have a copy of all disaster-recovery documentation stored at multiple locations as well as at the offsite data storage company. This provides redundancy if a recovery becomes necessary.

Allocating hardware and making the site ready to act as a failover site are simple tasks in concept, but the actual failover and failback process can be troublesome. Keep in mind that the preceding list applies to failover sites, not mirrored or redundant sites configured to provide load balancing.

Failing Over Between Sites

Before failing over between sites can be successful, administrators need to be aware of what services need to fail over and in which order of precedence. For example, before an Exchange server can be restored, Active Directory domain controllers, Global Catalog servers, and DNS servers must be available.

To keep such a cutover at a high level, the following tasks need to be executed in a timely manner:

1. Update Internet DNS records pointing to the Exchange server(s).

2. Restore any necessary Windows Server 2003 domain controllers, Global Catalog servers, and internal DNS servers.

3. Restore the Exchange server(s).

4. Test client connectivity, troubleshoot, and provide remote and local client support as needed.

Failing Back After Site Recovery

When the initial site is back online and available to handle client requests and provide access to data and networking services and applications, it is time to consider failing back the services. This can be a controversial subject because failback procedures are usually more difficult than the initial failover procedure. Most organizations plan on the failover and have a tested failover plan that might include database log shipping to the disaster-recovery site. However, they do not plan how they can get the current data back to the restored servers in the main or preferred site.

Questions to consider for failing back are as follows:

- Will downtime be necessary to restore databases between the sites?

- When is the appropriate time to fail back?

- Is the failover site less functional than the preferred site? In other words, are only mission-critical services provided in the failover site, or is it a complete copy of the preferred site?

The answers really lie in the complexity of the failed-over environment. If the cutover is simple, there is no reason to wait to fail back.

Providing Alternative Methods of Client Connectivity

When failover sites are too expensive and are not an option, that does not mean that an organization cannot plan for site failures. Other lower-cost options are available but depend on how and where the employees do their work. For example, many times users who need to access email can do so without physically being at the site location. Email can be accessed remotely from other terminals or workstations.

The following are some ways to deal with these issues without renting or buying a separate failover site:

- Consider renting racks or cages at a local ISP to colocate servers that can be accessed during a site failure.

- Have users dial in from home to a terminal server hosted at an ISP to access Exchange.

- Set up remote user access using Terminal Services or Outlook Web Access at a redundant site so that users can access their email, Calendar, and contacts from any location.

- Rent temporary office space, printers, networking equipment, and user workstations with common standard software packages such as Microsoft Office and Internet Explorer. You can plan for and execute this option in about one day. If this is an option, be sure to find a computer rental agency first and get pricing before a failure occurs and you have no choice but to pay the rental rates.

Recovering from a Disk Failure

Organizations create disaster-recovery plans and procedures to protect against a variety of system failures, but disk failures tend to be the most common in networking environments. The technology used to create processor chips and memory chips has improved drastically over the past couple decades, minimizing the failure of systemboards. And while the quality of hard drives has also drastically improved over the years, because hard drives are constantly spinning, they have the most moving parts in a computer system and tend to be the items of most failure.

Key to a disk fault-tolerant solution is creating hardware fault tolerance on key server drives that can be recovered in case of failure. Information is stored on system, boot, and data volumes that have varying levels of recovery needs.

Hardware-Based RAID Array Failure

Common uses of hardware-based disk arrays for Windows servers include RAID 1 (mirroring) for the operating system and RAID 5 (striped sets with parity) for separate data volumes. Some deployments use a single RAID 5 array for the OS, and data volumes for RAID 0/1 (mirrored striped sets) have been used in more recent deployments.

RAID controllers provide a firmware-based array-management interface, which can be accessed during system startup. This interface enables administrators to configure RAID controller options and manage disk arrays. This interface should be used to repair or reconfigure disk arrays if a problem or disk failure occurs.

Many controllers offer Windows-based applications that can be used to manage and create arrays. Of course, this requires the operating system to be started to access the Windows-based RAID controller application. Follow the manufacturer's procedures on replacing a failed disk within hardware-based RAID arrays.

> **NOTE**
>
> Many RAID controllers allow an array to be configured with a *hot spare disk*. This disk automatically joins the array when a single disk failure occurs. If several arrays are created on a single RAID controller card, hot spare disks can be defined as global and can be used to replace a failed disk on any array. As a best practice, hot spare disks should be defined for arrays.

System Volume

If a system disk failure is encountered, the system can be left in a completely failed state. To prevent this problem from occurring, the administrator should always try to create the system disk on a fault-tolerant disk array such as RAID 1 or RAID 5. If the system disk was mirrored (RAID 1) in a hardware-based array, the operating system will operate and boot normally because the disk and partition referenced in the boot.ini file will remain the same and will be accessible. If the RAID 1 array was created within the operating system using Disk Manager or `diskpart.exe`, the mirrored disk can be accessed upon bootup by choosing the second option in the `boot.ini` file during startup. If a disk failure occurs on a software-based RAID 1 array during regular operation, no system disruption should be encountered.

Boot Volume

If Windows Server 2003 has been installed on the second or third partitions of a disk drive, a separate boot and system partition will be created. Most manufacturers require that for a system to boot up from a volume other than the primary partition, the partition must be marked active before functioning. To satisfy this requirement without having to change the active partition, Windows Server 2003 always tries to load the boot files on the first or active partition during installation, regardless of which partition or disk the system files will be loaded on. When this drive or volume fails, if the system volume is still intact, a boot disk can be used to boot into the OS and make the necessary modification after changing the drive.

Data Volume

A data volume is by far the simplest of all types of disks to recover. If an entire disk fails, simply replacing the disk, assigning the previously configured drive letter, and restoring the entire drive from backup will restore the data and permissions.

A few issues to watch out for include these:

- Setting the correct permissions on the root of the drive

- Ensuring that file shares still work as desired

- Validating that data in the drive does not require a special restore procedure

Recovering from a Boot Failure

Occasionally, a Windows Server 2003 system can suffer a service or application startup problem that could leave a server incapable of completing a normal bootup sequence. Because the operating system cannot be accessed in this case, the system remains unavailable until this problem can be resolved.

Windows Server 2003 includes a few alternative bootup options to help administrators restore a server to a working state. Several advanced bootup options can be accessed by pressing the F8 key when the boot loader screen is displayed (see Figure 32.1). If the Recovery Console was previously installed, it is listed as an option in the boot loader screen. The advanced boot options include these:

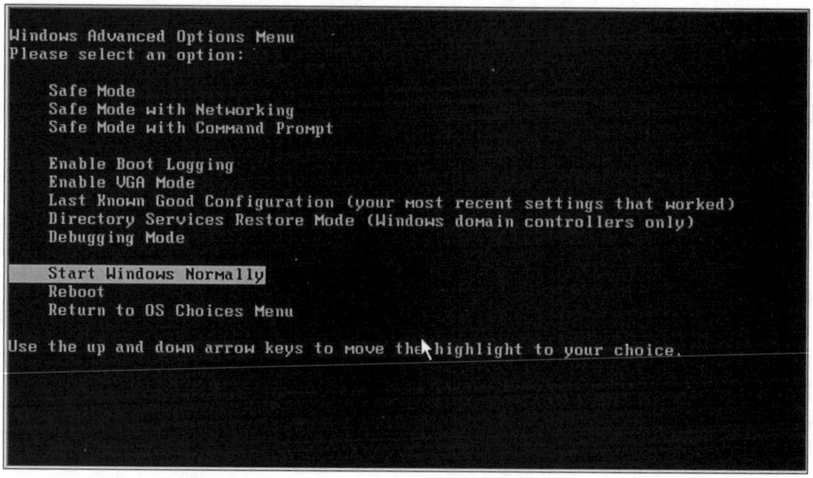

FIGURE 32.1 The advanced boot options of Windows 2003.

- **Safe Mode**   This mode starts the operating system with only the most basic services and hardware drivers, and disables networking. This allows administrators to access the operating system in a less functional state to make configuration changes to service startup options, some application configurations, and the system Registry.

- **Safe Mode with Networking**   This option is the same as Safe Mode, but networking drivers are enabled during operation. This mode also starts many more operating system services upon startup.

- **Safe Mode with Command Prompt**   This option is similar to the Safe Mode option; however, the Windows Explorer shell is not started by default.

- **Enable Boot Logging**   This option boots the system normally, but all the services and drivers loaded at startup are recorded in a file named ntbtlog.txt, located in the %systemroot% directory. The default location for this file is C:\Windows\ntbtlog.txt. To simplify reading this file, the administrator must delete the existing file before a bootup sequence is logged so that only the information from the last bootup is logged.

- **Enable VGA Mode**   This mode loads the current display driver, but it displays the desktop at the lowest resolution. This mode is handy if a server is plugged into a different monitor that cannot support the current resolution.

- **Last Known Good Configuration**   This mode starts the operating system using Registry and driver information saved during the last successful logon.

- **Directory Services Restore Mode**   This mode is only for domain controllers and allows for maintenance and restoration of the Active Directory database or the SYSVOL folder.

- **Debugging Mode** This mode sends operating system debugging information to other servers through a serial connection. This requires a server on the receiving end with a logging server that is prepared to accept this data. Most likely, standard administrators will never use this mode.

- **Start Windows Normally** As the name states, this mode loads the operating system as it would normally run.

- **Reboot** This option reboots the server.

- **Return to OS Choices Menu** This option returns the screen to the boot loader page so that the correct operating system can be chosen and started.

The Recovery Console

The Recovery Console provides an option for administrators to boot up a system using alternate configuration files to perform troubleshooting tasks. Using the Recovery Console, the bootup sequence can be changed, alternate boot options can be specified, volumes can be created or extended, and service startup options can be changed. The Recovery Console has only a limited number of commands that can be used, making it a simple console to learn. If Normal or Safe Mode bootup options are not working, the administrator can use the Recovery Console to make system changes or read the information stored in the boot logging file using the `type` command. The boot logging file is located at `C:\Windows\ntbtlog.txt` by default and exists only if someone tried to start the operating system using any of the Safe Mode options or the boot logging option.

Recovering from a Complete Server Failure

Because hardware occasionally fails and, in the real world, operating systems do have problems, a server-recovery plan is essential, even though it might never be used. The last thing any administrator wants is for a server failure to occur and to end up on the phone with Microsoft technical support asking for the server to be restored from backup when no plan is in place. To keep from being caught unprepared, the administrator should have a recovery plan for every possible failure associated with Windows Server 2003 systems.

Restoring Versus Rebuilding

When a complete system failure occurs, whether it is due to a site outage, a hardware component failure, or a software corruption problem, the method of recovery depends on the administrator's major goal. The goal is to get the server up and running, of course, but behind the scenes, many more questions should be answered before the restore is started:

- How long will it take to restore the server from a full backup?

- If the server failed due to software corruption, will restoring the server from backup also restore the corruption that actually caused the failure?

- Will reloading the operating system and Exchange manually followed by restoring the system state be faster than doing a full restore?

Loading the Windows Server 2003 operating system and Exchange Server 2003 software can be a relatively quick process. This ensures that all the correct files and drivers are loaded correctly and all that needs to follow is a system state restore to recover the server configuration and restore the data. One of the problems that can occur is that, upon installation, some applications generate Registry keys based on the system's computer name, which can change if a system state restore is performed.

Exchange Server 2003 has a `setup /disasterrecovery` installation option and does not need the server's system state restore—just the original computer name and domain membership, as long as computer and user certificates are not being used.

The key to choosing whether to rebuild or restore from backup is understanding the dependencies of the applications and services to the operating system, and having confidence in the server's stability at the time of the previous backups. The worst situation is attempting a restore from backup that takes several hours, only to find that the problem has been restored as well.

Manually Recovering a Server

When a complete server system failure is encountered and the state of the operating system or an application is in question, the operating system can be recovered manually. Locating the system's original configuration settings is the first step. This information is normally stored in a server build document or wherever server configuration information is kept.

Because each system is different, as a general guideline for restoring a system manually, perform the following steps:

1. Install a new operating system on the original system hardware and disk volume, or one as close to the original configuration as possible. Be sure to install the same operating system version—for example, Windows Server 2003 Enterprise or Standard Server.

2. During installation, name the system using the name of the original server, but do not join a domain.

3. Do not install additional services during installation, and proceed by performing a basic installation.

4. When the operating system completes installation, install any additional hardware drivers as necessary and update the operating system to the service pack and security patches that the failed server was expected to have installed. To reduce compatibility problems, install the service packs and updates as outlined in the server build document to ensure that any installed applications will function as desired. During a restore is not the time to roll out additional system changes. The goal is to get the system back online, not to upgrade it.

5. Using the Disk Management console, create and format disk volumes and assign the correct drive letters as recorded in the server build document.

6. If the server was originally part of a domain, join the domain using the original server name. Because many Windows Server 2003 services use the server name or require the service to be authorized in a domain, perform this step before installing any additional services or applications.

7. Install any additional Windows Server 2003 services as defined in the server build document.

8. Install Exchange Server 2003 using the same version of Exchange (Standard or Enterprise) that was originally installed. Apply any Exchange Service Packs and updates that were expected to be on the original server as well. When installing Exchange, use the `setup /disasterrecovery` installation process that will install Exchange but will not add new databases.

9. Restore Exchange data to the new server.

10. Test functionality, add this system to the backup schedule, and start a full backup.

> **NOTE**
>
> If certificates were issued to the previous server, the new server must enroll with the Certificate Authority (CA) for a new certificate before encrypted communication can occur.

Restoring a Server Using a System State Restore

The restoration of an Exchange Server 2003 system into an existing Active Directory domain does not require the installation of the system state because the procedures covered in the previous section will recover the server and database for the server replacement. However, if the failure of Exchange also included the loss of the Active Directory Global Catalog and there is no other Global Catalog in the organization, a system state restore of the Global Catalog needs to be performed before Exchange can be restored.

Exchange Server 2003 requires a valid Active Directory to be in place. This process might be required if the Exchange server was the only server in the network and, thus, the loss of the Exchange server also meant the loss of the only Global Catalog server. This also might be the case if there was a site failure and all servers, including the Exchange Server and Active Directory Global Catalog server, were lost.

To recover the system state, follow these steps:

1. Shut down the original server or build a new server hardware system.

2. Install a new copy of Windows 2003 on the system hardware and disk volume, or one as close to the original configuration as possible. Be sure to install the same

operating system version—for example, Windows Server 2003 Enterprise or Standard Server.

3. During installation, name the system using the name of the original server, but do not join a domain.

> **NOTE**
>
> If the machine is joined to the original domain during the clean installation, a new security iden-
> tifier (SID) will be generated for the machine account. A system state restore after this restores an
> invalid computer SID, and many services and applications will fail.

---

4. Do not install additional services during installation, and proceed by performing a basic installation.

5. When the operating system completes installation, install any additional hardware drivers as necessary and update the operating system to the latest service pack and security patches. To reduce compatibility problems, install the service packs and updates as outlined in the server build document, to ensure that any installed applications will function as desired.

6. Using the Disk Management console, create and format disk volumes and assign the correct drive letters as recorded in the server build document.

7. After the installation, restore any necessary drivers or updates to match the original configuration. This information should be gathered from a server configuration document (server build document). Then reboot as necessary.

After all the updates have been installed, restore the previously backed-up system state data; afterward, restore any additional application or user data.

System State Restore

This section outlines how to restore the system state to a member or standalone Windows Server 2003 system. To restore the system state, perform the following steps:

1. Click Start, All Programs, Accessories, System Tools, Backup.

2. If this is the first time you've run Backup, it opens in Wizard mode. Choose to run it in Advanced mode by clicking the Advanced Mode hyperlink.

3. Click the Restore Wizard (Advanced) button to start the Restore Wizard.

4. Click Next on the Restore Wizard welcome screen to continue.

5. On the What to Restore page, select the appropriate cataloged backup medium, expand the catalog selection, and check System State. Click Next to continue.

6. If the correct tape or file backup medium does not appear in this window, cancel the restore process. Then, from the Restore Wizard, locate and catalog the appropriate medium and return to the restore process from step 1.

7. On the Completing the Restore Wizard page, click Finish to start the restore. The restore will look something similar to Figure 32.2.

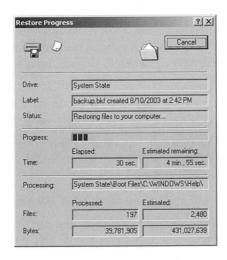

FIGURE 32.2   Performing a system state restore on an Exchange server.

8. When the restore is complete, review the backup log for detailed information and click Close on the Restore Progress window when finished.

9. Reboot the system as prompted.

10. When the system restarts, log in using an account with Local and/or Domain Administrator rights, as necessary.

11. After the system state is restored, Exchange Server 2003 can be installed.

Restoring a System Using an Automated System Recovery Restore

When a system has failed and all other recovery options have been exhausted, an Automated System Recovery (ASR) restore can be performed, provided that an ASR backup has been previously performed. The ASR restore will restore all disk and volume configurations, including redefining volumes and formatting them. This means that the data stored on all volumes needs to be restored after the ASR restore is complete. This restore brings a failed system back to complete server operation, except for certain applications that require special configurations after the restore. For example, the Remote Storage service data needs to be restored separately.

> **NOTE**
>
> An ASR restore re-creates all disk volumes, but if a new or alternate system is being used, each disk must be of equal or greater size to the disks on the original server. Otherwise, the ASR restore will fail.

To perform an ASR restore, follow these steps:

1. Locate the ASR floppy created for the failed node, or create the floppy from the files saved in the ASR backup medium. For information on creating the ASR floppy from the ASR backup medium, refer to Help and Support from any Windows Server 2003 Help and Support tool.

2. Insert the Windows Server 2003 operating system medium in the CD-ROM drive of the server you are restoring to, and start the installation from this CD.

3. When prompted, press F6 to install any third-party storage device drivers, if necessary. This includes any third-party disks or tape controllers that Windows Server 2003 will not natively recognize.

4. Press F2 when prompted to perform an Automated System Recovery.

5. Insert the ASR floppy disk into the floppy drive and press Enter when prompted. If the system does not have a local floppy drive, one must temporarily be added; otherwise, an ASR restore cannot be performed.

6. The operating system installation proceeds by restoring disk volume information and reformatting the volumes associated with the operating system. When this process is complete, the operating system will restart after a short countdown, the graphic-based OS installation will begin, and the ASR backup will attempt to reconnect to the backup medium automatically. If the backup medium is on a network drive, the ASR backup reconnection will fail. If it fails, specify the network location of the backup medium using a UNC path, and enter authentication information, if prompted.

7. When the medium is located, open the medium and click Next and then Finish to begin recovering the remaining ASR data.

8. When the ASR restore is complete, if any local disk data was not restored with the ASR restore, restore all local disks.

9. Click Start, All Programs, Accessories, System Tools, Backup.

10. If this is the first time you've run Backup, it opens in Wizard mode. Choose to run it in Advanced mode by clicking the Advanced Mode hyperlink.

11. Click the Restore Wizard (Advanced) button to start the Restore Wizard.

12. Click Next on the Restore Wizard welcome screen to continue.

13. On the What to Restore page, select the appropriate cataloged backup medium, expand the catalog selection, and check the desired data on each local drive. Click Next to continue.

14. On the Completing the Restore Wizard page, click Finish to start the restore. Because you want to restore only what ASR did not, you do not need to make any advanced restore configuration changes.

15. When the restore is complete, reboot the server, if prompted.

16. After the reboot is complete, log on to the restored server and check server configuration and functionality.

17. If everything is working properly, perform a full backup and log off the server.

Restoring the Boot Loader File

When a Windows Server 2003 system is recovered using an ASR restore, the boot.ini file might not be restored. This file contains the options for booting into different operating systems on multiboot systems and booting into the Recovery Console if it was previously installed. To restore this file, simply restore it from backup to an alternate folder or drive. Delete the boot.ini file from the C:\ root folder and move the restored file from the alternate location to C:\ or whichever drive the boot.ini file previously was located on.

Recovering Exchange Application and Exchange Data

To recover an Exchange Server, there are several different ways of rebuilding the core Exchange server and restoring the Exchange data. The restoration of Exchange databases must be done to a server with the exact same server name as the original server where the databases were backed up from.

After the Active Directory and base Windows server(s) have been installed, the first process is installing or restoring the Exchange application software; the second process is installing the data files for Exchange.

Recovering Using Ntbackup.exe

When program and data files are corrupt or missing, or a previously backed-up copy is needed, the information can be restored using Ntbackup.exe if a previous backup was performed using this utility. The following process should be followed:

1. Log on to the server using an account that has at least the privileges to restore files and folders. Backup Operators and Local Administrator groups have this right, by default.

2. Click Start, All Programs, Accessories, System Tools, Backup.

3. If this is the first time you've run Backup, it opens in Wizard mode. Click on Next to continue with a restore.

4. Select Restore Files and Settings, and then click Next.

5. On the What to Restore page, select the appropriate cataloged backup medium, expand the catalog selection, and select to restore all applicable volumes (C:, D:, E:, and so on) and the System State. Then click Next.

7. If the correct tape or file backup medium does not appear in this window, cancel the restore process. Then, from the Restore Wizard, locate and catalog the appropriate medium and return to the restore process from step 4.

8. On the Completing the Restore Wizard page, click Finish to start the restore.

9. When the restore is complete, review the backup log for detailed information, and click Close on the Restore Progress window when finished.

10. Reboot the server. The system should come up as a complete replacement of the original server system.

Performing a Restore of Only Exchange Database Files

If Exchange server program files have been corrupt or the restore of the full backup information from tape might restore corruption and server instability, an administrator can choose to install Exchange Server 2003 from scratch and restore just the database files. This process involves installing the Exchange program files from CD-ROM and then restoring a copy of the Exchange databases.

To install Exchange and restore the Exchange database files, do the following:

1. Log on to the server using an account that has administrative privileges to install application software as well as restore data from tape.

2. Ensure that the server has the exact same server name as it had before. Also make sure that the version of Windows is the same version.

3. Install Exchange Server 2003 using the setup /disasterrecovery command. When prompted, confirm the Disaster Recovery method of installation, as shown in Figure 32.3.

4. After Exchange Server 2003 has been installed, restore data files to the Exchange server.

Restoring Exchange Data Files from Tape

If the Exchange data files are stored on tape, restore just the Exchange database files by doing the following:

1. Click Start, All Programs, Accessories, System Tools, Backup.

2. If this is the first time you've run Backup, it opens in Wizard mode. Choose to run it in Advanced mode by clicking the Advanced Mode hyperlink.

3. Click the Restore Wizard (Advanced) button to start the Restore Wizard.

4. Click Next on the Restore Wizard welcome screen to continue.

5. On the What to Restore page, select the appropriate cataloged backup medium, expand the catalog selection, and select the *.edb and *.stm files for restoration.

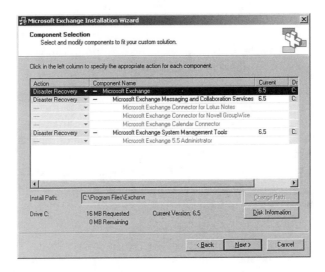

FIGURE 32.3   Selecting the Disaster Recovery method of installation.

> **NOTE**
>
> The Exchange database files for a server are typically `priv.edb`, and the public folder files are typically `pub.edb`. Exchange Server 2003 also has streaming message databases that are typically `priv.stm` and `publ.stm`. The files are typically stored in `\Program Files\Exchsrvr\mdbdata`; however, in Exchange Server 2003, administrators can name Exchange database files and specify folder locations differently than the default settings. Also, the Enterprise edition of Exchange Server 2003 allows for up to five databases for each storage group, with up to four storage groups on a server. So, an Exchange server could potentially have 20 different directories each with a *.edb and *.stm file for the databases stored.

6. If the correct tape or file backup medium does not appear in this window, cancel the restore process. Then, from the Restore Wizard, locate and catalog the appropriate medium and return to the restore process from step 4.

7. On the Completing the Restore Wizard page, click Finish to start the restore.

8. When the restore is complete, review the backup log for detailed information, and click Close on the Restore Progress window when finished. Reboot the Exchange server to restart all services. (Alternately, after a restore of data, the individual databases can just be mounted to get the Exchange server back and operational.)

Recovering from Database Corruption

If an Exchange database is corrupt, it is not extremely effective to restore the corrupt database to a production server. The server might continue to operate, but database corruption never goes away on its own, and you eventually will have to repair the database. In fact, when minor database corruption is not repaired, the corruption can get to the point that entire sections of the Exchange database become inaccessible.

A couple methods can be used to repair a corrupt Exchange database, or at least restore the database and extract good information from the database. Key to the successful recovery of as much information as possible is using the right tool. In many cases, administrators jump right into using the ESEUTIL /p repair command; instead of repairing the Exchange database to 100% condition, the utility finds a corrupt section of the database and deletes all information from that portion of the database on. So, although the Exchange system becomes 100% clean, the utility deleted 20–30% of the data that was in the database to get the database to a clean state. The ESEUTIL /P command is the task of last resort: Other tools work around corrupt database areas and allow the administrator to recover as much of the data as possible.

Going all the way back to the start of the chapter in the "What to Do Before Performing Any Server-Recovery Process" section, this is where having a complete backup of the databases in Exchange is really important. If a process to repair or recover information causes more harm to the database than good, there is still a backup copy to restore and start again.

Flat File Copying the Exchange Databases

One of the best techniques Exchange experts use when working to recover corruption in a database is to make a flat file copy of the Exchange databases. A flat file copy is merely an exact copy of the Exchange databases copied to another portion of the server hard drive or to another server. To do a manual copy of the databases, do the following:

1. Unmount the Exchange database stores by going into the Exchange System Manager. Traverse the tree past Administrative Groups, Servers, Storage Group. Right-click on the mailbox store and select Dismount Store.

2. Dismount the store for all mailbox stores you will be working on.

3. Copy (using Windows Explorer, or XCOPY) the *.edb and *.stm files to a safe location (usually the filenames are priv1.edb and priv1.stm and are stored in

`\Program Files\Exchsrvr\mdbdata\` for the default—however, as additional databases are created, the directory names and filenames can differ).

> **NOTE**
>
> If the databases need to be manually restored, a simple XCOPY (or Windows Explorer copy) of the databases back to the original subdirectories will bring the data back to the condition the databases were in at the time the databases were copied off the system. Inside the directories (`\Program Files\Exchsrvr\mdbdata` or the like) are other files, such as `tmp.edb`, *.log, files. These files are support files to the Exchange databases. These files could be copied off the system and then copied back if a restore is desired. The support files beyond the basic `priv1.edb`, `priv1.stm`, `pub1.edb`, and `pub1.stm` files typically need to be copied as a group. After maintenance is run on the main *.edb and *.stm files, the support files are typically unuseable because they are no longer associated with the master database files.

Moving Mailboxes to Another Server in the Site

One way of extracting mail from a corrupt database is to move the mailbox or mailboxes to a different server in the site. Instead of trying to run utilities to fix the corruption in the database, which can take several hours (or even days, depending on the size of the database and the amount of corruption that needs to be fixed), an administrator can set up another server in the Exchange site and move the mailboxes to a new server.

Moving mailboxes grabs all of the mail, Calendar, contacts, and other mailbox information from one server and moves the information to a new server. As the information is written to the new server, the information is automatically defragmented and corruption is not migrated. Additionally, mailboxes can be moved from one server to another without ever having to bring down the production server. A mailbox user must be logged out of Outlook and must not be accessing Exchange before the mailbox can be moved. However, if mailboxes are moved when individuals are out of the office or at lunch, or on weekends, the mailboxes can be moved without users ever knowing that their information was moved from one system to another.

The two caveats to moving mailboxes are these: Corrupt mailboxes will not move, and user Outlook profiles will be changed. For Outlook profiles, because a user's Outlook profiles point to a specific server, when a mailbox is moved from one server to another, the user's profile also needs to point to the new server. Fortunately, with Exchange and Outlook, when a user's mailbox is moved, Outlook tries to access the mailbox on the original server, and the server notifies Outlook that the mailbox has been moved to a new Exchange server. The user's Outlook profile automatically changes to associate the profile to the new server where the user's mailbox resides. So, as long as the old server remains operational and the user attempts to access email from the old server, the profiles will be automatically changed the next time the user tries to access email. Typically within 1–2 weeks after moving mailboxes from one server to another, the user profiles are all automatically changed.

As for corrupt mailboxes, unfortunately, Exchange typically does not move a corrupt mailbox. So, if a user's mailbox has been corrupted, the mailbox will remain on the old server. Moving the data from the corrupt mailbox will need to be handled in a manner specified in the following section, "Extracting Mail from a Corrupt Mailbox." However, if 80–90% of the user mailboxes can be moved to a new server, the administrators are trying to recover only a handful of mailboxes instead of all mailboxes on a server. This could mean far less downtime for all users who had mail on the server and could limit the exposure of data loss to a limited number of users.

To move mailboxes between servers in a site, do the following:

1. Open the Exchange System Manager.

2. Select the Administrative Group where the mailboxes to be moved reside.

3. Highlight the mailboxes to be moved.

4. From the Action menu, select the Exchange Tasks option and click the Next button on the welcome screen.

5. At the Available Tasks page, select Move Mailbox and click the Next button to continue.

6. Click the Mailbox Store option and choose the destination store where the mailboxes will be moved. Select Next when complete.

7. Configure the options for addressing corruption, and set the desired limits for this move. Select the Next button to begin the mailbox move.

8. Review the results of the mailbox move, and click Finish to complete the move.

Extracting Mail from a Corrupt Mailbox

When mailboxes cannot be moved between servers, either due to mailbox corruption or because the organization does not have a spare server to move mailboxes between, the exmerge.exe utility can be used to export mailboxes to a file. The ExMerge utility is freely downloadable from the Microsoft downloads page at www.microsoft.com/downloads (search for "ExMerge" or "Mailbox Merge Wizard").

ExMerge allows an administrator to select specific mailboxes and export the data from the mailbox into a PST file. The PST file can then be imported (using the ExMerge utility) into another server. Unlike the Move Mailbox tool, which is an all-or-nothing migration tool, ExMerge extracts information on an item-by-item basis. When corruption is found in a user's mailbox, the corrupted item is skipped and the balance of the user's information is extracted.

The ExMerge utility can be used to extract all mailboxes from a server and import the information back into a new server. However, because ExMerge extracts and imports information item by item, it could take more than an hour to extract 1GB of mail and another hour to import that 1GB of mail back into a new server. So, if the Move Mailbox tool can migrate the information directly from one server to another over the wire, the migration process of good mailboxes goes much faster. However, for corrupt mailboxes, the ExMerge method does skip corrupt portions of mailboxes and minimizes the loss of information.

To use the ExMerge utility, do the following:

1. Download the ExMerge utility from Microsoft.

2. Extract the `exmerge.exe` file (this explodes out four to five ExMerge utility files).

3. Copy the files into the `\Program Files\Exchsrvr\Bin` directory on the Exchange server.

4. Launch the `exmerge.exe` program and click Next through the welcome screen.

5. Choose Export or Import (Two-Step Procedure) and click Next.

> **NOTE**
>
> The ExMerge utility has an Export and Import (One-Step Procedure) option that exports the information from one server and imports the information into another server. Exchange experts do not commonly use this because they want to isolate the export and import functions to have better control over the results. If during the export or import processes an error occurs when performing both the export and import processes, it's harder to determine whether the problem was an export problem or an import problem. It's also harder to know where the problem faulted and where to pick up to complete the data-migration process. Using the two-step procedure ensures that a clean export can be successfully completed before an import is begun. Any problem in the export or import process also can more easily be identified.

6. Select Step 1 to extract data from an Exchange server, and click on Next.

7. Enter the name of the server where the information is being extracted; then click Next.

8. Select the storage group from which the mailboxes will be extracted; then select Next.

9. Choose the mailboxes that are to be extracted (hold down the Ctrl key to select individual mailboxes, or click on the Select All button to select all mailboxes to be extracted). Click on Next to continue.

> **NOTE**
>
> The ExMerge utility extracts information from the source server, but it leaves a copy of the information in the server. This allows information to be extracted without impacting the pre-existing state of information in the source server.

10. Select the default locale or language set used for the mailbox (for example, English US). Then click Next to continue.

11. Select the drive and subdirectory where the mailbox(es) should be extracted to; then click Next.

> **NOTE**
>
> Even if the data will ultimately reside on another server, if the server being extracted has ample disk space, it is faster to have the mailboxes extracted from the server to a local hard drive than to try to write the exported data across a LAN or WAN connection to another server. Remember, you might be extracting gigabytes of information, and it's a lot faster to extract the information to a local hard drive than over even a 100Mb Ethernet connection.

12. Choose to change the filenames during the extract process and to save the settings of the configuration information, or just leave them as the default and select Next to continue. A summary screen displays the results of the extraction, as shown in Figure 32.4.

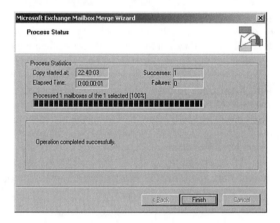

FIGURE 32.4   Extracting information from an Exchange database.

To import the ExMerge information to another server, the process is very similar. Do the following:

1. Launch the `exmerge.exe` program and click Next through the welcome screen.

2. Choose the Export or Import (Two-Step Procedure) option, and click Next.

3. Select Step 2 to import data into an Exchange server, and click on Next.

4. Enter the name of the server where the information will be imported, and then click Next.

32

5. Select the storage group into which the mailboxes will be imported; then select Next.

6. Choose the mailboxes that are to have data imported (hold down the Ctrl key to select individual mailboxes, or click on the Select All button to select all mailboxes to be extracted). Click on Next to continue.

7. Select the default locale or language set used for the mailbox (such as English US). Then click Next to continue.

8. Select the drive and subdirectory where the mailbox(es) should be imported from; then click Next.

> **NOTE**
>
> If the data currently resides on another server and there is a lot of information to import (more than 1GB), you might consider copying the files onto the hard drive of the server where the data will be imported from. This can drastically improve the import time because the file read is done on a message-by-message basis, and an XCOPY or Windows Explorer transfer of files is compressed.

9. Choose to change the filenames during the extraction process and to save the settings of the configuration information, or just leave them as default and select Next to continue. After completing, a summary screen displays the results of the import.

Running the ISINTEG and ESEUTIL Utilities

When a database is determined to be corrupt, usually an administrator is directed to run the built-in utilities on Exchange to run maintenance on the databases. The utilities are the ISINTEG ("eye-ess-in-tehg") and ESEUTIL ("ee-ess-ee-u-tihl"). However, depending on the condition of the database, a very corrupt database can take several hours to run, only to result in the loss of data. Some administrators are incorrectly told to never run the utilities because they will always result in loss of data. It's typically just a lack of knowledge of how the utilities work that leads to misunderstanding the potential results of the databases.

As noted in the previous two sections, there might be better options for recovering information from a corrupt database. Instead of trying to fix a known corrupt database, simply migrating the information off a server or extracting information from corrupt databases is frequently a better fix. However, if the determination is to run the utilities, a few things should be noted:

1. The ISINTEG utility is a high-level utility that checks the consistency of the database, validating the branches of the database that handle data, data directory tables, attachment objects, and the like. Fixing the database table makes way for a more intensive data integrity check of the database.

2. The ESEUTIL utility is a low-level utility that checks the data within the database. ESEUTIL does not differentiate between a corrupt section of the database and how that section impacts mailboxes or messages. So, when a complete repair is performed using ESEUTIL, entire mailboxes can be deleted or all attachments for the entire database can be eliminated to fix the corruption. This is why running ESEUTIL to repair a database is a function of last resort.

3. To run ISINTEG on a database takes around 1 hour for every 10GB being scanned for a moderately corrupt database. The repairs are done relatively quickly, and the database is ready for more extensive scanning.

4. Running ESEUTIL on a database takes anywhere from 1 hour for every 10GB to up to 1 hour per 1GB, depending on the level of repair being performed. It is not unreasonable to see a relatively corrupt 30GB database take more than 24 hours to complete the repair.

5. ISINTEG and ESEUTIL can be performed only offline, meaning that the Exchange server is offline during the process. Users cannot access their mailboxes during the ISINTEG and ESEUTIL processes. Thus, if it takes 20–40 hours of downtime to complete the repair of a database, the Move Mailbox method that can be run without bringing servers offline is frequently a more palatable solution.

6. However, if run on a regular basis, the ISINTEG and ESEUTIL utilities can clean up an Exchange database before serious corruption occurs. Administrators who get scared off performing maintenance because of the potential threat of losing data could actually minimize their chance of data corruption if the utilities are run regularly. See Chapter 19 for recommended maintenance practices.

The common parameters used for the ISINTEG and ESEUTIL utilities are as follows. For regular maintenance such as checking the database structure's integrity and performing defragmentation of the database, the following commands should be run:

```
isinteg -s SERVERNAME -test allfoldertests
```

```
eseutil /d priv1.edb
```

When run against an Exchange Server 2003 system, the ISINTEG utility produces a summary similar to the one in Figure 32.5.

> **NOTE**
>
> The ISINTEG and ESEUTIL utilities typically reside in the \Program Files\Exchsrvr\Bin directory of the Exchange server. The databases that are typically specified in ESEUTIL are the priv1.edb and pub1.edb. However, if an organization has multiple database and storage groups, several database might need to be checked separately for integrity.

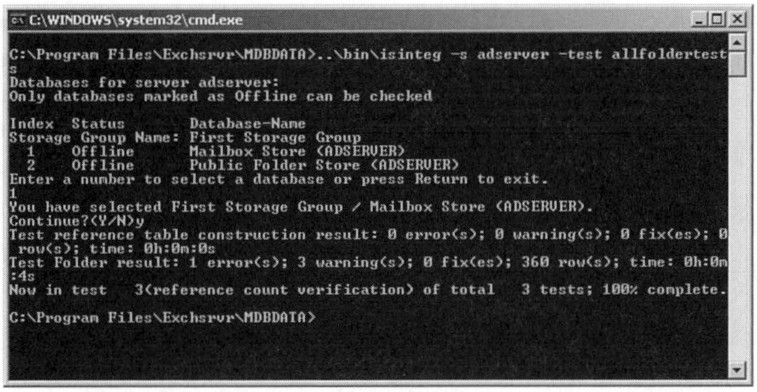

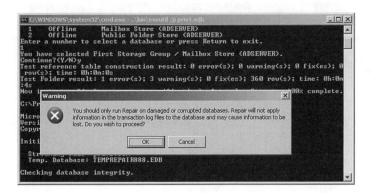

FIGURE 32.5   Results from an ISINTEG utility run.

When a database needs to be repaired, eseutil /p priv1.edb can be run. Beware: The /p repair command is a brute-force repair and deletes sections of the database to make the integrity of the database clean. A message provides an additional warning about ESEUTIL, as shown in Figure 32.6. When running the /p command in ESEUTIL, entire sections of the database might be deleted to repair and recover the state of the database.

FIGURE 32.6   ESEUTIL warning when a database repair (/p) is run.

Using the Recovery Storage Group in Exchange Server 2003

When an administrator wants to recover a mail message, a Calendar appointment, a contact, a folder, or entire user mailboxes, Exchange Server 2003 has a Recovery Storage Group function that provides a recovery mechanism. In the past, if an administrator wanted to recover a mailbox or information, the administrator would have to build a brand-new Exchange Server with the exact same server name in the lab and then restore a database to the lab server. After the restore, the administrator could run the ExMerge utility to export the desired mailbox or information, and then transfer the information to the production server and ExMerge the information back into the production server.

The recovery storage group in Exchange Server 2003 facilitates the restore of any database, including an Exchange 2000 SP3 or higher database from any server within an Administrative Group. So, an Exchange database can be restored to the recovery storage group, and then information can be extracted without ever having to bring up another server or shut down the production server.

Creating a Recovery Storage Group

A recovery storage group is created on any Exchange Server 2003 system in an Administrative Group where the original database resides. To create a recovery storage group, do the following:

1. Launch the Exchange System Manager utility.

2. Traverse the tree past the Administrative Group and past the servers. Right-click on the name of the server that will host the recovery storage group and select New, Recovery Storage Group, as shown in Figure 32.7.

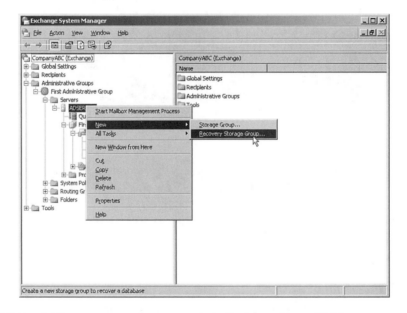

FIGURE 32.7   Adding a recovery storage group to Exchange Server 2003.

> **NOTE**
>
> The server that will host the recovery storage group must have enough disk space to allow for the full restore of the database that will be hosted on the system.

3. Specify the name of the recovery storage group as well as the location of the database and logs, or just select the defaults and click OK to continue. A recovery storage group container is added to the server.

4. Right-click on the recovery storage group container and select Add Database to Recover. Select the mailbox store you want to recover, and click OK.

5. Launch your tape software and restore the database you want to recover to a temporary subdirectory.

6. When the restore is complete, right-click on the mailbox store in the recovery storage group and select Mount Store.

7. Use the ExMerge utility covered in the section "Extracting Mail from a Corrupt Mailbox," earlier in this chapter.

Recovering Internet Information Services

When Internet Information Services (IIS) data is erased or the service is not functioning as desired, restoring the configuration might be necessary. To restore the IIS metabase data, perform the following steps:

1. Log on to the desired IIS server using an account with Local Administrator privileges.

2. Click Start, Programs, Administrative Tools, Internet Information Services (IIS) to start the IIS Manager.

3. Select the Web server in the left pane.

4. Select Action, All Tasks, Backup/Restore Configuration.

5. On the Configuration Backup/Restore page appears a listing of automatic backups that IIS has already performed. Select the desired backup and click the Restore button to perform a manual restore.

6. A pop-up window opens stating that all Internet services will be stopped to restore the data and restarted afterward. Click Yes to begin the restore.

7. When the restore is complete, a confirmation pop-up window is displayed. Click OK to close this window.

8. Click Close on the Configuration Backup/Restore page.

9. Back in the IIS Manager window, verify that the restore was successful, close the window, and log off the server when you're finished.

Backups are stored in `%systemroot%\system32\Inetsrv\MetaBack`, by default.

Recovering IIS Data and Logs

IIS Web and FTP folders are stored in the `C:\InetPub\` directory. The default location for the IIS logs is `C:\Windows\system32\LogFiles`. To recover the IIS Web site, FTP site, or IIS logs, restore the files using either shadow copy data or a backup/restore tool such as Ntbackup.exe.

Recovering the Cluster Service

Cluster nodes require that special backup and restore procedures be followed to ensure a successful recovery if a cluster failure is encountered. For detailed information on backing up and restoring a cluster node, refer to Chapter 30, or use the Windows Server 2003 Help and Support tool.

Recovering Windows Server 2003 Domain Controllers

When a Windows Server 2003 domain controller fails, the administrator needs to either recover this server or understand how to completely and properly remove this domain controller from the domain. The following are some questions to consider:

- Did this domain controller host any of the domain or forest Flexible Single Master Operations (FSMO) roles?

- Was this domain controller a Global Catalog (GC) server, and, if so, was it the only GC in a single Active Directory site?

- If the server failed due to Active Directory corruption, has the corruption been replicated to other domain controllers?

- Is this server a replication hub or bridgehead server for Active Directory site replication?

Using the preceding list of questions, the administrator can decide how best to deal with the failure. For example, if the failed domain controller hosted the PDC emulator FSMO role, the server could be restored or the FSMO role could be manually seized by a separate domain controller. If the domain controller was the bridgehead server for Active Directory site replication, recovering this server might make the most sense so that the desired primary replication topology remains intact. The administrator should recover a failed domain controller as any other server would be recovered, restore the OS from an ASR restore or build a clean server, restore the system state, and perform subsequent restores of local drive data as necessary.

Recovering Active Directory

When undesired changes are made in Active Directory or the Active Directory database is corrupted on a domain controller, recovering the Active Directory database might be necessary. Restoring Active Directory can seem like a difficult task, unless frequent backups are performed and the administrator understands all the restore options.

The Active Directory Database

The Active Directory database contains all the information stored in Active Directory. The Global Catalog information is also stored in this database. The actual filename is `ntds.dit` and, by default, is located in `C:\Windows\NTDS\`. When a domain controller is restored from server failure, the Active Directory database is restored with the system state. If no special steps are taken when the server comes back online, it will ask any other domain controllers for a copy of the latest version of the Active Directory database. This situation is called a **nonauthoritative restore** of Active Directory.

When a change in Active Directory needs to be rolled back or the entire database needs to be rolled back across the enterprise or domain, an authoritative restore of the Active Directory database is necessary.

Active Directory Nonauthoritative Restore

When a domain controller is rebuilt from a backup after a complete system failure, simply recovering this server using a restore of the local drives and system state is enough to get this machine back into the production network. When the machine is back online and establishes connectivity to other domain controllers, any Active Directory and SYSVOL updates will be replicated to the restored server.

Nonauthoritative restores are also necessary when a single domain controller's copy of the Active Directory database is corrupt and is keeping the server from booting up properly. To restore a reliable copy of the Active Directory database, the entire system state needs to be restored; if additional services reside on the domain controller, restoring the previous configuration data for each of these services might be undesirable. In a situation like this, the best option is to try to recover the Active Directory database using database maintenance and recovery utilities such as Esentutl.exe and Ntdsutil.exe. These utilities can be used to check the database consistency, defragment, and repair and troubleshoot the Active Directory database. For information on Active Directory maintenance practices with these utilities, refer to Windows Server 2003 Help and Support.

To restore the Active Directory database to a single domain controller to recover from database corruption, perform the following steps:

1. Power up the domain controller and press the F8 key when the boot loader is displayed on the screen.

2. When the advanced boot options are displayed, scroll down, select Directory Services Restore Mode, and then press Enter to boot the server. This mode boots the Active Directory database in an offline state. When you choose this boot option, you can maintain and restore the Active Directory database.

3. When the server boots up, log on using the username Administrator and the Restore mode password specified when the server was promoted to a domain controller. To

change the Restore mode password on a domain controller running in Normal mode, use the Ntdsutil.exe utility; this process is covered in Chapter 31.

4. Click Start, Run.

5. Type **Ntbackup.exe** and click OK.

6. When the Backup or Restore window opens, click the Advanced Mode hyperlink.

7. Select the Restore and Manage Media tab.

8. Select the appropriate backup medium, expand it, and check the system state. If the correct medium is not available, the file must be located or the tape must be loaded in the tape drive and cataloged before it can be used to restore the system state.

9. Choose to restore the data to the original location, and click the Start Restore button in the lower-right corner of the backup window.

10. A pop-up window indicates that restoring the system state to the original location will overwrite the current system state. Click OK to continue.

11. A confirm restore window opens in which you can choose advanced restore options. Click OK to initiate the restore of the system state.

12. When the restore is complete, a system restart is necessary to update the services and files restored during this operation. Because only a nonauthoritative restore of the Active Directory database is necessary, click Yes to restart the server.

13. After the server reboots, log in as a domain administrator.

14. Check the server event log and Active Directory information to ensure that the database has been restored successfully. Then log off the server.

Active Directory Authoritative Restore

When a change made to Active Directory is causing problems, or when an object is modified or deleted and needs to be recovered to the entire enterprise, an Active Directory Authoritative Restore is necessary.

To perform an authoritative restore of the Active Directory database, follow these steps:

1. Power up the domain controller and press the F8 key when the boot loader is displayed on the screen.

2. When the advanced boot options are displayed, scroll down, select Directory Services Restore Mode, and press Enter to boot the server. This mode boots the Active Directory database in an offline state. When you choose this boot option, you can maintain and restore the Active Directory database.

3. When the server boots up, log in using the username Administrator and the Restore mode password specified when the server was promoted to a domain controller. To

change the Restore mode password on a domain controller running in Normal mode, use the Ntdsutil.exe utility; this process is covered in Chapter 31.

4. Click Start, Run.

5. Type **Ntbackup.exe** and click OK.

6. When the Backup or Restore window opens, click the Advanced Mode hyperlink.

7. Select the Restore and Manage Media tab.

8. Select the appropriate backup medium, expand it, and check the system state. If the correct medium is not available, the file must be located, or the tape must be loaded in the tape drive and cataloged before it can be used to restore the system state.

9. Choose to restore the data to the original location, and click the Start Restore button in the lower-right corner of the backup window.

10. A pop-up window indicates that restoring the system state to the original location will overwrite the current system state. Click OK to continue.

11. A confirm restore window opens in which you can choose advanced restore options. Click OK to initiate the restore of the system state.

12. When the restore is complete, a system restart is necessary to update the services and files restored during this operation. Because only a nonauthoritative restore of the Active Directory database is necessary, click No.

13. Close the backup window and click Start, Run.

14. Type **cmd.exe** and click OK to open a command prompt.

15. At the command prompt, type **ntdsutil.exe** and press Enter.

16. Type **Authoritative restore** and press Enter.

17. Type **Restore Database** and press Enter to restore the entire database. The respective Active Directory partitions, such as the schema partition and the domain-naming context partition, are replicated to all other appropriate domain controllers in the domain and/or forest.

18. An authoritative restore confirmation dialog box appears; click Yes to start the authoritative restore.

19. The command prompt window displays whether the authoritative restore was successful. Close the command prompt and reboot the server.

20. Boot up the server in Normal mode, log in, and open the correct Active Directory tools to verify whether the restore was successful. Also, check on other domain controllers to ensure that the restore is being replicated to them.

21. When you're done, perform a full backup of the domain controller or at least the system state; then log off the server when the backup is complete.

Partial Active Directory Authoritative Restore

Most Active Directory authoritative restores are performed to recover from a modification or deletion of an Active Directory object. For example, a user account might have been deleted instead of disabled, or an Organizational Unit's security might have been changed and the administrator is locked out. Recovering only a specific object, such as a user account or an Organizational Unit or a container, requires the distinguished name (DN) of that object. To find the distinguished name, the administrator can use the Ntdsutil utility; however, if an LDIF dump of Active Directory exists, this file is more helpful. If no LDIF file exists and the DN of the object to be recovered is unknown, the recovery of the single object or container is not possible.

To simplify the steps to partial recovery, you will recover a single user account using the logon john that was previously contained in the Users container in the Companyabc.com domain. To restore the user account, follow these steps:

1. Power up the domain controller and press the F8 key when the boot loader is displayed on the screen.

2. When the advanced boot options are displayed, scroll down, select Directory Services Restore Mode, and press Enter to boot the server. This mode boots the Active Directory database in an offline state. When you choose this boot option, you can maintain and restore the Active Directory database.

3. When the server boots up, log in using the username Administrator and the Restore mode password specified when the server was promoted to a domain controller. To change the Restore mode password on a domain controller running in Normal mode, use the Ntdsutil.exe utility; this process is covered in Chapter 31.

4. Click Start, Run.

5. Type **Ntbackup.exe** and click OK.

6. When the Backup or Restore window opens, click the Advanced Mode hyperlink.

7. Select the Restore and Manage Media tab.

8. Select the appropriate backup medium, expand it, and check the system state. If the correct medium is not available, the file must be located, or the tape must be loaded in the tape drive and cataloged before it can be used to restore the system state.

9. Choose to restore the data to the original location, and click the Start Restore button in the lower-right corner of the backup window.

10. A pop-up window indicates that restoring the system state to the original location will overwrite the current system state. Click OK to continue.

11. A confirm restore window opens in which you can choose advanced restore options. Click OK to initiate the restore of the system state.

12. When the restore is complete, a system restart is necessary to update the services and files restored during this operation. Because only a nonauthoritative restore of the Active Directory database is necessary, click No.

13. Close the backup window and click Start, Run.

14. Type `cmd.exe` and click OK to open a command prompt.

15. At the command prompt, type `ntdsutil.exe` and press Enter.

16. Type `Authoritative restore` and press Enter.

17. Type `Restore Object "cn=John,cn=Users,dc=companyabc,dc=com"` and press Enter.

18. The success or failure status of the restore appears in the command prompt. Now type `quit` and press Enter. Repeat this step until you reach the `C:` prompt.

19. Close the command prompt windows and reboot the server.

20. Log on to the server with a Domain Administrator account, and verify that the account has been restored. Then log off the server.

Global Catalog

No special restore considerations exist for restoring a Global Catalog server other than those outlined for restoring Active Directory in the previous sections. The Global Catalog data is re-created based on the contents of the Active Directory database.

Restoring the SYSVOL Folder

The SYSVOL folder contains the system policies, Group Policies, computer startup/ shutdown scripts, and user logon/logoff scripts. If a previous version of a script or Group Policy Object is needed, the SYSVOL folder must be restored. As a best practice and to keep the process simple, the SYSVOL folder should be restored to an alternate location where specific files can be restored. When the restored files are placed in the SYSVOL folder, the File Replication Service recognizes the file as new or a changed version and replicates it to the remaining domain controllers. If the entire SYSVOL folder needs to be pushed out to the remaining domain controllers and the Active Directory database is intact, a primary restore of the SYSVOL is necessary.

To perform a primary restore of the SYSVOL folder, follow these steps:

1. Power up the domain controller and press the F8 key when the boot loader is displayed on the screen.

2. When the advanced boot options are displayed, scroll down, select Directory Services Restore Mode, and press Enter to boot the server. This mode boots the Active Directory database in an offline state. When you choose this boot option, you can maintain and restore the Active Directory database.

3. When the server boots up, log in using the username Administrator and the Restore mode password specified when the server was promoted to a domain controller. To change the Restore mode password on a domain controller running in Normal mode, use the Ntdsutil.exe utility; this process is covered in Chapter 31.

4. Click Start, Run.

5. Type **Ntbackup.exe** and click OK.

6. When the Backup or Restore window opens, click the Advanced Mode hyperlink.

7. Select the Restore and Manage Media tab.

8. Select the appropriate backup medium, expand it, and check the system state. If the correct medium is not available, the file must be located, or the tape must be loaded in the tape drive and cataloged before it can be used to restore the system state.

9. Choose to restore the data to the original location, and click the Start Restore button in the lower-right corner of the backup window.

10. A pop-up window indicates that restoring the system state to the original location will overwrite the current system state. Click OK to continue.

11. A confirm restore window opens in which you can choose advanced restore options. Click the Advanced button to view the advanced restore options.

12. Check the box labeled When Restoring Replicated Data Sets, Mark the Restored Data as the Primary Data for All Replicas, as shown in Figure 32.8.

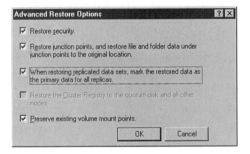

FIGURE 32.8   Choosing to perform a primary restore.

13. Click OK to return to the Confirm Restore page, and click OK to start the restore.

14. When the restore is complete, a system restart is necessary to update the services and files restored during this operation. Because only a nonauthoritative restore of the Active Directory database is necessary, click Yes to restart the server.

15. After the server reboots, log in using an account with Domain Administrator access.

16. Check the server event log and the SYSVOL folder to ensure that the data has been restored successfully. Log off the server when you're finished.

Summary

Recovering from a disaster in Exchange Server 2003 involves a variety of different options. Exchange Server 2003 provides several ways to recover from a variety of different disasters—not simply recovering an entire server in case of a major disaster, but also recovering information that was lost due to data corruption or simply because a user deleted a message or a folder. Disaster recovery takes several different forms and levels based on the recovery needs of the organization.

An important factor in any recovery is to have proper documentation on the configuration of the Exchange environment. Be sure to have documented server names, server configurations, and messaging routing information so that when a recovery process needs to be conducted, the administrators know the impact that a change in one site might have on other sites and locations.

When performing recovery of information in Exchange, the process needs to involve the isolation of the problem, whether the problem is specific to Exchange or is related to Active Directory or other network services. Because the Global Catalog in Active Directory is the core directory for Exchange, knowing how to recover the Active Directory Global Catalog is an important task for an Exchange administrator to understand.

And if the recovery process involves recovery due to database corruption, instead of jumping in and running Exchange utilities to repair the Exchange database, other alternatives can be used, such as migrating mailboxes off of production servers onto new servers within a site. The tools involve not only the Mailbox Move function, but also the ExMerge utility.

Finally, with tools such as the recovery storage group, the administrators of an Exchange environment can restore an Exchange database to a server without having to rebuild an entire server in the lab. Just restoring the data to a temporary server allows the administrator to extract the necessary information needed to recover information.

With all the tools available for recovery, an administrator of an Exchange Server 2003 environment has far more options available for recovery of a single message, folder, mailbox, or entire server than ever. By using the right tool for the right task, the administrator can provide a much better response to resolving Exchange server–related problems.

Best Practices

- When analyzing an Exchange recovery process, consider multiple alternatives beyond restoring an entire server or running the built-in Exchange utilities.

- Because Exchange Server 2003 uses Active Directory for the user directory, Exchange administrators should know about Active Directory recovery.

- Having good documentation on the Exchange environment makes for an easier time in recovering from system failures.

- Preplanning with a failover site can prepare an organization for a server or site failure, to provide faster response in system failure recovery.

- Recovering from a server failure can be done several different ways; the option of restoring a server versus recovering a server needs to be analyzed before proceeding with a process.

- Exchange Server 2003 systems can be recovered using the setup /disasterrecovery command for Exchange setup, greatly simplifying the recovery process in Exchange.

- Doing an XCOPY on a database before performing any maintenance can provide a backup copy of the Exchange databases in case a database restore needs to be performed.

- Moving mailboxes from an old server with corrupt databases to a new server in the same site can keep the Exchange system operational while data is moved off a failing environment.

- Extracting mail from an old server using the ExMerge utility to a new server can extract good data and leave corrupt portions of information on the old system, without having to do a server database repair.

- Running the ISINTEG and ESEUTIL utilities on a regular basis for maintenance helps maintain the integrity of Exchange databases.

- Using the ISINTEG and ESEUTIL utilities on corrupt databases can cause the loss of data because the utilities attempt to repair the Exchange database at all costs.

- A recovery storage group can simplify the recovery of information from backup by allowing data to be restored to a production server, without having to rebuild a new temporary server in a lab before data restore can even begin.

- Active Directory recovery is an important task; the process of restoring and recovering a failed directory should be tested in a lab and should be familiar.

CHAPTER 33

Capacity Analysis and Performance Optimization

Technology enhancements in Exchange Server 2003, in comparison to its predecessor, Exchange Server 2000, afford new optimization in performance. These enhancements can improve the messaging environment's reliability, availability, and scalability. In order to be able to make use of these features, however, you must carefully plan the deployment of Exchange Server 2003. This involves proper capacity planning and analysis of areas wherein a well-planned configuration can make an enormous difference in performance.

Capacity analysis and performance optimization processes and procedures are, most often, low-priority tasks. This is frequently because productivity is regularly measured by what can be achieved now and not always what can be properly planned or designed. The benefits of capacity analysis and performance monitoring can be obtained in the short term, but they are more important when established over longer periods of time. As a result, the main focus of most IT departments shifts to the more immediate and more tangible day-to-day processes and IT needs.

The results of capacity analysis and performance optimization save organizations of all sizes time, effort, and expenditures. This chapter is designed to provide best practices for properly and proactively performing capacity analysis and performance optimization so that IT personnel can work more effectively and efficiently, organizations can capture savings, and the Exchange Server 2003 infrastructure can optimally operate.

Examining Exchange Server 2003 Performance Improvements

Before delving into ways to tweak Exchange Server 2003 performance, it is important to have an understanding of the performance improvements that have been made since its predecessor, Exchange 2000. Although some of these performance improvements are more noticeable than others, Exchange Server 2003 has proven its ability to scale into the enterprise and beyond.

Communication Improvements

Exchange Server 2003 includes major improvements in the way it handles client/server communications. These improvements entail changes made to communication links between sites, servers, and users. Implemented changes translate into a fundamentally different approach toward how Exchange Server 2003 handles routing of messages from site to site as well as to and from the client computer.

Improvements in Link State Connections

In order to determine the best possible route to send a message between servers, Exchange uses **link state routing** technology. The best route is chosen based on the status and the cost of the connections. While routing messages between servers and sites, no alternate paths might be available to Exchange Server 2003 servers, or the existing connectors might be intermittently available. By determining whether there are alternate and available connections, Exchange Server 2003 significantly reduces the amount of traffic between servers.

Another performance improvement with Exchange Server 2003 analyzing links between servers is how it efficiently propagates link status information to other servers in and between sites. If no alternate paths are detected for a message to take, the available route is marked as always in service. Exchange will never change this state back to an out-of-service state unless an alternate path becomes available. As a result, propagation of link state information in and between sites is reduced, and consequently overall network traffic is optimized.

Synchronization and Replication Enhancements

Synchronization and replication enhancements available in Exchange Server 2003 can be analyzed from various viewpoints. Generally speaking, these enhancements include changes made to the Outlook client, Outlook Web Access client, and public folders.

Client-side Performance Enhancements

Among the new performance-enhancing features of Exchange Server 2003 and Outlook 2003 is the ability to collect client-side data by recording RPC errors that occur on the client. This information is then reported in the Event Viewer.

Outlook 2003 Client Synchronization

Significant reduction of Remote Procedure Calls (RPCs) to the Exchange Server from the Outlook 2003 client has resulted in noticeable improvements in client performance even in low-bandwidth conditions. This improvement was primarily made available through the employment of the following features:

- **Cached Exchange Mode** Cached Exchange Mode refers to the Outlook 2003 client keeping a local copy of the user's mailbox on the client computer. This is similar to an Offline Folder (OST) file in earlier versions of Exchange. There are some differences, however: This mode requires less configuration (as shown in Figure 33.1), uses the Offline Address Book (OAB) by default, and copies the entire mailbox rather than relying on the user to specify which folders to synchronize with Exchange Server 2003. Although this reduces the number of data requests sent to the server, this mode also determines whether or not the connection with Exchange is slow (128KB or less) and then adapts accordingly. For instance, if the user connects via the corporate LAN, the full message, including attachments, is copied to the local cached copy. If the user later connects using a 56KB modem, only headers are copied unless the user opens the message. This is done automatically and is transparent to the user.

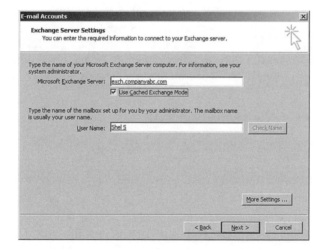

FIGURE 33.1 Cached Exchange Mode option.

- **Outlook Synchronization** Synchronization communication between the Outlook client and Exchange Server 2003 uses data compression to reduce traffic overhead. Changes that are made through the Outlook client are also sent to Exchange Server 2003 incrementally, thereby providing additional network traffic optimization.

Outlook Web Access (OWA) Performance Enhancements

An abundance of new features are available in OWA, and the biggest one by far is the interface. However, the following primary features contribute to performance enhancements:

- **Compression Support**   OWA compression uses GZip to keep bandwidth requirements low and improves response times even over dial-up or other low-bandwidth connections. Configuring OWA to use high compression (that is, compression of static and dynamic pages) can reduce bandwidth requirements as much as 50%. It is important to note that clients must use Internet Explorer (IE) 6 (or Netscape 6) or higher in order to take advantage of OWA compression.

- **Logon Options**   Outlook Web Access is now available in two configurations: Premium and Basic Experience. These two configurations are presented to users at the time of login and depending on available bandwidth, the user can choose which version of OWA to load, thus improving performance.

Improved Public Folder Store Replication

Public folder store replication has greatly improved in respect to the way Exchange Server 2003 handles the receipt of updates from various other servers. In Exchange 2000 Server, a server holding the largest number of needed updates would always be chosen regardless of its transport cost. When determining update status during the replication process, Exchange Server 2003 takes the following three main elements into account on a priority basis and calculates the replication algorithm based on the data gathered from these questions:

- Which server has the lowest transport cost?

- For servers with equal transport costs, which server is the newest version of Exchange?

- For servers with equal transport costs and versions, which server owns the greater number of updates?

This architecture enables reduction of replication traffic over slower links because lower-cost servers (servers in the same site) always take precedence over higher-cost servers (those located in remote sites).

Performance Scalability Improvements

Some of the Exchange Server 2003 enhancements to performance and scalability are

- **Improved Distribution List Member Caching**   The processing resources required to look up the membership of Distribution Lists has been greatly reduced by redesigning the cache rule in a way that lookups and insertions can be achieved by 60% fewer Distribution List–related queries made against Active Directory. Therefore a small AD performance optimization has been achieved by changes made to the cache rule.

- **Enhanced Internet Mail Delivery**   Exchange Server 2003 relies heavily on Windows Server 2003 DNS for message delivery, and the algorithms used relating to load-balanced DNS-based Internet delivery have been enhanced. In circumstances where the external DNS Server is not available or the network is experiencing latency, Exchange Server 2003 has greater tolerance, which results in a greater reliability of message delivery.

Analyzing Capacity

Capacity analysis for an Exchange Server 2003 environment requires a well-established understanding of the business and messaging needs of the organization and a well-documented outline of the organization's expectations of its messaging environment. Business constantly undergoes change, and so do capacity requirements and measurements of an organization.

The first step in capacity analysis is to grasp an understanding of these changes and define performance expectations. This can be done by establishing policies and service-level agreements. It is in these policies and service-level agreements that an administrator can outline acceptable performance thresholds and more accurately gauge the capacity needs of Exchange Server 2003. These thresholds can also be used to accurately establish performance baselines from which to analyze the requirements against available resources.

To help develop the policies and service-level agreements, use questionnaires, interviews, business objectives and the like along with performance measurements.

Establishing Baselines

The importance of establishing meaningful baselines of the messaging environment cannot be underscored enough. Baselines are particularly important in the sense that they are the measurable tools that can be used to balance what is required of Exchange Server 2003 with what resources are needed to fulfill those requirements. Achieving this balance can be made simpler if an administrator consults performance metrics, such as industry-standard benchmarks.

In order to establish an accurate baseline of Exchange Server 2003, there are a number of tools that can help an administrator in this process. These tools are discussed in detail in the following sections. Some of these capacity analysis tools are built into Windows Server 2003, and others are built into Exchange Server 2003. Many third-party tools and utilities are also available for the careful measurement of Exchange Server 2003 capacity requirements and performance analysis.

Monitoring Exchange Server 2003

A variety of built-in Microsoft tools is available to help an administrator establish the baseline of the Exchange Server 2003 environment. Among these, the Performance Monitor Microsoft Management Console (MMC) snap-in is one of the most common tools used to measure the capacity requirements of Exchange Server 2003.

Using the Performance Monitor Console

The Performance snap-in enables an in-depth analysis of every measurable aspect of the Exchange server. The information that is gathered using the Performance snap-in can be presented in a variety of forms—including reports, real-time charts, or logs—which add to the versatility of this tool. The resulting output formats enable an administrator to present a baseline analysis in real-time or through historical data. The Performance snap-in, shown in Figure 33.2, can be launched from the Start, Administrative Tools menu.

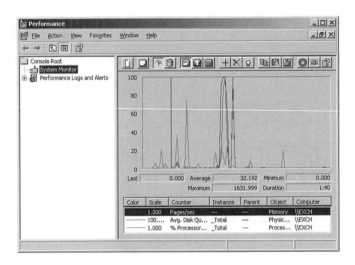

FIGURE 33.2 The Performance snap-in.

Using Network Monitor

The Network Monitor, as illustrated in Figure 33.3, is a reliable capacity-analysis tool used specifically to monitor network traffic. There are two flavors of the Network Monitor: one that is built into Windows Server 2003 and one that is provided in System Management Server (SMS). The one included with Windows Server 2003 is a more downscaled version. It is capable of monitoring network traffic to and from the local server on which it runs. The SMS version monitors network traffic coming to or from any computer on the network and enables you to monitor network traffic from a centralized machine. This facilitates gathering capacity analysis data, but it is also important to note that it could present possible security risks because of its ability to promiscuously monitor traffic throughout the network.

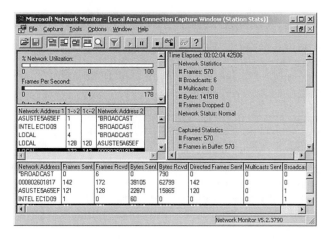

FIGURE 33.3 The Network Monitor interface.

Using Task Manager

Task Manager displays real-time performance metrics, so an administrator can quickly get an overall idea of how the Exchange Server 2003 is performing at any given time. Its biggest downfall, however, is that it does not store any historical data, so it not a suitable tool for capacity analysis purposes.

Simulating Stress with Jetstress

Jetstress is a tool written by the Microsoft Exchange product group to help IT personnel with capacity and performance analysis of the disk subsystem on an Exchange system prior to deploying in a production environment.

An administrator can put the Exchange server's disk subsystem to the test using simulated I/O workloads mimicking an Exchange environment. Jetstress is broken into two tests (Jetstress Disk Performance Test or the Jetstress Disk Subsystem Stress Test), which can be used to test Exchange storage or the entire disk subsystem. The tests run for 2 and 24 hours, respectively, and Microsoft recommends running both tests to adequately determine the Exchange Server 2003 disk subsystem configuration, performance, and reliability.

NOTE

Jetstress is a free utility that can be downloaded from Microsoft's Web site:

`http://www.microsoft.com/exchange/tools/2003.asp)`

It is recommended that you read the Jetstress documentation before installing and using this tool.

Analyzing and Monitoring Core Elements

The capacity analysis and performance optimization process can be intimidating because there can be an enormous amount of data to work with. In fact it can easily become unwieldy if not done properly. The process is not just about monitoring and reading counters; it is also an art.

As you monitor and catalog performance information, keep in mind that more information does not necessarily yield better optimization. Tailor the number and types of counters that are being monitored based on the server's role and functionality within the network environment. It's also important to monitor the four common contributors to bottlenecks: memory, processor, disk, and network subsystems. When monitoring Exchange Server 2003, it is equally important to understand the various Exchange roles to keep the number of counters being monitored to a minimum.

Memory Subsystem Optimizations

As with earlier versions of Windows, Windows Server 2003 tends to use the amount of memory that you throw at it. However, it outperforms its predecessors in terms of how efficiently memory is managed. Nevertheless, fine-tuning system memory can go a long way toward making sure that Exchange has adequate amounts of memory.

Memory management is performed by Windows Server 2003 and is directly related to how well applications such as Exchange Server 2003 perform. Exchange Server 2003 also has greatly enhanced memory management and the way it uses virtual memory. This reduces memory fragmentation and enables more users to be supported on a single server or cluster of servers.

> **TIP**
>
> Use the /3GB /USERVA=3030 parameters in boot.ini for any Exchange Server 2003 server with 1GB of memory or more installed. This enables Exchange Server 2003 to manage memory more efficiently and support a greater number of users.

With the Performance Monitor Console, there are a number of important memory-related counters that can help in establishing an accurate representation of the system's memory requirements. The primary memory counters that provide information about hard pages (pages that are causing the information to be swapped between the memory and the hard disk) are

- **Memory—Pages/sec** The values of this counter should range from 5–20. Values consistently higher than 10 are indicative of potential performance problems, whereas values consistently higher than 20 might cause noticeable and significant performance hits.

- **Memory—Page Faults/sec**   This counter, together with the Memory—Cache Faults/sec and Memory—Transition Faults/sec counters, can provide valuable information about page faults that are not committed to disk. They were not committed to disk because the memory manager allocated those pages to a standby list, also known as **transition faults**. Most systems today can handle a large number of page faults, but it is important to correlate these numbers with the Pages/sec counter as well to determine whether Exchange is configured with enough memory.

Figure 33.4 shows some of the various memory-related and process-related counters.

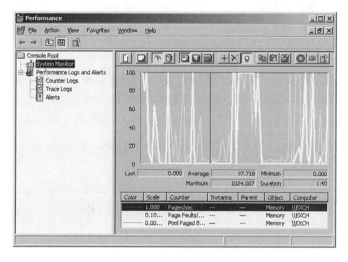

FIGURE 33.4   Memory-related counters in Windows Server 2003.

Improving Virtual Memory Usage

Calculating the correct amount of virtual memory is one of the more challenging parts of planning a server's memory requirements. While trying to anticipate growing usage demands, it is critical that the server has an adequate amount of virtual memory for all applications and the operating system. This is no different for Exchange Server 2003.

Virtual memory refers to the amount of disk space that is used by Windows Server 2003 and applications as physical memory gets low or when applications need to swap data out of physical memory. Windows Server 2003 uses 1.5 times the amount of RAM as the minimum paging file size by default, which for many systems is adequate. However, it is important to monitor memory counters to determine whether this amount is truly sufficient for that particular server's resource requirements. Another important consideration is the maximum size setting for the paging file. As a best practice, this setting should be at least 50% more than the minimum value to enable paging file growth, should the system require it. If the minimum and maximum settings are configured with the same value, there is a greater risk that the system could experience severe performance problems or even crash.

The most indicative sign of low virtual memory is the presence of 9582 warning events logged by the Microsoft Exchange Information Store service that can severely impact and degrade the Exchange Server's message-processing abilities. These warning events are indicative of virtual memory going below 32MB. If unnoticed or left unattended, these warning messages might cause services to stop or the entire system to crash.

> **TIP**
>
> Use the Performance snap-in to set an alert for Event ID 9582. This helps proactively address any virtual memory problems and possibly prevent unnecessary downtime.

To get an accurate portrayal of how Exchange Server 2003 is using virtual memory, monitor the following counters within the MSExchangeIS object:

- **VM Largest Block Size**   This counter should consistently be above 32MB.

- **VM Total 16MB Free Blocks**   This counter should remain over three 16MB blocks.

- **VM Total Free Blocks**   This value is specific to your messaging environment.

- **VM Total Large Free Block Bytes**   This counter should stay above 50MB.

Other important counters to watch closely are

- **Memory—Available Bytes**   This counter can be used to establish whether the system has adequate amounts of RAM. The recommended absolute minimum value is 4MB.

- **Paging File—% Usage**   % Usage is used to validate the amount of the paging file used in a predetermined interval. High usage values might be indicative of requiring more physical memory or needing a larger paging file.

Monitoring Processor Usage

Analyzing the processor usage can reveal invaluable information about system performance and provide reliable results that can be used for baselining purposes. There are three major Exchange-related processor counters that are used for capacity analysis of an Exchange Server 2003:

- **% Privileged Time**   This counter indicates the percentage of non-idle processor time spent in privileged mode. The recommended ideal for this value is under 55%.

- **% Processor Time**   This counter specifies the processor use of each processor or the total processor use. If these values are consistently higher than 50–60%, consider upgrade options or segmenting workloads.

Monitoring the Disk Subsystem

Exchange Server 2003 relies heavily on the disk subsystem and it is therefore a critical component to properly design and monitor. Although, the disk object monitoring counters are by default enabled in Windows Server 2003, it is recommended that these counters be disabled until such time that an administrator is ready to monitor them. The resource requirements can influence overall system performance. The syntax to disable and reenable these counters is as follows:

```
diskperf -n (to disable)
diskperf -y [\\computer_Name] (to reenable)
```

Nevertheless, it is important to gather disk subsystem performance statistics over time.

The primary Exchange-related performance counters for the disk subsystem are located within the Physical and Logical Disk objects. Critical counters to monitor include, but are not limited to, the following:

- **Physical Disk—% Disk Time**   This counter analyzes the percentage of elapsed time that the selected disk spends on servicing read or write requests. Ideally this value should remain below 50%.

- **Logical Disk—% Disk Time**   This counter displays the percentage of elapsed time that the selected disk spends fulfilling read or write requests. It is recommended that this value be 60–70% or lower.

- **Current Disk Queue Length (Both Physical and Logical Disk Objects)**   This counter has different performance indicators depending on the monitored disk drive (Database or Transaction Log volume). On disk drives storing the Exchange Database, this value should be below the number of spindled drives divided by 2. On disk drives storing transaction log data, this value should be below 1.

Monitoring the Network Subsystem

The network subsystem is one of the more challenging elements to monitor because there are a number of factors that make up a network. In an Exchange messaging environment, site topologies, replication architecture, network topologies, synchronization methods, the number of systems, and more are among the many contributing factors.

In order to satisfactorily analyze the network, all facets must be considered. This will most likely require using third-party network monitoring tools in conjunction with built-in tools such as the Performance snap-in and Network Monitor.

Properly Sizing Exchange Server 2003

Before delving into recommended configurations for Exchange Server 2003, it is essential to not only understand the fundamentals of this messaging system but also the dependencies and interactions those components have with the underlying operating system (that is, Windows Server 2003). Being a client-server messaging application, maximizing Exchange Server 2003 involves fine-tuning all of its core and extended components. Optimization of each of these components affects the overall performance of Exchange.

The core components of Exchange Server (for example, the information stores, connectors, transaction logs, and more) have a direct bearing on gauging resource requirements. The number of users in a messaging environment and the various Exchange functions are equally influential.

Optimizing the Disk Subsystem Configuration

There are many factors—such as the type of file system to use, physical disk configuration, database size, and log file placement—that need to be considered when you are trying to optimize the disk subsystem configuration.

Choosing the File System

Among the file systems supported by Windows Server 2003 (that is, FAT and NTFS), it is recommended to use only NTFS on all servers—especially those in production environments. NTFS provides the best security, scalability, and performance features. For instance, NTFS supports file and directory-level security, large file sizes (files of up to 16TB), large disk sizes (disk volumes of up to 16TB), fault tolerance, disk compression, error detection, and encryption.

Choosing the Physical Disk Configuration

Windows Server 2003, like its predecessors, supports RAID (Redundant Array of Inexpensive Disks). The levels of RAID supported by the operating system are

- RAID 0 (Striping)

- RAID 1 (Mirroring)

- RAID 5 (Striping with Parity)

There are various other levels of RAID that can be supported through the use of hardware-based RAID controllers.

The deployment of the correct RAID level is of utmost importance because each RAID level has a direct effect on the performance of the server. From the viewpoint of pure performance, RAID level 0 by far gives the best performance. However, fault tolerance and the reliability of system access are other factors that contribute to overall performance. The skillful administrator strikes a balance between performance and fault tolerance without sacrificing one for the other. The following sections provide recommended disk configurations for Exchange Server 2003.

> **NOTE**
>
> As mentioned earlier, there are various levels of RAID, but for the context of Exchange Server 2003 there are two recommended basic levels to use: RAID 1 and RAID 5. Other forms of RAID, such as RAID 0+1 or 1+0, are also optimal solutions for Exchange Server 2003. These more advanced levels of RAID are supported only when using a hardware RAID controller. As a result, only RAID 1 and 5 are discussed in this chapter.

Disk Mirroring (RAID 1)

In this type of configuration, data is mirrored from one disk to the other participating disk in the mirror set. Data is simultaneously written to the two required disks, which means read operations are significantly faster than systems with no RAID configuration or with a greater degree of fault tolerance. Write performance is slower, though, because data is being written twice—once to each disk in the mirror set.

Besides adequate performance, RAID 1 also provides a good degree of fault tolerance. For instance, if one drive fails, the RAID controller can automatically detect the failure and run solely on the remaining disk with minimal interruption.

The biggest drawback to RAID 1 is the amount of storage capacity that is lost. RAID 1 uses 50% of the total drive capacity for the two drives.

> **TIP**
>
> RAID 1 is particularly well suited for the boot drive and for volumes containing Exchange Server 2003 log files.

Disk Striping with Parity (RAID 5)

In a RAID 5 configuration, data and parity information is striped across all participating disks in the array. RAID 5 requires a minimum of three disks. Even if one of the drives fails within the array, the Exchange Server 2003 server can still remain operational.

After the drive fails, Windows Server 2003 continues to operate because of the data contained on the other drives. The parity information gives details of the data that is missing due to the failure. Either Windows Server 2003 or the hardware RAID controller also begins the rebuilding process from the parity information to a spare or new drive.

RAID 5 is most commonly used for the data drive because it is a great compromise among performance, storage capacity, and redundancy. The overall space used to store the striped parity information is equal to the capacity of one drive. For example, a RAID 5 volume with three 200GB disks can store up to 400GB of data.

Hardware Versus Software RAID

Hardware RAID (configured at the disk controller level) is recommended over software RAID (configurable from within the Windows Server 2003) because of faster performance, greater support of different RAID levels, and capability of recovering from hardware failures more easily.

Database Sizing and Optimization

As mentioned throughout this book, Exchange Server 2003 is available in two versions: Standard and Enterprise. The Standard Edition supports one storage group with one private and one public information store. The maximum information store (database) size is 16GB. The Enterprise Edition provides support for up to four storage groups with a combined total of 20 useable databases per server with practically unlimited database size.

The flexibility with the Enterprise Edition is beneficial not just in terms of growth but also performance and manageability. More specifically, the advantages for segmenting can include the following:

- Administrators are enabled to segment the user population on a single Exchange server.

- Multiple mailboxes can more evenly distribute the size of the messaging data and help prevent one database from becoming too large and possibly unwieldy for a given system.

- Multiple databases present greater opportunities for faster enumeration of database indexing.

- Multiple databases can be segmented onto different RAID volumes and RAID controller channels.

- Transaction logs can be segmented from other log files using separate RAID volumes.

- Failures such as database corruption affect a smaller percentage of the user population.

- Offline maintenance routines require less scheduled downtime, and fewer users are affected.

> **TIP**
>
> The recommended best practice is to keep database sizes in the 10–20GB range. An administrator can use this guideline to gauge or plan for the number of users each database should optimally contain. This best practice is also useful in determining the appropriate number of Exchange Server 2003 servers that are required to support the number of users in the organization.

Determining the number of storage groups and databases for Exchange Server 2003 should also be based on workload characterization. Users can be grouped based on the how they interact with the messaging system (for example, in terms of frequency, storage requirements, and more). Users placing higher demands on Exchange Server 2003 can be placed into a separate storage group and separate databases so that the greater number of read/write operations do not occur in the same database and are more evenly distributed.

Optimizing Exchange Logs

Similar to the previous versions of Exchange, transaction log files should be stored on separate RAID volumes. This enables significant improvements in disk input/output (I/O) operations. Transaction logs are created on a per storage group level rather than per database. Therefore, when you have multiple storage groups, multiple log files are created that enable simultaneous read and write operations. If the transaction logs are then placed on separate RAID volumes, there can be significant improvements to performance.

> **TIP**
>
> Because transaction logs are as important to Exchange Server 2003 as the data contained in the databases, the most suitable RAID configuration to use for transaction log files is RAID 1. This provides suitable performance without sacrificing fault tolerance.

Sizing Memory Requirements

The recommended starting point for the amount of memory an Exchange Server 2003 server is installed with is 256MB. The specific memory requirements naturally vary based on server roles, server responsibilities, and the number of users to support. In addition, some organizations define certain guidelines that must be followed for base memory configurations. A more accurate representation of how much memory is required can be achieved by baselining memory performance information gathered from the Performance snap-in or third-party tools during a prototype or lab testing phase.

Another important factor to take into consideration is when the organization adds functionality to Exchange Server 2003 or consolidates users onto fewer servers. This obviously increases resource requirements, especially in terms of adding more physical memory. In these scenarios, it is recommended to use the base amount of memory (for example, 256MB) and then add the appropriate amount of memory based on vendor specifications. It is also important to consult with the vendor to determine what the memory requirements may be on a per user basis. This way the organization can plan ahead and configure the proper amount of memory prior to needing to scale to support a larger number of users in the future.

Sizing Based on Server Roles

Server roles can have a considerable bearing on both the performance and capacity of Exchange Server 2003. Based on the various roles of the Exchange servers, the strategic placement of Exchange services and functionality can greatly improve performance of the overall messaging system while reducing the need for using additional resources. By the same token, a misplaced Exchange service or functional component can noticeably add to network traffic and degrade the overall performance of the messaging system.

Servers are generally divided into two sets of roles: front-end and back-end servers. Within these two sets of roles are several key roles that an Exchange Server 2003 server can serve, including, but not limited to, OWA, public folder, mailbox store, or bridgehead server.

Front-end servers are the first point of contact for client messaging requests. The servers proxy these requests to the back-end servers for processing. The front-end/back-end topology is recommended for organizations that use OWA, POP, or IMAP for employees accessing the messaging system over the Internet.

Another key difference between a front-end and back-end server is storage requirements. Back-end servers usually host mailbox or public folder stores, and front-ends have minimal requirements. Back-end servers, therefore, usually have much higher and greater storage requirements, as well as processing power and memory requirements.

Front-end Server Sizing

There are various factors that affect the performance of a front-end server, including the following:

- The number and type of protocols supported

- The number of users supported

- The authentication methods supported

- Encryption requirements

Tables 33.1 through 33.3 show the recommended resource requirements of various dedicated front-end servers. It is important to note that these guidelines are minimum recommendations, and actual requirements may vary depending upon the organization.

TABLE 33.1   Recommended Minimum POP3 Front-end Server Configurations

Resource	Description
RAM	256MB.
Processor	Pentium III 800MHz or higher processor.
Hard disk	RAID 1 for Windows Server 2003 and Exchange Server 2003 (assuming no mail is stored on the front-end server and logging is not enabled).
Network	100Mbps or higher NIC(s).
Other considerations	If connections to this server are over *SSL* consider using a NIC that offloads SSL processing.

TABLE 33.2   Recommended Minimum OWA or IMAP4 Front-end Server Configurations

Resource	Description
RAM	256MB plus 512KB of RAM per active, concurrent client connection.
Processor	Dual Pentium III 800MHz or higher processors.
Hard disk	RAID 1 for Windows Server 2003 and Exchange Server 2003 (assuming no mail is stored on the front-end server and logging is not enabled).
Network	100Mbps or higher NIC(s).
Other considerations	If connections to this server are over *SSL* consider using a NIC that offloads SSL processing.

TABLE 33.3   Recommended Minimum SMTP Front-end Server Configurations

Resource	Description
RAM	Recommended 512MB to manage large queues.
Processor	Dual Pentium III 800MHz or higher processors.
Hard disk	RAID 1 can be used for Windows Server 2003 and Exchange Server 2003. If large amounts of disk space are required for SMTP queues, a separate RAID 0+1 volume can be used.
Network	100Mbps or higher NIC(s).
Other considerations	Encrypting the SMTP traffic using *TLS* (Transport Layer Security) does not necessarily require significantly more memory or processing power.

> **TIP**
>
> Similar front-end servers can be combined for additional availability and performance requirements using Microsoft's Network Load Balancing (NLB).

Back-end Server Sizing

As mentioned earlier, back-end servers generally host mailbox and public folder stores. They can also provide various other functions, including features that are typically thought of as front-end functions.

The myriad of functionality options and other considerations (for example, the number of users to support, mailbox store size(s), incoming and outgoing message size restrictions, security requirements, and more) can make back-end server sizing a daunting task at best. As a best practice, it is recommended that an Exchange Server 2003 server be configured with a minimum of 512MB of memory and dual processors. Physical memory has been, and continues to be, an inexpensive component and is one of the easiest ways to upgrade a server. As such you might even consider using 1GB as a minimum standard for back-end servers. For the disk subsystem, it is recommended to implement three hardware-based RAID volumes: a RAID 1 volume for Windows Server 2003 and Exchange Server 2003 system-related files, a RAID 5 volume for the mailbox and public folder stores, and another RAID 1 volume for transaction logs. The number of volumes for the transaction logs may vary depending on the number of storage groups configured on the server.

> **TIP**
>
> Another best practice is to thoroughly test server configurations in a lab environment prior to deploying in production.

Optimizing Exchange Through Ongoing Maintenance

Through typical usage, Exchange databases become fragmented. This fragmentation gradually slows server performance and can also lead to corruption over extended periods of time. In order to ensure that an Exchange Server continues to service requests in an optimized manner and the chances of corruption are minimized, it is important to perform regular maintenance on Exchange.

Although Exchange Server 2003 performs online maintenance tasks on a nightly basis, this accounts for roughly only 60–70% of the maintenance tasks that are recommended. Offline maintenance, on the other hand, achieves the true optimization of the information stores, as well as prevents and fixes corruption. Offline optimization routines help keep the messaging server operating like a well-oiled engine and ensure that Exchange provides the highest serviceability and reliability.

> **CAUTION**
>
> It is of utmost importance to perform a full backup of Exchange Server 2003 prior to and immediately after running offline maintenance. After the backup has completed, it is equally important to verify the backups.

Because offline maintenance procedures require at least one database or that the entire server is offline, it is also important to schedule maintenance during the off-peak hours and notify the end users in advance.

> **NOTE**
>
> If Exchange Server 2003 Enterprise Edition is being used, you can perform maintenance on a single database and not affect other data that is stored within other databases. In addition, the entire server does not have to be offline.

The utilities to use for offline maintenance are ESEUTIL (ESEUTIL.EXE) and the Integrity Checker (ISINTEG.EXE). These utilities perform a number of functions, including, but not limited to, checking database and table integrity, identifying and correcting corruption, and defragmenting databases. For further information on the recommended best practices on maintaining Exchange Server 2003 and step-by-step instructions for offline maintenance, refer to Chapter 19, "Exchange Server 2003 Management and Maintenance Practices."

Monitoring Exchange with Microsoft Operations Manager

Microsoft Operations Manager (MOM) is an application that can be used to actively monitor Exchange Server 2003. Employing MOM in an Exchange messaging environment offers administrators the following benefits:

- MOM has the capability of detecting even the smallest of problems that, if gone unnoticed, can lead to more complicated issues. Early detection of problems enables an administrator to troubleshoot the problem areas well in advance.

- MOM can monitor all Exchange-related system health indicators.

- The Exchange Server 2003 Management Pack leverages all the new features of Exchange Server 2003.

- The Exchange Server 2003 Management Pack also includes the Microsoft Knowledge Base, which can be used for fast and reliable resolution of issues.

- MOM can centrally manage a large number of Exchange Server 2003 servers over widely dispersed deployments.

- MOM can actively monitor server availability by verifying that services are running, databases are mounted, messages are flowing, and users are able to logon.

- MOM can actively monitor server health by monitoring free disk space thresholds, mail queues, security, performance thresholds, and more.

- MOM provides detailed reports on database sizes, traffic analysis, and more.

- Alerts can be sent based on customized thresholds and events.

In short, MOM is an excellent tool that administrators can use to proactively monitor the Exchange environment from a centralized location.

Figure 33.5 shows the various Mail Queue performance counters.

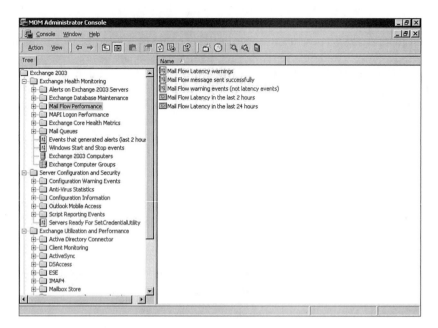

FIGURE 33.5   MOM Mail queue performance counters.

Summary

Despite all the performance, reliability, scalability, and availability enhancements of Exchange Server 2003, capacity analysis and performance optimization are still a necessity. The techniques and processes described in this chapter not only help you determine how to size a server or tweak it to operate optimally; they also reflect a methodology for continually monitoring a changing environment. By keeping one step ahead of the system, an organization can use resources more efficiently and effectively and in return save time, effort, and costs associated with supporting Exchange Server 2003.

Best Practices

The following are best practices from this chapter:

- Begin capacity analysis and performance optimization sooner rather than later.

- Create performance baselines in which to gauge the changing requirements and performance levels of Exchange Server 2003.

- Establish SLAs and other policies that reflect the business expectations of the messaging environment.

- Monitor only those counters that are pertinent to the server's configuration.

- Always monitor the four common contributors to bottlenecks: memory, disk subsystem, processor, and network.

- Run performance and stress tests in a lab environment prior to implementing in a production environment.

- Establish regular maintenance routines, including those for offline maintenance tasks.

- Set an alert for Event ID 9582 to proactively address any memory or virtual memory problems.

- Use the /3GB /USERVA=3030 parameters in boot.ini for any Exchange Server 2003 server with 1GB of memory or more installed.

- Keep Exchange Server 2003 database sizes in the 10–20GB range whenever possible.

- Use separate, hardware-based RAID 1 volumes for system files and transaction logs.

33

Index

NUMBERS

A

How can we make this index more useful? Email us at indexes@samspublishing.com

C

How can we make this index more useful? Email us at indexes@samspublishing.com

How can we make this index more useful? Email us at indexes@samspublishing.com

How can we make this index more useful? Email us at indexes@samspublishing.com

N

X - Y - Z

Your Guide to Computer Technology

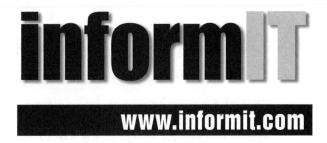

www.informit.com

Sams has partnered with **InformIT.com** to bring technical information to your desktop. Drawing on Sams authors and reviewers to provide additional information on topics you're interested in, **InformIT.com** has free, in-depth information you won't find anywhere else.

ARTICLES

Keep your edge with thousands of free articles, in-depth features, interviews, and information technology reference recommendations—all written by experts you know and trust.

POWERED BY
Safari

ONLINE BOOKS

Answers in an instant from **InformIT Online Books'** 600+ fully searchable online books. Sign up now and get your first 14 days **free**.

CATALOG

Review online sample chapters and author biographies to choose exactly the right book from a selection of more than 5,000 titles.

 www.samspublishing.com